Cardiovascular and Pulmonary PHYSICAL THERAPY

Evidence to Practice

FIFTH EDITION

Cardiovascular and Pulmonary PHYSICAL THERAPY

Evidence to Practice

Donna Frownfelter, PT, DPT, MA, CCS, RRT, FCCP
Assistant Professor and Program Director
Post Professional Doctor of Physical Therapy
College of Health Professions
Rosalind Franklin University of Medicine and Science
North Chicago, Illinois

Elizabeth Dean, PhD, PT
Professor
Department of Physical Therapy
Faculty of Medicine
University of British Columbia
Vancouver, Canada

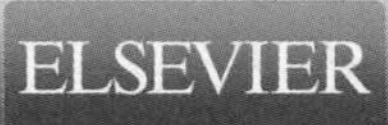

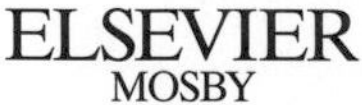

3251 Riverport Lane
St. Louis, Missouri 63043

CARDIOVASCULAR AND PULMONARY PHYSICAL THERAPY: EVIDENCE TO PRACTICE

ISBN: 978-0-323-05913-8

Notices

Knowledge and best practice in this field are constantly changing. As new research and experience broaden our understanding, changes in research methods, professional practices, or medical treatment may become necessary.

Practitioners and researchers must always rely on their own experience and knowledge in evaluating and using any information, methods, compounds, or experiments described herein. In using such information or methods they should be mindful of their own safety and the safety of others, including parties for whom they have a professional responsibility.

With respect to any drug or pharmaceutical products identified, readers are advised to check the most current information provided (i) on procedures featured or (ii) by the manufacturer of each product to be administered, to verify the recommended dose or formula, the method and duration of administration, and contraindications. It is the responsibility of practitioners, relying on their own experience and knowledge of their patients, to make diagnoses, to determine dosages and the best treatment for each individual patient, and to take all appropriate safety precautions.

To the fullest extent of the law, neither the Publisher nor the authors, contributors, or editors, assume any liability for any injury and/or damage to persons or property as a matter of products liability, negligence or otherwise, or from any use or operation of any methods, products, instructions, or ideas contained in the material herein.

Library of Congress Cataloging-in-Publication Data

Cardiovascular and pulmonary physical therapy: evidence to practice / [edited by] Donna Frownfelter, Elizabeth Dean. – 5th ed.
p. ; cm.
Includes bibliographical references and index.
ISBN 978-0-323-05913-8 (hardcover: alk. paper)
I. Frownfelter, Donna L. II. Dean, Elizabeth (Elizabeth W.)
[DNLM: 1. Lung Diseases–rehabilitation. 2. Physical Therapy Modalities. 3. Cardiovascular Diseases–rehabilitation. 4. Cardiovascular Diseases–therapy. 5. Lung Diseases–therapy. 6. Respiratory Therapy. WF 145]
616.1′06–dc23

2012000437

Executive Editor: Kathy Falk
Developmental Editor: Megan Fennell
Publishing Services Manager: Julie Eddy
Senior Project Manager: Celeste Clingan
Designer: Margaret Reid

Printed in the United States of America

Last digit is the print number: 9 8 7 6 5 4 3 2 1

Contributors

Michael Wade Baskin, PT, DPT, RRT
GT Physical Therapy
Louisville, Mississippi

Gary Brooks, PT, DrPH, CCS
Associate Professor
Department of Physical Therapy Education
Upstate Medical University
Syracuse, New York

Scotty Butcher, PhD, MSc, BScPT, ACSM-RCEP, CSCS
Assistant Professor
School of Physical Therapy
College of Medicine
University of Saskatchewan
Saskatoon, Canada

Diane E. Clark, PT, MBA, DScPT
Associate Program Director
Department of Physical Therapy
School of Health Professions
The University of Alabama at Birmingham
Birmingham, Alabama

Meryl I. Cohen, DPT, MS, CCS
Instructor
Department of Physical Therapy
Miller School of Medicine
Therapist
Sylvester Cancer Center
University of Miami Medical Group
Coral Gables, Florida
Adjunct Instructor
Department of Physical Therapy
Massachusetts General Hospital Institute of Health Professions
Boston, Massachusetts

Simone Dal Corso, PT, PhD
Physiotherapist of Respiratory Division
Respiratory Division
Federal University of São Paulo
São Paulo, Brazil

Carol M. Davis, DPT, EdD, MS, FAPTA
Professor Emerita
Department of Physical Therapy
University of Miami
Miller School of Medicine
Coral Gables, Florida

Anne Mejia-Downs, PT, MPH, CCS
Assistant Professor
Kannert School of Physical Therapy
College of Health Sciences
University of Indianapolis
Indianapolis, Indiana
Supplemental Physical Therapist and Cardiovascular and Pulmonary Specialist
Methodist Hospital Rehabilitation Services
Indiana University Health
Indianapolis, Indiana

Katherine Ennis, PT, DPT
Cadence Health
Delnor Hospital
Geneva, Illinois

Christian Evans, PhD, PT
Associate Professor
Physical Therapy Program
College of Health Sciences
Midwestern University
Downers Grove, Illinois

Eduard Gappmaier, PT, PhD
Associate Professor
Department of Physical Therapy
University of Utah
Salt Lake City, Utah

Rik Gosselink, PT, PhD
Professor Rehabilitation Sciences
Respiratory Rehabilitation
University Hospitals Leuven
Faculty of Kinesiology and Rehabilitation Sciences
Katholieke Universiteit Leuven
Leuven, Belgium

Willy E. Hammon, III, BSc, PT
Chief of Rehabilitative Services
Oklahoma University Medical Center
Oklahoma City, Oklahoma

Kelly Hawthorne, PT, DPT, GCS
Assistant Professor and Director of Clinical Education
Department of Physical Therapy
Rosalind Franklin University of Medicine and Science
North Chicago, Illinois

Gail M. Huber, PT, PhD
Assistant Professor
Department of Physical Therapy & Human Movement Sciences
Feinberg School of Medicine
Northwestern University
Chicago, Illinois

Patrick Knott, PhD, PA-C
Associate Dean
College of Health Professions
Professor and Associate Vice President for Academic Affairs
Physician Assistant Program
Rosalind Franklin University of Medicine and Science
North Chicago, Illinois

Stacy J. Laack, MS, PA-C
Physical Assistant Program
College of Health Professions
Rosalind Franklin University of Medicine and Science
North Chicago, Illinois

B.J. Lehecka, DPT
Adjunct Professor
Department of Physical Therapy
Wichita State University
Wichita, Kansas

John D. Lowman, PT, PhD, CCS
Assistant Professor
Department of Physical Therapy
The University of Alabama at Birmingham
Birmingham, Alabama

Mary Massery, PT, DPT
Massery Physical Therapy
Glenview, Illinois

Lisa Sigg Mendelson, RN, MS, CPAN
Senior Clinical Nurse
Ambulatory Surgery
Rush University Medical Center
Chicago, Illinois

Victoria A. Moerchen, PT, PhD
Assistant Professor
Department of Physical Therapy and Rehabilitation Science
University of Maryland School of Medicine
Baltimore, Maryland

Claire Peel, PT, PhD, FAPTA
Professor, Physical Therapy
University of Alabama at Birmingham
Birmingham, Alabama

Christiane Perme, PT, CCS
Senior Physical Therapist
Department of Physical Therapy and Occupational Therapy
The Methodist Hospital
Houston, Texas

Arthur V. Prancan
Associate Chair
Department of Pharmacology
Rush University Medical Center
Chicago, Illinois

Elizabeth J. Protas, PT, PhD, FACSM, FAPTA
Vice President and Dean
George T. Bryan Distinguished Professor
School of Health Professions
University of Texas Medical Branch
Galveston, Texas

Mary Rahlin, PT, DHS, PCS
Assistant Professor
Physical Therapy
Rosalind Franklin University of Medicine and Science
North Chicago, Illinois

Myriam D. Riboh, MS, PA-C
Instructor
College of Health Professions
Rosalind Franklin University of Medicine and Science
North Chicago, Illinois

Jennifer M. Ryan, PT, DPT, MS, CCS
Senior Physical Therapist
Rush University Medical Center
Chicago, Illinois

Susan Scherer, PT, PhD
Professor
School of Physical Therapy
Regis University
Denver, Colorado
Associate Dean
Rueckert-Hartman College for Health Professions
Regis University
Denver, Colorado

Alexandra J. Sciaky, PT, MS, CCS
Cardiopulmonary Clinical Specialist
Center Coordinator of Clinical Education
Physical Therapy Department
Veterans Administration Healthcare System
Ann Arbor, Michigan

Preface

Writing the Preface for a book or its revision is an opportunity to pause and reflect. As we take a collective breath seeing the next edition become an entity, we inevitably reflect on our vision for this edition, and the degree to which we have achieved this.

Our vision has always been an ambitious one. This is appropriate given the power of nondrug and nonsurgical approaches to health promotion and remediation of chronic conditions injury and illness. In this fifth edition, specifically, we have revised the title further to reflect changes in theory and practice, and knowledge translation. In the fourth edition, we changed the title from "Cardiopulmonary Physical Therapy: Evidence and Practice" to "Cardiovascular and Pulmonary Physical Therapy: Evidence and Practice" to align the title with the change in the name of the Cardiovascular and Pulmonary Section of the American Physical Therapy Association. In this revised edition, our intention was to further link evidence and practice with a minor yet important change, i.e., the replacement of "evidence and practice" with "evidence to practice"; thus, the revised title is now "Cardiovascular and Pulmonary Physical Therapy: Evidence to Practice."

The merits of the structure of the book and the interrelationship of its Parts and component chapters have held up well with intense scrutiny by external reviewers and users of the book. Therefore, we have concentrated on strengthening the emphasis on the epidemiological basis for content and lifestyle-related conditions given that most patients today have risk factors or manifestations of these conditions, and, in turn, these conditions invariably impact the cardiovascular and pulmonary systems either primarily or secondarily. In addition, contributors were committed to reporting the highest level of physiological and scientific evidence for overall management approaches and treatment interventions. Because of the international appeal of the book over its multiple editions, we remain committed to using boxes, tables, figures, appendices, and pictures as strategically and selectively as possible to best illustrate concepts, ideas, and management considerations. We have paid particular attention to these materials to ensure they reinforce the information in the text to the utmost degree. We take the book's reputation most seriously; therefore we have attempted to incorporate changes that meet the needs of as many stakeholders as possible including students, educators, clinicians across specialties and areas of care, specialists, and other health professionals. We are most appreciative of these stakeholders who have taken time to advise us in this revision.

In ensuring the appeal of the book to users, we have made several changes. First, we have further improved chapter flow and the consistency of their information with additional cross referencing. To enhance the learning experience for students we have contextualized the academic content wherever possible into a clinical framework, which in turn is further reinforced in the cases in the accompanying online Clinical Case Study Guide. Throughout editions, the book has been acknowledged for its user-friendly approach and continues to be a primary textbook in the field. Consistent with the needs in health care this century, we have attempted to broadly consider the impact of multisystem influences on the cardiovascular and pulmonary systems across the continuum of health and dysfunction (consistent with the International Classification of Functioning, Disability and Health [World Health Organization]). Our commitment to the content being both evidence-informed and evidence-based has led us to consider this perspective, in the selection of invited contributors and in the case examples in the accompanying online Clinical Case Study Guide. Each chapter has key terms and review questions to guide the reader in grasping central concepts and translating these into practice. In addition, to serve as an authoritative resource to colleagues developing specific programs such as pulmonary rehabilitation and cardiac rehabilitation that have established international standards, we have outlined the standards for these programs in an easy to use format in appendices for handy reference.

To meet the needs of busy faculty and instructors who need to keep up to date, we provide learning resources and outlines, PowerPoint slides for lectures, and review questions for group work. These resources complement the online Clinical Case Study Guide that accompanies the text. We have further responded to clinicians who need updated information on examination, evaluation, interventions, and outcomes for patients with cardiovascular and pulmonary limitations. In the literature, examination and evaluation tools focus increasingly on the use of standardized outcome measures and professional associations are increasingly encouraging clinicians and students to use these measures routinely and systematically. This is considered essential in contemporary practice to evaluate patients' progress objectively and in a clinically relevant manner. Further, such practice provides an indicator in deciding whether to treat a patient, for changing interventions or their parameters, and as a basis for discontinuing treatment or discharging the patient.

It has been a pleasure for us to reflect on our vision for this edition and how well we have achieved our goals. We sincerely hope the fifth edition meets and surpasses your expectations. With years in the field, we appreciate more than ever that "every patient is a cardiovascular and pulmonary patient" and hope that the information in the book will help ensure health is promoted in every patient, and also ensure we provide "the right treatment, for the right patient, at the right time" in pursuit of the best physical therapy outcomes based on best practice.

We very much look forward to your feedback and welcome suggestions for the sixth edition at any time.

Acknowledgments

The tenets of Hippocrates of "first do no harm" and "the function of protecting and developing health must rank even above that of restoring it when it is impaired" have provided an overarching philosophy and context of practice for this book. It is this perspective that I believe has largely distinguished its contribution and ongoing favorable reception by students, clinicians, and educators worldwide. Over the years, I have often reflected on the wisdom of Hippocrates and cite him frequently. It therefore seems fitting that I formally acknowledge him and his seminal work. The tenets of Hippocrates are as relevant today as they were more than two millennia ago in providing a context in which to address the pandemic of lifestyle-related conditions today. This vision has become blurred in a care arena with competing interests, e.g., a disproportionate emphasis on illness care than on health care and the lens of illness care as a lucrative business. We have attempted to do justice to the ideas and wisdom of Hippocrates in the context of today's health-care needs and priorities. In fact, as one of the leading established health professions and, of these, the primary profession committed to non invasive approaches, physical therapy is in a strategic position to lead in the pursuit of "health and participation for all."

As yet another edition of the book goes to press, I reflect on how we arrived here. No foreword material would be complete without primary acknowledgment of my long-time colleague and friend, the primary co-editor of the book, Donna Frownfelter. I think back to her first edition of the book, a best-seller in the field in North America. I continue to marvel at Donna's unwavering commitment to her original vision through each edition of the book, yet her ever willingness to adapt and change as the world and the needs of the profession evolve along with the demand for evidence-based practice. Thank you, Donna, for the opportunity to be on this journey with you. It has been a phenomenal one.

Few words can express my appreciation to my family, more recently new husband Lawrence Aronsen, and friends for your unending support, inquiries, and quality time. During book revisions, my conversation becomes rather single focused when asked "how are things?" Thank you for your forbearance and understanding and in seeing this project through once again. And, Lawrence, yourself having been through this process several times, your quiet implicit understanding and no-explanation-needed support were invaluable to me in moving things along each day.

My sincere appreciation to the Elsevier team. There are many people behind the scenes in a major undertaking such as the fifth edition of a major textbook. You have contributed in many ways to this new and improved edition. In particular, I would like to thank Kathy Falk, Megan Fennell, and Celeste Clingan. In each of your roles, I thank you for your commitment, support, and adaptability during this revision. You have added to its quality while supporting us and our vision.

Finally, I would like to express my gratitude to the international physical therapy community and my colleagues around the world for your insights and shared vision. In the preface of the fourth edition, I had said that "...by the fifth edition, physical therapists around the world will have increasingly made their mark as primary health care professionals and leaders in the assault on the diseases of civilization by being effective agents of change." Based on multiple international visits since that time, I am heartened to see the groundswell of change taking place in several countries at the levels of our professional bodies, entry-level physical therapy programs, educators, researchers, and clinicians, and their emerging impact on policy makers and ministries of health. By the sixth edition, I look forward to this groundswell becoming a tsunami with physical therapists making major inroads across all of these levels and collectively impacting global health.

I continue to look forward to working with international colleagues toward a shared vision of "health and participation for all." By collectively translating our substantial knowledge base to address the world's leading health-care challenges, we shall make a difference.

Elizabeth Dean, PT, PhD

Contents

Part I

Cardiovascular and Pulmonary Function in Health and Disease

PART I OUTLINE

Chapter 1

Epidemiology as a Basis for Informing Contemporary Physical Therapy Practice

Elizabeth Dean

KEY TERMS

Building healthy communities
Epidemiology
Global health
Healthy people
International Classification of Functioning, Disability and Health
Lifestyle-related conditions
Magic bullet
Noninvasive practitioner
Our village
Paradigm shift
World Health Organization

CHAPTER OUTLINE

This past century, health care priorities have shifted from the prevention and management of acute infectious diseases to the prevention and management of lifestyle-related conditions. These include ischemic heart disease (IHD), smoking-related conditions (including chronic obstructive pulmonary disease [COPD]), hypertension and stroke, diabetes, obesity, and cancer. Not only have the morbidity and mortality resulting from these conditions escalated to their current pandemic proportions, but the probability that an individual (child or adult) has at least one risk factor is high.

To address the gap between lifestyle practices and the body of knowledge on the relationship between lifestyle choices and health,[1] a societal commitment to reducing the number of patients rather than increasing the focus on biomedical care (drugs and surgery) has never been more urgent. Physical therapists are uniquely qualified and strategically positioned as health care professionals to lead in the translation of this well-established body of knowledge into daily practice.[2] A consideration of the risks of lifestyle-related conditions in every individual is consistent with a comprehensive model of best practice in the context of epidemiological trends—that is, evidence-based practice in the context of practice priorities that are themselves informed by evidence. This chapter expands these concepts and outlines principles for applying them proactively and as a priority in the health care of every patient. Physical therapists can have a major impact on the leading priorities of health care, one individual at a time.

What Is Health?

Consistent with the tenets of Hippocrates to which all health care professions aspire—"first do no harm" and "the function of protecting and developing health must rank even above that of restoring it when it is impaired"—the primary objective of health care is to promote health and wellness, to prevent illness and disability and, in the event that these occur, to exploit the least invasive interventions.

The World Health Organization (WHO) defines health as "a complete state of physical, emotional and social well-being"—not merely the absence of disease and impairment.[3] Although physical well-being contributes to health in the other dimensions, it does not ensure health. Thus emotional and social well-being should be assessed as systematically as is physical well-being in a model of care based on health. Collectively, these domains of health translate into an individual's capacity to perform activities that enable him or her to participate fully in life.[4] The WHO's definition of health has not been amended since 1948. Although having withstood time, this definition has failed to be incorporated as the primary goal of contemporary health care.

Over the past century, the primary determinants of improved health have been the provision of clean water, sanitation, basic nutrition, shelter, and security, rather than biomedical advances (other than mass vaccination programs). In addition, education and socioeconomic and employment status are independent determinants of health. Biomedical care has had particular success in controlling infection, providing symptomatic relief of acute problems, and providing emergency care. Such care, however, has not had the impact on health that the primary determinants of health have had overall, nor has biomedical care achieved major success in preventing, reversing, and managing chronic lifestyle-related conditions.

By the time an individual has entered the biomedical system, health care in its truest sense has failed. Without question, the need exists for invasive care (drugs and surgery), well-equipped hospitals, and highly qualified health care professionals. On the other hand, as practitioners committed to noninvasive care, physical therapists have the capacity to promote health and well-being in their practices, with the global goals of reducing the number of patients and minimizing the need for invasive care. The role of physical therapists in preventing and managing chronic lifestyle-related conditions is essential.

Because of widespread immigration, the cultural and ethnic demographic profiles of high-income countries such as those in North America and Europe are changing rapidly. Beliefs, attitudes, values, cultures, ethnicity, and traditions affect health, ill health, and their interactions, including how often individuals seek health care. For example, Asian immigrants to the United States report fewer stress-related and psychological problems than do non-Hispanic Caucasians.[5] With increasing time in the United States, however, reports of stress increase for Asian Americans. This may reflect a number of factors: cultural differences in the acceptability of reporting psychological distress (leading to underreporting by members of some cultural groups), sensitization to the definition and the awareness of stress with increasing duration of residence, or the compounding effect of increasing stress in the new culture. How best to reduce racial and ethnic disparities through culturally competent health care is a matter of debate and requires such outcomes as client satisfaction, improved health status, and culturally appropriate management and delivery across racial and ethnic groups.[6,7]

Since the psychobiological adaptation model was posited over 25 years ago,[8] the few models of physical therapy practice that have been reported have included psychosocial and other nonphysiological components.[9-11] Psychosocial components include health belief, self-efficacy, and perceived control. The Health Belief Model is useful in appreciating the ways in which belief may affect health, illness, and the responses and reactions to them (Table 1-1).[12] Assessment of self-efficacy provides an index of an individual's sense of mastery over his or her health and well-being. These concepts can be used in a clinician's practice setting. A few questions can help assess a patient's perception of susceptibility to risk or a condition. These concepts can provide a basis for health education that includes increasing the patient's awareness of the effects of lifestyle factors on health and of their consequences. The action necessary to avoid the condition or minimize its risk can be selectively targeted for each individual when the individual's context is known.

The International Classification of Functioning, Disability and Health advocated by the WHO interrelates body functions and structures, activity, and participation in life.[4] The biomedical model focuses on impairment (i.e., body functions and structures), with less attention to health and wellness,

Table 1-1 Concepts of the Health Belief Model

Concept	Definition	Application
Perceived susceptibility	One's belief of the chances of getting a condition	Define the population(s) at risk and their risk levels Personalize risk based on a person's traits or behaviors Heighten perceived susceptibility if too low
Perceived severity	One's belief of the seriousness of a condition and its consequences	Specify and describe consequences of the risk and the condition
Perceived benefits	One's belief in the efficacy of the advised action to reduce risk or seriousness of impact	Define action to take—how, where, when Clarify the expected positive effects Describe evidence of effectiveness
Perceived barriers	One's belief in the tangible and psychological costs of the advised behavior	Identify and reduce barriers through reassurance, incentives, and assistance
Cues to action	Strategies to activate "readiness"	Provide how-to information Promote awareness Provide reminders
Self-efficacy	Confidence in one's ability to take action	Provide training, guidance, and positive reinforcement

From Stretcher VJR, Rosenstock IM: The health belief model. In Glanz K, Lewis FM, Rimer BK, editors: *Health behavior and health education: theory, research and practice,* San Francisco, 1977, Jossey-Bass.

sickness impact, life satisfaction, and quality of life, which reflects an individual's participation in life and associated activities. One problem that occurs when the primary focus is on the remediation of limitations of function and structure in managing the leading health care priorities of our day (i.e., chronic lifestyle-related conditions) is that such limitations do not necessarily affect activity and participation—the essence of a meaningful life. These relationships need to be evaluated in each case rather than assumed.

The integration of health belief and motivational models has been a means of incorporating psychosocial dimensions of care, interventions, and outcomes so as to directly focus on an individual's limitations of activity and participation. As a result of this paradigm shift, an increasing number of measurement tools are available to assess the dimensions of health. These tools can be categorized as generic, as having general application across individuals and conditions, or as having specific application to a cohort of individuals, based on age, condition, or some other variable (see examples in Chapter 17). Many of these scales have been validated on a subset of these cohort groups. Physical therapists need to be able to use these tools knowledgeably and specifically to assess outcomes in their practices, just as they use conventional tools to assess and evaluate anatomic structure and physiological function. One such measure is the Short Form-36, which evaluates health-related quality of life and has become an established tool for general use and has been adapted cross-culturally.[13,14] Such tools can be used to evaluate the individual's perception of health improvement, which supplements conventional objective clinical measures.

The Paradox

People living in high-income countries (e.g., countries in North America and Europe, and some Asian countries) and, increasingly, in countries whose economies are growing are experiencing a paradox: an increase in the negative impact of a more Western lifestyle combined with an increase in advances in biomedicine. Technological and economic advances have been proposed as factors contributing to an obesity-conducive environment.[15] The effects of low activity (hypokinesis) and poor nutritional choices on health in Western countries have been reported to be synergistic and partially additive,[16] although a potent interaction may exist. The power of nonpharmacological interventions and solutions to affect global health priorities related to chronic lifestyle-related conditions can no longer be considered secondary to pharmacological solutions.[17,18] Rather, they may need to be considered foremost.

A nationwide, population-based strategy to improve lifestyle is the primary means of improving a country's overall health and minimizing morbidity and premature mortality from chronic lifestyle-related conditions with the least risk and cost.[19-21] Even a modest reduction in cardiac risk factors, for example, could save approximately three times as many life-years as invasive interventions.[22] Preserving and maximizing health in the most cost-effective, low-risk, and ethical manner warrant being universal health care priorities in the 21st century to stem the tide of chronic lifestyle-related conditions.

Lifestyle-Related Conditions

Poor nutritional choices and sedentary lifestyles combined with tobacco use, excessive alcohol consumption, and stress underpin chronic lifestyle-related conditions in high-income countries, and they pose the greatest threats to public health.[23-25] Eight major risk factors related to lifestyle and their documented impacts on health appear in Table 1-2. This trend has given rise to dramatic increases in a relatively newly defined condition, metabolic syndrome, which includes insulin resistance, high blood pressure, elevated triglycerides and cholesterol, and obesity. With industrialization and technological advances, lifestyle-related conditions are on the rise in low- and middle-income countries as well.[26,27] Despite their prevalence, however, the WHO has long proclaimed that lifestyle-related conditions are largely preventable.[28]

Table 1-2 Major Modifiable Risk Factors for Lifestyle-related Conditions

Risk Factor	Cardiovascular (IHD & Hypertension) and Peripheral Vascular Disease	Obstructive Lung Disease	Stroke	Type 2 Diabetes Mellitus	Cancer	Osteoporosis
Smoking	X	X	X	X	X*	X
Physical inactivity	X		X	X	X	X
Obesity	X	X	X	X	X	
Nutrition	X		X	X	X	X
High blood pressure	X		X	X		
Dietary fat†/blood lipids	X		X	X	X	
Elevated glucose levels	X		X	X	X	
Alcohol‡	X		?	X	X	X

*An increased risk of all-cause cancer. Smoking is not only related to cancer of the nose, mouth, airways, and lungs; smoking increases the risk of all-cause cancer.

†Partially saturated, saturated, and trans fats are the most injurious to health.

‡Alcohol can be protective in moderate quantities, red wine in particular.

Modified from the Heart and Stroke Foundation of Canada, 2003; Bradberry JC: Peripheral arterial disease: pathophysiology, risk factors, and role of antithrombotic therapy, *Journal of the American Pharmacy Association* 44(2 Suppl 1):S37–S44, 2004; Charkoudian N, Joyner MJ: Physiologic considerations for exercise performance in women, *Clinics in Chest Medicine* 25:247–255, 2004.

Atherosclerosis is the major common denominator and contributor to lifestyle-related conditions, including ischemic heart disease (IHD), hypertension, and stroke. Factor analysis supports a two-factor solution for heart disease and possibly for other lifestyle-related conditions: family history (factor 1) and lifestyle factors such as smoking, serum cholesterol, blood pressure, nutrition, exercise, and weight control (factor 2).[29] At the population level, choosing health—which includes smoking abstinence along with optimal nutrition and exercise throughout life—can enhance the quality of life, decrease the prevalence of chronic lifestyle-related conditions, and reduce the burden of these conditions on individuals, families, communities, and countries, including suffering and health care costs.[30-32]

Life Cycle and Lifestyle-Related Conditions

Lifestyle-related conditions have their foundation in childhood because their associated underlying health behaviors are rooted during this critical period. The latency period before developing significant signs and symptoms can be decades.

IHD secondary to atherosclerosis continues to be the leading cause of premature mortality and disability in industrialized countries. The prevention and management of risk factors of systemic atherosclerosis should be a primary target of contemporary care for children as well as for adults.[33-35] Ischemic cerebrovascular, coronary, and peripheral vascular conditions are manifestations of the same underlying pathological process, blood vessel narrowing caused by atherosclerosis and thrombosis. Smoking, a high-fat diet, and inactivity can precipitate damage to the endothelium and fat deposition within arterial walls. This common pathway has been associated with increased fibrinogen and C-reactive protein, markers of inflammation.[36] The focus of biomedical research has shifted to the role of inflammatory mediators and the contribution of low-density lipoproteins to atherosclerosis and away from the concept of degenerative vessel disease. Fibrinogen is an inflammation mediator and a clotting factor. People with cardiovascular disease have high fibrinogen levels, which further increase the risk for thrombosis and manifestations of circulatory disease. Inflammation has been implicated in a growing number of chronic conditions, such as IHD, stroke, asthma, gastrointestinal ulcers, cirrhosis of the liver, Alzheimer disease, cancer, and autoimmune conditions.[37,38] Unhealthy lifestyle choices have been thought to contribute to a proinflammatory state, giving rise to low-grade infection in various organ systems and leading to the signs and symptoms associated with various chronic degenerative processes.[39] Although this is an important finding, a proinflammatory milieu and inflammation are not the causes of the chronic conditions with which they have been associated but, rather, are precipitating effects of traumas resulting from lifestyle.

Promotion of a healthy lifestyle early in life transfers responsibility to the individual as much as possible and away from some inherent pathophysiological cause. Although conventional invasive biomedical care with medications and surgery may provide symptomatic relief, only fundamental changes in lifestyle can address the root cause in the majority of cases of chronic lifestyle-related conditions. The physical therapist as a contemporary health care provider can serve as an effective health coach in the care of children and adults.

Lifestyle-related conditions can no longer be considered adult conditions or age-related conditions. Children are exhibiting signs of cardiovascular disease, including arterial atherosclerotic streaking, hypertension, type 2 diabetes mellitus, and obesity.[40] Forty years ago, these conditions manifested in adults. With sedentary lifestyles, low activity, and poor nutrition, children are showing the results of accumulated injury to blood vessels and larger body frames and weights. As a consequence, children today are manifesting lifestyle-related conditions earlier than previous generations and are thus expected to die prematurely from these conditions and to have shorter life expectancies than their parents. Throughout their lives, these individuals can expect to have prolonged morbidity associated with these conditions, the secondary complications of these conditions, associated adverse responses to other health complaints, and increased iatrogenic problems (secondary to drugs and surgery).[41,42] Health promotion strategies directed toward parents and young children will help to offset the population's health threat of lifestyle-related conditions.

Life expectancy has almost doubled since 1900. The post–World War II baby-boom generation characterizes the demographics of many industrialized countries. This cohort has lived in prosperous times and up to that time was the longest living generation in history. Despite the prosperity seen by the baby boomers, this era was associated with more sedentary lifestyles and access to food products low in nutritional value. Although the manifestations of lifestyle-related conditions are associated with aging, they are not necessary consequences of aging. This is based on cross-cultural comparison studies. Optimal nutrition, exercise, stress control, smoking abstinence, and moderate alcohol consumption, if any, are central to reducing the probability of chronic lifestyle-related conditions and associated disability and maximizing quality of life as people age.[43] In particular, increased quality of life with a higher threshold for chronic lifestyle-related conditions and less morbidity toward the end of life is the objective. Figure 1-1 shows the theoretical increase in the threshold of these conditions with healthy lifestyle choices (i.e., not smoking,

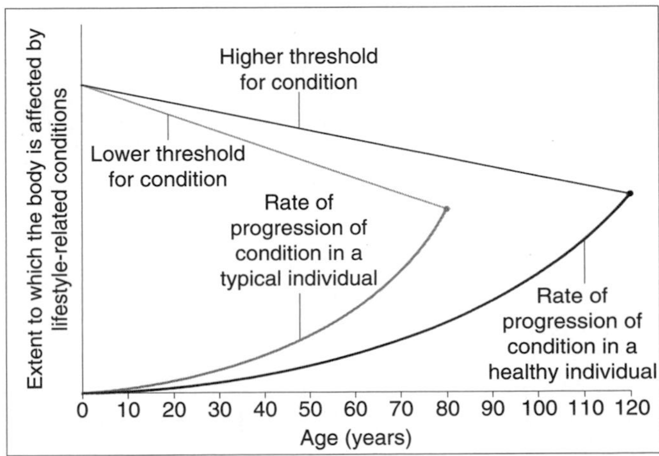

Fig. 1-1 Theoretical relationship between the threshold of lifestyle-related conditions and their rate of progression over the life cycle. *(From Dean E, Lomi C, Bruno S, et al: Addressing the common pathway underlying hypertension and diabetes in people who are obese: the ultimate knowledge translation gap,* International Journal of Hypertension *[in press].)*

optimal nutrition and weight control, regular physical activity and exercise, optimal sleep, and reduced stress) and reduced rate of progression of chronic conditions. Ostensibly, the net result is more "life to years" as well as more "years to life."

"First Do No Harm"

As primarily a noninvasive health care profession, physical therapy is uniquely positioned to have a primary role in promoting health and wellness, while also preventing, managing, and in some cases, reversing these pandemic lifestyle-related conditions, objectives that commonly coexist because they share a common pathway.[44] Integrating health promotion into practice would directly address the ultimate knowledge translation gap in health care (with respect to the benefits of healthy living).[45] Indeed, focusing on health promotion, in addition to directly addressing the risk factors and/or manifestations of secondary lifestyle-related conditions, may result in more favorable outcomes for a patient's presenting problem. Triage of individuals by both noninvasive practitioners and invasive practitioners would constitute a bold initiative in health care. Such triage could establish whether a patient's complaint is best managed in the short and long term wholly noninvasively, wholly invasively, or by some combination, with a view to weaning the patient off medications or minimizing the medication. Similarly, every effort should be made to avoid surgical intervention and its risks whenever possible (i.e., surgical intervention as a last resort rather than a first resort) by exploiting noninvasive interventions and strategies to restore health and promote lifelong health. When an individual enters the health care delivery system, her or his receptivity to health information is likely to be high. This is a prime opportunity to evaluate risk factors and prescribe a lifelong health plan.

The effectiveness of nonpharmacological treatments in the management of chronic lifestyle-related conditions has been well documented, but implementation has been poor.[46-48] As noninvasive practitioners, physical therapists have a primary role on the health team, which may include physicians and surgeons (i.e., invasive practitioners), nurses, nutritionists, pharmacists, social workers, psychologists, respiratory therapists, spiritual leaders, and others, depending on the requirements of each case. On a broader level, physical therapists can serve in a multisector capacity as consultants and work alongside health care policy makers, corporate business people, urban planners, and architects in developing healthy and safe homes, workplaces, recreational facilities, and communities. The role of the physical therapist clinician is shifting from hospital-based acute care and private practice to the community, schools, industry, home, workplace, and playing field.

Biomedical research that evaluates drugs and surgery often lacks control groups that are otherwise healthy or a comparative group in the research design that includes a potentially superior, noninvasively managed group where feasible. For example, a 12-month exercise program involving selected individuals with stable coronary artery disease has shown superior event-free survival and exercise capacity when compared with individuals who received percutaneous coronary intervention.[49] In another study, the mortality rate of individuals with heart disease has been estimated to be reduced by 20% to 25% with cardiac rehabilitation, which is comparable to the results of established therapies such as beta blockers.[50] Cardiac rehabilitation is noninvasive; thus it is cheaper and has few side effects. Management is focused on changing negative health behaviors and maximizing lifelong health rather than on simply altering a sign or a symptom.

Changing one's lifestyle can be more challenging than taking a drug or undergoing surgery. In both cases, the patient is a passive recipient of treatment. Being an effective agent of change and promoting active participation by clients in their own health are fundamental to the expertise of the physical therapist who specializes in noninvasive, long-term health and care. In societies with open and free marketplaces (such as in North American and European countries), people are presented with seemingly endless choices, many of which can be injurious to lifelong health. Thus physical therapists need superior skills in educating people regarding their lifestyle choices and promotion of health.

In contrast to biomedical advances, progress in these noninvasive yet high-impact interventions receives much less coverage and attention as lead articles in peer-reviewed medical journals or by the popular press. Yet these noninvasive advances show significant promise for having a major impact on the population's health and well-being, including increased probability of lifelong health at minimal cost, compared with the results of invasive interventions, which frequently do not address the causes or contributing factors. Such findings need to be integrated into contemporary practice to ensure that individuals are not subjected unnecessarily to the risks associated with prolonged courses of medication and invasive procedures, along with the high probability of repeated invasive procedures. Noninvasive interventions have a distinct advantage over drugs and surgery—they empower individuals to manage their own long-term health by learning skills that will change deleterious lifestyle habits and reduce the risks and costs of hospitalization and its recurrence. Considering the risks and costs of an invasive procedure such as revascularization, the advantages of noninvasive interventions are worthy of much greater attention.

Evidence-Informed Practice

Addressing the Health Care Priorities of the Day

Physical therapists treat individuals with chronic lifestyle-related conditions as either primary or secondary diagnoses. Smoking is currently the leading cause and contributor to chronic conditions and premature death in the United States, with poor diet and sedentary lifestyle anticipated soon to overtake tobacco use.[51] Television viewing, an indicator of sedentary living, is associated with obesity and is a marker of cardiovascular disease independent of total reported physical activity.[51] As noninvasive practitioners, physical therapists have a responsibility to manage these conditions and their risk factors in all patients so as to prevent or control their physical, psychosocial, economic, and societal impact and to promote health in their practices. By prioritizing health and addressing suboptimal health behaviors, regardless of a patient's primary complaint, the complaint may be mitigated, the rate and quality of recovery potentially improved, and the potential for recurrence reduced.

Our Village

Fundamental to the principle of evidence-informed practice is the fact that health care providers respond to epidemiological indicators and an understanding of the changing demographics and face of our "village." Lifestyle-related conditions are the leading killers in our village. Men can expect to live 75 years; women, 82 years.[52] Functional capacity, however, is estimated to decrease 10% per decade, and half of this decrement is due to sedentary living. Raising children to be healthy and physically active will promote a generation of healthy adults and will thereby delay their physical dependence by 10 to 20 years.

Health care workers with international health organizations are trained to manage the unique needs of their villages. This entails knowing the health priorities of the village and making decisions that positively affect the problems and reduce their impact on the community as a whole. In some parts of the world, a health care worker who focuses on malaria when intestinal parasites are the priority is a hindrance, rather than a help, to that village. Similarly, in our health care climate, physical therapists need to make it a priority to meet the leading needs of their "villages." Smoking abstinence, good nutrition, weight control, exercise, and stress management are evidence-based noninvasive interventions consistent with the needs of contemporary physical therapy practice; the therapeutic potential and impact of those elements on the health of our village are enormous. For example, each kilogram of weight loss has a dose-dependent effect on health outcomes. Further, as little as 30 minutes of moderately intense activity on most days of the week offsets the deleterious effects of sedentary living.[53] With the aging of the people of our village and the signs of lifestyle-related conditions now evident in children and young people, the burden of chronic conditions will be prolonged, particularly as individuals approach the end of life. It has been suggested that life expectancy will plateau or even decrease as a result.[42]

Indigenous peoples in North America and Australasia have unique health challenges and needs. They tend to be less well educated than the dominant culture, have fewer employment opportunities, experience more violent injuries and deaths, and have poorer health and shorter lives. They have significant health risks because of sociocultural factors and genetic predisposition, such as higher rates of IHD, stroke, type 2 diabetes mellitus, obesity, hypertension, tobacco use, and alcoholism. Large-scale intervention programs are needed for the Native American population based on studies of the health of its children.[54] The past few generations have witnessed a shift from indigenous foods to refined grains and foods high in fat and sugar and from active to inactive lifestyles. These trends have exacted an enormous toll in terms of personal and social health indicators.

As individuals age in industrialized countries, their activity levels tend to decline. With relatively long life expectancy in these countries, sedentary lifestyles may prolong end-of-life morbidity. A study of individuals who adhered to exercise programs and those who did not revealed the importance of variables such as self-efficacy, perceived fitness, social support, and enjoyment.[55] The results of this study have important implications for urban planning; they can inform the design of healthy communities, as well as individual activity and exercise programs.

A study of black Seventh-day Adventists has provided a unique opportunity to isolate the effects of lifestyle on African Americans. Seventh-day Adventists promote spiritual well-being and a healthy diet and lifestyle. As a result, the health of black Seventh-day Adventists is better and the incidence of chronic lifestyle-related conditions is lower than that of African Americans who are not Seventh-day Adventists.[56] In addition, based on the results of a study of a large cohort, Mormons tend to be fitter and have fewer risk factors for IHD than do other Americans.[57]

The physical activity profiles of African American women have been compared with recommendations for moderate levels of activity.[58] In this study, findings showed that few subjects met the recommended levels of daily physical activity. Exercise was performed on fewer than the recommended number of days per week and for less than the recommended 8 to 10 minutes per session. Attention to frequency and duration may be particularly important when counseling African American women about regular physical activity.

African American women have a higher risk for cardiovascular disease and stroke than do Caucasian American women.[59] Based on a cross-sectional study of 399 urban African American women, correlates of physical activity within this cohort were identified. Programs to promote physical activity should address the safety of the physical environment and psychosocial factors. Inactive women with less than a high school education and those who perceive themselves to be in poor health should be considered special target groups.

Latina women have a higher risk for cardiovascular disease and stroke than do Caucasian American women; this has been attributed to the higher incidence of obesity and type 2 diabetes mellitus among Latinas.[60] The facilitators and barriers to exercising in this cultural cohort have been examined in a cross-sectional study of 300 Latinas. Physical activity has been reported to be higher in younger women, in married women, and in women who had confidence that they could become more active, who saw people exercising in the neighborhood, and who attended religious services.[60] The church was recommended as a suitable community setting for initiating programs that provide women with the knowledge, skills, and motivation to become more active and to transmit this information to others in the community through their families.

The impact of gender is being increasingly appreciated in terms of health affliction, access to health care, and physiological responses and psychological reactions to illness.[61,62] In a Swedish cohort of older adult individuals, obesity-related health indicators and risk factors were reported to differ in men and women and also to differ on the basis of socioeconomic status.[63] In response to cardiac rehabilitation, gender-specific effects on high-density lipoprotein cholesterol have been documented.[64] Women demonstrate greater improvement in high-density lipoprotein than do men.

Urbanization, modernization, and immigration are affecting global health. Within industrialized countries, indigenous people are moving from rural to urban areas; this is occurring in the United States, Canada, Australia, New Zealand, and many African countries. Rather than seeing improvements in their health overall, relocated rural people are succumbing to lifestyle-related conditions. Middle-aged black men who move to urban areas from rural South Africa, for example, increase their risk for IHD and stroke.[65] One explanation for this observation is increased autonomic reactivity to the stress of relocation; however, other lifestyle factors may be implicated. These patterns have been reported for other groups as well; for example, Mexicans and Asians who move to affluent industrialized countries.[66] The typical health advantage for people who move to the West from certain Asian countries, such as Japan, is lost with increasing numbers of years in the new culture.[67]

Principles of Evidence-Informed Practice

The efficacy of the quick fix (drugs and surgery) in the management of chronic conditions, particularly lifestyle-related conditions, is being seriously questioned. With respect to long-term outcomes, noninvasive interventions may often be more successful.[68] Premature mortality can be significantly reduced with regular physical activity, optimal nutrition and weight control, and avoidance of smoking.[69] Relative to invasive care, noninvasive interventions associated with physical therapy (health education and exercise) are low in cost; yet access to these noninvasive measures is commonly more limited than access to invasive care.

The Priorities of Our Village

Health risks and the causes of premature death today are largely related to lifestyle-related conditions, namely:

- Ischemic heart conditions
- Smoking-related conditions, including COPD
- Hypertension and stroke
- Type 2 diabetes mellitus, obesity and metabolic syndrome
- Cancers

These conditions are frequently either the primary or the secondary diagnoses of the patients treated by physical therapists. This positions physical therapists favorably to make direct assaults on the risk factors of lifestyle-related conditions, as well as on their manifestations in patients. Physical therapists have the advantage of prolonged patient contact during treatments compared with other health care providers, and such contact can be exploited in targeting teachable moments and health education opportunities.

Although most people are aware of the positive benefits of healthy choices, what is less apparent to them is that small changes in health behaviors can result in major effect sizes. These effect sizes most often surpass those of medications targeted at a single sign or symptom. In a study of over 23,000 people between 35 and 65 years old, for example, Ford and his colleagues[70] showed that over an 8-year period, people who did not smoke, had a body mass index under 30, were physically active for at least 3.5 hours a week, and followed healthy nutritional principles had a 78% lower risk for developing a chronic lifestyle-related condition. Specifically, the risk for type 2 diabetes mellitus was reduced by 93%, myocardial infarction by 81%, stroke by 50%, and cancer by 36%. Even if not all four of these health factors were present, the risk for developing one or more chronic lifestyle-related conditions decreased commensurate with an increase in the number of positive lifestyle factors. Should a medication be found to have such potent benefits, it would be hailed as nothing short as miraculous.

The goal in health care is to exploit the benefits of lifestyle modification and supplement those benefits with medication only if necessary,[71] rather than the other way around (supplementing medication with lifestyle modification). A healthy lifestyle is the treatment of choice for lifestyle-related conditions; it is also the primary intervention for their prevention.[72] The translation of these research findings into health care practice is a priority.

Ischemic Heart Disease

The risk factors for IHD are well established.[73] They contribute to atherosclerotic deposits not only throughout coronary vessels but throughout the systemic arterial vasculature.[74] Nonmodifiable risk factors include age, sex, family history, and past history. Modifiable risk factors include increased cholesterol, increased homocysteine, smoking, inactivity, high blood pressure, diabetes, weight, and stress.[75-77] Less commonly acknowledged risk factors include elevated C-reactive proteins (markers of inflammation[37]), sharing a lifestyle with someone who has IHD,[78] and having overweight parents.[79] Further, a shared lifestyle confers increased evidence of IHD in and health risk for children.[80] Other emerging risk factors include passive smoking, level of education, depression, anger coupled with hostility, and social isolation.[81,82]

Based on epidemiological evidence, a 1% decrease in cholesterol reduces the risk for IHD by 3%, and a long-term reduction in diastolic blood pressure of 5 to 6 mm Hg reduces the risk by 20% to 25%.[83] Thus even modest changes can have a sizable impact on health. Most risk factors are associated with behavior choices and can be substantially modified.[84]

Risk factors for IHD are prevalent in the general population. When a cross section of people in their later middle-age years was screened, atherosclerosis involving the femoral artery affected two-thirds of them.[85] Further, a direct relationship existed between the degree of atherosclerosis and cardiovascular and general circulatory health. Individuals with peripheral artery disease have a several-fold increased risk for IHD; thus peripheral artery disease can be considered a marker of systemic atherosclerosis. It is estimated that optimal lifestyle could reduce cardiac events related to atherosclerosis by 70% to 80%. Regular walking has a significant effect on reducing the risk for IHD, as has vigorous activity.[86] In men with left ventricular hypertrophy, moderate physical activity reduces the risk for stroke by 49% compared with sedentary men who do not have left ventricular hypertrophy.[87] Type 2 diabetes mellitus has been reported to be a strong risk factor (and hypertension a less strong risk factor) for IHD in women when compared with men.[88]

Self-reported fitness has been reported to be independently related to fewer risk factors for IHD and angiographic evidence of IHD in women undergoing coronary angiography for suspected ischemia.[89] Measures of obesity are not independently associated with these outcomes. Thus fitness appears to be more important than body weight for cardiovascular risk in women. Physical activity and fitness warrant detailed assessment. They should be an integral part of the cardiovascular risk-factor stratification, and interventions should aim at long-term increases in physical activity and fitness. Assessment of physical activity and exercise programs should be included in the management of all people, particularly in women and those at risk for IHD.

Nutrition is a well-established determinant of health and an independent risk factor for lifestyle-related conditions and other chronic conditions. The average North American diet, which tends to be monotonous and unbalanced, has been thought to be a primary contributor to the prevalence of lifestyle-related conditions. Despite its unhealthy characteristics, the North American diet is increasingly being emulated in other parts of the world.

Mediterranean-type diets have been increasingly shown to have multiple health benefits and are superior to the North American diet in terms of food diversity and healthfulness. These diets are high in fish, fresh fruit and vegetables, and multigrains. Mediterranean-type diets are also low in added sugar and salt, and they favor unsaturated vegetable oil over saturated animal fats. When diet-related studies are evaluated, people who consume fish twice a week have a 47% reduced risk for cardiac mortality compared with those who eat fish less than once a month.[90] Cereal fiber (two whole-grain slices of bread daily) is associated with a 14% reduced risk for myocardial infarction or stroke. Cereal fiber consumption even later in life is associated with a reduced incidence of cardiovascular disease.[91] One alcoholic drink a day is associated with the least number of cerebrovascular abnormalities. Moderately and highly physically intense leisure-time activities predict 28% and 44% lower mortality rates, respectively, compared with little activity. Low, moderate, and high levels of exercise are associated with 30%, 37%, and 53% more years of healthy life, respectively. Aerobic training can reduce serum lipids even in older individuals; high-density lipoproteins increase and low-density lipoproteins decrease.[92] With lifestyle change, atherosclerosis can regress and associated cardiac events can be minimized.[93-96]

Psychosocial factors have been identified as risk factors for IHD. Difficulty in managing anger and hostility is one such risk factor, regardless of whether a person has a type A or a type B personality.[97] Stress is a risk factor that can be classified as minor daily hassles or as major negative events. Lipoprotein levels increase with both levels; however, coping style and subjective appraisal of stressors are powerful mitigating factors.[98] Cumulative daily hassles may be underestimated in terms of their impact on health compared with major life stressors. After an individual's first coronary event, avoidance strategies are inversely associated with healthy lifestyles, whereas positive reappraisal and problem solving are directly associated.[99] Positive reappraisal and problem solving, program participation, rather than adopting distancing and escape strategies predict a person's capacity to change lifestyle after a coronary episode. Stress management should consider the type of stressor and help to modify the individual's coping strategies and interpretation of stressors.

The risk for a cardiac event after the first one is high.[100,101] Thus there is a high prevalence of repeated revascularization procedures and the prescription of more drugs with increased potency to help offset worsening pathophysiological changes. Ornish[102] reported that 194 individuals with previous revascularization procedures avoided repeat procedures for at least 3 years (the duration of follow-up in the study) when they participated in a comprehensive lifestyle-change program. Compared with individuals who also had had a previous revascularization procedure but did *not* participate in the lifestyle-change program, those who did participate reported a level of angina comparable to that experienced with revascularization. The effects of noninvasive intervention can be considered long term, given their multisystem benefits. Revascularization focuses on the repair of an impairment and does not provide the additional multisystem benefits of the lifestyle-change program.

To date, efforts to champion aggressive modification of risk factors have been modestly successful. Optimal control of modifiable risk factors for coronary atherosclerosis, including cigarette smoking, dyslipidemia, hypertension, and sedentary lifestyle are well known to reduce the incidence of IHD and, in turn, revascularization procedures and health care utilization.[103] Our major health crisis can be addressed only by means of a system of care committed to health, wellness, aggressive risk-factor prevention, and lifestyle modification.

Smoking-Related Conditions

Smoking is the leading cause of preventable death in the United States, as well as the rest of the world.[51] Despite the well-documented health hazards, smoking remains prevalent in industrialized and nonindustrialized countries and is estimated to shorten life by 11 minutes for each cigarette smoked.[104] Thus smoking cessation is a primary health care goal, as well as a professional goal. (In 1996, the APTA adopted guidelines from the Agency for Health Care Policy and Research [AHCPR], which have subsequently been revised.[105]) The danger of smoking extends beyond COPD and cancer. Overall morbidity and all-cause mortality, including cancer of organs other than the respiratory tract, are higher in smokers.

Of the leading causes of mortality worldwide, COPD is typically among the top killers and is associated with the loss of a million years of life each year.[106] In the United States, COPD ranks fourth behind IHD, cancer, and stroke. Long-term smokers have higher incidences of all-cause morbidity and mortality (Table 1-3); thus smoking leads to life-threatening conditions that are systemic and are related not just to the respiratory tract.[90] Former and current smokers have 25% and 44% fewer healthy years of life, respectively, compared with lifelong nonsmokers. Smoking cessation is a priority for all individuals, not only those with lung disease, regardless of disease severity.[107] Smoking by children is highly associated with parental smoking; thus smoking by adults with young families has become a primary focus of public health initiatives.[79] Smoking is the single most important preventable cause of illness and death.

Pulmonary rehabilitation has demonstrated sustainability of smoking cessation and other health benefits in individuals with COPD;[108] thus its use is warranted as a preventive measure, as well as for the remediation and management of disease.[109] Rehabilitation programs have proven efficacy, independent of pharmacotherapy, so they should be considered primary interventions rather than priorities after conventional expensive medical care has failed.[110] Only with health coaching and follow-up can these individuals effect lifelong health behavior change to minimize exacerbations, reduce doctor and hospital visits, continue working, and reduce overall morbidity. Innovative smoking cessation programs warrant development so that they have maximal impact in the most significant window of opportunity and stage of readiness of a smoker to quit. One such program consisted of 5 weeks of counseling.[111] The mean time to deliver the intervention was 44 minutes. At 1 month, 70% of participants had

Table 1-3 Tobacco Facts and Multisystem Consequences of Smoking

Type/Area of Effects	Effects and Conditions That Are More Common in Smokers
Mortality from smoking	Tobacco causes 30% of all deaths of people between 35 and 69 years of age Tobacco reduces a person's life as follows: Ages 35 to 59 years: Those killed by tobacco lose about 27 years of life Ages 60 to 69 years: Those killed by tobacco lose about 16 years of life
Brain	Stroke
Mouth	Lip and oral cancers
Pharynx and larynx	Cancers of the pharynx and larynx
Esophagus	Cancer of the esophagus
Lungs	Cancer of the lungs
Heart	Ischemic heart disease, hypertension, and circulatory diseases
Chronic lung disease	Bronchitis and emphysema; 90% of deaths from chronic lung disease attributable to smoking Upper respiratory tract infections and increased days of absenteeism
Gastric and duodenal ulcers	Higher risk in smokers
Bladder and kidney cancers	Higher risk in smokers
Bone	Postmenopausal women who smoke have reduced bone density compared with nonsmokers Increased risk of bone fractures and delayed healing
Fertility and Pregnancy	Infertility Increased risk for spontaneous abortions, still births, pre-term deliveries, low-birth-weight babies, and sudden infant death syndrome Potential developmental and learning delays in children

Data from National Cancer Institute: Cancer Facts, 2010; U.S. Department of Health and Human Services: The health consequences of smoking: a report of the Surgeon General, U.S. Department of Health and Human Services, Centers for Disease Control and Prevention, National Center for Chronic Disease Prevention and Health Promotion, Office on Smoking and Health, 2004; Peto R, Lopez AD, Boreham J, et al: Mortality from tobacco in developed countries: indirect estimation based on national vital statistics, *Lancet* 339:1268–1278, 1992; Twardella D, Kupper-Nybelen J, Rothenbacher D, et al: Short-term benefit of smoking cessation in patients with coronary artery disease: estimates based on self-reported smoking data and serum cotinine measurements, *European Heart Journal* 25:2101–2108, 2004.

continued to abstain. The mean cost of the intervention was approximately $50 for each person.

Smoking cessation is the most cost-effective intervention for smokers with heart disease in terms of health protection and risk reduction. Further, treatment of hyperlipidemia and referral to cardiac rehabilitation are highly cost-effective per quality-adjusted life-year and are relatively cost-effective per year of life saved. Smoking is an established risk factor for ischemic stroke, subarachnoid hemorrhage, and intracerebral hemorrhage,[112] as well as for IHD. The risk is directly proportional to the amount smoked. Risk factor detection and management are the cornerstones of high-impact and high-quality care of cardiovascular disease.

Hypertension and Stroke

Stroke is a preventable tragedy for nearly 750,000 people in the United States annually; hypertension is the most common risk factor.[113] Although lowering blood pressure below 130/85 mm Hg is well accepted across ages, the success of blood pressure control has been reported to be less than 25% in the hypertensive population.[114] Stroke risk is far from being well controlled despite considerable understanding of its causes, and it remains a major health threat. Risk factors for stroke include previous stroke, hypertension, IHD, atrial fibrillation, hyperlipidemia, diabetes, abnormal ankle-to-brachial pressure index, reduced exercise endurance, retinopathy, albuminuria, autonomic neuropathy, smoking, alcohol consumption, and lack of exercise.[113,115-119]

Risk factors for hypertension and stroke can be accentuated by smoking, elevated cholesterol, glucose intolerance, inactivity, and obesity.[120] In addition to stroke, serious consequences of hypertension include hypertension heart disease and renal disease. Implicated as a cause of stroke is increased sympathetic reactivity.[121]

In the adult population between 60 and 74 years of age, almost 75% of African Americans and 50% of Caucasians have high blood pressure.[122] As with IHD, risk factors for high blood pressure consist of nonmodifiable and modifiable risk factors. Nonmodifiable risk factors include age, sex, race, and other genetic factors. Modifiable risk factors include diets high in sodium and low in potassium, alcohol consumption, reduced physical activity, and being overweight.[123] Obesity is a strong predictor of hypertension.[124] Although significant reduction of hypertension has been attributed to low-dose thiazide diuretics and beta blockers, the first line of defense to prevent high blood pressure and normalize blood pressure should be nutritional approaches, weight reduction, and regular physical activity and exercise.[125] In individuals whose hypertension is controlled, the combination of a Mediterranean diet and physical activity can reduce health risk substantially.[126] Like other lifestyle-related conditions, hypertension is increasingly common in American children; thus screening should be included in routine pediatric assessments.[127]

With respect to nutrition, high sodium and low potassium have been implicated in hypertension and stroke, as have lipids. The National Academy of Science has recently announced that reducing added salt by as little as one-third would reduce hypertension in the United States by 25% (11 million fewer cases). Low plasma vitamin C is associated with a several-fold increased risk for stroke, particularly in men who are overweight and hypertensive.[128] A minimal reduction in diastolic blood pressure (5 to 6 mm Hg) reduces the risk for stroke by 35% to 40%.[83] Thus weight control; regular exercise; a diet rich in fruits, vegetables, and whole-grain cereals; smoking cessation; and blood pressure control are central to stroke prevention, as well as to the comprehensive management of stroke.

Although weight reduction is an essential component of hypertension prevention and management, the protective effect of physical activity may be unrelated to the degree of obesity.[129] A 4% to 8% reduction in body weight can reduce blood pressure by 3 mm Hg, and physical activity can reduce blood pressure by 5/3 mm Hg.[130]

In normotensive African American men, aerobic exercise can attenuate an exaggerated blood pressure response.[131] Similarly, normotensive fit African American women have blunted blood pressure responses to experimental stressors.[132] One study reported no relationship between physical activity and hypertension, flow-mediated dilation of the brachial artery, or an index of angiogenesis assessed with plasma vascular endothelial growth factor (the latter two being indicators of endothelial dysfunction).[133] In this study, however, physical activity was based on self-report in a questionnaire rather than on fitness outcomes, so the results of the study are difficult to interpret.

Physical activity and optimal nutrition can reduce the risk for early atherosclerosis, a precursor to stroke, in lifelong nonsmokers.[134] Smokers benefit less from this protective effect. Physical activity seems not only to reduce the risk for stroke but also to provide a potent prophylactic strategy for increasing blood flow and reducing brain injury during cerebral ischemia.[135] A possible mechanism is augmented endothelium-dependent vasodilation via up-regulation of endothelial nitric oxide synthase throughout the vasculature. Aerobic exercise three times a week reduces cerebral infarct size and functional deficits in a mouse model and improves endothelium-dependent vasorelaxation.[135]

Assessment of risk for hypertension is an important component of each patient's assessment. The management strategy should be based on an analysis of the overall risk assessment rather than on blood pressure alone. The prevention of hypertension requires more than normalizing blood pressure if the deadly manifestations of high blood pressure including IHD are to be avoided. Because of the dire consequences of hypertension, the American Heart Association advocates stringent blood pressure limits—specifically, below 130/85 mm Hg, regardless of age.[136] Recommendations by the American Heart Association concerning physical activity and exercise guidelines for survivors of stroke concur that physical conditioning is a primary goal in these individuals, who must contend with both the pathological effects of stroke and the effects of deconditioning.[137] Walking as little as 2 hours a week can reduce the risk for stroke by 50%.[130] Improved conditioning may help to reduce limitations of activity and participation and hence improve quality of life. The burden of disease and disability and their risk factors may be correspondingly reduced.

To affect the health of the population, stroke prevention depends on the dissemination of these well-established and widely available interventions to a large number of people through public health policy. Advice given by a health provider to individuals with stroke for the purpose of prevention of a second stroke can have significant impact. In one study, individuals were simply advised to eat fewer high-fat and high-cholesterol foods and to exercise more.[138] Compared with a control group that received no advice, those receiving advice reported fewer days with limited activity, fewer days that "were not good physically," and more "healthy" days. The results of this study are compelling in that even simple advice by a health care provider can have a major impact on important health behaviors and on potential health outcomes.

Type 2 Diabetes Mellitus and Metabolic Syndrome

Type 2 diabetes mellitus is a serious multisystem condition that has rapidly become pandemic in Western countries and some other countries where its incidence was previously minimal. In addition to the serious physical and functional consequences of this condition, perceived health status and quality of life are also compromised.[139] By 2010, an estimated 250 million people will be affected worldwide.[140] Formerly known as adult-onset diabetes, type 2 diabetes mellitus is now being diagnosed in children, predisposing them to blindness, IHD, stroke, renal disease, peripheral neuropathies, vascular insufficiency, and amputations.[141,142] Inositol acts as a poison on the membranes of cells in the presence of high blood sugar, and it has been implicated in the deadly systemic consequences of diabetes. The primary consequences include pathological changes to the macro- and microvasculature and to the nerve endings. Impaired glucose tolerance is a marker of vascular complications in the large and small blood vessels, independent of an individual's progression to diabetes. Early detection of glucose intolerance allows intensive dietary and exercise modifications, which have been shown to be more effective than drug therapy in normalizing postprandial glucose and inhibiting progression to diabetes.[143] Diabetic autonomic neuropathy as an independent risk factor for stroke may reflect increased vascular damage and effect on the regulation of cerebral blood flow in individuals with diabetes.[115]

Individuals with type 2 diabetes mellitus have increased risk for cardiovascular disease compared with individuals without diabetes, so strict control is essential. Moderate physical activity (such as brisk walking[144]) along with weight loss is a powerful combination to reduce the risk for type 2 diabetes mellitus, as well as to reverse it. These interventions combined with a balanced diet can reduce the risk for developing diabetes among those who are at high risk by 50% to 60%.[86] Cigarette smoking is an independent risk factor for type 2 diabetes mellitus[145] and is particularly dangerous for individuals who already have diabetes.[141]

Metabolic syndrome refers to a virulent and lethal group of atherosclerotic risk factors, including dyslipidemia, obesity, hypertension, and insulin resistance, and it affects some 47 million people in the United States.[146] The incidence of the syndrome is increasing and warrants aggressive noninvasive management. Insulin sensitivity is predicted primarily by body mass index, smoking, age, and daily physical activity. Weight reduction counters the effects of metabolic syndrome and may counter the associated hypertension and dyslipidemia as well. Diet and exercise are primary components of the multifactorial approach to preventing and managing this lethal condition.

Obesity

Obesity has been increasing exponentially over recent decades; currently, 61% of the American population is overweight.[147] Obesity is becoming a global pandemic that rivals malnutrition as a health priority in some low-income countries,[148] and it contributes to health risks for all lifestyle-related conditions. The complications and risks for which each patient should be assessed include IHD, cardiac myopathy, and chronic heart and lung dysfunction; hypertension and stroke; some cancers;

insulin insensitivity and type 2 diabetes mellitus; gallbladder disease; dyslipidemia; osteoarthritis and gout; and pulmonary conditions, including alveolar hypoventilation and sleep apnea.[149-153] With each kilogram of weight above normal, the risk for hypertension, IHD, and type 2 diabetes mellitus increases proportionately. Obesity is commonly linked with insulin resistance and high blood pressure, which may reflect reduced activity and exercise. Reduced physical activity is a predictor of obesity.[154] Insulin resistance associated with lack of exercise in people who are overweight may be further compounded by insulin resistance associated with chronic inflammation observed in fat cells.[155] Abdominal obesity, lipid metabolism, and insulin resistance are interrelated markers for coronary artery disease.[156] In addition to cardiovascular and general health risk, being overweight affects quality of life.[157,158]

Comprehensive management of an individual who is overweight and has abnormal blood glucose levels includes normalizing blood glucose (with recommendations for low-glycemic foods and small, frequent snacks rather than infrequent large meals), weight reduction, restricted intake of trans fats and saturated fats, strict blood pressure and lipid control, regular physical activity and exercise, and avoidance of tobacco.[159]

Nutritional habits during childhood are associated with lifestyle-related conditions in adulthood.[160] Obesity in children is associated with parental obesity.[79] Maintaining weight within a healthy body mass index range throughout life is recommended for optimal health. Although body mass index may be limited with respect to assessing adiposity because it fails to discriminate between muscle and fat and identify regional adipose depositions, it remains a useful supplementary clinical index.[161] Physical therapy has a primary role in preventing and managing overweight and obesity in every client or patient, regardless of age, given obesity's serious multisystem consequences, psychosocial sequelae, and threat to life participation and satisfaction.[162]

Cancer

The risk factors for cancer are well documented and include environmental and behavioral factors such as nutrition (fats and refined foods), inactivity, poor air quality and smoking, psychological factors, and ingestion of and exposure to chemicals. Cancer, hallmarked by an overgrowth of cells, eventually compromises normal organ function.

Cancers associated with the highest mortality rates include lung, colorectal, and pancreatic cancer.[163] Smoking has been implicated as a risk factor for many cancers, not only those involving the respiratory tract. The role of lifestyle factors in cancer remission has not been studied in detail.

Cancer prevention and rehabilitation have become a specialty area, requiring an integrated knowledge of pathophysiology, psychosocial implications, and management interventions.[164,165] Routine assessment of health behaviors and risk factors and healthy living recommendations may help avert the diagnosis of many cancers or mitigate their effects. To date, evidence that walking is an effective strategy to prevent cancer has been best established for colon cancer,[86] although breast cancer and prostate cancer have also been reported to be positively affected by regular aerobic exercise including walking.[166,167]

Musculoskeletal Health

Osteoporosis and arthritis contribute to considerable morbidity and secondarily to mortality. Because both of these conditions have lifestyle components, a lifestyle risk factor review should be included in every initial assessment to establish a baseline of musculoskeletal health. Moderate levels of physical activity, including walking, are associated with a substantially lower risk for hip fractures in postmenopausal women.[168] Thus assessment of both nonmodifiable and modifiable risks is a major component of the health assessment as a means of minimizing morbidity and potential mortality.[9] Osteoporosis and associated morbidity, particularly in older age groups, is a serious health issue that warrants monitoring. Establishing baseline information on bone health in every patient is prudent, given the relationship between bone health and lifestyle behaviors (e.g., activity and nutrition—smoking and heavy consumption of meat, alcohol, and coffee). Although older, postmenopausal women have been the focus of bone health studies, other groups are also at risk for osteoporosis and should not be overlooked: older men; inactive children, particularly girls; and individuals with chronic conditions who may be less able to undertake weight-bearing activities and physical activity. In a study of the development of bone mass and strength in girls and young women, only exercise (not daily calcium intake) was associated with bone density and strength.[169] This finding stresses the singular importance of bone building in young people to help offset osteoporosis later in life and associated decrement in quality of life.

Psychological Health

Mental health problems and depression are prevalent in Western society despite its affluence. Based on one descriptive study, individuals with mental health conditions such as schizophrenia tend to have poor physical health and die prematurely from cardiovascular disease.[170] Compared with women who have schizophrenia, men with the condition consumed less fruit, vegetables, whole grains, and rice than recommended. Further, the incidence of smoking and obesity in both sexes was higher than in the general population. Cholesterol levels were high and activity levels low. This study suggested cause for concern about both the physical and psychological well-being of individuals with mental health conditions and indicated the need for further investigation of the physical health and well-being of people with mental challenges.

Dementia and Alzheimer disease appear to be increasing. Aging has been countered as a primary argument for this trend in favor of lifestyle-related influences including nutrition, specifically, processed meat consumption. Recently, Alzheimer disease has been associated with the consumption of meat from animals that have been fed nonnatural foods. This has been thought to lead to misfolding of DNA, thus affecting cognitive function in people who have consumed such products over many years.[171] Other factors that have been associated with the condition include decreased cerebral blood flow.[172] Understanding the vascular component of this condition along with food-related explanations will be an important advance in its prevention and management. In a cohort of older African Caribbean individuals, vascular risk has been associated with cognitive impairment and physical activity is inversely related to impaired cognition.[173] Exercise training has been reported to improve physical health and depression in individuals with Alzheimer disease.[174] Whether this reflects a vascular component of the pathogenesis of the disease that is offset by exercise warrants elucidation.

Dental Health

Periodontitis, characterized by low-grade infection of the gums, is widespread and may be associated with serious systemic health problems. In a study of 39,461 men, periodontitis risk decreased with increased physical activity, independent of such risk factors as age, smoking, diabetes, body mass index, alcohol consumption, and total calories.[175] Inactivity and the typical Western diet have been described as proinflammatory. Whether the benefits of a physically active lifestyle and an optimal diet can extend to dental health warrants investigation.

Promoting Healthy Living: The Contemporary Physical Therapist's Role

Assessment of health behaviors and recommendations for healthy living can be put into practice in every patient interaction[176] and, in turn, help reduce the population's health risk and mitigate the economic cost of lifestyle-related conditions.[177] Increased consumption of meat, fat, and sugar has contributed to the increased prevalence of lifestyle-related conditions in low- and middle-income countries, as well as in high-income countries.[178] An associated increase in the prevalence of insulin-resistance syndromes is further increasing the incidence of cardiovascular disease.[179] Anthropologists have argued that food abundance and inactivity may be altering evolutionary processes and that these factors contribute to the current pandemic of chronic conditions.[180] Attitudes toward factors contributing to lifestyle-related conditions reflect the values and behaviors of society. Optimal control will be achieved only with widespread public health policy, social action involving health care providers, and an increase in individual responsibility.

Why Physical Therapists Need to Understand and Advocate Optimal Nutrition

Physical therapists use exercise as a primary intervention to prevent, remediate, or mitigate the effects of disease and disability. As clinical exercise physiologists, they need substantial understanding of healthy nutrition, nutritional assessment, and nutritional regimens that will maximize human performance in patient populations. Such populations are comparable to athletes in that they need to meet the metabolic demands of their day (or event), as well as maximizing their health overall. Without such knowledge, assessment and exercise prescription are suboptimal and, in turn, therapeutic outcomes are suboptimal.

Given that an association has been established between diet and chronic lifestyle-related conditions, the question of what is the optimal nutritional regimen for humans has been widely debated. Of note is that the anatomic structure and physiological (endocrine) function of humans are consistent with an organism designed for a largely plant-based diet—that is, having hands rather than claws, a particular tooth type and skin type, salivary glands, acidity in the saliva, ptyalin in the saliva, a specific level of hydrochloric acid in the stomach, and an intestinal tract of a certain length.[181]

Cultures that consume a diet based primarily on plants tend to have superior health outcomes. The diets of octogenarians in Asia and of centenarians in general tend to be high in fiber and low in saturated and trans fats, refined sugar, and salt compared with the typical diet of Western people.[182] The Mediterranean diet, which includes plentiful fruits, vegetables, fish, and vegetable oil, has shown health benefits and is associated with lower incidence of chronic disability and premature death compared with the typical Western diet.[87,126] Cultures in the Mediterranean region also tend to have higher activity levels, which influences metabolism and physiological responses to food.

Weight-loss diets are a multibillion-dollar industry in Western cultures. Many of these diets are unsubstantiated or may theoretically work but are not well balanced in terms of the macro- and micronutrients needed daily for optimal health. Low-carbohydrate diets have been popular, but weight loss associated with these diets results from calorie restriction and the duration of the diet rather than from a reduction in carbohydrate consumption.[183] Weight control is achieved by the balance between optimal caloric and nutrient content consumed and optimal energy expenditure. Given the pandemic of obesity in industrialized countries, physical therapists need to understand the normal physiological adaptations to poor food choices and sedentary lifestyles—weight distribution, endocrine changes, cardiovascular and pulmonary changes, and musculoskeletal changes—in order to prescribe the best lifelong management programs.

Overweight and obesity constitute a life-threatening pandemic that warrants management before the manifestation of one or more of its life-threatening consequences, in addition to its associated psychosocial and economic consequences. Along with obesity, glucose intolerance may complicate the picture, or the patient may have subclinical intolerance. Central adiposity, in particular, has been associated with a high incidence of insulin resistance, which may explain the high rates of dyslipidemia, hypertension, and type 2 diabetes mellitus in these individuals.[184] Thus the physical therapist has a primary role in basic nutrition counseling, commensurate with the promotion of optimal health, and in providing information about nutrition (related to exercise energetics and glucose control) to support a prescribed dosage of regular exercise and physical activity. A nutritionist may need to be consulted to provide nutrition counseling beyond fundamental needs, especially in complicated cases.

Nutrition guidelines have been revised by the U.S. Department of Health and Human Services[185] and Health Canada.[186] Compared with previous versions, the revisions appear to be better aligned with the literature than with the interests of lobby groups from the food industry and producers of so-called nutritional supplements. Some authorities have argued that the current pandemic of lifestyle-related conditions reflects adherence to guidelines over which food-industry lobbyists had influence, rather than lack of adherence by consumers. Current consumption of fats, refined foods, and vegetables in North America, for example, has failed to meet the recommended revised guidelines. Diets high in salt, saturated fat, and refined foods, and low in servings of vegetables and fruit have been implicated in lifestyle-related conditions.

The revised guidelines are more evidence based and have been designed to optimize health and reduce the risk for chronic conditions. Earlier guidelines fell short with respect to this objective. Adherence to established dietary guidelines for Americans as assessed by the healthy eating index was only weakly associated with risk for major chronic conditions in men[187] and was not associated at all with risk for major chronic conditions in women.[188] Thus dietary guidelines and the healthy eating index require refining to achieve more favorable outcomes and to allow them to be assessed.

An optimal food pyramid, on which the revised nutrition guidelines are based, is shown in Figure 1-2, *A*. The pyramid illustrates general guidelines for maximizing health in the general public, and these guidelines have been shown to offset lifestyle-related conditions.[189] Each individual's diet should conform with these guidelines for optimal lifelong health. The nutrition food pyramid emphasizes abundant servings of vegetables at the base; followed by vegetable or lean-meat protein sources and dairy; beans, lentils, and whole grains; and low-glycemic foods. Red meat and eggs, positioned at the top of the pyramid, are to be consumed most sparingly. The typical Western diet is short on vegetables, fruits, and fiber (particularly insoluble fiber)[190-192] and includes excess salt, sugar, highly refined foods, and saturated and trans fats.[193] Diets high in grain-based foods are associated with reduced cardiovascular risk, independent of other behaviors.[193,194] The food pyramid has recently been revised as a plate icon where 2-3 servings of vegetables cover half the plate, a quarter carbohydrates (multigrains) and the remaining quarter vegetable protein or animal protein Figure1-2, *B*. Unless a person has an objectively identified deficit, there is no evidence that nutrient supplementation adds benefit to a daily nutritious diet.

Attention to nutrition is important not only in relation to body weight. Cholesterol and triglycerides are risk factors for IHD.[195] To address this major health threat, lipid-lowering drugs have glutted the pharmaceutical market and one-stop coronary cholesterol clinics have been advertised. However, a cardioprotective diet, which has been well described in the literature, should be the goal, in conjunction with lipid-lowering agents in selected cases. Even when medications are used, weaning individuals off them as lipids and cholesterol are lowered by noninvasive means is an important goal of physical therapy, in conjunction with a lifelong program of exercise, good nutrition, no smoking, moderate alcohol consumption, and stress management.

With respect to body mass, risk factors increase as body mass increases beyond a healthy range. Studies recommend that a healthy waist girth (low risk) is <84 cm (33 in) for women and <89 cm (35 in) for men.[196] Further, waist-to-hip ratio has been shown to be a better predictor of myocardial risk than body weight alone.[197] Thus measures of height and weight to calculate body mass index, as well as waist and hip girth, are simple standardized assessment tools and outcomes that can be used diagnostically and as tools to evaluate response to interventions such as dietary education and exercise to achieve optimal weight.

Finally, Western diets have excessive salt content—hence the pandemic of hypertension. Measures need to be taken to legislate the salt added in food production and processing. An overriding simple solution at the individual level is restricting added salt to foods. A one-third reduction of salt intake by the average American (from 3400 mg to 2300 mg daily) would reduce cases of hypertension (the second-leading cause of death in the United States), by 11 million and would lower health care costs by $17.8 billion.[198]

Why Physical Therapists Need to Understand Exercise in the Context of Population Health

The physical activity and exercise pyramid is illustrated in Figure 1-2, *B*. This pyramid shows a physically active lifestyle at the base, followed by aerobic exercise three to five times a week, followed by strengthening exercise and flexibility, with rest and inactivity at the top.

Sedentary behavior has been a recent focus of study with the recognition that reducing sedentary behavior is not necessarily synonymous with increasing physical activity. The literature supports that prolonged periods of being sedentary are associated with greater health risk than multiple short periods of sedentary behavior (i.e., breaks in sedentary time).[199,200] Sedentary activity is common today; people often sit for long periods in front of a television or computer, and children and adolescents are increasingly consumed with screen-based activities. Recommendations for breaks in sedentary behavior are complementary to those for increasing physical activity. Sedentary behavior in early childhood is associated with such behavior in adolescence and adulthood.[201] Encouraging physical activity in adults and children regularly throughout the day requires not only individualized education about exercise, but structuring neighborhoods, transportation systems, recreational facilities, homes, and workplaces that are health promoting.

The physical activity pyramid, like the food pyramid, is a reminder of the importance of lifestyle choices for optimal health.[202] Generally, walking 10,000 steps a day is consistent with an active lifestyle and good health in an adult,[203] whereas fewer than 5000 steps a day would be considered a sedentary lifestyle. Walking 7500 to 9999 steps a day is consistent with a somewhat active lifestyle, and more than 12,500 steps a day would be consistent with a highly active lifestyle.

With increased physical activity, the risks for IHD, stroke, and colon cancer are reduced. The precise dosage-response relationships between physical activity and health and between physical fitness and health have yet to be clarified and may differ among people.[204] Moderate physical activity, which does not have to be strenuous or prolonged, includes leisure activities such as walking and gardening and is associated with marked health benefits.[145] Even light to moderate physical activity in middle and old age confers marked benefit to cardiovascular health and is protective against all-cause mortality.[205] The U.S. Surgeon General recommends 30 minutes of moderately intense exercise on most days, with an accumulated duration of 180 minutes a week.[206]

Exercise has a profound effect on the endothelial function of blood, which has been implicated in atherosclerosis, IHD, cerebrovascular disease, and gastrointestinal conditions, and could explain exercise's multisystem benefits. Moderate levels of physical activity reduce the risk for stroke, independent of other factors.[207] In addition to dietary habits, reduced physical activity has been implicated in most lifestyle-related conditions including osteoporosis, and exercise is recognized as an essential component in the primary prevention of these conditions. Even mild physical activity has an important role in the primary prevention of type 2 diabetes mellitus through its

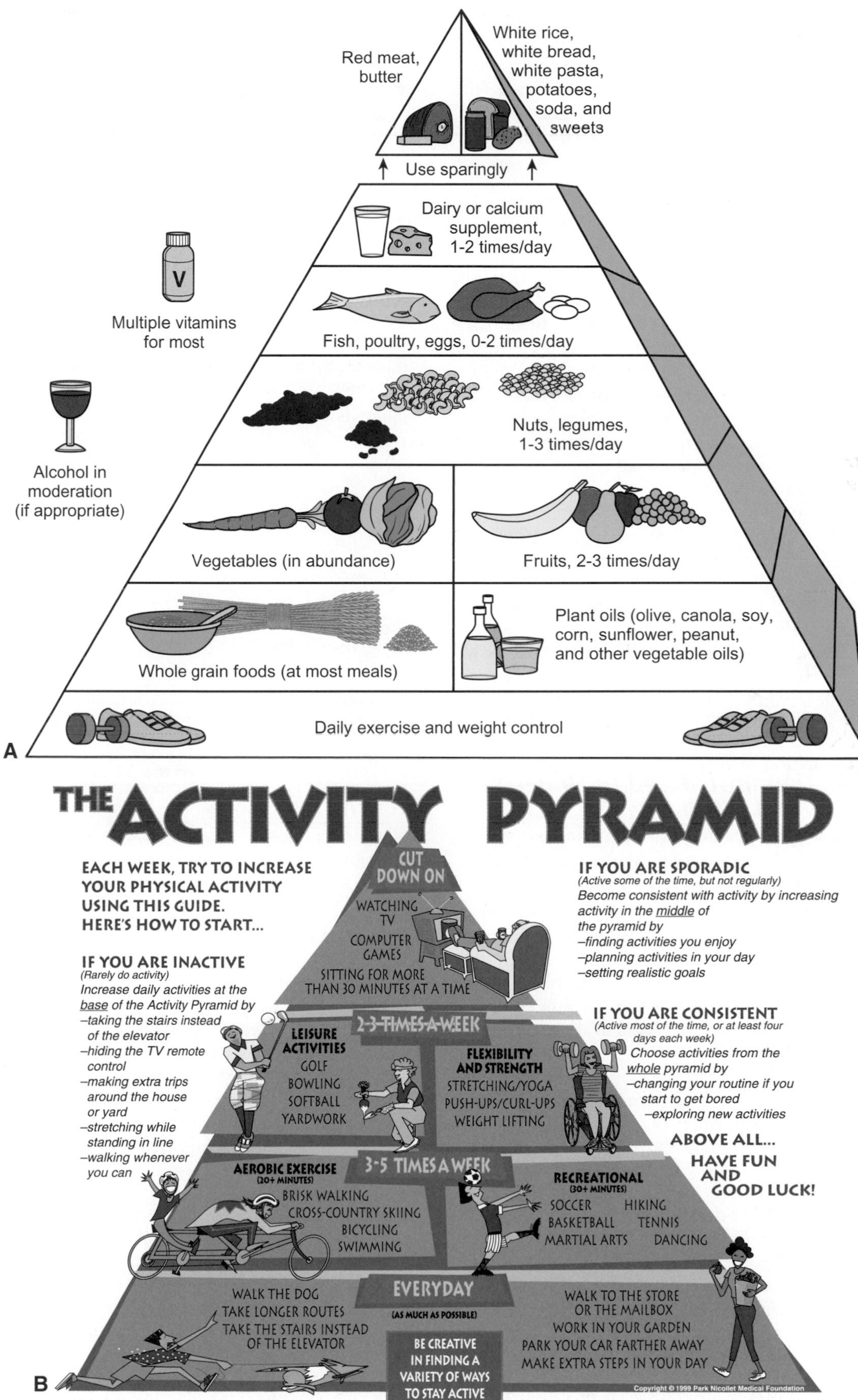

Fig. 1-2 Nutrition and activity pyramid guides. **A,** An alternative Food Guide Pyramid based on the latest research on optimal nutrition. **B,** The Activity Pyramid. *(**A** from Clayton BD:* Basic Pharmacology for Nurses, *ed 15, St Louis, 2010, Mosby.* ***B*** *from Park Nicollet Health Source Institute for Research and Education, Minneapolis, Minn.)*

direct effect on increased tissue sensitivity to insulin.[208] Nonpharmacological interventions for preventing and managing hypertension have been strongly advocated to maximize their therapeutic benefit and minimize the risks associated with medications.[209] Furthermore, in older people, regular physical activity has an important role in preventing chronic conditions and prolonged end-of-life suffering.[210]

Why Physical Therapists Should Promote Smoking Cessation

Smoking is the leading cause of premature death. It results in premature death and higher rates of all-cause death.[50] Although Caucasian Americans have a higher rate of smoking than do African Americans, African Americans and women who smoke have respiratory problems at a younger age, despite having started smoking later and having a lower overall pack-year smoking history.[211] Men with a strong intention to quit have been reported to have a more favorable attitude toward quitting and a stronger sense of perceived control than those with a less strong intention to quit. In addition, men who have a strong intention to quit smoking have greater success.[212] With a view to promoting lifelong health, advocating smoking reduction and cessation is an important responsibility of the physical therapist regardless of the patient's problems.

Over time, smoking cessation can reverse many of the lethal effects of smoking (Table 1-4; also see Table 1-3). For smokers unable to quit, advocating "competing" health strategies has been proposed.[213] Improved diets and increased physical activity and exercise, however, do not counter the negative effects of smoking.[134]

Table 1-4 Health Benefits of Quitting Smoking

	Benefits
Immediate Benefits	Family: Quitting smoking removes harmful environmental tobacco smoke that pollutes nonsmokers' breathing space Individual: Your body starts to heal itself; the levels of carbon monoxide and nicotine in your system decline rapidly; heart rate and blood pressure drop quickly; peripheral circulation improves
Benefits after 1 Year	Increased risk for ischemic heart disease decreases 50%
Benefits after 3 Years	Risk for heart disease declines to levels similar to those of lifelong nonsmokers
Benefits after 5 Years	Risk for cancers of the oral cavity and esophagus reduced by 50% Risk for bladder cancer reduced by about 50% Risk for stroke can return to levels similar to those of nonsmokers Risk for cervical cancer is significantly reduced
Benefits after 10 Years	Risk for lung cancer decreases 50% to 70%
Benefits after 15 Years	Risk for ischemic heart disease is similar to that of lifelong nonsmokers Risk for death is similar to that of lifelong nonsmokers

Data from the American Cancer Society, 2004; U.S. Department of Health and Human Services. The Health Consequences of Smoking: A Report of the Surgeon General. U.S. Department of Health and Human Services, Centers for Disease Control and Prevention, National Center for Chronic Disease Prevention and Health Promotion, Office on Smoking and Health, 2004; American Lung Association. www.lungusa.org/site/pp.asp?c=dvLUK9O0E&b=22938; Manson JE, Tosteson H, Ridker PM, et al: The primary prevention of myocardial infarction, *New England Journal of Medicine* 326:1406–1416, 1992.

Why Physical Therapists Need to Understand Ethnic and Cultural Differences

Industrialized countries are becoming increasingly ethnically and culturally diverse as people migrate around the globe, particularly to high-income countries where lifestyle-related conditions are prevalent. With birth rates on the decline in these countries, immigration is being encouraged. Thus it is important to understand the role and impact of ethnicity and culture as important factors influencing health, ill health, use of health care services, the types of health education that are needed, and the ways in which they should be disseminated.[214]

The prevalence of COPD and its associated mortality increase with age, rates being higher in Caucasians than in other ethnic groups in North America.[211] Among people with advanced COPD, however, African Americans and women are more prone than other groups to the adverse effects of tobacco. Cardiovascular disease in Mexican Americans and Native Americans is a particular concern and has implications for optimal care and service delivery.[54,215,216] Obesity, hypertension, and metabolic syndrome are also more prevalent in these groups, so their special needs should be recognized by physical therapists. Currently, Eastern Europe, the Middle East, and Asia have the highest smoking prevalence in the world.

The health advantages that people of other cultures enjoy in their homelands (Asians, for example) are compromised when they immigrate to Western countries and adopt Western dietary and exercise habits.[67,217,218] Although they may benefit from improved health services and access, lifestyle-related conditions exact more of a toll on new immigrants with each passing year. The physical therapist has a unique role as health educator in promoting optimal lifestyle practices in new immigrants, as well as in long-term residents.

People from Utah, 72% of whom are Mormon by faith and follow a strict lifestyle code, have among the best health indexes in the country and some of the lowest rates of chronic disease,[57] but ethnic minorities in Utah are at increased risk for heart disease and stroke, among other conditions. Designing preventive and management strategies requires responding to the needs of different groups. A training program designed specifically for African Americans with stroke and complex comorbidities can be highly effective in improving fitness and reducing risk for further disease and disability.[219] Racial differences have been documented with respect to the interactions of obesity, hypertension, and diabetes between African American and European American women.[220] Greater emphasis needs to be placed on targeting risk factors in various ethnic and cultural groups. For example, alcohol consumption in Caucasian Americans and weight control in African Americans and Caribbean groups are among the targeted priorities.[221] For each individual, the severity of the problem, the risks, and the willingness to change needs to be assessed to effectively target management strategies. Sensitivity to cultural, as well as to individual, differences when designing health-education strategies is essential to the long-term success of the intervention.

Cultural differences in self-reports of body functioning have been reported.[222] These differences, along with low education status, are thought to explain the overrating of functional status in self-reports as compared with objective measures of performance. These observations support the need for greater cultural sensitivity and awareness in the clinic, particularly when the patient belongs to a minority group and the physical therapist is part of the dominant Caucasian American group. These findings support the need for objective functional assessment in addition to self-reported functional status.

Another important cultural factor in health care is the reporting of exertion, discomfort, and pain, which affect activity and participation. Studies have examined the expression of pain and the responses of health care providers to the pain expressed by people from cultures different from those of the health care provider. In addition to cultural differences in pain expression, patients from cultures that are highly expressive in expressing discomfort and pain have been reported to receive less medication and fewer pain control interventions than individuals who are less expressive, a characteristic consistent with the dominant culture.[223,224]

Physical Therapists as Drivers of Change in Health Behaviors

Direct patient access is fast becoming a reality for physical therapists worldwide. With this trend comes the additional responsibility of knowing whom *not* to treat as well as whom to treat. The physical therapist may be the entry to health care for many patients, so she or he needs to consider the patient's overall health and risk factors in addition to focusing on the specific physical problem that brought the patient to physical therapy. Even if the patient has been referred for physical therapy, the therapist has a responsibility to ensure that the patient's health status is optimal so as to maximize the patient's response to treatment and to address factors contributing to the patient's other complaints, which may be the more serious and important considerations. In a direct-access model of health care delivery, the physical therapist needs to know what is not amenable to noninvasive physical therapy management and, in such cases, have the patient referred to or managed concurrently with an invasive medical care practitioner.

Based on the discordance between the extant knowledge of lifestyle-related conditions and health-promoting lifestyles, health care has failed to significantly reduce the prevalence of these diseases and their risk factors. The issue of why people do not always make appropriate lifestyle choices is of central importance to their health and to the practice of the health care provider. Patients may be more inclined to make follow-up visits to their health care providers than to change their lifestyles.[225] One explanation for the failure of conventional models of health education[226-232] is that traditionally they have been based on a unidirectional model of information delivery—that is, from the health care provider (a dominant person) to the individual or patient (a subordinate person) in the form of brochures, books, videos, magazine articles, and television and radio announcements. These formats typically are not well targeted to a specific demographic or to the needs of the learner. Smoking cessation programs, for example, have been reported to be more effective when targeted to the specific needs of middle-aged men, including resources that promote a perceived sense of control over health behavior.[233] Changes in behavior are effected most successfully in a personal, bidirectional model, including rapport building, trust, commitment, and follow-up. Other important factors include receptivity, susceptibility, beliefs, timing, message delivery, barriers, reinforcers, and external stimulus-control factors.[234] Such a strategy is the so-called AIM approach: *A*ssess the learner, *I*dentify barriers to learning, and *M*otivate the individual to make change.[235]

Cardiovascular disease is the leading cause of death in women, particularly those over 60 years of age. This cohort of women believes they are at low risk for heart attack, yet 82% of coronary events in women are explained by the absence of a low-risk lifestyle.[236] Although women may respond favorably to risk-reduction initiatives, their awareness of risk factors and prevention strategies may be poor.[237] When health information (with respect to a low-fat plant-based diet, exercise, smoking cessation, and stress management) is delivered in a supportive group environment, in innovative multiple formats (e.g., a retreat and group meetings), people make sustainable lifestyle changes that reduce health-risk factors, decrease the need for medication, and improve their quality of life.[238,239] Furthermore, health education is more effective when cultural differences that affect health beliefs, attitudes, and behaviors are considered.[240-242]

Understanding poor adherence to health behavior change is as important as understanding the factors contributing to good adherence. In healthy middle-aged men at risk for IHD, for example, poor adherence to the recommendation to increase dietary fiber is related to smoking, hostility, perception of barriers to diet change, and poor knowledge of risk factors.[243] Poor adherence to following a low-fat diet is related to smoking, young age, and having no family members or friends with IHD. Poor adherence to an exercise program is associated with young age and having young children at home. Such information for various target groups is important in planning effective health-education interventions. The results of studies, however, are based on group outcomes. Individual assessments are needed to determine the barriers to and facilitators of learning for each person. The physical therapist needs to anticipate that these may change for an individual over time.

Education is a common component of the management of every patient with the exception of those who are unconscious, severely mentally challenged, or cognitively incapable of responding to the information. Even in these cases, education of the attending health care providers and caregivers can be the priority. The success of health education reflects the individual's expectations.[244] Most physical therapists and other health care providers have little background in assessing expectations. Physical therapists would benefit from formal education in assessing the learners' needs and wants, expectations, and readiness to learn and implement positive changes in their behaviors. Varying expectations may be particularly important when the patient is from a culture different from that of the physical therapist.

Various theories have been proposed to explain people's health choices and to promote improved choices. One such theory is that of reasoned action or planned behavior.[245] Based on this theory, an individual's decision to engage in a healthy behavior such as exercise is based on his or her intention. Intention is a function of the person's attitudes, perceived control and self-efficacy, and social factors. The elements of the McEwen model of health motivation are comparable and have been used, for example, to effect positive lifestyle changes in individuals participating in cardiac rehabilitation.[246] The assessment includes the individual's current knowledge, perceived severity, perceived susceptibility, perceived value of action, background variables, internal and external aids and hindrances, and the catalyst factors. Understanding the factors that affect an individual's lifestyle choices is vital for targeting health education so as to produce sustained outcomes.

The transtheoretical model of "readiness to change behavior"[247] outlines several behavioral-change stages, including precontemplative, contemplative, preparation, action, and maintenance. In designing health promotion education programs, this model helps to identify the stage of readiness to change, so that interventions can be tailored to and timed with an individual's readiness to interact with the information, thereby enhancing outcomes. The five stages of change are shown in Box 1-1. Key questions can be asked to establish an individual's stage of readiness to change (Box 1-2).

A study of change in exercise behavior employing the transtheoretical model in sedentary women compared psychological variables and the capacity for a moderate or vigorous exercise program, either at home or at a center, to effect change in their exercise habits over 18 months.[248] Self-efficacy for exercise competence increased as women moved from the contemplative to the action stage and was particularly marked in the groups involved in vigorous exercise. Almost half of the women shifted from the action stage to the maintenance stage. The intervention was effective regardless of the setting and the intensity of the exercise program.

When patients are in the preparation and action stages, the physical therapist can teach a range of self-monitoring skills and recording strategies along with information about circulatory and heart conditions, risk factors, and prevention. Blood pressure self-monitoring can be taught, provided the equipment is calibrated and checked by the physical therapist, standardized procedures are used, and the patient's measurement proficiency is evaluated.[249]

Psychological principles, including cognitive and behavior-modification strategies, are central to behavior change; they include the stimulus environment and events before the behavior, the reinforcement of the behavior, and consequent events.[250] Shaping, feedback, and reinforcement schedules are

Box 1-1 Prochaska's Stages of Readiness to Change*

Precontemplation

- Not currently engaged in the target behavior
- Not seriously thinking of change in the next 6 months
- Unaware of the need to change or denies the need to change

Contemplation

- Not currently engaged in the behavior
- Seriously considering making a change within the next 6 months
- Acknowledges that the behavior is unhealthy
- Seeks out information regarding the pros and cons of changing

Preparation

- Planning to change within the next 30 days
- Has attempted to change in the previous year
- On the verge of taking action to change behavior
- Begins to reevaluate self in light of the new behavior

Action

- Engaged in the desired behavior
- Has implemented the change only in the past 6 months
- Tries the behavior but is at high risk for relapse

Maintenance

- Has maintained the behavior for 6 months

*An individual can be at different stages for different health behaviors.
From Prochaska JJ, Spring B, Nigg CR: Multiple health behavior change research: an introduction and an overview, Preventive Medicine *46:181–188, 2008.*

Box 1-2 Assessing Readiness to Change by Using a Quiz

The Stages of Readiness to Change model is designed to help people adopt new health behaviors. Knowing where you are in the stages of readiness to change helps you to understand the steps you should take to move to subsequent stages to achieve lifelong sustainable health behaviors.

Circle a response to each question using the "Y" or the "N."

Y = Yes, I meet my health objective on this question.

N = For each "N" you circle, circle the readiness-to-change number that applies:

1 = Not thinking about change at this time (precontemplative)

2 = Thinking about change (contemplative)

3 = Preparing to change (preparation)

Readiness to Change Checklist	Response		Readiness to Change		
Do you exercise moderately intensely at least 3 times a week for 20 to 40 minutes?	Y	N	1	2	3
Are you physically active during your average day (walk, walk briskly, take stairs)?	Y	N	1	2	3
Is your weight within normal range?	Y	N	1	2	3
Do you eat at least 5 servings of fruit and vegetables daily?	Y	N	1	2	3
Do you minimize the trans and saturated fats in your diet?	Y	N	1	2	3
Do you minimize highly refined carbohydrates in your diet (sugar and white flour)?	Y	N	1	2	3
Do you drink alcohol less often than 5 times a week?	Y	N	1	2	3
Are you a nonsmoker?	Y	N	1	2	3
Are you generally relaxed during your day and do you feel in control?	Y	N	1	2	3

powerful strategies. Complex behaviors such as lifestyle behaviors may be shaped by the introduction of small, progressive, easily achievable steps toward a larger goal, a process comparable to the integrated stepwise approach used to improve dietary habits.[96] These principles can be incorporated into a model of lifestyle modification that incorporates factors such as culture.[234,250]

Education and effecting change in health behaviors are perhaps the most important components of the physical therapist's expertise because such change dramatically affects the lifelong health of each individual patient. Preventive health messages stated by a health care provider can be powerful, and they are a strong predictor of change in health behaviors.[230,251-253] However, preventive health messages are delivered to a relatively small number of patients by their health care providers. Thus lifestyle recommendations should be delivered as a holistic management priority to every patient, in a structured, conscious manner comparable to the rigor and precision of a prescribed treatment program. The cumulative time the physical therapist spends with each patient over days, weeks, and years translates into numerous teachable moments. Multiplying this time spent annually in teachable moments by the number of physical therapists in the world indicates that the potential for having a societal impact and making a global assault on lifestyle-related conditions is enormous.

Sending a patient home with a brochure on exercise or telling a patient not to smoke has a low probability of producing lasting results—or any results at all. The educational needs of the patient, in terms of receptivity to new information and to the styles of teaching and learning that are being used, need to be established; otherwise, both the clinician and the patient are wasting their time. Educational needs are multifactorial; they include health beliefs, self-efficacy, readiness to change, and motivation. The transtheoretical model[247] of readiness to change (see Boxes 1-1 and 1-2) is valuable in demonstrating how to determine the patient's stage through appropriate questions and how to devise strategies for moving a patient from one stage to the next in a progression toward preparation, action, and maintenance. Self-efficacy is an important determinant of readiness to change and of one's capacity to effect and maintain a behavioral change.[254] If the stage of readiness to change is considered when promoting healthy lifestyles, health coaching can be successful even if brief.[255] The level of importance a person ascribes to a behavior and that person's sense of confidence that she or he can effect the change are the main determinants in whether the person will achieve the threshold level and make the change. Factors that contribute to this decision should be integral components of the assessment; they can be examined systematically, as outlined in Table 1-5. The individual is asked to weigh the benefits and costs of changing a given lifestyle behavior as opposed to not changing that behavior at that point in time. Decision balance analysis involves having the patient identify the benefits and costs of making a lifestyle change *and* of not making the change. This information is useful to the practitioner in directing and planning interventions that will effect changes in health behavior in an individual.

People in need of care such as hospitalized patients are a receptive and captive audience. They present prime opportunities for identifying teachable moments. Even if older, these individuals are motivated to better understand their risk factors and to change their lifestyles.[256]

Table 1-5 **Health Behavior Change: Decision Balance Analysis**

Change	**No Change**
Benefits	Benefits
1.	1.
2.	2.
3.	3.
4.	4.
Costs	Costs
1.	1.
2.	2.
3.	3.
4.	4.

Modified from Rollnick S, Mason P, Butler C: *Health behavior change: a guide for practitioners,* Philadelphia, 2002, Churchill Livingstone.

The impact of the physical therapist as a driver of change may reflect her or his capacity to serve as a role model. Physicians who exercise, for example, are more likely to advise that their patients exercise, as well as to advocate other positive health behaviors.[257,258] Thus as a health care professional, practicing what one preaches may have a powerful effect on patient adherence to lifestyle change and health recommendations.

Evidence-Based Practice

Evidence-based practice has become a major thrust in the physical therapy profession; it ensures that our practice has both a physiological and a scientific basis. An important source of evidence that has shaped cardiovascular and pulmonary physical therapy over the past 50 years has been systematic, methodologically rigorous studies in the physiological and clinical sciences.

Knowledge into Action

With the advent of Sackett's rules of evidence[259] and schemes for grading the quality of scientific studies and critical-appraisal topics,[260] physical therapists have had to learn to be discriminating consumers of research. In addition, systematic reviews and metaanalyses have emerged to examine areas of practice where there are discrepancies in the literature regarding a treatment's effect and to answer specific clinical questions. The levels of evidence and the grading recommendations for the quality of studies are shown in Table 1-6.

In becoming an evidence-based practitioner, the physical therapist needs to know what is *not* known in the field, as well as what is known. The therapist should distinguish this knowledge from what is known inconclusively and from areas in which no studies have been done. The physical therapist needs to be comfortable with uncertainty when applying interventions and receptive to integrating new information as it emerges.

Table 1-6 **Basis for Clinical Recommendations Based on Levels of Evidence and Grading of Recommendations**

Level of Evidence	Type of Evidence
I	Evidence is obtained from meta-analysis of multiple, well-designed, controlled studies. Randomized trials with low false-positive and low false-negative errors (high power). Evidence is obtained from at least one well-designed experimental study.
II	Randomized trials with high false-positive and/or negative errors (low power).
III	Evidence is obtained from well-designed, quasi-experimental studies, such as nonrandomized, controlled single group, pre-post, cohort, time, or matched case-control series.
IV	Evidence is from well-designed, nonexperimental studies such as comparative and correlational descriptive and case studies.
V	Evidence from case reports and clinical examples.
Grade	**Grading of Recommendations**
A	There is evidence of type I or consistent findings from multiple studies of types II, III, or IV.
B	There is evidence of types II, III, or IV and findings are generally consistent.
C	There is evidence of types II, III, or IV but findings are inconsistent.
D	There is little or no systematic empirical evidence.

From Cook DJ, Guyatt GH, Laupacis A, et al: Rules of evidence and clinical recommendations on the use of antithrombotic agents, *Chest* 102(4 Suppl): 305S–311S, 1992.

The effectiveness of exercise-based interventions in the prevention and remediation of lifestyle-related conditions has been documented for the components of such interventions and at the highest levels of evidence. Physical therapy has to ensure that its practices are based on the literature and that the profession assumes a leadership role in promoting exercise for the development and maintenance of health, for the prevention of disease and disability, and for the remediation of illness and injury.

Physical Therapists as Drivers of Change

Physical therapists are health care professionals well qualified to bridge the gap between knowledge and practice in health care and its delivery. Our role is to increase the number of people at low risk for lifestyle-related conditions rather than focus primarily on high-risk individuals. The biomedical model is being replaced by a broader health model that views the individual in the context of his or her life and culture.

Strategies of behavioral change such as the transtheoretical model[261] are being adopted with increasing frequency for the purpose of promoting healthy lifestyle change. Implementation of such a program in the workplace has been shown to increase physical activity in previously sedentary adults, to reduce the number of reported barriers to such activity, and to increase muscle endurance, predicted $\dot{V}O_2$, and flexibility.[262]

Refocusing and Expanding the Clinical Repertoire of Physical Therapists

Today's health care system is complex, and multiple forces drive the direction of types of services and their delivery. The reductionist perspective of the human body in the biomedical model largely predominates as the model underlying illness care. (Reductionism is the belief that the whole can be understood by the examination of small parts, that is, that treatment focuses on the disease rather than the mind and body as a whole.) Such illness care has been increasingly influenced by economic forces and directed care based on economic factors, such as drug prescription, rapid discharge from the hospital, and focus on process and functional outcomes.[263] The absence of health promotion and wellness initiatives on a patient-by-patient basis before hospital discharge results from economic priorities, yet is a lost window of opportunity at a time when an individual may be receptive to information relating to changes in health behaviors—the teachable moment.[263] Preventive information about nutrition, exercise, smoking cessation, and excessive alcohol consumption is not receiving the attention it deserves from health care providers or from patients.

As noninvasive practitioners, physical therapists are positioned professionally to be leaders in effecting health behavior change. Knowledge of physiology, pathophysiology, and clinical medicine and surgery is not sufficient for the physical therapist to be able to address complex, contemporary, population-wide health problems. To implement effective prevention and interventions with sustainable outcomes, the physical therapist has to consider the interface of treatments and recommendations for each individual. Establishing rapport, exploring the patient's perception of the importance of change in health behavior, building confidence, exchanging information, and reducing resistance are key interpersonal skills needed to promote sustainable health-behavior change.[264-266]

The medical literature abounds with consensus statements of policies and procedures for treating specific conditions. Physical therapy has the expertise to develop parallel guidelines for noninvasive interventions, which in many instances, should be considered before invasive interventions or at least concurrently with them. The medical literature supports invasive care, so often it is not balanced with noninvasive interventions. For example, the report of the Sixth American College of Chest Physicians Consensus Conference on Antithrombotic Therapy has been cited in recommendations for patients following total hip arthroplasty.[267] Physical therapy has a primary perioperative role in the prophylaxis and management of the potentially lethal effects of thrombosis after surgery. This perspective is relatively obscure in the position statement compared with the emphasis on drugs and other options; yet it is highly effective, has an excellent cost-benefit ratio, and results in minimal side effects compared with the systemic risks of antithrombotic therapy.

The time has come for a call to action within the physical therapy profession concerning the ill health that plagues our village. It is time to take a leadership role in the prevention of lifestyle-related conditions and their reversal, as well as remediation. In the pursuit of health and participation for all, physical therapists have a primary role in health care policy making, including the health of communities and countries, and should become involved in urban and environmental health initiatives, in community health planning,[268-270] and in health and wellness programs, as well as continuing to provide vital one-on-one care to people. Physical therapists can be leaders in promoting community-based programs such as community-based tai chi programs[270] and programs for individuals with physical challenges, including stroke.[271,272] Community-based programs have been shown to be effective if they are well planned and supervised.

Translating sustainable health behavior from the hospital or clinic to the home cannot be assumed; rather, it is a unique skill that should be based on psychosocial teaching and learning factors. Although center- and clinic-based care is convenient for the health care provider, transitioning to home and community is fundamental to the process. The closer-to-home philosophy allows skills to be generalized from one setting to another. Closer-to-home health care delivery has attracted interest largely for economic reasons. However, the fact that better care and longer-lasting sustainable health behaviors may result is also a major reason to promote such care. Cardiac rehabilitation, for example, when initiated in the home environment in low-risk individuals, shows more sustainable physical and psychosocial benefits over time than when initiated in a facility.[273] Community-based programs have to be adapted to the cultural and socioeconomic conditions of that community to promote optimal buy-in from the participants and to maximize their success.[221,274]

Continuing Professional Education

With the ongoing need to be up to date, physical therapists must accrue continuing education credits. With the plethora of opportunities in the open marketplace, courses and workshops need to be stringently evaluated regarding the evidence base of their content and the qualifications of their instructors.

Practice evolves dynamically. Physical therapists can expect that what they learn during their professional education will be challenged and refined over time, with the advancement of knowledge. The practitioner should identify research gaps and help to support research activity, even if not directly engaged in research. Being receptive to changes in practice and serving as a driver of change are characteristics of the contemporary physical therapist. The work of clinicians and scientists should be closely interwoven, and ongoing partnerships must exist between them. Only in this way can clinically important questions be addressed and practice be changed on the basis of advances and discoveries. This approach is subsumed in so-called participatory action research, which aims to unite the needs of the researchers and the stakeholders (patients and clinicians).

Another component of staying up to date through continuing education is reading the professional literature. Knowing what to read and understanding how to read the literature are as important to the clinician as clinical skills, and both skills have to be refined throughout the practitioner's career. Table 1-7 rates the levels of quality of common publications and reading materials accessed by clinicians. Box 1-3 identifies important factors that should be considered when reading in order to enhance professional expertise. Journal clubs in the profession have become a popular means of sharing and discussing published information.

Table 1-7 Sources of Health Information and Quality Rating

Information Source	Quality Rating
Scientific/Professional	Usually externally peer-reviewed journals (blind or nonblinded); although not infallible, information in journals has the highest probability of containing credible information, compared with other sources
Monographs	May or may not be peer reviewed
Books	Usually not peer reviewed
Professional newsletters	Typically not reviewed
Magazines	Highly variable
Newspapers	Highly variable
Television and radio	Highly variable
Internet	Highly variable

Every Patient Is a Case Study

The randomized controlled clinical trial (RCCT) has become the gold standard for evaluating clinical interventions. Despite the scientific rigor involved, the limitations of the RCCT need to be appreciated by clinicians. Because of these limitations, Simon[275] has argued that the clinical relevance of the RCCT may be overestimated and would be better described as a "silver standard." The designs of RCCTs and their statistical analyses are based on probability theory. Because of this, results can be generalized only to comparable groups, not to an individual—the focus of the clinical situation. The results of RCCTs homogenize the outcomes for individuals who responded to treatment, failed to respond, or had negative outcomes. As clinical practitioners, we are interested in knowing how a particular individual with a given presentation will respond to a given treatment. The clinician needs to exercise a high level of clinical reasoning and judgment in determining the probability of a favorable response to a given treatment regimen in a given individual, based on studies of groups. Thus the physical therapist needs to understand the differences between the responders (favorable and unfavorable) in an RCCT and the nonresponders. This information is seldom detailed in published articles.

Another limitation of RCCTs is that in the real world, individuals seen by physical therapists have multiple comorbidities. In the interest of experimental control, conditions that confound the patient's presentation and treatment response

Box 1-3 Factors to Consider When Reading to Enhance Professional Expertise

Clinical Studies: Extracting Information and Translating the Findings into Practice

- What is the source of the information and its credibility?
- Was the work reviewed objectively by leaders in the field?
- Are the reviewers unbiased and free of any conflict of interest in reviewing the work (no financial or other gain from reviewing the work favorably or unfavorably)?
- Is the information based on a sound study?
- Is the research question derived from the existing literature appropriately?
- Is the study designed appropriately to address the question?
- What type of clinical trial? Is there a control group?
- Are subjects randomly selected and randomly assigned to groups?
- Do the methods control for all confounding variables?
- Are the methods standardized?
- How valid and reliable are the measures?
- Is the statistical analysis appropriate for the research design and research question?
- Is the sample size appropriate?
- Could the outcomes have been influenced by the outcome testers? Are the testers blind to the intervention group that each subject is assigned to?
- Are the results appropriately interpreted (neither over- or understated)?
- Do the results support the hypotheses or answer the research questions?
- Is the interpretation of the results and their clinical implications stated appropriately?

Physiological Studies: Extracting Information and Translating the Findings into Practice

- How sound is the physiological rationale?
- Are the methods rigorous and sound?
- How credible is the generalization to patient populations in the clinical setting?

are selectively eliminated, or the groups are randomized so that they are relatively equivalent in this dimension. Rarely can the findings of a study that compares groups be applied perfectly to a given clinical situation.

The clinical decision-making process is iterative and time limited.[9] Physical therapy diagnoses are derived from detailed histories and assessments. Clinical hypotheses are formulated, and the physical therapist systematically evaluates them to establish the cause of the complaints and factors that contribute to them. The physical therapist selects valid and reliable measures and outcomes and conducts them in a standardized manner. The patient's treatment response and prognosis are predicted so as to establish a timeline for treatment. Based on the assessment, each treatment intervention is prescribed (e.g., with respect to exercise, the type, intensity, duration, frequency, and course). Periodic reevaluation with established standardized outcomes measures are conducted to determine whether the patient has achieved the treatment objective and may be discharged or whether the prescriptions need to be modified and, if so, in what way. The relevant outcomes and outcome measures are identified at the start of treatment, and the treatment responses are evaluated over time until the predetermined outcomes are achieved within the predetermined time frame.

Aligning practice with research requires that the physical therapist apply research tools in practice, or at least have an understanding of them and their impact on drawing conclusions about the effect of treatment. For example, patients often improve spontaneously with time. This phenomenon is called "regression toward the mean." Physical therapy often involves an eclectic treatment approach involving multiple interventions. Because of this, individual treatment effects cannot be isolated. Rather, the physical therapist has to conclude that treatments A, B, and C may have resulted in some improvement; however, the effect of spontaneous improvement with time can be determined only in a controlled clinical trial or on the basis of a prolonged unchanging baseline in the patient's symptoms. Confounding variables such as medications and improvement with time need to be isolated so that it is possible to say that they may have contributed to the outcome, even if they cannot be ruled out. Confounding variables, which result from inadequate experimental control, cloud the interpretation of cardiovascular and pulmonary physical therapy studies.[276] The effect of placebo also plays a major role in treatment outcome. This effect reflects such factors as patient expectancy. Once maligned and considered a characteristic of the hypochondriac, the placebo effect is now known to be a potent and clinically important self-healing effect that warrants being promoted. To date, there is little scientific evidence about how to exploit the power of the placebo effect systematically to promote self-healing.

A typical example of an individual with comorbidities seen by the physical therapist is the person with acute back pain who is also overweight, has high blood pressure, and has a family history of IHD. In such cases, the physical therapist may have to introduce interventions in a stepwise manner. Even though immediate relief needs to be provided for the acute back discomfort, the comorbidities, as well as the low back pain, contribute significantly to the state of the individual's health and well-being at present and figure importantly in the future (with respect to prolonged morbidity and premature death). Thus for maximal and sustainable health, a lifelong health program needs to be implemented. To do this effectively, the practitioner needs a stepwise, paced approach that engages other members of the health care team as needed. The first goal is to provide physical relief of acute pain. Then a weight-reduction and exercise program plan is introduced commensurate with the individual's needs and wants. A nutritionist may need to be consulted not only to assist with weight loss but also to educate the patient about dietary principles to address hypertension (e.g., salt restriction) and minimize the risk for type 2 diabetes mellitus. Weight reduction, improved core and general strength, and aerobic conditioning may eliminate the cause of the low back pain or may attenuate it significantly over the long term. These interventions can also reduce blood pressure and help maintain blood glucose levels within normal limits, considering that the patient is at risk for diabetes. Follow-up is implemented to monitor progress and maintain psychosocial supports so as to ensure the long-term sustainability and success of the lifestyle changes. Such a regimen overcomes the limitations of a conventional course of analgesia and musculoskeletal physical therapy. Although the latter may produce short-term results, it does not necessarily address the underlying problem or eliminate the likelihood of recurrence of the primary problem and related health-behavior risks over time.

Health promotion practice needs to be modified to the needs of a patient based on his or her cultural background and affiliation. Cultural competence in practice is geared toward augmenting clinical outcomes by adapting communication style, assessments, and treatments. Differences in people with respect to culture, traditions, and religion or faith can affect health, illness, health reporting, beliefs, and expectations about treatment intervention, as well as adherence to the treatment program. For example, the holy month of Ramadan requires creativity in managing the needs of Muslims. During Ramadan, Muslims fast from dawn to dusk, and the fast may include abstinence from water as well as from food. Sedentary people show greater adverse physiological effects during this period, both when at rest and during exercise, than do active people.[277] Body weight drops in a predictable manner. The respiratory exchange ratio decreases during exercise, reflecting increased fat metabolism. Serum iron and platelets decrease, particularly in sedentary people, and fluid balance is better maintained in active people. Exercise, particularly whole-body exercise, may have to be curtailed or modified during fasting. This is especially true when Ramadan falls during the hot summer months.

Adapting lifestyle and treatment recommendations to the needs of the people physical therapists serve is fundamental to a successful outcome. The parameters of exercise prescription for optimal health benefits have been well documented (see Chapter 18). Prolonged adherence to physical activity and exercise programs, however, is poor. Understanding the factors that sustain health behaviors is as critical as the physiological basis for them. One study compared the effects of conventional aerobic training with the effects of a program designed to increase strength, endurance, and mind-body coordination but designed also for "comfort," so that the program would be more appealing to people unused to exercise. After training, participants in the latter group had superior endurance compared with those in the conventional group, and they reported more comfort and less exertion. This preliminary study supported the idea that an exercise program modified for comfort and enjoyment still resulted in a greater capacity to adapt to increased physiological demands. Such programs should be extended so that adherence over time can be evaluated. In addition, readiness to change as described in the transtheoretical model needs to be considered in studies of long-term lifestyle change.[278]

Physical Therapy's Role: Participation in Health Promotion Practice

Healthy lifestyle choices (specifically, not smoking, optimal nutrition, maintaining an optimal weight, not being sedentary, being physically active and exercising regularly, sleeping well and avoiding undue stress) can prevent lifestyle-related conditions. Should the risk factors or manifestations of lifestyle-related conditions emerge, adopting healthy living practices can reverse the risk factors or manifestations in some cases, as well as prevent future signs and symptoms. Given the established prevalence of lifestyle-related conditions, a primary clinical competency of physical therapy in the 21st century is multiple health behavior change.[261,278] In addition to promoting health and wellness one on one, physical therapists need to present a high profile in health promotion and illness prevention by developing and writing physical therapy publications throughout the various levels of their professional associations. They can participate in consensus groups within these associations to issue physical therapy position statements, broadcast television and radio public service announcements, and set up information booths in shopping malls, community centers, and other strategic places within the community. Innovative wellness and prevention programs such as heart camps and retreats should be established.[279] Such active leadership and participation by physical therapists enables them to exploit a range of avenues for effective communication and education strategies directed to the general public in addition to traditional one-on-one contact with patients.

Capitalizing on public health and condition-specific initiatives (e.g., Heart Month and Cancer Month) can reinforce existing community, state or province, national, and global health initiatives. The physical therapist needs to be proactive and function as a role model for health as a community leader by acknowledging these important initiatives and arranging activities to support them. Formal acknowledgment of the initiatives strengthens the profession's identity and its responsibility regarding the conditions being addressed. It also educates the public and reinforces physical therapy's role in the prevention, primary management, and in some cases, reversal of these conditions in the minds of the public, insurers, health care policy makers, health care colleagues, legislators, and others. For example, to address the serious pandemic of type 2 diabetes, the state of Tennessee has initiated statewide action. Schools and communities have been selected as primary prevention targets for the promotion of healthy food choices and activity programs.[280] The initiative is multidisciplinary and multisectorial, and health profession organizations, government, churches, schools, and employers across the state are participating. The World Health Organization has several important annual health markers, including May 31 of each year, which has been designated as World No Tobacco Day. These occasions should be publicized and supported collectively by the physical therapy community globally.

Physical Therapy's Role: Participation in Population-Wide Health Initiatives

As primary health care professionals, physical therapists are uniquely positioned to develop, support, and promote innovative health programs, thereby strengthening the health of communities en masse as well as doing so one person at a time in the clinic. Several excellent resources are available on the subject of building healthy neighborhoods and communities; they are highly recommended to physical therapists as bases for practicing at the levels of the village and community as well as the individual.[281,282]

Multicomponent, multiprofessional wellness and preventive health programs have been proposed to be components of each hospital department, including the emergency department. Hospital-based programs can be successfully implemented in diverse geographic areas and can be focused on each region's needs.[267] Despite the compelling benefits of home- and community-based care, their effectiveness cannot be assumed. Programs need to be judiciously targeted with due consideration given to the purpose of care, the target population, the congruence of the care and individuals' needs and wants, and outcomes at the individual and societal levels.[283]

The Groningen Active Living Model is an example of a behavior change model that has been developed to encourage sedentary adults to be physically activity.[55] The variables that were examined to determine program success included perceived fitness, social support, self-efficacy, and enjoyment. The outcomes were program adherence and physical activity. With respect to adherence, task self-efficacy was an important mediating variable in this cohort, followed by self-efficacy in overcoming barriers, in social support, and in enjoyment. Perceived physical ability and fitness were relatively less important mediators.

The Hearts for Life community-based program has shown positive outcomes with respect to risk reduction and improvement of knowledge.[284] The Choose to Move physical activity program for women provides an important model for public health and participatory research organizations of targeted, low-cost self-help programs that support the *Healthy People 2020*[285] objectives for physical activity, nutrition, and cardiovascular health.[286] Women who completed the program increased their physical activity, reduced their consumption of high-fat foods, and increased their knowledge and awareness of cardiovascular risk and its symptoms. Schools and workplaces are also sites for innovative health programs in the community. Preventive cardiology programs for children, such as HeartPower!, show some success in nutritional domains.[287] Such programs, however, could benefit from the expertise of a physical therapist with respect to developing, coordinating, integrating, and evaluating a physical activity and an exercise component. Low-income families in particular have an increased risk for inactivity and obesity. A school program for children of low-income families used the Internet, videos, provision of health snacks, and participation in a gym lab to promote exercise and healthy food choices.[288] This program resulted in reduced fat intake and increased physical activity by the children.

One medium through which a physical therapist can assume the role of health coach has been through telerehabilitation. Telerehabilitation has come of age and is a major vehicle that can be exploited by physical therapists for targeted education of patients in the community[289] and for general preventive health. Home-based education about nutrition and exercise has been reported as a means of targeting individuals with obstructive sleep apnea and promoting lifestyle change.[290]

Marketing research methods have been investigated as a means of improving population health outcomes and making their success rates comparable to those that have been well established in business marketing. Mass media promotion has been used to communicate an innovative physical activity and exercise resource called Small Steps.[291] Callers responded to a mass publication campaign to promote Small Steps. People phoned toll free to a call-in center where trained screeners recruited members of the public into a controlled trial, identified their stage of readiness to change based on a few structured questions, and sent out the Small Steps kit, which provided information about being physically active and exercising, along with a workbook. More than 80% of the callers were women. The prospect of making small steps toward improving their health was as compelling for men as for women. At the 3-month follow-up, self-reported current levels of physical activity (main outcome) had changed substantially. Thus the results supported the idea that with the use of mass media, people who are in the preparation stage of being more physically active can shift to the action stage. Long-term studies are needed to establish the long-term benefits of this program and its translation into health outcomes. The reasons given for calling the resource center included the appeal of taking small steps when undertaking health behavior changes, improving nutrition, becoming more active, learning new things, and assisting others to improve their diets and activity levels.

Implications of Epidemiology and Health Care Trends for Physical Therapy Practice

In the 21st century, the impact of noninvasive physical therapy outcomes will be reflected in part by the number of individuals who quit smoking, lose weight, consume healthier foods, exercise, and manage life stress (including moderate use of alcohol), regardless of patients' primary diagnoses. Addressing these priorities first can also alleviate musculoskeletal and neuromuscular problems or at least offset their consequences (such as low back pain). Weight loss, for example, can reduce the energy cost of walking in individuals with stroke, heart disease, or lung disease by optimizing biomechanical efficiency. Furthermore, addressing these priorities reduces the need for use of the health care system (doctor- and hospital-based care) and helps to avoid or minimize the need for drugs and surgery. Such a strategy will enable the profession collectively to address the leading population-wide health priorities of our time one patient at a time—and to affect health globally.

Implications of Epidemiology and Health Care Trends for Physical Therapy Professional Education

Physical therapy professional curricula need to be continuously reviewed with respect to their congruence with epidemiology and health care trends and the provision of evidence-based practice in this context, that is, being informed by epidemiological indicators amenable to noninvasive interventions. Physical therapy in the 21st century requires a high level of expertise in multiple health behavior change, including smoking cessation and counseling for basic nutrition, as well as the prescription of exercise. Patient education needs to be based on the assessment of the patient's learning style and readiness to change. To be effective, health education requires prioritizing goals, delivering health information, evaluating outcomes, and promoting lifelong behavior changes. Physical therapists' capacities to teach and promote learning should be formally evaluated just as are their capacities to prescribe exercise or other physical therapy interventions. A cross-sectional study of health care providers and their provision of health information to patients reported considerable disparities among providers. For instance, the provider's gender and that of the patient influenced whether education was attempted and, if so, what type. Female providers tend to include health education more often than their male counterparts.

The Magic Bullet and the Fountain of Youth

A "magic bullet" and a "fountain of youth" are not just myths. They exist, but they are not to be found in a pill or in surgery. For almost a century of documented physical therapy practice, education and exercise have been the hallmarks of the profession[292-294] and the elixirs that add years to life and life to years. These "drugs" have been at the core of the practice of the physical therapist, who is distinguished from invasive-medicine practitioners primarily by the use of noninvasive "drugs" as opposed to the invasive interventions of pharmacotherapy and surgery. In addition to providing preventive health benefits, lifestyle changes such as smoking cessation, optimal nutrition, and exercise can enhance the quality of life[295] and increase the probability of long-term health.

Given the epidemiological changes in global health, this is physical therapy's moment on the world health care stage, a time to promote health and wellness in every patient and to prevent, manage, and in some cases, reverse lifestyle-related conditions that are contributing to enormous social and economic burdens globally. The profession is uniquely and strategically positioned to lead the assault on lifestyle-related conditions by integrating health promotion into practice. The benefits of noninvasive strategies such as physical activity and exercise and healthy living are clear. If a drug could offer these same benefits and similarly improve public health, it would be heralded as nothing short of a miracle remedy. Although public perception of the benefits of noninvasive intervention is on the rise, much work remains to be done. The role of health coach for every patient could be one of the most rewarding competencies for physical therapists of the 21st century as they strive to make a positive impact on public health, one patient at a time.

Summary

This chapter describes the pivotal role of the noninvasive practitioner—namely, the physical therapist—within the contemporary framework of health in the 21st century. With the pandemic of lifestyle-related conditions, physical therapists need to consider the underlying risk factors for these conditions in every individual, regardless of the physical therapist's particular specialties or areas of practice and regardless of the patient's primary reasons for the consultation. A patient's low back pain or tennis elbow, for example, may be mere inconvenience compared with his or her smoking, excessive body weight, inactivity, high blood pressure, high cholesterol, or abnormal blood sugar. Physical therapists are uniquely qualified professionally and are strategically well positioned to address the leading health priorities of our time by using the profession's primary "drugs"—education and exercise—in diverse settings, one individual at a time or in groups. In addition, physical therapists need to identify risk factors in all patients, irrespective of presenting problems and diagnoses, so that they can prescribe optimal treatment, including exercise, to address lifestyle risk factors and monitor the patient for therapeutic and safety reasons. Physical therapists pride themselves on their communication skills, which are fundamental to building rapport with people and effecting lifelong behavior change. This expertise can be exploited because physical therapists not only spend more time with people during visits than most health professionals, but also see them over repeated visits. As effective drivers of change, physical therapists can exert considerable influence on their patients over time, given the potential teachable moments through the course of care. In the 21st century, physical therapy's impact will be reflected in outcomes associated with prevention, potential reversal, and management of lifestyle-related conditions, over and above the conventional practice of physical therapists across clinical areas and settings.

Review Questions

1. Describe lifestyle-related conditions.
2. How do lifestyle-related conditions affect every patient seen by the physical therapist? Relate your answer to the World Health Organization's International Classification of Functioning, Disability and Health.
3. Distinguish physical therapy's role in the promotion of health and wellness versus prevention, management, and in some cases, cure.
4. Describe the physical therapist in her or his role as a consumer of research.
5. Describe the concept of evidence-based practice in the context of evidence-informed practice.
6. Describe how you, as a physical therapist, are a driver of change.
7. Describe how the profession of physical therapy is uniquely positioned to assume a leadership role in addressing the leading health problems of our time.
8. You are in dialogue with a physician colleague about a patient who may be a candidate for hip replacement. The patient is obese, has hypertension, and is at high risk for diabetes. How would you describe the power of noninvasive practice as opposed to or in conjunction with invasive practice in effecting maximal health outcomes for the patient?
9. Reference is made in the chapter to the "magic bullet" and the "fountain of youth." Describe these fabled constructs in the context of 21st-century physical therapy practice.

References

1. Steptoe A, Kerry S, Rink E, et al: The impact of behavioral counseling on stage of change in fat intake, physical activity, and cigarette smoking in adults at increased risk of coronary artery disease. *American Journal of Public Health* 91(2):265–269, 2001.
2. Smith SC, Jr: Need for a paradigm shift: the importance of risk factor reduction therapy in treating patients with cardiovascular disease. *American Journal of Cardiology* 82(10B):10T–13T, 1998 Nov 26.
3. World Health Organization: Definition of health. www.who.int/about/definition/en/print.html; retrieved January 2011.
4. World Health Organization: International Classification of Functioning, Disability and Health, 2002. www.sustainable-design.ie/arch/ICIDH-2PFDec-2000.pdf; retrieved January 2011.
5. Uppaluri CR, Schumm LP, Lauderdale DS: Self-reports of stress in Asian immigrants: effects of ethnicity and acculturation. *Ethnicity and Disease* 11(1):107–114, 2001.

6. Anderson LM, Scrimshaw SC, Fullilove MT, et al: Culturally competent healthcare systems: a systematic review. *American Journal of Preventive Medicine* 24(3 Suppl):68–79, 2003.
7. Cappell J, Veenstra G, Dean E: Cultural competence in healthcare: Critical analysis of the construct: Its assessment and implications. *Journal of Theory Construction and Testing* 11:30–37, 2007.
8. Dean E: A psychobiologic adaptation model of physical therapy practice. *Physical Therapy* 65(7):1061–1068, 1985.
9. American Physical Therapy Association: *Guide to physical therapist practice*, ed 2, Physical Therapy, 81:1–746. Washington, DC, 2003, American Physical Therapy Association.
10. Cott C, Finch E, Gasner D, et al: The movement continuum theory of physical therapy. *Physiotherapy Canada* 47(2):87–95, 1995.
11. Darrah J, Loomis J, Manns P, et al: Role of conceptual models in a physical therapy curriculum: Application of an integrated model of theory, research, and clinical practice. *Physiotherapy Theory and Practice* 22:239–250, 2006.
12. Stretcher VJR, Rosenstock IM: The health belief model. In Glanz K, Rimer BK, Viswanath K, editors: *Health behavior and health education: theory, research and practice*, San Francisco, 2008, Jossey-Bass.
13. Mitani H, Hashimoto H, Isshiki T, et al: Health-related quality of life of Japanese patients with chronic heart failure: assessment using the Medical Outcome Study Short Form 36. *Circulation Journal* 67:215–220, 2003.
14. Ware JE, Jr, Sherbourne CD: The MOS36-item short-form health survey (SF-36): conceptual framework and item selection. *Medical Care* 30:473–483, 1992.
15. Franklin BA: The downside of our technological revolution? An obesity-conducive environment. *American Journal of Cardiology* 87:1093–1095, 2001.
16. Vuori IM: Health benefits of physical activity with special reference to interaction with diet. *Public Health Nutrition* 4:517–528, 2001.
17. Kingsley CM, Gupta SC: How to reduce the risk of coronary artery disease: teaching patients a healthy life-style. *Postgraduate Medicine* 91:147–150, 153–154, 157–160, 1992.
18. Sorrentino MJ: Cholesterol reduction to prevent CAD: what do the data show? *Postgraduate Medicine* 108:40–42, 45–46, 49–52, 2000.
19. Kavanagh T: Exercise in the primary prevention of coronary artery disease. *Canadian Journal of Cardiology* 17:155–161, 2001.
20. Wahlqvist ML: Chronic disease prevention: a life-cycle approach which takes account of the environmental impact and opportunities of food, nutrition and public health policies—the rationale for an eco-nutritional disease nomenclature. *Asia Pacific Journal of Clinical Nutrition* 11(Suppl):S759–S762, 2002b.
21. Wood D: Asymptomatic individuals—risk stratification in the prevention of coronary artery disease. *British Medical Journal* 59:3–16, 2001.
22. Critchley JA, Capewell S, Unal B: Life-years gained from coronary artery disease mortality reduction in Scotland: prevention or treatment? *Journal of Clinical Epidemiology* 56:583–590, 2003.
23. Bijnen FC, Caspersen CJ, Mosterd WL: Physical inactivity as a risk factor for coronary artery disease: a WHO and International Society and Federation of Cardiology position statement. *Bulletin World Health Organization* 72:1–4, 1994.
24. Musaiger AO: Diet and prevention of coronary heart disease in the Arab Middle East countries. *Medical Principles and Practice* 11(Suppl 2):9–16, 2002.
25. World Health Organization: Technical Report Series. *Geneva, Switzerland: World Health Organization* 916:i-viii1–149, 2003.
26. Cheng TO: Price of the modernization of China. *Circulation* 103:E131–E133, 2001.
27. Ebrahim S, Smith GD: Exporting failure? Coronary heart disease and stroke in developing countries. *International Journal of Epidemiology* 30:201–205, 2001.
28. World Health Organization: *Annual Health Reports 1999–2003*, Geneva, Switzerland, 1993–2003, World Health Organization.
29. Wright L, Murcer S, Adams K, et al: The factor analysis structure of seven physical CHD risk factors: a replication study. *Journal of Clinical Psychology* 50:216–219, 1994.
30. Cheng A, Braunstein JB, Dennison C, et al: Reducing global risk for cardiovascular disease: using lifestyle changes and pharmacotherapy. *Clinical Cardiology* 25:205–212, 2002.
31. Ebrahim S: Cost-effectiveness of stroke prevention. *British Medical Bulletin* 56:557–570, 2000.
32. Mann JI: Diet and risk of coronary heart disease and type 2 diabetes. *Lancet* 360:783–789, 2002.
33. McCrindle BW: Cardiovascular risk factors in adolescents: relevance, detection, and intervention. *Adolescent Medicine* 12:147–162, 2001.
34. Misra A: Risk factors for atherosclerosis in young individuals. *Journal of Cardiovascular Risk* 7:215–229, 2000.
35. Zafari AM, Wenger NK: Secondary prevention of coronary heart disease. *Archives of Physical Medicine and Rehabilitation* 79:1006–1017, 1998.
36. Sakakibara H, Fujii C, Naito M: Plasma fibrinogen and its association with cardiovascular risk factors in apparently healthy Japanese students. *Heart Vessels* 19:144–148, 2004.
37. Anonymous: Your heart attack risk: inflammation counts. *Harvard Women's Health Watch* 10:1–3, 2003.
38. Brod SA: Unregulated inflammation shorts human functional longevity. *Inflammation Research* 49:561–570, 2000.
39. Packer L: *Oxidative stress and inflammatory mechanisms in obesity, diabetes, and the metabolic syndrome*, Boca Raton, FL, 2007, CRC Press.
40. Berenson GS, Srinivasan SR, Bao W, et al: Association between multiple cardiovascular risk factors and atherosclerosis in children and young adults. *New England Journal of Medicine* 338:1650–1656, 1998.
41. Katz D: The basic (care) and feeding of homo sapiens: consensus, controversy, and cluelessness. Toronto, Ontario, 2003, Proceedings of the Canadian Cardiovascular Congress.
42. Olshansky SJ, Passaro DJ, Hersow RC, et al: A potential decline in life expectancy in the United States in the 21st century. *New England Journal of Medicine* 352:1138–1145, 2005.
43. Woo J: Relationships among diet, physical activity and other lifestyle factors and debilitating diseases in the elderly. *European Journal of Clinical Nutrition* 54(Suppl 3):S143–S147, 2000.
44. Dean E, Al-Obaid S, Dornelas de Andrade A, et al: The First Physical Therapy Summit on Global Health: Implications and recommendations for the 21st century. *Physiotherapy Theory and Practice* (In press), 2011a.
45. Dean E, Lomi C, Bruno S, et al: Addressing the common pathway underlying hypertension and diabetes in people who are obese: The ultimate knowledge translation gap. *International Journal of Hypertension* doi:10.4061/2011/835805, 2011b.
46. Clini E, Costi S, Lodi S, Rossi G: Non-pharmacological treatment for chronic obstructive pulmonary disease. *Medical Science Monitor* 9:300–305, 2003.
47. Dean E: Physical therapy in the 21st century (Part I): Toward practice informed by epidemiology and the crisis of lifestyle conditions. *Physiotherapy Theory and Practice* 25:330–353, 2009a.
48. Dean E: Physical therapy in the 21st century (Part II): Evidence-based practice within the context of evidence-informed practice. *Physiotherapy Theory and Practice* 25:354–368, 2009b.
49. Hambrecht R, Walther C, Mobius-Winkler S, et al: Percutaneous coronary angioplasty compared with exercise training in patients with stable coronary artery disease: a randomized trial. *Circulation* 109:1371–1378, 2004.
50. Marota Montero JM, Velasco Rami JA: Cardiac rehabilitation and secondary prevention in ischemic cardiopathy. *Revista Espanda de Cardiologia* 48(Suppl 1):85–89, 1995.
51. Jakes RW, Day NE, Khaw KT, et al: Television viewing and low participation in vigorous recreation are independently associated with obesity and markers of cardiovascular disease risk: EPIC-Norfolk population-based study. *European Journal of Clinical Nutrition* 57:1089–1096, 2003.
52. National Vital Statistics Reports: United States Life Tables (2004). Estimated life expectancy at birth in years, by race and sex. *Center for Disease Control* 56:9, 2007.
53. Varo Cenarruzabeita JJ, Martinez Hernandez JA, Martinez-Gonzalez, MA: Benefits of physical activity and harms of inactivity. *Medical Clinics (Barcelona)* 121:665–672, 2003.
54. Storey M, Stevens J, Himes J, et al: Obesity in American-Indian children: prevalence, consequences, and prevention. *Preventive Medicine* 37(Suppl)S3–S12, 2003.
55. Stevens M, Lemmink KA, van Heuvelen MJ, et al: Groningen Active Living Model (GALM): stimulating physical activity in sedentary older adults' validation of the behavioral change model. *Preventive Medicine* 37:561–570, 2003.
56. Nyenhuis DL, Gorelick PB, Easley C, et al: The black Seventh-day Adventist exploratory health study. *Ethnicity and Disease* 13:208–212, 2003.
57. LaMonte MJ, Eisenman PA, Adams TD, et al: Cardiorespiratory fitness and coronary heart disease risk factors: the LDS Hospital Fitness Institute cohort. *Circulation* 102:1623–1628, 2000.
58. Whitt M, Kumanyika S, Bellamy S: Amount and bouts of physical activity in a sample of African-American women. *Medicine and Science in Sports and Exercise* 35:1887–1893, 2003.

59. Wilbur J, Chandler PJ, Dancy B, et al: Correlates of physical activity in urban Midwestern African-American women. *American Journal of Preventive Medicine* 25:45–52, 2003a.
60. Wilbur J, Chandler PJ, Dancy B, Lee, H: Correlates of physical activity in urban Midwestern Latinas. *American Journal of Preventive Medicine* 25:69–76, 2003b.
61. Charkoudian N, Joyner MJ: Physiologic considerations for exercise performance in women. *Clinics in Chest Medicine* 25:247–255, 2004.
62. Holund U, Thomassen A, Boysen G, et al: Importance of diet and sex in prevention of coronary artery disease, cancer, osteoporosis, and overweight or underweight: a study of attitudes and practices of Danish primary care physicians. *American Journal of Clinical Nutrition* 65:2004S–2006S, 1997.
63. Cabrera C, Wilhelmson K, Allebeck P, et al: Cohort differences in obesity-related indicators of 70-year-olds, with special reference to gender and education. *European Journal of Epidemiology* 18:883–890, 2003.
64. Savage PD, Brochu M, Ades PA: Gender alters the high-density lipoprotein cholesterol response to cardiac rehabilitation. *Journal of Cardiopulmonary Rehabilitation* 24:248–254, 2004.
65. van Rooyen JM, Huisman HW, Eloff FC, et al: Cardiovascular reactivity in black South-African males of different age groups: the influence of urbanization. *Ethnicity and Disease* 12:69–75, 2002.
66. Suh I, Oh KW, Lee KH, et al: Moderate dietary fat consumption as a risk factor for ischemic heart disease in a population with a low fat intake: a case-control study in Korean men. *American Journal of Clinical Nutrition* 73:722–727, 2001.
67. Goel MS, McCarthy EP, Phillips RS, et al: Obesity among US immigrant subgroups by duration of residence. *Journal of the American Medical Association* 292:2860–2867, 2004.
68. Simonds AK: Ethics and decision making in end-stage lung disease. *Thorax* 58:272–277, 2003.
69. Woo J, Ho SC, Yu AL: Lifestyle factors and health outcomes in elderly Hong Kong Chinese aged 70 years and over. *Gerontology* 48:234–240, 2002.
70. Ford ES, Bergmann MM, Kroger J, et al: Healthy living is the best revenge. *Archives of Internal Medicine* 169:1355–1362, 2009.
71. Haskell WL: Cardiovascular disease prevention and lifestyle interventions: effectiveness and efficacy. *Journal of* 18:245–255, 2003.
72. Gibbons LW, Clark SM: Exercise in the reduction of cardiovascular events: lessons from epidemiologic trials. *Cardiology Clinics* 19:347–355, 2001.
73. Williams MA, Fleg JL, Ades PA, et al: Secondary prevention of coronary heart disease in the elderly (with emphasis on patients > or = 75 years of age): an American Heart Association scientific statement from the Council on Clinical Cardiology Subcommittee on Exercise, Cardiac Rehabilitation, and Prevention. *Circulation* 105:1735–1743, 2002.
74. Bradberry JC: Peripheral arterial disease: pathophysiology, risk factors, and role of antithrombotic therapy. *Journal of the American Pharmacy Association* 44(2 Suppl 1):S37–S44, 2004.
75. Keller C, Fleury J, Mujezinovic-Womack M: Managing cardiovascular risk reduction in elderly adults: by promoting and monitoring healthy lifestyle changes, health care providers can help older adults improve their cardiovascular health. *Journal of Gerontological Nursing* 29:18–23, 2003.
76. Shapiro JS: Primary prevention of coronary artery disease in women through diet and lifestyle. *New England Journal of Medicine* 343:16–22, 2000.
77. Twisk JW, Kemper HC, van Mechelen W, et al: Which lifestyle parameters discriminate high- from low-risk participants for coronary heart disease risk factors: longitudinal analysis covering adolescence and young adulthood. *Journal of Cardiovascular Risk* 4:393–400, 1997.
78. Macken LC, Yates B, Blancher S: Concordance of risk factors in female spouses of male patients with coronary artery disease. *Journal of Cardiopulmonary Rehabilitation* 20:361–368, 2000.
79. Paterno CA: Coronary risk factors in adolescence. The FRICELA study. *Revista Espanda de Cardiologia* 56:452–458, 2003. (English abstract).
80. Gidding SS: Preventive pediatric cardiology: tobacco, cholesterol, obesity, and physical activity. *Pediatric Clinics of North America* 46:253–262, 1999.
81. Graves KD, Miller PM: Behavioral medicine in the prevention and treatment of cardiovascular disease. *Behavior Modification* 27:3–25, 2003.
82. Panagiotakos DB, Pitsavos C, Chrysohoou C, et al: Risk stratification of the coronary heart disease in Greece: final results from the CARDIO2000 Epidemiological Study. *Preventive Medicine* 35:548–556, 2002.
83. Sleight P: Cardiovascular risk factors and the effects of intervention. *American Heart Journal* 121:990–994, 1991.
84. Sebregts EH, Falger PR, Bar FW: Risk factor modification though nonpharmacological interventions in patients with coronary artery disease. *Journal of Psychosomatic Research* 48:425–441, 2000.
85. Leng GC, Papacosta O, Whincup P, et al: Femoral atherosclerosis in an older British population: prevalence and risk factors. *Atherosclerosis* 152:167–174, 2000.
86. Bauman AE: Updating the evidence that physical activity is good for health: an epidemiological review 2000–2003. *Journal of Science in Medicine and Sport* (1 Suppl):6–19, 2004.
87. Pitsavos C, Panagiotakos DB, Chrysohoou C, et al: Physical activity decreases the risk of stroke in middle-age men with left ventricular hypertrophy: 40-year follow-up (1961–2001) of the Seven Countries Study (the Corfu Cohort). *Journal of Human Hypertension* 18:495–501, 2004.
88. Burkman RT, Jr: Strategies for reducing cardiovascular risk in women. *Journal of Reproductive Medicine* 36(3 Suppl):238–246, 1991.
89. Wessel TR, Arant CB, Olson MB, et al: Relationship of physical fitness vs body mass index with coronary artery disease and cardiovascular events in women. *Journal of the American Medical Association* 292:1179–1187, 2004.
90. Mozaffarian D, Fried LP, Burke GL, et al: Lifestyles of older adults: can we influence cardiovascular risk in older adults? *American Journal of Geriatric Cardiology* 13:153–160, 2004.
91. Mozaffarian D, Kumanyika SK, Lemaitre RN, et al: Cereal, fruit, and vegetable fiber intake and the risk of cardiovascular disease in elderly individuals. *Journal of the American Medical Association* 289:1659–1666, 2003.
92. Park SK, Park JH, Kwon YC, et al: The effect of long-term aerobic exercise on maximal oxygen consumption, left ventricular function and serum lipids in elderly women. *Journal of Physiologic Anthropology and Applied Human Science* 22:11–17, 2003.
93. Haskell WL, Alderman EL, Fair JM, et al: Effects of intensive multiple risk factor reduction on coronary atherosclerosis and clinical cardiac events in men and women with coronary artery disease. The Stanford Coronary Risk Intervention Project (SCRIP). *Circulation* 89:975–990, 1994.
94. Niebauer J, Hambrecht R, Velich T, et al: Attenuated progression of coronary artery disease after 6 years of multifactorial risk intervention: role of physical exercise. *Circulation* 96:2534–2541, 1997.
95. Ornish D: Avoiding revascularization with lifestyle changes: The Multicenter Lifestyle Demonstration Project. *American Journal of Cardiology* 82:72T–76T, 1998.
96. Srinath U, Jonnalagadda SS, Naglak MC, et al: Diet in the prevention and treatment of atherosclerosis: a perspective for the elderly. *Clinical Geriatric Medicine* 11:591–611, 1995.
97. Anonymous: Overcoming the threat of anger: more than type A behavior, hostility raises health risks. *Heart Advisor* 7:6, 2004.
98. Twisk JW, Snel J, Kemper HC, van Mechelen W: Changes in daily hassles and life events and the relationship with coronary heart disease risk factors: a 2-year longitudinal study in 27–29-year-old males and females. *Journal of Psychosomatic Research* 46:229–240, 1999.
99. Henrichon C, Robichaud-Ekstrand S: Adaptive strategies and adaptation after participation in an education program after a first coronary event. *Recherche et Soins Infirmerie* 70:39–65, 2002, (English abstract).
100. Hannan EL, Kilburn H, O'Donnel JF: Adult open heart surgery in New York State: an analysis of risk factors and hospital mortality rates. *Journal of the American Medical Association* 264:1768–1774, 1990.
101. Weintraub WS, Jones EL, Morris DC, et al: Outcome of reoperative coronary bypass surgery versus coronary angioplasty after previous bypass surgery. *Circulation* 95:868–877, 1997.
102. Ornish D, Scherwitz LW, Billings JH, et al: Intensive lifestyle change for reversal of coronary heart disease. *Journal of the American Medical Association* 280:2001–2007, 1998.
103. Squires RW: Preventive rehabilitation cardiology: the Mayo Clinic approach. *Medical Interface* 9:62–68, 1996.
104. Shaw M, Mitchell R, Dorling D: Time for a smoke? One cigarette reduces your life by 11 minutes. *British Medical Journal* 36:297–298, 2000.
105. AHCPR Supported Clinical Practice Guidelines: Treating tobacco use and dependence: 2008 Update. http://www.ncbi.nlm.nih.gov/bookshelf/br.fcgi?book=hsahcpr&part=part1.bxml; retrieved January 2011.
106. Pierson DJ: Translating new understanding into better care for the patient with chronic obstructive pulmonary disease. *Respiratory Care* 49:99–109, 2004.
107. Yohannes AM, Hardy CC: Treatment of chronic obstructive pulmonary disease in older patients: a practical guide. *Drugs and Aging* 20:209–228, 2003.
108. Calverley PM, Walker P: Chronic obstructive pulmonary disease. *Lancet* 362:1053–1061, 2003.
109. Ockene IS, Miller NH: Cigarette smoking, cardiovascular disease, and stroke: a statement for healthcare professionals from the American Heart Association. American Heart Association Task Force on Risk Reduction, *Circulation* 96:3243–3247, 1997.

110. Maltais F, Bourbeau J: Medical management of emphysema. *Chest Surgery Clinics of North America* 5:673–689, 1995.
111. McDaniel AM: Assessing the feasibility of a clinical practice guideline for inpatient smoking cessation intervention. *Clinical Nurse Specialist* 13:228–235, 1999.
112. Kurth T, Kase CS, Berger K, et al: Smoking and the risk of hemorrhagic stroke in men. *Stroke* 34:1151–1155, 2003.
113. Kirshner HS: Medical prevention of stroke, 2003. *Southern Medical Journal* 96:354–358, 2003.
114. Chalmers J, Chapman N: Challenges for the prevention of primary and secondary stroke: the importance of lowering blood pressure and total cardiovascular risk. *Blood Pressure* 10:344–351, 2001.
115. Cohen JA, Estacio RO, Lundgren RA, et al: Diabetic autonomic neuropathy is associated with an increased incidence of strokes. *Autonomic Neuroscience* 108:73–78, 2003.
116. Cucchiara BL, Kasner SE: Atherosclerotic risk factors in patients with ischemic cerebrovascular disease. *Current Treatment Options in Neurology* 4:445–453, 2002.
117. Hart RG, Halperin JL: Atrial fibrillation and thromboembolism: a decade of progress in stroke prevention. *Annals of Internal Medicine* 131:688–695, 1999.
118. Kurl S, Laukkanen JA, Rauramaa R, et al: Cardiorespiratory fitness and the risk of stroke in men. *Archives of Internal Medicine* 163:1682–1688, 2003.
119. Piravej K, Wiwatkul K: Risk factors for stroke in Thai patients. *Journal of the Medical Association of Thailand* 86:S291–S298, 2003.
120. Shinton R: Lifelong exposures and the potential for stroke prevention: the contribution of cigarette smoking, exercise, and body fat. *Journal of Epidemiology and Community Health* 51:138–143, 1997.
121. Everson SA, Lynch JW, Kaplan GA, et al: Stress-induced blood pressure reactivity and incident stroke in middle-aged men. *Stroke* 32:1263–1270, 2001.
122. Chobanian AV, Bakris GL, Black HR, et al: Seventh report of the joint national committee on prevention, detection, evaluation, and treatment of high blood pressure. *Hypertension* 42:1206–1252, 2003.
123. Slama M, Susic D, Frolich ED: Prevention of hypertension. *Current Opinions in Cardiology* 17:531–536, 2002.
124. Shaper AG: Obesity and cardiovascular disease. *Ciba Foundation Symposium* 201:90–103, 1996.
125. Hamilton BP, Hamilton JH: Hypertension in elderly persons. *Endocrine Practice* 3:29–41, 1997.
126. Pitsavos C, Panagiotakos DB, Chrysohoou C, et al: The effect of the combination of Mediterranean diet and leisure time physical activity on the risk of developing acute coronary syndromes, in hypertensive subjects. *Journal of Human Hypertension* 16(7):517–524, 2002.
127. National Institutes of Health: *Average blood pressure on the rise among American children/teenagers*, Washington, DC, 2004, U.S. Department of Health and Human Services.
128. Kurl S, Tuomainen TP, Laukkanen JA, et al: Plasma vitamin C modifies the association between hypertension and risk of stroke. *Stroke* 33:1568–1573, 2002.
129. Hu G, Barengo NC, Tuomilehto J, et al: Relationship of physical activity and body mass index to the risk of hypertension: a prospective study in Finland. *Hypertension* 43:25–30, 2004.
130. Costa FV: Non-pharmacological treatment of hypertension in women. *Journal of Hypertension* 20(Suppl 2):S57–S61, 2002.
131. Bond V, Stephens Q, Adams RG, et al: Aerobic exercise attenuates an exaggerated exercise blood pressure response in normotensive young adult African-American men. *Blood Pressure* 11:229–234, 2002.
132. Jackson EM, Dishman RK: Hemodynamic responses to stress among black women: Fitness and parental hypertension. *Medicine and Science in Sports and Exercise* 34: 1097–1104, 2002.
133. Felmeden DC, Spencer CG, Blann AD, et al: Physical activity in relation to indices of endothelial function and angiogenesis factors in hypertension: a substudy of the Anglo-Scandinavian Cardiac Outcomes Trial (ASCOT). *Journal of Internal Medicine* 2003.
134. Luedemann J, Schminke U, Berger K, et al: Association between behavior-dependent cardiovascular risk factors and asymptomatic carotid atherosclerosis in a general population. *Stroke* 33:2929–2935, 2002.
135. Endres M, Gertz K, Lindauer U, et al: Mechanisms of stroke protection by physical activity. *Annals of Neurology* 54:582–590, 2003.
136. American Heart Association: Blood pressure guidelines. www.americanheart.org/presenter.jhtml?identifier=4450; retrieved January 2011, 2010.
137. Gordon NF, Gulanick M, Costa F, et al: Physical activity and exercise recommendations for stroke survivors: an American Heart Association scientific statement from the Council on Clinical Cardiology, Subcommittee on Exercise, Cardiac Rehabilitation, and Prevention; the Council on Cardiovascular Nursing; the Council on Nutrition, Physical Activity, and Metabolism; and the Stroke Council. *Circulation* 109:2031–2041, 2004.
138. Greenland KJ, Giles WH, Keenan NL, et al: Physician advice, patient actions, and health-related quality of life in secondary prevention of stroke through diet and exercise. *Stroke* 33:565–570, 2002.
139. Gregg EW, Mangione CM, Cauley JA, et al: Diabetes and incidence of functional disability in older women. *Diabetes Care* 25:61–67, 2002.
140. Turtle JR: The economic burden of insulin resistance. *International Journal of Clinical Practice* (Suppl):23–28, 2000.
141. Abraham WT: Preventing cardiovascular events in patients with diabetes mellitus. *American Journal of Medicine* 116(Suppl 5A):39S–46S, 2004.
142. Ten S, MacLaren N: Insulin resistance syndrome in children. *Journal of Clinical Endocrinology and Metabolism* 89:2526–2539, 2004.
143. Singleton JR, Smith AG, Russell JW, et al: Microvascular complications of impaired glucose tolerance. *Diabetes* 52:2867–2873, 2003.
144. Hu FB, Stampfer MJ, Solomon C, et al: Physical activity and risk for cardiovascular events in diabetic women. *Annals of Internal Medicine* 134:96–105, 2001.
145. Wannamethee SG, Shaper AG, Perry IJ: Smoking as a modifiable risk factor for type 2 diabetes in middle-aged men. *Diabetes Care* 24:1590–1595, 2001.
146. Scott CL: Diagnosis, prevention, and interventions for the metabolic syndrome. *American Journal of Cardiology* 92:35–42, 2003.
147. Keller KB, Lemberg L: Obesity and the metabolic syndrome. *American Journal of Critical Care* 12:167–170, 2003.
148. World Health Organization: *Obesity: preventing and managing the global epidemic*, Geneva, Switzerland, 2000, World Health Organization.
149. Anonymous: Obesity: preventing and managing the global epidemic. Report of a WHO consultation. *World Health Organization Technical Report Series* 894:i–xii 1–253, 2000.
150. Grundy SM: Obesity, metabolic syndrome, and coronary atherosclerosis. *Circulation* 105:2696–2698, 2002.
151. Hu FB: Overweight and obesity in women: health risks and consequences. *Journal of Women's Health* 12:163–172, 2003.
152. Kannel WB, Wilson PW, Nam BH, et al: Risk stratification of obesity as a coronary risk factor. *American Journal of Cardiology* 90:697–701, 2002.
153. Tanaka K, Nakanishi T: Obesity as a risk factor for various diseases: necessity of lifestyle changes for healthy aging. *Applied Human Science* 15:139–148, 1996.
154. Wenche DB, Holmen J, Kruger O, et al: Leisure-time physical activity and change in body mass index: an 11-year follow-up study of 9357 normal weight healthy women 20–49 years old. *Journal of Women's Health* 13:55–62, 2004.
155. Xu H, Barnes GT, Yang Q, et al: Chronic inflammation in fat plays a crucial role in the development of obesity in the development of obesity-related insulin resistance. *Journal of Clinical Investigation* 112:1821–1830, 2003.
156. Frayne KN: Insulin resistance, impaired postprandial lipid metabolism and abdominal obesity: a deadly triad. *Medical Principles and Practice* 11(Suppl 2):31–40, 2002.
157. Eckel RH, Krauss RM: American Heart Association call to action: obesity as a major risk factor for coronary artery disease. AHA Nutrition Committee. *Circulation* 97:2099–2100, 1998.
158. Trakas K, Oh PI, Singh S, et al: The health status of obese individuals in Canada. *International Journal of Obesity* 25:662–668, 2001.
159. Wilson PW, Kannel WB: Obesity, diabetes, and risk of cardiovascular disease in the elderly. *American Journal of Geriatric Cardiology* 11:119–123, 125, 2002.
160. Caballero B: Early nutrition and risk of disease in the adult. *Public Health and Nutrition* 4:1335–1336, 2001.
161. Liu S, Manson JE: What is the optimal weight for cardiovascular health? *British Medical Journal* 322:631–632, 2001.
162. Racette SB, Deusinger SS, Deusinger, RH: Obesity: overview of prevalence, etiology, and treatment. *Physical Therapy* 83:276–288, 2003.
163. Centers for Disease Control and Prevention: Recent trends in mortality rates for four major cancers, by sex and race/ethnicity—United States, 1990–2000. *MMWR Weekly* 51:49–53, 2002. www.cdc.gov/mmwr/preview/mmwrhtml/ss5303a1.htm; retrieved January 2011.
164. Glassman SJ, Rashbaum IG, Walker WC: Cardiopulmonary rehabilitation and cancer rehabilitation. 1. Cardiac rehabilitation. *Archives of Physical Medicine and Rehabilitation* 82(3 Suppl 1):S47–S51, 2001.
165. Rashbaum IG, Walker WC, Glassman SJ: Cardiopulmonary rehabilitation and cancer rehabilitation. 2. Cardiac rehabilitation in disabled

populations. *Archives of Physical Medicine and Rehabilitation* 82(3 Suppl 1):S52–S55, 2001.
166. Pastakia K, Kumar S: Exercise parameters in the management of breast cancer: a systematic review of randomized controlled trials. *Physiotherapy Research International Wiley Online Library* 2010 DOI: 10:1002/pri505.
167. Galvao DA, Taaffe DR, Newton RU: Physical activity and genitourinary cancer survivorship. *Recent Results in Cancer Research* 186:217–236, 2011.
168. Feskanich D, Willett W, Colditz G: Walking and leisure-time activity and risk of hip fractures in postmenopausal women. *Journal of the American Medical Association* 288:2300–2306, 2002.
169. Lloyd T, Petit MA, Lin HM, Beck TJ: Lifestyle factors and the development of bone mass and bone strength in young women. *Journal of Pediatrics* 144:776–782, 2004.
170. McCreadie RG: Diet, smoking and cardiovascular risk in people with schizophrenia: descriptive study. *British Journal of Psychiatry* 183:534–539, 2003.
171. Waldman W, Lamb M: *Dying for a hamburger. Modern meat processing and the epidemic of Alzheimer's disease*, Toronto, 2004, McClelland & Stewart Ltd.
172. Krill JJ, Halliday GM: Alzheimer's disease: its diagnosis and pathogenesis. *International Review of Neurobiology* 48:167–217, 2001.
173. Stewart R, Richards M, Brayne C, Mann A: Vascular risk and cognitive impairment in an older, British, African-Caribbean population. *Journal of the American Geriatric Society* 49:263–269, 2001.
174. Teri L, Gibbons LE, McCurry SM, et al: Exercise plus behavioral management in patients with Alzheimer disease: a randomized controlled trial. *Journal of the American Medical Association* 290:2015–2022, 2003.
175. Merchant AT, Pitiphat W, Rimm EB, et al: Increased physical activity decreases periodontal risk in men. *European Journal of Epidemiology* 18:891–898, 2003.
176. Giannuzzi P, Mezzani A, Saner H, et al: Physical activity for primary and secondary prevention: position paper of the Working Group on Cardiac Rehabilitation and Exercise Physiology of the European Society of Cardiology. *Journal of Cardiovascular Risk* 10:19–27, 2003.
177. Fletcher GF, Balady G, Blair SN, et al: Statement on exercise: benefits and recommendations for physical activity programs for all Americans. A statement for health professionals by the Committee on Exercise and Cardiac Rehabilitation of the Council on Clinical Cardiology, American Heart Association. *Circulation* 94:857–862, 1996.
178. Larsen CS: Animal source foods and human health during evolution. *Journal of Nutrition* 133(11 Suppl 2):3893S–3897S, 2003.
179. Nesto RW: The relation of insulin resistance syndromes to risk of cardiovascular disease. *Reviews in Cardiovascular Medicine* 4(Suppl 6):S11–S18, 2003.
180. Chakravarthy MV, Booth FW: Eating, exercise, and "thrifty" genotypes: connecting the dots toward an evolutionary understanding of modern chronic disease. *Journal of Applied Physiology* 96:3–10, 2004.
181. Sorenson M: Herbivorous by design. In *Mega health*, Ivins, Utah, 1992, National Institute of Fitness.
182. Sanders TA: High- versus low-fat diets in human diseases. *Current Opinions in Clinical Nutrition and Metabolic Care* 6:151–155, 2003.
183. Astrup A, Larsen TM, Harper A: Aktins and other low-carbohydrate diets: hoax or an effective tool for weight loss? *Lancet* 364:897–899, 2004.
184. Ferreira SR, Lerario DD, Gimeno SG, et al: Obesity and central adiposity in Japanese immigrants: role of the Western dietary pattern. *Journal of Epidemiology* 12:431–438, 2002.
185. United States Department of Health and Human Services, Consumer Information Center: The food guide pyramid. www.usda.gov; retrieved January 2011.
186. Health Canada: Office of Nutrition Policy and Promotion. Revision of Canada's Food Guide to Health Eating. www.hc-sc.gc.ca; retrieved January 2011.
187. McCullough ML, Feskanich D, Rimm EB, et al: Adherence to the Dietary Guidelines for Americans and risk of major chronic disease in men. *American Journal of Clinical Nutrition* 72:1223–1231, 2000a.
188. McCullough ML, Feskanich D, Stampfer MJ, et al: Adherence to the Dietary Guidelines for Americans and risk of major chronic disease in women. *American Journal of Clinical Nutrition* 72:1214–1222, 2000b.
189. Polidori MC: Antioxidant micronutrients in the prevention of age-related diseases. *Journal of Postgraduate Medicine* 49:229–235, 2003.
190. Liu S, Manson JE, Lee IM, et al: Fruit and vegetable intake and risk of cardiovascular disease: the Women's Health Study. *American Journal of Clinical Nutrition* 72:922–928, 2000a.
191. Liu S, Manson JE, Stampfer MJ, et al: Whole grain consumption and risk of ischemic stroke in women: a prospective study. *Journal of the American Medical Association* 284:1534–1540, 2000b.
192. Shike M: Diet and lifestyle in the prevention of colorectal cancer: an overview. *American Journal of Medicine* 106:11S–15S, 1999.
193. McBurney ML: Candidate foods in the Asia-Pacific region for cardiovascular protection: relevance of grains and grain-based foods to coronary artery disease. *Asia Pacific Journal of Clinical Nutrition* 10:123–127, 2001.
194. McKeown NM, Meigs JB, Liu S, et al: Whole-grain intake is favorably associated with metabolic risk factors for type 2 diabetes and cardiovascular disease in the Framingham Offspring Study. *American Journal of Clinical Nutrition* 76:390–398, 2002.
195. Giles PD, Ramachandran S, Whitaker AJ, et al: The one-stop coronary cholesterol clinic: a multidisciplinary approach to implementing evidence-based treatment. *Postgraduate Medicine Journal* 72:744–748, 1996.
196. Janssen I, Katzmarzyk PT, Ross R: Waist circumference and not body mass index explains obesity-related health risk. *American Journal of Clinical Nutrition* 79:379–384, 2004.
197. Yusuf S, Hawken S, Ôunpuu S, et al: Obesity and the risk of myocardial infarction in 27 000 participants from 52 countries: a case-control study. *The Lancet* 366:1640–1649, 2005.
198. Report of the Institute of Medicine of the National Academy of Sciences. IOM report declares high blood pressure a neglected disease, calls for strategies to change Americans' lifestyles and diets to curb hypertension. Washington, DC, February 22, 2010.
199. Healy GN, Dunstan DW, Salmon J, et al: Breaks in sedentary time. Beneficial associations with metabolic risk. *Diabetes Care* 31:661–666, 2008.
200. Thorp AA, Healy GN, Owen N, et al: Deleterious associations of sitting time and television viewing time with cardiometabolic risk biomarkers. *Diabetes Care* 33:327–334, 2010.
201. Biddle SJH, Pearson N, Ross GM, Braithwaite R: Tracking of sedentary behaviors of young people: a systematic review. *Preventive Medicine* 51:345–351, 2010.
202. Foss M, Merle L, Keteyian S: *Fox's physiologic basis for exercise and sport*, ed 6, Boston, 1998, McGraw-Hill.
203. Tudor-Locke C, Bassett DR, Jr: How many steps/day are enough? Preliminary pedometer indices for public health. *Sports Medicine* 34:1–8, 2004.
204. Blair SN, Cheng Y, Holder JS: Is physical activity or physical fitness more important in defining health benefit? *Medicine and Science in Sports and Exercise* 33(6 Suppl):379–399, 2001.
205. Katzmarzyk PT, Gledhill N, Shepherd RJ: The economic burden of physical inactivity in Canada. *Canadian Medical Association Journal* 163:1435–1440, 2000.
206. Gunnarsson OT, Judge JO: Exercise in midlife: how and why to prescribe it for sedentary patients. *Geriatrics* 52:71–72, 77–80, 1997.
207. Lee CD, Blair SN: Cardiopulmonary fitness and stroke mortality in men. *Medicine and Science in Sports and Exercise* 34:592–595, 2002.
208. Sato Y: Diabetes and life-styles: role of physical exercise for primary prevention. *British Journal of Nutrition* 84(Suppl):S187–S190, 2000.
209. Orozco-Valero M: Large therapeutic studies in elderly patients with hypertension. *Journal of Human Hypertension* 16(Suppl 1):S38–S43, 2002.
210. Messinger-Rapport BJ, Sprecher D: Prevention of cardiovascular diseases: coronary artery disease, congestive heart failure, and stroke. *Clinical Geriatric Medicine* 18:463–483, 2002.
211. Chatila WM, Wynkoop WA, Vance GG, Criner GJ: Smoking patterns in African Americans and whites with advanced COPD. *Chest* 125:15–21, 2004.
212. Nguyen MN, Beland F, Otis J: Is the intention to quit smoking influenced by other heart-healthy lifestyle habits in 30- to 60-year-old men? *Addiction and Behavior* 23:23–30, 1998.
213. Naslund GK, Fredrikson M, Hellenius ML, et al: Effect of diet and physical exercise intervention programmes on coronary artery disease risk in smoking and non-smoking men in Sweden. *Journal of Epidemiology and Community Health* 50:131–136, 1996a.
214. Kromhout D, Menotti A, Keseloot H, Sans S: Prevention of coronary heart disease by diet and lifestyle: evidence from prospective cross-cultural, cohort, and intervention studies. *Circulation* 105:893–898, 2002.
215. Luepker RV: Cardiovascular disease among Mexican Americans. *American Journal of Medicine* 110:147–148, 2001.
216. North KE, Howard BV, Welty TK, et al: Genetic and environment contributions to cardiovascular disease risk in American Indians: the Strong Heart Family Study. *American Journal of Epidemiology* 157:303–314, 2003.
217. Egusa G, Watanabe H, Ohshita K, et al: Influence of the extent of westernization of lifestyle on the progression of preclinical atherosclerosis

in Japanese subjects. *Journal of Atherosclerosis and Thrombosis* 9:299–304, 2002.
218. Wahlqvist ML: Asian migration to Australia: food and health consequences. *Asia Pacific Journal of Clinical Nutrition* 11:S562–S568, 2002a.
219. Rimmer JH, Riley B, Creviston T, et al: Exercise training in a predominantly African-American group of stroke survivors. *Medicine and Science in Sports and Exercise* 32:1990–1996, 2000.
220. Dubbert PM, Carithers T, Sumner AE, et al: Obesity, physical inactivity, and risk for cardiovascular disease. *American Journal of Medical Science* 324:116–126, 2002.
221. Dundas R, Morgan M, Redfern J, et al: Ethnic differences in behavioural risk factors for stroke: implications for health promotion. *Ethnicity and Health* 6:95–103, 2001.
222. Owens PL, Bradley EH, Horwitz SM, et al: Clinical assessment of function among women with a recent cerebrovascular event: a self-reported versus performance-based measure. *Annals of Internal Medicine* 136:802–811, 2002.
223. Cleeland CS, Gonin R, Baez L, et al: Pain and treatment of pain in minority patients with cancer. The Eastern Co-operative Oncology Group Minority Outpatient Pain Study. *Annals of Internal Medicine* 127:813–816, 1997.
224. Todd KH, Samaroo N, Hoffman JR: Ethnicity as a risk factor for inadequate emergency department analgesia. *Journal of the American Medical Association* 269:1537–1539, 1993.
225. Bergman E, Bertero C: You can do it if you set your mind to it: a qualitative study of patients with coronary artery disease. *Journal of Advances in Nursing* 36:733–741, 2001.
226. Baxter AP, Milner PC, Hawkins S, et al: The impact of heart health promotion on coronary heart disease lifestyle risk factors in school children: lessons learnt from a community-based project. *Public Health* 111:231–237, 1997.
227. Cupples ME, McKnight A: Five year follow up of patients at high cardiovascular risk who took part in randomized control trial of health promotion. *British Medical Journal* 319:687–688, 1999.
228. Egan F: Cardiac rehabilitation in the new millennium. *Intensive Critical Care Nursing* 15:163–168, 1999.
229. Joseph LN, Babikian VL, Allen NC, et al: Risk factor modification in stroke prevention: the experience of a stroke clinic. *Stroke* 30:16–20, 1999.
230. Nisbeth O, Klausen K, Andersen LB: Effectiveness of counseling over 1 year on changes in lifestyle and coronary heart disease risk factors. *Patient Education and Counseling* 40:121–131, 2000.
231. Rausch M, Turkoski B: Developing realistic treatment standards in today's economic climate: stroke survivor education. *Journal of Advances in Nursing* 30:329–334, 1999.
232. Sumanen M, Koskenvuo M, Immonen-Raiha P, et al: Secondary prevention of coronary artery disease is disappointing among patients of working age. *Family Practice* 21:304–306, 2004.
233. Nguyen MN, Beland F, Otis J, et al: Diet and exercise profiles of 30- and 60-year-old male smokers: implications for community heart health programs. *Journal of Community Health* 21:107–121, 1996.
234. Guiese BJ: Behavioral medicine strategies for heart disease prevention: the example of smoking cessation. *Preventive Cardiology* 3:10–15, 2000.
235. Kingsbury K: Taking AIM: how to teach primary and secondary prevention effectively. *Canadian Journal of Cardiology* 14(Suppl):22A–26A, 1998.
236. Carlsson CM, Stein JH: Cardiovascular disease and the aging woman: overcoming barriers to lifestyle changes. *Current Women's Health Report* 2:366–372, 2002.
237. McPherson R: Coronary artery disease and women: applying the guidelines for risk factor management. *Canadian Journal of Cardiology* 16(Suppl A):5A–10A, 2000.
238. Billings JH: Maintenance of behavior changes in cardiorespiratory risk reduction: a clinical perspective from the Ornish Program for reversing coronary heart disease. *Health Psychology* 19(1 Suppl):70–75, 2000.
239. Toobert DJ, Glasgow RE, Radcliffe JL: Physiologic and related behavioral outcomes from the Women's Lifestyle Heart Trial. *Annals of Behavioral Medicine* 22:1–9, 2000.
240. Khattab MS, Abolfotouh MA, Alakija W, et al: Risk factors of coronary artery disease: attitude and behaviour in family practice in Saudi Arabia. *Eastern Mediterranean Health Journal* 5:35–45, 1999.
241. Kok FJ, Matroos AW, van den Ban AW, et al: Characteristics of individuals with multiple behavioral risk factors for coronary artery disease: the Netherlands. *American Journal of Public Health* 72:986–991, 1982.
242. Nakamura J, Amano W, Araki Y, et al: Coronary risk factor management in primary practice in Shibuya, Tokyo. *Journal of Cardiology* 42:207–212, 2003. (English abstract).
243. Naslund GK, Fredrikson M, Hellenius ML, et al: Determinants of compliance in men enrolled in a diet and exercise intervention trial: a randomized, controlled study. *Patient Education and Counseling* 29:247–256, 1996b.
244. Lau-Walker, M: Cardiac rehabilitation: the importance of patient expectations—a practitioner survey. *Journal of Clinical Nursing* 13:177–184, 2004.
245. Azjen I: From intention to actions: a theory of planned behavior. In Kuhl J, Beckmann J, editors: (1985). *Action control: from cognition to behavior*, Berlin and New York, 1983, Springer.
246. Demarais A, Robichaud-Ekstrand S: McEwen's conceptual model in cardiac rehabilitation. *Canadian Nurse* 94:40–46, 1998. (English abstract).
247. DiClemente CC, Prochaska JO: Toward a comprehensive, transtheoretical model of change—stages of change and addictive behaviors. In Miller WR, Heather N, editors: (1998). *Treating addictive behaviors*, ed 2, New York, 1998, Springer.
248. Cox KL, Gorely TJ, Puddey IB, et al: Exercise behavior change in 40- to 65-year-old women: the SWEAT Study (Sedentary Women Exercise Adherence Trial). *British Journal of Health Psychology* 8(Pt 4):477–495, 2003.
249. Mengden T, Chamontin B, Phong Chau N, et al: User procedure for self-management of blood pressure. First International Consensus Conference on Self Blood Pressure Measurement. *Blood Pressure Monitoring* 5:111–129, 2000.
250. Wierenga ME, Oldham KK: Weight control: a lifestyle-modification model for improving health. *Nursing Clinics of North America* 37:303–313, 2002.
251. Thomas RJ, Kottke TE, Brekke MJ, et al: Attempts at changing dietary and exercise habits to reduce risk of cardiovascular disease: who's doing what in the community? *Preventive Cardiology* 5:102–108, 2002.
252. Tresch DD, Aronow WS: Smoking and coronary artery disease. *Clinics in Geriatric Medicine* 12:23–32, 1996.
253. Winslow E, Bohannon N, Brunton SA, et al: Lifestyle modification: weight control, exercise, and smoking cessation. *American Journal of Medicine* 101:25S–31S, 1996.
254. Meland E, Maeland JG, Laerum E: The importance of self-efficacy in cardiovascular risk factor change. *Scandinavian Journal of Public Health* 27:11–17, 1999.
255. Steptoe A, Wardle J, Cui W, et al: Trends in smoking, diet, physical exercise, and attitudes toward health in European university students from 13 countries, 1990–2000. *Preventive Medicine* 35:97–104, 2002.
256. Gariballa SE, Peet SM, Fotherby MD, et al: The knowledge of hospital patients about vascular disease and their risk factors. *Postgraduate Medical Journal* 72:605–608, 1996.
257. Abramson S, Stein J, Schaufele M, et al: Personal exercise habits and counseling practices of primary care physicians: a national survey. *Clinical Journal of Sports Medicine* 10:40–44, 2000.
258. Wells KB, Lewis CE, Leake B, et al: Do physicians preach what they practice? A study of physicians' health habits and counseling practices. *Journal of the American Medical Association* 252:2846–2848, 1984.
259. Sackett DL, Straus SE, Richardson WC, et al: *Evidence-based medicine: how to practice and teach EBM*, Edinburgh, New York, 2000, Churchill Livingstone.
260. Maher CG, Sherrington C, Herbert RD, et al: Reliability of the PEDro scale for rating quality of randomized controlled trials. *Physical Therapy* 83:713–721, 2003.
261. Prochaska JO, DiClemente CC: Transtheoretical therapy: toward a more integrative model of change. *Psychotherapy: Theory, Research and Practice* 19:276–288, 1982.
262. White JL, Ransdell LB: Worksite intervention model for facilitating changes in physical activity, fitness, and psychological parameters. *Perceptual and Motor Skills* 97:461–466, 2003.
263. Guilmette TJ, Motta SI, Shadel WG, et al: Promoting smoking cessation in the rehabilitation environment. *Archives of Physical Medicine and Rehabilitation* 80:560–562, 2001.
264. Mason P, Rollnick S, Butler C: *Health behavior change: a guide for practitioners*, Edinburgh. New York, 2010, Churchill Livingstone/Elsevier.
265. Rollnick S, Heather N, Bell A: Negotiating behaviour change in medical settings: the development of brief motivational interviewing. *Journal of Mental Health* 1:25–37, 1992.
266. Rollnick S, Butler CC, Stott N: Helping smokers make decisions: the enhancement of brief intervention for general medical practice. *Patient Education and Counseling* 31:191–203, 1997.

267. Koertge J, Weidner G, Elliott-Edler M, et al: Improvement in medical risk factors and quality of life in women and men with coronary artery disease in the Multicenter Lifestyle Demonstration Project. *American Journal of Cardiology* 91:1316–1322, 2003.
268. Bean JF, Vora A, Frontera WR: Benefits of exercise for community-dwelling older adults. *Archives of Physical Medicine and Rehabilitation* 85(Suppl 3):S31–S42, 2004.
269. Campbell I: The obesity epidemic: can we turn the tide? *Heart* 89(Suppl 2):ii22–24, 2003.
270. Jones AYM, Dean E, Scudds R: Effectiveness of a community-based Tai Chi program and implications for public health initiatives. *Archives of Physical Medicine and Rehabilitation* 86:619–625, 2005.
271. Ada L, Dean CM, Hall JM, et al: A treadmill and overground walking program improves walking in persons residing in the community after stroke: a placebo-controlled, randomized trial. *Archives of Physical Medicine and Rehabilitation* 84:1486–1491, 2003.
272. Eng JJ, Chu KS, Kim CM, et al: A community-based group exercise program for persons with chronic stroke. *Medicine and Science in Sports and Exercise* 35:1271–1278, 2003.
273. Smith KM, Arthur HM, McKelvie RS, et al: Differences in sustainability of exercise and health-related quality of life outcomes following home or hospital-based cardiac rehabilitation. *European Journal of Cardiovascular Prevention and Rehabilitation* 11:313–319, 2004.
274. Clark AM, Barbour RS, McIntyre PD: Preparing for change in the secondary prevention of coronary heart disease: a qualitative evaluation of cardiac rehabilitation within a region of Scotland. *Journal of Advances in Nursing* 39:589–598, 2002.
275. Simon SD: Is the randomized clinical trial the gold standard of research? *Journal of Andrology* 22:938–943, 2001.
276. Dean E: Invited commentary on "Are incentive spirometry, intermittent positive pressure breathing, and deep breathing exercises effective in the prevention of postoperative pulmonary complications after upper abdominal surgery?" A systematic overview and meta-analysis. *Physical Therapy* 74:10–15, 1994.
277. Ramadan J, Telahoun G, Al-Zaid NS, et al: Responses to exercise, fluid, and energy balances during Ramadan in sedentary and active males. *Nutrition* 15:735–739, 1999.
278. Prochaska JO: Multiple health behavior research represents the future of preventive medicine. *Preventive Medicine* 46:281–285, 2008.
279. Song R, Lee H: Managing health habits for myocardial infarction (MI) patients. *International Journal of Nursing Studies* 38:375–380, 2001.
280. Bailey JE, Gibson DV, Jain M, et al: QSource quality initiative: reversing the diabetes epidemic in Tennessee. *Tennessee Medicine* 96:559–563, 2003.
281. Kawachi I, Berkman LF, editors: *Neighborhoods and health*, New York, 2003, Oxford University Press.
282. Minkler M, editor: *Community organizing and community building for health*, New Brunswick, NJ, 2005, Rutgers University Press.
283. Smith BJ, McElroy HJ, Ruffin RE, et al: The effectiveness of coordinated care for people with chronic respiratory disease. *The Medical Journal of Australia* 177:481–485, 2002.
284. Kirk-Gardner R, Steven D: Hearts for Life: a community program on health promotion. *Canadian Journal of Cardiovascular Nursing* 13:5–10, 2003.
285. Healthy People 2020. www.healthypeople.gov/2020/default.aspx; Retrieved January 2011.
286. Koffman DM, Bazzarre T, Mosca L, et al: An evaluation of Choose to Move 1999: an American Heart Association physical activity program for women. *Archives of Internal Medicine* 161:2193–2199, 2001.
287. Skybo TA, Ryan-Wenger N: A school-based intervention to teach third-grade children about the prevention of heart disease. *Pediatric Nursing* 28:223–229, 235, 2002.
288. Frenn M, Malin S, Bansal N, et al: Addressing health disparities in middle school students' nutrition and exercise. *Journal of Community Health Nursing* 20:1–14, 2003.
289. Lai JC, Woo J, Hui E, et al: Telerehabilitation—a new model for community-based stroke rehabilitation. *Journal of Telemedicine and Telecare* 10:199–205, 2004.
290. Oki Y, Shiomi T, Sasanable R, et al: Multiple cardiovascular risk factors in obstructive sleep apnea syndrome patients and an attempt at lifestyle modification using telemedicine-based education. *Psychiatry and Clinical Neuroscience* 53:311–313, 1999.
291. Poscente N, Rothstein M, Irvine MJ: Using marketing research methods to evaluate a stage-specific intervention. *American Journal of Health Behavior* 26:243–251, 2002.
292. Colson JRC: *Progressive exercise therapy in rehabilitation and physical education*, Bristol, UK, 1983, John Wright & Sons Ltd.
293. Gardiner MD: *The principles of exercise therapy*, ed 4, London, 1981, G. Bell & Hyman.
294. Tidy NM: *Massage and remedial exercise*, Baltimore, MD, 1933, Wood and Company.
295. Hellenius ML, Dahlof C, Aberg H, et al: Quality of life is not negatively affected by diet and exercise intervention in healthy men with cardiovascular risk factors. *Quality of Life Research* 4:13–20, 1995.

Chapter 2

Oxygen Transport: The Basis of Cardiovascular and Pulmonary Physical Therapy

Elizabeth Dean

KEY TERMS

Cellular respiration
Exercise stress
Gravitational stress
Oxygen transport pathway

CHAPTER OUTLINE

Oxygen transport is essential to life, activity, and participation in life consistent with the International Classification of Functioning, Disability and Health (ICF).[1] Maximizing the efficiency of the oxygen transport pathway promotes optimal mobility and independence, the cornerstones of quality of life and well-being. Attention to oxygen transport—its deficits and threats to it—is the concern of physical therapists, irrespective of the primary clinical area of their practices. This is particularly true given the trend toward physical therapists' direct access to patients and the prevalence of lifestyle-related conditions, all of which affect oxygen transport either directly or indirectly.

Cardiovascular and pulmonary physical therapy consists of noninvasive interventions that can reverse or mitigate insults to oxygen transport. It can eliminate, delay, or reduce the need for medical interventions, such as supplemental oxygen, intubation, mechanical ventilation, suctioning, bronchoscopy, chest tubes, surgery, and medications. To achieve these outcomes, the physical therapist must fully assess oxygen transport and prescribe optimal treatment interventions. This is possible only with a comprehensive understanding of oxygen transport and the factors that determine and influence it.

This chapter details the oxygen transport system (including the pathway and its component steps), which provides a conceptual basis for cardiovascular and pulmonary physical therapy practice. Oxygen transport is the basis of life. Treatment of impaired or threatened oxygen transport (i.e., cardiovascular and pulmonary dysfunction) is a physical therapy priority.

In a healthy person, the oxygen transport system is perturbed by movement and activity, changes in body position, and emotional state. In a person with pathology, disruption of or threat to this system is a medical priority because of the threat to life or the impairment of functional capacity.

The fundamental steps in the oxygen transport pathway, as well as their function and interdependence, are described. Special attention is given to cellular respiration and the body's use of oxygen during metabolism at the cellular level in muscle. The factors that perturb oxygen transport in health are described—namely, gravitational stress secondary to changes in body position, exercise stress secondary to increased oxygen demand of the working muscles, and emotional stress and arousal. A thorough understanding of the effects of those factors that normally perturb oxygen transport is essential in

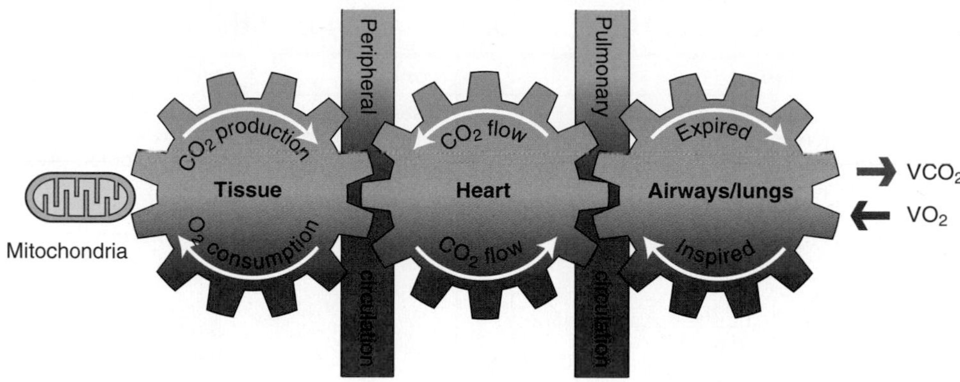

Fig. 2-1 Scheme of components of ventilatory-cardiovascular-metabolic coupling underlying oxygen transport. *(Modified from Wasserman KK, Hansen JE, Sue DY, et al:* Principles of exercise testing and interpretation including pathophysiology and clinical applications, *ed 4, Philadelphia, 2005, Lippincott Williams & Wilkins.)*

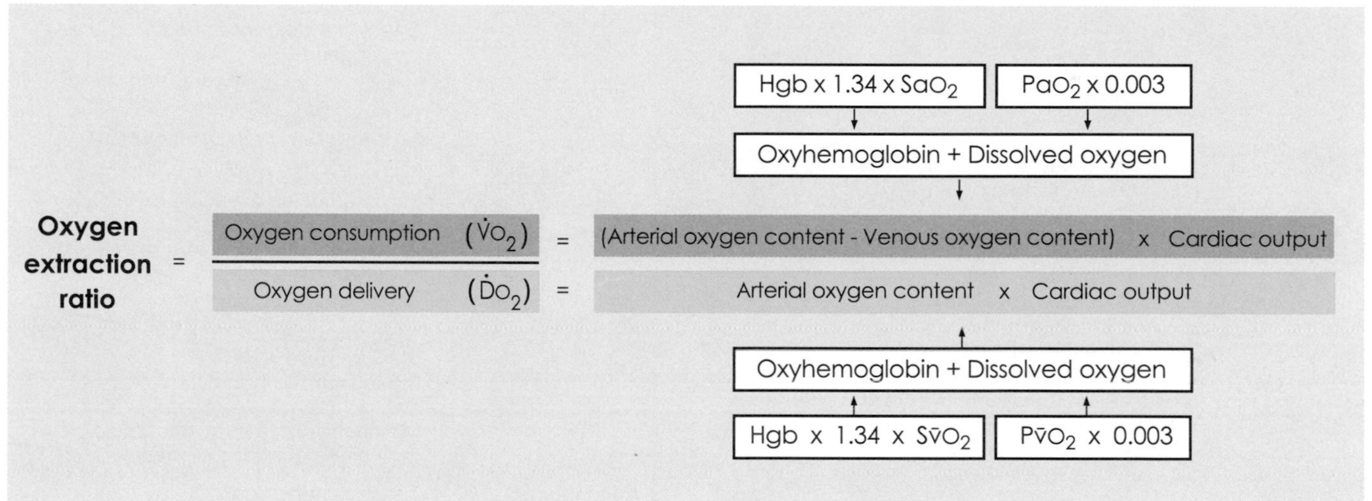

Fig. 2-2 Formulas for determining oxygen delivery (DO_2), oxygen consumption ($\dot{V}O_2$), and oxygen extraction ratio (OER). *(Modified from Epstein CD, Henning RJ: Oxygen transport variables in the identification and treatment of tissue hypoxia,* Heart Lung *22:328–348, 1993.)*

order to accurately assess and treat deficits in oxygen transport.

Oxygen Transport

Oxygen transport refers to the delivery of fully oxygenated blood to peripheral tissues, cellular uptake of oxygen, use of oxygen within the tissue, and the return of partially desaturated blood to the lungs. The oxygen transport pathway consists of multiple steps ranging from the ambient air to the perfusion of peripheral tissues with oxygenated arterial blood (Figure 2-1). Oxygen transport has become the basis for conceptualizing cardiovascular and pulmonary function and diagnosing and managing cardiovascular and pulmonary dysfunction.[2-8]

Oxygen transport variables include oxygen delivery (DO_2), oxygen consumption ($\dot{V}O_2$), and the oxygen extraction ratio (OER), the utilization coefficient. Oxygen demand is the amount of oxygen required by the cells for aerobic metabolism. Oxygen demand is usually reflected by $\dot{V}O_2$; however, in cases of severe cardiovascular and pulmonary dysfunction and compromise to oxygen transport, $\dot{V}O_2$ can fall short of the demand for oxygen. Oxygen transport variables, including the components of DO_2, $\dot{V}O_2$, and OER, are shown in Figure 2-2. DO_2 is determined by arterial oxygen content and cardiac output, $\dot{V}O_2$ by the arteriovenous oxygen content difference and cardiac output, and oxygen extraction by the ratio of DO_2 to $\dot{V}O_2$.

Measures and indexes of oxygen transport that reflect the function of the component steps of the oxygen transport pathway are shown in Table 2-1.

Energy Transfer and Cellular Oxidation

Cellular metabolism and survival depend on the continuous synthesis and degradation of adenosine triphosphate (ATP), the major source of energy for biological work. Work is

Table 2-1 Measures and Indexes of the Function of the Steps in the Oxygen Transport Pathway

Variable	Measure or Index
Control of Ventilation	PO.1 (central drive to breathe) Ventilatory responses of hypoxia and hypercapnia Pao_2 and Sao_2 responses to exercise
Inspired Gas	Alveolar oxygen pressure Alveolar carbon dioxide pressure Alveolar nitrogen pressure Hemoglobin Plasma proteins and their concentrations Red blood cells and count White blood cells and count Platelets Clotting factors Clotting times Hematocrit Pao_2 $PaCO_2$ (end tidal CO_2) $P(A\text{-}a)o_2$ Cao_2 $C\bar{v}o_2$ $C(a\text{-}\bar{v})o_2$ difference HCO_3 Sao_2 pH PAo_2/Pao_2 Pao_2/Fio_2 Serum lactate
Pulmonary Variables	Minute ventilation Tidal volume Respiratory rate Dead space volume Alveolar volume Alveolar ventilation Distribution of ventilation Static and dynamic lung compliance Airway resistance Functional residual capacity Closing volume Vital capacity Forced expiratory volumes and flows Other pulmonary volumes, capacities, and flow rates Inspiratory and expiratory pressures Work of breathing Respiratory muscle strength and endurance
Pulmonary Hemodynamic Variables	Cardiac output Total perfusion Distribution of perfusion Anatomical shunt Physiological shunt Systolic and diastolic pulmonary artery pressures Pulmonary capillary blood flow Pulmonary capillary wedge pressure Pulmonary vascular resistance Pulmonary vascular resistance index
Systemic Hemodynamic Variables	Heart rate Electrocardiogram (ECG) Systemic blood pressure Mean arterial blood pressure Systemic vascular resistance Systemic vascular resistance index Central venous pressure Pulmonary artery pressure Wedge pressure Blood volume Cardiac output Cardiac index Stroke volume Stroke index Shunt fraction Ejection fraction Left ventricular work Right ventricular work Fluid balance Renal output Creatinine clearance and blood urea nitrogen (BUN)
Diffusion	$D(A\text{-}a)o_2$ Diffusing capacity Diffusing capacity/alveolar volume
Gas Exchange	Oxygen consumption ($\dot{V}o_2$) Carbon dioxide production ($\dot{V}CO_2$) Respiratory exchange ratio ($\dot{V}CO_2/\dot{V}o_2$) Ventilation and perfusion matching Pao_2/Pao_2 $P(A\text{-}a)o_2$
Oxygen Extraction and Use	Oxygen extraction ratio ($\dot{V}o_2/Do_2$) $C(a\text{-}\bar{v})o_2$ difference $P(a\text{-}\bar{v})o_2$ difference $S\bar{v}o_2$ Metabolic enzymes at the cellular level Oxyhemoglobin dissociation
Adequacy of Tissue Perfusion and Oxygen Transport	Tissue oxygenation Tissue pH

performed in biological systems for contraction of skeletal, cardiac, and smooth muscle (e.g., exercise, digestion, glandular secretion, and thermoregulation) and for nerve impulse transmission (Box 2-1). These processes require a continuous supply of ATP, which is made available primarily by aerobic (oxygen-requiring) processes. In the event that oxygen delivery is inadequate, nonaerobic (anaerobic, or non–oxygen-requiring) energy-transferring processes can also supply ATP. Supplying energy anaerobically, however, is more costly metabolically; that is, it is not efficient, is limited, and cannot be sustained because of the disruptive effects of lactate (a cellular byproduct of anaerobic metabolism) on physiological processes. Metabolic acidosis is a consequence of lactate accumulation. In patients who are critically ill, the presence of metabolic acidosis secondary to anaerobic metabolism can be life threatening. Prolonged anaerobic metabolism is lethal in

Box 2-1 Biological Work Requiring Continuous Oxygen Supply

- Contraction of skeletal muscle
- Contraction of cardiac muscle
- Contraction of smooth muscle
- Nerve impulse transmission
- Active cellular metabolic processes
- Active cellular pumping mechanisms

two respects. First, the patient is increasingly dependent on anaerobic metabolism because of inadequate DO_2 to peripheral tissues; second, acidosis interferes with normal cellular processes and homeostasis, which require an optimal pH of 7.40.

The ATP molecule consists of an adenine and a ribose molecule with three phosphates attached. The splitting of the terminal phosphate bond or the two terminal phosphate bonds generates a considerable amount of energy. This energy is used to power various chemical reactions associated with metabolism. These metabolic processes take place in specialized organelles in the cells called mitochondria. The primary pathways that are responsible for the formation of ATP are the Krebs cycle and the electron transfer chain.

The Krebs cycle and the electron transfer chain are the biochemical pathways in the mitochondria of the cell responsible for harnessing oxygen for aerobic metabolism and ensuring a continuous supply of oxygen for this process. Initially, glucose is phosphorylated to produce two molecules of ATP (glycolysis). Glucose is oxidized to produce two molecules of pyruvic acid, yielding a net gain of two molecules of ATP per molecule of glucose. The two pyruvate molecules enter the Krebs cycle, where they are oxidized to CO_2 and water. This process yields 30 ATP molecules. Hydrogen ions released in the process are transferred to the electron transfer chain, yielding 4 ATP molecules for cellular metabolism. Electrons are removed from hydrogen and funneled down the electron transport chain by specialized electron carrier molecules, cytochromes 1 to 5. Only the last of these cytochromes, cytochrome oxidase, can reduce molecular oxygen to water. This process is driven by a gradient of high-to-low potential energy. This energy, transferred as electrons, is passed from H_2 to O_2 and is trapped and conserved as high-energy phosphate bonds. Oxygen is involved in these metabolic pathways only at the end of the electron transfer chain, where oxygen is the final electron acceptor and combines with H_2 to form H_2O. More than 90% of ATP synthesis takes place through the electron transfer chain by means of the oxidative reactions associated with oxidative phosphorylation. An individual's peak aerobic capacity is determined by the availability of oxygen at the end of the electron transport chain.

For each molecule of glucose that is metabolized, 36 molecules of ATP are produced: 4 molecules by substrate phosphorylation (anaerobic) and 32 by oxidative phosphorylation (aerobic). The low ATP yield from anaerobic metabolism explains why anaerobic metabolism can serve only as a short-term energy source.

The complex, enzymatically controlled chemical reactions of metabolism are designed to form and conserve energy through the Krebs cycle and the electron transfer chain and then use this energy for biological work.[9,10] Carbohydrates, fats, and proteins ingested from foodstuffs in the diet are oxidized to provide the energy for phosphorylation of adenosine diphosphate (ADP) (i.e., the formation of ATP by combining ADP with phosphate). These substances are broken down, and they access the Krebs cycle at the pyruvic acid or acetyl coenzyme A (CoA) levels (Fig. 2-3). Some amino acids can enter the Krebs cycle directly.

The Krebs cycle degrades acetyl CoA to carbon dioxide (CO_2) and hydrogen (H_2) atoms. The primary purpose of this cycle is to generate hydrogen ions for the electron transfer chain by two principal electron acceptors, nicotinamide adenine dinucleotide (NAD) and flavin adenine dinucleotide (FAD). Many acids catalyze the numerous reactions of the Krebs cycle.

Cellular oxidation, or respiration, refers to the function of the electron transfer chain to release energy in small amounts and to conserve energy in the formation of high-energy bonds. It is this process that ensures a continual energy supply to meet the needs of metabolism (Fig. 2-4).

Three major systems of energy transfer exist to supply energy during all-out exercise over varying durations.[10] Although these systems are discrete, they overlap. Cellular ATP and creatine phosphate (CP) are immediate energy sources for the first 10 seconds of exercise. From 30 to 60 seconds, glycolysis provides a short-term energy source. The ATP-CP system and the glycolytic system are anaerobic processes. As exercise persists for several minutes, the long-term aerobic system predominates. Thus, for sustained physical activity and exercise, energy is provided primarily by aerobic metabolism. For this process, oxygen is provided by the oxygen transport pathway. Carbon compounds that enter the body in the form of carbohydrate, fat, and protein undergo oxidative metabolism in the form of aerobic glycolysis in the mitochondria in the cytoplasm of cells.

Muscle Contraction and Metabolism

The basic mechanism for muscle contraction is excitation contraction coupling.[11,12] Action potentials mediated centrally or through the spinal cord depolarize the muscle cell membrane (the sarcolemma) and stimulate the release of calcium from the lateral sacs of the sarcoplasmic reticulum. The sarcoplasmic reticulum is an extensive network of invaginations and tubular channels encasing the muscle fibers (myofibrils). The calcium floods over the myofilaments of the myofibrils within the sarcomere. Myofilaments consist of thin actin fiber and thick myosin fiber protein, which interdigitate with each other, giving the typical striated appearance to skeletal muscle (Fig. 2-5). Actin is a helical molecule with tropomyosin intertwined along its length. Tropomyosin normally inhibits the interaction of actin and myosin. Calcium causes a conformational change of the tropomyosin molecule that enables troponin, also distributed along the actin molecule, to combine with calcium. The combining of calcium and troponin triggers the interdigitation of actin and myosin (the sliding-filament theory of muscle contraction). Contraction involves myosin heads (cross bridges) attaching to and detaching from actin in a cyclical manner that causes the actin and myosin filaments to slide past each other. In this way, the muscle is shortened without shortening of the myofilaments.

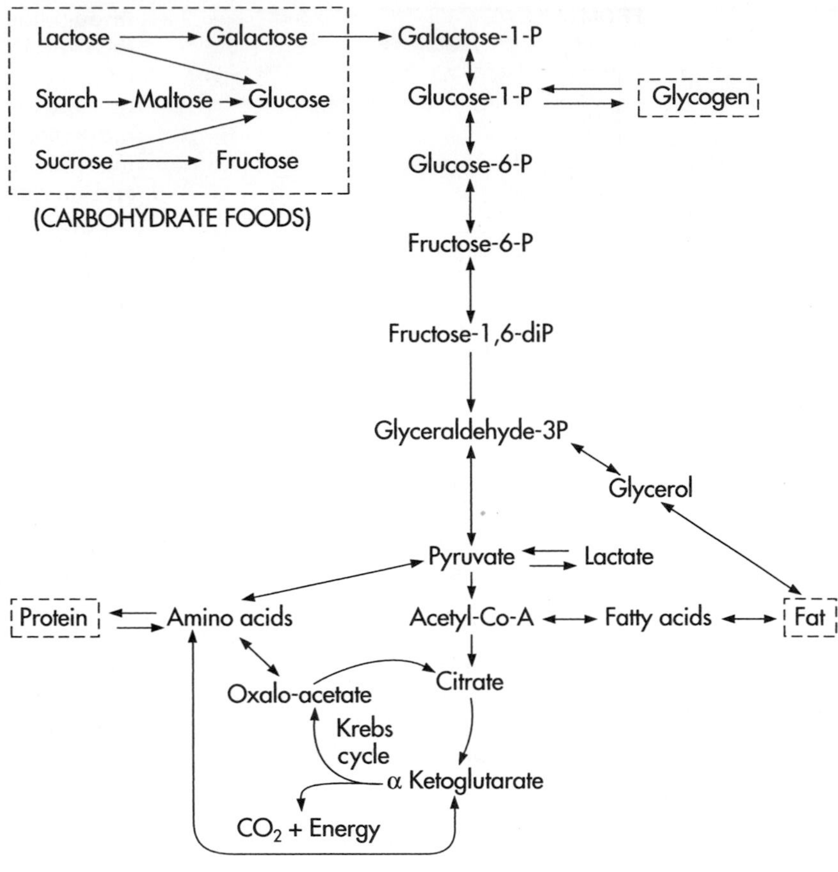

Fig. 2-3 Interrelationships among carbohydrate, fat, and protein metabolism and their points of entry into the Krebs cycle. *(From Mougios V: Exercise biochemistry, Champaign, Ill, 2006, Human Kinetics.)*

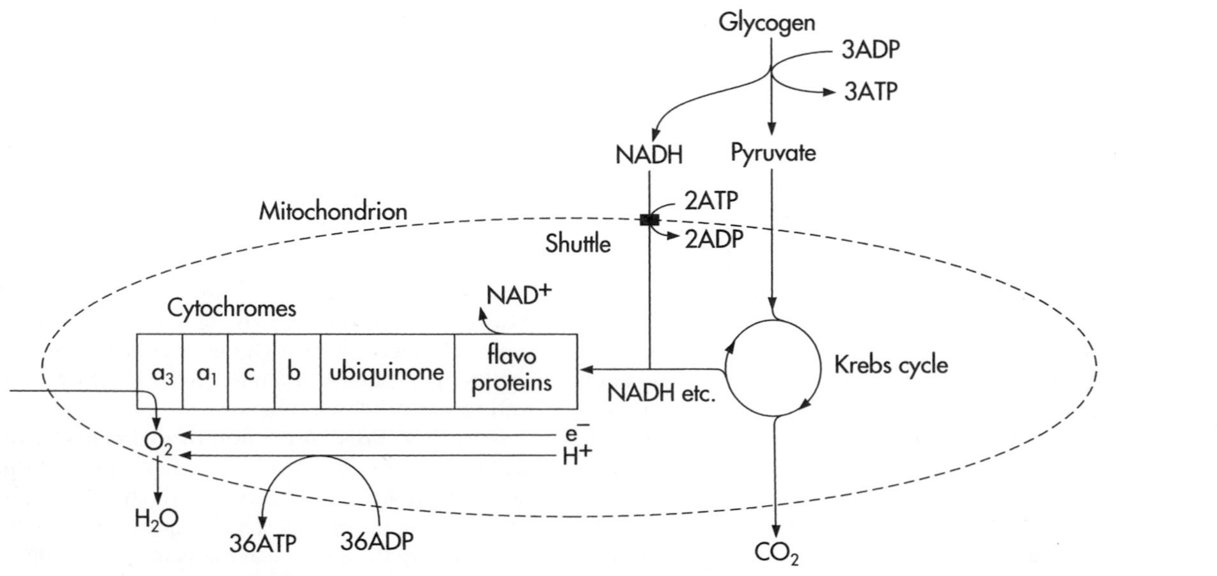

Fig. 2-4 Electron transfer chain and its relationship with the Krebs cycle. *(From Mougios V: Exercise biochemistry, Champaign, Ill, 2006, Human Kinetics).*

The energy for muscle contraction in the form of adenosine triphosphate (ATP) is generated within the mitochondria of the myofibrils. Myosin ATPase splits ATP so that the transfer of this energy can be used for muscle contraction. Specifically, the enzyme ATPase is activated when actin and myosin are joined. ATP is then available to bind with the cross bridge, causing it to detach from actin. Relaxation occurs with the cessation of electrical excitation and the rapid removal or sequestration of calcium into the lateral sacs of the sarcoplasmic reticulum.

The specific metabolic properties of muscle depend on the constituent muscle fiber types.[13] The three primary muscle fiber types are fast-twitch fibers, slow-twitch fibers, and intermediate fibers, which have the properties of both fast-twitch

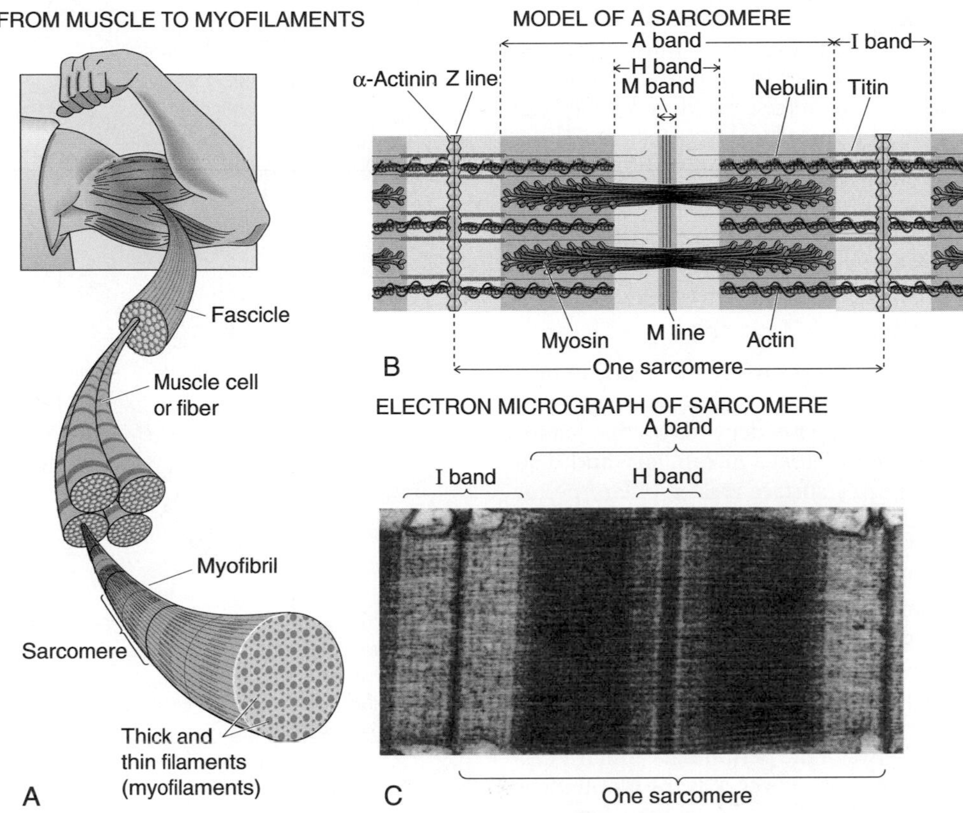

Fig. 2-5 Structure of the sarcomere. *(From Boron WF:* Medical physiology, *St Louis, 2005, Saunders.)*

and slow-twitch fibers. The fast-twitch fibers (fast glycolytic fibers) are recruited during short-term, sprint-type exercise that relies mainly on anaerobic metabolism. These fibers are well adapted for rapid, forceful contractions because they have large amounts of myosin ATPase, rapid calcium release and uptake, and a high rate of cross-bridge cycling. Slow-twitch fibers (slow oxidative fibers) are recruited during prolonged aerobic exercise. These fibers have large amounts of myoglobin, mitochondria, and oxidative enzymes. Compared with the fast-twitch fibers, slow-twitch fibers are fatigue resistant. The intermediate fibers have both anaerobic and aerobic metabolic enzymes, which makes these fibers capable of both types of muscle work. Although the characteristics of the fiber types are distinct, activity and exercise recruit both types of fibers. Depending on the particular activity or exercise, one fiber type may be preferentially recruited over the others.

Principles of Oxygen Transport

Individuals need a continuous supply of oxygen to meet moment-to-moment demands for oxygen commensurate with changing metabolic demands for energy at the cellular level as well as basal metabolic demands.[14,15] Oxygen transport occurs by convection or diffusion. Convection of oxygen refers to the movement of oxygen from the alveoli to the tissue capillaries and is determined primarily by hemoglobin concentration, oxygen saturation, and cardiac output. The diffusion of oxygen refers to the movement of oxygen from the capillaries to the mitochondria and is determined by metabolic rate, vascular resistance, capillary recruitment, and tissue oxygen consumption and extraction.

Normally, DO_2 is regulated by tissue metabolism and the overall demand for oxygen. At rest, DO_2 is three to four times greater than oxygen demand, and $\dot{V}O_2$ is not directly dependent on DO_2. In a healthy individual, the increased metabolic demands of exercise constitute the greatest challenge to the oxygen transport system; $\dot{V}O_2$ can increase 20 times. In response to increased muscle metabolism, blood flow increases to the peripheral muscles through vasodilation and capillary recruitment, thereby increasing the availability of oxygen to working tissues and its extraction from the arterial blood. As DO_2 and $\dot{V}O_2$ increase, venous return, stroke volume, and heart rate also increase, thereby increasing cardiac output (CO). CO can increase by more than five times during strenuous exercise. The capacity to increase CO reflects a person's overall aerobic power.

At rest, regional differences in the proportion of CO normally delivered to the body organs reflect differences in organ functions and are not necessarily matched to the metabolic rate.[16] For example, the distribution of CO to the kidneys is 20%; to the mesenteric, splenic, and portal tissues, 20% to 30%. Comparatively, muscle at rest receives 10% and the brain and myocardium receive less than 5% each.

Oxygen Content of the Blood

The majority of oxygen is transported in arterial blood to the tissues. Oxygen is largely combined with hemoglobin (98%) compared with a relatively minimal amount that is dissolved in the blood (2%). The oxyhemoglobin dissociation curve represents the relationship between the affinity of hemoglobin for oxygen and the arterial oxygen tension. The affinity of hemoglobin for oxygen depends on the tissues' oxygen demand. In a healthy individual, exercising muscle increases the demand for oxygen. The heat of the working muscles and the acidic environment during exercise result in reduced oxyhemoglobin affinity and increased oxygen release. This is reflected by a shift to the right of the oxyhemoglobin dissociation curve (see Chapter 4). The affinity of hemoglobin and oxygen is increased with the cessation of exercise, which is reflected by a leftward shift of the curve.

Oxygen Delivery to the Tissues

The final steps in oxygen transport involve the dissociation of oxygen from hemoglobin and the diffusion of oxygen from the capillaries to the cells.[17] Diffusion depends on the quantity and rate of blood flow, the difference in capillary and tissue oxygen pressures, the capillary surface area, capillary permeability, and diffusion distance.[18] With increased metabolic demand by the tissues, capillary dilation and recruitment increase capillary surface area and reduce vascular resistance to flow, diffusion distance is decreased, the movement of oxygen into the cell is facilitated, and the tissue oxygen tension is increased.

Two diffusion gradients determine effective oxygen transport: one occurs between the pulmonary capillaries and the alveoli; the other occurs between the peripheral capillaries and the tissue cells. Diffusion of oxygen occurs as the blood moves from the aorta to the arterioles. The mean oxygen tension in the aorta is about 95 mm Hg and in the arterioles is 70 to 80 mm Hg. The oxygen gradient between the arterioles and the cells is the steepest. The mean oxygen pressure is less than 50 mm Hg in the capillaries. The oxygen tension in the capillaries determines the rate of diffusion to the cells. An optimal diffusion gradient maintains the oxygen tension in the cell at between 1 and 10 mm Hg; oxygen tension is less than 0.5 mm Hg in the mitochondria.[16] This decremental PaO_2 profile down the oxygen transport pathway, from the airways to the tissues, is termed the oxygen cascade (Figure 2-6).

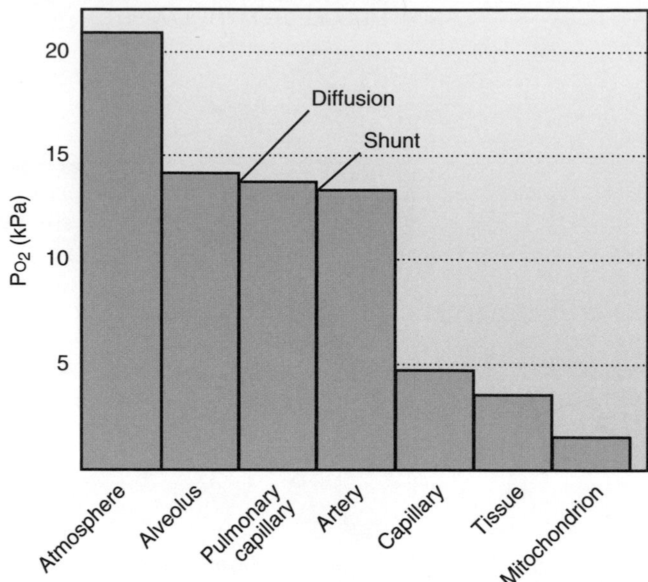

Fig. 2-6 Scheme of oxygen partial pressures from air to tissue. The cascade reflects the removal of oxygen by the pulmonary capillary blood and the tissues. Depressions caused by the effects of diffusion and shunt are also illustrated. *(From Ronco C, Bellomo R, Kellum J:* Critical Care Nephrology, *ed 2, Philadelphia, 2009, Saunders.)*

Cardiac Output

In addition to arterial oxygen content, CO is a primary determinant of DO_2.[14] The transport of oxyhemoglobin to the tissues is dependent on convective blood flow by way of CO. CO is the volume of blood pumped from the right or left ventricle per minute. The components of CO are stroke volume (SV) and heart rate (HR) (i.e., CO = SV × HR). SV is the amount of blood ejected from the left ventricle during each ventricular systole or heartbeat and is determined by the preload, myocardial distensibility, myocardial contractility, and afterload. DO_2 is optimized in patients by increasing CO through the therapeutic manipulation of preload, myocardial contractility, afterload, and heart rate.

Preload

Preload is the end-diastolic muscle fiber length of the ventricles before systolic ejection. On the left side it reflects the left ventricular end-diastolic volume (LVEDV). The LVEDV is dependent on venous return, blood volume, and left atrial contraction. An increase in ventricular volume stretches the myocardial fibers and increases the force of myocardial contraction (the Starling effect) and stroke volume. This effect is limited by the physiological limits of distension of the myocardium. Excessive stretching, as in fluid overload of the heart, leads to suboptimal overlap of the actin and myosin filaments, thus impairing rather than enhancing contractility.

Afterload

Afterload is the resistance to the ejection of blood during ventricular systole. Afterload of the left ventricle is determined primarily by four factors: the distensibility of the aorta, the vascular resistance, the patency of the aortic valve, and the viscosity of the blood.

Myocardial Contractility

Myocardial contractility reflects actin-myosin coupling during contraction and is assessed by the ejection fraction, the rate of circumferential muscle fiber shortening, the pressure-volume relationships, and the rate of change of ventricular pressure over time.

Oxygen Debt

Tissue oxygen debt, or recovery oxygen consumption, is the difference between oxygen demand and oxygen consumption. In healthy individuals, oxygen debt can be sustained for short periods during intense exercise. Anaerobic metabolism is stimulated to produce ATP under these conditions. In patients who are critically ill, the degree of oxygen debt is correlated with survival.[19]

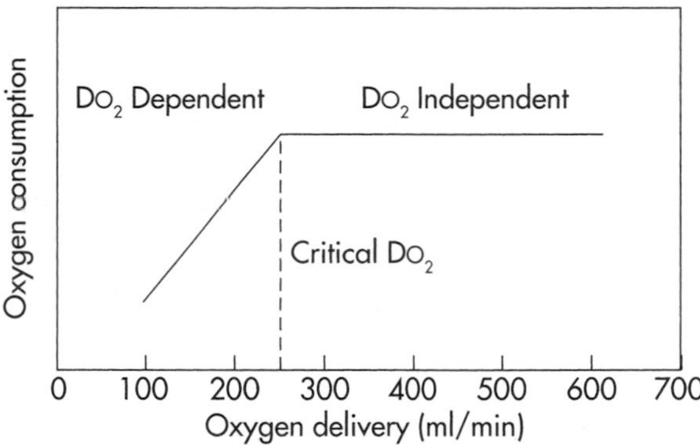

Fig. 2-7 Relationship between oxygen consumption ($\dot{V}O_2$) and oxygen delivery (DO_2). The DO_2-independent phase represents the normal metabolic state. The DO_2-dependent phase represents the dependency of $\dot{V}O_2$ on DO_2 when DO_2 falls below the critical DO_2. *(Modified from Phang PT, Russell JA: When does $\dot{V}O_2$ depend on DO_2?* Respiratory Care *38:618–630, 1993.)*

Oxygen Extraction Ratio or Utilization Coefficient

The oxygen extraction ratio, or utilization coefficient, reflects the proportion of oxygen delivered to that consumed. OER is calculated by dividing $\dot{V}O_2$ by DO_2. Normally, OER is 23% at rest.

Supply-Dependent Oxygen Consumption

Normally, a decrease in DO_2 does not reduce $\dot{V}O_2$.[20] With a decrement in DO_2, the tissues extract a commensurate amount of oxygen from the blood. In patients who are critically ill, DO_2 may be limited to the point where basic metabolic needs for oxygen (300 mL/min/M²) are not met.[20-23] The critical level at which $\dot{V}O_2$ falls is associated with tissue anaerobic metabolism and the development of lactic acidosis and decreased pH (Fig. 2-7).[19,24] Serum lactates correspondingly increase and provide a valid index of anaerobic metabolism in patients with multiorgan system failure. When oxygen transport data are analyzed, the effect of sedation may suggest a dependency between DO_2 and $\dot{V}O_2$, so the impact of medication in this relationship must be considered.[25]

Oxygen Transport Pathway

Oxygen transport is dependent on several interconnecting steps, ranging from inhalation of oxygen-containing air through the nares to oxygen extraction at the cellular level in response to metabolic demand (see Fig. 2-1). These steps provide the mechanism for ventilatory, cardiovascular, and metabolic coupling. In addition, blood is responsible for transporting oxygen within the body; thus its constituents and consistency directly affect this process.

Quality and Quantity of Blood

Although not considered a discrete step in the oxygen transport pathway, blood is the essential medium for transporting oxygen. To fulfill this function, blood must be delivered in an adequate yet varying amount, proportional to metabolic demands, and must have the appropriate constituents and consistency. Thus consideration of the characteristics of the circulating blood volume is essential to any discussion of oxygen transport.

Blood volume is compartmentalized within the intravascular compartment such that 70% is contained within the venous compartment, 10% in the systemic arteries, 15% in the pulmonary circulation, and 5% in the capillaries.[26] The large volume of blood contained within the venous circulation permits adjustments to be made as CO demand changes. The veins constrict, for example, when CO needs to be increased. When blood volume is normal and body fluids are appropriately distributed between the intravascular and extravascular compartments, fluid balance is considered normal. When they are disrupted, a fluid balance problem exists. In addition, fluid imbalance affects the concentration of electrolytes, particularly sodium, which is present in the highest concentration in the extracellular fluid. Four primary fluid problems that have implications for oxygen transport are water deficit, water excess, sodium deficit, and sodium excess (see Chapter 16). Other ions that are affected often in fluid and electrolyte imbalance deficits include potassium, chloride, calcium, and magnesium. These electrolyte disturbances also contribute to impaired oxygen transport by affecting the electrical and mechanical behavior of the heart and blood vessels, thereby also affecting CO and the distribution of oxygenated arterial blood to the periphery.

Blood is a viscous fluid composed of cells and plasma. Because 99% of blood consists of red blood cells, the white blood cells play almost no role in determining the physical characteristics of blood.

Hematocrit refers to the proportion of red blood cells in the plasma. The normal hematocrit is 38% for women and 42% for men. Blood is several times more viscous than water, which increases the difficulty with which blood is pumped through the heart and flows through vessels; the greater the number of cells, the greater the friction between the layers of blood, which results in increased viscosity. Thus the viscosity of the blood increases significantly with increases in hematocrit. An increase in hematocrit, as in polycythemia, increases blood viscosity several times. The concentration and types of protein in the plasma can also affect viscosity, but to a lesser extent.

In adults, red blood cells are produced in the marrow of the membranous bones, such as the vertebrae, sternum, ribs, and pelvis. The production of red blood cells at these sites diminishes with age. Tissue oxygenation is the basic regulator of red blood cell production. Hypoxemia stimulates red blood cell production through erythropoietin production in bone.[26]

Viscosity of the blood has its greatest effect in the small vessels. Blood flow is considerably reduced in small vessels, which results in aggregates of red blood cells adhering to the vessel walls. This effect is not offset by the tendency of the blood to become less viscous in small vessels (a result of the alignment of the blood cells flowing through these vessels, which minimizes the frictional forces between layers of flowing blood cells). In small capillaries, blood cells can become stuck, particularly where the nuclei of endothelial cells protrude and momentarily obstruct blood flow.

The major function of the red blood cells is to transport hemoglobin, which in turn carries oxygen from the lungs to the tissues. Red blood cells also contain a large quantity of carbonic anhydrase, which catalyzes the reaction between CO_2 and H_2O. The rapidity of this reaction makes it possible for blood to react with large quantities of CO_2 to transport it from the tissues to the lungs for elimination.

Hemoglobin is contained within red blood cells in a concentration of up to 34 g/dL of cells. Each gram of hemoglobin is capable of combining with 1.34 mL of oxygen (see Figure 2-2). In healthy women, 19 mL of oxygen can be carried in the blood (given that the whole blood of women contains an average of 14 g/100 mL of blood); in healthy men, the blood can carry 21 mL of oxygen (assuming the average concentration in the whole blood of men is 16 g/dL).

The clotting factors of the blood are normally in a proportion that does not promote clotting. Factors that promote coagulation (procoagulants) and factors that inhibit coagulation (anticoagulants) circulate in the blood. In the event of a ruptured blood vessel, prothrombin is converted to thrombin, which catalyzes the transformation of fibrinogen to fibrin threads. This fibrin mesh captures platelets, blood cells, and plasma to form a blood clot.

The extreme example of abnormal clotting is disseminated intravascular coagulation (DIC), when both hemorrhage and coagulation occur simultaneously. The acute form of this syndrome occurs in patients who are critically ill and undergoing multiorgan system failure. The mechanism appears to involve tissue factors, factors that damage the blood vessel walls, and factors that increase platelet aggregation. The chronic form of DIC occurs in chronic conditions such as neoplastic disease.

Plasma is the extracellular fluid of the blood and contains 7% proteins—namely, albumin, globulin, and fibrinogen. The primary function of albumin and, to a lesser extent, globulin and fibrinogen, is to create osmotic pressure at the capillary membrane and to prevent fluid leaking into the interstitial spaces. Globulins transport substances in the blood and provide immunity as the antibodies that fight infection and toxicity. Fibrinogen is fundamental to blood clotting. Most blood proteins, including hemoglobins, are also excellent acid-base buffers and are responsible for 70% of all the buffering power of whole blood.

Blood flow (Q) depends on a pressure gradient (P) and vascular resistance (R) (i.e., $Q = P/R$). Thus blood flow equals the pressure gradient divided by resistance. The length of a given blood vessel and the viscosity of the blood are also determinants of blood flow.

The average blood volume is 5000 mL. Approximately 3000 mL of this is plasma and 2000 mL is red blood cells. These values vary according to gender, weight, and other factors. Normally, changes in blood volume reflect fluid imbalances (deficits and excesses) created by losses through the skin and respiratory tract, as well as through urinary, sweat, and fecal losses. Exercise and hot weather are major challenges to fluid balance in health.

Plasma contains large quantities of sodium and chloride ions and small amounts of potassium, calcium, magnesium, phosphate, sulfate, and organic acid ions. Plasma also contains a large amount of protein. The large ionic constituents of plasma are responsible for regulating intracellular and extracellular fluid volumes, as well as the osmotic factors that cause shifts of fluid between the intracellular and extracellular compartments.

Oxyhemoglobin Dissociation

Demand for oxygen at the cellular level changes from moment to moment. The properties of oxyhemoglobin dissociation ensure that there is a continuous supply of oxygen at the cellular level. Oxygen combines with hemoglobin molecules in the pulmonary circulation and then is released in the tissue capillaries in response to a reduced arterial oxygen tension. The S-shaped oxyhemoglobin dissociation curve (see Chapter 4) shifts to the right in response to reduced tissue pH, increased CO_2, increased temperature, and increased diphosphoglycerate (DPG), a constituent of normal blood cells.

Blood delivery and its ability to transport oxygen effectively are central to all steps in the oxygen transport pathway and must be considered at each stage in clinical problem solving and decision making.

Steps in the Oxygen Transport Pathway

Step One: Inspired Oxygen and Quality of the Ambient Air

In healthy individuals, the concentration of inspired oxygen is relatively constant at 21%. If an individual is at a high altitude, the fraction of inspired oxygen is reduced as elevation increases.

Atmospheric air consists of 79% nitrogen, 20.97% oxygen, and 0.03% CO_2. Because nitrogen is an inert gas and is not absorbed in the lungs, it has a crucial role in keeping the alveoli open. The constituents of the air have become an increasingly important social, environmental, and health issue because of environmental hazards, pollution, and the thinning of the ozone layer, which result in deterioration of air quality, an increase in toxic oxygen-free radicals, and a reduction in atmospheric oxygen pressure.

Many factors influence air quality: geographical region, season, urban versus rural area, high versus low elevation, home environment, work environment, indoor versus outdoor ambience, level of ventilation, presence of air conditioning, buildings that are closed, areas with high levels of particulate matter, areas with gaseous vapors and toxic materials that can be inhaled, and smoke-filled versus smoke-free environments. Poor air quality may overwhelm the filtering ability of the upper respiratory tract and the sensitivity of the airways, causing lung damage, both acutely and over time. Chronic irritation of the lungs by poor air quality can lead to allergies, chronic inflammatory reactions, fibrosis, and alveolar capillary membrane thickening. At the alveolar level, the inspired air is saturated with water vapor. In dry environments, however, the upper respiratory tract may become dehydrated, lose its protective mucous covering, become eroded, and provide a portal for infection even though the air is adequately humidified by the time it reaches the lower airways and alveoli.

Step Two: Airways

The structures of the airways throughout the respiratory tract differ according to their functions. The main airway, the trachea, consists of cartilaginous rings, connective tissue, and small amounts of smooth muscle. This structure is essential to provide a firm and relatively inflexible conduit for air to pass from the nares through the head and neck to the lungs while avoiding airway collapse. As the airways become smaller and branch throughout the lung tissue, they consist primarily of smooth muscle. Airway narrowing, or obstruction, and the resulting increased resistance to airflow can be caused by a variety of factors, including edema, mucus, foreign objects, calcification, particulate matter, and space-occupying lesions, as well as by hyperreactivity of bronchial smooth muscle. The airways are lined with cilia, which are fine, microscopic, hair-like projections responsible for wafting debris, cells, and microorganisms away from the lungs into larger airways to be removed and evacuated. The airways are also lined with mucus, which consists of two layers, the upper gel layer and the lower sol layer, with which the cilia communicate.

Step Three: Lungs and Chest Wall

Air entry into the lungs depends on the integrity of the respiratory muscles, in particular the diaphragm, the lung parenchyma, and the chest wall. The contraction and descent of the diaphragm generate a negative intrapleural pressure that inflates the lungs. The distribution of ventilation is determined primarily by the negative intrapleural pressure gradient down the lungs. The negative intrapleural pressure gradient results in uneven ventilation down the lungs and in interregional differences (see Chapter 4). There are, however, other factors that contribute to uneven ventilation within regions of the lung. These intraregional differences reflect regional differences in lung compliance and airway resistance.[27] In patients with partially obstructed airways, reduced lung compliance and increased airway resistance increase the time needed for alveolar filling. Gas exchange is compromised if there is inadequate time for alveolar filling or emptying (i.e., increased time constants).[18] Different time constants across lung units contribute to uneven patterns of ventilation during inspiration. A lung unit with a long time constant is slow to fill and empty, and it may continue filling when surrounding units are emptying. Another factor that contributes to uneven ventilation is altered diffusion distance. In diseases in which diffusion distance is increased, ventilation among lung units is uneven.

The lungs and the parietal pleura are richly supplied with thin-walled lymphatic vessels.[16] Lymphatic vessels have some smooth muscle and thus can actively contract to propel lymph fluid forward. This forward motion is augmented by valves along the lymphatic channels. The rise and fall of the pleural pressure during respiration compress lymphatic vessels with each breath, which promotes a continuous flow of lymph. During expiration and increased intrapleural pressure, fluid is forced into the lymphatic vessels. The visceral pleura continuously drains fluid from the lungs. This creates a negative pressure in the pleural space, which keeps the lungs expanded. This pressure exceeds the elastic recoil pressure of the lung parenchyma, which counters the tendency of elastic recoil to collapse the lungs.

The peritoneal cavity of the abdomen consists of a visceral peritoneum containing the viscera and a parietal peritoneum lining the abdominal cavity. Numerous lymphatic channels interconnect the peritoneal cavity and the thoracic duct; some arise from the diaphragm. With cycles of inspiration and expiration, large amounts of lymph are moved from the peritoneal cavity to the thoracic duct of the venous drainage system. High venous pressures and vascular resistance through the liver can interfere with normal fluid balance in the peritoneal cavity. This leads to the transudation of fluid with high protein content into the abdominal cavity. Such an accumulation of fluid is referred to as ascites. Large volumes of fluid can accumulate in the abdominal cavity and compromise cardiovascular and pulmonary function secondary to increased intraabdominal pressure on the underside of the diaphragm.

Optimal diaphragmatic excursion requires a balance between thoracic and intraabdominal pressures. Increases in abdominal pressure secondary to factors such as fluid accumulation can impair diaphragmatic descent and chest wall expansion. Other factors include gas entrapment, gastrointestinal obstruction, space-occupying lesions, and paralytic ileus.

Step Four: Diffusion

Diffusion of oxygen from the alveolar sacs to the pulmonary arterial circulation depends on four factors: the area of the alveolar capillary membrane, the diffusing capacity of the alveolar capillary membrane, the pulmonary capillary blood volume, and the ventilation and perfusion ratio.[9] The transit time of blood at the alveolar capillary membrane is also an important factor that determines diffusion. The blood remains in the pulmonary capillaries for 0.75 second at rest. Within 0.25 second, one-third of that time, the blood is completely saturated. This provides a safety margin during exercise or other conditions in which CO is increased and pulmonary capillary transit time is reduced. The blood can normally be fully oxygenated even with reduced transit time.

Step Five: Perfusion

The distribution of blood perfusing the lungs is primarily gravity dependent, so the dependent lung fields are perfused to a greater extent than are the nondependent lung fields. In upright lungs, the bases are better perfused than the apices (see Chapter 4). Ventilation and perfusion matching is optimal in the midzones of upright lungs.[18] In healthy individuals, the ventilation-to-perfusion ratio is a primary determinant of arterial oxygenation. In upright lungs, this ratio is 0.8 in the midzone.

Step Six: Myocardial Function

Optimal myocardial function and CO depend on the synchronized coupling of electrical excitation of the heart and its mechanical contraction. The sinoatrial node, located in the right atrium, is the normal pacemaker for the heart and elicits the normal sinus rhythm with its multiple-component P-QRS-T configuration (see Chapter 12). This wave of electrical excitation spreads throughout the specialized neural conduction system of the atria, the interventricular septum, and the ventricles and is followed by the contraction of the atria and then of the ventricles. The contraction of the right and left ventricles ejects blood into the pulmonary and systemic circulations, respectively.

CO depends on several factors in addition to the integrity of the conduction system and the adequacy of myocardial depolarization (dromotropic effect). The amount of blood returned to the heart (preload) determines the amount ejected (the Starling effect). The distensibility of the ventricles to accommodate this blood volume must be optimal—neither too stiff nor too compliant. The force and contractility of the myocardial muscle must be sufficient to eject the blood (inotropic effect and chronotropic effect, respectively). CO is determined by the aortic pressure needed to overcome peripheral vascular resistance and the capacity of the ventricles to eject blood into the pulmonary and systemic circulations (afterload).

The pericardial cavity, like the pleural and peritoneal cavities, is a potential space containing a thin layer of fluid. The space normally has a negative pressure. During expiration, pericardial pressure is increased and fluid is forced out of the space into the mediastinal lymphatic channels. This process is normally facilitated by increased volumes of blood in the heart and each ventricular systole.

Step Seven: Peripheral Circulation

When oxygenated blood is ejected from the heart, the peripheral circulation provides a conduit to supply this blood to metabolically active tissue. Blood vessels throughout the body are arranged both in series and in parallel. The arteries and capillaries are designed to advance blood and thus perfuse the tissues with oxygenated blood. The architecture of the vasculature is such that the proximal large arteries have a higher proportion of connective tissue and elastic elements than do the distal medium and small arteries, which have a progressively higher proportion of smooth muscle. This structure enables the large proximal arteries to withstand high pressure when blood is ejected during ventricular systole. Considerable potential energy is stored within the elastic walls of these blood vessels as the heart contracts. During diastole the forward propulsion of blood is facilitated by the elastic recoil of these large vessels. The thin-walled muscular arterioles serve as the stopcocks of the circulation and regulate blood flow through regional vascular beds (e.g., of the skin, gut, muscle, and organs) and maintain peripheral vascular resistance to regulate systemic blood pressure. Blood flow through these regional vascular beds is determined by neural and humoral stimulation (exogenous) and by local tissue factors (endogenous). Blood pressure control is regulated primarily by neural stimulation of the peripheral circulation and regional vascular beds.

The microcirculation consists of the precapillary arterioles, capillaries, and venules. The Starling effect governs the balance of hydrostatic and oncotic pressures within the capillaries and surrounding tissues. The balance of these pressures is 0.3 mm Hg; its net effect is a small outward filtration of fluid from the microvasculature into the interstitial spaces (see Chapter 4). Any excess fluid or loss of plasma protein is drained into the surrounding lymphatic vessels, which usually have a small negative pressure, as does the interstitium. Integrity of the microcirculation is essential to regulate the diffusion of oxygen across the tissue capillary membrane and removing CO_2 and waste products.

The greater the muscular component of blood vessels, the greater their responsiveness to both exogenous neural stimulation and endogenous stimulation via circulating humoral neurotransmitters, such as catecholamines and local tissue factors. This responsiveness is essential for the moment-to-moment regulation of the peripheral circulation with respect to tissue perfusion and oxygenation, commensurate with tissue metabolic demands and control of total peripheral resistance and systemic blood pressure.

Step Eight: Tissue Extraction and Use of Oxygen

Perfusion of the tissues with oxygenated blood commensurate with metabolic demand is the principal goal of the oxygen transport system.[3] Oxygen is continuously being used by all cells in the body; thus it diffuses rapidly out of the circulation and through cell membranes to meet varying metabolic needs. Diffusion occurs down a gradient from areas of high to low oxygen pressure. The distances between capillaries and cells are variable, so a significant safety factor is required to ensure adequate arterial oxygen tensions. Intracellular PO_2 ranges from 5 to 60 mm Hg, with an average of 23 mm Hg.[16] Given that only 3 mm Hg of oxygen pressure is needed to support metabolism, 23 mm Hg of oxygen pressure provides an adequate safety margin. These mechanisms ensure an optimal oxygen supply over a wide range of oxygen demands during healthy functioning and in the event of impaired oxygen delivery because of illness. Normally, the rate of oxygen extraction by the cells is regulated by the oxygen demand of cells (i.e., the rate at which ADP is formed from ATP) rather than by the availability of oxygen.

Adequate quality and quantity of mitochondrial enzymes required for the Krebs cycle and electron transfer chain, along with the availability of myoglobin, may be limiting factors in the oxygen transport pathway secondary to nutritional deficits and muscle enzyme deficiencies. Myoglobin is a protein comparable to hemoglobin and is localized within muscle mitochondria. Myoglobin combines reversibly with oxygen to provide an immediate source of oxygen when there are increased metabolic demands and to facilitate oxygen transfer within the mitochondria.

Normally the amount of oxygen extracted by the tissues at rest is 23% (i.e., the ratio of oxygen consumed to oxygen delivered). This ratio ensures that greater amounts of oxygen can be extracted during periods of increased metabolic demand.

To detect tissue hypoxia, particularly in patients who are critically ill, regional assessments such as gastric mucosal PCO_2 and pH have been proposed as being superior to global assessment of $\dot{V}O_2$ and DO_2.[28] Regional measures of oxygenation could help to enhance the specificity of treatment based on tissue indicators.[29]

Step Nine: Return of Partially Desaturated Blood and CO_2 to the Lungs

Partially desaturated blood and CO_2 are removed from cells via the venous circulation to the right side of the heart and lungs. CO_2 diffuses across the alveolar capillary membrane and is eliminated from the body through the respiratory system, and deoxygenated venous blood is reoxygenated. The oxygen transport cycle is sensitively tuned to adjust to changes in the metabolic demand of the various organ systems, such as digestion in the gastrointestinal system and cardiac and skeletal muscle work during exercise.

Factors that interfere with tissue oxygenation and the capacity of the tissue to use oxygen include abnormal oxygen demands, reduced hemoglobin and myoglobin levels, edema, and poisoning of the cellular enzymes.[30]

Factors that Normally Perturb Oxygen Transport

Basal metabolic rate (BMR) reflects the rate of metabolism for an individual in a completely rested state: no food intake within several hours, a good night's sleep, no arousing or distressing emotional stimulation, and a comfortable ambient temperature. Normally, the BMR is constant within and among individuals if measured under standardized conditions. BMR reflects the energy expended by the body's cells to maintain resting function and includes the work of breathing; heart, renal, and brain function; and thermoregulation.

Normally, over the course of the day, the human body is exposed to fluctuations in ambient temperature and humidity, ingestion states, activity and exercise levels (exercise stress), body positions and body position changes (gravitational stress), emotional states (emotional stress), and states of arousal. These factors significantly influence $\dot{V}O_2$ and energy expenditure from moment-to-moment and thus increase rate of metabolism.

Several factors related to disease can significantly increase oxygen consumption and metabolic rate over and above the BMR. Such factors include fever, the disease process itself, the process of healing and recovery from injury or disease, thermoregulatory disturbance, reduced arousal, increased arousal resulting from anxiety or pain, sleep loss, medical and surgical interventions, fluid imbalance, and medications.[5] These factors may contribute to a systemic increase in the BMR or may reflect local changes in tissue metabolism. Autoregulation of the regional vascular beds promotes increased regional blood flow in accordance with their local tissue metabolic demand.

Because gravitational stress and exercise stress are fundamental to normal cardiovascular and pulmonary function and oxygen transport, the effects of gravity and exercise are highlighted. These two factors augment arousal through stimulation of the reticular activating system in the brainstem and the autonomic nervous system (ANS), which, when depressed, significantly compromises oxygen transport. Emotional stress also has a marked effect on the stimulation of the ANS (the fight-or-flight response) and hence on oxygen transport. These concepts and their clinical implications are described in detail in Chapters 18 and 19.

Gravitational Stress

Humans are designed to function in a 1-g gravitational field. Given that 60% of the body weight is fluid contained within the intravascular and extravascular compartments and that this fluid has considerable mass, changes in body position result in significant instantaneous fluid shifts that can threaten hemodynamic stability.[6,31] To maintain consciousness and normal body function during changes in body position, the heart and peripheral vasculature are designed to detect these fluid shifts and accommodate quickly to avoid deleterious functional consequences (e.g., reduced SV, CO, circulating blood volume, and cerebral perfusion). Preservation of the fluid-regulating mechanisms is essential to counter the hemodynamic effects of changing body position. This capacity is impaired with recumbency, which has long been associated with bed rest deconditioning in patients and older populations.[32,33] Restoration of adaptation to gravitational stress by upright positioning of a patient is the only means by which these fluid-regulating mechanisms can be maintained and orthostatic intolerance and its short- and long-term sequelae averted.

Exercise Stress

Exercise constitutes the greatest perturbation to homeostasis and oxygen transport in humans. CO can increase by five times to adjust to the metabolic demands of exercise stress. All steps in the oxygen transport pathway are affected by exercise stress. Ventilation is increased, and ventilation and perfusion matching is optimized to maximize oxygenation of blood. Heart rate and stroke volume are increased to effect greater CO of oxygenated blood to the tissues. At the tissue level, oxygen extraction is enhanced.

Emotional Stress

The body responds to emotional stress much as it does to exercise stress—by undergoing the sympathetic stress reaction (the fright-fight-flight reaction). Perceived threat, the basis of emotional stress, can also trigger the fright-fight-flight reaction and a series of sympathetically mediated physiological responses. This reaction, which prepares the body for fight or for flight, includes an increase in circulating stress hormones, heart rate, blood pressure, CO, blood glucose, muscle strength, mental alertness, cellular metabolism, and local blood flow to specific muscle groups, as well as inhibition of involuntary function.

Summary

This chapter describes the oxygen transport system, a system that is essential to life, activity, and social participation. Its component steps and their interdependence are highlighted. This framework provides a conceptual basis for the practice of cardiovascular and pulmonary physical therapy.

The oxygen transport system is designed to deliver oxygen from the ambient air to every cell in the body to support cellular respiration (i.e., metabolic use of oxygen at the cellular level). Blood is the essential medium in which cellular and noncellular components transport oxygen from the cardiovascular and pulmonary unit to the peripheral tissues. The fundamental components in the oxygen transport pathway are described. These components include the quality of the ambient air, the airways, lungs, chest wall, pulmonary circulation, lymphatic circulation, heart, peripheral circulation, and peripheral tissues of the organs of the body.

In healthy individuals, the most significant factors that perturb oxygen transport are changes in gravitational stress secondary to changes in body position, exercise stress secondary to the increased oxygen demand of working muscles, and arousal and emotional stress. A thorough understanding of the normal effects of gravitational and exercise stress and arousal is essential to understanding deficits in oxygen transport. Numerous factors can impair and threaten oxygen transport, including underlying pathophysiology, restricted mobility, recumbency, factors related to the patient's care, and factors related to the individual (see Chapters 2 and 17). The physical therapist needs a detailed understanding of these concepts to diagnose such threats and deficits, to understand their impact on activity and participation, and to prescribe effective treatments.

Review Questions

1. Describe the clinical implications of limitations of oxygen transport at three levels: structure and function, activity, and participation (consistent with the International Classification of Functioning, Disability and Health).
2. Describe the oxygen transport pathway, its steps and their interdependence.
3. Describe the physiological processes of energy transfer and cellular oxidation.
4. Explain oxygen transport with respect to oxygen delivery, uptake and extraction, and the interrelationship among these processes.
5. Outline the factors that perturb oxygen transport in health.

References

1. World Health Organization: International Classification of Functioning, Disability and Health. www.sustainable-design.ie/arch/ICIDH-2PFDec-2000.pdf; retrieved September 2010, 2000.
2. Dantzker DR: The influence of cardiovascular function on gas exchange. *Clin Chest Med* 4(2):149–159, 1983.
3. Dantzker DR: Adequacy of tissue oxygenation. *Critical Care Medicine* 21:S40–S43, 1993.
4. Dantzker DR, Boresman B, Gutierrez G: Oxygen supply and utilization relationships. *American Review of Respiratory Disorders* 143:675–679, 1991.
5. Dean E: Oxygen transport: a physiologically based conceptual framework for the practice of cardiopulmonary physiotherapy. *Physiotherapy* 80:347–355, 1994.
6. Dean E, Ross J: Discordance between cardiopulmonary physiology and physical therapy. *Chest* 101:1694–1698, 1992a.
7. Goldring RM: Specific defects in cardiopulmonary gas exchange. *American Review of Respiratory Disorders* 129:S57-S59, 1984.
8. Ross J, Dean E: Integrating physiological principles into the comprehensive management of cardiopulmonary dysfunction. *Physical Therapy* 69:255–259, 1989.
9. Barrett KE, Barman SM, Boitano S, Brooks HL: *Ganong's review of medical physiology*, ed 23, New York, 2009, McGraw-Hill Professional Publishing.
10. McArdle WD, William D, Katch FI, Katch VL: *Essentials of exercise physiology*, ed 3, Baltimore, 2006, Lippincott Williams & Wilkins.
11. Kirchberger MA: Excitation and contraction of skeletal muscle. In West JB, Best CH, Taylor NB, editors: *Best and Taylor's physiological basis of medical practice*, ed 12, Baltimore, 1991, Williams & Wilkins.
12. Tortora GJ, Derrickson B: *Principles of anatomy and physiology*, ed 12, Hoboken, NJ, 2008, John Wiley and Sons, Inc.
13. Foss ML, Keteyian SJ, Fox EL: *Fox's physiological basis for exercise and sport*, ed 6, Madison, Wis, 1998, William C Brown Pub.
14. Dantzker DR, Scharf SM: *Cardiopulmonary critical care*, ed 3, Philadelphia, 1998, Saunders.
15. Ehrman JK, Gordon PM, Visich PS, Keteyian SJ, editors: *Clinical exercise physiology*, ed 2, Champaign, Ill, 2009, Human Kinetics.
16. Hall JE: *Guyton and Hall textbook of medical physiology*, ed 12, Philadelphia, 2010, Elsevier.
17. Schumaker PT, Samsel RW: Oxygen delivery and uptake by peripheral tissues: physiology and pathophysiology. *Critical Care Clinics* 5:255–269, 1989.
18. West JB: *Respiratory physiology—the essentials*, ed 8, Philadelphia, 2008, Lippincott Williams & Wilkins.
19. Mizock BA, Falk JL: Lactic acidosis in critical illness. *Critical Care Medicine* 20:80–93, 1992.
20. Phang PT, Russell JA: When does $\dot{V}O_2$ depend on DO_2? *Respiratory Care* 38:618–630, 1993.
21. Fenwick JC: Increased concentrations of plasma lactate predict pathologic dependence of oxygen consumption on oxygen delivery in patients with adult respiratory distress syndrome. *Journal of Critical Care* 5:81–86, 1990.
22. Lorente JA, Renes E, Gomez-Agunaga MA, Landin L, de la Morena J, Liste O: Oxygen delivery–dependent oxygen consumption in acute respiratory failure. *Critical Care Medicine* 19:770–775, 1991.
23. Myles PS, McRae R, Ryder I, Hunt JO, Buckland MR: Association between oxygen delivery and consumption in patients undergoing cardiac surgery. Is there supply dependence? *Anaesthesiology and Intensive Care Medicine* 24:651–657, 1996.
24. Schumaker PT, Cain SM: The concept of critical oxygen delivery. *Intensive Care Medicine* 13:223–229, 1987.
25. Boyd O, Grounds M, Bennett D: The dependency of oxygen consumption on oxygen delivery in critically ill postoperative patients is mimicked by variations in sedation. *Chest* 101:1619–1624, 1992.
26. Sandler H, Vernicos J: Cardiovascular effects of inactivity. In Sandler H, Vernikos J, editors: *Inactivity: Physiological Effects*, Orlando, Fla, 1986, Academic Press.
27. Ross J, Dean E: Body positioning. In Zadai CC, editor: *Clinics in physical therapy. Pulmonary management in physical therapy*, New York, 1992, Churchill Livingstone.
28. Baigorri F, Russell JA: Oxygen delivery in critical illness. *Critical Care Clinics* 12:971–994, 1996.
29. Maizes JS, Murtuza M, Kvetan V: Oxygen transport and utilization. *Respiratory Care Clinics in North America* 6:473–500, 2000.
30. Kariman K, Burns SR: Regulation of tissue oxygen extraction is disturbed in adult respiratory distress syndrome. *American Review of Respiratory Diseases* 132:109–114, 1985.
31. Dean E, Ross J: Oxygen transport: the basis for contemporary cardiopulmonary physical therapy and its optimization with body positioning and mobilization. *Physical Therapy Practice* 1:34–44, 1992b.
32. Chase GA, Grave C, Rowell LB: Independence of changes in functional and performance capacities attending prolonged bed rest. *Aerospace Medicine* 37:1232–1237, 1966.
33. Winslow EH: Cardiovascular consequences of bed rest. *Heart Lung* 14:236–246, 1985.

Cardiovascular and Pulmonary Anatomy

Elizabeth Dean

KEY TERMS

Cardiovascular and pulmonary unit
Heart
Lymphatic circulation
Parenchyma
Peripheral circulation
Pulmonary circulation
Respiratory muscles
Thoracic cavity
Tracheobronchial tree

CHAPTER OUTLINE

The heart lies in series with the lungs, constituting the cardiovascular and pulmonary unit, the central component of the oxygen transport pathway.[1,2] Virtually all the blood returned to the right side of the heart passes through the lungs and is delivered to the left side of the heart for ejection into the systemic, coronary, and bronchopulmonary circulations. Because of this interrelationship, changes in lung function can exert changes in heart function and vice versa. A detailed understanding of the anatomy of the heart and lungs and how these organs work synergistically is essential to the practice of cardiovascular and pulmonary physical therapy.

This chapter presents the anatomy of the cardiovascular and pulmonary systems, including the skeletal features of the thoracic cavity; muscles of respiration; anatomy of the tracheobronchial tree; lung parenchyma; basic anatomy of the heart; and peripheral, pulmonary, and lymphatic circulations.[3-11]

Thorax

The bony thorax covers and protects the principal organs of respiration and circulation as well as the liver and the stomach (Fig. 3-1). The anterior surface is formed by the sternum and the costal cartilage. The lateral surfaces are formed by the ribs. The posterior surface is formed by the 12 thoracic vertebrae and the posterior part of the 12 ribs. At birth, the thorax is nearly circular, but during childhood and adolescence it becomes more elliptical. In adulthood, the transverse diameter of the chest wall is greater than the anteroposterior diameter.

Sternum

The sternum, or breastbone, is a flat bone with three parts: manubrium, body, and xiphoid process. The manubrium is the widest and thickest bone of the sternum. Its upper border is scalloped by a central jugular notch, which can be palpated, and by two clavicular notches that house the clavicles. Its lower

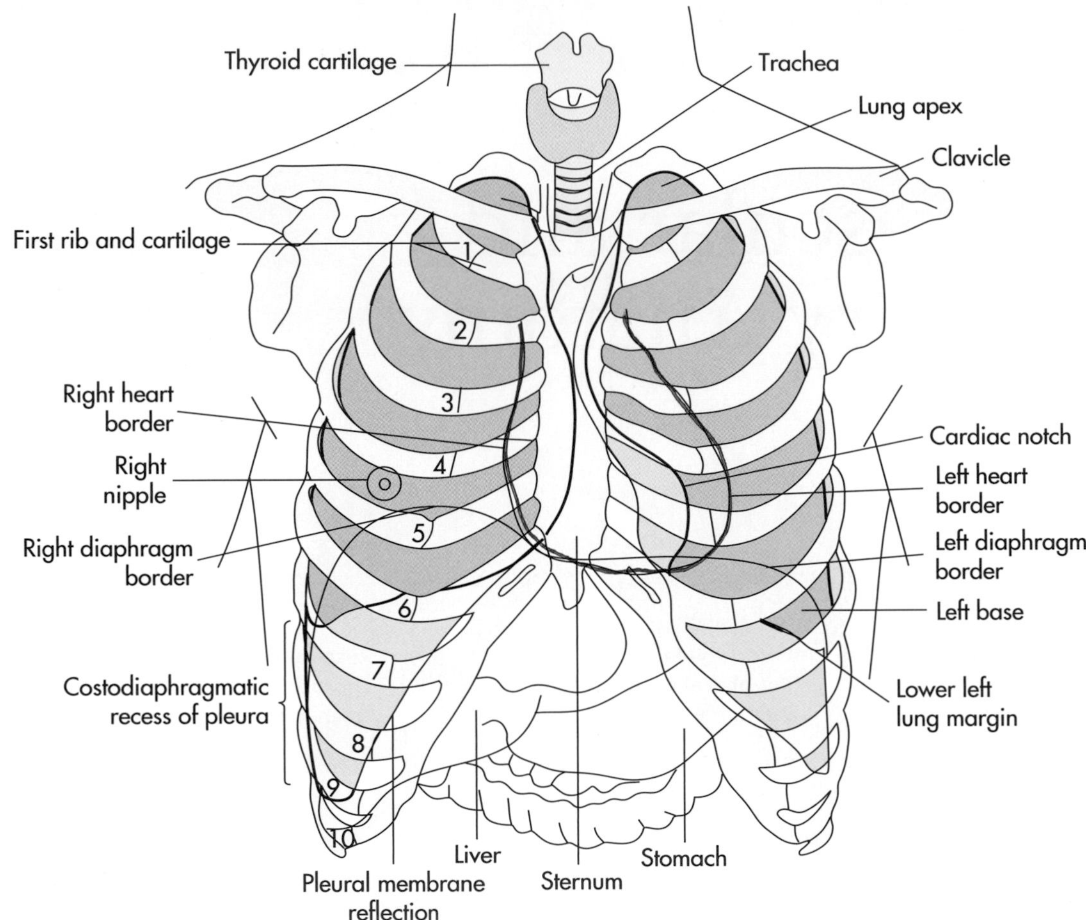

Fig. 3-1 The lungs in relationship to the rib cage and other thoracic structures. *(From Beachey W:* Respiratory care anatomy and physiology: foundations for clinical practice, *ed 2, Philadelphia, 2008, Mosby.)*

border articulates with the upper border of the body at a slight angle, the sternal angle or angle of Louis. This angle, which is easily palpated, is a landmark located between thoracic vertebrae T4 and T5, and is on a level with the second costal cartilages. The bifurcation of the trachea into the right and left main stem bronchi also occurs at the sternal angle. The manubrium and body are joined by fibrocartilage, which may ossify in later life.

The body of the sternum is twice as long as the manubrium. It is a relatively thin bone and can be easily pierced by needles for bone marrow aspirations. The heart is located beneath and to the left of the lower third of the body of the sternum. Although it is attached by cartilage to the ribs, this portion of the sternum is flexible and can be depressed without breaking. This maneuver is used, with care, in closed cardiac massage to artificially circulate blood to the brain and extremities. The lower margin of the body is attached to the xiphoid process by fibrocartilage. This bone is the smallest of the three parts of the sternum and usually fuses with the body of the sternum in later life.

Ribs

A large portion of the bony thoracic cage is formed by 12 ribs located on either side of the sternum. The first seven ribs connect posteriorly with the vertebral column and anteriorly through costal cartilages with the sternum. These are known as the true ribs. The remaining five ribs are known as the false ribs. The first three have their cartilage attached to the cartilage of the rib above. The last two are free or floating ribs. The ribs increase in length from the first to the seventh rib and then decrease to the 12th rib. They also increase in obliquity until the ninth rib and then decrease in obliquity to the 12th rib.

Each rib has a small head and a short neck that articulate with two thoracic vertebrae. The shaft of the rib curves gently from the neck to a sudden sharp bend, the angle of the rib. Fractures often occur at this site. A costal groove is located on the lower border of the shaft of the ribs. This groove houses the intercostal nerves and vessels. Chest tubes and needles are inserted above the ribs to avoid these vessels and nerves. The ribs are separated from each other by the intercostal spaces that contain the intercostal muscles.

Movements of the Thorax

The frequency of movement of the bony thorax joints is greater than that of almost any other combination of joints in the body. Two types of movements have been described: the pump-handle movement and the bucket-handle movement (Fig. 3-2).[12] The upper ribs are limited in their ability to move.

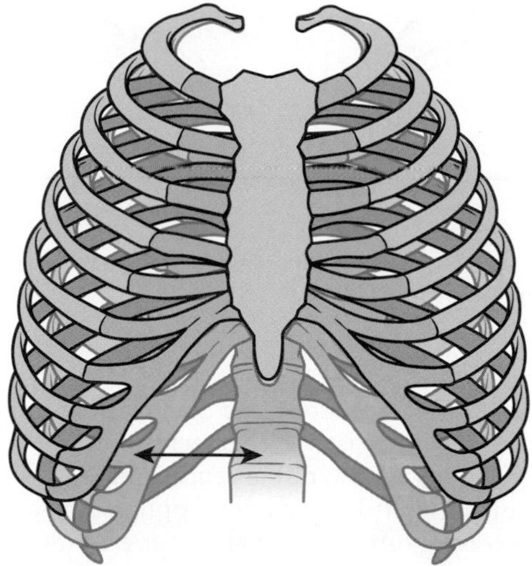

Fig. 3-2 The movements of the ribs. **A,** "Bucket handle," lower rib. **B,** "Pump handle," first rib.

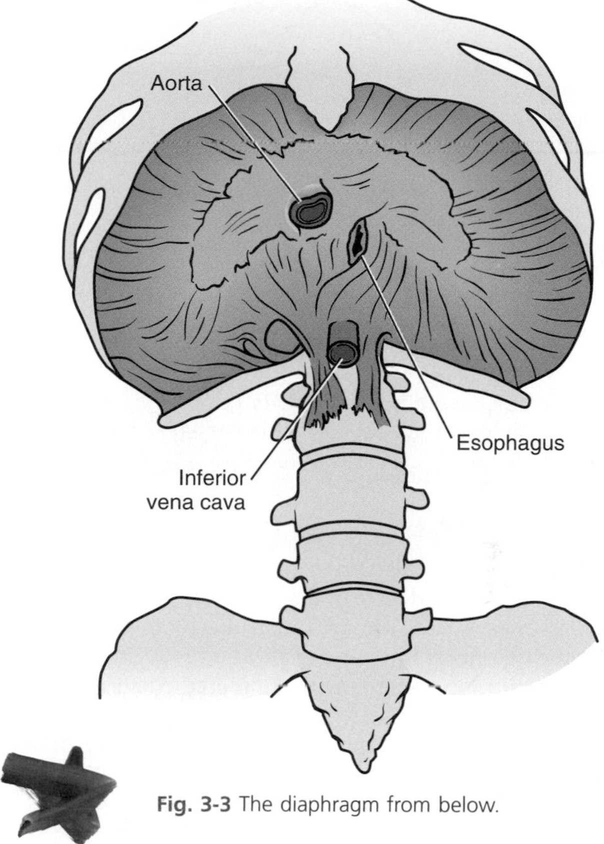

Fig. 3-3 The diaphragm from below.

Each pair swings like a pump handle, with elevation thrusting the sternum forward. This forward movement increases the anteroposterior diameter and the depth of the thorax and is called the pump-handle movement. In the lower ribs, there is little anteroposterior movement. During inspiration, the ribs swing outward and upward, each rib helps to elevate the rib above it. This bucket-handle movement increases the transverse diameter of the thoracic cage. Thus during inspiration, the thorax increases its volume by increasing its anteroposterior and transverse diameters.

Muscles of Respiration

Inspiration

Inspiration is an active movement involving the contraction of the diaphragm and intercostal muscles. Additional muscles may come into play during exertion in a healthy person. In disease, the role of these accessory muscles of inspiration may have an important role even at rest. The accessory muscles include the sternocleidomastoids, scalenes, serratus anterior, pectoralis major and minor, trapezius, and erector spinae. The degree to which these accessory muscles are recruited by the patient depends on the severity of cardiovascular and pulmonary distress.

Diaphragm

The diaphragm is the principal muscle of respiration. During quiet breathing, the diaphragm contributes approximately two-thirds of the tidal volume in the sitting or standing positions and approximately three-fourths of the tidal volume in the supine position. Approximately two-thirds of the vital capacity in all positions is contributed by the diaphragm.

The diaphragm is a large, dome-shaped muscle that separates the thoracic and abdominal cavities. Its upper surface supports the pericardium (with which it is partially blended), heart, pleurae, and lungs. Its lower surface is almost completely covered by the peritoneum and overlies the liver, kidneys, suprarenal glands, stomach, and spleen (Fig. 3-3). This large muscle can be divided into right and left halves. Each half is made up of three parts: sternal, lumbar, and costal. These three parts insert into the central tendon, which lies just below the heart. The sternal part arises from the back of the xiphoid process and descends to the central tendon. On each side is a small gap, the sternocostal triangle, which is located between the sternal and costal parts. It transmits the superior epigastric vessels and is often the site of diaphragmatic hernias. The costal parts form the right and left domes. They arise from the inner surfaces of the lower four ribs and the lower six costal cartilages, then interdigitate and transverse the abdomen to insert into the anterolateral part of the central tendon, the central part of the diaphragm. The lumbar part arises from the bodies of the upper lumbar vertebrae and extends upward to the central tendon. The central tendon is a thin, strong aponeurosis situated near the center of the muscle, somewhat closer to the front of the body. It resembles a trefoil leaf, with its three divisions or leaflets. The right leaflet is the largest, the middle is the next largest, and the left leaflet is the smallest.

Major vessels traverse the diaphragm through one of three openings (see Fig. 3-3). The vena caval opening is located to the right of the midline in the central tendon and contains branches of the right phrenic nerve and the inferior vena cava. The esophageal opening is located to the left of the midline and contains the esophagus, the vagal nerve trunks, and branches of the gastric vessels. The aortic opening is located in the midline and contains the aorta, the thoracic duct, and sometimes the azygos vein. The diaphragm is also pierced by branches of the left phrenic nerve, small veins, and lymph vessels.

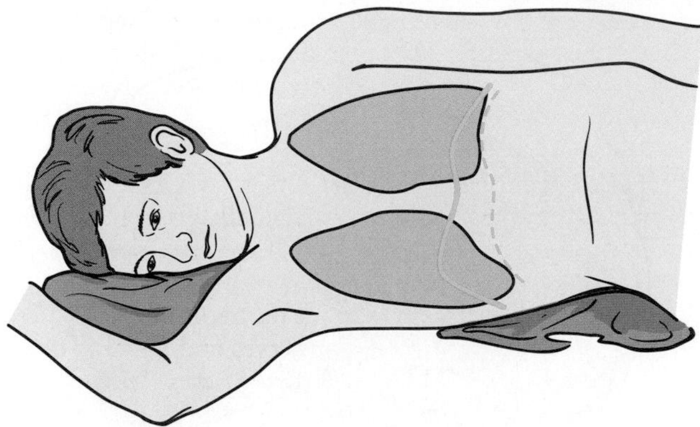

Fig. 3-4 When the patient is lying on his or her side, the dome of the diaphragm on the lower side rises farther in the thorax than the dome on the upper side.

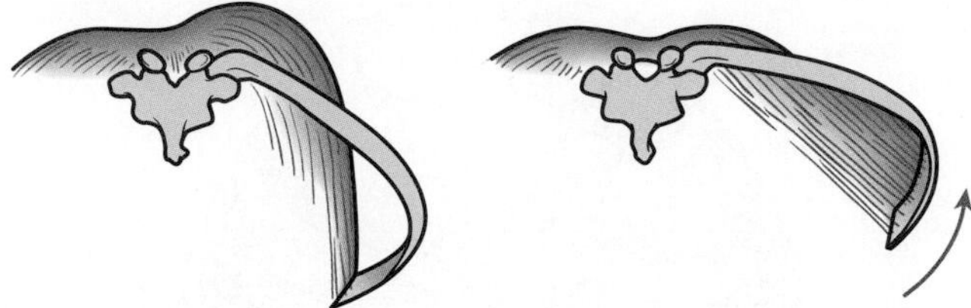

Fig. 3-5 Contraction of the costal fibers of the diaphragm causes rib eversion and elevation.

The position of the diaphragm and its range of movement vary with posture, the degree of distention of the stomach, size of the intestines, size of the liver, and obesity. Average movement of the diaphragm in quiet respiration is 12.5 mm on the right and 12 mm on the left. This can increase to a maximum of 30 mm on the right and 28 mm on the left during increased ventilation. An individual's posture determines the position of the diaphragm. In the supine position, the resting level of the diaphragm rises. The greatest respiratory excursions during normal breathing occur in this position; however, the lung volumes are decreased because of the elevated position of the abdominal organs within the thoracic cavity. In a sitting or upright position, the dome of the diaphragm is pulled down by the abdominal organs, allowing a larger lung volume. For this reason, individuals who are short of breath are more comfortable sitting than reclining. In a side-lying position, the dome of the diaphragm on the lower side rises farther into the thorax than the dome on the upper side (Fig. 3-4). The abdominal organs tend to be displaced forward in a side-lying position, allowing greater excursion of the dome on the lower side. In contrast, the upper side moves little with respiration. On radiograph, the position of the diaphragm can indicate whether the film was taken during inspiration or expiration and may also indicate pathology in the lungs, pleurae, or abdomen.

Each half of the diaphragm is innervated by a separate nerve—the phrenic nerve on that side. Although the halves contract simultaneously, it is possible for half of the muscle to be paralyzed without affecting the other half. Generally, the paralyzed half remains at the normal level during rest. With deep inspiration, however, the paralyzed half is pulled up by the negative pressure in the thorax.

Contraction of the diaphragm increases the thoracic volume vertically and transversely. The central tendon is drawn down by the diaphragm as it contracts. As the dome descends, abdominal organs are pushed forward as far as the abdominal walls will allow. When the dome can descend no farther, the costal fibers of the diaphragm contract to increase the thoracic diameter of the thorax. This occurs because the fibers of the costal part of the diaphragm run vertically from their attachment at the costal margin. Thus contraction of these fibers elevates and everts the ribs (Fig. 3-5). If the diaphragm is in a low position, it will change the angle of pull of the muscle's costal fibers. Contraction of these fibers creates a horizontal pull, which causes the lateral diameter to become smaller as the ribs are pulled in toward the central tendon.

As the diaphragm descends, it compresses the abdominal organs, increasing intraabdominal pressure. At the same time, the intrathoracic pressure decreases as the lung volume is increased by the descending diaphragm. Inspiratory airflow occurs as a result of this decrease in intrathoracic pressure (see Chapter 4). The pressure gradient between the abdominal and thoracic cavities also facilitates the return of blood to the right side of the heart.

Movement of the diaphragm can be controlled voluntarily to some extent. Vocalists spend years learning to manipulate their diaphragms so they can produce controlled sounds when singing. The diaphragm momentarily ceases movement when a person holds his or her breath. The diaphragm is involuntarily involved in parturition, bearing down in bowel movements, and laughing, crying, and vomiting. Hiccups are spasmodic, sharp contractions of the diaphragm that can indicate disease (e.g., a subphrenic abscess) if they persist.

Intercostals

The external intercostals extend down and forward from the tubercles of the ribs (above) to the costochondral junction of the ribs (below), where they become continuous with the anterior intercostal membrane (Fig. 3-6). This membrane extends the muscle forward to the sternum. There are 11 external intercostal muscles on each side of the sternum. They are thicker posteriorly than anteriorly and thicker than the internal intercostal muscles. They are innervated by the intercostal nerves, and contraction draws the lower rib up and out toward the upper rib. This action increases the volume of the thoracic cavity.

There are 11 internal intercostals on each side. These are considered primarily expiratory in function. The intercartilaginous or parasternal portion of the internal intercostals contracts with the external intercostals during inspiration to help elevate the ribs. In addition to their respiratory functions, the intercostal muscles contract to prevent the intercostal spaces from being drawn in or bulged out during respiratory activity.

Sternocleidomastoid

The sternocleidomastoid (SCM) muscles are strong neck muscles arising from two heads, one from the manubrium and one from the medial part of the clavicle (see Fig. 3-6). These two heads fuse into one muscle mass that inserts behind the ear into the mastoid process. It is innervated by the accessory

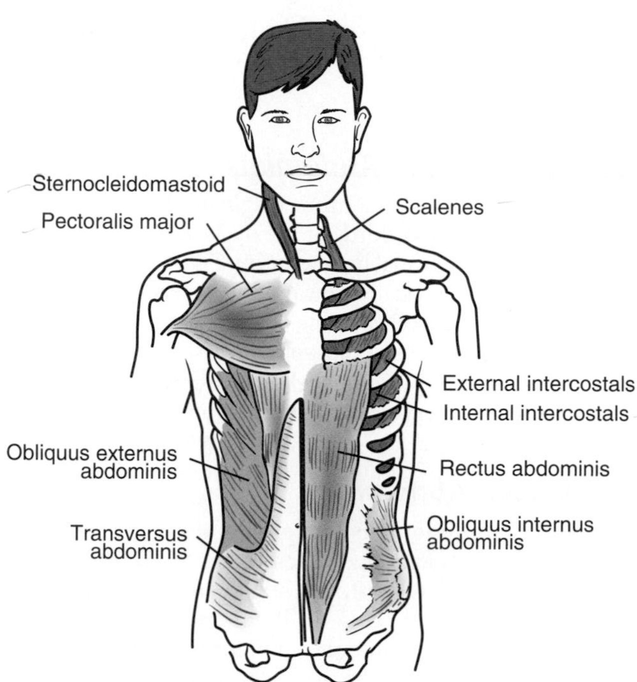

Fig. 3-6 Respiratory muscles (anterior view).

nerve and the second cervical nerve. There are two of these muscles, one on each side of the neck. When one SCM contracts, it tilts the head toward the shoulder of the same side and rotates the face toward the opposite shoulder. If the two SCM muscles contract together, they pull the head forward into flexion. When the head is fixed, the muscles assist in elevating the sternum, increasing the anteroposterior diameter of the thorax.

The SCMs are the most important accessory muscles of inspiration. Their contractions can be observed in all patients during forced inspiration and in all patients who are dyspneic. These muscles become visually predominant in patients who are chronically dyspneic (see Chapter 5).

Scalenes

The anterior, medial, and posterior scalenes are three separate muscles that are considered a functional unit. They are attached superiorly to the transverse processes of the lower five cervical vertebrae and inferiorly to the upper surface of the first two ribs (see Fig. 3-6). They are innervated by their corresponding cervical spinal nerves. These muscles are primarily supportive neck muscles, but they can assist in respiration through reverse action. When their superior attachment is fixed, the scalenes act as accessory respiratory muscles and elevate the first two ribs during inspiration.

Serratus Anterior

The serratus anterior arises from the outer surfaces of the first eight or nine ribs. It curves backward, forming a sheet of muscle that inserts into the medial border of each scapula. It is innervated by the long thoracic nerve (cervical nerves C5, C6, and C7). There are two of these muscles, one on each side of the body. Normally they assist in forward pushing of the arm (as in punching). When the scapulae are fixed, the serratus anterior muscles act as accessory respiratory muscles and elevate the ribs to which they are attached.

Pectoralis Major

The pectoralis major is a large muscle arising from the clavicle, the sternum, and the cartilages of all the true ribs (see Fig. 3-6). This muscle spreads across the anterior chest and inserts into the intertubercular sulcus of the humerus. It is innervated by the lateral and medial pectoral nerves and cervical nerves C5, C6, C7, C8, and T1. There are two of these muscles, one on each side of the body. This muscle rotates the humerus medially and draws the arm across the chest. During climbing and pull-ups, it draws the arms toward the trunk. During forced inspiration when the arms are fixed, it draws the ribs toward the arms, thereby increasing thoracic diameter.

Pectoralis Minor

The pectoralis minor is a thin muscle originating from the outer surfaces of the third, fourth, and fifth ribs near their cartilages. It inserts into the coracoid process of the scapula. It is innervated by the pectoral nerves (cervical nerves C6, C7, and C8). There are two of these muscles, one on each side of the body. They contract with the serratus anterior to draw the scapulae toward the chest. During deep inspiration, they contract to elevate the ribs to which they are attached.

Trapezius

The trapezius consists of two muscles that form an extensive diamond-shaped sheet extending from the head down the back and out to both shoulders (Fig. 3-7). Its upper belly originates from the external occipital protuberance, curves around the side of the neck, and inserts into the posterior border of the clavicle. The middle part of the muscle arises from a thin diamond-shaped tendinous sheet, the supraspinous ligaments, and the spines of the upper thoracic region; it then runs horizontally and inserts into the spine of the scapula. Its lower belly arises from the supraspinous ligaments and the spines of the lower thoracic region, runs upward, and inserts into the lower border of the spine of the scapula. This large muscle is innervated by the external or spinal part of the accessory nerve and cervical nerves C3 and C4. Its main function is to rotate the scapulae during arm elevation and control gravitational descent of the arms. It also braces the scapulae and raises them, as when shrugging the shoulders. Its ability to stabilize the scapulae makes it an important accessory muscle in respiration. This stabilization enables the serratus anterior and pectoralis minor to elevate the ribs.

Erector Spinae

The erector spinae is a large muscle extending from the sacrum to the skull (see Figure 3-7). It originates from the sacrum, the iliac crest, and the spines of the lower thoracic and lumbar vertebrae. It separates into a lateral iliocostalis, an intermediate longissimus, and a medial spinalis column. This muscle mass inserts into various ribs and vertebral processes all the way up to the skull. It is innervated by the corresponding spinal nerves. These muscles extend, laterally flex, and rotate

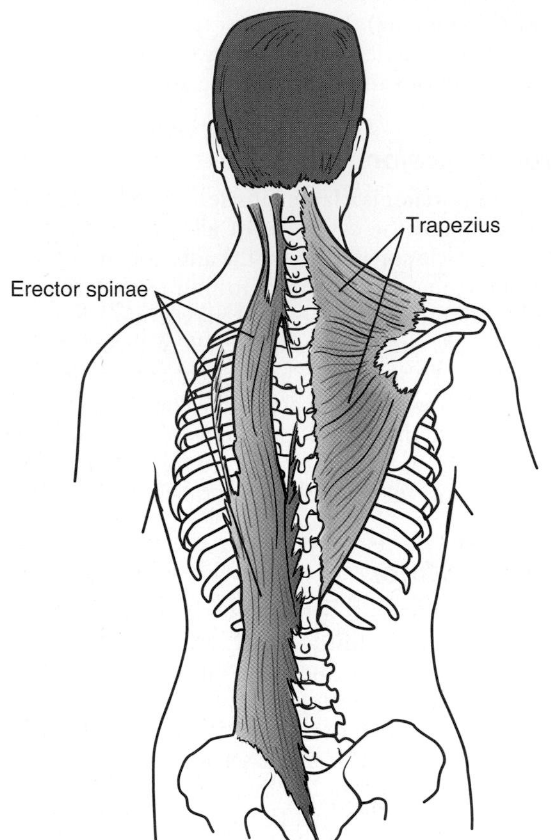

Fig. 3-7 Respiratory muscles (posterior view).

the vertebral column. They are considered accessory respiratory muscles through their extension of the vertebral column. In deep inspiration, these muscles extend the vertebral column, allowing further elevation of the ribs.

Expiration

Expiration is a passive process that occurs when the intercostals and diaphragm relax. Relaxation of the intercostals and diaphragm allows the ribs to drop to their preinspiratory position and the diaphragm to rise. These activities compress the lungs, which then raises intrathoracic pressure above atmospheric pressure and contributes to air flow out of the lungs.

Rectus Abdominis

The rectus abdominis rises from the pubic crest, extends upward, and inserts into the xiphoid process and the costal margin of the fifth, sixth, and seventh costal cartilages (see Fig. 3-6). It is innervated by corresponding spinal nerves and its action is considered within the context of the other abdominal muscles.

Obliquus Externus Abdominis

The obliquus externus abdominis arises in an oblique line from the fifth costal cartilage to the 12th rib (see Fig. 3-6). Its posterior fibers attach in an almost vertical line with the iliac crest. The other fibers extend down and forward and attach to the front of the xiphoid process, the linea alba, and the pubic symphysis. It is innervated by the lower six thoracic spinal nerves.

Obliquus Internus Abdominis

The obliquus internus abdominis originates from the lumbar fascia, the anterior two-thirds of the iliac crest, and the lateral two-thirds of the inguinal ligament (see Fig. 3-6). Its posterior fibers run almost vertically upward and insert into the lower borders of the last three ribs. The other fibers join an aponeurosis attached to the costal margin above, the linea alba in the midline, and the pubic crest below. It is innervated by the lower six thoracic nerves and the first lumbar spinal nerves.

Transversus Abdominis

The transversus abdominis arises from the inner surface of the lower six costal cartilages, the lumbar fascia, the anterior two-thirds of the iliac crest, and the lateral one-third of the inguinal ligament (see Fig. 3-6). It runs across the abdomen horizontally and inserts into the aponeurosis, extending to the linea alba. It is innervated by the lower six thoracic nerves and the first lumbar spinal nerves.

Action of the Abdominal Muscles

The four muscles of the abdomen work together to provide a firm but flexible wall to keep the abdominal viscera in position. The abdominal muscles exert a compressing force on the abdomen when the thorax and pelvis are fixed. This force can be used in defecation, urination, parturition, and vomiting. In forced expiration, the abdominal muscles help force the diaphragm back to its resting position and thus force air from the lungs. If the pelvis and vertebral column are fixed, the obliquus externus abdominis aids expiration further by depressing and compressing the lower part of the thorax. Patients with chronic obstructive pulmonary disease (COPD) have difficulty in exhalation, which causes them to trap air in their lungs. The continued contraction of the abdominal muscles throughout exhalation helps them force this air from the lungs. The abdominal muscles also play an important role in coughing. First, a large volume of air is inhaled, and the glottis is closed. The abdominal muscles then contract, raising intrathoracic pressure. When the glottis opens, the large difference in intrathoracic and atmospheric pressure causes the air to be expelled forcefully at tremendous flow rates (tussive blast). Individuals with weak abdominal muscles (from neuromuscular diseases, paraplegia, quadriplegia, or extensive abdominal surgery) often have ineffective coughs (see Chapters 6 and 32).

The four abdominal muscles have many other nonrespiratory functions, both individually and as a group; these functions are not discussed here.

Internal Intercostals

There are 11 internal intercostal muscles on each side of the thorax. Each muscle arises from the floor of the costal groove and cartilage, passes inferiorly and posteriorly and inserts on the upper border of the rib below. These internal intercostals extend from the sternum anteriorly, around the thorax to the posterior costal angle. They are generally divided into two parts: the interosseous portion, located between the sloping parts of the ribs, and the intercartilaginous portions, located between costal cartilages. The intercartilaginous portions are considered inspiratory in function. Contraction of the interosseous portions of the intercostals depresses the ribs and may aid in forceful exhalation. These muscles are innervated by the adjacent intercostal nerves.

Overview of the Process of Breathing

During quiet inspiration, the diaphragm, external intercostals, and intercartilaginous portions of the internal intercostals are the primary muscles that contract. The diaphragm contracts first and then descends, enlarging the thoracic cage vertically. When the abdominal contents prevent further descent of the diaphragm, the costal fibers of the diaphragm contract, which causes the lower ribs to swing up and out to the side (bucket-handle movement). This lateral rib movement is assisted by the external intercostals and the intercartilaginous portion of the internal intercostals. The transverse diameter of the thorax is increased by this bucket-handle movement. Finally, the upper ribs move forward and upward (pump-handle movement), also through contraction of their external intercostals and the intercartilaginous portions of the internal intercostals. This increases the anteroposterior diameter of the thorax. The epigastric area protrudes, then the ribs swing up and out laterally, and finally the upper ribs move forward and upward.

Quiet expiration is passive and involves no muscular contraction, although some electrical activity can be detected with electromyography. The inspiratory muscles relax, which raises intrathoracic pressure as the ribs and diaphragm return to their preinspiratory positions and compress the lungs. This increased pressure allows airflow from the lungs.

During forced inspiration, an additional number of accessory muscles may contract along with the muscles involved in quiet inspiration. The erector spinae contract to extend the vertebral column. This extension permits greater elevation of the ribs during inspiration. Various back muscles (e.g., erector spinae, trapezius, and rhomboids) contract to stabilize the vertebral column, head, neck, and scapulae. This enables accessory respiratory muscles to assist inspiration through reverse action. The SCM raises the sternum. The scalenes elevate the first two ribs. The serratus anterior, pectoralis major, and pectoralis minor assist bilateral elevation of the ribs. All these accessory muscles tend to elevate the ribs, thus increasing the anteroposterior diameter but not the transverse diameter of the thorax. (The transverse diameter does increase slightly as a result of the increased strength of the contraction of the normal inspiratory muscles.) The marked increase in anteroposterior diameter in relation to transverse diameter creates an impression of en bloc breathing in a patient using accessory muscles.

During forced expiration, the interosseous portion of the internal intercostals and the abdominal muscles contract to force air out of the lungs. Forced expiration can be slow and prolonged (as in patients with COPD) or rapid and expulsive (as in a cough). If the abdominal contractions are strong enough, the trunk flexes during exhalation. This flexion further compresses the lungs, forcing more air from them.

Upper Airways

Nose

Noses vary in size and shape among individuals. The nose is composed of bony and cartilaginous parts. The upper one-third is primarily bony and contains the nasal bones, the frontal processes of the maxillae, and the nasal part of the frontal bone. Its lower two-thirds are cartilaginous and contain the septal, lateral, and major and minor alar nasal cartilages. The nasal cavity is divided into right and left halves by the nasal septum. This cavity extends from the nostrils to the posterior apertures of the nose in the nasopharynx. The lateral walls of the cavity are irregular as a result of projecting superior, middle, and inferior nasal chonchae. There is a meatus located beneath or lateral to each choncha through which the sinuses drain. The chonchae increase the surface area of the nose for maximum contact with inspired air. The superior chonchae and adjacent septal wall are referred to as the olfactory region. They are covered with a thin, yellow olfactory mucous membrane consisting of bipolar nerve cells that are olfactory in function. Only a portion of inspired air reaches the olfactory region to provide a sense of smell. When people smell something specific, they sniff. This action lifts the inspired air so that more of it comes into contact with the olfactory region.

The anterior portion (vestibule) of the nasal cavity (Fig. 3-8) is lined with skin and coarse hairs (vibrissae) that entrap inhaled particles. The rest of the cavity and sinuses (with the exception of the olfactory region) are lined with respiratory mucous membrane. This membrane is composed of pseudostratified columnar ciliated epithelium (Fig. 3-9). It contains goblet cells, as well as mucous and serous glands that produce mucus and serous secretions. These secretions entrap foreign particles and bacteria. This mucus is then swept to the nasopharynx by the cilia at a rate of 5 to 15 mm/min, where it is swallowed or expectorated. The mucous membrane is vascular, with arterial blood supplied by branches of the internal and external carotid arteries. Venous drainage occurs through the anterior facial veins. The mucous membrane is thickest over the chonchae. As air is inhaled, it passes around and over the chonchae, whose vascular moist surfaces heat, humidify, and filter the inspired air. The mucous membrane may become swollen and irritated as a result of upper respiratory infections and may secrete copious amounts of mucus. Because this membrane is continuous with sinuses, auditory tubes, and lacrimal canaliculi, people with colds often complain of sinus headaches, watery eyes, earaches, and other symptoms. Secretions can be so copious that the nasal passages become completely blocked.

Pharynx

The pharynx is an oval fibromuscular sac located behind the nasal cavity, mouth, and larynx. It is approximately 12 to 14 cm long and extends from the base of the skull to the esophagus below, at the level of the cricoid cartilage opposite the sixth cervical vertebra. The pharynx has three compartments: the nasal cavity (nasopharynx), mouth (oropharynx), and larynx (laryngopharynx). The pharyngeal walls are lined with ciliated respiratory mucous membrane in the nasal portion and with stratified squamous membrane in the oral and laryngeal parts.

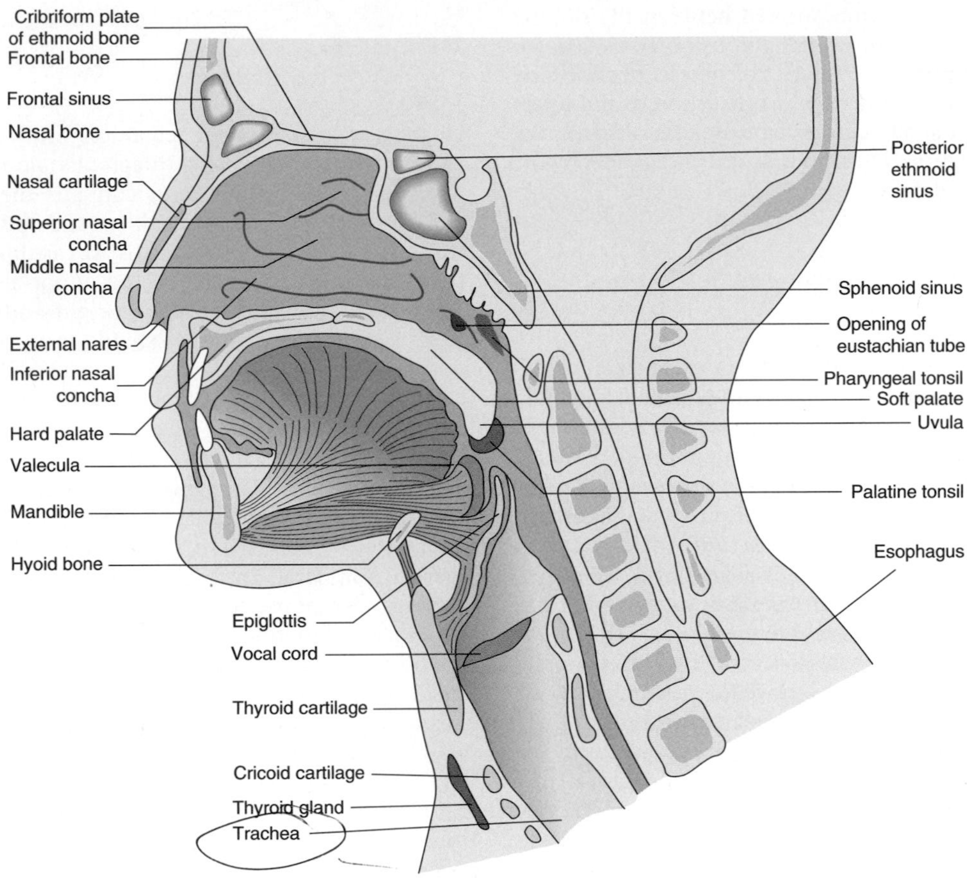

Fig. 3-8 Sagittal section of the head and neck. *(From Hicks GH:* Cardiopulmonary anatomy and physiology, *Philadelphia, 2000, WB Saunders.)*

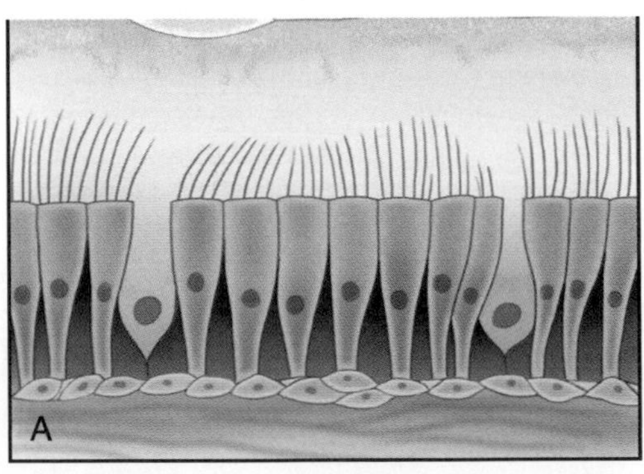

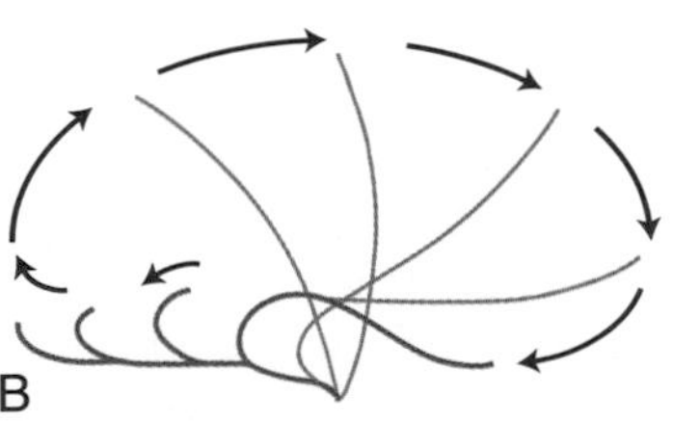

Fig. 3-9 A, Pseudostratified columnar ciliated epithelium. **B,** Normal movements of cilia.

The nasopharynx is a continuation of the nasal cavities (see Fig. 3-8). It lies behind the nose and above the soft palate. With the exception of the soft palate, its walls are immovable, so its cavity is never obliterated as are the oropharynx and laryngopharynx. The nasopharynx communicates with the nasal cavity anteriorly through the posterior apertures of the nose. It communicates with the oropharynx and laryngopharynx through an opening, the pharyngeal isthmus, which is closed by elevations of the soft palate during swallowing.

The oropharynx extends from the soft palate to the epiglottis (see Fig. 3-8). It opens into the mouth anteriorly through the oropharyngeal isthmus. Its posterior walls lie on the bodies of the second and third cervical vertebrae. Laterally, two masses of lymphoid tissue—the palatine tonsils—may be seen. These tonsils form part of a circular band of lymphoid tissue surrounding the opening into the digestive and respiratory tracts.

The laryngopharynx lies behind the larynx and extends from the epiglottis above to the inlet of the esophagus below (see Fig. 3-8). The fourth to sixth cervical vertebrae lie behind the laryngopharynx. In front of the laryngopharynx are the epiglottis, the inlet of the larynx, and the posterior surfaces of the arytenoid and cricoid cartilages.

Larynx

The larynx is a complex structure composed of cartilages and cords moved by sensitive muscles (Fig. 3-10). It is located between the trachea and laryngopharynx, for which it forms an anterior wall. With its rapid closure it acts as a sphincteric valve, preventing food, liquids, and foreign objects from entering the airway. It controls airflow and at times closes so that thoracic pressure may be raised and the upper airways cleared by a propulsive cough when the larynx opens. Expiratory airflow vibrates as it passes over the contracting vocal chords, producing the sounds used for speech. (The larynx is not essential for speech. Humans can speak by learning to dilate the upper part of the esophagus so that air vibrates as it passes over that area; this is called esophageal speech.)

In adult men, the larynx is situated opposite the third, fourth, and fifth cervical vertebrae; it is situated somewhat higher in women and children. The larynx is essentially the same in children, but at puberty, the male larynx increases in size considerably until its anteroposterior diameter has almost doubled. All the cartilages enlarge, and the thyroid cartilage becomes prominent anteriorly.

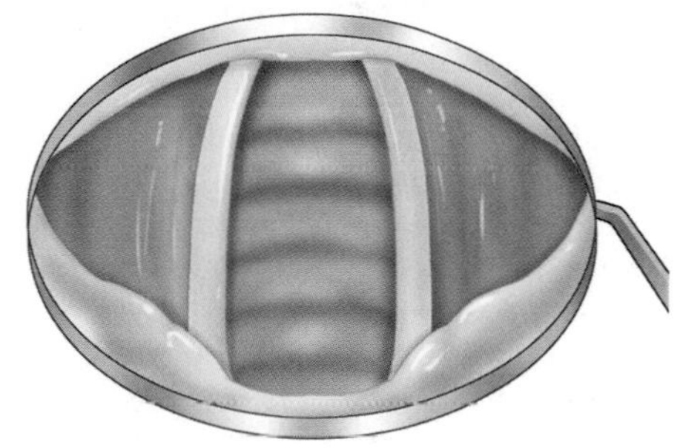

Fig. 3-10 Visualization of the larynx via a laryngoscope.

Vocal cord adductor contraction results in approximation of the vocal cords and narrowing of the glottis. The adductors of the cords are important in protecting the lower airways. Their contraction prevents fluids, food, and other substances from being aspirated. All the intrinsic laryngeal muscles are innervated by the recurrent laryngeal nerve (a branch of the vagus nerve), with the exception of the cricothyroid muscle, which is supplied by the external branch of the superior laryngeal nerve (also a branch of the vagus nerve).

Lower Airways

Trachea

The trachea is a semirigid cartilaginous tube approximately 10 to 11 cm long and 2.5 cm wide. It lies in front of the esophagus and descends with a slight inclination to the right from the level of the cricoid cartilage (Fig. 3-11; see also Fig. 3-10). It travels behind the sternum into the thorax to the sternal angle (opposite the fifth thoracic vertebra), where it divides to form the right and left main stem bronchi. The tracheal wall is strengthened by 16 to 20 horseshoe-shaped cartilaginous rings. The open parts of the tracheal rings are completed by fibrous and elastic tissue and unstriated transverse muscle. This highly flexible part of the ring is positioned posteriorly. It indents or curves inward during coughing, which increases the velocity of expelled air. The cartilaginous rings lie horizontally one above the other, separated by narrow bands of connective tissue. The trachea is lengthened during hyperextension of the head; during swallowing, which raises the trachea; and during inspiration, when the lungs expand and

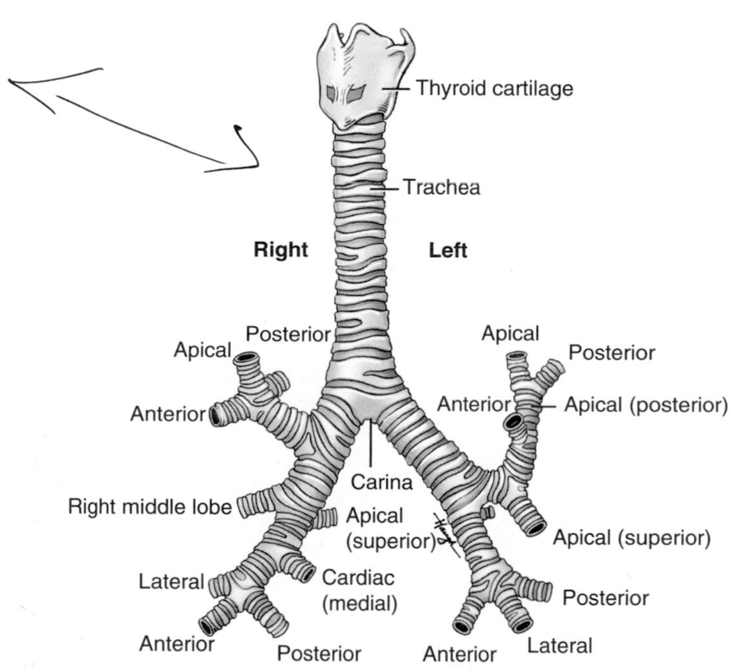

Fig. 3-11 Tracheobronchial tree (a three-quarter view, rotated toward the right side).

pull the trachea downward. Its cross-sectional area becomes smaller with contraction of the unstriated transverse muscle fibers that complete the tracheal rings.

The mucous membrane of the trachea contains columnar ciliated epithelium and goblet cells. Each ciliated epithelial cell contains approximately 275 cilia. These structures beat rapidly in a coordinated and unidirectional manner, propelling a sheet of mucus toward the head, from the lower respiratory tract to the pharynx, where it is swallowed or expectorated. The cilia beat in this layer of mucus with a forceful forward stroke followed by an ineffective backward stroke that returns the cilia to their starting position. Mucociliary escalation propelling of mucus by the cilia toward the upper trachea for clearance, is essential. When cilia are paralyzed by smoking, alcohol, dehydration, anesthesia, starvation, or hypoxia, mucus begins to accumulate in distal, gravity-dependent airways, causing infiltrates and eventually localized areas of lung collapse referred to as atelectasis.

The number of mucus-containing goblet cells is approximately equal to the number of ciliated epithelial cells. Reserve cells lie beneath the ciliated and goblet cells. These reserve cells can differentiate into either goblet cells or ciliated cells. Beneath the reserve cells lie the gland cells. There are approximately 40 times more gland cells than goblet cells. Mucus is composed of 95% water, 2% glycoprotein, 1% carbohydrate, trace amounts of lipid, deoxyribonucleic acid (DNA), dead tissue cells, phagocytes, leukocytes, erythrocytes, and entrapped foreign particles. Mucus lines the airways from the trachea to the alveoli. Two separate layers have been observed: the sol layer, which lies on the mucosal surface and contains high concentrations of water, and the gel layer, which is more superficial and viscous because of its lower concentration of water.

The right main stem bronchus is an extension of the trachea and is wider, shorter, and more vertical than the left main stem bronchus. Greater width and more vertical course cause a majority of aspirated foreign material to pass through the right main stem bronchus. The azygos vein arches over the right main stem bronchus; the right pulmonary artery lies beneath it. The right main stem bronchus divides to form the right upper lobe bronchus, the right middle lobe bronchus, and the right lower lobe bronchus. The right upper lobe divides into three segmental bronchi: apical, posterior, and anterior. The apical bronchus runs almost vertically toward the apex of the lung. The posterior bronchus is directed posteriorly in a horizontal direction, and the anterior bronchus is directed anteriorly in an almost horizontal direction. The right middle lobe bronchus divides about 10 mm below the right upper lobe bronchus and descends anterolaterally. The right lower lobe bronchus divides into five segmental bronchi. The apical or superior bronchus runs almost horizontally, posteriorly. The medial or cardiac bronchus descends medially toward the heart. The anterior basal bronchus descends anteriorly. The lateral basal bronchus descends laterally, and the posterior bronchus descends posteriorly. Each segment describes its anatomic position.

The left main stem bronchus is narrower and runs more horizontally than the right main stem bronchus. The aortic arch passes over it, and the esophagus, descending aorta, and thoracic duct lie behind it. The left pulmonary artery lies anteriorly and above the left main stem bronchus. The left main stem bronchus has two major divisions: the left upper lobe bronchus and the left lower lobe bronchus. The left upper lobe bronchus has three major segmental bronchi. The anterior bronchus ascends at approximately a 45-degree angle. The apical-posterior bronchus has two branches: one runs vertically and the other posteriorly toward the apex of the left lung. The lingular bronchus descends anterolaterally, much the same as does the right middle lobe bronchus of the right lung. The right lower lobe bronchus divides into four segmental bronchi. The superior or apical bronchus runs posteriorly in a horizontal direction. The anterior bronchus descends anteriorly. The lateral bronchus descends laterally, and the posterior bronchus descends posteriorly. The segments describe their anatomic position.

The bronchi of the airways continue to divide until there are approximately 23 generations (Table 3-1). The main, lobar, and segmental bronchi are made up of the first four generations. The walls contain U-shaped cartilage in the main bronchi. This cartilage becomes less well defined and more irregularly shaped as the bronchi continue to divide. In the segmental bronchi, the walls are formed by irregularly shaped helical plates with bands of bronchial muscle. The mucous membrane in these airways is essentially the same as that in the trachea, but the cells become more cuboidal in the lower divisions.

The subsegmental bronchi extend from the fifth to the seventh generation. Although the diameter of these airways becomes progressively smaller, the total cross-sectional area increases because of the increased number of divisions. The mucous membrane is essentially the same, and helical cartilaginous plates and cilia become sparser. These changes continue throughout the 8th to 11th generations, which are referred to as bronchioles.

The terminal bronchioles extend from the 12th to the 16th generation. The diameter of these airways is approximately 1 mm. Cartilage is no longer present to provide structural rigidity. The airways are embedded directly in the lung parenchyma, and it is the elastic properties of this parenchyma that keep these lower airways open. Strong helical muscle bands are present and their contraction forms longitudinal folds in the mucosa that sharply decrease the diameter of the airways. The epithelium of the terminal bronchioles is cuboidal and no longer ciliated. The cross-sectional area of the airways increases sharply at this level. All the airways to this level (generations 1 to 16) are considered conducting airways because their purpose is to transport gas to the respiratory bronchioles and alveoli, where gas exchange occurs. The conducting airways receive their arterial blood from the bronchial circulation (branches of the descending aorta). Airways below this point receive their arterial blood from the pulmonary arteries.

The respiratory bronchioles extend from the 17th to the 19th generation. They are considered a transitional zone between bronchioles and alveoli. Their walls contain cuboidal epithelium interspersed with some alveoli. The number of alveoli increases with each generation. The walls of the bronchioles are also buried in the lung parenchyma. The airways depend on traction of this parenchyma to maintain their lumen. Muscle bands are also present between alveoli.

Alveolar ducts extend from the 20th to the 22nd generation. Their walls are composed entirely of alveoli, which are separated from one another by their septae. Septae contain smooth muscle, elastic and collagen fibers, nerves, and capillaries.

Alveolar sacs make up the 23rd generation of air passages. They are essentially the same as alveolar ducts, except that they

Table 3-1 Structural Characteristics of the Air Passages

	Generation (mean)	Number	Mean Diameter (mm)	Area Supplied	Cartilage	Muscle	Nutrition	Placement	Epithelium
Trachea	0	1	18	Both lungs	U-shaped		From inferior thyroid, thoracic, and branches of bronchial arteries		
Main bronchi	1	2	13	Individual lungs				Within connective tissue sheath alongside arterial vessels	
Lobar bronchi	2 ↓ 3	4 ↓ 8	7 ↓ 5	Lobes	Irregular shape and helical plates	Helical bands	From the bronchial circulation		Columnar, ciliated
Segmental bronchi	4	16	4	Segments					
Small bronchi	5 ↓ 11	32 ↓ 2000	3 ↓ 1	Secondary lobules					
Bronchioles and terminal bronchioles	12 ↓ 16	4000 ↓ 65,000	1 ↓ 0.5			Strong helical muscle bands		Embedded directly in the lung parenchyma	Cuboidal
Respiratory bronchioles	17 ↓ 19	130,000 ↓ 500,000	0.5	Primary lobes		Muscle band between alveolar thin bands in alveolar septa	From the pulmonary circulation		Cuboidal to flat between the alveoli
Alveolar ducts	20 ↓ 22	1,000,000 ↓ 4,000,000	0.3	Alveoli				Lung parenchyma	Alveolar epithelium
Alveolar sacs	23	8,000,000	0.3					Lung parenchyma	Alveolar epithelium

Adapted from Weibel ER: Morphometry of the human lung. *New York, 1963, Springer.*

end as blind pouches. Communication occurs between blind pouches in the form of the pores of Kohn, which are channels in alveolar walls, and the Lambert canals, which are communications between bronchioles and alveoli. These communications are thought to be responsible for the rapid spread of lung infection. They also provide collateral ventilation to alveoli whose bronchi are obstructed. Although this ventilation does little to arterialize blood, it does help prevent collapse of these alveoli. Each alveolar sac contains approximately 17 alveoli. There are about 300 million alveoli in an adult man, 85% to 95% of which are covered with pulmonary capillaries. Alveolar epithelium is composed of two cell types. Type I cells, squamous pneumocytes, have broad thin extensions that cover about 95% of the alveolar surface. Type II cells, the granular pneumocytes, are more numerous than type I cells but occupy less than 5% of the alveolar surface. This is because of their small, cuboidal shape. These cells are responsible for the production of surfactant, a phospholipid that lines the alveoli. Surfactant keeps alveoli expanded by lowering their surface tension. Type II cells have been shown to be the primary cells involved in repair of the alveolar epithelium. Type III cells, alveolar brush cells, are rare and found only occasionally in humans.

An additional type of cell, the alveolar macrophage, is found within the alveoli. These cells are thought to originate from stem cell precursors in the bone marrow and reach the lung through the blood stream. They are large, mononuclear, ameboid cells that roam in the alveoli, alveolar ducts, and alveolar sacs. Macrophages contain lysosomes, which are capable of killing engulfed bacteria. They are especially effective in neutralizing inhaled gram-positive organisms. They also engulf foreign matter and are transported to the lymphatic system or migrate to the terminal bronchioles, where they attach themselves to the mucus. Macrophages are carried by the mucus to larger airways and eventually to the pharynx. Because cilia are not present below the 11th generation of air passages, clearance of foreign matter and bacteria from these areas is largely dependent on macrophages.

Other cells located in the distal airways that are important in the defense of the lung are the lymphocytes and polymorphonuclear leukocytes. Immunoglobulins (IgA, IgG, and IgM) in the blood serum enhance the engulfing activity of the macrophages. Two types of lymphocytes are found in the lung: the B lymphocyte and the T lymphocyte. The B lymphocytes produce gamma globulin antibodies to fight lung infections, whereas the T lymphocytes release a substance that attracts macrophages to the site of the infection. The polymorphonuclear leukocytes are important in engulfing and killing blood-borne gram-negative organisms.

Lungs

Two lungs (each covered with its pleurae—the visceral pleura and the parietal pleura), lie within the thoracic cavity. Each lung is attached to the heart and the trachea by its root and the pulmonary ligament. The lungs are otherwise free in the thoracic cavity. The lungs are light, soft, spongy organs whose color darkens with age as they become impregnated with inhaled air pollutants. They are covered with the visceral pleura, a thin, glistening serous membrane that covers all surfaces of the lungs. The visceral pleura extends to the mediastinum and inner thoracic wall, where it becomes known as the parietal pleura. The space between the two pleurae maintains a negative pressure at all times and is therefore termed a potential space. This negative pressure maintains lung inflation. A small amount of pleural fluid lubricates the two pleurae as they slide over each other during breathing. In disease, fluid, tumor cells, or air can invade the pleural space and collapse the underlying lung.

Each lung has an apex, a base, and three surfaces (costal, medial, and diaphragmatic). There are also three borders (anterior, inferior, and posterior). Each lung is divided by fissures into separate lobes. In the right lung, the oblique fissure separates the lower lobe from the middle, whereas the horizontal fissure separates the upper lobe from the middle. The right lung is heavier and wider than the left lung. It is also shorter because of the location of the right lobe of the liver. The left lung is divided into upper and lower lobes by the oblique fissure. It is longer and thinner than the right lung because the heart and pericardium are located in the left thorax. Numerous structures enter the lung at the hilus, or root of the lung, including the main stem bronchus, the pulmonary artery, pulmonary veins, bronchial arteries and veins, nerves, and lymph vessels. The root, or hilus, of the lungs lies opposite the bodies of the fifth, sixth, and seventh thoracic vertebrae. The lungs are connected to the upper airways by the trachea and main stem bronchi.

Surface Markings

Surface markings of the lungs can be outlined on the chest with a basic knowledge of bony landmarks and of the gross anatomy of each lung (Table 3-2 and Fig. 3-12). The apices of both lungs extend 2 or 3 cm above the clavicles at the medial ends. The anteromedial border of the right lung runs from the sternoclavicular joint to the sternal angle and downward to the xiphisternum. The inferior border runs from the xiphisternum laterally to the sixth rib in the midclavicular line, the eighth rib in the midaxillary line, and the 10th rib in the midscapular line. The midscapular line runs downward from the inferior angle of the scapula with the arm at rest. The inferior border joins the posterior medial border of the lung 2 cm lateral to the tenth thoracic vertebra. The posterior medial border runs 2 cm lateral to the vertebral column from the seventh cervical vertebra to the tenth thoracic vertebra.

The left lung is generally smaller than the right and accommodates the position of the heart. The medial border on the anterior aspect runs from the sternoclavicular joint to the middle of the sternal angle, down the midline of the sternum to the fourth costal cartilage. A lateral indentation of about 2 to 3 cm forms the cardiac notch at the level of the fifth and sixth costal cartilages. The courses of the inferior and medial borders on the posterior aspect are similar in the left and right lungs. In the left lung, however, the inferior border crosses at the level of the 10th thoracic vertebra, not the 12th, as is observed in the right lung.

The position of the fissures of the lungs can be outlined over the chest wall. In both lungs, the oblique fissure begins between the second to fourth thoracic vertebrae. This can be roughly estimated by following a line continuous with the medial border of the abducted scapula around the midaxillary line at the fifth rib and terminating at the sixth costal cartilage anteriorly. The horizontal fissure of the right lung originates

Table 3-2 **Anatomic Arrangement of the Bronchopulmonary Segments**

Lobe	Right Lung: Bronchopulmonary Segments	Lobe	Left Lung: Bronchopulmonary Segments
Upper	Apical: Extends above the clavicle anteriorly; smaller area posteriorly Anterior: Occupies area between the clavicle and horizontal fissure Posterior: Remainder of upper lobe on the posterior aspect down to the oblique fissure	Upper	Apical posterior: Extends above the clavicle anteriorly; occupies area comparable to that of the apical and posterior segments of the right lung Anterior: Occupies area between the clavicle and the border of the lingula (line comparable to the horizontal fissure of the right lung)
Middle	Lateral: Extends medially from junction of the two fissures at the third intercostal space to occupy one-third of the anterior surface of the lobe Medial: Occupies the remaining anterior surface of the lobe	(Lingula)[‡]	Superior: Occupies upper half of the lingula Inferior: Occupies lower half of the lingula
Lower (Base)	Anterior: Occupies basal area beneath the oblique fissure anteriorly Superior: Occupies half the area from the oblique fissure downward* on the posterior aspect Lateral: Extends from the junction of the middle lobe over the midaxillary area to occupy one-third the area inferior to the superior segment on the posterior aspect Posterior: Occupies two-thirds of the area posteriorly beneath the superior segment Medial: Occupies a space on the inner aspect of the right base[†]	Lower (Base)	Anterior: Occupies area inferior to the oblique fissure anteriorly Superior: Occupies one-third of the basal area posteriorly from the oblique fissure downward Lateral: Occupies the lateral half of the remaining two-thirds of the left lower lobe beneath the superior segment on the posterior aspect Posterior: Occupies the medial portion of the remaining two-thirds of the left lower lobe beneath the superior segment on the posterior aspect

*This segment is best drained when the patient lies prone. Superior segments also called apical segments.

[†]Medial basal segment has no direct exposure to the chest wall; therefore it cannot be directly auscultated. This segment is best drained when the patient is positioned for the left lateral basal segment because of the comparable angle of its bronchus.

[‡]Lingula is not an area that is anatomically distinct from the right middle lobe; rather, it is anatomically part of the left upper lobe.

from the oblique fissure at the level of about the fourth intercostal space in the midaxillary line and courses medially and slightly upward over the fourth rib anteriorly. The left lung has no horizontal fissure.

Bronchopulmonary Segments

The bronchopulmonary segments lie within the three lobes of the right lung and the two lobes of the left lung. There are 10 bronchopulmonary segments on the right and 8 on the left. Brief anatomic descriptions of the position of each lobe are provided in Table 3-2. Figure 3-12, *A*, illustrates the surface markings on the anterior view of the lungs and the position of the various bronchopulmonary segments within the major anatomic divisions provided by the fissures. Figure 3-12, *B*, shows some of these features from the lateral views. Figure 3-12, *C*, illustrates the surface markings and bronchopulmonary segments of the posterior aspect of the lungs.

Heart

The heart is a conical, hollow muscular pump enclosed in a fibroserous sac, the pericardium. Its size is closely related to body size and corresponds remarkably to the size of an individual's clenched fist. It is positioned in the center of the chest behind the lower half of the sternum. The largest portion of the heart lies to the left of the midsternal line; the apex is found approximately 9 cm to the left, in the fifth intercostal space.

The surface markings of the heart can be traced by joining four points over the anterior chest wall. On the right, the heart extends from the third to the sixth costal cartilage at a distance of about 10 to 15 mm from the sternum. On the left, the heart extends from the second costal cartilage to the fifth intercostal space, 12 to 15 mm and 9 cm from the left sternal border, respectively. Joining the two points on the left side outlines the left atrium and ventricle. The heart is rotated to the left in the chest, so the right side of the heart is foremost. Joining the two uppermost points outlines the level of the atria, and joining the two lower points represents the margin of the right ventricle.

The heart as a whole is freely movable within the pericardial cavity and changes position during both contraction and respiration. During contraction, the apex moves forward, strikes the chest and imparts the chest-and-apex beat, which may be felt and seen. Abnormal positioning of the apex beat can indicate cardiac enlargement or displacement. During breathing, the movements of the diaphragm determine the position of the heart. This is because of the attachment of the central tendon of the diaphragm to the pericardium. Changes in position during quiet breathing are hardly noticeable, but with deep inspirations, the downward excursion of the diaphragm causes the heart to descend and rotate to the right. The opposite occurs during expiration. Pathology of the lungs can also change the position of the heart. Atelectasis shifts the heart to

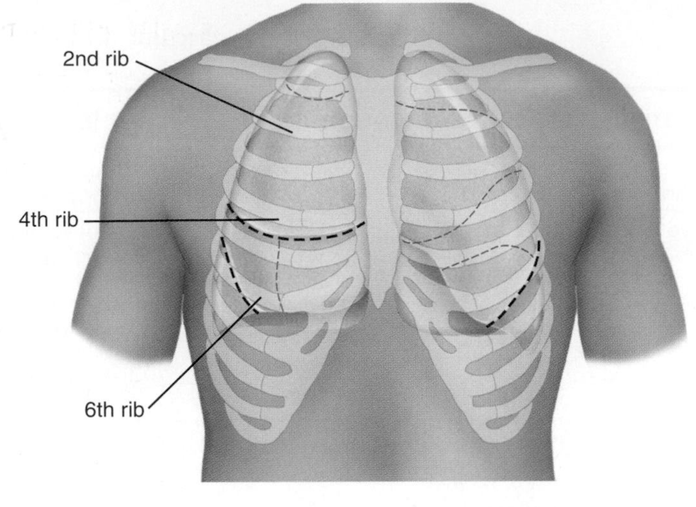

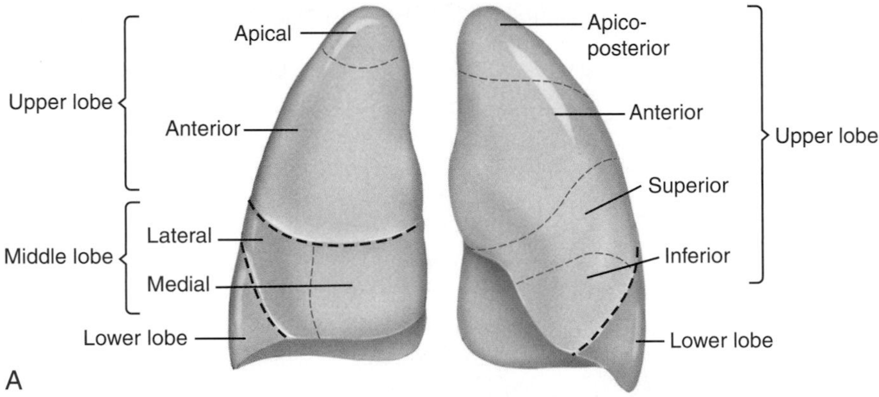

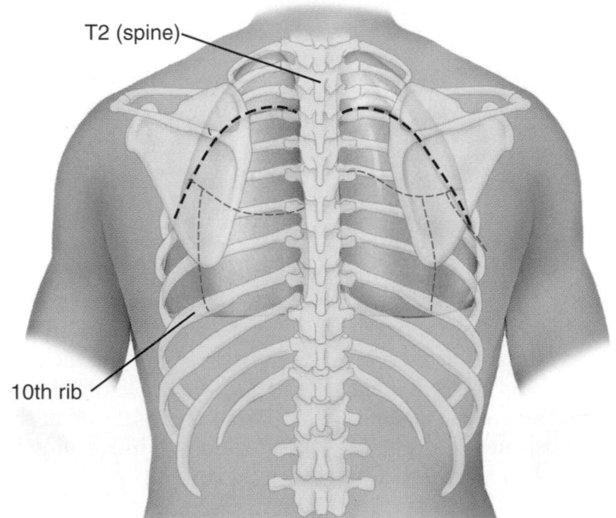

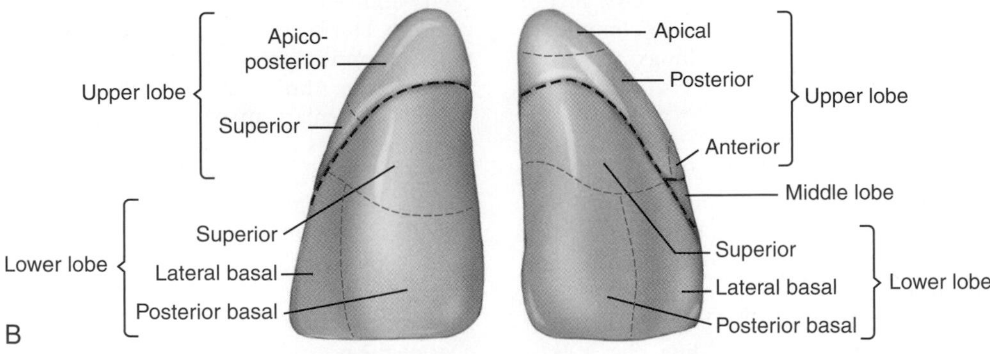

Fig. 3-12 Surface markings of the lungs (anterior **[A]**, posterior **[B]**, and lateral **[C]** aspects). The underlying bronchopulmonary segments are also shown. *(Modified from Cherniak RM, Cherniack L:* Respiration in health and disease, *ed 3, Philadelphia, 1983, WB Saunders.)*

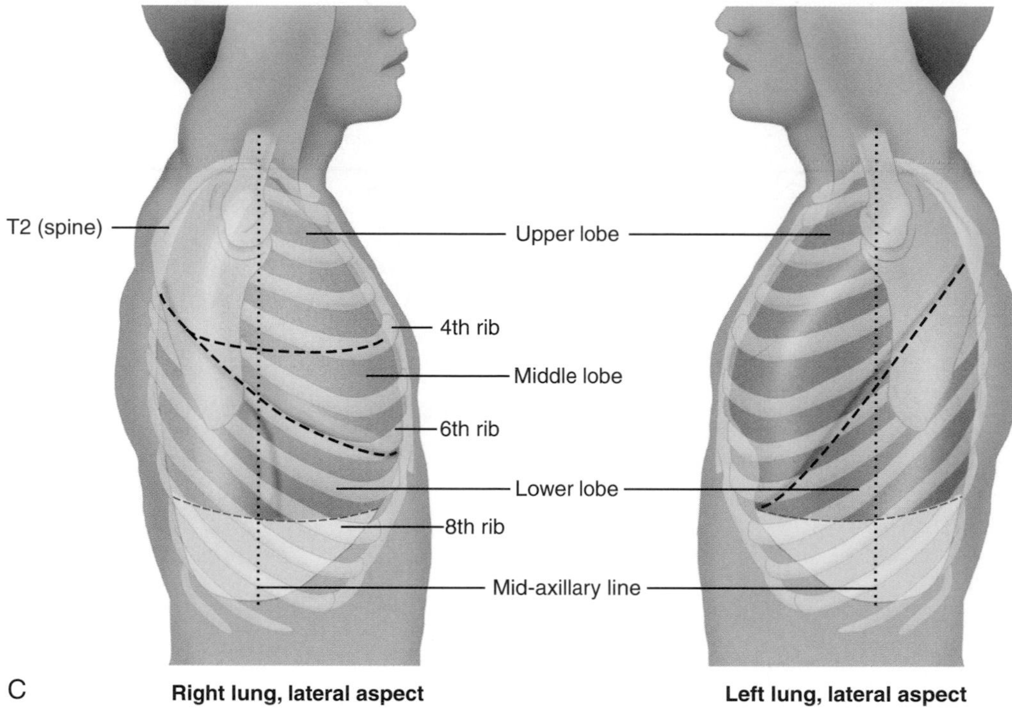

Fig. 3-12, cont'd

the same side. In tension pneumothorax, where air enters the chest (usually through an opening in the chest wall) and cannot escape, the positive pressure shifts the heart away from the side of the pathology.

The heart is enclosed by the pericardium, whose two surfaces can be visualized by visualizing the heart as a fist plunged into a large balloon. The outer surface, a tough fibrous membrane, is called the fibrous pericardium. It encases the heart as well as the organs and terminations of the great vessels. This membrane is so unyielding that when fluid accumulates rapidly in the pericardial cavity, it can compress the heart and impede venous return. When this occurs often, a window is cut in the pericardium, allowing the fluid to escape. The inner surface, the serous pericardium, is a serous membrane that lines the fibrous pericardium. Between 10 and 20 mL of clear pericardial fluid separates and moistens the two pericardial surfaces. The pericardium, with its fluid, minimizes friction during contraction. It also holds the heart in position and prevents dilation. The serous pericardium consists of an outer layer (the parietal layer) and an inner layer (the visceral layer or epicardium).

The heart is divided into right and left halves by an obliquely placed longitudinal septum (Fig. 3-13, *A*). Each half has two chambers: the atrium, which receives blood from veins, and the ventricle, which ejects blood into the arteries. The superior vena cava, inferior vena cava, and intrinsic veins of the heart deposit venous blood into the right atrium. Blood then passes through the tricuspid valve to the right ventricle. The right ventricle ejects the blood through the pulmonary valve into the pulmonary arteries, which are the only arteries in the body that contain deoxygenated blood. Pulmonary veins return the blood to the left atrium, and from there it passes through the mitral valve to the left ventricle. From the left ventricle it is ejected through the aortic valve into the main artery of the body, the aorta.

The heart is divided into three layers: the epicardium, myocardium, and endocardium. The outermost layer, the epicardium, is visceral pericardium and is often infiltrated with fat. The coronary blood vessels that nourish the heart run in this layer before entering the myocardium. The myocardium consists of cardiac muscle fibers. The thickness of the layers of cardiac muscle fibers is directly proportional to the amount of work they perform. The ventricles do more work than the atria; hence their walls are thicker. The pressure in the aorta is higher than that in the pulmonary trunk. This requires greater work from the left ventricle, so its walls are twice as thick as those of the right ventricle. The innermost layer, the endocardium, is the smooth endothelial lining of the interior of the heart.

Heart Valves

The four valves of the heart, although delicate in appearance, are designed to withstand repetitive closures against high pressures. Normally, they operate properly for more than 80 years without need of repair or replacement. The tricuspid and mitral valves function differently from the other valves of the heart. Being located between the atria and ventricles, they must effect a precise closure within a contracting cavity.

During diastole, the two leaflets or cusps of the mitral valve and the three cusps of the tricuspid valve relax into the cavities of the ventricles, allowing blood to flow between the two chambers. As the ventricular chambers fill with blood, the cusps of the valves are forced up into a closed position. Fibrous cords, the chordae tendinae, are located on the ventricular surfaces of these cusps. These cords connect the cusps of the valve with the papillary muscles of the ventricular walls. As pressure builds in the ventricular chambers, contraction of these muscles prevents the cusps from being forced up into the atria. Dysfunction or rupture of the chordae tendinae or

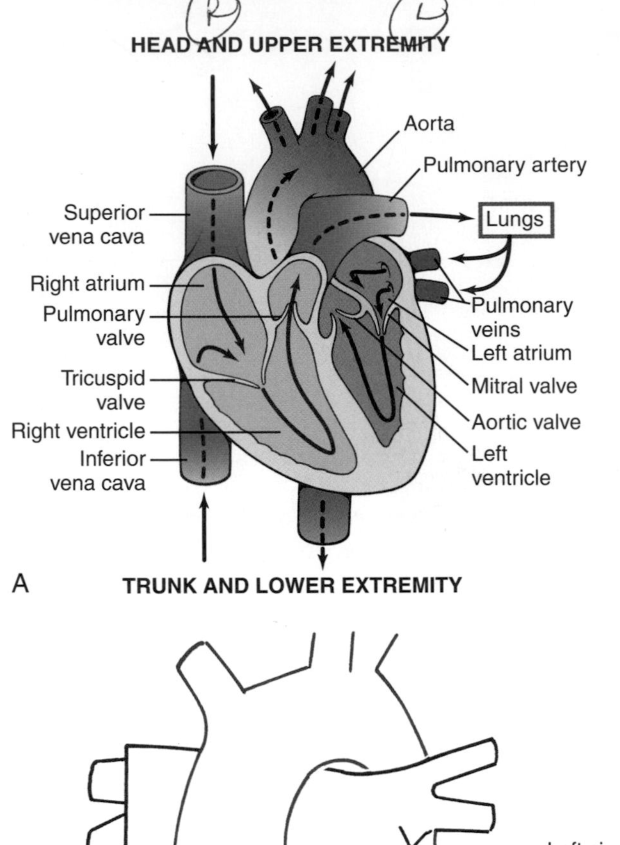

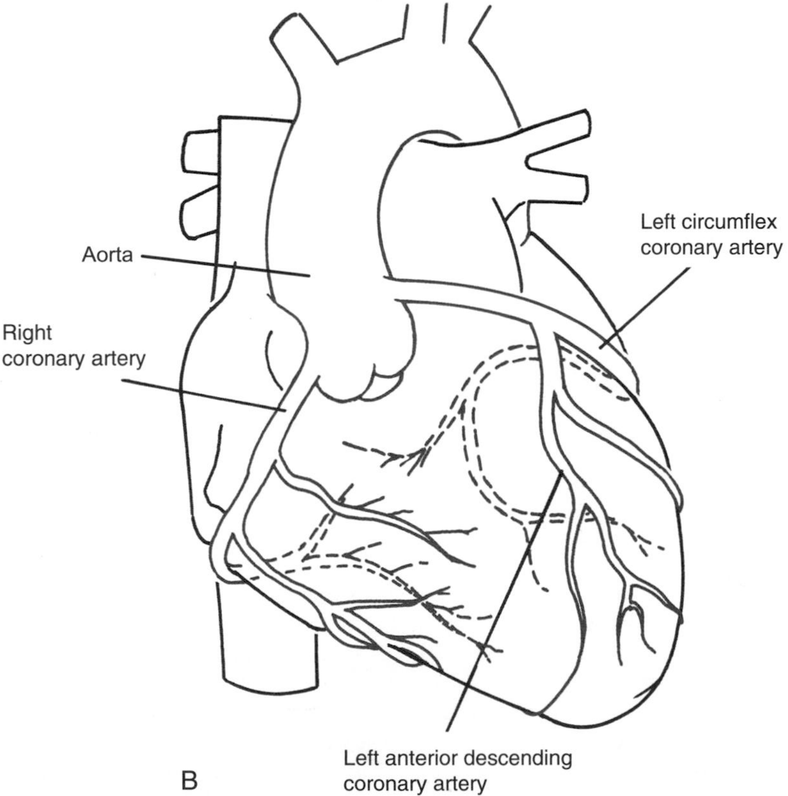

Fig. 3-13 Blood flow through the heart. **A,** The three major coronary arteries that supply blood to the heart. **B,** Blood flow through internal structures. (***A,*** *from Hall J:* Guyton and Hall textbook of medical physiology, *ed 12, Philadelphia, 2011, Saunders.* ***B,*** *from Goldberger:* Clinical electrocardiography: a simplified approach, *ed 7, Philadelphia, 2009, Mosby.)*

the papillary muscles may undermine the support of one or more valve cusps, producing regurgitation from the ventricles to the atria.

The pulmonic and aortic valves are similar in appearance, but the aortic cusps are slightly thicker than the pulmonic cusps. Each valve has three fibrous cusps, the bases of which are firmly attached to the root of the aorta or the pulmonary artery. The free edges of these valves project into the lumen of the vessels. At the end of systole, blood in the aorta and pulmonary artery forces the cusps of the valves shut. These valves are attached in such a manner that they cannot be everted into the ventricles by increased pressure in the vessels. During diastole, the cusps support the column of blood filling the ventricles. Contraction of the ventricles during systole increases pressure within the ventricular chambers, forcing the cusps to open and allow blood flow into the vessels.

The arterial supply of the heart muscle is derived from the right and left coronary arteries, which arise from the aortic

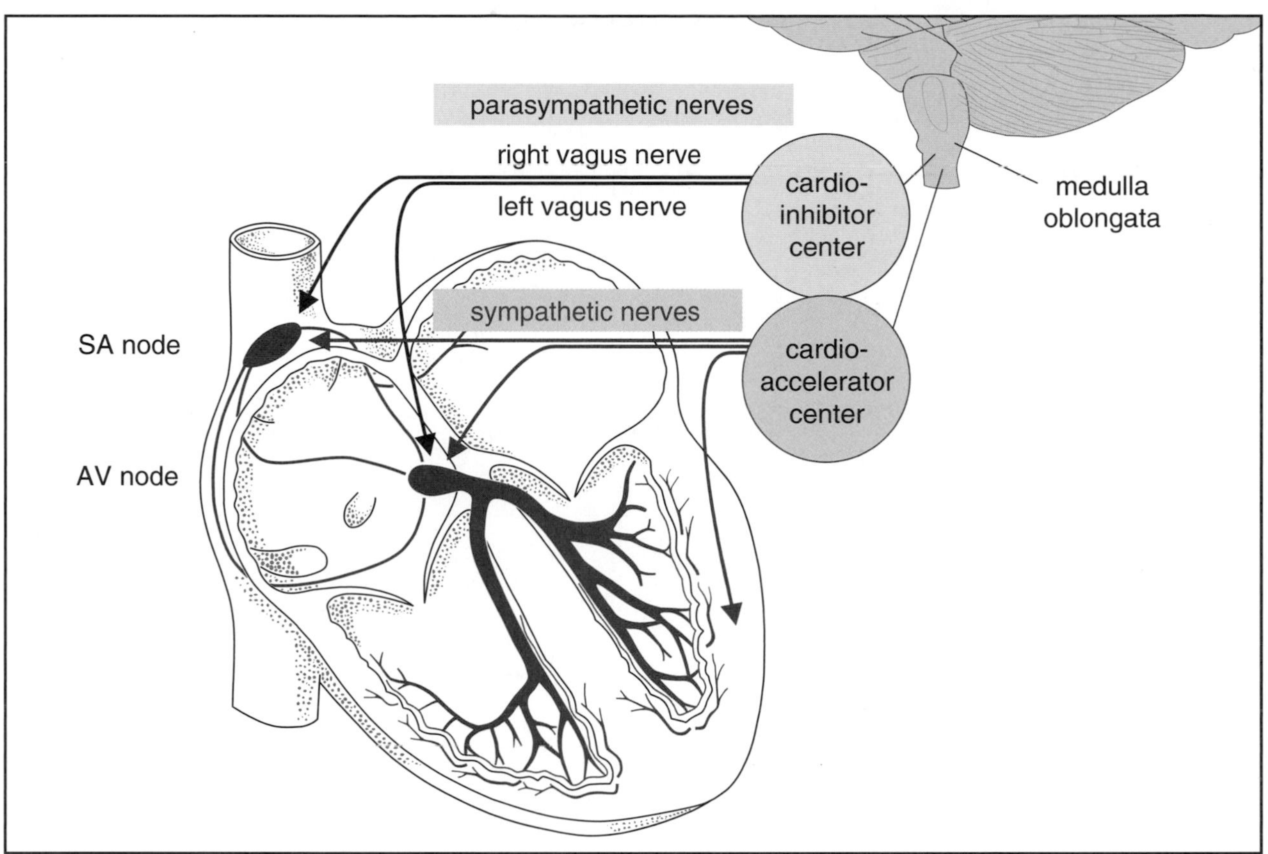

Fig. 3-14 Sympathetic and parasympathetic innervation of the heart. *(From Huszar RJ:* Basic dysrhythmias: interpretation and management*, ed 3, Philadelphia, 2007, Mosby.)*

sinuses (Fig. 3-13, *B*). The left coronary artery (LCA) divides into the anterior descending artery and the left circumflex artery. These arteries supply most of the left ventricle, the left atrium, most of the ventricular septum, and in 45% of people, the sinoatrial (SA) node. The right coronary artery (RCA) supplies most of the right ventricle, the atrioventricular (AV) node, and in 55% of people, the SA node. Infarction of these arteries or their branches can cause interruption or cessation of the conduction system and death of the myocardial muscle in the area supplied by the artery. The severity of the infarction is dependent on the size of the artery and the importance of the area it supplies.

The heart is drained by a number of veins. Most of the veins of the heart enter the coronary sinus, which then empties into the right atrium. A small number of veins, the thebesian veins, empty directly into the right and left ventricles.

Innervation

Innervation of the heart involves a complex balance between its intrinsic automaticity and extrinsic nerves (Fig. 3-14). The SA and AV nodes provide the heart with an inherent ability for spontaneous rhythmic initiation of the cardiac impulse. The rate of this impulse formation is regulated by the autonomic nervous system (ANS), which also influences other phases of the cardiac cycle. It controls the rate of spread of the excitation impulse and the contractility of both atria and ventricles.

The ANS extends its influence to the heart via the vagus nerve (parasympathetic) and upper thoracic nerves (sympathetic). These nerves mingle around the root and arch of the aorta near the tracheal bifurcation, forming the cardiac plexus. Extensions from the cardiac plexus richly supply the SA and AV nodes. They are so well mingled that scientists are unable to determine which nerves supply which parts of the heart. Stimulation of the sympathetic nervous system causes acceleration of the discharge rate in the SA node, an increase in AV nodal conduction, and an increase in the contractile force of both atrial and ventricular muscles. Stimulation of the vagus nerve causes cardiac slowing and decreased AV nodal conduction. Thus the parasympathetic system decelerates heart rate, and the sympathetic system accelerates heart rate.

Intrinsic innervation of the heart centers around the SA node, which lies near the junction of the superior vena cava and the right atrium. It is the normal pacemaker of the heart, sending concentric waves of excitation throughout the atrium. Without neural influence, impulse formation from this node would be greater than 100 beats per minute. Vagal influence, however, decreases the impulse formation to 60 to 90 beats per minute. The SA node paces the heart as long as it generates impulses at a faster rate than any other part of the myocardium and as long as these impulses are rapidly conducted from the atria to the ventricles. Normal impulse formation may be interrupted by vascular lesions (occlusion of the coronary arteries) or by cardiac disease (pericarditis). The SA node is especially susceptible to pericarditis and all other surface

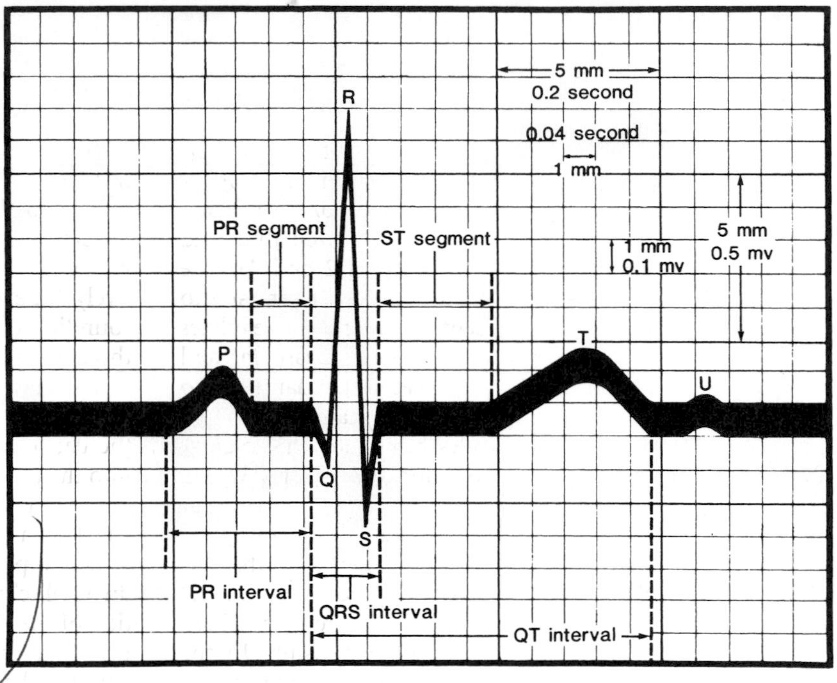

Fig. 3-15 A normal ECG showing characteristic waves, intervals, and segments.

cardiac diseases because of its superficial position immediately beneath the epicardium.

The muscle fibers of the heart are self-excitatory, which enables the heart to contract rhythmically and automatically. The normal pacemaker of the heart, the SA node, is located in the posterior wall of the right atrium. The concentric waves of excitation sent out by the SA node must travel through the AV node to reach the ventricles. This node is located in the floor of the right atrium, just above the insertion of the tricuspid valve. Its main function is to cause a 0.04-second delay in impulse transmission. This delay is beneficial for two reasons: it postpones ventricular excitation until the atria have had time to eject their contents into the ventricles, and it limits the number of signals that can be transmitted by the AV node. The AV node also has its own inherent rhythmicity, firing at a much slower rate than the SA node (40 to 60 beats per minute). Its main pathology is a result of occlusion of the right coronary artery, which supplies the AV node in 90% of cases. From the AV node arises a triangular group of fibers known as the AV bundle, or bundle of His. This bundle divides in the ventricular septum into two branches: the left bundle branch and the right bundle branch. Each of these bundles continues to divide into many fine nerve fibers that spread throughout the ventricles and terminate in the Purkinje fibers, which are continuous with the cardiac muscle. The waves of excitation pass through the bundle of His, down the bundle branches, and through the Purkinje fibers, which permeate the ventricles and cause them to contract. This wave of depolarization gives rise to the normal P-QRS-T configuration of the electrocardiogram (ECG) tracing (Fig. 3-15) (see Chapter 12). The P wave indicates atrial depolarization, the QRS complex indicates ventricular depolarization, and the T wave indicates ventricular repolarization. There is no wave indicating atrial repolarization because atrial repolarization is embedded in the QRS complex[13,15] (see Physiology of the Electrical Excitation of the Heart and ECG Interpretation, Chapter 12).[14,15]

Systemic Circulation

The systemic vascular system is a complex series of branching blood vessels throughout the body. It provides nutrition and oxygen to, and removes waste products from, all tissues of the body. The driving force for this system is the heart. The vascular system has two major components: the peripheral and the pulmonary circulations.[5]

Blood vessels are designed to forward oxygenated blood from the heart during systolic ejection from the left ventricle, perfuse the vascular beds commensurate with their metabolic needs, and remove metabolic waste. Anatomically, the proximal vessels have a higher proportion of connective tissue and elastin so as to withstand high pulse pressures (e.g., the aorta, which carries blood to the head, viscera, and limbs). In addition, potential energy is stored in the walls of the larger vessels during systole. During diastole, the elastic recoil of these vessels maintains the forward motion of the blood between ventricular systoles. The medium-size blood vessels have proportions of connective tissue and elastin comparable to smooth muscle. As the blood vessels become smaller, smooth muscle predominates. The arterioles are primarily smooth muscle, so their diameter can alter significantly. They regulate the blood flow to regional tissue beds and are also responsible for regulating total peripheral resistance and systemic blood pressure. They are called the stopcocks of the circulation. Many factors (e.g., nervous impulses, hormonal stimulation, drugs, oxygen, and carbon dioxide concentrations) determine the degree of contraction of vascular smooth muscle and whether contraction occurs locally or throughout the entire body.

Arterioles branch to form the smallest vessels, capillaries, which consist of a single layer of endothelial cells forming lumen just large enough for red blood cells to pass. The capillary bed is enormous, with a capacity far exceeding 5 L. In active tissue such as muscle and brain, the capillary network is finer and denser; the network is less dense in less active tissue such as tendon. Gas exchange occurs in the capillary bed, where red blood cells give up their oxygen and blood plasma transudes capillary walls, carrying nutrition to tissue.

The microcirculation specifically consists of the metarterioles, the capillary bed, and the venules. The capillary wall is a semipermeable membrane that is responsible for the transfer of oxygen, nutrients, and waste between the circulation and tissue via the interstitial fluid (see Chapters 2 and 4). The capillary pores selectively allow molecules of different size to pass through them. This is an essential feature that regulates the movement of fluid in and out of the intravascular and extravascular compartments. This process is fundamental to maintaining and regulating normal hemodynamics.

Capillaries give rise to the venules, which are the smallest veins. These veins branch and become increasingly larger. Blood flow through the veins is largely dependent on muscular or visceral action or pressures. These pressures are intermittent and, were it not for double-cusp valves located within the veins, blood would flow backward with fluctuation in the pressure gradient and cessation of flow. In the extremities, muscular contractions move blood into the trunk. In the pelvic and abdominal region, blood flow is dependent on intraabdominal pressure exceeding intrathoracic pressure. Veins in the trunk become increasingly larger until they finally enter the superior and inferior vena cavae.

Pulmonary Circulation

The vena cavae empty directly into the right atrium. Blood flow from the right side of the heart through the lungs is known as pulmonary circulation. The quantity of blood flowing through pulmonary circulation is approximately equal to that flowing through systemic circulation. Blood flows from the right ventricle into the pulmonary artery, which divides into right and left branches 4 cm from the ventricle. These branches then separate, one to each lung, where they continue to divide into smaller arteries. The pulmonary arteries and arterioles are much shorter, have thinner walls and larger diameters, and are more distensible than their systemic counterparts. This gives the pulmonary system compliance as great as that of the systemic arterial system, thereby allowing the pulmonary arteries to accommodate the stroke volume output of the right ventricle. Pulmonary vascular resistance and arterial pressure are one-sixth that of the systemic system (pulmonary arterial pressure is 20/10 mm Hg compared with 120/80 mm Hg systemically).

Pulmonary capillaries are short and arise abruptly from larger arterioles. They form a dense network over the walls of the alveoli to minimize the distance over which gas exchange occurs. The pulmonary veins are also very short but have distensibility characteristics similar to those of veins in the systemic system. Unlike systemic veins, however, pulmonary veins have no valves. Pulmonary veins act as a capacitance vessel, or a blood reservoir, for the left atrium. Contraction of smooth muscle in the veins makes the reservoir constrict. This increases blood volume in relation to the internal volume of the vessels. The pulmonary veins become larger until they converge into two veins from each lung, which then carry oxygenated blood to the left atrium.

Lymphatic Circulation

The lymphatic circulation provides an additional route for fluid to be returned from the interstitium to the systemic circulation and thus has a central role in the regulation of interstitial fluid dynamics. Lymph, the fluid that flows in the lymphatic channels, is interstitial fluid with a composition similar to that of tissue fluid. The vessels of the lymphatic system move excess fluid, large proteins, and other large molecules away from the interstitial spaces. Although relatively little protein leaks from the capillaries into the surrounding tissue, the absence of its immediate removal is life threatening.

Virtually all areas of the body drain into a network of lymphatic channels. From the lower portion of the body and from the left head and neck, excess tissue fluid and protein drain into the thoracic duct, which empties into the venous circulation at the junction of the left internal jugular vein and the subclavian vein. Lymph from the right side of the head, neck, arm, and parts of the right thorax drain into the right lymph duct, which empties into the venous circulation at the junction of the right internal jugular vein and the subclavian vein. Lymph from the lower part of the body drains into the inguinal and abdominal lymphatic channels. The pressure in the lymphatic system is usually slightly negative, which helps to keep the interstitium "dry." The lymph vessels are thin walled and have some smooth muscle, so they can contract to propel their contents. In addition, lymph vessels have valves to facilitate forward motion and minimize retrograde movement of lymph.

Summary

This chapter reviews the anatomy of the cardiovascular and pulmonary systems. The anatomic features of the respiratory pump are described with respect to the structures of the bony thorax, of the muscles of respiration associated with the chest wall, and of the diaphragm. The upper and lower respiratory tracts are described, as is the relationship of the tracheobronchial tree to the lung parenchyma. The lung parenchyma is defined anatomically in terms of discrete bronchopulmonary segments contained within three major divisions of each lung. The specific surface markings defined by the lung fissures and the landmarks of the bronchopulmonary segments are outlined. The basic anatomy of the heart is described. The structures of the peripheral and pulmonary circulations are also presented. Special reference is made to the lymphatic circulation and its central role in the regulation of capillary fluid dynamics. A detailed understanding of cardiovascular and pulmonary anatomy is fundamental to the knowledge base underlying the assessment and management by physical therapists of cardiovascular and pulmonary dysfunction and impaired oxygen transport.

Review Questions

1. Describe the cardiovascular and pulmonary unit and why it is a more useful classification than describing either the heart or lungs separately.
2. Describe the thorax and its movements.

3. Describe the respiratory muscles and their functions.
4. Explain the pathway of oxygen from the atmosphere to the alveolar capillary membrane.
5. Describe the movement of blood returning from the periphery through the heart to the pulmonary and peripheral circulations.
6. Describe the movement of deoxygenated blood from the periphery back to the heart.
7. Explain the role of the lymphatic circulation and its physiological significance.
8. Describe the interdependence between the lungs and the heart in relation to its clinical implications.

References

1. Scharf SM, Cassidy SS, editors: *Heart-lung interactions in health and disease*, ed 42, New York, 2001, Informa Healthcare.
2. Weber KT, Janicki JS, Shroff SG, et al: The cardiopulmonary unit: the body's gas transport system. *Clinics in Chest Medicine* 4:101–110, 1983.
3. Barrett KE, Brooks H, Boitano S, et al: *Ganong's Review of medical physiology*, ed 23, New York, 2009, McGraw-Hill Professional Publishing.
4. Berne RM, Levy MN: *Cardiovascular physiology*, ed 8, Philadelphia, 2000, Elsevier.
5. Fuster V, Alexander WR, O'Rourke RA, et al: *Hurst's the heart*, ed 12, New York, 2007, McGraw-Hill.
6. Gray H, Bannister LH, Berry MM, et al, editors: *Gray's anatomy: the anatomical basis of medicine and surgery*, ed 38, Philadelphia, 1995, Elsevier.
7. Hall, JE: *Guyton and Hall textbook of medical physiology*, ed 12, Philadelphia, 2010, Elsevier.
8. Katz AM: *Physiology of the heart*, ed 4, Philadelphia, 2005, Lippincott Williams & Wilkins.
9. Lumb AB, Pearl RG: *Nunn's applied respiratory physiology*, ed 6, Philadelphia, 2005, Butterworth Heinemann.
10. Mason RJ, Broaddus VC, Martin T, et al: *Murray and Nadel's textbook of respiratory medicine*, ed 5, Philadelphia, 2010, Elsevier.
11. West JB: *Respiratory physiology: The essentials*, ed 8, Baltimore, 2008, Williams & Wilkins.
12. Cherniack RM, Cherniack L: *Respiration in health and disease*, ed 3, Philadelphia, 1983, WB Saunders.
13. Kinney MR, Packa DR: *Andreoli's comprehensive cardiac care*, ed 8, Philadelphia, 1996, Elsevier.
14. Dubin, D: *Rapid interpretation of EKGs: a programmed course*, ed 6, Tampa, Fla, 2000, Cover Publishing.
15. Wagner, GS: *Marriott's practical electrocardiography*, ed 11, Philadelphia, 2007, Lippincott Williams & Wilkins.

Chapter 4

Cardiovascular and Pulmonary Physiology

Elizabeth Dean

KEY TERMS

Control of breathing
Control of the heart
Diffusion
Electromechanical coupling
Gas exchange
Oxyhemoglobin dissociation
Mechanics of breathing
Ventilation and perfusion matching

CHAPTER OUTLINE

This chapter reviews basic cardiovascular and pulmonary physiology. A thorough understanding of normal physiology provides a basis for understanding the deficits in cardiovascular and pulmonary function (in the context of limitation of activity and social participation, as well as structure and function) and the adaptations to changing physiological and pathophysiological demands. This knowledge provides the foundation for conducting a thorough assessment and prescribing treatment.[1-8]

Cardiovascular Physiology

Control of the Heart

The mechanical activity of the heart is precisely regulated in accordance with the electrical activity of the heart to effect optimal cardiac output to the organs of the body.[9,10] The electrical activity of the heart, based on electrocardiography, in both health and pathology, is described in detail in Chapter 12. The electrical and mechanical events of the cardiac cycle and their coupling (electromechanical coupling) are summarized in Figure 4-1. These events include the spread of the wave of electrical excitation throughout the myocardium; the resulting sequence of contraction of the atria and ventricles, followed by dynamic changes in blood pressure and volume in the heart chambers; the heart sounds; and the timing of these events. The cardiac cycle takes 0.8 second in a heart beating at 75 beats per minute. Ventricular systole or ejection takes about one-third of this time. Its onset and termination are marked, respectively, by the closing and opening of the atrioventricular valves (mitral and tricuspid). Diastole, or the period between successive ventricular systoles, in which the ventricles fill with blood, takes two-thirds of the 0.8 second of each cardiac cycle.

Phases of Systole and Diastole

Ventricular systole normally has three phases: the isovolumetric contraction period, the rapid ejection period, and the slower ejection period. Ventricular diastole also has three phases: the passive rapid-filling phase, the slower filling phase (diastasis), and the active rapid-filling phase.

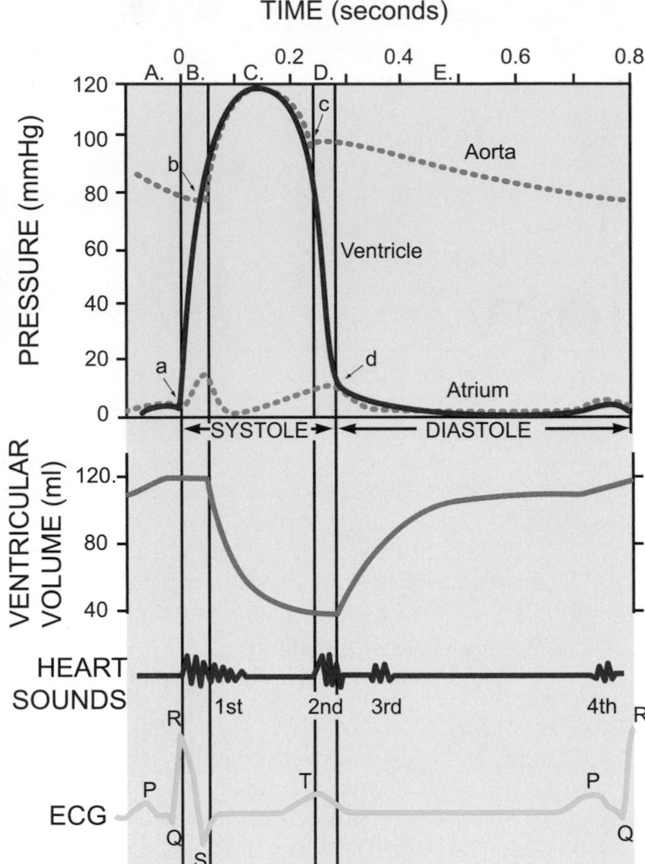

Fig. 4-1 Summary of electrical and mechanical events of the heart. *A,* Atrial systole. *B,* Isovolumetric contraction. *C,* Ejection. *D,* Isovolumetric relaxation. *E,* Rapid inflow, diastasis, and active rapid filling. Note the relationship between ventricular pressure and volume: *a,* closure of the atrioventricular valves; *b,* opening of the semilunar valves; *c,* closure of the semilunar valves; *d,* opening of the atrioventricular valves.

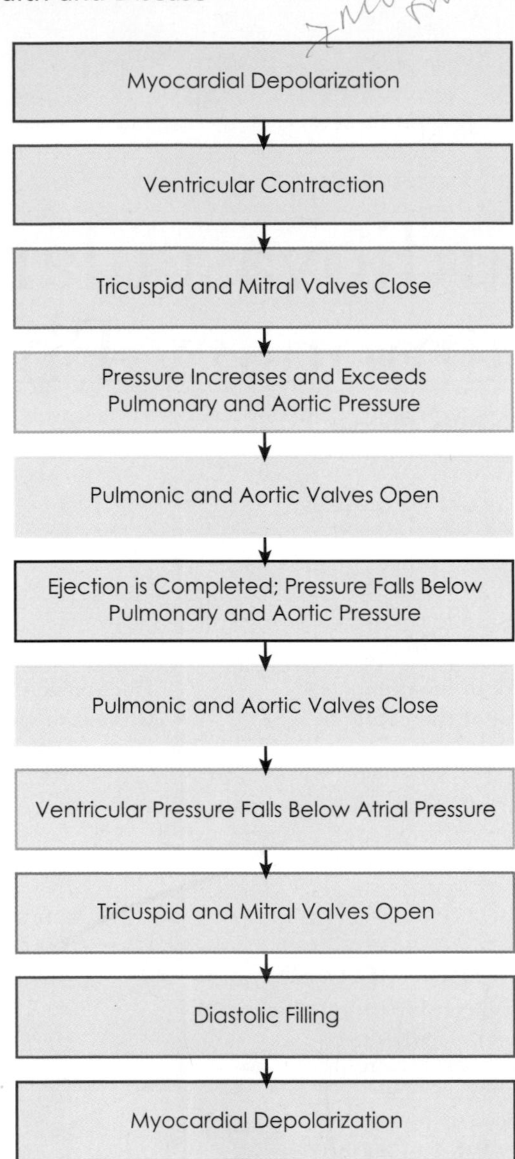

Fig. 4-2 The sequence of pressure changes in the heart during the cardiac cycle.

Cardiac Reflexes

The heart behaves automatically and is therefore termed a functional syncytium. Three primary reflexes enable the heart to increase stroke volume and cardiac output with moment-to-moment changes in myocardial demand.

The first reflex is the Starling effect, which refers to the increased force of contraction that occurs with increased venous return (preload). The second reflex, the Anrep effect, refers to the increase in ventricular contractile force as a result of an increase in aortic pressure (afterload). The third reflex, the Bowdich effect, refers to the corresponding increase in heart rate when myocardial contractile force increases. The integrated function of these three reflexes ensures that cardiac output adjusts as demands on the heart change (i.e., in healthy individuals, primarily in response to exercise, body position, and emotional stress).

Volume and Pressure Changes

Changes in the ventricular volume curve and aortic pressure wave reflect changes in atrial and ventricular pressures during systole and diastole. The sequence of events appears in a flow chart in Figure 4-2. Pressure gradients within the heart are responsible for the opening and closing of the valves. Coordinated valve opening and closure are important to promote the forward movement of blood and prevent mechanical inefficiency of the heart pump resulting from valvular regurgitation of blood during ventricular contraction. Regurgitation of blood in the retrograde direction gives rise to heart murmurs that are audible on auscultation of the heart.

Heart Sounds

The heart sounds are described as a low-pitched, long-duration sound (S_1) followed by a higher pitched, slower duration sound (S_2) that resembles the phonic sounds of LUB-dub. S_1 is associated with the closure of the atrioventricular valves. S_2 is associated with the closure of the semilunar valves. In inspiration, the aortic valve closes several milliseconds before the pulmonic valve, resulting in a splitting of the second heart sound, S_2. During inspiration, intrathoracic pressure becomes more negative, and venous return and right heart volume increase; hence pulmonary ejection is prolonged in this situation, and closure of the pulmonary valve is delayed. Other variations in splitting of S_2 occur with pathology. The presence of a third (S_3) or fourth (S_4) heart sound is usually considered abnormal. S_3 is usually associated with the passive rapid-filling phase and S_4 with the active rapid-filling phase.

Peripheral Circulation

The purpose of the peripheral circulation, including the microcirculation at the tissue level, is to provide saturated oxygenated blood and remove partially desaturated blood. The microcirculation within each organ regulates the blood flow both exogenously, via the neurological system, and endogenously, via the humoral system, commensurate with the metabolic needs of that tissue bed (see Chapter 3). The four principal factors that determine the movement of fluid in the microcirculation are the following:

1. The capillary hydrostatic pressure from the blood pressure, which tends to move blood across the capillary membrane and out of the circulation into the interstitium
2. The capillary oncotic pressure from the proteins within the blood vessels, which tends to retain fluid in the circulation
3. The interstitial hydrostatic pressure, which tends to move fluid back into the circulation
4. The interstitial oncotic pressure, which tends to draw fluid out of the circulation and into the interstitium

The net forces acting on the capillary fluid are nearly in equilibrium, with a slight tendency for fluid to be filtered out of the systemic circulation into the interstitium. Box 4-1 illustrates the mean pressures that determine normal fluid dynamics across capillary membranes.

Transport of Oxygen

Once oxygen reaches the blood, it rapidly combines with hemoglobin to form oxyhemoglobin. A small proportion of oxygen is dissolved in the plasma. The use of the hemoglobin molecule as an oxygen carrier allows for greater availability and efficiency of oxygen delivery to the tissues in response to metabolic demand. Saturation of the oxygen-carrying sites on the hemoglobin molecule is curvilinearly related to the partial pressure of oxygen in the tissues. This relationship is called the oxyhemoglobin dissociation curve and is a sigmoid, or S-shaped, curve (Fig. 4-3). The hemoglobin of arterial blood is 99%, or almost completely saturated with oxygen. Under normal circumstances, arterial blood is mixed with a small proportion of venous blood from the coronary and pulmonary circulation, resulting in arterial saturation slightly less than 100%. The graph shows a range of partial pressures of oxygen that may exist in the tissues. At relatively high arterial oxygen pressures, the oxygen saturation is high. This reflects high association or low dissociation between oxygen and hemoglobin. Saturation does not fall significantly until the partial pressure of oxygen falls below 80 mm Hg. Even at PO_2 levels of 40 to 50 mm Hg, arterial saturation is still 75%. This suggests that the oxyhemoglobin dissociation system has an enormous capacity to meet the varying needs of different tissues without severely compromising arterial saturation. A PO_2 of less than 50%, for example, has a profound effect on arterial saturation. This demonstrates an adaptive response of hemoglobin dissociation to respond to low oxygen tissue pressures by greater dissociation of oxygen from hemoglobin as the need arises. As PO_2 improves with increased supply of oxygen or decreased demand, the affinity between oxygen and hemoglobin increases, and arterial saturation increases. Thus oxygen is not released unless there is a need for greater oxygen delivery to the tissues.

Various conditions can increase or decrease hemoglobin's affinity for oxygen and thereby cause a shift in the oxyhemoglobin dissociation curve (see Fig. 4-3). A shift to the right results in decreased oxygen affinity and greater dissociation of oxygen and hemoglobin. In this instance, for any given partial pressure of oxygen, there is a lower saturation than normal. This means that there is more oxygen available to the tissues. Shifts in the curve to the right occur with increasing concentration of hydrogen ions (i.e., decreasing pH), increasing PCO_2, increasing temperatures, and increasing levels of 2,3-DPG (diphosphoglycerate), a byproduct of red blood cell metabolism. West suggests that "a simple way to remember these shifts is that an exercising muscle (increased metabolic demand), is acid, hypercapnic and hot, and it benefits from increased unloading of oxygen from its capillaries."[8]

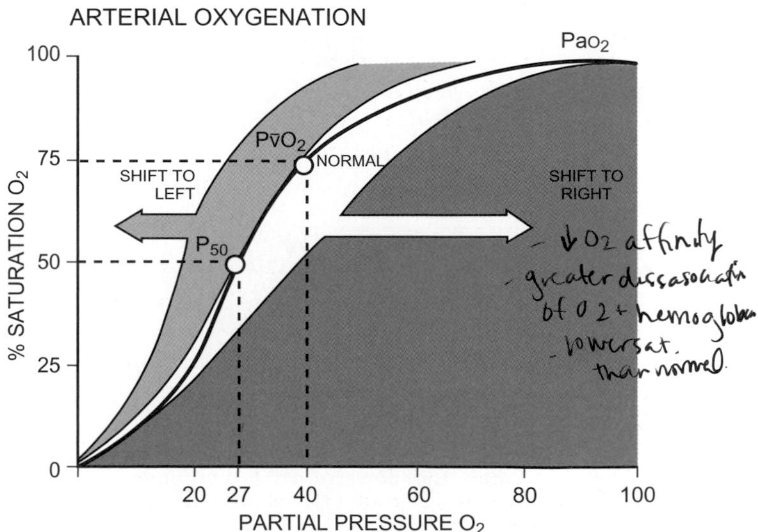

Fig. 4-3 The oxyhemoglobin dissociation curve.

Box 4-1 Balance of Forces Moving Fluid into and out of the Capillary

Mean Forces Moving Fluid out of the Capillary

Mean capillary pressure	17.0 mm Hg
Negative interstitial pressure	6.3 mm Hg
Oncotic interstitial pressure	5.0 mm Hg
Total outward pressure	28.3 mm Hg

Mean Forces Moving Fluid into the Capillary

Plasma oncotic pressure	28.0 mm Hg
Total inward pressure	28.0 mm Hg

Net Outward Pressure

28.3 (outward pressure) − 28.0 (inward pressure) = 0.3 mm Hg

A shift of the curve to the left results in increased oxygen affinity. Thus for any given partial pressure of oxygen, there is a higher saturation than normal. This means that there is less oxygen available to the tissues. This occurs in alkalemia, hypothermia, and decreased 2,3-DPG.

Anemia (reduced red blood cell count and hemoglobin) and polycythemia (excess red blood cell count and hemoglobin) produce changes in the oxygen content of the blood, as well as in its saturation. Anemia shifts the curve to the right and lowers the maximal saturation achievable. Polycythemia has the opposite effect. The curve is shifted to the left, and maximal saturation approaches 100%.

Transport of Carbon Dioxide

Carbon dioxide (CO_2) is an acid produced by cells as a result of cell metabolism. It is carried in various forms by venous blood to the lungs, where it is eliminated. Most of the CO_2 added to plasma diffuses into the red blood cells, where it is buffered and returned to the plasma to be carried to the lungs. The buffering mechanism is so effective that large changes in dissolved CO_2 can occur with small changes in blood pH.

The transport of CO_2 has an important role in the acid-base status of the blood and maintenance of normal homeostasis. The lung excretes 10,000 mEq of carbonic acid per day. (Carbonic acid is broken down into water and CO_2. The CO_2 is buffered and eliminated through the lungs.) The kidney can excrete only 100 mEq of acid per day. Therefore alterations in alveolar ventilation can have profound effects on the body's acid-base status. A decrease in the lung's ability to ventilate causes a sharp rise in P_{CO_2} and a drop in pH. This causes acute respiratory acidosis. If this change occurs gradually, the pH will remain within normal limits while the P_{CO_2} is elevated. This is known as a compensated respiratory acidosis. Hyperventilation or excessive ventilation causes rapid elimination of CO_2 from the blood. This results in a decreased P_{CO_2} and an increased pH and is known as acute respiratory alkalosis. Again, if the change occurs gradually, the pH remains within normal limits, even though the P_{CO_2} is decreased. This is a compensated respiratory alkalosis.

Cardiopulmonary Physiology

Ventilation

Ventilation is the process by which air moves into the lungs. The volume of air inhaled can be measured with a spirometer. The various lung capacities and volumes are defined in Chapter 9.

Regional differences in ventilation exist throughout the lung. Studies using radioactive inert gas with a radiation counter over the chest wall have shown that when the gas is inhaled by an individual in the seated position and measurements are taken, radiation counts are greatest in the lower lung fields, intermediate in the midlung fields, and lowest in the upper lung fields. This effect is position or gravity dependent. In the supine position, the apices and bases are ventilated comparably, and the lowermost lung fields are better ventilated than the uppermost lung fields. Similarly, in the lateral, or side-lying, position, the lower lung fields are preferentially ventilated compared with the upper lung fields (see Chapter 19).

The causes of regional differences in ventilation can be explained in terms of the anatomy of the lung and the mechanics of breathing. An intrapleural pressure gradient exists down the lung. In the upright position, intrapleural pressure tends to be more negative at the top of the lung and becomes progressively less negative toward the bottom of the lung. This pressure gradient is thought to reflect the weight of the suspended lung. The more negative intrapleural pressure at the top of the lung results in relatively greater expansion of that area and a larger resting alveolar volume. The expanding pressure in the bottom of the lung, however, is relatively small, so there is a smaller resting alveolar volume in the bottom. This distinction between the upper and lower lung fields is fundamental to understanding differences in regional ventilation. Regional differences in resting alveolar volume should not be confused with regional differences in ventilation volume. Ventilation refers to volume change as a function of resting volume. The relatively higher resting volume in the upper lung fields renders them stiffer, or less compliant, than the lower lung fields, where there are low lung volumes and greater compliance. The lower lung fields, therefore, exhibit a greater volume change in relation to resting volume, and that effects greater overall ventilation, compared with the upper lung fields. Ventilation is favored in the lowermost lung fields, regardless of body position.

Diffusion

Once air has reached the alveoli, it must cross the alveolar-capillary (A-C) membrane (Fig. 4-4). Gases, specifically oxygen entering the lungs and carbon dioxide leaving the lungs, must cross through the surfactant lining, the alveolar epithelial membrane, and the capillary endothelial membrane. Oxygen then has to travel through a layer of plasma, the erythrocyte membrane, and intracellular fluid in the erythrocyte, until it encounters a hemoglobin molecule. This distance is actually small in normal lungs, but in disease states it may increase. The alveolar wall and the capillary membrane often become thickened. Fluid, edema, or exudate may separate the two membranes. These conditions are often first detected when arterial P_{O_2} becomes chronically lower than normal. Oxygen diffuses slowly through the A-C membrane in comparison to CO_2 diffusion. As a result, patients with diffusion problems frequently have hypoxemia with a normal P_{CO_2}. Sarcoidosis, asbestosis, scleroderma, and pulmonary edema are conditions that decrease the diffusing capacity of the gases. The capacity may also decrease in emphysema because of a decrease in total surface area for gas exchange.

Perfusion

Perfusion of the lungs refers to the blood flow of the pulmonary circulation available for gas exchange. The pulmonary circulation operates at relatively low pressures compared with the systemic circulation. For this reason, the walls of the blood vessels in the pulmonary circulation are thinner than comparable vessels in the systemic circulation. Compared with the systemic circulation, the lungs have little requirement for marked regional differences in perfusion.

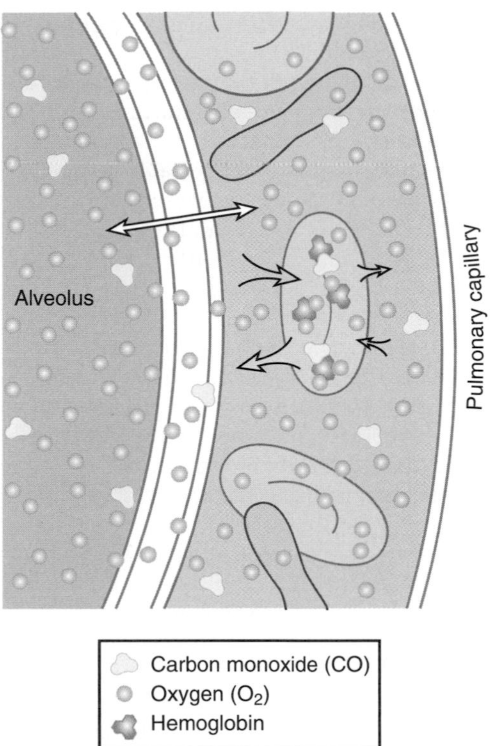

Fig. 4-4 The transfer of carbon monoxide and oxygen molecules across the alveolar-capillary membrane, through plasma, and across the red blood cell membrane. Also represented is the reaction with hemoglobin. *(From Mason RJ, Broaddus VC, Martin T, et al:* Murray and Nadel's textbook of respiratory medicine, *ed 5, Philadelphia, 2011, Saunders.)*

Hydrostatic pressure has a significant effect on the perfusion of the lower lobes. Hydrostatic pressure reflects the effect of gravity on the blood and tends to favor perfusion of the lower lung fields. This fact has been substantiated using radioactive tracers in the pulmonary circulation and measuring radiation counts over the lung fields. The nonuniformity of perfusion reflects the interaction of alveolar, arterial, and venous pressures down the lung. Normally blood flow is determined by the arteriovenous pressure gradient. In the lungs there are regional differences in alveolar pressure that can exert an effect on the arteriovenous pressure gradient. For example, in the upper lung fields, alveolar pressure approximates atmospheric pressure, which overrides the arterial pressure and effectively closes the pulmonary capillaries. In the lower lung fields, the opposite occurs. The relatively low volume of air in the alveoli is overridden by the greater capillary hydrostatic pressure. Thus the capillary pressure effectively overcomes the alveolar pressure.

Pulmonary blood vessels constrict in response to low arterial pressures of oxygen. This is termed hypoxic vasoconstriction. Hypoxic vasoconstriction in the lung is believed to serve as an adaptive mechanism for diverting blood away from underventilated or poorly oxygenated lung areas. Although hypoxic vasoconstriction may have an important role in improving the efficiency of the lungs as a gas exchanger, it may be potentially deleterious to a patient who has reduced arterial oxygen pressure secondary to pulmonary pathology.

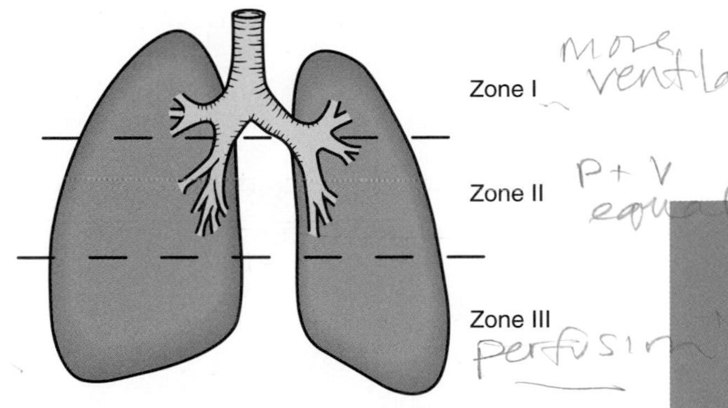

Fig. 4-5 The perfusion of the lungs is dependent on posture. In the upright position, three areas can be seen. Zone III has perfusion in excess of ventilation. In zone II, perfusion and ventilation are fairly equal. In zone I, ventilation occurs in excess of perfusion.

The acid-base balance of the blood also affects pulmonary blood flow. A low blood pH, or acidemia, for example, potentiates pulmonary vasoconstriction. Thus, impaired ventilatory function can disturb blood-gas composition and, in turn, acid-base balance. This effect can be amplified because of the cyclical reaction of pH on pulmonary vasoconstriction. Consideration of these basic physiological mechanisms is paramount to optimize physical therapy intervention.

Ventilation and Perfusion Matching

As discussed previously, gravity tends to pull blood into the dependent positions of the lung (Fig. 4-5). In erect humans, therefore, there is greater blood flow at the bases of the lung. In places, the arterial blood pressure exceeds the alveolar pressure and causes compression or collapse of the airways (Fig. 4-6). Blood flow to the apices is decreased because of gravity. Alveoli in this region are more fully expanded as a result of high transmural pressures and may further decrease blood flow by compressing blood vessels. It follows that the areas of optimal gas exchange occur where there is the greatest amount of perfusion and ventilation. This occurs toward the base of the lungs in erect humans. Changes in posture cause changes in perfusion and ventilation. Generally, greater air exchange occurs toward the gravity-dependent areas. In side-lying, there is greater gas exchange in the dependent lung (Fig. 4-7).

In normal lungs there is an optimal ratio, or matching of gas and blood. This ratio of ventilation to perfusion (V/Q) is 0.8 to maintain normal blood gas values of PO_2 and PCO_2. Therefore the lungs must be able to supply four parts ventilation to about five parts perfusion. When the ratio is not uniform throughout the lung, the arterial blood cannot contain normal blood-gas values. Regions with low ratios (perfusion in excess of ventilation) act as shunts, whereas regions with high ratios (ventilation in excess of perfusion) act as dead space (Fig. 4-8). Hypoxemia results if regions of abnormal V/Q predominate. An elevation in arterial PCO_2 may also occur unless the patient increases ventilation.

Physical therapists who are positioning patients with cardiovascular and pulmonary pathology may find that their patients experience greater distress when placed in certain positions. Such position-dependent distress can be explained

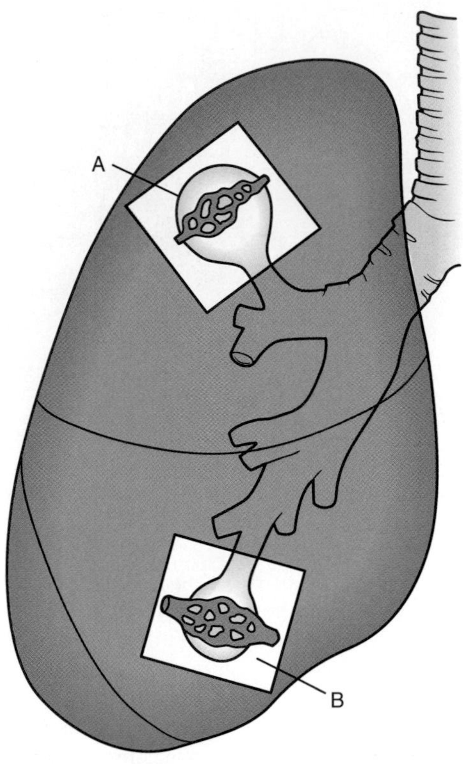

Fig. 4-6 The relationship between the size of the airways and the amount of perfusion in the area when lungs are in the upright position. **A,** Perfusion is decreased in the apices because of gravity. This enables the alveoli to expand fully. This expansion may compress blood vessels and thereby further decrease blood flow. **B,** Perfusion is increased in the bases of the lungs because of gravity. The enlarged vessels prevent full expansion of alveoli and may, in fact, compress them to a smaller size.

by ventilation-perfusion inequalities that cause poor gas exchange in the dependent lung.

The relationship of ventilation and perfusion in the lung is summarized in the following figures. Figure 4-9 shows increases in ventilation and perfusion down the upright lung. When optimal ventilation and perfusion match, V/Q occurs in the midlung zones. In the upright position, ventilation is in excess of perfusion in the apices, and perfusion is in excess of ventilation in the bases. Figure 4-10 illustrates the effects of shunt and physiological dead space on V/Q matching in the upright lung and shows their effect on alveolar gas. Specifically, Figure 4-10 shows a schematic representation of regional differences in ventilation and perfusion in the upper, middle, and lower zones of the upright lung. These gradients are reflected in the alveolar Po_2 and Pco_2 levels associated with alveolar dead space in the apices, appropriate V/Q matching in the midlung, and shunt in the bases.

Pulmonary Physiology

Control of Breathing

The act of breathing is a natural process to which most of us give little thought. Breathing unconsciously adjusts to varying degrees of activity while maintaining optimum arterial levels of Po_2 and PCO_2, whether we are resting or physically active. Sighing, yawning, hiccoughing, laughing, and vomiting are all involuntary acts that use respiratory muscles. Breathing can also be done under voluntary control. A person can stop breathing momentarily by breath holding or increase breathing by rapidly panting until he or she faints (from cerebral vascular constriction due to a decrease in arterial PCO_2).

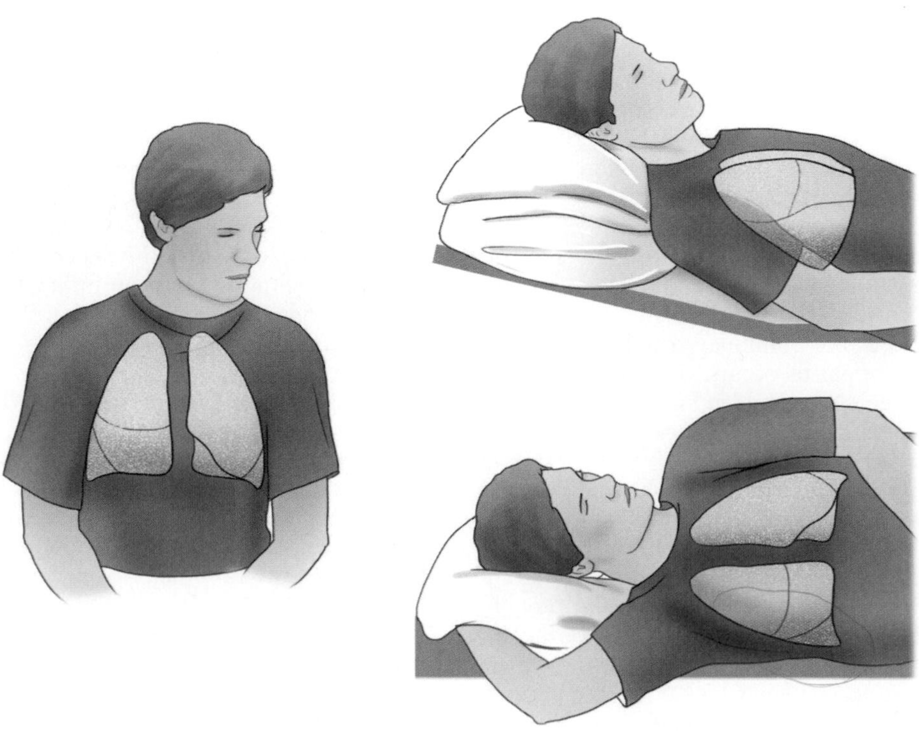

Fig. 4-7 The effect of positioning on the perfusion of the lung. Note that gravity-dependent segments have the greatest amount of perfusion.

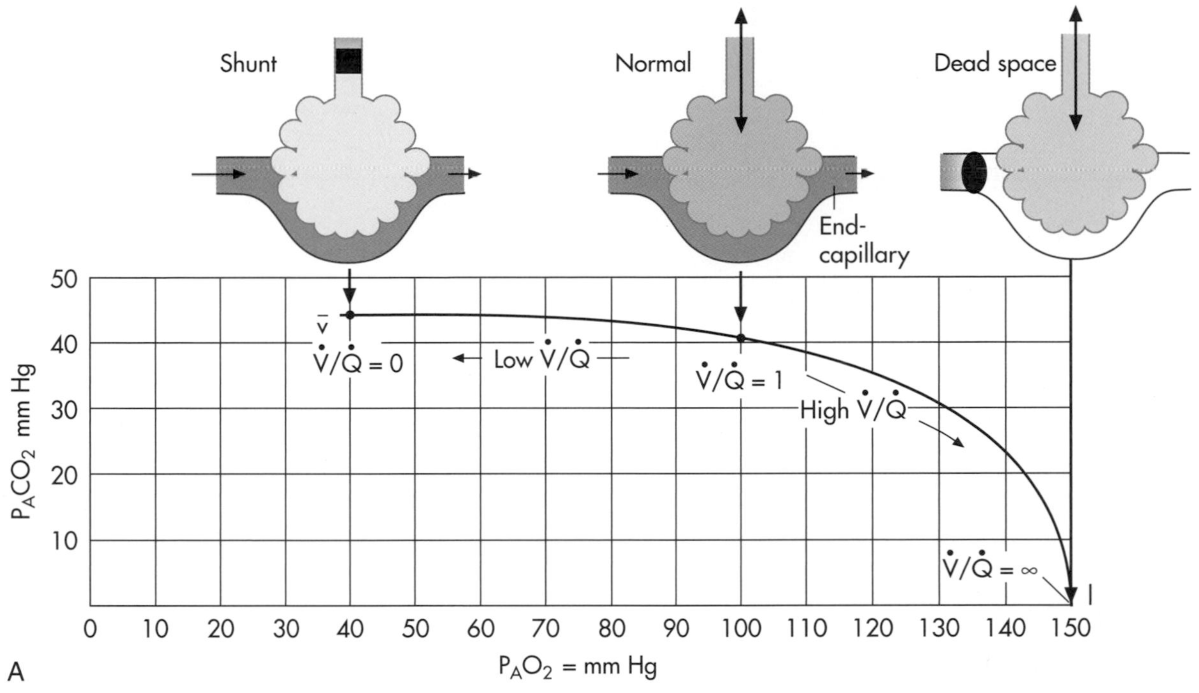

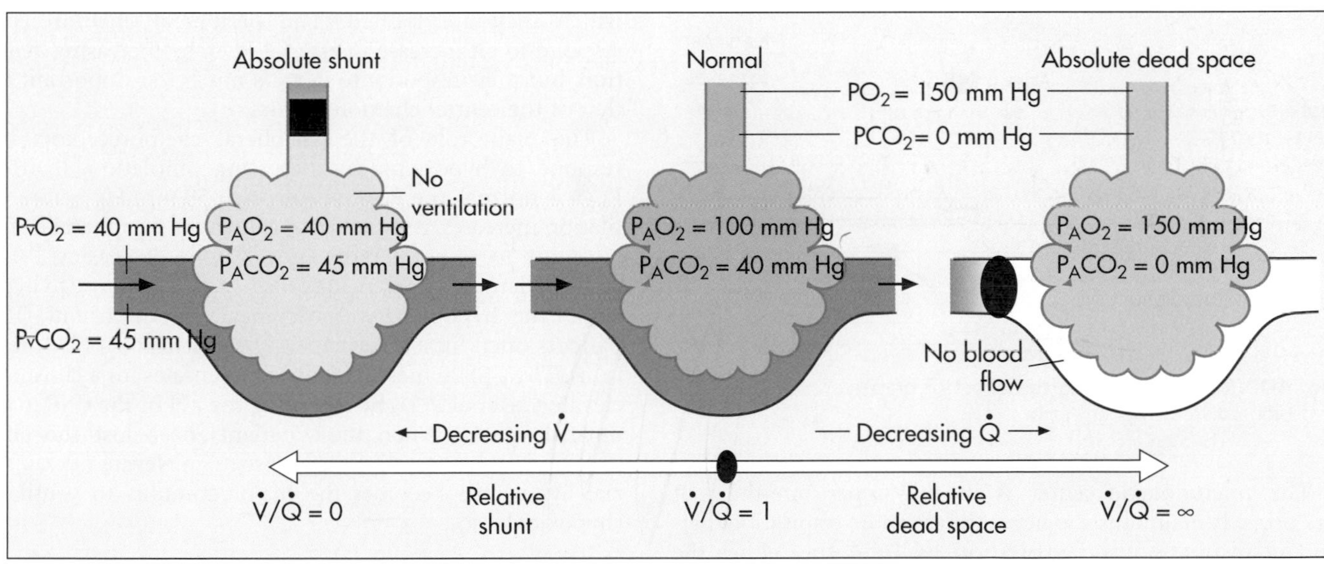

Fig. 4-8 A, The oxygen–carbon dioxide diagram. The diagonal line represents all possible PaO_2-$PaCO_2$ combinations from absolute shunt to absolute dead space in a single alveolus. The diagonal line also represents end-capillary PO_2 and PCO_2 values. $\bar{v}$ represents mixed venous blood composition; ∞ represents inspired gas composition; I represents inspired tracheal gas composition. **B,** The shunt–dead-space continuum. *(From Beachey W:* Respiratory Care Anatomy and Physiology: Foundations for Clinical Practice, *ed 2. Philadelphia, 2008, Mosby.)*

Exhalation is used in singing, speaking, coughing, and blowing, whereas inspiration is used for sniffing and sucking. Parturition, defecation, and the Valsalva maneuver are all performed while voluntarily holding one's breath. These activities are regulated by control centers located in the brain. The centers integrate a multitude of chemical, reflex, and physical stimuli before transmitting impulses to the respiratory muscles. The cerebral hemispheres control voluntary respiratory activity, whereas involuntary respiratory activity is controlled by centers located in the pons and medulla of the midbrain (Fig. 4-11).

Medullary and Pontine Respiratory Centers

The respiratory center in the medulla is in the reticular formation. It contains the minimum number of neurons necessary for the basic sequence of inspiration and expiration. Although this center is capable of maintaining some degree of respiratory activity, these respirations are not normal in character.

The apneustic center is in the middle and lower pons. If uncontrolled by the pneumotaxic center, prolonged inspiratory gasps (apneustic breathing) occur.

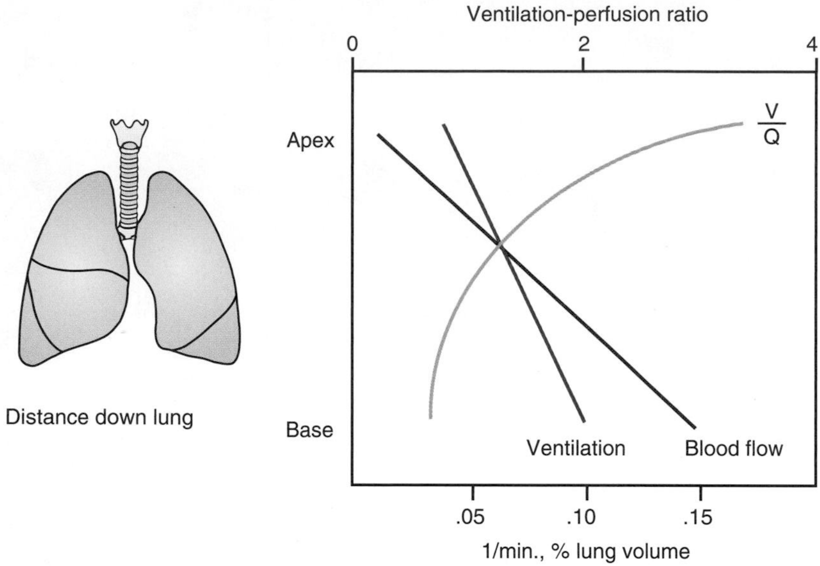

Fig. 4-9 The effect of gravity on ventilation, perfusion, and ventilation-perfusion matching (V/Q ratio).

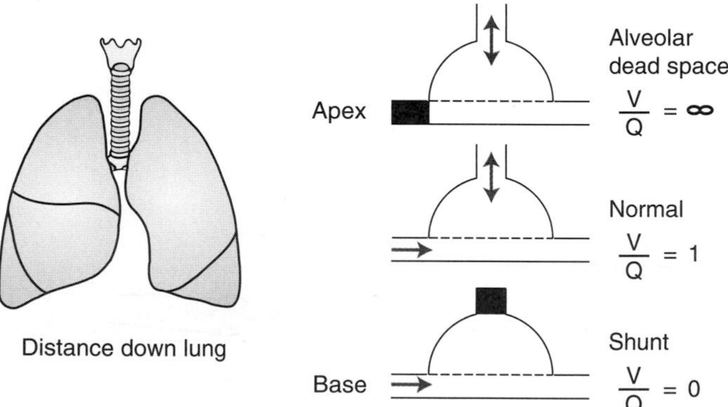

Fig. 4-10 Schemata showing the effect of gravity on ventilation and perfusion down the upright lung.

The pneumotaxic center is in the upper one-third of the pons. It maintains the normal pattern of respiration, balancing inspiration and expiration by inhibiting either the apneustic center or the inspiratory component of the medullary center.

Central Chemoreceptors

Central chemoreceptors are located on the ventral lateral surfaces of the upper medulla. They are bathed in the cerebrospinal fluid (CSF), which is separated from the blood by the blood-brain barrier. Although this barrier is relatively impermeable to hydrogen (H^+) and bicarbonate (HCO_3) ions, carbon dioxide (CO_2) diffuses through the barrier. Increased stimulation of central chemoreceptors by a rising arterial PCO_2 results in increased depth and rate of ventilation.

Peripheral Chemoreceptors

Peripheral chemoreceptors are located in the carotid bodies, which lie in the bifurcations of the common carotid artery and the aortic bodies above and below the aortic arch. These bodies receive blood from small branches of the vessels on which they are located. The peripheral chemoreceptors respond to an increase in arterial PCO_2 by increasing ventilation, but their response to PCO_2 is much less important than that of the central chemoreceptors.

The main role of the peripheral chemoreceptors is to respond to hypoxemia by increasing ventilation. If arterial PCO_2 is normal, the PO_2 must drop to 50 mm Hg before ventilation increases. A rising PCO_2 causes the peripheral chemoreceptors to respond more quickly to a decreasing PO_2. In some patients with severe lung disease, this response to hypoxemia (the hypoxic drive) becomes very important. These patients often have a permanently elevated PCO_2 (CO_2 retention). The CSF in these patients compensates for a chronically elevated arterial PCO_2 by returning the pH of the CSF to near normal values. When these patients have lost the ability to stimulate ventilation in response to an elevated PCO_2, arterial hypoxemia becomes the major stimulus to ventilation (hypoxic drive).

Reflexes

Hering-Breuer Reflex

In the late 1800s, Hering and Breuer noted that distention of anesthetized animal lungs caused a decrease in the frequency of inspiration and an increase in expiratory time. Receptors for this reflex are thought to lie in the smooth muscle of airways from the trachea to the bronchioles. More than 800 mL of lung volume above functional residual capacity are needed to activate the reflex and delay the next breath.

Cough Reflex

Mechanical or chemical stimuli to the larynx, trachea, carina, and lower bronchi result in a reflex cough and bronchoconstriction. The high velocity created by the cough sweeps mucus and other irritants up toward the pharynx (see Chapter 23).

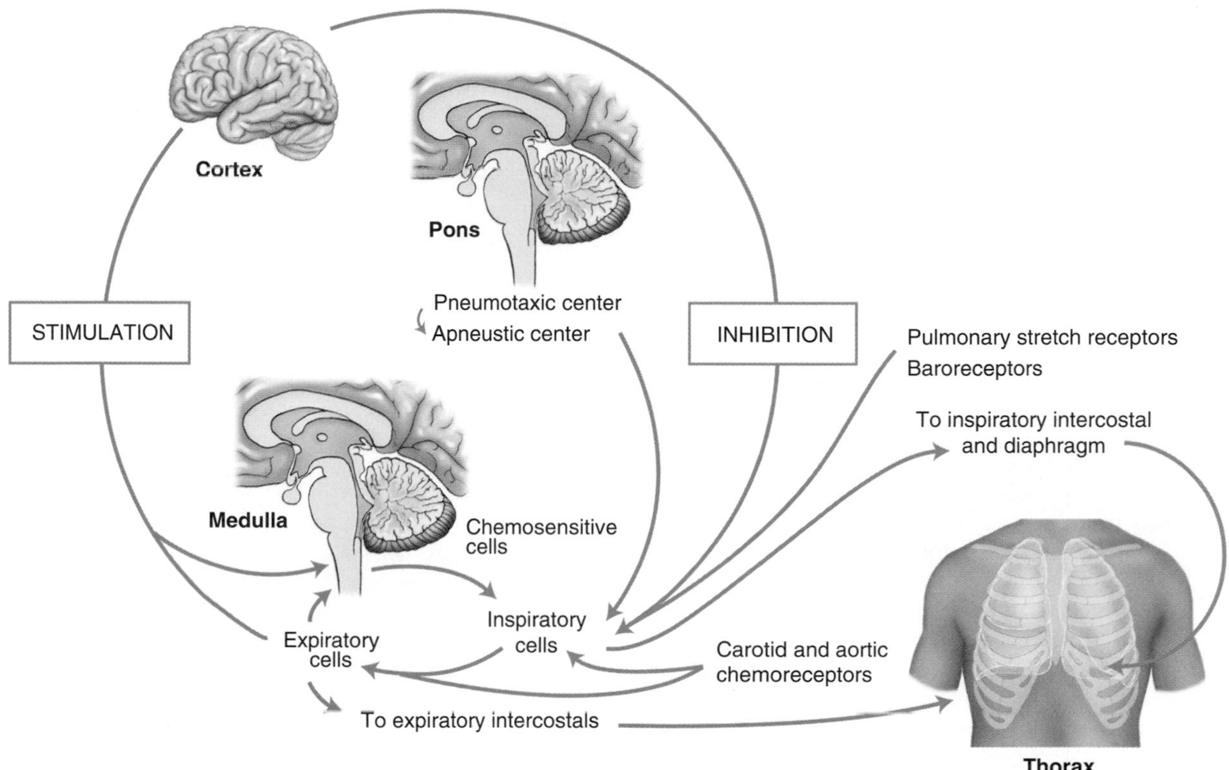

Fig. 4-11 Control of breathing.

Stretch Reflex

The intercostal muscles and the diaphragm contain sensory muscle spindles that respond to elongation. A signal is sent to the spinal cord and anterior horn motor neurons. These neurons signal more muscle fibers to contract (recruitment) and thus increase the strength of the contraction. Theoretically, such a stretch reflex may be useful when there is an increase in airway resistance or a decrease in lung compliance. Stretching the ribs and the diaphragm may activate the stretch reflex and help the patient take a deep breath. The fundamental pathways of the stretch reflex are shown in Figure 4-12. Research is needed, however, to establish the therapeutic role of proprioceptive neurofacilitation techniques based on stretch reflex theory in altering pulmonary function.

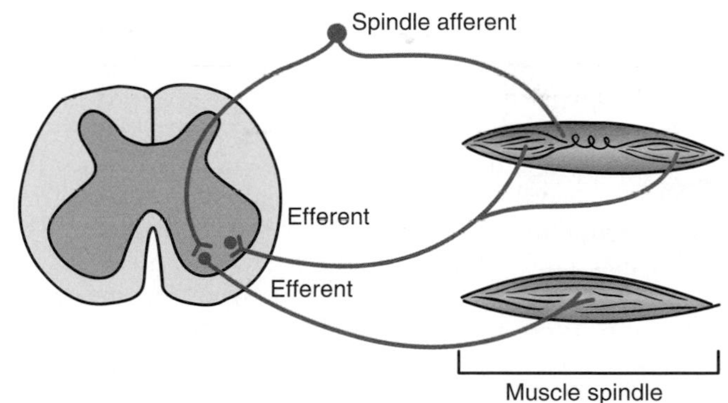

Fig. 4-12 Stretch reflex.

Joint and Muscle Receptors

Peripheral joints and muscles of the limbs are believed to have receptors that respond to movement and enhance ventilation in preparation for activity. Ventilation has also been shown to be stimulated by a similar reflex in humans and anesthetized animals in response to passive movement of the limbs. The precise pathways for these reflexes have not been well established.

Mechanoreceptors

Changes in systemic blood pressure cause corresponding changes in pressure receptors in the carotid and aortic sinuses. Increase in blood pressure causes mechanical distortion of the receptors in these sinuses, producing reflex hypoventilation. Conversely, a reduction in blood pressure can result in hyperventilation.

Mechanical Factors in Breathing

The flow of air into the lungs is a result of pressure differences between the lungs and the atmosphere. In normal breathing, inspiration occurs when alveolar pressure is less than atmospheric pressure. Muscular contraction of the respiratory muscles lowers alveolar pressure and enlarges the thorax. The decreased pressure causes air to flow from the atmosphere into the lungs. Patients who are unable to create adequate negative pressure may have to be mechanically ventilated. The ventilators create a positive pressure (greater than atmospheric pressure) that forces air into the lungs, where there is atmospheric pressure. The iron lung used during the poliomyelitis epidemic of the 1950s assisted ventilation by using cycles of negative pressure to inflate the lungs.

Exhalation occurs when alveolar pressure is greater than atmospheric pressure. At the cessation of inspiration, the respiratory muscles return passively to their resting positions.

The diaphragm rises, compressing the lungs and thereby increasing alveolar pressure. As the intercostals relax, the ribs resume their preinspiratory position, further compressing the lungs and increasing alveolar pressure. The increased alveolar pressure contributes to air flowing from the lungs. Normally, expiration is a passive process reflecting the elastic recoil of the lung parenchyma.

Resistance to Breathing

COMPLIANCE

The inner wall of the thorax, which is lined with parietal pleura, and the parenchyma of the lung, which is enclosed in visceral pleura, lie close to each another. The pleurae are separated by a potential space containing a small amount of pleural fluid. Muscular contraction of the intercostals and the diaphragm mechanically enlarges the thorax. The lungs are enlarged at this time because of their close proximity to the thorax. The healthy lung resists this enlargement and tries to pull away from the chest wall. The ease with which the lungs are inflated during inspiration is known as compliance and is defined as the volume change per unit of pressure change. Normal lungs are very distensible or compliant. They can become more rigid and less compliant as a result of diseases that cause alveolar, interstitial, or pleural fibrosis, or alveolar edema. Compliance increases with age and in emphysema, because of the loss of elastin.

The elastic recoil or compliance of the lung is also dependent on a surface fluid called surfactant, which lines the alveoli. This fluid increases alveolar compliance by lowering the surface tension, thereby reducing the muscular effort necessary to ventilate the lungs and keep them expanded. It is a complex lipoprotein that is produced in type II alveolar cells (see Chapters 2 and 4). A decrease in surfactant causes the alveoli to collapse. Reexpanding these alveoli requires a tremendous amount of work on the part of the patient. The patient may become fatigued and need mechanical ventilation. This occurs in respiratory distress syndrome in premature infants (previously called hyaline membrane disease) and in acute respiratory distress syndrome in adults. In another disease, alveolar proteinosis, there is excessive accumulation of protein in the alveolar spaces. This may be because of excessive production of surfactant or deficient removal of surfactant by alveolar macrophages.

The elastic properties of the lungs tend to collapse them if not counterbalanced by external forces. The tissues of the thoracic wall also have elastic recoil, which causes them to expand considerably if unopposed. These two forces oppose each other, keeping the lungs expanded and the thoracic cage in a neutral position. If these forces are interrupted (as in pneumothorax), the lung collapses and the thoracic wall expands (Fig. 4-13). Similarly, the overinflated, barrel-shaped chest of a patient with chronic obstructive pulmonary disease (COPD) is caused by the elastic tension of the chest wall being unopposed by the usual elastic forces of the lungs, which have been damaged by disease.

Pressure-Volume Relationships

Pressure-volume curves help define the elastic properties of the chest wall and lungs. The elasticity of the respiratory system as a whole is the sum of its two major components, the lungs and the chest wall. The so-called relaxation pressure curve is shown in Figure 4-14. The curve illustrates the static pressure of the lungs and chest wall and the combination of the two measured at given lung volumes. Functional residual capacity (FRC) reflects the balance of elastic forces exerted by the chest wall and the lungs and has significant implications for the clinical presentation and management of patients with cardiovascular and pulmonary dysfunction.

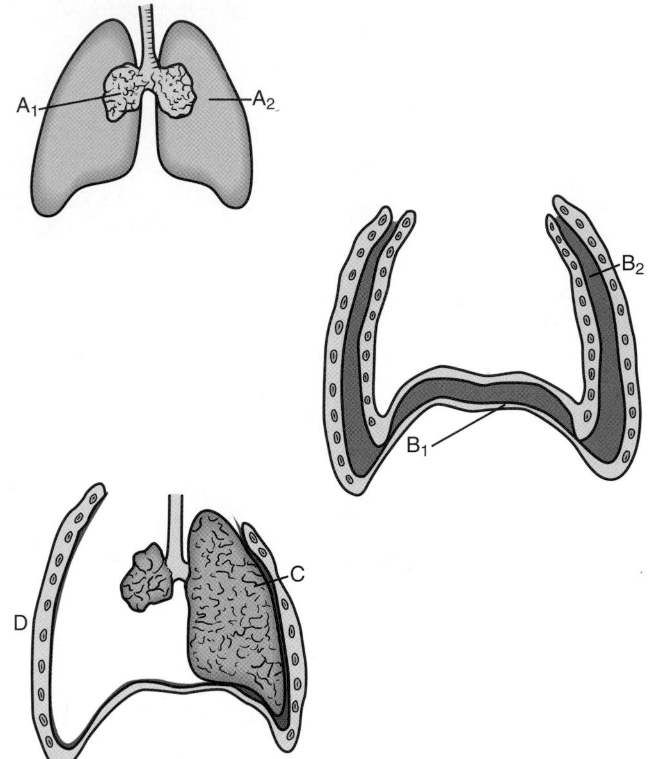

Fig. 4-13 Various relationships between the lungs and the thorax. *A_1*, The size the lungs would assume if they were not acted on by the elastic recoil of the thoracic wall. *A_2*, The normal size of lungs within the thorax. *B_1*, The size the thorax would assume if it were not acted on by the elastic recoil of the lungs. *B_2*, The normal position of the chest wall when acted on by the elastic recoil of the lungs. *C*, The normal relationship of lungs to thorax. *D*, The positions assumed by the lungs and thorax in a tension pneumothorax.

The relaxation pressure curve represents static pressure measurements. This means that the respiratory muscles are inactive, and the volume in the lungs at a given point in the respiratory cycle is determined by the balance of forces between the chest wall and the lungs. The chest wall and lungs exert elastic forces that oppose each other. The chest wall attempts to pull the lung out, and the lungs attempt to recoil and pull the chest wall in. The curves labeled "lung" and "chest wall" (see Fig. 4-14) are theoretical and illustrate the elastic force exerted by each when it is permitted to act unopposed by the other. Normally these two forces are exerted together, producing the pressure-volume relaxation curve. At FRC, these forces are in equilibrium; therefore this capacity constitutes the resting volume of the respiratory system.

In lung disease, the balance between chest wall and lung forces is disrupted.[11] More work and energy are required to sustain the respiratory effort.[12] The patient is less able to rely on normal elastic recoil of the chest wall, lungs, or both.

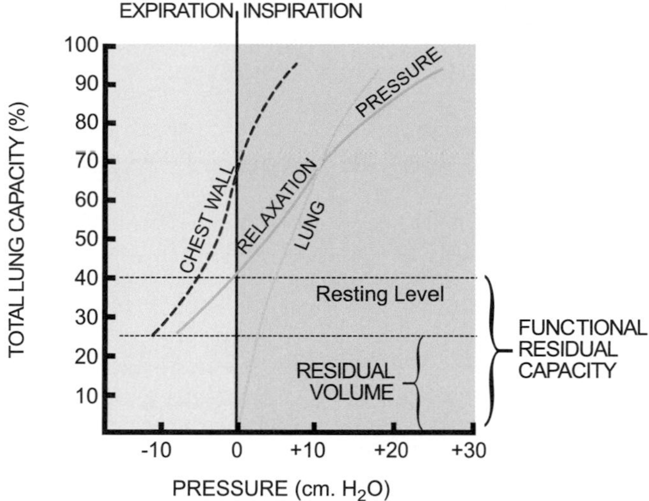

Fig. 4-14 The relaxation pressure curve. The pressure in the lungs at any volume reflects the elastic forces of the lungs and chest wall.

Therefore the patient must expend more energy to effect equivalent respiration. The limits of respiratory excursion are determined by both elastic and muscular forces. At total lung capacity, the elastic forces of the respiratory system are balanced by the inspiratory muscle force. At residual volume, the elastic forces of the chest wall are balanced by the maximum expiratory muscle force. This volume excursion from total lung capacity to residual volume reflects vital capacity.

Although the curves representing the elastic forces of the lungs and chest wall are theoretical, they are helpful in understanding the effect of lung dysfunction on pulmonary function and on the clinical presentation of the patient.[11] For example, in individuals with COPD, the characteristic barrel chest reflects the unopposed elastic forces of the chest wall as it succeeds in increasing the excursion of the chest as a result of reduced elastic recoil of the lungs. At the other extreme is the effect on the chest wall of a puncture wound, which disrupts the intrapleural pressure gradient that normally keeps the lung expanded and the chest wall contained. The result of such a puncture is to produce a pneumothorax in which the lung collapses down to the hilum and the chest wall springs outward (see Fig. 4-13).

AIRWAY RESISTANCE

The flow of air into the lungs depends on pressure differences and on the resistance to flow in the airways. Resistance is defined as the pressure difference required for one unit flow change. The air passages are divided into upper and lower airways (see Chapter 3). The upper airways are responsible for 45% of airway resistance. The resistance to airflow by the lower airways depends on many factors and is therefore difficult to predict. The branching of the lower airways is irregular, and the diameter of the lumen may vary because of external pressures and because of the contraction or relaxation of bronchial or bronchiolar smooth muscle. The lumen diameter may also decrease as a result of edema or mucus. Any of these changes in the airway diameter may cause an increase in airway resistance. Flow of air through these airways can be either laminar or turbulent (Fig. 4-15). Laminar flow is a

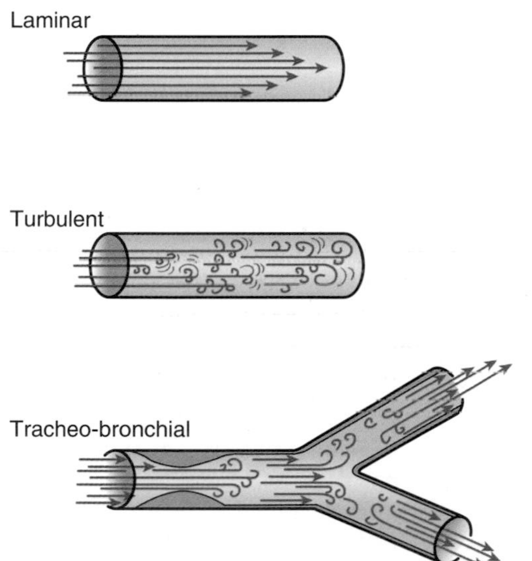

Fig. 4-15 The different types of airflow seen within the tracheobronchial tree.

streamlined flow in which resistance occurs mainly between the sides of the tubes and the air molecules. It tends to be cone shaped, with the molecules in contact with the walls of the tubes moving more slowly than the molecules in the middle of the tube. Turbulent flow occurs when there are frequent molecular collisions in addition to the resistance of the sides of the tubes. This type of flow occurs at high flow rates and in airways where there are irregularities caused by mucus, exudate, tumor, or other obstructions. In normal lungs, airflow is a combination of laminar and turbulent flow and is known as tracheobronchial flow.

The airways are distensible and compressible and thus susceptible to outside pressures. As these pressures compress the airways, they alter airway resistance. Transmural pressure is the difference between pressures in the airways and pressures surrounding the airways. In erect humans, there is a higher transmural pressure at the apices of the lungs than at the bases. This expands the alveoli at the apices relative to those at the bases. Although the alveoli in the apices have a greater volume at end expiration, the alveoli in the bases are better ventilated. This is because the alveoli in the bases operate at lower transmural pressures and can therefore accommodate a greater volume during inspiration than those at higher pressures.

Airway resistance decreases during inspiration as a result of the widening of the airways. During expiration, airways narrow, which increases resistance. The positive alveolar pressure that occurs during expiration partially compresses the airways. If these airways have lost their structural support as a result of disease, they may collapse and trap air distally (as in emphysema).

Summary

This chapter presents an overview of cardiovascular and pulmonary physiology with respect to breathing control and the central and peripheral mechanisms, such as muscle, joint, and lung and chest wall stretch receptors, involved in the regulation of respiration. The mechanics of breathing, chest wall and lung compliance, and airway resistance are described. The elastic properties of the respiratory system (i.e., chest wall and lungs) are reflected in the pressure-volume relaxation curve. This curve enables the physical therapist to better understand the efficiency and energy requirement of the respiratory system in their patients with cardiopulmonary dysfunction. Ventilation and perfusion matching is the basis of gas exchange and the adequacy of lung function. Many factors in addition to disease, however, can affect ventilation and perfusion matching, including age, body position, exercise, breathing at low lung volumes, and smoking history. The function of the heart is to provide adequate cardiac output, hence, adequate oxygen delivery to the vital organs and peripheral tissues. The optimal coupling of electrical and mechanical events in the heart to effect cardiac output is described.

Arterial Po_2 and Pco_2 are normally maintained within certain prescribed limits. In healthy individuals, oxyhemoglobin dissociation ensures adequate oxygen delivery to the tissues once oxygen has diffused through the alveolar capillary membrane into the circulation. Transport of CO_2 and its buffering mechanisms are central to acid-base balance and normal homeostasis.

Review Questions

1. Describe the control of breathing.
2. Explain the mechanics of breathing with respect to the chest wall and lung compliance.
3. Describe the distributions of ventilation, perfusion, and diffusion.
4. Explain the determinants of ventilation and perfusion matching.
5. Describe electromechanical coupling in the heart.
6. Describe the oxyhemoglobin dissociation curve and its clinical implications.

References

1. Barrett KE, Barman SM, Boitano S, et al: *Ganong's review of medical physiology*, ed 23, New York, 2009, McGraw-Hill.
2. Berne RM, Levy MN: *Cardiovascular physiology*, ed 8, St Louis, 2001, Mosby.
3. Fuster V, O'Rourke RA, Walsh R, et al: *Hurst's the heart*, ed 12, New York, 2008, McGraw-Hill.
4. Hall JE: *Guyton and Hall textbook of medical physiology*, ed 12, Philadelphia, 2010, Elsevier.
5. Katz AM: *Physiology of the heart*, ed 4, Philadelphia, 2005, Lippincott Williams & Wilkins.
6. Lumb AB, Pearl RG: *Nunn's applied respiratory physiology*, ed 6, Philadelphia, 2004, Butterworth Heinemann.
7. Mason RJ, Broaddus VC, Martin T, et al: *Murray and Nadel's textbook of respiratory medicine*, ed 5, Philadelphia, 2010, Saunders.
8. West JB: *Respiratory Physiology: The essentials*, ed 8, Baltimore, 2008, Lippincott Williams & Wilkins.
9. Dubin D: *Rapid interpretation of EKGs: a programmed course*, ed 6, Tampa, Fla., 2000, Cover Publishing.
10. Kinney MR, Packa DR: *Andreoli's comprehensive cardiac care*, ed 8, Philadelphia, 1996, Elsevier.
11. West JB: *Pulmonary pathophysiology: The essentials*, ed 7, Philadelphia, 2007, Lippincott Williams and Wilkins.
12. Jones AYM, Dean E, Chow CCS: Comparison of the oxygen cost of breathing exercises and spontaneous breathing in patients with chronic obstructive pulmonary disease. *Physical Therapy*, 83:424–431, 2003.

Cardiovascular and Pulmonary Pathophysiology

Elizabeth Dean

KEY TERMS

Acute coronary syndromes
Anemia
Angina
Athletic heart syndrome
Bronchiectasis
Chronic bronchitis
Coronary artery disease
Emphysema
Hypertension
Lung cancer
Myocardial infarction
Noncardiovascular and pulmonary conditions
Obstructive lung disease
Restrictive lung disease
Scleroderma
Syncope
Tuberculosis

CHAPTER OUTLINE

Because cardiovascular and pulmonary conditions are among the leading causes of morbidity and premature mortality, they often present clinically to the physical therapist as secondary as well as primary diagnoses. In addition, patients commonly have one or more risk factors for one or both of these broad categories of conditions. Thus physical therapists need a thorough understanding of these conditions, their prevention, their presentation, and their management. Lifestyle and environmental factors are primary causes and contributors (see Chapter 1); thus prevention and reversal of symptoms are aimed at modifying these factors wherever possible.

Smoking is a principal contributor to cardiovascular disease and the primary cause of chronic obstructive pulmonary disease (COPD). Abstinence from smoking is the only intervention that can prevent the majority of cases of COPD, and smoking cessation is the only intervention to retard its progression. Thus cessation of smoking is a primary health care goal at the community, societal, and individual levels,[1,2] and it should be a primary intervention by the physical therapist in any patient who smokes (see Chapter 1).

Risk factors for cardiovascular and pulmonary conditions should be assessed in every patient, irrespective of the reason for physical therapy referral or management. An individual with an overt history of cardiovascular or pulmonary conditions is managed based on the related signs and symptoms. However, if a patient comes to the physical therapist with dysfunction of the musculoskeletal, neuromuscular, or other system and happens to have a secondary diagnosis of a cardiovascular or pulmonary condition, this diagnosis must be considered in overall management and the interventions modified accordingly. Because it is life-threatening, a secondary diagnosis of a cardiovascular or pulmonary condition may be more clinically important for the physical therapist to manage than the primary diagnosis (e.g., low back pain, osteoarthritis, or Parkinson syndrome).

Recent advances in understanding the pathophysiology of cardiovascular and pulmonary conditions have highlighted a common denominator: inflammation of the endothelium of the blood vessels and the epithelium of the airways. With increasing severity of the condition, proteins alter their structure, and repair is required to maintain their essential structure and function with the upregulation of reparative proteins.[3] Activation of this defense system is triggered by ischemia, hypoxemia, and inflammation.

Myopathic changes have been observed in the peripheral muscles of people with chronic cardiovascular conditions and lung conditions (see Chapters 24 and 31). People with COPD, for example, have increased muscle fibrosis compared with age-matched people without the disease, and the cross-sectional area of type IIX muscle fibers is smaller.[4]

Some common causes underlying COPD have been proposed. The Dutch hypothesis explaining the development of both asthma and chronic obstructive lung disease proposes that environmental factors (e.g., smoking and air pollutants) are superimposed upon and interact with allergic and airway hyperresponsiveness components (genetic components). Smoking and airway hyperresponsiveness are the major risk factors for these conditions.[5]

It has been reported that gender plays a role in susceptibility to cardiovascular and pulmonary dysfunction, as well as in the severity of the dysfunction and the response to its management. This is reflected in the finding that women with COPD have an almost three-fold greater death rate than men. Specifically, women are more susceptible to the long-term adverse effects of smoking. Compared with men, they develop pathological changes more readily and have more severe symptomatology for a given long-term exposure to tobacco.[6]

The Global Initiative for Chronic Obstructive Lung Disease (GOLD) has proposed universal guidelines for the classification of COPD[7] on the basis of both spirometry and clinical symptoms to define stage of disease (Table 5-1). Serum or tissue markers are being sought to provide a basis for an objective diagnosis and refine intervention strategies.[8]

Objective measures of limitations of structure and function or impairments associated with cardiovascular and pulmonary conditions are not necessarily closely associated with health-related quality of life. Outcome measures of health-related quality of life and life satisfaction are supplemental to structure and function outcomes and are now being included in the overall clinical assessment of people with these conditions.[9] Thus management programs focus on interprofessional rehabilitation consisting of multiple components to address the complexity of the limitations associated with these conditions rather than traditional primary focus on limitations of functions and structures (see Chapters 1 and 17).[10]

Table 5-1 Universal Guidelines for the Classification of COPD

	Predicted FEV_1/FVC	FEV_1
Mild COPD	<70%	≥80%
Moderate COPD	<70%	<50% to 80%
Severe COPD	<70%	<30%

From Crapo RO, Morris AH, Gardner RM: Reference spirometric values using techniques and equipment that meet ATS recommendations, Am Rev Respir Dis *123:659-664, 1981.*

This chapter describes common pathophysiology of the cardiovascular and pulmonary systems and some common conditions that affect these systems secondarily.

The first part of this chapter describes the pathophysiology of common cardiovascular conditions. CAD is manifested in various clinical syndromes and most commonly results from atherosclerosis in the coronary arteries, which ultimately affects heart performance (i.e., stroke volume and heart rate, hence, cardiac output). The causes of clinical syndromes associated with CAD and the medical management and prognoses are briefly reviewed.

The two classic types of lung pathophysiology (obstructive and restrictive) are then presented. Interdependent pathophysiology of these lung pathologies, which invariably affects the heart as well as the lung, is described in Chapters 6 and 31 (also in Chapters 16, 34, and 36, which are related to critical care). The structure and function of the cardiovascular and pulmonary systems are interdependent (see Chapters 2, 3, 4, 5 and 6).[11] Dysfunction in one system can affect the function of the other.

Obstructive pulmonary conditions are characterized by a reduced expiratory airflow rate due to increased airway resistance. Restrictive pulmonary conditions are marked by the reduced inspiratory capacity of the lungs. Often, however, overlap exists between the two categories.

Coronary Artery Disease

Hypercholesterolemia

Although hypercholesterolemia is a primary risk factor for the development of atherosclerosis, increased cholesterol affects cardiac function independently in the absence of atherosclerosis and primary ischemic heart disease.[12] Elevated cholesterol levels change the structure and function of cell membranes, which in turn, affects myocardial contractility, excitability, and conduction properties. In addition, smooth muscle and endothelial dysfunction occurs, and enzyme activity and cation transporters are disrupted throughout the cardiovascular system. Thus the consequences of hypercholesterolemia are pervasive and warrant assessment even in the absence of overt atherosclerosis and ischemic heart disease.

Atherosclerosis

Pathophysiology

Atherosclerosis is triggered by trauma to the intima of the arterial wall. The trauma may be related to various primary cardiac risk factors, such as high blood pressure and cigarette smoking. Oxidative stress has been identified as the common denominator for atherogenesis, acute myocardial infarction (MI), and heart failure.[13] Healthy endothelium is central to optimal vascular control. High blood pressure has been identified as a trauma inducer because increased pressure and turbulence can damage the endothelial cells of the intima of the blood vessel wall, thus exposing the media to the circulation. The media, which consists primarily of smooth muscle, is thought to be the origin of the atherosclerotic lesion.

Cigarette smoking has also been identified as a potential inducer of trauma in the blood vessel wall. The hypothesized mode of injury appears to be different from that observed with increased blood pressure. Cigarette smoke is high in carbon monoxide and hydrocarbons that are carried by the red blood cells and the plasma. The hydrocarbons and carbon monoxide are thought to bind to the endothelial cells, causing damage to and possibly death of these cells.

Diabetes is another risk factor for cardiovascular disease of the myocardium and of the peripheral arteries.[14] The reduced contractility of the heart in people with diabetes is attributed to reduced calcium handling in the sarcoplasmic reticulum of muscle.

Once the media is exposed to the circulation, the process of atherosclerosis is initiated and this predisposes an individual to thromboembolic events, in even mild cases. Platelets aggregate at the injury site and release substances that induce endothelial and smooth muscle cell replication. It is at this site that fatty streaks and fibrous plaques develop. The cause of fatty-streak development is the deposition of low-density lipoproteins (LDLs) into the smooth muscle of the media. Why this occurs is unknown, but it appears to be related to smooth muscle cell proliferation and perhaps to increased energy demands. The initial fatty streaks are generally raised only slightly and do not impede circulation. When a fibrous plaque develops, however, impingement on the vessel lumen occurs. The plaque is relatively hard and consists of connective scar-like tissue, smooth muscle, and fat. Finally, the plaque may undergo calcification or may lead to hemorrhaging if the vessel wall necroses. The result is decreased blood flow (ischemia) and oxygenation (hypoxia) or complete lack of blood flow and oxygen (anoxia) to the target organ.

Atherothrombosis is a generalized and diffuse progressive process affecting multiple vascular beds.[15,16] The clinical consequences include the acute coronary syndromes, ischemic stroke, and peripheral arterial disease. Thus these conditions can be viewed as diverse manifestations of a common underlying pathology. The time course of these conditions is unpredictable; yet they can be life-threatening.

Thyroid is an important regulator of cardiac function and cardiovascular hemodynamics.[17] The effects of the physiologically active form of thyroid hormone triiodothyronine (T_3) on the systemic vasculature include relaxation of the vascular smooth muscle, hence reduced resistance and diastolic blood pressure. In hypothyroidism, cardiac contractility and cardiac output are decreased and systemic vascular resistance is increased, whereas the opposite occurs in hyperthyroidism. Cardiac dysfunction is associated with low levels of T_3.

Because of the current appreciation and understanding of the involvement of inflammation and endothelial injury in cardiovascular dysfunction, endothelial function biomarkers have been proposed as a sensitive means of evaluating cardiovascular disease.[18,19]

Risk Factors

As described earlier, high blood pressure, cigarette smoking, and hyperlipidemia are direct or primary risk factors for atherosclerosis. Secondary risk factors include age, gender, race, obesity, stress, and activity level. Modifiable risk factors include hypertension, hyperlipidemia, smoking, obesity, abnormal glucose tolerance and diabetes, stress level, and activity level. Homocysteine levels have a strong relationship with atherothrombotic disease and venous thromboembolism, and elevated levels may indicate thrombotic tendencies in individuals, particularly those who are younger, in the absence of other established risk factors.[20] Homocysteine levels can be reduced and regulated through diet by increasing fruit and vegetable intake. Recently, the tendency to panic has been implicated as a risk factor for cardiovascular disease,[21] and depression can result in a worse outcome.[22]

Vascular calcification is an established marker of atherosclerosis, which leads to increased arterial stiffness and reduced compliance and increased pulse pressure. Vascular calcification is highly correlated with mortality resulting from cardiovascular disease, particularly if diabetes or renal disease complicates the clinical presentation.[23,24] The three primary risk factors—diet, hypertension, and smoking—are modifiable by the individual, and altering the diet alone can reduce the probability of CAD five- to ten-fold.[25,26,27]

A proposed and potentially underestimated risk factor for cardiovascular disease is related to circadian rhythms.[28] It has been well established that people with heart failure have a higher rate of mortality in the early morning hours. This probably reflects diurnal variations in neurohumoral factors, including the activity of the sympathetic nervous system. The cardiac circadian clock synchronizes the response of the heart to the diurnal variations in the environment. Impairment of this mechanism could contribute to the pathogenesis of cardiovascular disease.

Aging has been implicated in lowering the threshold for the manifestation of cardiovascular disease.[29] Stiffening of the arteries increases afterload and alters left ventricular architecture. Left ventricular diastolic function changes, whereas systolic function remains unchanged.

Angina Pectoris

Angina pectoris is defined as chest pain that is related to ischemia of the myocardium. Ischemic pain, however, may be referred to the left shoulder, neck, jaw, or between the shoulder blades. In fact, pain anywhere above the umbilicus could be related to coronary ischemia. Angina can be classified as stable, unstable, or variant. People with chest pain but normal coronary arteries on angiography tend to be women, and this presentation is not as benign as previously believed.[30] With the advent of the ability to assess endothelial function, those at risk may be more readily identified and managed.

Stable Angina

Stable angina generally occurs during physical effort but may be related to stress. The individual is able to describe what type and intensity of activity causes the angina. Stable angina is characterized by substernal, usually nonradiating pain lasting between 5 and 15 minutes after relief from the initiating trigger, such as a given physical or psychological stressor. Sublingual nitrates and cessation of the activity causing the angina are indicated. Usually, the angina subsides completely with treatment. Angina brought about by emotional stress is more difficult to treat because stress cannot be stopped as easily as exercise.

Unstable Angina

Unstable angina occurs during physical exertion or psychological stress. The major difference between stable and unstable angina is the frequency, duration, and intensity of the pain. In unstable angina, the episodes are more frequent and the duration of each event is usually greater than 15 minutes. In addition, the intensity of the pain may be more severe. Unstable angina is usually an indicator of the progression of coronary artery disease. Individuals with unstable angina are at increased risk for MI. Unstable angina is less responsive to treatment with rest and sublingual nitrates. Often the individual needs to be hospitalized and treated with intravenous nitrates.

Variant Angina

Variant angina occurs while the individual is at rest, usually during waking and at the same hour. Exertion does not influence variant angina. This type of angina may benefit from rest and sublingual nitrates. Like unstable angina, the pain is intense and prolonged and can lead to infarction. In addition, dysrhythmias occur more commonly in individuals who have variant angina than in those with exertional angina (i.e., stable and unstable angina). Stable and unstable anginas reflect progressive arterial stenosis and ischemia. Variant angina is caused by a combination of stenosis and coronary artery spasm and is successfully treated with calcium channel blockers.

Prognosis of Angina

Individuals do not die of angina per se. The progression of atherosclerosis of the coronary arteries is reflected in the clinical changes that occur between the experience of angina and an MI. Even though there is no risk of mortality as a result of angina, an individual's lifestyle can change drastically. People with angina may be fearful of being active and may deny that they are having exertional chest pain. Denial, depression, anger, and hostility are common psychosocial correlates.[31] Depression and further reduction in physical activity can be associated with angina (diagnosed or undiagnosed and denied). Although restricted activity is an important component of initial treatment, low levels of activity can modify several risk factors and arrest the progression of atherosclerosis.[32] In addition, diet and exercise have been documented to reverse atherosclerosis.[25,26,33]

Obstructive Sleep Apnea Syndrome

Obstructive sleep apnea (OSA) has a greater incidence in individuals with atherosclerosis, cardiac dysrhythmias, and hypertension than in those without.[34] This has been explained in part by the presence of proinflammatory and prothrombotic factors.[35] OSA is characterized by the repetitive closing and opening of the posterior pharynx that are synchronized with breathing while sleeping, usually when recumbent. Apneic periods and arterial desaturation are also common to the syndrome. Additional pathologies common to OSA and atherosclerosis include endothelial dysfunction, increased C-reactive protein, fibrinogen, reduced fibrinolytic activities, and increased platelet activity and aggregation. OSA is now considered a risk factor for cardiovascular disease. The complications of sleep apnea syndrome are exacerbated by autonomic dysfunction as well. Sleep apnea often coexists undiagnosed in people with cardiovascular disease, activates mechanisms known to aggravate and advance cardiovascular injury, and contributes to resistance to therapeutic interventions.[34]

Myocardial Infarction

MI is defined as necrosis of a portion of the myocardium. The death of the myocardium occurs as a result of ischemia and anoxia. The vessels affected by occlusion are the right and left coronary arteries and their anterior and posterior descending branches. The right coronary artery supplies the posterior section and portions of the inferior section of the left ventricle. The left coronary artery branches and forms the circumflex and anterior descending arteries. The circumflex supplies the lateral portion of the left ventricle, and the anterior descending artery supplies the anterior portion. In addition, the right coronary artery supplies the right atrium atrioventricular bundle and the right ventricle. The left coronary artery supplies the left atrium and the primary portion of the conduction pathway. Generally, the clinical symptoms are similar to those of angina, with emphasis on extreme pressure as well as tightness over the sternal region. In addition, pain can radiate to the jaw, upper back, and shoulders (on the left more often than on the right).

MIs are categorized by location, size, and degree of involvement of the myocardial wall. The terms *small* and *large* are often used to describe MIs. Degrees of complication are also used in conjunction with size. MIs can be described as uncomplicated and complicated, based on the size of the MI and the patient's recovery. Location indicates the area of the heart involved and the coronary artery or branches that are involved. The anatomic areas of the heart are differentiated as anterior, posterior, lateral, and inferior. Finally, MIs are classified by the extent of damage to the wall. A transmural (or full-wall) infarct extends from the endocardium to the epicardium, whereas only some involvement of the ventricle wall may occur, for example, just beneath the epicardium (subepicardial) or just beneath the endocardium (subendocardial).

Silent ischemia is particularly prevalent in patients with high cardiac risk and is associated with a poor outcome.[36] Silent MIs can be detected when a patient has undergone ECG investigation or imaging for other problems.

Uncomplicated Myocardial Infarction

An uncomplicated MI is described as a small infarction with no complications during recovery. Usually the result is full recovery without a significant decrease in cardiac performance at rest and during minimal to moderate activity.[37] Location and the extent of the MI are critical with respect to outcome. MIs located in the inferior portion of the heart are considered the least clinically significant, and partial-wall-thickness MIs are less significant than transmural MIs.

TREATMENT

Initially, the treatment of a patient with an uncomplicated MI is comparable to that of a patient with a complicated MI, so the patient is cared for in a coronary care unit. The medical treatment is designed to decrease myocardial work and oxygen demand. Patients receive supplemental oxygen and are administered coronary vasodilators (nitroglycerin) to increase myocardial blood flow and analgesics to reduce ischemic pain. In addition, calcium channel blockers or beta blockers are administered to reduce the contractility and work of the myocardium. Antidysrhythmia medication may be prescribed if an aberrant cardiac rhythm is present or likely to occur.

Because the clinical course is uncomplicated, a patient's stay in the coronary care unit may be only a couple of days, with a total hospital stay of 3 to 5 days. Once the patient's condition is stabilized, management is oriented toward increasing physical activity and educating the patient and family with respect to risk factor reduction (see Chapters 29, 30, and 31).[38] This process is described as cardiac rehabilitation, phase I (see Chapter 30).

Complicated Myocardial Infarction

A complicated MI is distinct from an uncomplicated case because the patient may have one, a combination, or all four of the following complications: dysrhythmia, heart failure, thrombosis, and damage to heart structures.

DYSRHYTHMIAS

Dysrhythmias occur in 95% of patients with MIs. The type and severity of the dysrhythmia is dependent on the location and extent of the myocardial damage. Imbalance in autonomic regulation has been implicated in dysrhythmogenesis and sudden cardiac death.[39] Blunted heart rate variability has been established as a marker of sympathovagal imbalance and can serve as an indicator of cardiac risk.

The risk for serious or frequent dysrhythmias is lower in a patient with an uncomplicated MI because a small area of the myocardium is involved. Dysrhythmias that are life-threatening include complete AV heart block, ventricular-paced dysrhythmia, and ventricular tachycardia including ventricular flutter and fibrillation. In these conditions, either heart rate (comprising stroke volume, ejection fraction, and overall cardiac output) is too slow and cardiac output is impaired, or heart rate is too fast. Treatment of these conditions is immediate and requires drugs. If refractory to conservative management, cardioversion or electric shock (for flutter and fibrillation) is indicated. If a normal rhythm cannot be restored and maintained by the patient's own inherent pacemaker, an artificial pacemaker may have to be implanted.

Dysrhythmias may be present in the absence of overt myocardial ischemia or heart damage. Common dysrhythmias are presented in Chapter 4, and their clinical implications are presented in Chapter 12. One conduction abnormality that is receiving increasing attention is atrial fibrillation.[40] This dysrhythmia warrants management, given its association with thromboemboli and stroke (see Chapters 6 and 32). Furthermore, atrial fibrillation is the most common dysrhythmia associated with cardiac surgery (25% to 60%), and it leads to increased postoperative morbidity and mortality and to associated health care costs.[41,42] Atrial fibrillation has been reported to be more common in men—and also to be better tolerated by them than by women.[43]

HEART FAILURE

Another complication after MI is cardiac insufficiency and failure. Heart failure is a condition in which the heart is weakened by myocardial damage and is unable to provide cardiac output to meet the body's metabolic needs for oxygen, nutrition, and removal of waste products. When the heart experiences ischemia, the myocardium contracts with less force and conduction abnormalities may alter the mechanics of the contraction. If an area of the heart is infarcted, the affected myocardium does not contract, thus affecting overall cardiac output. Another type of heart failure not directly related to ischemia and infarction is congestive heart failure (described in the next section).

Recent terminology regarding the classification of heart failure differentiates diastolic and systolic heart failure.[44-47] Diastolic heart failure refers to the presence of the symptoms of heart failure in the absence of left ventricular dysfunction, the hallmark of systolic heart failure. Diastolic heart failure in which the left ventricle is stiff (reduced compliance and impaired relaxation resulting in increased end diastolic pressure) has been estimated to account for 40% to 50% of all cases of heart failure.[48] Diastolic dysfunction has been of increasing interest in nonprimary heart disease such as systemic sclerosis, and it appears to be more common than previously thought.[49] The two types of heart failure must be distinguished on the basis of Doppler echocardiography because their signs and symptoms are comparable. Both types are associated with marked morbidity and mortality.

Immediately post-MI, cardiac output is markedly reduced. The compensatory response of the body is to increase sympathetic and renin-angiotensin-aldosterone stimulation, resulting in increased heart rate and myocardial contractility. The result of this compensation is to normalize cardiac output to normal resting values. If myocardial damage is extensive, the kidneys compensate by retaining sodium and water to improve circulatory volume and venous return. Depending on the amount of myocardial tissue death, the individual may survive, but with resulting chronic congestive heart failure through persistent fluid retention and hypotension. If more than 40% of the left ventricle is infarcted, the result is usually cardiogenic shock followed by the death of the individual. Renin-angiotensin-aldosterone activation contributes to left ventricular remodeling, which is further augmented by vascular endothelial dysfunction, resulting in decreased nitric oxide bioavailability.[50]

Diabetic cardiomyopathy leads to heart failure independent of underlying coronary artery disease.[51] Both structural and functional abnormalities associated with diabetic cardiomyopathy have been linked to an underlying metabolic disorder. Other factors include myocardial fibrosis due to an inflammatory process, small blood vessel pathology, cardiac autonomic neuropathy, and insulin resistance.[52]

THROMBOSIS

Deep vein thrombosis (DVT) and related pulmonary emboli are largely preventable clinical complications, and when they do occur, their diagnosis may be missed in hospitalized patients.[53,54] These life-threatening complications are serious and warrant early detection. Mortality resulting from thrombi that migrate to the lungs (pulmonary emboli) is greatest initially after an acute MI. DVTs can be challenging to detect because of the lack of specificity of their clinical presentation. Another complication is increased incidence of thrombosis originating in deep leg veins and in the damaged heart itself. Thrombosis that starts in deep leg veins occurs because of lower limb inactivity and circulatory stasis. This is a complication that can be observed in patients after surgery. Emboli from a deep leg vein thrombus usually cause pulmonary complications. If the emboli are large or numerous, the result can be pulmonary tissue infarction and death. The incidence of pulmonary emboli has been reduced because patients now are usually ambulated soon after a medical event or surgery. Nonetheless, a pulmonary embolus must be considered a distinct possibility in all patients after an MI, surgery, or major trauma.

Heart, or mural wall, thrombosis can lead to an embolus lodging in the brain, intestine, kidney, artery to the extremities, or any location in the systemic arterial circulation. Usually, mural thrombi do not affect the pulmonary system because the small fragments become lodged in the capillaries and fail to access the venous system.

STRUCTURAL DAMAGE

Structural damage to the myocardium is another serious complication of MI. If the neural conduction pathway (bundle branch) located primarily within the septum is damaged, dysrhythmias result. In addition, papillary muscles that regulate heart valve closure can be infarcted. Valve incompetence leads to regurgitation and retrograde flow of blood from the ventricles, thus impeding the forward movement of blood through the heart and decreasing cardiac output. Full-thickness damage to the myocardial wall from atherosclerotic plaques significantly compromises normal cardiac function. Heart wall damage can result in ventricular aneurysms or ventricular wall rupture. Ventricular aneurysm, or the bulging of the weakened ventricular wall, occurs in transmural (full-wall-thickness) infarcts. Ventricular wall rupture, which can occur acutely after transmural infarction but is more common in the first to second week post-MI after an aneurysm, is usually fatal. Therefore, after an MI, it is critical to determine whether an aneurysm has occurred within the myocardium so that appropriate surgical intervention can be performed.

Risk factors for cardiac rupture include being female, being older, having hypertension, and experiencing the first cardiac event.[55] Clinical signs of rupture include syncope, chest pain, and jugular venous distention. In addition, defective ventricular remodeling may predispose the heart to rupturing.

TREATMENT

The treatment of a complicated MI is initially like that of an uncomplicated MI, where the patient is cared for in the coronary care unit. Similarly, medical treatment is designed to decrease myocardial work and oxygen demand. Patients receive supplemental oxygen and coronary vasodilators (nitroglycerin) to increase myocardial blood flow and analgesics to help further reduce ischemic pain. Myocardium calcium channel blockers or beta blockers are administered to reduce contractility. Finally, antidysrhythmia medication is prescribed to stabilize the electrical conduction system of the heart or if an aberrant cardiac rhythm is present.

Patients with complicated MIs require longer stays in the coronary care unit, and their total hospital stay times are longer than those of patients with uncomplicated MIs. The time in coronary care and total hospital stay are dependent on the complications that occur after the MI. Individuals with heart failure, thrombolytic events, or structural damage requiring surgery may be in the coronary care unit for a couple of weeks. Total hospital-stay times for patients with complicated MIs may exceed this length of time. Treatment after discharge from the intensive care unit, however, is similar to that of the patient with an uncomplicated MI; the goal is to increase physical activity and educate the patient and family in risk-factor reduction. The major difference in phase I cardiac rehabilitation for patients with complicated rather than uncomplicated MIs is the intensity, duration, and frequency of the initial exercise workload (i.e., a much lighter workload is prescribed for patients with complicated MI).[56] These patients also require closer monitoring. Progression is more conservative because patients are at higher risk after a complicated MI than after an uncomplicated MI.[56]

Prognosis after a Myocardial Infarction

After an MI, the prognosis depends on many factors. Compared with the patient's premorbid status, cardiovascular performance is reduced, unless the structural damage to the ventricle is minor (as in the case of many patients with uncomplicated MIs). The most important factor is the extent of ventricular damage. With early detection of transmural infarction and improvement in surgical intervention and coronary care, however, the number of acute post-MI deaths has been reduced.[38] Other critical factors include remaining cardiac capacity and cardiac status and risk factors. Even though CAD mortality has declined in the United States, the disease remains the leading cause of death in adults.

Severe infarction can necessitate emergency or elective revascularization surgery. Emergency surgery for an acute MI complicated by cardiogenic shock is associated with satisfactory long-term survival; however, perioperative risk is high.[57]

Congestive Heart Failure

Congestive heart failure (CHF) is a leading cause of hospitalization and death. It is characterized by the inability of the heart to maintain adequate cardiac output. The incidence of congestive heart failure appears to be increasing because of the prevalence of injurious lifestyle behaviors, aging, and improved survival after acute cardiac episodes.[58]

Almost half of all patients with congestive heart failure are women.[59] Smoking, diabetes, and high blood pressure are stronger risk factors for CHF in women than in men. Peripartum cardiomyopathy, which is unique to women in their childbearing years, occurs either in the late stages of pregnancy or within several months after giving birth.

The causative factors of heart failure are usually ischemia and MI secondary to ischemic heart disease. For the heart to maintain optimal blood flow to the pulmonary and systemic circulations, heart rate and stroke volume must be adequate. If heart rate is regular and within an acceptable range, stroke volume is the critical factor for maintaining adequate cardiac output. Stroke volume is a function of the amount of blood in the left ventricle at the end of diastole (preload); the amount of pressure and resistance the heart must overcome to eject blood into the systemic circulation (afterload); and myocardial contractility, which is the amount of force the left ventricle can apply to the blood within the chamber. If any one of these three variables is adversely affected, cardiac output is reduced. Progressive deterioration of myocardial contractility and dilation and fluid overload precipitate heart failure.

Dyspnea is the primary complaint of people with congestive heart failure. It can be challenging to distinguish between dyspnea resulting from CHF and dyspnea resulting from pulmonary causes. B-type natriuretic peptide (BNP) is synthesized, stored, and released in the ventricular myocardium, and it is stimulated by changes in ventricular wall tension and stretch.[60] The use of BNP holds some promise as a marker for congestive heart failure and a guide to clinical management.

Congestive heart failure is a major contributor to progressive renal dysfunction and anemia.[61] Anemia is observed in one-third of all patients with CHF. Conversely, chronic renal dysfunction can cause severe cardiac injury and is often associated with anemia. Thus congestive heart failure, chronic renal insufficiency, and anemia create a vicious circle that warrants aggressive medical management to attenuate the progression of the three conditions.

Acute Heart Failure

If an individual has a significant MI, the contractility and pumping ability of the heart is immediately reduced. The initial result is decreased cardiac output and the damming of blood in the veins. (The damming of blood in the pulmonary circulation leads to congestive heart failure, as discussed earlier.) The result is increased systemic venous pressure. This acute phase, which may reduce cardiac output to 40% of normal resting values, is short-lived, lasting only a few seconds before the sympathetic nervous system is stimulated, and the parasympathetics become reciprocally inhibited. Sympathetic innervation causes an increase in the contractility of viable myocardial tissue, and the increase in cardiac output may be 100%. In addition, sympathetic innervation increases venous return because the tone of blood vessels is increased. The result is increased systemic filling pressure and, thus, increased preload. The sympathetic reflex after MI becomes maximally operational within 30 seconds; therefore, except for some pain and fainting, individuals experiencing mild MIs may not know they have suffered a heart attack. The sympathetic response can continue if cardiac output is maintained at an adequate level at rest. Ischemic pain, however, may persist and warrants treatment.

Chronic Heart Failure

After an MI, several physiological responses occur along with sympathetic reflex compensation. The kidneys retain fluid almost immediately after an MI. A decrease in glomerular pressure secondary to decreased cardiac output is implicated. In addition, there is an increase in renin output and therefore an increase in angiotensin production. Angiotensin promotes reabsorption of water and salt from the renal tubules. The effect of moderate fluid retention is an increase in blood volume and venous return. This increases preload, hence cardiac output. If the MI was severe, however, the result can be excessive fluid retention. This results in systemic edema and overstretching of the heart due to excessive blood volume and venous return. In the chronic state, this condition is termed chronic heart failure.

Recovery of the damaged myocardium occurs after MI. New collateral arteries are formed to supply the peripheral portions of the infarcted region. This revascularization can assist marginally active cells to become fully functional again. In addition, the unaffected myocardial cells hypertrophy. In a mild to moderate MI, such recovery can result in major improvement in cardiac function and can take 6 weeks to several months, depending on extent of injury.

Gas transfer across the alveolar-capillary membrane is impeded in CHF. This may be explained by the pressure and volume overloading, which injures the alveolar blood-gas barrier, hence impairing the diffusion of blood across it.[62] In the short term these changes may be reversible. If the membrane is chronically challenged, however, the anatomic and physiological integrity of the membrane is remodeled. These changes have been associated with worsened symptoms and exercise tolerance. Further, these changes may be prognostic of patient outcome.

Cardiac remodeling is a central feature of heart-failure progression.[63] Remodeling refers to the alteration of the structure and geometry of the heart in response to myocardial insult or pressure or volume overload. Such remodeling reflects the adaptation that is needed to maintain adequate heart function with changing conditions. Increased muscle mass is one of the primary adaptations, and it usually involves left ventricular hypertrophy.[64] Adaptive hypertrophy of the left ventricle is clinically important in that it is associated with increased morbidity and mortality rates.[65] A further consequence of adaptive cardiac hypertrophy is the potential for reduced responsiveness to the metabolic and functional effects of insulin, which further contributes to the heart's hypoeffectiveness.[66] Pharmacological studies have been conducted to examine the role of drugs on the remodeling process in individuals with heart failure. Studies of the role of nonpharmacological interventions, including exercise, in cardiac remodeling have not been made.

A reciprocal relationship between CHF and diabetes has been well established.[67] People with CHF may be at increased risk for diabetes due to reduced physical activity, cellular metabolic defects, reduced muscle perfusion, and poor nutrition. The increased sympathetic stimulation associated with CHF increases insulin resistance and decreases insulin release from the beta cells of the pancreas. Both factors contribute to glucose intolerance and diabetes, which in turn lead to hyperglycemia and increased risk for cardiovascular and metabolic complications.

Even in patients with chronic heart failure, regular exercise may be associated with a protective metabolic phenotype.[68] This effect of exercise could explain why fit people have less severe MIs than nonfit people.

Compensated and Decompensated Heart Failure

Compensated heart failure is the final stage after the acute, then chronic, physiological compensation for cardiac dysfunction. In this state the heart can pump blood effectively but at a reduced cardiac output compared with the pre-MI condition. The individual's cardiac reserve, that is, the difference between maximum and resting cardiac output, is greatly reduced. With even small increases in metabolic demand through exercise, symptoms of acute failure reappear because the limits of compensation are exceeded. These symptoms include rapid heart rate, pallor, and diaphoresis.

Decompensated heart failure affects 5 million Americans and is associated with a 5-year mortality rate of almost 50%.[69] Decompensated failure occurs when the heart is so severely damaged or weakened that normal cardiac output cannot be attained. This type of failure is defined as a sustained deterioration of at least one New York Heart Association functional class, usually with evidence of sodium retention.[70] Cardiac output is insufficient to maintain normal renal function. Fluid continues to accumulate so the heart is stretched and weakened further, permitting only moderate to low quantities of blood to be pumped. In unilateral heart failure, the left ventricle may fail while the right ventricle continues to pump vigorously. Blood volume and pulmonary capillary pressure increase. If this occurs, fluid filters into the interstitial spaces of the alveoli, resulting in pulmonary edema, impaired gas exchange, and suffocation. As the heart weakens, not only is systemic blood flow compromised, so is the coronary system. The area most affected is the subendocardial region. As these cells become infarcted, the heart weakens further until other regions of the heart also become ischemic and infarcted.

Prognosis

End-stage cardiac disease without effective pharmaceutical or surgical intervention, including revascularization or heart transplantation, results in death. Intermediate measures to avert deterioration have emerged, including cardiac resynchronization therapy through biventricular pacing.[71] The addition of implantable cardioverter defibrillators may help to minimize the occurrence of sudden death in people with CHF. Left-ventricle assistance devices may be used to support the function of the failing heart until it responds to conservative management or until surgery is scheduled.[72] Surgical ventricular restoration holds some promise for reversing inappropriate remodeling of the myocardium after infarction and restoring its normal elliptical shape.[73] The primary pharmaceutical interventions used to mitigate heart failure include diuretics to reduce fluid overload and cardiac glycosides such as digitalis to improve myocardial contractility. These interventions are combined with modification of salt and fluid intake. Other factors can predict a poor outcome. Sleep apnea syndrome, for example, is common in people with CHF and is associated with a poor prognosis. As ejection fraction is decreased, the risk for thrombus formation and stroke increases.[74]

In cases where the heart has compensated poorly and remains weak and the cardiac output is minimal, heart transplant is the only recourse. Because organ donors are not readily available, the number of individuals who need new hearts far exceeds the available donor organs. Posttransplant prognosis is related to the recipient's surgical suitability and the health of the donor organ. The prognosis will also reflect the amount of cardiac reserve.

Valvular Heart Disease

Heart valve incompetence is classified as being either congenital or acquired (i.e., after a bacterial or viral infection of the heart valves) and can affect any one of the four heart valves. Surgical repair or replacement of defective mitral valves, tricuspid valves, and aortic valves constitutes a significant proportion of cardiac surgeries. Mitral and aortic valve disease is particularly common in people over 65 years of age.[75,76] In this age group, symptoms can be masked by such comorbidities as cardiovascular disease, pulmonary disease, and hypertension. Surgical repair is associated with favorable short- and long-term outcomes. Some valve defects are benign and treatment is not indicated. Some people can tolerate heart valve defects as children, but they become symptomatic with age. Currently, these types of valve defects are often corrected at birth or early in life.

One common valve defect is prolapse of the mitral valve, which is more common in women than in men and may warrant repair.

Cardiac defects may be present as secondary diagnoses in an individual being managed by a physical therapist. Such defects need to be considered in terms of an individual's capacity to respond to exercise, as well as the condition's overall effect on the individual's life. Exercise limitation secondary to heart valve disease may mask limitations due to other causes, or vice versa.

Athletic Heart Syndrome

Although physical fitness is associated with innumerable health benefits (see Chapters 1 and 18), cardiovascular adaptation to intense exercise in athletes (athletic heart syndrome) can mimic disease processes associated with cardiovascular disease.[77] Sudden cardiac death in athletes is often associated with cardiac hypertrophy, dysrhythmias, or both. In addition, cardiac episodes in athletes may reflect the manifestation of congenital abnormalities in electrical activity or mechanical function of the heart. Thus screening athletes for cardiovascular adaptation is warranted. Physical therapists involved with sports teams need to be vigilant regarding risk factors associated with the athletic heart syndrome to detect and avoid untoward events.

Systemic Hypertension

Systemic hypertension, or wide pulse pressure hypertension, has become increasingly prevalent and is implicated in multiorgan dysfunction, not only in cardiac dysfunction and failure (see Chapter 1). Systolic hypertension syndrome refers to a complex of hemodynamic maladaptations, including stiff central arteries, normal peripheral arteries, arteriolar constriction, metabolic abnormalities, cardiac hypertrophy, and increased blood pressure variability.[78] In addition to the conventional measures of hemodynamic status, measures of arterial mechanics, including arterial compliance, elastic modulus, impedance, pulse wave velocity, and pulse pressure amplification, are used for diagnosis and management.

Hypertension is strongly implicated in cardiovascular disease and stroke.[79] When systemic hypertension syndrome advances to heart disease, the prognosis is poor.[80]

Obesity is considered a primary risk factor for hypertension, as well as for heart disease, stroke, and renal dysfunction. Mechanisms that have been proposed for obesity-related hypertension include insulin resistance, hyperinsulinemia, dyslipidemia, increased sympathetic activity, sodium and water retention, cardiac dysfunction, and endothelial dysfunction.[81] To adapt to an increasing workload, the heart enlarges. When it can no longer adequately compensate, the heart begins to fail, and that is usually coupled with respiratory failure. Myocardial hypertrophy is considered an independent risk factor for cardiovascular disease in people who are obese and is a strong predictor of heart failure.

The occurrence and clinical implications of myocardial fibrosis in people with hypertension are well established.[82] The rennin-angiotensin-aldosterone system and contributions of mineralocorticoids and endothelin have been implicated in the development of myocardial fibrosis.

Thyroid hormone has well-documented effects on cardiovascular function, including blood pressure.[17] In hyperthyroidism, pulse pressure is increased, whereas in hypothyroidism, pulse pressure is narrowed. Adaptations of the cardiovascular system alter blood pressure to accommodate new demands on the system. The effects of thyroid hormone on blood pressure, therefore, are mediated both directly and indirectly.

Pulmonary Hypertension

Pulmonary hypertension is increasingly recognized as a pathology that can occur secondary to some other pulmonary condition or with no apparent cause (idiopathic pulmonary hypertension). By definition, pulmonary hypertension exists when the mean pulmonary pressure is greater than 25 mm Hg at rest and greater than 30 mm Hg during exercise.[83] Pulmonary blood pressure can increase in response to increased pulmonary vascular resistance, blood flow, and pulmonary artery wedge pressure. The cause of pulmonary hypertension has shifted from being attributed to vasoconstrictive dysfunction to being attributed to angioproliferative dysfunction.[84] Endothelial dysfunction has been implicated.[85] Although the prognosis is variable, with some people surviving months and others decades, guidelines have been recommended to assess the prognosis for individuals with pulmonary artery hypertension and to institute appropriate intervention expeditiously.[86]

Obstructive Lung Disease

COPD is also known as chronic obstructive lung disease (COLD), chronic obstructive airway disease (COAD), and chronic airway or airflow obstruction (CAO).[87] Exacerbations characterize these conditions and contribute largely to their associated morbidity and mortality.[88] COPD is common worldwide and contributes to major disability, as well as to economic and social burdens.

More than 30 million Americans have COPD.[89] The first part of this chapter describes chronic bronchitis, emphysema, asthma, and bronchiectasis. A patient usually presents with more than one of these conditions. Most people with COPD have a combination of chronic bronchitis, emphysema, and airway hyperactivity. The typical presentation includes episodic wheezing along with a variable degree of chronic bronchitis and emphysema.[90] A radiograph typically shows hyperinflated lungs, flattened diaphragms, and an enlarged right ventricle as a result of hypoxemia and increased pulmonary artery pressure. Other findings vary from patient to patient, depending on the predominant disease process contributing to the COPD.

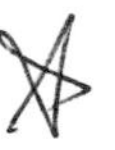

Inflammation of the bronchial wall is typically present through the course of the disease, with increasing inflammation during exacerbations. In addition to destruction of the lung parenchyma in emphysema, small airways are affected (obstructive bronchiolitis). Chronic inflammation leads to the remodeling and narrowing of the small airways. The destruction of lung parenchyma and the inflammation cause loss of elasticity. The two principal theories about the pathophysiological causes of COPD include oxidative stress and an imbalance between proteinases and antiproteinases. Chronic inflammation of the lung parenchyma associated with COPD can be associated with systemic inflammation and further chronic degenerative dysfunction. Because of the prominence of inflammation in the underlying pathophysiology in COPD, interest in the use of inflammatory markers in clinical assessment is considerable.[91,92]

The symptoms of individuals with COPD can be accentuated during sleep. The mechanisms can originate centrally, as well as peripherally (i.e., in lower airways and the chest wall).[93] Adverse effects include hypoventilation, cardiac dysrhythmias, and pulmonary hypertension, all of which can predispose an individual to nocturnal death. Evaluation of sleep is therefore an essential component of the overall assessment.

Chronic Bronchitis

Chronic bronchitis is a condition associated with chronic swelling and inflammation of the bronchi and bronchioles. The diagnosis is based on report of a cough producing sputum on most days for 3 months during 2 consecutive years when other conditions have been ruled out.[94] The degree of airway narrowing is assessed with spirometry.

Pathologically, an increase in the size of the tracheobronchial mucous glands (increased Reid index) occurs, along with goblet cell hyperplasia.[95] Mucous cell metaplasia of bronchial epithelium results in a decreased number of cilia. Ciliary dysfunction and disruption of the continuity of the mucous blanket are common. In the peripheral airways, bronchiolitis, bronchiolar narrowing, and increased amounts of mucus are observed.[96]

Chronic bronchitis results from long-term irritation of the tracheobronchial tree. The most common cause of irritation is cigarette smoking.[97] Regular exposure to the inhaled toxic particles and gases in cigarette smoke causes inflammation in the epithelium of the central airways (larger than 4 mm in internal diameter). This inflammatory process is associated with an increased production of mucus by the goblet cells and mucous glands. Smoking inhibits ciliary action and destroys cilia. The hypersecretion of mucus and the loss and impairment of cilia lead to a chronic productive cough. The fact that smokers secrete an abnormal amount of mucus predisposes them to respiratory infection and prolonged recovery from such infection. The irritation of smoke in the tracheobronchial tree causes bronchoconstriction. Although smoking is the most common cause of chronic bronchitis, other triggers include air pollution, bronchial infections, and occupations in which air quality is affected.

Patients with chronic bronchitis often appear blue as a result of hypoxemia. Although many patients have a high arterial partial pressure of carbon dioxide ($Paco_2$), the pH is normalized by renal retention of bicarbonate (Hco_3). The bone marrow compensates for chronic hypoxemia by increasing the production of red blood cells, leading to polycythemia.[90] Polycythemia increases blood viscosity and the work required by the heart to pump and circulate the blood through the lungs and systemic vasculature. Long-term hypoxemia leads to hypoxic pulmonary vasoconstriction, increased pulmonary artery pressure and, potentially, right ventricular hypertrophy.

Individuals with bronchitis often expectorate mucoid sputum. In an exacerbation, usually from infection, they have an even greater amount of purulent sputum. Ventilation-perfusion abnormalities are common, and they increase hypoxemia and $Paco_2$ retention. The respiratory rate increases, as does the use of accessory muscles. Oxygen demand by these muscles and production of carbon dioxide (CO_2) increase beyond the capacity of the ventilatory system. The work of breathing increases disproportionately. This contributes to a further decrease in the arterial partial pressure of oxygen (Pao_2) and an increase in $Paco_2$. The hypoxemia and respiratory acidemia increase pulmonary artery constriction, which further increases pulmonary artery pressure and right ventricular strain. During an exacerbation, these patients are usually treated with intravenous fluids, antibiotics, bronchodilators, and low-flow oxygen. Corticosteroids may be administered. Diuretics and digitalis are used to treat right ventricular failure.

Emphysema

Emphysema is defined as "a condition of the lung characterized by abnormal permanent enlargement of airspaces distal to the terminal bronchiole, accompanied by destruction of their walls."[98] There are two main types of emphysema: centrilobular and panlobular.[99] Centrilobular emphysema is 20 times more common than panlobular emphysema, although both types often coexist in the same patient.

Centrilobular emphysema is characterized by inflammation, edema, thickened bronchiolar walls, and destruction of the respiratory bronchioles. These changes are common and are marked in the upper lobes and the superior segments of the lower lobes.[100] Centrilobular emphysema is more common in men than in women, is rare in nonsmokers, and is common in patients with chronic bronchitis.

Panlobular emphysema, characterized by destructive enlargement of the alveoli, affects primarily the lower lobes (Fig. 5-1). This type of emphysema is characteristic of alpha$_1$-antitripsin deficiency, which involves an imbalance between the elastin and elastase in the lung parenchyma. The emphysematous lung develops secondary to loss of radial traction on the bronchioles and loss of the elastic recoil of the alveoli. When individuals without pulmonary dysfunction inhale, the airways are stretched open by the enlarging elastic lung. In exhalation, the airways are narrowed as a result of the decreasing stretch of the lung. The lungs of people with panlobular emphysema have decreased elasticity because of the destruction of surrounding alveolar walls. Thus the bronchioles lack tethering and support, which exposes them to collapse even during normal exhalation.

Bullae, emphysematous spaces larger than 1 cm in diameter, are commonly present in patients with emphysema (Fig. 5-2).[101,102] Bullae develop from a coalescence of adjacent areas of emphysematous lung or because of an obstruction of the conducting airways that permits the flow of air into the alveoli during inspiration but impedes the outflow of air during expiration. The alveoli become hyperinflated and eventually the walls are damaged, leading to an enlarged air space in the lung parenchyma. These bullae can exceed 10 cm in diameter and they compromise the function of the remaining lung tissue (Fig. 5-3). Surgical intervention to remove bullae may be indicated. Pneumothorax, a serious complication, can result from their rupture.

There are several long-term structural and functional changes in the lungs of people with emphysema. The diagnosis is based on these changes. Chronic airflow obstruction

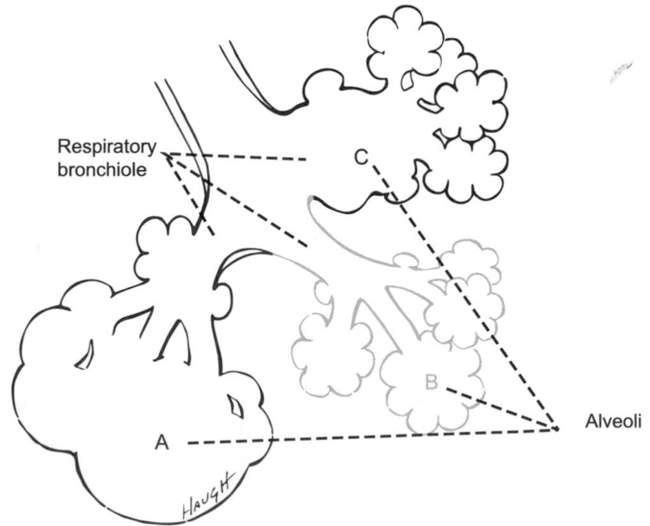

Fig. 5-1 *A,* Panlobular emphysema is characterized by a destructive enlargement of the alveoli. *B,* A normal respiratory bronchiole and alveoli. *C,* Centrilobular emphysema is characterized by a selective enlargement and destruction of the respiratory bronchiole.

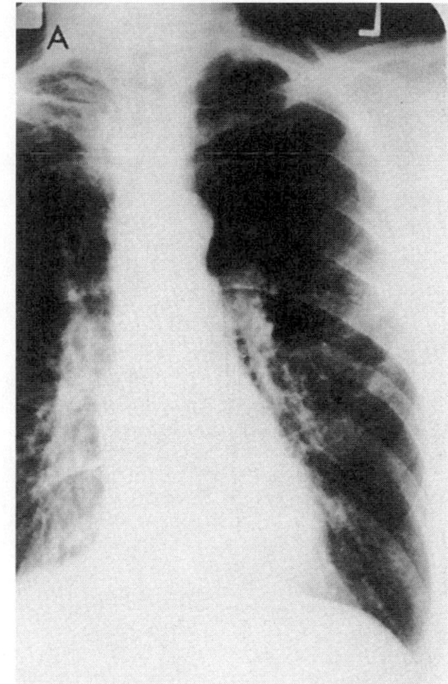

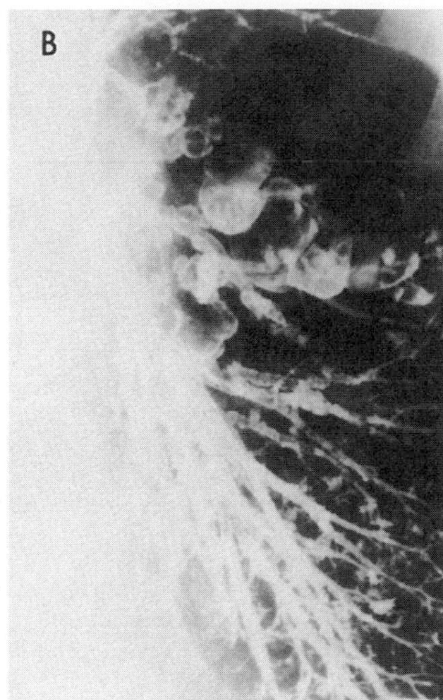

Fig. 5-2 A, AP chest film reveals bullous emphysema with multiple, thin, rounded fibrotic lucencies. **B,** The spot film bronchogram of the left midlung field shows intact bronchi and distal emphysematous blebs. *(Courtesy TH Johnson, MD.)*

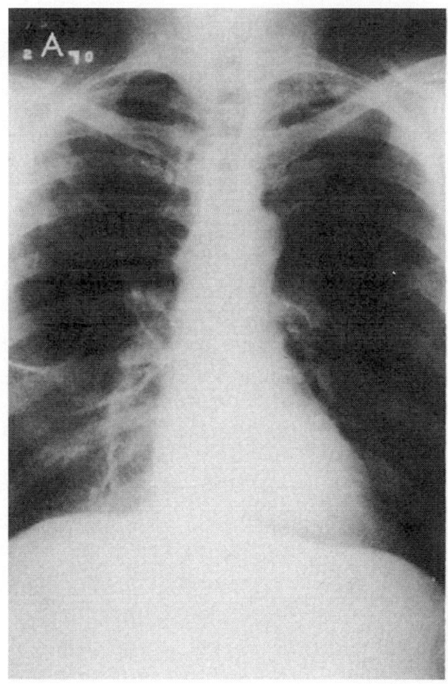

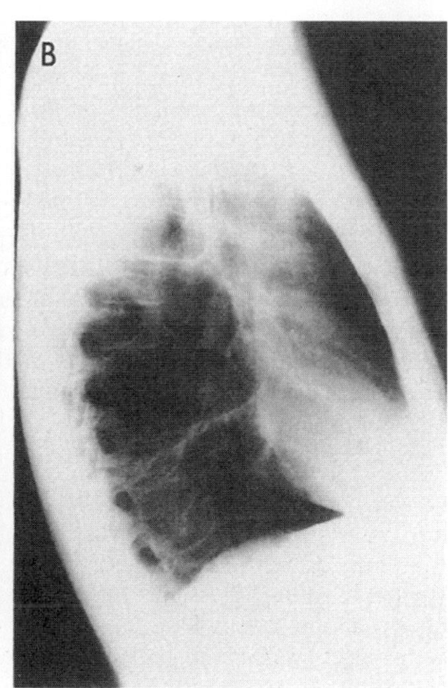

Fig. 5-3 A, AP view, and **B,** lateral view, of the chest of a patient with advanced bullous emphysematous changes. Note the bullae in the upper lung fields. The lateral film reveals an increased AP diameter of the thorax, a flattening of the diaphragm, and an increased anterior clear space. *(Courtesy TH Johnson, MD.)*

reflects both the effect of chronic inflammation of the small airways (contributing to obstructive bronchiolitis) and parenchymal destruction (emphysema). The latter contributes to the loss of alveolar tethering and attachment, resulting in increased lung compliance (reduced elastic recoil) of the affected lung regions. The airways lose their ability to remain open during expiration, which contributes to dynamic airway closure.

Shortness of breath is the most common complaint of a person with emphysema, and it reflects psychological factors, as well as pulmonary impairment.[103] Dyspnea is persistent (present daily) and worsens with exertion and during respiratory infections. These patients appear thin and have elevated shoulders and an increased anteroposterior chest diameter. They tend to breathe with the accessory muscles of respiration. These patients tend to lean forward when distressed, resting their forearms on their knees or sitting with their arms extended at their sides and pushing down against the bed or chair, to elevate their shoulders and improve the efficiency of the accessory muscles to support breathing. They may breathe through pursed lips during the expiratory phase of breathing.

On auscultation, breath sounds are reduced throughout most or all lung fields. Radiographs show overinflated lungs, flattened hemidiaphragms, and elongated hearts (Fig. 5-4). Pulmonary function tests show decreased vital capacity, FEV_1, maximum voluntary ventilation, and diffusing capacity. The total lung capacity increases as a result of greater anatomic

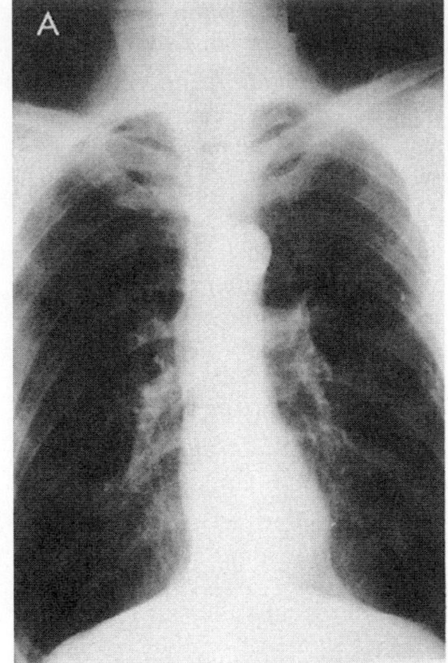

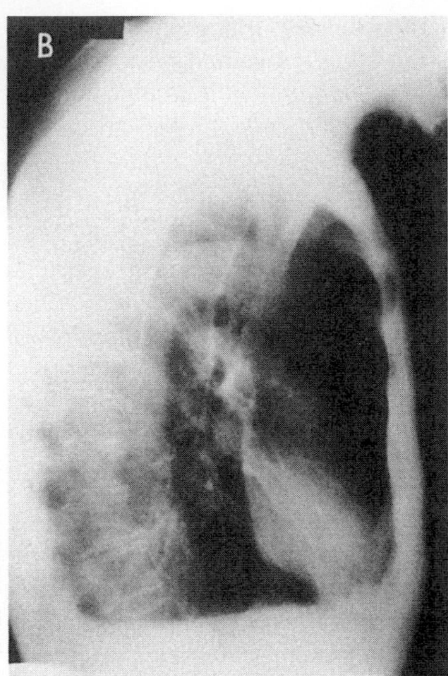

Fig. 5-4 A, AP chest film reveals the increased lucency of lung fields and the flattening of the diaphragm in emphysema. The vascular structures are crowded medially. **B,** Lateral chest film reveals an increased AP diameter and flattening of the diaphragms. There is an increase in the anterior clear space. These are all findings in emphysema. *(Courtesy TH Johnson, MD.)*

dead space caused by hyperinflation, whereas the residual volume and functional residual capacity increase even more. Arterial blood gases reflect a mildly or moderately low Pa_{O_2}, a normal or slightly elevated Pa_{CO_2}, and a normal pH. At the end stage of disease, these patients develop heart failure (Fig. 5-5).

COPD is often associated with sodium retention, leading to massive edema and the development of right-sided heart failure.[104] Cardiac output can remain remarkably normal, suggesting that the pathology is related to fluid overload. Underfilling of the arterial side of the circulation has been proposed for stimulating the sodium-retaining mechanism in right-sided heart failure.

Exacerbations of the disease are more frequent and severe with increased severity of lung pathology and impairment of baseline pulmonary function.[105] The principal cause of an acute exacerbation of COPD is infection, which may be of viral or bacterial origin. The infection causes an inflammatory response, which causes an increased production of mucus and airflow obstruction. If hospitalization is required, treatment usually includes IV fluids, antibiotics, and low-flow oxygen.[90] Some patients may receive bronchodilators, corticosteroids, diuretics, and digitalis. Theophylline is often prescribed as a bronchodilator in COPD, but it also has other important benefits. Theophylline has been shown to improve respiratory muscle strength and endurance, mucociliary clearance, respiratory drive, and cardiac function.[106,107] Pursed-lip breathing can relieve dyspnea and improve arterial blood gases in some people with COPD.[108] The majority of people with COPD report symptoms consistent with asthma, bronchitis, or both, which explains why inhaled corticosteroids reduce symptoms and improve survival in some patients.[106,109,110]

Individuals with COPD who are hypoxemic when awake become more hypoxemic during sleep, with desaturation most marked during REM sleep.[111] The mechanism is thought to reflect alveolar hypoventilation and ventilation-perfusion mismatch. Diminished ventilation during sleep also increases the risk for cardiac dysrhythmias.[93] If COPD is associated with obstructive sleep apnea, patients have increased risk for respiratory insufficiency and failure. During acute exacerbations, these effects can be augmented, thus contributing to nocturnal death.

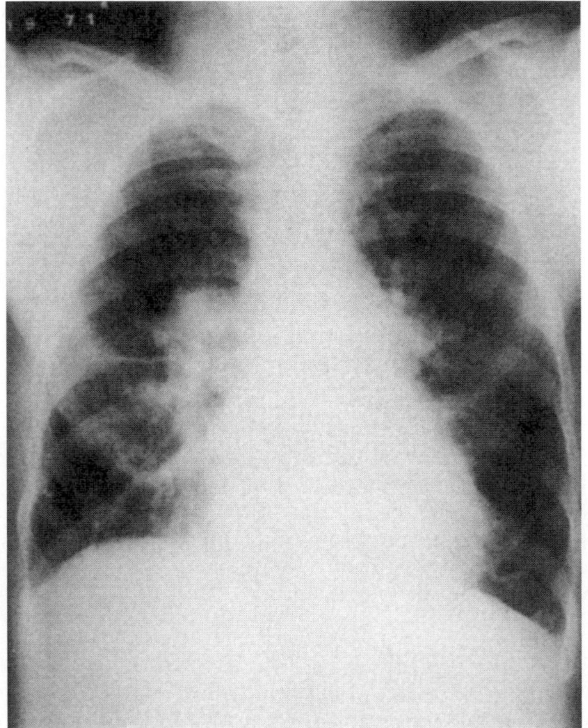

Fig. 5-5 The chest film reveals peripheral emphysematous lucency. The hilar areas are tremendously enlarged by the pulmonary arteries in a typical cor pulmonale configuration. Cardiomegaly is also present. *(Courtesy TH Johnson, MD.)*

Risk factors for emphysema include smoking, a history of chronic bronchitis, and increasing age.[94] The risk for developing COPD is 30 times greater in smokers than in nonsmokers.[99,100] The relatively rare form of inherited emphysema, $alpha_1$-antitrypsin deficiency, develops fairly early in life and is unrelated to smoking history. Repeated lower respiratory tract infections can play a role.

COPD is associated with clinically important extrapulmonary effects, including peripheral skeletal muscle dysfunction, muscle wasting, and osteoporosis.[91] Recent literature supports the theory that chronic lung and heart conditions share a common myopathy (see Chapters 24 and 31).[112-114] Both muscle wasting and altered muscle protein metabolism have been implicated in the muscle adaptation to COPD.[115] This finding has important implications for rehabilitation.

Respiratory muscle weakness and fatigue are associated with the severity of COPD.[116] Muscle weakness results from structural ventilatory impairments, adaptations to the chronic mechanical load imposed by the underlying pathology, and deconditioning. A delicate balance exists between respiratory muscle overload and adaptation. Respiratory muscle strength and endurance are fundamental to assessment, evaluation, treatment prescription, and prognosis.

Venous thromboembolism poses major risk to individuals with COPD, particularly during acute exacerbations, when blood volume may be relatively reduced in the presence of normally elevated hematocrit and, during an exacerbation, these patients are less active.[117] Even though pharmacologic prophylaxis has been advocated for high-risk patients, the physical therapist should institute prophylactic measures for all patients.

For comprehensive evaluation of the functional status of individuals with chronic lung disease, exercise testing provides an integrated perspective of organ-system function and can be used to prescribe physical activity and a structured exercise program (see Chapter 24). Exercise testing data provide supplemental information in the assessment because resting pulmonary function is not necessarily closely associated with functional capacity.

COPD progresses from respiratory insufficiency to failure. The two categories of failure are lung failure, resulting in hypoxemia, and pump failure, resulting in alveolar ventilation and hypercapnia.[118] These two conditions are managed differently based on their underlying pathophysiological mechanisms and varying clinical manifestations.

Prognosis of Chronic Bronchitis and Emphysema

Without cessation of smoking and with chronic respiratory irritation, progressive loss of lung function and worsening of symptoms will progress in people with chronic bronchitis and emphysema.[119]

Smoking cessation is the only effective intervention for preventing or reducing the life-threatening effects of COPD.[120] The decline in pulmonary function (FEV_1) is decelerated, supporting the theory that inflammation and remodeling of the airways are positively affected. Histopathological studies, however, support the idea that inflammation can persist after cessation of smoking. Longitudinal studies are needed to identify the time course and other factors that may contribute to this negative sequela and its remediation.

Individuals with COPD are at risk for tissue catabolism and associated weight loss. Poor nutrition is associated with increased morbidity. Diets are optimized, and nutritional supplements are recommended on the basis of consultation with a nutritionist. The physical therapist pays particular attention to nutrition because interventions that include exercise impose energetic demands. Diet and exercise confer considerable benefits to the functional status of people with COPD that cannot be duplicated by pharmacological interventions.[121]

The life-threatening complications of COPD are associated with prolonged hypoxemia, leading to oxidative stress on the individual, which is manifested by ischemia affecting the organ systems. This causes dysfunction of the brain, heart, kidneys, and lungs. The most common causes of death in patients with COPD are congestive heart failure, respiratory failure, pneumonia, bronchiolitis, and pulmonary embolism. The basic mechanism underlying acute respiratory dysfunction is ventilation-perfusion mismatching with increased anatomical and physiological dead space that leads to hypercapnia and acidosis.[122]

With increasing severity of disease, the load on the heart increases as a result of several factors. COPD leads to sodium retention, volume overload, edema, and right-sided heart dysfunction.[97] Cardiac output, however, can remain relatively normal. Total peripheral vascular resistance falls, with reduced effective circulating blood volume.

An individual with end-stage COPD is severely compromised and may be unable to engage in much meaningful activity. Lung-volume reduction surgery has demonstrable long-term (at least 5 years) objective and subjective benefits in selected patients with disease of the upper lobes and impaired exercise tolerance.[123,124]

Asthma

Asthma is a chronic inflammatory condition of the airways that is characterized by an increased responsiveness of the airway smooth muscle to various stimuli (due to a lowering of the threshold of airway smooth muscle reactivity). It is manifested by widespread narrowing of the airways that reverses either spontaneously or as a result of treatment.[125-127] During an asthma attack, the lumens of the airways are narrowed or occluded by a combination of bronchial smooth muscle spasm, inflammation of the mucosa, and overproduction of viscous mucus.[128-130] Specifically, eosinophilic inflammation is prevalent, and airway remodeling of the bronchial airways occurs over time.[131,132] Clinically, peak expiratory flow rates are sensitive to subtle changes in airway status, which may be detected before the onset of symptoms.[133] This early objective sign can be useful in anticipating an asthma attack.

Asthma is a widespread condition that affects 5% to 10% of the population of the United States.[134] Asthma is prevalent in individuals under 25 years of age, where estimates of prevalence vary from 5% to 15%.[135] Approximately 80% of children with asthma do not have asthma after 10 years of age.

Asthma that begins before the age of 35 is usually allergic or extrinsic. Asthma attacks are precipitated when an individual comes into contact with a substance to which she or he is sensitive, such as pollens or household dust (Box 5-1). Commonly, people with asthma are allergic to multiple allergens.[126]

Box 5-1 Factors That Can Precipitate an Asthma Attack

Allergic or Extrinsic Asthma	Nonallergic or Intrinsic Asthma
Pollen (especially ragweed)	Inhaled irritants
Animals	Cigarette smoke
Feathers	Dust
Molds	Pollution
Household dust	Chemicals
Food	Weather
	High humidity
	Cold air
	Respiratory infections
	Common cold
	Bacterial bronchitis
	Drugs
	Aspirin
	Emotions
	Stress
	Exercise

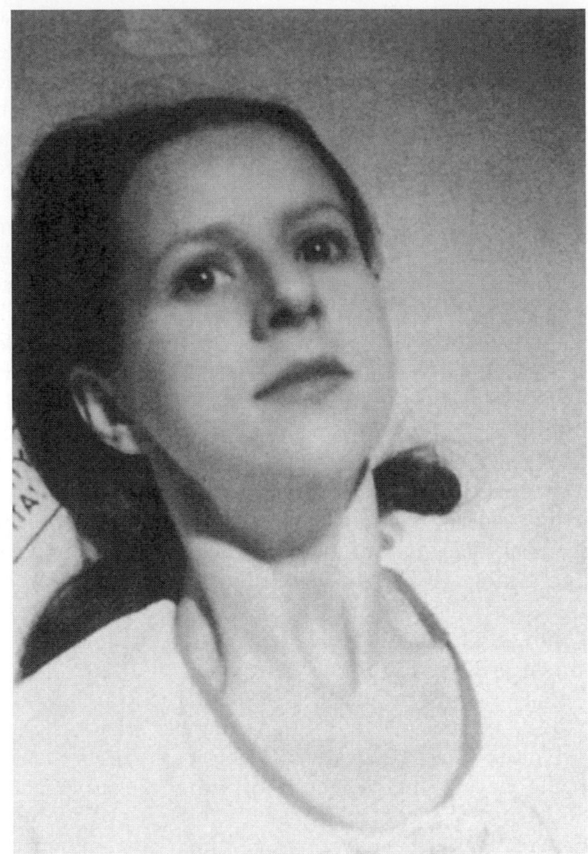

Fig. 5-6 A patient in respiratory distress during an acute asthma attack. Note the marked use of the sternocleidomastoids and other accessory muscles during inspiration.

Exercise-induced asthma (EIA) is prevalent in school children as well as in competitive athletes. EIA appears to result from hyperosmolar changes or exposure to temperature changes in the airways.[136] The condition can often be well controlled medically.

If a person's first asthma attack occurs after 35 years of age, there is usually evidence of chronic airway obstruction with intermittent episodes of acute bronchospasm. These individuals whose attacks are not triggered by specific substances are referred to as having nonallergic or intrinsic asthma (see Box 5-1). Chronic bronchitis is commonly found in this group, and this type of individual is often seen in the hospital setting.

Individuals with acute asthma attacks often report being awakened at night or early in the morning with one or more symptoms, including cough, dyspnea, wheezing, and chest tightness.[95] Waking at night is so common in the patient with asthma that its absence from the history may cast doubt on its diagnosis. The patient has a rapid rate of breathing and is using the accessory respiratory muscles (Fig. 5-6). The expiratory phase of breathing is prolonged with audible wheezing. As the lungs become increasingly hyperinflated, however, the breath sounds diminish. The patient may cough often, though unproductively, and may complain of chest tightness. Radiologically, the lungs may appear hyperinflated or may show small atelectatic areas caused by retained secretions. Tachypnea, hyperinflation, accessory muscle use, sitting upright, and pulsus paradoxus (difference in systolic blood pressure during inspiration and expiration) are useful guides for determining the severity of airway obstruction present.[129,137] Early in the attack, arterial blood gases reflect slight hypoxemia and a low $Paco_2$ (from hyperventilation). As the attack progresses, the Pao_2 continues to fall and the $Paco_2$ increases. As obstruction becomes severe, deterioration of the patient occurs, evidenced by a high $Paco_2$, a low Pao_2, and a pH below 7.30. Optimal monitoring of the patient's status is based on flow-volume loops and clinical judgment.[138]

The goals of medical management of acute asthma include maintenance of adequate arterial oxygen saturation, relief of airway obstruction, and reduction of airway inflammation.[129] Patients who are hospitalized usually require intravenous fluids, bronchodilators, supplemental oxygen, and corticosteroids.

A severe asthma attack that persists for hours and is unresponsive to medical management is referred to as status asthmaticus. The patient may appear dehydrated, cyanotic, and near exhaustion due to labored breathing. In contrast to the audible wheezing heard early in the attack, the lung sounds can be greatly diminished or absent. Status asthmaticus has a significant death rate, so it is a medical emergency. Bilateral manual lower chest compression can assist expiration and may have value as an emergency treatment of asthma. Patients in respiratory failure require mechanical ventilation. Averting the adverse consequences of dynamic hyperinflation is the goal.[139]

On autopsy, the lungs of people with asthma are hyperinflated and fail to deflate when the thorax is opened.[140] The airway mucosa is inflamed and edematous, and the basement membrane is thickened. The mucous glands are enlarged, and the number of goblet cells is increased. Bronchospasm is evidenced by airway smooth muscle hypertrophy. The lumens of the bronchioles are filled with viscous, sticky mucus, which can precipitate death by asphyxiation (Fig. 5-7). Secretions in the tracheobronchial tree of a patient with asthma are a combination of mucus, secreted by the mucous glands, and an exudate from the dilated capillaries beneath the basement membrane.[141] Cilia fail to sweep the mucoserous fluid as effectively as they sweep mucus alone. In addition, sheets of ciliated epithelium can be shed into the bronchial lumens, further contributing to airway obstruction. Although the alveoli are overinflated, the permanent destructive changes associated with emphysema are not present.

Prognosis of Asthma

Early detection of an exacerbation of asthma is imperative. Mortality has been attributed to the failure to detect severity early.[129] As a chronic inflammatory condition, asthma may result in irreversible lung damage if untreated.[142] Antiinflammatory medications such as inhaled corticosteroids have a role in controlling mild to moderate cases of asthma. In severe disease that requires heavier doses, the adverse effects of long-term corticosteroid use become prevalent— namely, osteoporosis and glaucoma.[137] Guidelines for the prevention and management of asthma have been well established.[143]

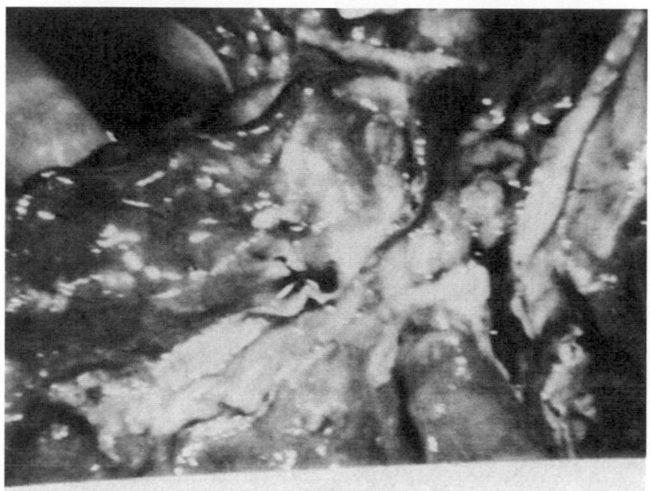

Fig. 5-7 Gross specimen of lung showing large mucus plug within the bronchial tree of a patient who died of status asthmaticus. *(Courtesy JJ Coalson, PhD.)*

Bronchiectasis

Bronchiectasis is defined as an abnormal dilation of medium-sized bronchi and bronchioles (about the fourth to ninth generations) and generally associated with a previous, chronic necrotizing infection within these airways. Ordinarily, there is sufficient cartilage within the walls of the larger bronchi to protect them from dilation.

The airway deformities can be classified into three types.[90] Cylindrical (or longitudinal) bronchiectasis is the most common type, with a uniform dilation of the airways. Varicose bronchiectasis refers to a greater dilation than in cylindrical bronchiectasis, causing the bronchial walls to resemble varicose veins (Fig. 5-8). Saccular (or cystic) bronchiectasis refers to airways that have intermittent spherical ballooning (Fig. 5-9).

Bronchiectasis is usually localized to a few segments or an entire lobe of one lung and has a predilection for the basal segments of the lower lobes. Some 40% to 50% of cases are bilateral. When the left lower lobe is involved, it is not unusual to find bronchiectasis in the lingula of the left upper lobe as well. It is interesting to note that bronchiectasis of the right middle lobe is relatively common in older adults and can contribute to both hemoptysis and repeated infections of this lobe. Upper lobe bronchiectasis generally involves the apical and posterior segments and is usually caused by tuberculosis or bronchopulmonary aspergillosis.

Pathologically, the mucosa appears edematous and ulcerated. Destruction of the elastic and muscular structures of the airway walls is evident with resultant dilation and fibrosis. The walls are lined with hyperplastic, nonciliated, mucus-secreting cells that have replaced the normal ciliated epithelium. This change is significant because it interrupts the mucociliary

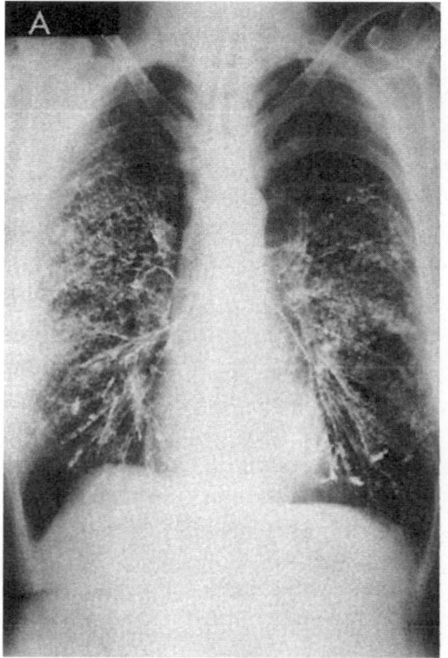

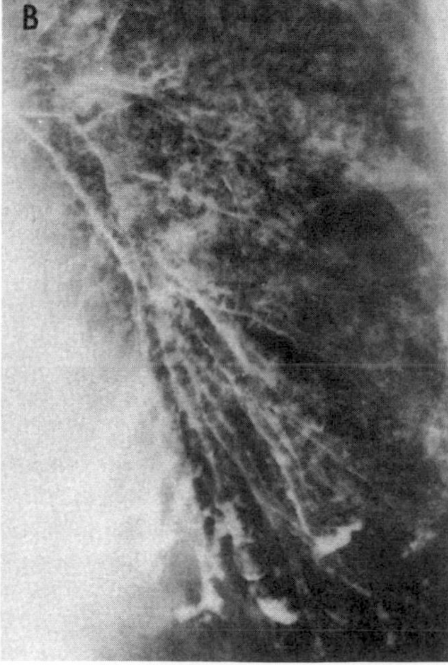

Fig. 5-8 A, AP chest film of a bronchogram with cylindrical and varicose bronchiectasis in the lower lung fields. **B,** Close-up view of cylindrical and varicose bronchiectatic changes in the left lower lobe. *(Courtesy TH Johnson, MD.)*

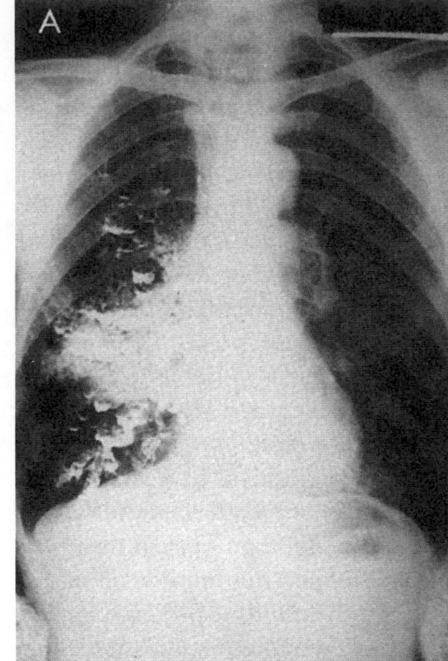

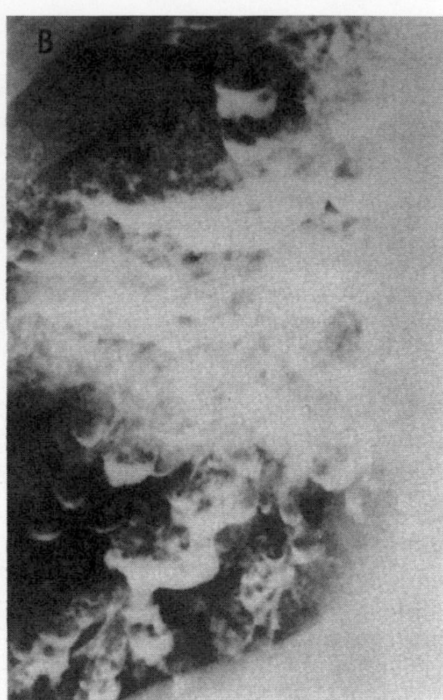

Fig. 5-9 **A,** AP chest film of a bronchogram shows saccular bronchiectasis. **B,** Close-up view of bronchiectatic areas with grapelike saccular bronchiectasis. *(Courtesy TH Johnson, MD.)*

blanket and causes the pooling of infected secretions, which further damages and irritates the bronchial walls.[144]

The cause of bronchiectasis is related to obstruction of the airways and respiratory infections.[90,144] Some 60% of cases of bronchiectasis are preceded by acute respiratory infections. The infection involves the bronchial walls. Portions of the mucosa are destroyed and replaced by fibrous tissue. The radial traction of the lung parenchyma on the damaged bronchi causes the involved airways to become permanently dilated and distorted. These areas, devoid of normal ciliated cells, contain secretions that eventually become chronically infected.

Obstruction can cause bronchiectasis by collapsing lung tissue (atelectasis) distal to the obstruction.[144] The increased negative pressure in the chest (resulting from the collapsed lung) increases the traction on the airways causing them to expand and become distorted. Secretions are retained and, if the obstruction is prolonged, infection may destroy the walls of the bronchi. Infection control with antibiotics has markedly decreased the incidence of bronchiectasis.

Sputum volume during a 24-hour period can be used as an indicator of severity of disease to categorize patients with bronchiectasis. Those producing less than 10 mL per day have been categorized as having mild bronchiectasis, 10 to 150 mL as having moderate bronchiectasis, and more than 150 mL as having severe bronchiectasis.

It is now relatively uncommon for people to have severe, diffuse, long-standing bronchiectasis. Those who do have it appear physically emaciated, and as many as 25% of them may have clubbed fingers. A chronic cough with expectoration of unpleasant-tasting purulent sputum is typical in these patients. Changes in body position while sleeping or on arising often stimulate coughing as secretions drain from the small peripheral to the large central airways. These individuals may have right-sided heart failure due to fibrosis that extends into and involves the pulmonary capillary bed. Patients with widespread bronchiectasis appear dyspneic and must work hard to breathe because of hypoxemia and hypercapnia due to ventilation-perfusion mismatching. Anastomosis of the bronchial and pulmonary vascular systems causes shunting of the systemic blood from the hypertrophied bronchial arteries.[145]

Most patients have a chronic productive cough. Some patients complain of relatively few symptoms except during a respiratory infection, when they have increased cough and sputum production. The amount of sputum expectorated and the severity of the cough vary from patient to patient according to the amount of involvement. Hemoptysis does occur in about half of older patients, evidently because of the erosion of enlarged bronchial arteries that accompany the dilated bronchi. Other common symptoms include dyspnea, wheezing, and pleuritic chest pain.[144]

Pulmonary function tests of patients with localized bronchiectasis show few or no abnormalities. In more widespread disease, however, there is a reduction in the FEV_1, maximum midexpiratory flow rate, maximal voluntary ventilation (MVV), and diffusing capacity and an increase in the residual volume.[90,95]

Prognosis of Bronchiectasis

Before the era of antibiotics, the prognosis for individuals with bronchiectasis was poor. Infection was usually the precipitating cause of death. Today, with advances in medical management, the prognosis for patients is much better.[144] Most patients can lead relatively normal lives. Right-sided heart failure, a complication of diffuse, long-standing bronchiectasis, can lead to death. Pneumonia and hemorrhage are less common causes of death. Repeated bronchopulmonary infections can contribute to worsening pulmonary function and an earlier death. Before the antimicrobial era, most patients with untreated, widespread, severe bronchiectasis died within 25 years. Prognosis depends on the extent of the disease process at the time of diagnosis and on optimal medical management. Patients with moderate, localized disease, with timely intervention, can expect a relatively normal life expectancy.

Restrictive Lung Disease

Environmental factors play a major role in the etiology of primary restrictive lung conditions. Recently, smoking, which has been largely implicated in COPD and has been associated with all-cause cancer, has been reported to have an associated restrictive pulmonary component in some people.[146] Primary restrictive lung disease is characterized by stiffening of the lung parenchyma, which prevents the lungs from expanding fully. Normally, as the diaphragm descends during inspiration, the dimensions of the chest wall increase and the alveoli expand. A decrease in the compliance of the lung parenchyma, as in interstitial fibrosis, sarcoidosis, pneumoconiosis, and scleroderma, can produce this defect. Pleural abnormalities such as pleural effusion due to alveolar compression prevent the lungs from expanding fully. Thoracic changes such as kyphoscoliosis and ankylosing spondylitis restrict lung expansion by restricting chest wall movement. Obesity and ascites restrict lung expansion by limiting diaphragmatic displacement.

The pulmonary function of individuals with interstitial lung dysfunction has characteristic features.[147] Vital capacity, inspiratory capacity, and total lung capacity are reduced. Residual volume can be normal or reduced. If the restriction is pulmonary in origin, the lung compliance and diffusing capacity are reduced. Reduced exercise tolerance is associated with marked arterial desaturation.

Common restrictive lung conditions are described below. Multisystem conditions that can predispose an individual to restrictive lung dysfunction are common and are presented in Chapter 6.

Diffuse Interstitial Pulmonary Fibrosis

Pulmonary fibrosis is a common response to various types of lung injuries.[148] Numerous acute and chronic lung conditions are associated with fibroproliferation, inflammation, or both, predisposing an individual to fibrosis. These are collectively known as interstitial lung disease.

The hypothesis that inflammation causes the development of interstitial pulmonary fibrosis is being challenged by a growing body of evidence suggesting that an abnormal wound-healing response to multiple microscopic sites of acute alveolar injury occurs, progressing to fibrosis.[135,149] The resolution of the fibroproliferation response to irritation and injury is essential to patient survival. More than 130 types of interstitial lung disease have been described. Diffuse interstitial pulmonary fibrosis represents a common histological response to a wide variety of insults.[150] Initially, an insult or injury to the pulmonary parenchyma causes an influx of inflammatory and immune cells, resulting in a diffuse inflammatory process distal to the terminal bronchiole (alveolitis).[151] This can progress to subacute interstitial disease with the presence of acute and chronic inflammatory cells. Chronic disease is manifest by thickened alveolar walls and progression to fibrosis and scarring. A role for circulating cells of hematopoietic origin has been proposed as a causal factor.[150] In addition, apoptosis has been implicated in the pathophysiology of pulmonary fibrosis.[152]

The known causes of pulmonary fibrosis include occupational or environmental exposure to inorganic dusts (e.g., silica and coal), toxic gases, and certain drugs or poisons.[153,154] In addition, interstitial lung disease is associated with rheumatoid arthritis and systemic sclerosis.[155] Twins, siblings, and other family members have been reported to have a higher incidence of diffuse interstitial pulmonary fibrosis, which supports the idea that there is a genetic link. Less commonly, interstitial pulmonary fibrosis has been reported in individuals with Raynaud's phenomenon and ulcerative colitis.

Idiopathic pulmonary fibrosis (IPF), or cryptogenic fibrosing alveolitis, is a chronic, progressive, irreversible disease of unknown cause.[148,149] The median survival time after diagnosis is approximately 3 years. Idiopathic interstitial pneumonia is associated with idiopathic pulmonary fibrosis and is a type of chronic fibrosing interstitial pneumonia with the histiologic appearance of usual interstitial pneumonia (UIP).[87] It is a condition that occurs primarily in individuals over 50 years of age. Risk factors include cigarette smoking, use of antidepressants, chronic aspiration, and exposure to metal and wood dusts.

The most common early symptoms of IPF are fatigue, dyspnea on exertion, and chronic unproductive cough. As the disease progresses, the patient becomes more dyspneic and cyanotic. On auscultation, crackles are noted, chest expansion is reduced, and clubbing of the fingers may be present.

Chest radiograph usually indicates diffuse reticular markings that show prominently in the lower lung fields. High-resolution computerized tomography is often used because it is more sensitive than a radiograph; it usually reveals patchy, predominantly peripheral reticular abnormalities in the bases. It is used to evaluate the extent of parenchymal involvement and to monitor disease progression.

Pulmonary function tests show reduced lung volumes and capacities, maintained flows, and abnormal gas exchange.[156] Compliance is markedly reduced to less than half of the predicted value. Reduced diffusing capacity is the earliest and most consistent change. Initially, arterial PaO_2 may be normal at rest but may decrease markedly with exercise. $PaCO_2$ is reduced as a result of hyperventilation, and pH is maintained by renal compensation. Later, the PaO_2 is greatly reduced because of the thickened alveolar membrane and ventilation-perfusion mismatching.

Bronchoalveolar lavage (BAL) may be used to assess the amount of inflammation and the accumulation of immune effector cells and proteins in the alveoli.[157] The technique consists of wedging a fiberoptic bronchoscope into a sublobar airway, then infusing 20 to 50 mL aliquots of saline into the peripheral airway. The saline is immediately aspirated by syringe. A total of 150 to 300 mL is instilled and recovered. The fluid and cells are analyzed. High-intensity alveolitis is defined by the presence of 10% or more polymorphonuclear granulocytes (PMNs) in BAL cell differential counts; low-intensity alveolitis consists of 10% PMNs or less.[158]

Lung biopsies that demonstrate an abundance of inflammatory cells suggest early disease, whereas a prevalence of fibrosis is indicative of advanced disease. A distinct category of IPF has been described and may be clinically useful.[154] Desquamous interstitial pneumonitis (DIP) is characterized by the intraalveolar accumulation of mononuclear cells, relatively intact alveolar walls without destruction or fibrinous exudates (numerous inflammatory cells with little or no fibrosis). This pattern has correlated with a more benign course and a better response to corticosteroids. Because a pattern of

DIP is commonly seen with UIP and IPF, DIP may represent an earlier, more easily reversible stage of IPF.

Corticosteroids are the mainstay of treatment for diffuse interstitial pulmonary fibrosis,[154,159] although their efficacy is being questioned for treatment of IPF because the favorable response rate is only 25% to 30% and there is a high incidence of adverse effects.[160,161] Regardless, a trial of immunosuppressive therapy is usually prescribed for a short period. Objective measures such as blood counts, erythrocyte sedimentation rate, pulmonary function testing, exercise tests with measurement of arterial oxygen desaturation and diffusing capacity, BAL fluid analysis, and the patient's symptoms should demonstrate improvement; otherwise, the medication is likely to be discontinued. Individuals who are not responsive to corticosteroids may be placed on antiinflammatory medications such as colchicines[160] or immunosuppressive drugs such as cyclophosphamide, azathioprine, or penicillamine.[148,161,162] Penicillamine is more effective in patients with connective tissue diseases and interstitial fibrosis other than IPF.

Patients should stop smoking. Supplemental oxygen is important, along with exercise, because there is a characteristic significant fall in arterial oxygen tension (PaO_2).[162] Individuals who require more than a 4-L flow per minute by nasal prongs may prefer direct administration of oxygen into the trachea. In addition to supplying higher concentrations of oxygen to the lungs, many patients prefer not to wear conspicuous nasal prongs.

Patients who have refractory restrictive lung disease may be candidates for single or double lung transplantation. Outcomes of transplantation surgery have been improving (see Chapter 40).

Most individuals with acute interstitial pneumonia and diffuse alveolar damage die within 6 months.[148] Patients with the chronic form who are treated with steroids can survive for years. Untreated, these patients commonly die within 1 to 4 years. The cause of death is usually related to respiratory or heart failure, although some die of adenocarcinoma and undifferentiated or alveolar cell carcinoma of the lung.

Pulmonary Infiltrates with Eosinophilia

Eosinophils are commonly present in lung tissue as part of the body's cellular response to a variety of agents and systemic immunological diseases.[95] They are present in the airways and lung tissue of patients with idiopathic pulmonary fibrosis. In interstitial lung disease that appears to have an allergic component (e.g., hypersensitivity pneumonitis, drug-induced lung syndromes, and sarcoidosis), eosinophils are minor components of the tissue reaction. In certain primary or systemic diseases, however, eosinophils can be the most conspicuous inflammatory cell present in the lung. These conditions can be grouped together and referred to as eosinophilic syndromes. Considerable overlapping exists among these syndromes because their causes and pathogenesis remain poorly understood.[162]

Simple Pulmonary Eosinophilia

Simple pulmonary eosinophilia is a self-limiting disease in which chest radiographs demonstrate migratory, fleeting areas of pulmonary infiltrates located in the periphery of the lungs, along with minimal respiratory symptoms and blood eosinophilia. Certain drugs such as sulfonamides have been implicated as a cause.[162] This disease is also referred to as Loeffler pneumonia and as the PIE syndrome (peripheral infiltrates with blood eosinophilia). If the disease is related to an allergic response to microfilaria, human parasites (e.g., *Ascaris lumbriocoides, Strongyloides stercoralis*), or cat and dog parasites (ascarids) that produce visceral larva migrans, it is termed tropical eosinophilia.

Prolonged Pulmonary Eosinophilia

Prolonged pulmonary eosinophilia is more chronic than the simple form and is associated with a more severe symptom complex. Over time, it can result in a form of diffuse interstitial pulmonary fibrosis that reveals honeycombed lung changes on chest radiograph and a restrictive pattern on pulmonary function tests.

The condition is more common in women. Symptoms include an acute respiratory illness with fever, night sweats, weight loss, and dyspnea. Prolonged pulmonary eosinophilia can be confused with tuberculosis, but patients with prolonged pulmonary eosinophilia deteriorate when treated with antituberculosis drugs. This disease must also be differentiated from eosinophilic granuloma and the desquamative form of idiopathic interstitial pneumonitis. Dense infiltrates located in the periphery of the lung on chest radiographs provide an important clue. Often a lung biopsy is necessary to confirm the diagnosis. Corticosteroids markedly improve the patient's symptoms and the appearance of the chest radiograph within weeks. Months or years of treatment may be required.[154]

Eosinophilic Granuloma

Eosinophilic granuloma (or histiocytosis X) can be either a unifocal disease affecting the lungs only or a multifocal disease involving the bones of the skull, mandible, vertebrae, pelvis, ribs, and extremities. Lung involvement is characterized by an interstitial granuloma composed of moderately large, pale histiocytes and eosinophils, and arteriolitis with eosinophils. The histiocytic process with eosinophils then involves bronchioles, alveolar ducts, and alveolar septae, which leads to their destruction. The proliferative endarteritis causes necrosis.

This disease most commonly affects men in their 30s or 40s. They usually have symptoms of fatigue, malaise, weight loss, a nonproductive cough, dyspnea on exertion, and chest pain, sometimes related to a pneumothorax or rib lesions. The chest radiograph often indicates a diffuse micronodular and interstitial infiltrate initially involving the middle and lower lung fields. In more advanced disease, small cystic areas develop in the infiltrate, producing a honeycomb pattern. Spontaneous pneumothorax is a complication in approximately 25% of cases.

The course of the disease varies.[154] Spontaneous regression with residual symptoms occurs in 10% to 25% of cases. In many patients, the disease stabilizes or "burns out," leaving them with a moderate pulmonary impairment as a result of fibrosis, cystic lung changes, and a restrictive defect on pulmonary function tests. Dyspnea on exertion is common. Some patients have persistent bronchitis. Corticosteroids are not particularly effective. Treatment is mainly symptomatic, with judicious use of antibiotics and bronchodilators. Occasionally, progressive pulmonary disease leads to right-sided heart failure and respiratory failure.

Pulmonary Alveolar Proteinosis

Pulmonary alveolar proteinosis (PAP) is an uncommon condition of unknown origin that is characterized by alveoli filled with lipid-rich "proteinaceous" material (i.e., surfactant phospholipids) in the absence of defects of the alveolar wall, interstitial spaces, conducting airways, or pleural surfaces. Most commonly, men between the ages of 30 and 50 are affected, although people of all ages and both sexes can be affected. There are three clinical types of PAP. The most common type (>90%) is acquired PAP, which is considered an autoimmune response. Hematopoietic growth factor (granulocyte-macrophage colony-stimulating factor [GM-CSF]) is essential for local regulation of surfactant homeostasis in the lungs. People with acquired PAP have a circulating, neutralizing GM-CSF antibody. The remaining two types are congenital PAP and secondary PAP; the latter is associated with environmental factors, immunological disorders, malignancies, and hematopoietic disorders.[163]

The most common symptoms are progressive dyspnea and weight loss, with cough; hemoptysis and chest pain are reported less frequently. Chest radiographs reveal diffuse bilateral (commonly perihilar) opacities (Fig. 5-10). Physical findings may include fine inspiratory crackles, dullness to percussion, and in the later stages, cyanosis and finger clubbing. Pulmonary function studies show reduced vital capacity, functional residual capacity, and diffusing capacity. Arterial blood gases indicate a low Pa_{O_2}, especially during exercise, with normal Pa_{CO_2}, and pH.[95]

The treatment of choice for patients with moderate to severe dyspnea on exertion due to alveolar proteinosis is whole-lung lavage.[164] In the operating room, after general anesthesia and the placement of a double-lumen tube (which isolates each lung), the patient is positioned in the lateral decubitus position, with the lung that is to be lavaged in the lowermost position. The double-lumen tube enables the patient to be ventilated to functional residual capacity by the uppermost lung while the lower lung is filled with saline. An additional 300 to 500 mL saline is alternately allowed to run in and out of the lung in response to gravity. As the saline flows out, manual percussion is performed over the lavaged lung, which increases the amount of proteinaceous material washed from the affected lung. The effectiveness of mechanical percussion, manual vibration, and manual percussion in removing material from involved lungs has been compared, and manual percussion has been found to be superior.[165,166] In this procedure the affected lung is lavaged with 20 to 70 L saline. The patient may be positioned prone during the administration of the final 10 to 15 L of the lavage. After the procedure, the patient is transported to the recovery room and, once stabilized, to the ward. After a few days, the procedure may be repeated in the opposite lung.

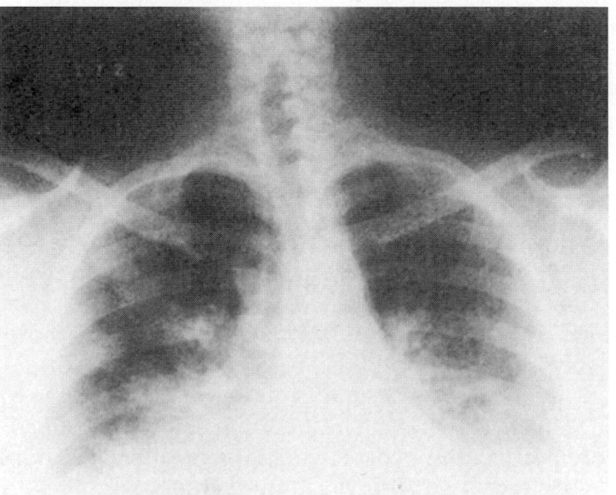

Fig. 5-10 Pulmonary alveolar proteinosis. AP chest film demonstrates an irregular, patchy, poorly defined confluence of acinar shadows that are symmetrical in both lower lung fields. The appearance is very similar to that of pulmonary edema. *(Courtesy TH Johnson, MD.)*

Most patients show significant clinical improvement after whole-lung lavage, including improved Pa_{O_2}, diffusing capacity, and vital capacity.[164,166] Many also show an improved radiograph. After lavage, patients must be followed up, because the material may reaccumulate over time. Some patients do have spontaneous remissions without undergoing lavage.

The use of limited lobar lavage through a bronchoscope has shown some benefit.[167] Half of patients who have acquired PAP with subcutaneous GM-CSF show improvement, but they show a lower rate of improvement than is seen after whole-lung lavage.[164]

Before whole-lung lavage became standard treatment, almost all children with alveolar proteinosis died and 20% to 25% of adults died within a few years, usually because of respiratory failure, right-sided heart failure, or uncontrolled infection. The majority of patients now improve greatly or recover.[164]

Sarcoidosis

Sarcoidosis is one of the most common causes of interstitial pulmonary disease.[95,168] It is a granulomatous disorder of unknown origin that can affect multiple organ systems.[169] Initial findings can include bilateral hilar adenopathy, pulmonary infiltration, and skin or eye lesions.[170] The lungs are the organs most often involved, and in such cases, 20% to 50% of patients seek medical attention because of respiratory symptoms. African Americans are affected 10 to 20 times more often than Caucasians, and women are affected twice as often as men. It usually occurs in the third or fourth decade of life.

The intrathoracic changes can be classified into four stages.[95] In the first stage, the patient is asymptomatic, with the chest radiograph showing bilateral hilar adenopathy and right paratracheal adenopathy (Fig. 5-11, *A*). In the second stage, a diffuse pulmonary infiltration is found, along with the bilateral hilar adenopathy. Interstitial infiltration or fibrosis, without hilar adenopathy, characterizes the third stage (Fig. 5-11, *B*). In the fourth stage, emphysematous changes, cysts, and bullae occur.

About one-third of people with sarcoidosis involving the lungs have spontaneous regressions with some residual fibrosis. The remaining two-thirds have progressive pulmonary impairment, along with a variable degree of impairment to the heart, liver, spleen, lymph nodes, muscles, bones, and central nervous system. Most people with sarcoidosis need no treatment. Corticosteroids, although controversial, have shown benefit.

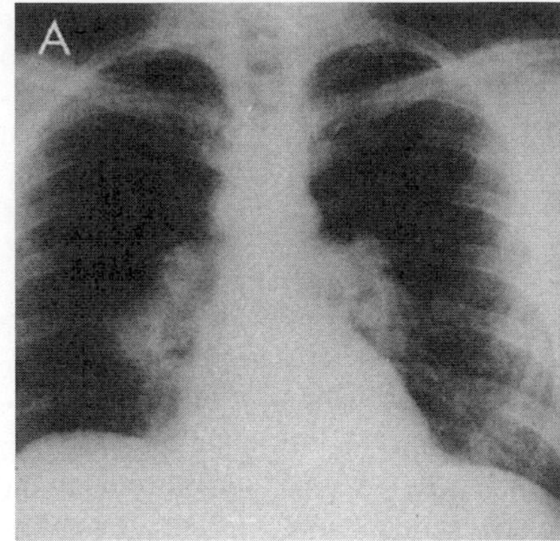

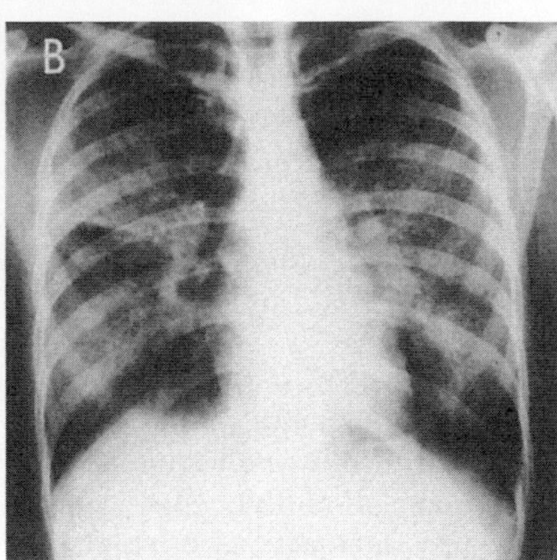

Fig. 5-11 A, Sarcoidosis in its first stage is manifested by bilateral hilar adenopathy. Usually, there are no significant physical symptoms. **B,** Disseminated sarcoidosis (third stage) reveals widespread parenchymal changes with scarring. The hilar adenopathy is usually decreased. *(Courtesy TH Johnson, MD.)*

Rheumatoid Arthritis

Rheumatoid arthritis (RA) is a systemic disease that involves the joints but can affect the lungs, pleurae, and heart. The most common thoracic complication in RA is pleuritis, with or without pleural effusions. Although RA occurs twice as often in women, pleuritis has a striking predilection for men.[162] Pleural disease is one manifestation of RA, occasionally causing fibrothorax and restrictive lung disease that requires decortication.

Interstitial lung disease, indicated by abnormal pulmonary function tests demonstrating a restrictive ventilatory impairment and a reduced ventilatory capacity, is evident in about 40% of people with RA. It is also more prevalent in men. The chest radiograph shows diffuse interstitial infiltrates, especially in the lung bases. Pulmonary nodules, which are pathologically identical to the subcutaneous nodules found in RA, may also occur and may cavitate.[155]

Coal miners with RA may have chest radiographs that demonstrate rounded densities that evolve rapidly and undergo cavitation (Caplan syndrome) in contrast to the massive fibrosis found in coal miners' pneumoconiosis.

Systemic Lupus Erythematosus

Although systemic lupus erythematosus (SLE) is a systemic collagen vascular disease, 50% to 90% of patients have pleural or pulmonary involvement. Pleuritic chest pain often signals polyserositis associated with SLE. Pleural effusions are a manifestation of polyserositis and are present in 40% to 60% of individuals with SLE. Often they are bilateral.

Chronic interstitial pneumonitis is found in 3% to 13% of people with SLE, and acute lupus pneumonitis occurs in 1% to 4%.[171] Patients with pulmonary involvement have dyspnea on exertion and a cough productive of mucoid sputum.[155] Although rare, complaints of supine dyspnea suggest diaphragmatic paresis or a diffuse myopathy of the diaphragm.[171] The chest radiograph usually indicates patchy, nonspecific densities, basilar linear or plate-like atelectasis, or both. Pleural effusions and pulmonary infiltrates are common, whereas diffuse interstitial fibrosis is rare. Pulmonary function tests often indicate a restrictive pattern with a decreased diffusing capacity and reduced arterial oxygen saturation.

Progressive Systemic Sclerosis (Scleroderma)

Progressive systemic sclerosis, also called scleroderma, is an uncommon condition that causes thickening and fibrosis of the connective tissue throughout the body and replacement of many elements of the connective tissue by colloidal collagen. Although the skin is most often involved, the lungs, heart, kidney, bones, and other parts of the body can also be affected. Approximately two-thirds of people with progressive systemic sclerosis have pulmonary involvement.[155,162]

Many of these patients with pulmonary involvement are asymptomatic, although symptoms can include weight loss, progressive dyspnea, low-grade fever, and cough (sometimes producing mucoid sputum). Chest radiographs show a characteristic fibrosis of the middle and lower lung fields. Auscultation often reveals bibasilar crackles. Pulmonary function tests reveal a restrictive defect with impaired diffusion.

The form of treatment for pulmonary involvement in patients with progressive systemic sclerosis is controversial, but usually involves corticosteroids, cyclophosphamide, or both.[155]

The prognosis for patients with only skin and joint involvement is much better than for those with involvement of the heart, lungs, and kidneys. Those with kidney involvement have a poor prognosis and a survival rate of only several years. Women have a poorer prognosis than men.

Tuberculosis

Tuberculosis (TB), a highly infectious bacterial disease, was prominent in the first half of the 1900s. With improved sanitation and medical care, TB was largely controlled. A recent resurgence of the disease has been documented, however, probably resulting from the migration patterns of people globally and the poor becoming poorer in high-income countries. TB affects many organ systems, including the lungs, and is more prevalent in people living in poor sanitary conditions with poor health. Mycobacterium tuberculosis is highly contagious but responds well to medication.[87,172] The resurgence of tuberculosis in high-income countries has become a significant public health concern.

Lung Cancer

Lung cancer is by far the leading cause of death due to cancer in both men and women.[173] The growth and division of cells is regulated by the DNA within every cell. When the DNA is damaged, which is estimated to be the result of lifestyle behaviors and environmental factors at least 50% of the time, cell division becomes uncontrolled. Cancer-causing agents, or carcinogens, related to lung disease include oxygen radicals and toxins in cigarette smoke. Although lung cancer is associated primarily with smoking, the occurrence of many other cancers is also higher in smokers. Thus the risk for cancer in general is increased in smokers. A physical therapist needs to understand the pathophysiology of all cancers, particularly lung cancer, and their medical and surgical management, as well as the impact of the natural history of a given cancer and the stage of a particular cancer on an individual's health-related quality of life. Lung cancer, as all cancers, tends to have multisystem consequences that must be understood by the physical therapist and considered during management. The physical therapist has a primary role in cancer prevention, in its early detection (by recognizing the seven warning signs of cancer), and in its management during conservative and surgical phases of care and over the long term.

End-Stage Lung Disease

Lung transplantation may be indicated in end-stage lung disease. Bronchiolitis obliterans syndrome is a serious complication of lung transplantation, but its cause is uncertain.[174]

Anemia

Anemia usually results from blood loss or from acute or chronic dysfunction of red blood cell production. The adaptive responses of the oxygen transport system involve the cardiovascular system and an increase in cardiac output and redistribution of blood flow to favor coronary and cerebral circulations at the expense of the splanchnic vascular beds.[175] These adaptations can maintain tissue oxygenation with hematocrit levels as low as 21%.[176]

Anemia is also commonly seen clinically in patients after orthopedic surgery, in renal failure, and in patients undergoing chemotherapy for cancer. Patients may be treated with blood transfusion or erythropoietin. Mild anemia may be managed by dietary measures and over-the-counter vitamin and mineral tablets alone. Moderate anemia may require mineral supplements. Anemia compromises recovery. Optimal management augments responses to rehabilitation and recovery, reduces fatigue, and improves exercise capacity, muscle strength, and performance of the activities of daily living.[177] Whether there is a critical hemoglobin level that allows for optimal participation and activity performance is unclear. The presence of CAD may mitigate hemodynamic compensation to blood loss and other causes of anemia and may attenuate treatment responses.[178]

Sickle cell anemia is a genetic condition that is common in African Americans and characterized by an abnormal shape of the red blood cell, which impedes its movement through the capillary beds. Patients with sickle cell anemia have a low anaerobic threshold in the presence of a high heart rate reserve, but they have no gas exchange abnormalities.[179] Patients may have restrictive lung pathology, increased alveolar dead space, and hypoxemia. Increased dead space may reflect impaired pulmonary capillary perfusion due to the sickle cells. Exercise hyperventilation is thought to be associated with increased anaerobiosis.

Type 2 Diabetes Mellitus

Type 2 diabetes mellitus is increasing in prevalence worldwide (see Chapter 1). Insulin resistance and glucose intolerance result from the additive effect of poor diets and inactivity. Diabetes is a multisystem condition; however, cardiovascular disease is the leading cause of morbidity and mortality in people with diabetes.[180] Organ system dysfunction results from hyperglycemia and the deposition of sorbitol on cell membranes. The toxicity of sorbitol leads to the vascular and neurological complications of this life-threatening condition. Recent evidence supports the theory that the metabolic defects associated with diabetes (impaired glucose tolerance, insulin resistance, and proinflammatory and prothrombotic states) lead to endothelial dysfunction and acceleration of atherosclerosis.[181] Hyperglycemia is associated with changes in the myocardium that lead to diabetic cardiomyopathy and heart failure. These changes can occur even in the absence of hyperglycemia, which has been linked with cardiovascular remodeling.[182] Erectile dysfunction in men has been associated with atherosclerosis and with high fasting blood glucose.[15] A diagnosis of erectile dysfunction can lead to the detection of diabetes. Adequate control of diabetes is essential to minimize these consequences.

Metabolic Syndrome

People with metabolic syndrome are at increased risk for cardiac, pulmonary, and metabolic dysfunction and diabetes. The syndrome results from deleterious body weight, inactive lifestyle, atherogenic diet, or some combination thereof.[183] Assessment is based on elevated triglycerides, low high-density lipoprotein cholesterol, elevated fasting blood glucose, elevated blood pressure, and increased abdominal circumference. At least three of these findings must be present for a diagnosis of metabolic syndrome.

Syncope

Syncope is a syndrome hallmarked by a short period of loss of consciousness resulting from a transient reduction of blood flow to the brain. Although systemic hypotension is the most common cause, it may result from a combination of factors. Syncope occurs mostly in people with cardiovascular dysfunction and in older people. Cardiovascular-related causes include orthostatic factors related to standing upright, cardiac dysrhythmia, and structural cardiac and pulmonary causes.[184] Less common forms of syncope include neurally mediated reflex syncope and syncope resulting from cerebrovascular disorders. A patient complaining of light-headedness, dizziness, grayouts, blackouts, or fainting episodes needs a thorough multisystem assessment to establish and manage the precise causes.

Cardiac Dysfunction in Noncardiac Conditions

Cardiovascular and pulmonary consequences of noncardiovascular and pulmonary conditions are described in Chapter 6. Although their effects can be subtle, cardiovascular and pulmonary manifestations of these conditions can be serious and even life-threatening. These consequences need to be addressed by the physical therapist during the assessment to guide and modify management. Tools such as ECG are essential in detecting cardiovascular abnormalities at rest and during exercise in patients with noncardiovascular and pulmonary conditions such as electrolyte disturbance, pulmonary embolism, esophageal disorders, drug-related conditions, and neuromuscular conditions.[185]

The connective tissue disorders, including systemic sclerosis, have cardiovascular consequences.[49] Because the heart is significantly involved, scleroderma can manifest as myocardial dysfunction, conduction abnormalities, and pericardial disease. The cardiovascular system can also be involved secondarily because of involvement of the lungs and kidneys.

Myocardial and cardiovascular dysfunction is well recognized as a leading cause of morbidity and mortality in people with neuromuscular conditions, and it can be a major complication in their management.[186,187] Early detection and management of such dysfunction are keys to lifelong health, reduced incidence and severity of associated morbidity, and modification of rehabilitation in this cohort of individuals.

Obesity is an independent risk factor for heart failure.[188] The cellular changes reflect the increased metabolic strain mediated by increased mechanical strain and work of the heart.

Renal disease can lead to heart failure or result from it. In addition, anemia is implicated in both conditions. The triad of these conditions has been termed the cardiorenal anemia syndrome.[189] Anemia increases the severity of CHF and mortality, and renal disease causes anemia. Both renal dysfunction and anemia worsen heart complications. Epoetin (recombinant human erythropoietin), which is used to correct anemia associated with renal dysfunction, also decreases the compensatory increase in left ventricular muscle mass, thereby reducing associated cardiac morbidity and mortality.[190]

Summary

Knowledge of the pathophysiology of primary and secondary cardiovascular and pulmonary dysfunction is essential to the practitioner for relating the underlying pathophysiology to the clinical signs and symptoms and to the appropriate treatment goals and interventions. The cardiovascular and pulmonary systems are interdependent anatomically and physiologically. The physical therapist must distinguish the contribution of cardiovascular or pulmonary pathology to an individual's limitations on participation in life and ability to perform life's requisite activities. In addition, this knowledge is essential in prescribing interventions and appropriately monitoring the patient.

This chapter first distinguishes the pathophysiology related to the structure and function of obstructive and restrictive lung conditions. Obstructive conditions are characterized by decreased airflow during expiration (as a result of increased airway resistance), airway obstruction, and hyperinflation of the lungs. Restrictive conditions are characterized by increased lung stiffness or chest wall rigidity that limits inspiration. Both types of lung pathology progressively limit functional capacity. Second, the essential pathophysiological features of atherosclerosis, ischemic heart disease, coronary artery disease, and related syndromes are described. The pathophysiological consequences of hypertension, diabetes mellitus, anemia, and syncope on oxygen transport are highlighted. Finally, cardiac dysfunction secondary to noncardiac conditions is addressed and linked to discussion of this topic covered in Chapter 6.

Review Questions

1. Describe the role of smoking in the incidence of cardiovascular and pulmonary conditions. Or consider, if smoking had never existed, what would be the epidemiological impact on cardiovascular and pulmonary disease?
2. Describe how lung dysfunction can lead to cardiac dysfunction and provide examples.
3. Describe how cardiac dysfunction can lead to lung dysfunction and provide examples.
4. Distinguish obstructive from restrictive pulmonary pathology and how each manifests clinically.
5. Obstructive and restrictive lung pathology seldom exist alone. Describe how these types of pathology can coexist.
6. Describe tuberculosis and explain why it must be a concern to the contemporary physical therapist.
7. Describe the process of atherosclerosis and the ways in which it is injurious to life.
8. Evaluate the relative contributions of acquired cardiovascular disease and congenital cardiovascular disease to your role as a physical therapist.
9. Describe the pathophysiological progression of cardiac insufficiency to failure and death. Describe how lifestyle changes recommended by the physical therapist as part of comprehensive management could stall such progression.
10. Describe the implications of hypertension, anemia, diabetes mellitus, and syncope on your practice as a physical therapist across clinical settings, including working in the community and working with healthy seniors.
11. What is meant by the term *athletic heart syndrome*? What are the implications in regard to your role as a physical therapist with a sports team?

Acknowledgment

The author gratefully acknowledges the contributions of Willy E. Hammon III to early versions of this chapter.

References

1. Dhala A, Pinsker K, Prezant DJ: Respiratory health consequences of environmental tobacco smoke. *Medical Clinics of North America* 88:1535–1552, 2004.
2. Kamholz SL: Pulmonary and cardiovascular consequences of smoking. *Medical Clinics of North America* 88:1415–1430, 2004.
3. Sartori C, Scherrer U: Turning up the heat in the lungs: a key mechanism to preserve their function. *Advances in Experimental Medical Biology* 543:263–275, 2003.
4. Gosker HR: Myopathological features in skeletal muscle of patients with chronic obstructive pulmonary disease. *European Respiratory Journal* 22:280–285, 2003.
5. Postma DS, Boezen HM: Rationale for the Dutch hypothesis: allergy and airway hyperresponsiveness as genetic factors and their interaction with environment in the development of asthma and COPD. *Chest* 126(2 Suppl):96S–104S, 2004.
6. Chapman KR: Chronic obstructive pulmonary disease: are women more susceptible than men? *Clinics in Chest Medicine* 25:331–341, 2004.
7. Global Initiative for Chronic Obstructive Pulmonary Disease. GOLD Patient Guide. May 2002. http:/www.goldcopd.com; retrieved February 2011.
8. Pauwels R, Calverley P, Buist AS, et al: COPD exacerbations: the importance of a standard definition. *Respiratory Medicine* 98:99–107, 2004.
9. Tomas LH, Varkey B: Improving health-related quality of life in chronic obstructive pulmonary disease. *Current Opinions in Pulmonary Medicine* 10:120–127, 2004.
10. World Health Organization. International Classification of Functioning, Disability and Health. http://www.who.int/classifications/icf/wha-en.pdf; retrieved February 2011, 2002.
11. Meyer FJ, Schoene AM, Borst MM: Pathophysiological aspects of cardiopulmonary interaction. *Clinical Nephrology* 60(Suppl 1):S75-S80, 2003.
12. Saini HK, Arneja AS, Dhalla NS: Role of cholesterol in cardiovascular dysfunction. *Canadian Journal of Cardiology* 20:333–346, 2004.
13. Molavi B, Mehta JL: Oxidative stress in cardiovascular disease: molecular basis of its deleterious effects, its detection, and therapeutic considerations. *Current Opinions in Cardiology* 19:488–493, 2004.
14. Belke DD, Dillmann WH: Altered cardiac calcium handling in diabetes. *Current Hypertension Report* 6:424–429, 2004.
15. Foresta C, Caretta N, Aversa A, et al: Erectile dysfunction: symptom or disease? *Journal of Endocrinological Investigation* 27:80–95, 2004.
16. Munger MA, Hawkins DW: Atherothrombosis: epidemiology, pathophysiology, and prevention. *Journal of the American Pharmaceutical Association* 44(2 Suppl 1):S5–S12, 2004.
17. Danzi S, Klein I: Thyroid hormone and blood pressure regulation. *Current Hypertension Report* 513–520, 2003.
18. Szmitko PE, Wang CH, Weisel RD, et al: Biomarkers of vascular disease linking inflammation to endothelial activation: part II. *Circulation* 108:2041–2048, 2003.
19. Verma S, Buchanan MR, Anderson TJ: Endothelial function testing as a biomarker of vascular disease. *Circulation* 108:2054–2059, 2003.
20. Kaira DK: Homocysteine and cardiovascular disease. *Current Atherosclerosis Report* 6:101–106, 2004.
21. Katerndahl D: Panic plaques: panic disorder and coronary artery disease in patients with chest pain. *Journal of the American Board of Chest Physicians* 17:114–126, 2004.
22. Kemp DE, Malhotra S, Franco KN, et al: Heart disease and depression: don't ignore the relationship. *Cleveland Clinic Journal of Medicine* 70:749–754, 2003.
23. Giachelli CM: Vascular calcification mechanisms. *Journal of the American Society of Nephrology* 15:2959–2964, 2004.
24. Verma S, Szmitko PE, Anderson TJ: Endothelial function: ready for prime time? *Canadian Journal of Cardiology* 20:1335–1339, 2004.
25. Ornish D: Avoiding revascularization with lifestyle changes: The Multicenter Lifestyle Demonstration Project. *American Journal of Cardiology* 82:72T–76T, 1998.
26. Ornish D, Brown SE, Scherwitz LW, et al: Can lifestyle changes reverse coronary heart disease? The Lifestyle Heart Trial. *Lancet* 336:129–133, 1990.
27. Ornish D, Scherwitz LW, Billings JH, et al: Intensive lifestyle change for reversal of coronary heart disease. *Journal of the American Medical Association* 280:2001–2007, 1998.
28. Young ME: Circadian rhythms in cardiac gene expression. *Current Hypertension Report* 5:445–453, 2003.
29. Oxenham H, Sharpe N: Cardiovascular aging and heart failure. *European Journal of Heart Failure* 5:427–434, 2003.
30. Bugiardini R, Bairey Merz CN: Angina with "normal" coronary arteries: a changing philosophy. *Journal of the American Medical Association* 293:477–484, 2005.
31. Beckham JC: Pain coping strategies in patients referred for evaluation of angina pectoris. *Journal of Cardiopulmonary Rehabilitation* 15:173–180, 1994.
32. Niebauer J, Hambrecht R, Schlierf G, et al: Five years of physical exercise and low fat diet: effects on progression of coronary artery disease. *Journal of Cardiopulmonary Rehabilitation* 15:47–64, 1995.
33. Schuler G, Hambrecht R, Schlierf G, et al: Myocardial perfusion and regression of coronary artery disease in patients on a regimen of intensive physical exercise and low fat diet. *Journal of the American College of Cardiology* 19:34–42, 1992.
34. Shamsuzzaman AS, Gersh BJ, Somers VK: Obstructive sleep apnea: implications for cardiac and vascular disease. *Journal of the American Medical Association* 290:1906–1914, 2003.
35. Parish JM, Somers VK: Obstructive sleep apnea and cardiovascular disease. *Mayo Clinic Proceedings* 79:1036–1046, 2004.
36. Solomon H, DeBusk RF: Contemporary management of silent ischemia: the role of ambulatory monitoring. *International Journal of Cardiology* 96:311–319, 2004.
37. Cahalin LP: Exercise tolerance and training for healthy persons and patients with cardiovascular disease. In Hasson S, editor: *Clinical exercise physiology*, St. Louis, 1994, Mosby.
38. Wenger N: Early ambulation physical activity: myocardial infarction and coronary artery bypass surgery. *Heart Lung: The Journal of Critical Care* 1:14–17, 1984.
39. Sztajel J: Heart rate variability: a noninvasive electrocardiographic method to measure the autonomic nervous system. *Swiss Medical Weekly* 134:514–522, 2004.
40. Waldo AL: Mechanisms of atrial fibrillation. *Journal of Cardiovascular Electrophysiology* 14(12 Suppl):S267–S274, 2004.
41. Knotzer H, Dunser MW, Mayr AJ, et al: Postbypass arrhythmias: pathophysiology, prevention, and therapy. *Current Opinions in Critical Care* 10:330–335, 2004.
42. Palin CA, Kailasam R, Hogue CW, Jr: Atrial fibrillation after cardiac surgery: pathophysiology and treatment. *Seminars in Cardiothoracic and Vascular Anesthesia* 8:175–183, 2004.
43. Peters RW, Gold MR: The influence of gender on arrhythmias. *Cardiology in Review* 12:97–105, 2004.
44. Banajee P, Clark AL, Nikitin N, et al: Diastolic heart failure: paroxysmal or chronic? *European Journal of Heart Failure* 6:427–431, 2004.
45. Gutierrez C, Blanchard DG: Diastolic heart failure: challenges of diagnosis and treatment. *American Family Physician* 69:2609–2616, 2004.
46. Paul S: Diastolic dysfunction. *Critical Care Nursing Clinics in North America* 15:495–500, 2003.
47. Thohan V: Prognostic implications of echocardiography in advanced heart failure. *Current Opinions in Cardiology* 19:238–249, 2004.
48. Khouri SJ, Maly GT, Suh DD, et al: A practical approach to the echocardiographic evaluation of diastolic function. *Journal of the American Society of Echocardiography* 17:290–297, 2004.
49. Steen V: The heart in systemic sclerosis. *Current Rheumatology Reports* 6:137–140, 2004.
50. Bauersachs J, Schafer A: Heart failure, platelet activation and inhibition of the rennin-angiotensin-aldosterone system. *Archives des Maladies du Coeur et des Vaisseaux* 97:889–893, 2004.
51. Hayat SA, Patel B, Khattar RS, et al: Diabetic cardiomyopathy: mechanisms, diagnosis and treatment. *Clinical Science (London)* 107:539–557, 2004.
52. Fang ZY, Prins JB, Marwick TH: Diabetic cardiomyopathy: evidence, mechanisms, and therapeutic implications. *Endocrine Review* 25:543–567, 2004.
53. Goldhaber SZ, Elliott CG: Acute pulmonary embolism: part 1: epidemiology, pathophysiology, and diagnosis. *Circulation* 108:2726–2729, 2003.
54. Tapson VF: Acute pulmonary embolism. *Cardiology Clinics* 22:353–365, 2004.
55. Wehrens XH, Doevendans PA: Cardiac rupture complicating myocardial infarction. *International Journal of Cardiology* 95:295–392, 2004.
56. Rowe MH: Effect of rapid mobilization on ejection fractions and ventricular volumes after myocardial infarction. *American Journal of Cardiology* 63:1037–1041, 1989.
57. Vitali E, Colombo T, Garatti A, et al: Surgical treatment of acute myocardial infarction. *Italian Heart Journal* 5(Suppl 6):92S–99S, 2004.
58. Murray-Thomas T, Cowie MR: Epidemiology and clinical aspects of congestive heart failure. *Journal of the Renin Angiotensin Aldosterone System* 4:131–136, 2003.

59. Pijna IL, Buchter C: Heart failure in women. *Cardiology in Review* 11:337–344, 2003.
60. Maisel AS, McCullough PA: Cardiac natriuretic peptides: a proteomic window to cardiac function and clinical management. *Review of Cardiovascular Medicine* 4(Suppl 4):S3–S12, 2003.
61. Silverberg D, Wexler D, Blum M, et al: The cardio-renal anaemia syndrome: does it exist? *Nephrology, Dialysis and Transplantation* 18(Suppl 8):viii7–12, 2003.
62. Guazzi M: Alveolar-capillary membrane dysfunction in heart failure: evidence of pathophysiologic role. *Chest* 124:1090–1102, 2003.
63. Sharpe N: Cardiac remodeling in coronary artery disease. *American Journal of Cardiology* 93:17B–20B, 2004.
64. Titcomb CP, Jr: LVH: consequences associated with cardiac remodeling. *Journal of Insurance in Medicine* 36:42–46, 2004.
65. Maron BJ, McKenna WJ, Danielson GK, et al: A Report of the American College of Cardiology Foundation Task Force on Clinical Expert Consensus Documents and the European Society of Cardiology Committee for Practice Guidelines. *Journal of the American College of Cardiology* 42:1687–1713, 2003.
66. Allard MF, Wambolt RB, Longnus SL, et al: Hypertrophied rat hearts are less responsive to the metabolic and functional effects of insulin. *American Journal of Endocrinology and Metabolism* 279:E487–E493, 2000.
67. Tenenbaum A, Fisman EZ: Impaired glucose metabolism in patients with heart failure: pathophysiology and possible treatment strategies. *American Journal of Cardiovascular Drugs* 4:269–280, 2004.
68. Burelle Y, Wambolt RB, Grist M, et al: Heart and circulatory physiology, *American Journal of Physiology* 287: H1055–H1063, 2004.
69. Peacock WF, Allegra J, Ander D, et al: Management of acute decompensated heart failure in the emergency department. *Congestive Heart Failure* Sept-Oct(Suppl 1):3–18, 2003.
70. Mills RM, Hobbs RE: Drug treatment of patients with decompensated heart failure. *American Journal of Cardiovascular Drugs* 1:119–125, 2001.
71. Gura MT, Foreman L: Cardiac resynchronization therapy for heart failure management. *American Academy of Cardiac Nurses Clinical Issues* 15:326–339, 2004.
72. Hirsch DJ, Cooper JR, Jr: Cardiac failure and left ventricular assist devices. *Anesthesiology Clinics in North America* 21:625–638, 2003.
73. Conti JV: Surgical ventricular restoration: techniques and outcomes. *Congestive Heart Failure* 10:248–251, 2004.
74. Pulerwitz T, Rabbani LE, Pinney SP: A rationale for the use of anticoagulation in heart failure management. *Journal of Thrombosis and Thrombolysis* 17:87–93, 2004.
75. Segal BL: Valvular heart disease, part 1: diagnosis and surgical management of aortic valve disease in older adults. *Geriatrics* 58:31–35, 2003.
76. Segal BL: Valvular heart disease, part 2: mitral valve disease in older adults. *Geriatrics* 58:26–31, 2003.
77. Vasamreddy CR, Ahmed D, Gluckman TJ, Blumenthal RS: Cardiovascular disease in athletes. *Clinics in Sports Medicine* 23:455–471, 2004.
78. Izzo JL, Jr: Arterial stiffness and the systolic hypertension syndrome. *Current Opinions in Cardiology* 19:341–352, 2004.
79. Mayet J, Hughes A: Cardiac and vascular pathophysiology in hypertension. *Heart* 89:1104–1109, 2003.
80. Kostis JB: From hypertension to heart failure: update on the management of systolic and diastolic dysfunction. *American Journal of Hypertension* 16:18S–22S, 2003.
81. Sharma AM: Is there a rationale for angiotensin blockade in the management of obesity hypertension? *Hypertension* 44:12–19, 2004.
82. Moncrieff J, Lindsay MM, Dunn FG: Hypertensive heart disease and fibrosis. *Current Opinions in Cardiology* 19:326–331, 2004.
83. Simonneau G, Galiè N, Rubin LJ, et al: Clinical classification of pulmonary hypertension. *Journal of the American College of Cardiology* 43:5–12, 2004.
84. Voelkel NF, Cool C: Pathology of pulmonary hypertension. *Cardiology Clinics* 22:343–351, 2004.
85. Budhiraja R, Tuder RM, Hassoun PM: Endothelial dysfunction in pulmonary hypertension. *Circulation* 109:159–165, 2004.
86. McLaughlin VV, Presberg KW, Doyle RL, et al: Prognosis of pulmonary arterial hypertension: ACCP evidence-based clinical practice guidelines. *Chest* 126(Suppl 1):78S–92S, 2004.
87. American Thoracic Society: Official statement of the American Thoracic Society and the Centers for Disease Control and Prevention adopted by the ATS Board of Directors. Diagnostic Standards and Classification of Tuberculosis in Adults and Children. *American Journal of Respiratory and Critical Care Medicine* 161:1376–1395, 2000.
88. Sethi S, Murphy TF: Acute exacerbations of chronic bronchitis: new developments concerning microbiology and pathophysiology: impact on approaches to risk stratification and therapy. *Infectious Disease Clinics of North America* 18:861–882, 2004.
89. Evans SE, Scanlon PD: Current practice in pulmonary function testing. *Mayo Clinical Proceedings* 78:758–763, 2003.
90. Mason RJ, Broaddus VC, Martin T, et al: *Murray and Nadel's Textbook of Respiratory Medicine*, ed 5, Philadelphia, 2010, Saunders.
91. Andreassen H, Vestbo J: Chronic obstructive pulmonary disease as a systemic disease: an epidemiological perspective. *European Respiratory Journal* 46(Suppl):2S–4S, 2003.
92. Oudijk EJ, Lammers JW, Koenderman L: Systemic inflammation in chronic obstructive pulmonary disease. *European Respiratory Journal* 46(Suppl): 5S–13S, 2003.
93. McNicholas WT: Impact of sleep on ventilation and gas exchange in chronic lung disease. *Monaldi Archives of Chest Diseases* 59:212–215, 2003.
94. American Thoracic Society: http://www.thoracic.org/clinical/copd-guidelines/resources/copddoc.pdf; retrieved February 2011, 2005.
95. Crapo JD, Glassroth J, Karlinsky J, et al, editors: *Baum's textbook of pulmonary diseases*, ed 7, Philadelphia, 2004, Lippincott Williams Wilkins
96. Wright JL, Cagle P, Churg A, et al: Diseases of the small airways. *American Review of Respiratory Disease* 146:240–262, 1992.
97. United States Department of Health and Human Services: Reducing Tobacco Use: A Report of the Surgeon General: 2000. www.cdc.gov/tobacco; retrieved February 2011.
98. National Heart, Lung, and Blood Institute: The definition of emphysema. Report of a National Heart, Lung, and Blood Institute Division of Lung Diseases Workshop. *American Review of Respiratory Disease* 132:182–185, 2003.
99. Hogg JC, Senior RM: Chronic obstructive pulmonary disease 2: pathology and biochemistry of emphysema. *Thorax* 57:830–834, 2002.
100. Hogg JC: Pathophysiology of airflow limitation in chronic obstructive pulmonary disease. *Lancet* 364:709–721, 2004.
101. Celli BR: Pathophysiology of chronic pulmonary disease. In Cherniack NS, Altose MD, Homma I, editors: *Rehabilitation of the patient with respiratory disease*, New York, 1999, McGraw-Hill.
102. Thurlbeck WM, Wright JL: *Thurlbeck's chronic airflow obstruction*, ed 2, Hamilton, 1998, BC Decker.
103. De Peuter S, Van Diest I, Lemaigre V, et al: Dyspnea: the role of psychological processes. *Clinical Psychological Review* 24:557–581, 2004.
104. De Leeuw PW, Dees A: Fluid homeostasis in chronic obstructive lung disease. *European Respiratory Journal* 46(Suppl):33S–40S, 2003.
105. Wouters EF: Management of severe COPD. *Lancet* 364:883–895, 2004.
106. Sutherland ER, Martin RJ: Airway inflammation in chronic obstructive pulmonary disease: comparisons with asthma. *Journal of Allergy Clinical Immunology* 112:819–827, 2003.
107. Ziment I: Theophylline and mucociliary clearance. *Chest* 92(Suppl 38S):38S–43S, 1987.
108. Dechman G, Wilson C: Evidence underlying breathing retraining in people with stable chronic obstructive pulmonary disease. *Physical Therapy* 84:1189–1197, 2004.
109. Mapel DW: Treatment implications on morbidity and mortality in COPD. *Chest* 126(Suppl 2):150S–158S, 2004.
110. Sciurba FC: Physiologic similarities and differences between COPD and asthma. *Chest* 126(Suppl):117S–124S, 2004.
111. Weitzenblum E, Chaouat A: Sleep and chronic obstructive pulmonary disease. *Sleep Medical Review* 8:281–294, 2004.
112. Polla B, D'Antona G, Bottinelli R, et al: Respiratory muscle fibers: specialization and plasticity. *Thorax* 59:808–817, 2004.
113. Troosters T, Gosselink R, Decramer M: Chronic obstructive pulmonary disease and chronic heart failure: two muscle diseases? *Journal of Cardiopulmonary Rehabilitation* 24:137–145, 2004.
114. Warburton DER, Mathur S: Skeletal muscle training in people with chronic heart failure or chronic obstructive pulmonary disease. *Physiotherapy Canada* 56:143–157, 2004.
115. Jogoe RT, Engelen MP: Muscle wasting and changes in muscle protein metabolism in chronic obstructive pulmonary disease. *European Respiratory Journal* 46(Suppl):52S–63S, 2003.
116. Orozco-Levi M: Structure and function of the respiratory muscles in patients with COPD: impairment or adaptation? *European Respiratory Journal* 46(Suppl):41S–51S, 2003.
117. Ambrosetti M, Ageno W, Spanevello A, et al: Prevalence and prevention of venous thromboembolism in patients with acute exacerbations of COPD. *Thrombosis Research* 112:203–207, 2003.
118. Roussos C, Koutsoukou A: Respiratory failure. *European Respiratory Journal* 47(Suppl):3S–14S, 2003.

119. Keller CA: Pathophysiology and classification of emphysema. *Chest Surgery Clinics in North America* 13:589–613, 2003.
120. Willemse BW, Postma DS, Timens W, et al: The impact of smoking cessation on respiratory symptoms, lung function, airway hyperresponsiveness and inflammation. *European Respiratory Journal* 23:464–476, 2004.
121. Berry JK, Baum C: Reversal of chronic obstructive pulmonary disease associated weight loss: are there pharmacological treatment options? *Drugs* 64:1041–1052, 2004.
122. Calverley PM: Respiratory failure in chronic obstructive pulmonary disease. *European Respiratory Journal* 47(Suppl):26S–30S, 2003.
123. Martinez FJ, Flaherty KR, Iannettoni MD: Patient selection for lung volume reduction surgery. *Chest Surgery Clinics in North America* 13:669–685, 2003.
124. Trow TK: Lung-volume reduction surgery for severe emphysema: an appraisal of its current status. *Current Opinions in Pulmonary Medicine* 10:128–132, 2004.
125. Peters SP: Heterogeneity in the pathology and treatment of asthma. *American Journal of Medicine* 115(Suppl 3A):49S–54S, 2003.
126. Tarlo SM, Boulet L, Cartier A, et al: Canadian Thoracic Society Guidelines for occupational asthma. *Canadian Respiratory Journal* 5:289–300, 1998.
127. Wagner CW: Pathophysiology and diagnosis of asthma. *Nursing Clinics of North America* 38:561–570, 2003.
128. Minoguchi K, Adachi M: Pathophysiology of asthma. In Cherniak NS, Altose MD, Homma I, editors: *Rehabilitation of the patient with respiratory disease*, New York, 1999, McGraw-Hill.
129. Rodrigo G, Rodrigo C, Hall J: Acute asthma in adults: a review. *Chest* 125:1081–1102, 2004.
130. Rogers DF: Airway mucus hypersecretion in asthma: an undervalued pathology? *Current Opinions in Pharmacology* 4:241–250, 2004.
131. Cohn L, Elias JA, Chupp GL: Asthma: mechanisms of disease persistence and progression. *Annual Reviews in Immunology* 22:789–815, 2004.
132. Wenzel S: Mechanisms of severe asthma. *Clinical Experimental Allergy* 33:1622–1628, 2003.
133. Lung CL, Lung ML: General principles of asthma management: symptom monitoring. *Nursing Clinics of North America* 38:585–596, 2003.
134. Bowler RP: Oxidative stress in the pathogenesis of asthma. *Current Allergy and Asthma Reports* 4:116–122, 2004.
135. Kamp DW: Idiopathic pulmonary fibrosis: the inflammatory hypothesis revisited. *Chest* 12:1187–1189, 2003.
136. Storms WW: Review of exercise-induced asthma. *Medicine and Science in Sports and Exercise* 35:1464–1470, 2003.
137. Woolcock A: Asthma. In Mason RJ, Broaddus, VC, Martin, T, et al, editors: *Murray and Nadel's Textbook of Respiratory Medicine*, ed 5, Philadelphia, 2010, Saunders.
138. Brand PL, Roorda RJ: Usefulness of monitoring lung function in asthma. *Archives of Diseases in Children* 88:1021–1025, 2003.
139. Shapiro JM: Management of respiratory failure in status asthmaticus. *American Journal of Respiratory Medicine* 1:409–416, 2002.
140. Saetta M, Di Stefano A, Rosina C, et al: Quantitative structural analysis of peripheral airways and arteries in sudden fatal asthma. *American Review of Respiratory Disease* 143:138–143, 1991.
141. Kuyper LM, Pare PD, Hogg JC, et al: Characterization of airway plugging in fatal asthma. *American Journal of Medicine* 115:6–11, 2003.
142. DeKorte CJ: Current and emerging therapies for the management of chronic inflammation in asthma. *American Journal of Health Systems in Pharmacy* 60:1949–1959, 2003.
143. Guidelines and Protocols Advisory Committee: Asthma—Diagnosis and Management. http://www.bcguidelines.ca/gpac/guideline_asthma.html; retrieved February 2011, 2010.
144. Barker AF: Bronchiectasis. *New England Journal of Medicine* 346:1383–1393, 2002.
145. West JB: *Pulmonary pathophysiology: the essentials,* ed 7, Philadelphia, 2008, Lippincott Williams and Wilkins.
146. Flaherty KR, Martinez FJ: Cigarette smoking in interstitial lung disease: concepts for the internist. *Medical Clinics of North America* 88:1643–1653, 2004.
147. Chetta A, Marangio E, Olivieri D: Pulmonary function testing in interstitial lung diseases. *Respiration* 71:209–213, 2004.
148. American Thoracic Society: Idiopathic pulmonary fibrosis: diagnosis and treatment. International Consensus Statement. American Thoracic Society and the European Respiratory Society. *American Journal of Respiratory and Critical Care Medicine* 161:646–664, 2000.
149. Selman M: Idiopathic pulmonary fibrosis: challenges for the future. *Chest* 120:8–10, 2001.
150. Garantziotis S, Steele MP, Schwartz DA: Pulmonary fibrosis: thinking outside of the lung. *Journal of Clinical Investigation* 114:319–321, 2004.
151. Thannickal VJ, Toews GB, White ES, et al: Mechanisms of pulmonary fibrosis. *Annual Reviews in Medicine* 55:395–417, 2004.
152. Kuwano K, Hagimoto N, Nakanishi Y: The role of apoptosis in pulmonary fibrosis. *Histology and Histopathology* 19:867–881, 2004.
153. Higenbottam T, Kuwano K, Nemery B, et al: Understanding the mechanisms of drug-associated interstitial lung disease. *British Journal of Cancer* 91(Suppl 2):S31–S37, 2004.
154. Panos RJ, King TE: Pathophysiology of interstitial lung disease. In Cherniack NS, Altose MD, Homma I, editors: *Rehabilitation of the patient with respiratory disease*, New York, 1999, McGraw-Hill.
155. Strange C, Highland K: Interstitial lung disease in the patient who has connective tissue disease. *Clinics in Chest Medicine* 25:549–559, 2004.
156. Khalil N, O'Connor R: Idiopathic pulmonary fibrosis: current understanding of the pathogenesis and the status of treatment. *Canadian Medical Association Journal* 171:153–160, 2004.
157. Kavuru M: Therapeutic whole lung lavage: a stop-gap therapy for alveolar proteinosis. *Chest* 122:1123–1124, 2002.
158. Reynolds H: Bronchoalveolar lavage. *American Review of Respiratory Disease* 135:250–263, 1987.
159. Raghu G, Chang J: Idiopathic pulmonary fibrosis: current trends in management. *Clinics in Chest Medicine* 25:621–636, 2004.
160. Douglas WM, Ryu JH, Shroeder DR: Idiopathic pulmonary fibrosis: impact of oxygen and colchicine, prednisone or no therapy on survival. *American Journal of Respiratory and Critical Care Medicine* 161:1172–1178, 2000.
161. Flaherty KR, Toews GB, Lynch JP, 3rd, et al: Steroids in idiopathic pulmonary fibrosis: a prospective assessment of adverse reactions, response to therapy and survival. *American Journal of Medicine* 110:278–282, 2001.
162. Reynolds H, Matthay R: Diffuse interstitial and alveolar inflammatory disease. In George RB, Light RW, Matthay MA, et al, editors: *Chest medicine: essentials of pulmonary and critical care medicine*, ed 5, Philadelphia, 2005, Lippincott Williams Wilkins.
163. Venkateshiah SB, Thomassen MJ, Kavuru MS: Pulmonary alveolar proteinosis: clinical manifestations and optimal treatment strategies. *Treatments in Respiratory Medicine* 3:217–227, 2004.
164. Seymour J, Presnelli J: Pulmonary alveolar proteinosis: progress in the first 44 years. *American Journal of Respiratory and Critical Care Medicine* 166:215–235, 2002.
165. Hammon W, McCaffree D, Cucchiara A: A comparison of manual to mechanical chest percussion for clearance of alveolar material in patients with pulmonary alveolar proteinosis (phospholipidosis). *Chest* 103: 1409–1412, 1993.
166. Perez A, Rogers R: Enhanced alveolar clearance with chest percussion therapy and positional changes during whole-lung lavage for alveolar proteinosis. *Chest* 125:2351–2356, 2004.
167. Cheng SL, Chang HT, Lau HP, et al: Pulmonary alveolar proteinosis: treatment by bronchofiberoptic lobar lavage. *Chest* 122:1480–1485, 2002.
168. Baughman RP: Pulmonary sarcoidosis. *Clinics of Chest Medicine* 25: 521–530, 2004.
169. Wu JJ, Schiff KR: Sarcoidosis. *American Family Physician* 70:312–322, 2004.
170. Sharma OP: A clinical picture of sarcoidosis: treatment and prognosis. *Resident and Staff Physician* 23:123, 1997.
171. Keane M, Lynch J: Pleuropulmonary manifestations of systemic lupus erythematosus. *Thorax* 55:159–166, 2000.
172. American Thoracic Society: American Thoracic Society/ Centers for Disease Control and Prevention/Infectious Diseases Society of America: Treatment of Tuberculosis. *Journal of Respiratory and Critical Care Medicine* 167:603–662, 2003.
173. American Cancer Society: *Cancer facts and figures*. Atlanta, 2010, American Cancer Society. http://www.cancer.org/acs/groups/content/@nho/documents/document/acspc-024113.pdf; retrieved February 2011.
174. Corris PA: Lung transplantation. Bronchiolitis obliterans syndrome. *Chest Surgery Clinics of North America* 13:543–557, 2003.
175. Hebert PC, Van der Linden P, Biro G, et al: Physiologic aspects of anemia. *Critical Care Clinics* 20:187–212, 2004.
176. Morisaki H, Sibbald WJ: Tissue oxygen delivery and the microcirculation. *Critical Care Clinics* 20:213–223, 2004.
177. Carson JL, Terrin ML, Jay M: Anemia and postoperative rehabilitation. *Canadian Journal of Anaesthesiology* 50(Suppl):S60–S64, 2003.
178. Nappi J: Anemia in patients with coronary artery disease. *American Journal of Health-System Pharmacy* 60(14 Suppl 3):S4–S8, 2003.
179. Callahan LA, Woods KF, Mensah GA, et al: Cardiopulmonary responses to exercise in women with sickle cell anemia. *American Journal of Respiratory and Critical Care Medicine* 165:1309–1316, 2002.

180. Candido R, Srivastava P, Cooper ME, et al: Diabetes mellitus: a cardiovascular disease. *Current Opinions and Investigations and Drugs* 4:1088–1094, 2003.
181. Nesto RW: Correlation between cardiovascular disease and diabetes mellitus: current concepts. *American Journal of Medicine* 116(Suppl 5A):11S–22S, 2004.
182. Giles TD: The patient with diabetes mellitus and heart failure: at-risk issues. *American Journal of Medicine* 115(Suppl 8A):107S–110S, 2003.
183. Wagh A, Stone NJ: Treatment of metabolic syndrome. *Expert Review of Cardiovascular Therapy* 2:213–228, 2004.
184. Benditt DG, van Dijk JG, Sutton R, et al: Syncope. *Current Problems in Cardiology* 29:152–229, 2004.
185. Van Mieghem C, Sabbe M, Knockaert D: The clinical value of the ECG in noncardiac conditions. *Chest* 125:1561–1576, 2004.
186. Bhakta D, Groh WJ: Cardiac function tests in neuromuscular diseases. *Neurology Clinics* 22:591–617, 2004.
187. Pathak A, Senard JM: Pharmacology of orthostatic hypotension in Parkinson's disease: from pathophysiology to management. *Expert Review of Cardiovascular Therapy* 2:393–403, 2004.
188. Coviello JS, Nystrom KV: Obesity and heart failure. *Journal of Cardiovascular Nursing* 18:360–366, 2003.
189. Silverberg D, Wexler D, Blum M, et al: The association between congestive heart failure and chronic renal disease. *Current Opinions in Nephrology and Hypertension* 13:163–170, 2004.
190. London GM: Left ventricular hypertrophy: why does it happen? *Nephrology, Dialysis, and Transplantation* 18(Suppl 8):viii2–6, 2003.

Chapter 6

Cardiovascular and Pulmonary Manifestations of Systemic Conditions

Elizabeth Dean

KEY TERMS

Connective tissue conditions
Endocrine conditions
Gastrointestinal conditions
Hematological conditions
Hepatic conditions
Immunological conditions
Malnutrition
Musculoskeletal conditions
Neurological conditions
Obesity
Renal conditions
Rheumatoid conditions
Systemic conditions

CHAPTER OUTLINE

This chapter describes the cardiovascular and pulmonary consequences of systemic conditions. Systemic conditions can affect oxygen transport, either directly or in combination with primary cardiovascular and pulmonary dysfunction. Although these effects can be as catastrophic as those resulting from primary cardiovascular and pulmonary dysfunction or conditions, their presentation is often subtle and may elude detection until impairment is apparent. The pulmonary and pleural complications of cardiac disease and the cardiac complications of pulmonary disease are described first. The cardiovascular and pulmonary complications of conditions involving the following systems are then described: musculoskeletal, connective tissue, neurological, gastrointestinal (GI), hepatic, renal, hematological, endocrine, and immunological. Finally, the cardiovascular and pulmonary manifestations of nutritional disorders, specifically obesity and starvation (anorexia nervosa), are presented.

To maximize the effectiveness of their treatment prescriptions, physical therapists need to be able to predict the impact of systemic conditions on oxygen transport in a given patient.[1] Complications due to systemic conditions are increasingly prevalent. This may reflect both the aging of the population and the improved survival rate and prognosis of patients with multisystem comorbidity. In addition, it is becoming more common for physical therapists to treat patients without referral, in which case no referring practitioner is alerting the physical therapist about the presence and significance of underlying systemic conditions. In their role as clinical exercise physiologists, physical therapists must be able to identify all factors that compromise or threaten oxygen transport so that treatment interventions can be prescribed effectively and with minimal risk. In addition, untoward exercise responses need to be explained; thus the physical therapist needs a comprehensive understanding of how morbidity affects oxygen transport in general. In some instances, untoward exercise responses may alert the physical therapist to some previously undetected problem warranting referral to the patient's physician.

Diagnosis and Assessment

A comprehensive assessment of all factors that affect or threaten oxygen transport is essential, particularly for patients who are not obviously at risk (i.e., those without overt cardiovascular and pulmonary conditions). The physical therapist must be able to "red-flag" a patient with an underlying problem for which physical therapy may be contraindicated or an untoward treatment response may be anticipated. Alternatively, treatment may have to be modified or treatment responses monitored more often.

Specific diagnosis of the factors that contribute to or threaten cardiovascular and pulmonary dysfunction is paramount to effective treatment across all physical therapy specialties. The overall capacity of the oxygen transport system should be established to ensure that it can adequately respond to changes in metabolic demand (including those imposed by physical therapy treatment—specifically, exercise) and changes in body position in patients who are acutely ill. Even if cardiovascular and pulmonary dysfunction is not a patient's primary condition, it may be a secondary problem, which could seriously limit a patient's response to exercise. Such assessment will establish whether treatment, specifically exercise, should be modified to avert an incident or whether it is contraindicated altogether.

Oxygen transport can be affected by dysfunction of virtually any one of the major organ systems of the body (Box 6-1). The pulmonary and pleural complications of heart disease and the cardiac complications of pulmonary disease are usually predictable and therefore are most readily detected clinically. However, the cardiovascular and pulmonary complications of conditions affecting other organ systems can be more subtle, if not more devastating.

Cardiovascular Conditions

The pulmonary complications of heart disease and the cardiac complications of pulmonary disease have been well documented for several decades.[2] A mechanically inefficient heart disrupts the normal forward propulsion of deoxygenated and oxygenated blood to and from the lungs. Because the right and left sides of the heart function in series, a problem on one side inevitably has some effect, which can lead to a problem, on the other side. For these reasons, the heart and lungs should be thought of as a single functioning unit. Disruption of the cardiovascular and pulmonary circuit leads to the backlogging of blood and an increased volume of blood in the capacitance vessels or the veins. Right heart failure contributes to increased central venous pressure (i.e., right atrial pressure) and, if sufficiently severe, leads to bilateral peripheral edema in the dependent body parts. Because blood is not forwarded to the lungs adequately, hypoxemia can result. In turn, hypoxic vasoconstriction of the pulmonary circulation leads to increased pulmonary vascular resistance and, hence, to increased right ventricular afterload and work.

Left heart failure can result in inadequate forward movement of blood through the left heart, resulting in backlogging in the pulmonary circulation and cardiogenic pulmonary edema. Pulmonary edema alters lung mechanics and lymphatic drainage, and in turn, these effects contribute to an increased risk for infection secondary to impaired macrophage function and bacterial growth. Excess pulmonary fluid around the alveolar capillary membrane creates a diffusion defect. If fluid accumulation is extreme, backlogging may be transmitted to the right side of the heart and to the periphery. Comparable to excess fluid in the lungs, backup of fluid in the peripheral circulation can impair tissue perfusion. Other cardiovascular conditions such as systemic hypertension increase systemic afterload; this, in turn, increases the work of the heart, thereby reducing its mechanical efficiency.

Pulmonary function can be altered in cardiac disease. Left heart failure, for example, is associated with accumulation of fluid in the pulmonary interstitium. This leads to reduced caliber of the airways and early airway closure, air trapping, and increased residual volume. The fluid can produce reflex constriction of bronchial smooth muscle, leading to the syndrome of cardiac asthma. The combination of airway collapse and bronchoconstriction decreases total lung capacity, flow rates, and forced expiratory volumes. Ventilation and perfusion abnormalities are also associated with cardiac disease. Ventilation of underperfused lung zones contributes to increased ventilatory dead space, and perfusion of underventilated lung zones leads to a right-to-left shunt. In left heart failure, reduced lung compliance may contribute to inhomogeneous ventilation and perfusion.

In left heart failure, the normal pattern of increased ventilation to the bases may be reversed (i.e., the apices of the lungs may be better ventilated).[3] If pulmonary edema complicates the clinical picture, the alveoli become flooded, resulting in reduced ventilation and ventilation and perfusion mismatching. The alveolar-arterial oxygen (A-aO_2) gradient is then increased, diffusing capacity is decreased, and arterial partial pressure of oxygen (PaO_2) is decreased. Lung compliance is inversely related to pulmonary artery pressures and interstitial fluid accumulation.[4] The net effect of these abnormalities is both obstructive and restrictive pathophysiological patterns of lung dysfunction (i.e., reduced forced expiratory volumes and vital capacity and an overall increase in the work of breathing).

Pleural effusions can result from heart disease, in particular, congestive heart failure. Changes in intravascular pressures lead to transudative pleural effusions, and cardiac injury leads to exudative effusions. Comparable to fluid balance in other parts of the circulation, fluid balance in the lung is dependent on Starling forces (i.e., hydrostatic and oncotic pressures). In healthy individuals, several liters of fluid a day are absorbed

Box 6-1 Dysfunctions That May Affect the Cardiovascular and Pulmonary Systems and Oxygen Transport

- Musculoskeletal conditions
- Connective tissue (including collagen vascular) conditions
- Neurological conditions (CNS, PNS, or ANS)
- Gastrointestinal conditions
- Hepatic conditions
- Renal conditions
- Hematological conditions
- Endocrinological conditions
- Immunological conditions

from the pleural space, so when the balance of these forces is disrupted in disease, considerable fluid can accumulate in the pleural space. Impaired alveolar expansion due to pleural effusions is of clinical concern. Small effusions displace rather than compress the lung.

Pulmonary Conditions

Lung conditions can contribute to cardiac dysfunction in several ways. They invariably threaten oxygen transport by their effects on respiratory mechanics and ventilation-perfusion matching. To compensate, the heart attempts to increase cardiac output, which produces a corresponding increase in cardiac work. Overall, ventilation and oxygen transport are less efficient. Hypoxemia secondary to inadequate ventilation-perfusion matching may predispose the patient to cardiac dysrhythmias.

Pleural complications can arise from lung disease as well as from heart disease. Both heart and lung function can be compromised by altered fluid balance in the pleurae. Fluid balance in the pleural space is comparable, in terms of its regulation, to that in the alveolar space. Both are determined by Starling forces. Specifically, hydrostatic pressure pushes fluid into the pleural space while oncotic pressure counters the effect of these forces. The net effect of these filtration and absorption forces is a minimal net filtration pressure. When the balance of these forces is disrupted, heart and lung function can be threatened. Excessive fluid floods the space, usually reflecting both excessive hydrostatic pressure and diminished oncotic pressure. The lymphatic vessels become overwhelmed and are unable to keep the pleural space dry. Pleural fluid accumulates and either displaces lung tissue (in small to moderate effusions) or restricts the opening of adjacent alveolar sacs, causing atelectasis (severe effusions),[5] which, if sufficiently severe, may restrict cardiac filling. Pleural fluid accumulation poses a unique threat to oxygen transport as a result of its direct physical effect on the lungs, heart, or both, so it warrants special attention by physical therapists.

Pulmonary lymphatics control fluid balance within the lung parenchyma. Lymphatic vessels arise within the pleurae and not within the alveolar capillary space. They drain fluid from the interlobular septae and subpleural areas into the hilar vessels and the primary tracheobronchial lymph nodes. Problems arising within the heart or lungs can contribute to imbalances in the major lymphatic inflow and outflow channels. This contributes to fluid accumulation, stagnation, and physical compression of the myocardium and lungs.[6]

Both heart and lung disease can produce deleterious hematological changes to compensate for hypoxemia. Increases in the number of red blood cells raise the hematocrit and viscosity of the blood. This phenomenon increases the work of the heart further. In addition, viscous blood increases the probability of thromboemboli. This risk is superimposed on the existing risk for thromboemboli in hypoeffective hearts.

A thorough understanding of the interrelationship of the heart and lungs is essential for diagnosis and optimal management. In addition, the cardiovascular and pulmonary manifestations of other primary organ systems must be recognized and anticipated, particularly in patients with multisystem conditions.

Musculoskeletal Conditions

Musculoskeletal conditions impact cardiovascular and pulmonary function secondary to their effects on muscle (in particular, the diaphragm, muscles of the chest wall, oropharynx, larynx, and abdomen) and bones and joints (e.g., arthritis, ankylosing spondylitis, kyphoscoliosis, and deformities secondary to neuromuscular diseases and chronic lung diseases) (Table 6-1). Additional effects are imposed by inactivity (i.e., muscle wasting, joint rigidity, and deformity). Increased joint rigidity limits the amount of physical activity a patient may perform, which contributes to cardiovascular and pulmonary compromise, in addition to the local effect of increased chest wall rigidity and compromised bucket-handle and pump-handle motions. The normal three-dimensional movement of the chest wall and normal pulmonary circulation and lymphatic function are compromised (Chapter 23). The cardiovascular and pulmonary manifestations of musculoskeletal conditions are summarized in Table 6-1.

The cardiovascular and pulmonary deficits associated with musculoskeletal disorders of the chest wall include reduced and potentially asymmetric lung volumes consistent with pulmonary restriction, reduced flow rates, reduced inspiratory and expiratory pressures, atelectasis, dynamic airway compression, ventilation-perfusion mismatching, inefficient breathing pattern, impaired cough and gag reflexes, increased risk for aspiration, increased risk for obstruction secondary to

Table 6-1 Cardiovascular and Pulmonary Manifestations of Musculoskeletal Conditions

	Impairment	Factors that Potentially Contribute to Impairment
General Manifestations	Decreased alveolar ventilation	Altered respiratory mechanics Chest wall rigidity Decreased chest wall excursion
	Impaired mucociliary transport	Airflow obstruction Pulmonary restriction Atelectasis Inspissated secretions
	Increased work of breathing	Inefficient breathing pattern
	Increased work of the heart	Inefficient breathing pattern Constrictive pericarditis
	Decreased aerobic capacity	
Manifestations in Specific Conditions	Rheumatoid arthritis	Pleuritis Diffuse interstitial pneumonitis and fibrosis Pulmonary arteritis Bronchiolitis Pleural effusions
	Ankylosing spondylitis	Upper lobe fibrobullous disease Chest wall restriction

impaired mucociliary clearance, restricted mobility, compression of mediastinal structures and heart, and impaired lymphatic drainage, which depends on normal expiratory and inspiratory cycles.[7] Osteoporotic fractures also compromise normal chest wall configuration, hence, pulmonary function.[8]

Autoimmune conditions that have musculoskeletal manifestations can be associated with systemic conditions. Rheumatoid arthritis, for example, is associated with accelerated atherosclerosis.[9]

Connective Tissue Conditions

Connective tissue, or collagen, vascular disorders (e.g., scleroderma, systemic lupus erythematosus, and systemic sclerosis) invariably affect the cardiovascular and pulmonary systems (Box 6-2).[10] Inflammation and tissue injury can affect the airway, lung parenchyma, pulmonary vasculature, pleurae, respiratory muscles, heart, and pericardium. Shrinking-lung syndrome associated with chronic connective tissue changes is a feature of advanced disease and is characterized by loss of alveolar surface area, diffusion capacity, and lung volumes. Fibrotic changes increase the elasticity of the lung parenchyma and reduce lung compliance, thereby increasing the work of breathing. These changes are comparable to those in idiopathic pulmonary fibrosis. Both the electrical conduction system of the heart and its mechanical behavior are adversely affected by systemic connective tissue changes. Furthermore, connective tissue changes in the skin can lead to chest wall restriction. Renal-pulmonary syndrome has been associated with connective tissue conditions.[11] The cardiovascular and pulmonary manifestations of connective tissue conditions are summarized in Box 6-2.

Connective tissue conditions contribute to blood vessel changes and have been implicated in secondary pulmonary arterial hypertension.[12,13]

Neurological Conditions

Cardiovascular and pulmonary consequences of neurological conditions reflect the pathophysiological mechanisms involved.[14] There are three basic patterns of pathology: dysfunction of the central nervous system (CNS), dysfunction of the peripheral nervous system, and dysfunction of the autonomic nervous system. The cardiovascular and pulmonary manifestations of neurological conditions are summarized in Table 6-2.

Box 6-2 Cardiovascular and Pulmonary Manifestations of Connective Tissue/Collagen Vascular Conditions

General Manifestations	Specific Manifestations in Scleroderma
Acute injury to the alveolar-capillary unit	Restrictive ventilatory impairment
Alveolar hemorrhage	Decreased diffusing capacity
Interstitial pneumonitis	Diaphragmatic dysfunction
Interstitial pulmonary fibrosis	Gastroesophageal reflux and aspiration
Pulmonary hypertension	
Respiratory muscle dysfunction	
Pulmonary edema	
Pulmonary infection	
Abnormal diffusing capacity	
Chest wall restriction	

Dysfunction of the Central Nervous System

The primary centers for breathing control and control of the heart are seated in the midbrain. The generator for breathing control produces a regular respiratory rate through modulation of inspiratory and expiratory inhibitory and excitatory neurons.

Activity of the central generator is affected by arousal and the general alerting reaction of the reticular activating system. In addition, breathing control is influenced by the hypothalamus, orbital cortex, forebrain, and amygdala.[15]

Insult to the CNS can result in cardiovascular responses that precipitate neurogenic pulmonary edema. Such responses include systemic hypertension, pulmonary hypertension, intracranial hypertension, and bradycardia. The medulla may mediate the cardiovascular responses associated with neurogenic pulmonary edema. Marked sympathetic stimulation, catecholamine release, and vagotonia appear to precipitate neurogenic pulmonary edema and the resulting leaking of the alveolar capillary membrane and alveolar flooding.[16]

Cortical disturbances may have a direct effect on cardiovascular and pulmonary function. Among the most common disturbances seen clinically are cortical infarction and seizures. Hemispheric infarction can lead to contralateral weakness of the diaphragm and other respiratory muscles. Epileptic seizures disrupt breathing, which causes hypoxemia, respiratory acidosis, and a metabolic acidosis secondary to extreme muscle contraction and lactate accumulation. The associated increase in sympathetic stimulation can precipitate cardiac dysrhythmias and pulmonary edema.

Demyelinating diseases such as multiple sclerosis result in progressive deterioration of neuromuscular function. The muscles of respiration become increasingly involved, resulting in respiratory insufficiency due to weakness.[17,18] In addition, with increasing debility, cardiovascular and pulmonary conditioning is reduced. Weakness of the pharyngeal musculature contributes to loss of airway protection in addition to the loss of cough and gag reflexes. Aspiration is problematic for these patients as the disease advances.

Patients with stroke may have central dysfunction that affects cardiovascular and pulmonary regulation and function, including reduced electrical activity of the respiratory muscles or peripheral dysfunction such that weakness, spasticity, impaired biomechanics, and gait directly affect respiratory muscle function and chest wall excursion. Hemiparesis of the diaphragm on the affected side can occur. Abdominal muscle weakness contributes to impaired cough effectiveness. Pharyngeal weakness contributes to sleep apnea in these patients. The common clinical presentation of unilateral dysfunction leads to a posture characterized by listing to the affected side when recumbent or sitting and during ambulation. This posture impairs ventilation and chest wall expansion on the affected side. Abdominal muscle dysfunction directly affects intraabdominal pressure and the efficiency of diaphragmatic descent during contraction (i.e., should the abdominal muscles

Table 6-2 **Cardiovascular and Pulmonary Manifestations of Neurological Conditions**

Manifestation Type	Impairment	Factors that Potentially Contribute to Impairment
General	Impaired mucociliary transport	Decreased physical mobility Cilia dyskinesia Increased mucus accumulation Decreased cough and gag reflexes Impaired airway protection Increased airway resistance Increased risk for airway obstruction Impaired glottic closure Increased risk for aspiration
	Impaired alveolar ventilation	Decreased lung volumes and capacities, as well as flow rates Weakness of pharyngeal and laryngeal structures Respiratory muscle weakness Decreased respiratory muscle endurance
	Increased work of breathing	
	Decreased aerobic capacity and deconditioning	
Specific	Multiple sclerosis	Respiratory muscle weakness Impaired ventilation secondary to spasm Increased oxygen consumption secondary to spasm Increased oxygen consumption secondary to impaired posture and gait Impaired gag and cough reflexes Ineffective cough
	Cerebral palsy	Increased oxygen consumption secondary to increased muscle tone Decreased mobility and activity Impaired movement economy Impaired swallowing Impaired saliva control Decreased gag and cough reflexes Impaired coordination of thoracic and abdominal motion during respiration Ineffective cough and airway clearance mechanisms
	Stroke	Decreased movement economy Spasticity and increased oxygen demands Flaccidity of respiratory muscles Impaired respiratory muscle strength Impaired pulmonary function Asymmetric chest wall Weak and ineffective cough
	Parkinson syndrome	Increased oxygen consumption secondary to increased muscle tone Decreased movement economy Chest wall restriction and impaired pulmonary function Ineffective cough

become flaccid, the efficiency of diaphragmatic contraction is reduced). Lung volumes and flow rates are reduced proportionately, causing a restrictive pattern of lung function. Muscle spasticity contributes to chest wall restriction and increased metabolic cost. Reduced activity and exercise around the time of the stroke contribute to reduced cardiovascular and pulmonary conditioning and capacity of the oxygen transport system. A high proportion of patients with strokes are hypertensive and older, a population with a higher prevalence of heart disease and atherosclerosis.[19,20]

Cerebral palsy is associated with increased muscle tone, which correspondingly increases basal and exercise oxygen consumption, resulting in increased oxygen demands. Even though the demands are increased in this condition, oxygen delivery is compromised. For example, thoracic deformity and spasm of the muscles of the chest wall and abdomen impair the breathing pattern and its efficiency. Minimizing secondary scoliosis is a priority.[21] The airways of patients with cerebral palsy are vulnerable to obstruction because of poor gag, cough, and swallowing reflexes. In addition, these patients often have poor saliva control, which further increases the risk for aspiration. Mental retardation often complicates the presentation of cerebral palsy and prevents these patients from responding adequately to their hydration needs and being able to cooperate with life-preserving treatments. These patients may harbor numerous microorganisms, adding further to their general risk for infection. Of clinical importance is the fact that pulmonary function can be substantially improved with adaptive seating and postural control.[22]

Patients with Parkinson syndrome also exhibit cardiovascular and pulmonary deficits.[23] Oxygen demand is increased commensurate with increased muscle tone. Patients with Parkinson syndrome have reduced cardiovascular and pulmonary conditioning levels as a result of compromised agility and ability to be independently mobile. These patients have a restrictive pattern of lung disease in which most lung volumes and capacities are reduced. Chest wall rigidity impairs the normal pump-handle and bucket-handle movements, so breathing efficiency is reduced. The energy cost of breathing is correspondingly increased. Respiratory insufficiency in Parkinson syndrome likely reflects increases in tone of the respiratory muscles, chest wall rigidity, and parasympathetic tone and resulting airway obstruction. Parkinson syndrome can be associated with cardiac sympathetic denervation,[24] which has implications for the assessment, monitoring during exercise, and exercise prescription.

Patients with a history of poliomyelitis, with or without cardiovascular and pulmonary complications at onset, may exhibit pulmonary limitation several decades later.[25,26] These individuals are at risk for developing respiratory insufficiency as a result of respiratory and abdominal muscle weakness, chest wall deformity, minor infection, and periods of relative immobility; or secondary to medical interventions, such as anesthesia and sedation. Further, because of prolonged reduced physical activity, patients with chronic poliomyelitis may be overweight.

Diseases and lesions involving the brainstem can lead to various abnormal breathing patterns. Some common breathing aberrations are Cheyne-Stokes respiration, central neurogenic hyperventilation, apneustic breathing, and ataxic breathing. Cerebellar and basal ganglia lesions may produce respiratory muscle discoordination and dyspnea.

Spinal cord lesions have a variable effect on cardiovascular and pulmonary function, depending on the level of the lesion. Cervical lesions result in a high mortality rate due to cardiovascular and pulmonary complications. All lung volumes are diminished with the exception of total lung capacity (TLC), which over time returns to normal; tidal volume (TV), which is usually preserved (10% of TLC); and residual volume (RV), which is increased.[27] Patients with quadriplegia tend to have a greater diaphragmatic contribution to tidal ventilation than people without such injury. In addition, these patients have impaired cough as a result of the loss of innervation and paresis of the diaphragm, in some cases, and of abdominal and intercostal muscles. The contribution of accessory muscle activity to ventilation varies considerably. In quadriplegia in which only the accessory muscles and diaphragm have been spared, platypnea (increased dyspnea when upright) may occur.[28] In the upright position, the diaphragm is flattened and less efficient when moved downward by reduced abdominal pressures.

Thoracic lesions tend to have less effect on pulmonary function (vital capacity and forced expiratory volumes, in particular) than do cervical lesions, and the significance of this effect is reduced as the level of the lesion is reduced. Lumbar lesions may have minimal or no effect on pulmonary function; however, dysfunction of the abdominal muscles may limit cough effectiveness.

Dysfunction of the Peripheral Nervous System

Disorders of the peripheral nervous system include those of the motor neuron, peripheral nerve, neuromuscular junction, and muscle. Neuromuscular disorders of the larynx, pharynx, and tongue can lead to upper airway obstruction and increased airway resistance and can interfere with maintaining a clear airway. Aspiration is a common and serious problem associated with impaired motor control of the larynx, pharynx, and tongue.

Dysfunction of the Autonomic Nervous System

Cardiovascular and pulmonary consequences of disorders of the autonomic nervous system have been documented. Of those conditions with an autonomic component, autonomic neuropathies, diabetes, and alcoholism have been the most thoroughly studied. Multiple-system atrophy accompanies autonomic failure affecting multiple systems. Because of the anatomic proximity of the autonomic, respiratory, and hypnogenic neurons and the degeneration of these structures in this condition, dysfunction of the respiratory control mechanisms parallels autonomic and somatic dysfunction. The respiratory dysrhythmias that are seen in multiple-system atrophy include central and upper airway obstruction; irregular rate, rhythm, and amplitude of respiration, with or without oxygen desaturation; transient uncoupling of the intercostal and diaphragmatic muscle activity; prolonged periods of apnea; Cheyne-Stokes respiration; inspiratory gasps; and transient sudden respiratory arrest.[29]

Patients with diabetes and autonomic neuropathies exhibit variable cardiovascular and pulmonary dysfunction. Postural hypotension is a complication of diabetic autonomic neuropathy and efferent sympathetic vasomotor denervation. Norepinephrine levels are generally reduced in these patients. The splanchnic and peripheral circulations fail to constrict in response to standing, so cardiac output falls. The postural effect is exacerbated by reduced cardiac acceleration in patients with diabetes. Insulin has been associated with cardiovascular effects, including reduced plasma volume, increased peripheral blood flow secondary to vasodilation, and increased heart rate. In the presence of autonomic neuropathies, insulin can induce postural hypotension. Diabetic diarrhea secondary to abnormal gut motility can contribute to fluid loss and its sequelae. Cardiovascular and pulmonary changes associated with autonomic neuropathy secondary to diabetes include altered ventilatory responses to hypoxia and hypercapnia, altered respiratory pattern and apneic episodes during sleep, altered bronchial reactivity, and impaired cough.[29] Impaired peripheral perfusion and tissue nutrition are also consequences of diabetes and autonomic neuropathies, which will be described later in this chapter (see Endocrine Conditions).

Gastrointestinal Conditions

The cardiovascular and pulmonary manifestations of gastrointestinal (GI) dysfunction are summarized in Table 6-3. Inflammatory bowel disease and pancreatitis are principal examples of GI dysfunction affecting cardiovascular and pulmonary function. Aspiration is a significant cause of morbidity and mortality in patients with GI dysfunction, so it should be prevented or detected early. The pathophysiology, management, and outcome depend on the nature of the aspirate. Several predisposing factors produce aspiration pneumonia, including a decreased level of consciousness, disorders of pharyngeal and esophageal motility, altered anatomy, disorders of gastric and intestinal motility, and iatrogenic factors such as surgery, nasogastric intubation, and general anesthesia.

Inflammatory bowel disease can lead to the following cardiovascular and pulmonary pathologies: vasculitis, fibrosis,

Table 6-3 **Cardiovascular and Pulmonary Manifestations of GI Conditions**

Impairment	Factors that Potentially Contribute to Impairment
Risk for aspiration	Gastroesophageal reflux
Increased airway resistance	Bronchospasm
Decreased lung volumes	Elevated hemidiaphragms Compression atelectasis
Arterial hypoxemia	Alveolar capillary leak and V/Q mismatch Alveolar hemorrhage and consolidation worsen shunt Increased pulmonary vascular resistance

Box 6-3 **Cardiovascular and Pulmonary Manifestations of Liver Conditions**

- Intrapulmonary vascular dilation
- Pulmonary hypertension
- Expiratory airflow obstruction
- Chest wall deformity
- Pleural effusions
- Panacinar emphysema
- Pleuritis
- Bronchitis
- Bronchiectasis
- Hypoxic vasoconstriction
- Interstitial pneumonitis
- Pulmonary fibrosis

granulomatous disease, and pulmonary thromboembolism. Bronchitis and bronchiectasis have also been associated with inflammatory bowel disease; however, their occurrence is not related to disease severity or therapy. Biopsy specimens have shown basement membrane thickening, thickening of the epithelium, and infiltration of the underlying connective tissue with inflammatory cells.[30]

The pulmonary manifestations of acute pancreatitis are among the most important sequelae of this disease and often the cause of premature death. Problems include elevated hemidiaphragms, particularly on the right side; basal atelectasis; diffuse pulmonary infiltrates that appear more commonly on the right side than on the left side; pleural effusions that occur more commonly on the left side than on the right side; and pneumonitis. These findings are not specific for pancreatitis and are probably secondary to localized peritonitis, subphrenic collections, ascites, pain, and abdominal distension. In chronic pancreatitis, abdominal symptoms may be reduced and thoracic symptoms such as dyspnea, chest pain, and cough may predominate. Chronic effusions may result in pleural thickening.

Hepatic Conditions

Both acute and chronic liver conditions can predispose a patient to cardiovascular and pulmonary and cardiovascular complications (Box 6-3). Hepatic dysfunction can lead to hypoxemia secondary to intrapulmonary vascular dilation and noncardiogenic pulmonary edema. Hepatopulmonary syndrome, hallmarked by intrapulmonary vascular dilation, produces both diffusion and perfusion defects in the lungs and is the principal reason for severe hypoxemia.[31]

Such pulmonary vasodilation is associated with excess perfusion with respect to ventilation.[32] Arterial oxygenation may range from an asymptomatic increase in alveolar-arterial oxygen pressure difference to extreme breathlessness secondary to severe hypoxemia. Of relevance to the physical therapist is that oxygenation in these patients is frequently worse when the patient is standing compared with lying supine (orthodeoxia). In severe cases, pulmonary edema may occur secondarily to hepatic encephalopathy and cerebral edema.[33]

With respect to chronic liver conditions, cardiovascular and pulmonary manifestations have been associated with cirrhosis and hepatitis. The most common pulmonary abnormalities associated with these conditions are intrapulmonary vascular dilation with and without shunt, pulmonary hypertension, airflow obstruction, chest wall deformity, pleural effusions, panacinar emphysema, pleuritis, bronchitis, bronchiectasis, hypoxic vasoconstriction, interstitial pneumonitis, and fibrosis. Hypoxemia results from shunting, ventilation-perfusion mismatching, and diffusion abnormalities.

Pleural effusions and ascites interfere with diaphragm function and present unique problems in a patient with liver disease. Rich lymphatic connections exist between the abdominal and thoracic cavities, so ascitic fluid can flow into the pleural space. This effect is enhanced during inspiration, when the intraabdominal pressure is relatively positive and the intrapleural space is negative.

The liver is a primary organ for the production of procoagulants and anticoagulants in the blood, both of which are carefully regulated to maintain optimal balance. Liver dysfunction can disrupt the production of these complementary agents and lead to a tendency to bleed or clot. Disseminated intravascular coagulation refers to an extreme imbalance between these vasoactive agents in which bleeding and clotting problems occur simultaneously, resulting in serious consequences to the patient. With respect to central dysfunction, recently impaired myocardial contractility has been reported in patients with cirrhosis.[34]

Renal Conditions

Cardiovascular and pulmonary complications can result from renal dysfunction and from the category of disorders referred to as renal-pulmonary syndromes (Box 6-4).[35,36] The pathophysiological characteristics of these disorders include alveolar hemorrhage, interstitial and alveolar inflammation, and dysfunction of the pulmonary vasculature. Pulmonary function testing may detect both obstructive and restrictive abnormalities as a result of bronchial complications and as a result of inflammation and hemorrhage, respectively.

In systemic illness, pathology of the lungs and kidneys often coexist. Physical therapy warrants being aggressive, given the course of the renal-pulmonary syndromes and the potential for relapses and irreversible organ damage. Notwithstanding the serious medical implications of renal dysfunction, even

Box 6-4 Cardiovascular and Pulmonary Manifestations of Renal Conditions

- Alveolar hemorrhage
- Airway obstruction
- Decreased lung volumes
- Decreased diffusing capacity

Box 6-5 Cardiovascular and Pulmonary Manifestations of Hematological Conditions

General Cardiovascular Pulmonary Manifestations	Abnormalities of the Fluid Portion of the Blood	Abnormalities of the Cellular Portion of the Blood
Hemorrhage	Abnormal blood volume	Abnormal red blood cell count
Edema	Abnormal fluid balance (water excesses and deficits)	Abnormal red blood cells
Polycythemia	Abnormal electrolytes	Abnormal deformability of the red blood cells
Anemia	Abnormal plasma proteins	Abnormal hemoglobin
Infection	Abnormal procoagulants and anticoagulants	Abnormal oxyhemoglobin dissociation (e.g., carbon monoxide poisoning)
	Abnormal clotting times	Abnormal white blood cells and antibodies
		Blood dyscrasias

simple measures such as dietary salt restriction need to be advocated, even for patients on dialysis.[37]

Hematological Conditions

Hematological disorders that can manifest cardiovascular and pulmonary symptoms include abnormalities of the fluid and cellular components of the blood, as well as coagulopathies.[38] Cardiovascular and pulmonary manifestations of hematological conditions are summarized in Box 6-5. The primary underlying mechanisms by which these conditions disrupt gas exchange include hemorrhage, infection, edema, anemia, fibrosis, and malignancies.

Abnormalities related to red blood cells and their ability to transport hemoglobin and oxygen may produce signs resembling pulmonary pathology (e.g., tachypnea, dyspnea, and cyanosis). Abnormalities of the deformability of red blood cells alter blood viscosity and pulmonary blood flow. The interstitium can be disrupted by such factors as hemorrhage and malignancies. Coagulopathies disrupt the normal hemostasis and clotting mechanisms of the blood. Pulmonary hemorrhage and hemoptysis are common sequelae. The most common causes of pulmonary hemorrhage include vitamin K deficiency, hemophilia, hepatic failure, and disseminated intravascular coagulation. Pharmacological agents such as platelet inhibitors and anticoagulants can also result in pulmonary hemorrhage. Pulmonary thromboemboli are common events; symptoms include pleuritic chest pain, dyspnea, and hemoptysis.

Of the erythrocyte disorders, sickle cell anemia is probably the most common, and its manifestations largely reflect erythrocyte rigidity and vasoocclusion.[39] Acute chest infection and thrombosis leading to pulmonary infarction may occur with clinical symptoms such as fever, pleuritic chest pain, cough, and pulmonary infiltrates. The pulmonary function of patients with sickle cell anemia is abnormal; there is likely to be a reduction in TLC, vital capacity, diffusing capacity, arterial oxygen tensions, and exercise capacity.

The hematological malignancy disorders that can affect pulmonary function include the leukemias and Hodgkin disease. The three primary mechanisms by which these disorders can affect pulmonary function include direct infiltration, increased risk for opportunistic infection, and secondary effects of treatment, such as interstitial pneumonitis and fibrosis.

Disorders of plasma proteins can have significant effects on the Starling forces that maintain normal fluid balance within the tissue vascular beds. Depending on the amount of plasma protein, particularly albumin, fluid is retained in or lost from circulation. With reduced protein and oncotic pressure within the vasculature, more fluid is filtered out of the circulation into the interstitium. In catabolic states in which protein is broken down in the body, more protein leaks through the capillaries and takes water with it, thus leading to edema.

Endocrine Conditions

Endocrine and metabolic disorders can be associated with cardiovascular and pulmonary complications (Box 6-6).[6,40] Disorders of the thyroid gland, pancreas (diabetes mellitus), and adrenal glands are examples that are often seen clinically. Thyroid hormone influences surfactant synthesis and the central drive to breathe. Hypothyroidism can lead to sleep apnea, pleural effusions secondary to altered capillary permeability, and pericardial effusions. Decreases in vital capacity have also been reported secondary to muscle weakness. Individuals with hypothyroidism have exercise intolerance.[41] Hyperthyroidism increases cellular oxidative metabolism (the metabolic rate), leading to an increase in oxygen consumption and CO_2 production and an overall increase in minute ventilation.[41] Vital capacity, lung compliance, and diffusion capacity can be reduced. In addition, maximal inspiratory and expiratory pressures can be reduced secondary to muscle weakness. In thyroid dysfunction, cardiorespiratory function can be normal at rest, but dysfunction can be unmasked during exercise stress.

Individuals with diabetes may lose their pulmonary reserve capacity.[42] Although this may present as a subclinical finding, such loss can manifest with stress, aging, chronic hypoxia secondary to lung disease, or volume overload secondary to cardiac and renal failure.

People with diabetes are prone to aspiration and respiratory infections. Late complications of diabetic neuropathy include renal failure, which may be accompanied by pleural effusions and pulmonary edema. Autonomic neuropathy may affect vagal activity and airway tone and the vasomotor tone of the blood vessels. Ischemic heart disease and cardiomyopathies

Box 6-6 Cardiovascular and Pulmonary Manifestations of Endocrine Conditions

Thyroid Disorders
Hypothyroidism
Hypometabolism
- Fatigue and excessive sleeping
- Decreased aerobic conditioning
- Decreased vital capacity secondary to muscle weakness
- Sleep apnea
- Decreased heart rate
- Decreased cardiac output
- Decreased blood volume
- Pleural effusions
- Pericardial effusions

Hyperthyroidism
- Hypermetabolism
- Decreased vital capacity and diffusing capacity
- Fluid loss (diarrhea)
- Respiratory muscle weakness
- Fatigue and inability to sleep
- Decreased aerobic conditioning

Pancreatic Disorders (Diabetes)
Increased pulmonary endothelial thickness
Decreased TLC
Decreased vital capacity and forced expiratory volumes
Decreased airway vagal tone
Increased risk for aspiration
Possible reduced elastic recoil
Impaired hypoxic and hypercapnic responses
Impaired ventilatory response to exercise
Defective neutrophil production
Colonization with gram-negative bacilli
Pleural effusions and pulmonary edema with diabetic nephropathy
Increased sensitivity to increases in inspiratory resistive loading
Accelerated atherosclerotic vascular and cardiac changes
Increased ischemic heart disease
Cardiomyopathy
Increased risk for infection

Adrenal Insufficiency
Orthostatic symptoms
Decreased aerobic capacity secondary to anorexia, weakness, and fatigue
Impaired breathing mechanics secondary to GI symptoms
Increased tendency to retain fluid

are common in patients with diabetes and may cause congestive heart failure and cardiogenic pulmonary edema. Patients with diabetes have been reported to have reduced sensitivity to inspiratory loading,[43] which may impair their subjective responses to exercise. Peripheral perfusion can be compromised, resulting in diabetes. Limbs are endangered by reduced perfusion and reduced sensation. Severe cases result in limb ischemia, gangrene, and surgical amputation. Infection rates are high in patients with diabetes.

Adrenal insufficiency can also compromise oxygen transport.[40] Reduced aerobic capacity results from symptoms of weakness and fatigue and associated muscle and joint complaints. Orthostatic intolerance primarily reflects reduced inotropic capacity of the heart and reduced systemic vascular resistance.

Immunological Conditions

Congenital and acquired defects in the immunological status of the lungs lead to cardiovascular and pulmonary dysfunction, including inflammation and infection. Acquired immunodeficiency syndrome (AIDS), an example of a primary disorder of cell-mediated immunity, has reached epidemic proportions over the past 20 years. This syndrome leads to lymphocyte death. The most serious pulmonary infection associated with AIDS is *Pneumocystis carinii* pneumonia.[44] The fact that a patient with the human immunodeficiency virus (HIV) is likely to have recurrent pneumonia suggests that the infecting organisms persist in the lung despite treatment.[45] The clinical presentation includes diffuse pulmonary infiltrates, cough, dyspnea, and hemoptysis. These patients can also have symptoms of upper airway obstruction.

Nutritional Disorders

The two most common nutritional disorders seen in Western countries are obesity and anorexia nervosa, which is akin to starvation. Two-thirds of the U.S. population is now categorized as being overweight and at risk for its sequelae. Obesity contributes in several ways to impaired oxygen transport.[46] Alveolar hypoventilation and impaired PaO_2 and gas exchange result from chest wall restriction. Systemic and pulmonary blood pressures are increased. In addition, large abdomens and abdominal contents impinge on diaphragmatic motion and can restrict diaphragmatic descent. This can lead to compression of the dependent lung fields. Obesity is associated with elevated C-reactive protein, a marker for inflammation and elevated cardiovascular health risk.[47] Recumbency can induce respiratory insufficiency (positional respiratory failure). Individuals who are obese have a higher incidence of snoring and obstructive sleep apnea secondary to weakness and increased compliance of the postpharyngeal structures. In addition, these patients often have weak, ineffectual coughs resulting from expiratory muscle weakness and the mechanical inefficiency of these muscles. The work of breathing is markedly increased. Furthermore, in chronic cases, reactive pulmonary vasoconstriction in response to chronic hypoxemia contributes to right ventricular insufficiency and increased work of the heart and cardiomegaly. Individuals who are obese tend to be less active and aerobically deconditioned, with reduced efficiency of oxygen transport overall and increased risk for thromboemboli. Hypertension is also a serious sequela of obesity.

In addition to the direct effects obesity has on oxygen transport, central obesity has been strongly linked with metabolic syndrome. Additional risk factors include increased blood pressure, dyslipidemia (raised triglycerides and lowered high-density lipoprotein cholesterol), increased fasting glucose and type 2 diabetes mellitus.[48] In any patient who is overweight, these risk factors need to be assessed, not only so that treatment can be prescribed accordingly, but to facilitate referral of the patient to other health care professionals, if necessary. Abdominal fat, although associated with aging, is more closely linked with health risk than subcutaneous fat. Conventional measures of body composition may not estimate health risk sufficiently (e.g., insulin resistance and cardiovascular disease).[49]

The major cardiovascular and pulmonary manifestations of anorexia nervosa relate to generalized weakness and reduced

Box 6-7 Cardiovascular and Pulmonary Manifestations of Nutritional Disorders

Obesity

Alveolar hypoventilation
Obstructive sleep apnea
Decreased outward recoil of the chest wall
Increased abdominal contents
Increased mass of the abdominal wall
Decreased functional residual capacity
Decreased expiratory reserve volume
Decreased lung volumes, arterial oxygen tension (Pa_{O_2}), and saturation (Sa_{O_2}) in recumbency
Basal airway closure and resulting decrease in Pa_{O_2}
Marked pulmonary abnormalities during sleep
Decreased ventilatory responses to CO_2
Cardiomegaly
Rotation and horizontal position of the heart
Axis deviation on ECG
Decreased myocardial pumping efficiency
Decreased aerobic conditioning and oxygen transport reserve capacity

Starvation or Anorexia Nervosa

Generalized weakness, debility, decreased cardiopulmonary conditioning
Impaired mucociliary transport
Ineffective cough
Fluid and electrolyte disturbances
Cardiac dysrhythmias
Respiratory muscle weakness

endurance of all muscles, including the respiratory muscles. Cough effectiveness is correspondingly compromised. Oxygen transport reserve is minimal. Because of poor nutrition and fluid intake, the patient is at risk for anemia, fluid and electrolyte imbalances, and cardiac dysrhythmias.[50] Common manifestations of nutritional disorders are summarized in Box 6-7.

Summary

This chapter describes the cardiovascular and pulmonary consequences of common systemic conditions. Oxygen transport, the purpose of the cardiovascular and pulmonary system, can be significantly affected by dysfunction in virtually all organ systems of the body. The pathophysiological consequences of conditions of the following systems of oxygen transport are presented: cardiac, pulmonary, musculoskeletal, connective tissue/collagen vascular, neurological, gastrointestinal, hepatic, renal, hematological, endocrine, and immunological. In addition, the cardiovascular and pulmonary manifestations of nutritional disorders, including obesity and anorexia nervosa, are described.

Knowledge of these effects is essential to the practice of physical therapy across all specialties because of the prevalence of systemic conditions either singly or in combination. The presentation of the cardiovascular and pulmonary consequences of systemic conditions is often subtle or obscured and is associated with a poor prognosis, so early detection and appropriate management are essential.

Physical therapists must be able to diagnostically distinguish cardiovascular and pulmonary manifestations of systemic conditions in order to appropriately identify indications for physical therapy, contraindications, side effects, and unusual treatment responses. In addition, detailed assessment of the patient's problems ensures that problems amenable to physical therapy are appropriately treated and that those that are not are referred back to a physician. These skills are particularly important given the advent of direct-access practice and the fact that a high proportion of patients being treated by physical therapists have systemic conditions as secondary, as well as primary, diagnoses. Further, cardiovascular and pulmonary manifestations of systemic diseases may not have been previously diagnosed, but may be identified on the physical therapy assessment or manifested by the patient during exercise stress.

Review Questions

Describe (a) the cardiovascular and pulmonary manifestations and (b) the clinical implications for the physical therapists when a patient has one or more of the following types of dysfunction or conditions affecting the associated system:

1. Musculoskeletal dysfunction (chest wall and peripheral)
2. Connective tissue dysfunction; rheumatoid conditions
3. Neurological dysfunction
4. Hepatic dysfunction
5. Renal dysfunction
6. Hematological dysfunction
7. Endocrine dysfunction
8. Obesity
9. Malnutrition (e.g., anorexia nervosa)

References

1. Cavallaro Goodman C, Fuller KS: *Pathology: Implications for the physical therapist*, ed 3, St. Louis, 2009, Elsevier.
2. Scharf SM, Cassidy SS: *Heart-lung interactions in health and disease*, New York, 1989, Marcel Dekker.
3. James AE, Cooper M, White RI, et al: Perfusion changes on lung scans in patients with congestive heart failure. *Radiology* 100:99–106, 1971.
4. Saxton GA, Rabinowitz W, Dexter L, et al: The relationship of pulmonary compliance to pulmonary vascular pressures in patients with heart disease. *Journal of Clinical Investigation* 35:611–618, 1956.
5. Brown NE, Zamel N, Aberman A: Changes in pulmonary mechanics and gas exchange following thoracentesis. *Chest* 74:540–542, 1978.
6. Hall JE: *Guyton and Hall textbook of medical physiology*, ed 12, Philadelphia, 2010, Elsevier.
7. Mason RJ, Broaddus VC, Martin T, et al: *Murray and Nadel's textbook of respiratory medicine*, ed 5, Philadelphia, 2010, Elsevier.
8. Schlaich C, Minne HW, Bruckner T, et al: Reduced pulmonary function in patients with spinal osteoporotic fractures. *Osteoporosis International* 8:261–267, 1990.
9. Szekanecz Z, Kerekes G, Der H, et al: Accelerated atherosclerosis in rheumatoid arthritis. *Annals of the New York Academy of Sciences* 1108: 349–358, 2007.
10. Carmier D, Marchand-Adam S, Diot P, et al: Respiratory involvement in systemic lupus erythematosus. *Revue des Maladies Respiratoires* 27:e66–e78, 2010.
11. Bar J, Ehrenfeld M, Rozenman J, et al: Pulmonary-renal syndrome in systemic sclerosis. *Seminars in Arthritis and Rheumatism* 30:403–410, 2001.
12. Fagan A, Badesch DB: Pulmonary hypertension associated with connective tissue disease. *Progress in Cardiovascular Diseases* 45:225–234, 2002.
13. Raeside DA, Chalmers G, Clelland J, et al: Pulmonary artery pressure variation in patients with connective tissue disease: 24 hour ambulatory pulmonary artery pressure monitoring. *Thorax* 53:857–862, 1998.
14. Gilchrist JM: Overview of neuromuscular disorders affecting respiratory function. *Seminars in Respiratory and Critical Care Medicine* 23:191–200, 2002.

15. Barrett KE, Barman SM, Boitano S, et al: *Ganong's review of medical physiology*, ed 23, New York, 2009, McGraw Hill Companies.
16. Baumann A, Audibert G, McDonnell J, et al: Neurogenic pulmonary edema. *Acta Anaesthesiologica Scandinavica* 51:447–455, 2007.
17. Cooper CB, Trend PS, Wiles CM: Severe diaphragm weakness in multiple sclerosis. *Thorax* 40:631–632, 1985.
18. Smeltzer SC, Utell MJ, Rudick RA, et al: Pulmonary function and dysfunction in multiple sclerosis. *Archives of Neurology* 45:1245–1249, 1988.
19. Chimowitz MI, Mancini GBJ: Asymptomatic coronary artery disease in patients with stroke. *Current Concepts of Cerebrovascular Diseases and Stroke* 26:23–27, 1991.
20. Wolf PA, D'Agostino RB, Belanger AJ, et al: Probability of stroke: a risk profile from the Framingham Study. *Stroke* 22:312–318, 1991.
21. Saito N, Ebara S, Ohotsuka K, et al: Natural history of scoliosis in spastic cerebral palsy. *The Lancet* 351:1687–1692, 1998.
22. Nwaobi OM, Smith PD: Effect of adaptive seating on pulmonary function of children with cerebral palsy. *Developmental Medicine & Child Neurology* 28:351–354, 1986.
23. Mehta AD, Wright WB, Kirby B: Ventilatory function in Parkinson's disease. *British Medical Journal* 1:1456–1457, 1978.
24. Goldstein DS, Holmes C, Li ST, et al: Cardiac sympathetic denervation in Parkinson disease. *Annals of Internal Medicine* 133:338–347, 2000.
25. Dean E, Ross J, Road JD, et al: Pulmonary function in individuals with a history of poliomyelitis. *Chest* 100:118–123, 1991.
26. Steljes DG, Kryger MH, Kirk BW, et al: Sleep in postpolio syndrome. *Chest* 98:133–140, 1990.
27. Almenoff PL, Spungen AM, Lesser M, et al: Pulmonary function survey in spinal cord injury: Influences of smoking and level and completeness of injury. *Lung* 173:297–306, 1995.
28. Dantzker DR, Schay SM, Fletcher J: *Cardiopulmonary critical care*, ed 3, Philadelphia, 1997, Elsevier.
29. Bannister R, Mathais CJ: *Autonomic failure*, ed 4, New York, 2002, Oxford University Press.
30. Higenbottam T, Cochrane GM, Clark TJH, et al: Bronchial disease in ulcerative colitis. *Thorax* 35:581–585, 1980.
31. Sherlock S: The liver lung interface. *Seminars in Respiratory Medicine* 9:247–253, 1988.
32. Krowka MJ, Wiseman GA, Burnett OL, et al: Hepatopulmonary syndrome. A prospective study of relationships between severity of liver disease, PaO_2 response to 100% oxygen, and brain uptake after 99mTc MAA lung scanning. *Chest* 118:615–624, 2000.
33. Gill R, Sterling RK: Acute liver failure. *Journal of Clinical Gastroenterology* 33:191–198, 2001.
34. Laffi G, Barletta G, La Villa G, et al: Altered cardiovascular responsiveness to active tilting in nonalcoholic cirrhosis. *Gastroenterology* 113:891–898, 1997.
35. Matthay RA, Bromberg SI, Putman CE: Pulmonary renal syndromes: a review. *Yale Journal of Biology and Medicine* 53:497–523, 1980.
36. Rankin JA, Matthay RA: Pulmonary renal syndromes. II. Etiology and pathogenesis. *Yale Journal of Biology and Medicine* 55:11–26, 1982.
37. Ok E, Mees EJ: Unpleasant truths about salt restriction. *Seminars in Dialysis* 23:1–3, 2010.
38. Bromberg PA, Ross DW: The lungs and hematologic disease. In Murray JF, Nadel J, editors: *Textbook of respiratory medicine*, ed 3, Philadelphia, 2000, WB Saunders.
39. Rees DC, Williams TN, Gladwin MT: Sickle-cell disease. *The Lancet* 376:2018–2031, 2010.
40. Kirby RR, Taylor RW, Civetta JM: *Handbook of critical care*, ed 2, Philadelphia, 1996, Lippincott Williams & Wilkins.
41. Kahaly GJ, Kampmann C, Mohr-Kahaly S: Cardiovascular dynamics and exercise tolerance in thyroid disease. *Thyroid* 12:473–481, 2002.
42. Hsia CCW, Raskin P: Lung function changes related to diabetes mellitus. *Diabetes Technology & Therapeutics* 9(Suppl 1): S73–S82, 2007.
43. O'Donnell CR, Friedman LS, Russomanno JH, et al: Diminished perception of inspiratory-resistive loads in insulin-dependent diabetics. *New England Journal of Medicine* 319:1369–1373, 1988.
44. Hughes WT: *Pneumocystis carinii* pneumonia. *Seminars in Pediatric Infectious Diseases* 12:309–314, 2001.
45. Shelhamer JH, Ognibene FP, Macher AM, et al: Persistence of Pneumocystis carinii in lung tissue of acquired immunodeficiency syndrome patients treated for pneumocystis pneumonia. *American Review of Respiratory Diseases* 130:1161–1165, 1984.
46. Aronee LJ: Classification of obesity and assessment of obesity-related health risks. *Obesity Research* 10:105S–115S, 2002.
47. Bastard JP, Jardel C, Delattre J, et al: Evidence for a link between adipose Tissue interleukin-6 content and serum C-reactive protein concentrations in obese subjects. *Circulation* 99:2219–2222, 1999.
48. Alberti KGMM, Eckel RH, Grundy SM, et al: Harmonizing the metabolic syndrome. A Joint Interim Statement of the International Diabetes Federation Task Force on Epidemiology and Prevention; National Heart, Lung, and Blood Institute; American Heart Association; World Heart Federation; International Atherosclerosis Society; and International Association for the Study of Obesity. *Circulation* 120:1640–1645, 2009.
49. Kuk JL, Saunders TJ, Davidson LE, et al: Age-related changes in total and regional fat distribution. *Ageing Research Review* 8:339–348, 2009.
50. Kasper DL, Braunwald E, Fauci A, et al, editors: *Harrison's principles of internal medicine*, ed 16, St. Louis, 2004, McGraw-Hill.

Part II

Cardiovascular and Pulmonary Physical Therapy: Assessment

PART II OUTLINE

Measurement and Documentation

Claire Peel, John D Lowman, and Diane Clark

KEY TERMS

Documentation	Tests and measures	Validity
HIPAA Guidelines	Reliability	Outcomes

CHAPTER OUTLINE

Measurement and documentation are critical components in the process of providing patient care. Measurements (numerical or categorical assignments based on testing or measuring) form the basis for deciding intervention strategy and therefore influence patient response to therapeutic interventions.[1] Measurements are also used during treatment sessions to determine rate of progression and appropriateness of exercise prescriptions. Typically, therapists obtain a series of measures and, in combination with those made by other health care professionals, formulate a clinical hypothesis. The hypothesis includes both physical and psychosocial aspects. If parts of the hypothesis are incorrect because of inaccurate measures, interventions may be misdirected, which can result in treatment that is either not effective or unsafe. Consequently, knowledge of the qualities of measurements that relate to the cardiovascular and pulmonary systems is essential for effective patient care.

Documentation, interpretation of measurements, and the patient plan of care are also important for reimbursement and to ensure communication among health care team members. Timely and appropriate sharing of information on physiological responses to activity is often critical for optimal medical management. Documentation must be written clearly and concisely and include objective findings that will facilitate efficient and continuous care from all members of the health care team.

This chapter provides a discussion of types and characteristics of measurements that are common to cardiopulmonary physical therapy, followed by a discussion of the process of selecting and performing tests and measures, and interpreting the results. A discussion of the purposes and recommended terminology for documentation follows, including suggestions for providing objective and outcome-oriented information and supporting skilled and medically necessary physical therapy services in this population.

Characteristics of Measurements and Outcomes

The purpose of performing a measure is to assess or evaluate a characteristic or attribute of an individual. The characteristic to be measured must first be defined, and the purpose of performing each measure must be clear. Therapists can then select the most appropriate method of measuring, given the available resources and their clinical skills.

Table 7-1 Examples of Commonly Used Measurements and Their Respective Level of Measurement

Patient Characteristic	Test or Other Measure	Level of Measurement
Gender	Male/female	Nominal
Range of motion	Goniometry	Ratio
Muscle strength	Manual muscle testing (MMT) Isokinetic dynamometry	Ordinal Interval
Functional status	Functional independence measure Timed Up and Go (TUG)	Ordinal Ratio
Angina	Angina rating scale Borg CR10	Ordinal Ratio
Dyspnea	MRC scale Borg CR10 Visual Analog Scale	Ordinal Ratio Ratio

Table 7-2 Angina Rating Scale

Rating	Description
1	Mild, barely noticeable
2	Moderate, bothersome
3	Moderately severe, very uncomfortable
4	Most severe or intense pain ever experienced

From American College of Sports Medicine: *ACSM's guidelines for exercise testing and prescription.* Philadelphia, 2010, Lippincott Williams & Wilkins.

Box 7-1 Etiology of Congestive Heart Failure

Hypertension
Coronary artery disease (myocardial ischemia)
Cardiac dysrhythmias
Renal insufficiency
Cardiomyopathy
Heart valve abnormality
Pericardial effusion
Pulmonary embolism
Pulmonary hypertension
Spinal cord injury
Age-related changes

From Cahalin LP: Cardiac muscle dysfunction. In Hillegass EA, editor: Essentials of cardiopulmonary physical therapy, *ed 3, St Louis, 2011, Saunders.*

Levels or Types of Measurements

Measurements can be described according to their type or level of measurement. There are four levels of measurements: nominal, ordinal, interval, and ratio (Table 7-1).[2] Recognizing the level of measurement aids understanding and interpretation of the result.

Nominal

Objects or people are often placed in categories according to specific characteristics. If the categories have no rank or order, then the measurement is considered nominal. An example of a nominal measurement is the classification of patients with pulmonary disease into those with obstructive lung disease, restrictive lung disease, or a combination of obstructive and restrictive disease. The categories are mutually exclusive (i.e., all patients fit into one and only one category). Nominal categories are unranked, in that an individual with obstructive lung disease would not necessarily have a worse prognosis than an individual with restrictive lung disease.

The categories of a nominal measurement scale are defined using objective indicators that are universally understood. For example, the classification of patients with heart failure could be based on the primary cause for the development of the condition (Box 7-1). In each case, the cause would be determined by diagnostic testing such as angiography or echocardiography. Clear descriptions of the criteria for inclusion in each category are necessary to facilitate clinicians' agreement on the assignment of patients to categories. A high percentage of agreement indicates high interrater reliability.

Ordinal

Ordinal measurements are similar to nominal measurements with the exception that the categories are ordered or ranked. The categories in an ordinal scale indicate more or less of a certain attribute. The scale for rating angina is an example of an ordinal scale (Table 7-2). Each category is defined, and a rating of grade 1 angina is less than a rating of grade 4. In an ordinal scale, the differences between consecutive ratings are not necessarily equal. The difference between grade 1 angina and grade 2 is not necessarily the same as between grade 3 and grade 4 angina. Consequently, if numbers are assigned to categories, they can be used to represent rank but cannot be subjected to mathematical operations. Averaging angina scores is incorrect because averaging assumes that there are equal intervals between categories. A group of ordinal data could be reported as a percentage of each response (i.e., 80% of clients reported exercise-induced angina as 3 before a cardiac rehabilitation program.)

Categorical measurements are considered ordinal if being assigned to a specific category is considered better than or worse than being in another category. For example, patients with angina could be classified as having either stable or unstable angina. This measurement would be considered ordinal, because stable angina is considered a better condition to have compared with unstable angina.[3]

Interval

Interval measurements have units on a scale with equal distance between consecutive measurements and are differentiated from ratio measurements because the zero point is arbitrary rather than absolute. An arbitrary zero point is one that does not mean an absence of the characteristic that is being measured. Temperature, for example, can be measured using either an interval or a ratio scale. The Celsius temperature scale (interval measurement) assigns the zero point to the temperature at which water freezes, whereas the Kelvin scale (ratio measurement) assigns the zero point to an absence of heat.

The original Borg Ratings of Perceived Exertion (RPE) scale is considered an interval level of measurement.[4] This scale, ranging from 6 to 20, has been shown to be linear with oxygen consumption and heart rate.[4]

Measuring force production using an isokinetic dynamometer is an example of an interval measurement commonly used in physical therapy. Patients may generate muscle tension and move an extremity but register a score of zero because they cannot move as fast as the dynamometer. Interval measurements can have negative values and can be subjected to some arithmetic operations. Adding and subtracting values is logical. A patient who generates 10 ft-lb of torque at one session and 20 ft-lb at the following session increased her torque production by 10 ft-lb. However, interval values cannot be subjected to division or multiplication. It cannot be stated that the patient generated twice as much torque on the second session compared with the first session because it cannot be assumed that a reading of zero indicates no torque production.

Ratio

Ratio measurements have scales with units that are equal in size and have a zero point that indicates absence of the attribute being measured. Examples of ratio measurements that are used in cardiopulmonary physical therapy include heart rate, cardiac output, oxygen consumption, and 6-minute walk distance (6-MWD). Ratio measurements are always positive values and can be subjected to all arithmetic operations. For example, an aerobic capacity of 4 L/min is twice as great as an aerobic capacity of 2 L/min. The Borg CR10 scale and visual analogue scales are also examples of ratio level measurements.[4,5] The zero point of these scales is "nothing at all" or no perception of exertion. The CR10 scale may be preferable for use with patients who experience strong symptoms during testing or training.[6]

When deciding whether a measurement is a ratio or interval, the attribute that is being measured is defined. If the zero point indicates absence of the attribute, then the scale would be considered ratio. For example, cardiac output can be defined as the amount of blood in liters ejected from the left ventricle over a 1-minute period. A measurement of zero cardiac output would be absence of the characteristic, or no blood ejected from the left ventricle.

Reliability and Validity of Measurements

For a measurement to be of value to the therapist, the measure should be both reliable (reproducible) and valid (meaningful). When selecting and performing tests and measures, it is important to remember that measures can be reliable but not valid for a specific application.[7]

Reliability

Reliability is defined as the consistency or reproducibility of a measurement. Ideally, when attempting to measure a specific attribute, the value of the measurement should change only when the attribute changes. All measures, however, have some element of error that contributes to the variability of the measurement. When the error is relatively high, the value of the measurement can change even when the attribute does not change. Believing that a change has occurred when it has not can result in an inaccurate clinical decision related to intervention planning or progression.

Many factors contribute to measurement variability. The characteristic being measured may demonstrate a certain degree of variability. Blood pressure and heart rate vary depending on mental and physical factors such as body position, hydration level, anxiety, and time of day. For these attributes, multiple measurements often are used to provide the best estimate of the patient's true heart rate and blood pressure.

Another factor that contributes to the variability of a measurement is a change in the testing instrument. Testing instruments may vary in their readings because of changes in environmental conditions or malfunction of instrument parts. Instruments should be calibrated (i.e., compared with a known standard) on a regular basis to assure accuracy of the readings. Some instruments are relatively easy to calibrate. For example, values obtained using aneroid blood pressure devices can easily be compared with values obtained using mercury manometers. Values obtained using either palpation or a heart rate monitor can be compared with values obtained from electrocardiograph (ECG) recordings. The mercury manometer and the ECG would be considered the instruments that provided the best estimates of the characteristic being measured. Other devices, such as cycle ergometers, are more difficult to calibrate, and the usual approach is to rely on the manufacturer's specifications regarding the accuracy of the work rate readings.

A third factor contributing to measurement variability is the difference in the methods therapists use to obtain measurements. If a measurement is consistent when the same therapist repeats a test, then the measurement is said to have high intrarater reliability. Measurements that are consistent when multiple therapists perform the test under the same conditions are said to have high interrater reliability. Often, measurements have high intrarater reliability but lower interrater reliability because of variations in the specific methods used by therapists to attain the same measurement. Auscultation of breath sounds, a commonly used method of assessing patients in cardiopulmonary settings, has been shown to have only poor to fair interrater reliability.[8] Interrater reliability is important in clinical settings in which a patient may be evaluated and treated by more than one therapist. If the interrater reliability of a measurement is low, changes in the patient over time may not be accurately reflected. Interrater reliability for auscultation of breath sounds can be improved through education of the persons performing the measurements.[8]

Validity

Valid measurements are those that provide meaningful information and accurately reflect the characteristic for which the measure is intended. For a measure to be useful in a clinical setting, it must possess a certain degree of validity. Measurements can be reliable but not valid. For example, the ankle-brachial index (ABI) is reliable but not necessarily valid in all populations.[9]

There are various types of validity. Of importance in clinical practice are concurrent, predictive, and prescriptive validity. Concurrent validity is when a measurement accurately reflects measurements made with an accepted standard. Comparing a measurement made with a heart rate monitor with an ECG recording is an example of determining concurrent validity. In this example, the ECG recording would be considered the gold or accepted standard. Another example is using pulse oximetry during exercise testing. Yamaya and colleagues (2002)[10] compared pulse oximetry versus directly measured arterial oxygen saturation (the gold standard) and reported that a forehead sensor was more valid than a finger sensor. Measurements with predictive validity can be used to estimate the probability of occurrence of a future event. Screening tests often involve measurements that are used to predict future events. For example, identifying people with risk factors for coronary artery disease (CAD) leads to a prediction that their likelihood of developing CAD is higher than normal. Measures with prescriptive validity provide guidance to the direction of treatment. The categorical measurement of determining a person's risk for a future coronary event is a measurement that would need to have prescriptive validity. By classifying patients into high- versus low-risk categories on the basis of results of a diagnostic exercise test, the intensity and rate of progression of treatment is determined.

Sensitivity and Specificity

Accuracy of various types of exercise tests often is described by reporting sensitivity and specificity. Sensitivity is the ability of a measurement to identify individuals who are positive, or who have the characteristic that is being measured. If a test produces a high number of false-positive results, then the sensitivity will be low. A false-positive result means that the test result was positive but the characteristic was absent. Young women often have positive stress test results but do not have coronary artery disease. The consequence of a false-positive test result could be unnecessary treatment or further diagnostic testing. Specificity is the ability of a measurement to identify individuals who are negative, or who do not have the characteristic. A high number of false-negative results would produce a low specificity. A false-negative result has a negative test result even though the disease or characteristic is present. The consequence of a false-negative test result is not receiving treatment when it is indicated. Use of the Homans' sign to screen for deep vein thrombosis (DVT) is no longer advocated because the test lacks both sensitivity and specificity.[11,12]

Objective and Subjective Measurements

Measurements vary in degree of subjectivity versus objectivity. Subjective measurements are those that are affected in some way by the person obtaining the measurement (i.e., the measurer must make a judgment as to the value assigned). The assessment of a patient's breath sounds is influenced by many factors, including the therapist's choice of terminology for describing the findings, perception of normal breath sounds, and hearing acuity. The grading of functional skills may be influenced by the therapist's interpretation of what constitutes minimal versus moderate assistance. Because of the influence of the person performing the measure, subjective measurements usually have lower interrater reliability compared with objective measurements.[2]

Objective measurements are not affected by the person performing the measure (i.e., these measures do not involve judgment of the measurer). Heart rate measured by a computerized ECG system is an example of an objective measurement. Other examples include measuring blood pressure using an intraarterial catheter and oxygen consumption using a metabolic system. Objective measurements are not necessarily accurate but usually have high interrater reliability.[2]

Clinical Decision Making

The Hypothesis-Oriented Algorithm for Clinicians II (HOAC-II) intertwines the examination, evaluation, and diagnosis elements into an organized algorithm for clinical decision making.[13] Using the HOAC-II, initial data collection (e.g., data from the medical record and patient interview) during the examination allows for generation of patient-identified problems (PIPs) and an initial set of hypotheses that will guide the formulation of an examination strategy (i.e., selection and ordering of tests and measures). These initial measurements help refine the hypotheses and additional measurements are obtained to help confirm or deny the initial set of hypotheses, leading to an eventual hypothesis/physical therapy diagnosis (i.e., an idea of the underlying cause of the patient's problem), and/or a decision to consult with other health care practitioners. For instance, early in the examination process the therapist may suspect a proximal DVT; the Wells clinical decision rule can aid in deciding whether or not to refer the patient for further testing.[14]

Selecting Tests and Measures

Many factors influence the therapist's choice, including information obtained from the medical record, patient interview, and knowledge of available treatment options. Selected tests and measures should be relevant as measured by their potential ability to impact the direction of the examination and intervention. Tests and measures should be limited to those that are necessary to establish a clinical hypothesis, make decisions about appropriate interventions, and determine the effectiveness of the intervention. Therapists also must strive for efficiency and not repeat tests that have been performed by other health care professionals. Characteristics or qualities of measurements, such as reliability and validity, also influence the therapist's decision.

Another factor that influences the selection of tests and measures is the risk-benefit ratio. How do the risks of obtaining a measurement relate to the value of the information gained? Subjecting a patient to a symptom-limited graded exercise test during the acute stage of post-myocardial infarction (MI) could provide information to formulate an exercise prescription; however, the risks of performing this procedure at this phase of the recovery period likely outweigh the benefits.

Measurements selected need to be appropriate to the specific health condition (disorder or disease), severity of the condition, and other contextual (i.e., environmental and personal) factors specific to the patient.[15] Tests and measures that do not help optimize or assess patient-centered outcomes are an inefficient use of the therapist's time and add unnecessary costs to health care.

Performing Tests and Measures

General Principles

When performing tests and measures, therapists must take care to use procedures that can be replicated for future comparisons (i.e., there must be acceptable intrarater/interrater reliability). Time must be taken to ensure that conditions are optimal and that the patient is informed of his or her part in the activity. For example, measuring blood pressure in a noisy treatment area immediately when the patient arrives for an appointment may not provide an accurate measurement of resting blood pressure. Documenting the conditions in which a measure was made is also important. Conditions may include, but are not limited to, time of day, room temperature, recent activities performed by the patient (including medication administration), and type and model of measuring device (e.g., specific treadmill, sphygmomanometer, pulse oximeter, etc.). Also, if the patient needs supplemental oxygen, it is vital to document the oxygen flow rate or fraction of inspired oxygen and the oxygen delivery device (e.g., nasal cannula, Venturi mask, etc.) for proper test interpretation. For example, a patient's walking distance may not have improved, but if the patient used less oxygen, then a meaningful outcome was achieved.

Measures should be made with an objective and open mind (i.e., without anticipating the result of the measurement). A measure that is approached with a preconceived idea of the outcome may be affected by the therapist's expectations. Having confidence in the results of one's measurements is important and develops as clinical skills develop.

In clinics where more than one therapist is likely to evaluate or treat a patient, written procedures for performing measurements are necessary. Therapists also need to review the written procedures on a regular basis and practice performing the measures as a group. Practicing together is especially important for therapists who are new to the clinic. Interrater reliability for commonly used measures can be determined. If the reliability is low, written procedures may need to be revised to ensure optimal consistency of measurement. Many commonly used tests and measures, such as blood pressure and 6-minute walk test, have standardized methodology.[16,17]

Examination

Initial data collection from referral information or the medical record regarding the patient's current medical stability and functional status will help guide the examination strategy. For example, tests and measures will differ for a patient with an acute MI compared to a patient who is 3 weeks post-MI. Other factors to consider include the size of the infarction and associated complications such as dysrhythmias, heart failure, or angina. Other initial data collected during the interview may also guide the examination strategy. For example, if a patient becomes anxious when discussing walking on a treadmill, then perhaps a "field test," such as the 6-minute walk test (6-MWT), would be more prudent.

The examination begins with and is centered on the patient's self-identified problems that may reflect specific impairments, limitations in activity, and/or restrictions in patient-identified roles at home, work, and the community. The patient's goals for physical therapy should be reported. Documentation of examination findings should reflect the physical therapist's clinical reasoning in determining what impairments may underlie the patient's limitation in activity.

The history section may include information related to the current and past medical/surgical diagnoses, previous functional levels, lifestyle choices, living environment, medications, laboratory values, or diagnostic imaging results. The patient's perception of his or her cardiac or pulmonary condition is important, as are descriptions of pain or discomfort that may be associated with either a cardiac event or a pulmonary complication. Other systems, such as the musculoskeletal, neurological, and integumentary systems are briefly examined to identify concerns that may influence the patient's readiness or ability to participate in certain interventions.

Tests can be categorized as measuring impairments, activity limitations, or participation restrictions as defined by the World Health Organization's International Classification of Functioning, Disability and Health (ICF) model,[18] which was recently adopted by the American Physical Therapy Association (APTA).[19] A body function or body structure impairment is an abnormality of physiological function or anatomic structure at the tissue, organ, or body system level.[15] Examples of impairments include pain, dyspnea, decreased muscle strength or range of motion, abnormal heart rate and blood pressure values, and impaired aerobic capacity. Measurements of impairments are important because they assist therapists in deciphering the causes or reasons for limitations in activity. Activity limitations are difficulties an individual has in performing a task or action.[15] Activity limitations can be attributed to physical, social, cognitive, or emotional factors. Examples of activity limitations include the inability to dress, transfer, walk long distances, or climb stairs. Improvements in activity levels usually are of primary interest to patients and families and to those who reimburse for health care. Participation restrictions are those problems that an individual may experience in life situations, such as performing a job requirement or playing a sport.[15] Figure 7-1 illustrates a patient's condition using the ICF model.

When examining patients with cardiopulmonary disorders, therapists often assess responses to activity. Specific information on the activity and on the physiological responses should be included:

- Mode of activity (corridor or track walking, lower extremity cycling)
- Intensity, work level, or rate of activity (mph, percent grade, estimated MET (metabolic equivalent) level)
- Duration of activity at each intensity level

The description of activities should be written clearly so that the workload can be reproduced. Responses to activity include changes in heart rate and rhythm, blood pressure, respiratory rate, oxygen saturation levels, and heart and breath sounds from pre-activity to either during or immediately after activity. Subjective signs of exercise intolerance, such as changes in skin color, decrease in coordination, and sweating,

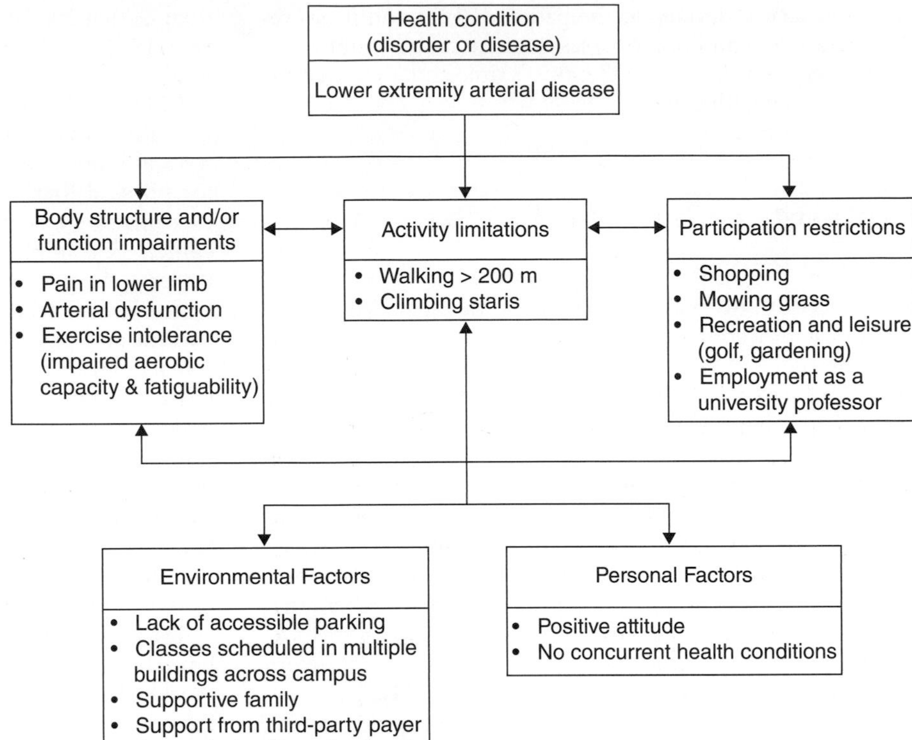

Fig. 7-1 Use of the ICF model to document a patient's condition and demonstrate various levels that need to be measured. The diagram illustrates how a person's health condition and body structure/function impairments affect participation in the community. Contextual factors (i.e., environmental and personal factors) interact at various levels to facilitate or hinder a person's health condition and level of function.

also need to be documented. Whether the patient used oxygen during treatment or required physical assistance should be noted. By objectively recording the activity performed and the physiological responses, therapists can estimate the patient's activity tolerance.

Evaluation and Interpretation of Findings

The evaluation process involves using the results of the examination to make clinical judgments. Therapists state their "clinical hypothesis," or explanation of reasons for activity limitations and/or participation restrictions. Evaluation reports provide the foundational support to confirm why the patient requires the skilled services of a physical therapist and why the services are medically necessary at this time. Examination findings may indicate the need for referral of the patient to other health care professionals or to community services.

Interpreting measurements often is challenging. Usually patients' problems are understood not by reviewing results of a single measure but by viewing relationships between results of several measures. For example, the finding that blood pressure does not increase with activity may not be considered abnormal by itself if the activity level is low or the patient is taking a beta-receptor antagonist medication (e.g., metoprolol); however, the finding of no increase in blood pressure with signs and symptoms of exercise intolerance (e.g., shortness of breath, dizziness, fatigue, etc.) during moderate-level activity in another patient may be indicative of cardiovascular pump dysfunction.

Knowledge of what is "normal" is important to interpret measurements accurately. For some measurements, normal values are well defined. Measurements of resting blood pressure, cholesterol, and blood glucose have defined categories of normal, borderline, and elevated. For other measurements, population normative standards are not specifically defined. For example, what is the normal increase in heart rate when walking at 3.5 mph on a level surface? Values for individuals differ depending on age, medications, fitness level, and walking efficiency. Results must be interpreted by considering these factors and pathological conditions, if present. Each individual has his or her own "normal" or usual response, and variations from this value could be considered abnormal.

Interpreting measurements is similar to putting the pieces of a puzzle together to create a picture of the patient and his or her activity limitations and participation restrictions. Data are collected from several sources, including the medical record, patient interview, and physical therapy examination. Measures performed and interpreted by other health care professionals can be obtained from the medical record; these include measures such as chest radiographs, blood tests, echocardiography, angiography, and ventilation-perfusion scans. During an interview, patients report information about their current and past medical problems and especially specific patient-identified problems. It is important to be sensitive to patient's feelings about their condition, noting their stage of emotional recovery. Detecting attitudes related to changing lifestyle habits is also important. After the interview, the therapist should have a sense of the patient as a person and begin to plan an intervention strategy for improving body structure and function impairments, and optimizing activity and participation.[13]

Measures made during the physical examination may include physiological responses to activity, breathing patterns, ventilatory capacity, and breath sounds. These measurements are integrated with results collected during the chart review and evaluated in the context of the patient-identified problems and the goals for each problem. As therapists refine their hypothesis, they develop a picture of the severity of the cardiopulmonary condition, stage of recovery, and presence of coexisting conditions. An intervention strategy is developed on the basis of the final clinical hypothesis/diagnosis. The intervention strategy is implemented, and measurements are regularly obtained during treatment sessions to reassess existing problems and goals. Because of the dynamic nature of many of the conditions that affect the cardiovascular and pulmonary systems, each treatment session can be viewed as a reassessment of the hypothesis and progress toward patient goals.

Minimal Clinically Important Difference

To help facilitate evidence-based practice related to interpreting outcome measurements, a minimal clinically important difference (MCID)—that is, "the minimal level of change required in response to an intervention before the outcome would be considered worthwhile in terms of a patient/client's function or quality of life"[20]—has been determined for several endurance/aerobic capacity tests and measures used by physical therapists. Examples include the 6-MWT (54 m[21] or 10% improvement[22]), modified shuttle test (40 m[23]), and the Borg CR10[4] and visual analog scale ratings of dyspnea (1 point and 10-20 mm [Table 7-3], respectively[24]). The MCID for various tests and measures can be used for setting relevant goals, as well as interpreting progress toward outcomes.

Physical Therapy Diagnosis, Prognosis, and Plan of Care

The physical therapy diagnosis serves to drive the selection of interventions. A physical therapy diagnosis may be written in the form of a problem list that may include both impairments and activity limitations. Problems can be listed in order of priority and stated in functional terms. For example, stating "patient unable to climb stairs because of abnormal ECG responses and dizziness," rather than "abnormal ECG response during activity" is recommended. Alternatively, physical therapy–related classification systems such as the Practice Patterns found in the Guide to Physical Therapist Practice[25] may be tailored to reflect the individual's physical therapy diagnosis.

Based on the results from a 6-MWT, or another appropriate test, a tentative physical therapy diagnosis of impaired aerobic capacity/endurance impairment could be made if the measurement falls outside the reference values for healthy adults.[26] Concurrent or complementary measures (e.g., respiratory rate, heart rate and blood pressure response, pulse oximetry, heart and lung sounds, ankle brachial index) could help further refine the hypothesis and determine whether the impaired endurance was more likely due to cardiac, peripheral vascular, or pulmonary impairments.

After identifying the patient's problems and determining a diagnosis for physical therapy, a plan of care that includes prognosis is developed. The plan of care includes goals and anticipated outcomes, specific interventions to be used, and the recommended frequency and duration of the interventions. The prognosis is the predicted level of improvement and the amount of time needed to reach that level. Providing additional data related to positive and/or negative contextual factors to justify prognosis is important to reinforce the skilled nature of services. Positive factors may include family support, previous functional levels, or the acuity of the condition. Negative factors may include the severity or chronicity of the condition, barriers in living environments, or lack of financial resources.

Goals are the outcomes to be achieved by participating in a physical therapy program and are generated by the therapist and patient in collaboration. Goals should have baseline measurements documented from the examination, be related to the identified problems, and be supported by statements in the evaluation section. Goals should highlight cardiovascular and pulmonary impairments that are thought to be linked to the activity limitations. Goals are stated in functional terms and concern what the patient will be able to do at discharge. For example, a goal could be "patient will be able to walk up two flights of stairs with appropriate heart rate and rhythm responses, within 2 weeks." Without documenting the associated cardiovascular and pulmonary impairments, the goal may not support the individual's need for skilled or medically necessary services by physical therapy.

To determine whether a goal has been met, the therapist must be able to observe or measure the activity. Therapists also estimate the time it will take to achieve the outcome. In a discharge or follow-up note, it is stated whether each goal has been met. If a goal has not been achieved, an explanation is provided.

The plan provides a description of the approach that will be taken to assist the patient in achieving the stated goals. The plan may include a description of treatment that can be provided, education for the patient and/or family, and referrals to other services. Descriptions of inpatient, outpatient, or home programs should be included in the plan. The plan of care also includes discharge planning.

Intervention

Interventions are physical therapy procedures and techniques designed to produce changes in the patient's condition. Procedures typically used by therapists treating patients with cardiopulmonary disorders include therapeutic exercise (i.e.,

Table 7-3 MRC Dyspnea Scale

Grade	Degree of Breathlessness Related to Activities
1	Not troubled by breathlessness except on strenuous exertion
2	Short of breath when hurrying on level ground or walking up a slight hill
3	Walks slower than contemporaries on level ground because of breathlessness, or has to stop for breath after ≈1 mile (or after 15 min) when walking at own pace
4	Stops for breath after walking about 100 yards (or after a few minutes) on level ground
5	Too breathless to leave the house, or breathless after dressing or undressing

Modified by permission from BMJ Publishing Group Limited. From Fletcher CM, Elmes PC, Wood CH: The significance of respiratory symptoms and the diagnosis of chronic bronchitis in a working population, *Br Med J* 1:257-266, 1959.

aerobic, resistance, breathing exercises), functional training (i.e., work hardening and work conditioning), and airway clearance techniques. The specific intervention selected by the therapist will be influenced by the severity of the cardiopulmonary disorder and the presence of complications. In some cases, the intervention mode and intensity can be derived from the measurement obtained. For instance, 6-MWD can predict peak VO_2 in patients with COPD[27] and heart failure;[28] with this predicted value, converted to METs, the physical therapist can develop an appropriate exercise prescription and guide the patient in selecting physical activities that would fall within a safe and therapeutic range. In addition, a treadmill or overground walking program could be established on the basis of the mean walking velocity during the 6-MWT.[29] Likewise, physical activity/exercise intensity could be set based on measurements of perceived exertion or dyspnea obtained during an exercise test.

Patient and family and/or caregiver instruction is part of all physical therapy interventions. Communication with other health care disciplines involved in the patient's care is essential to ensure efficient and effective health care. For example, for a patient who is being discharged from the hospital after cardiac surgery, the therapist may need to coordinate with the social worker to ensure that the patient receives home services that he or she needs for assistance with activities of daily living.

Documentation is an essential part of intervention. It is important to record the patient's responses to interventions, including changes in heart rate, blood pressure, and heart and lung sounds, recovery time after exercise, and reports of angina, dyspnea, or fatigue. A description of the intervention is recorded so that another therapist or physical therapist assistant can continue the program. Details related to dosage, such as frequency, intensity, and duration of each intervention should be clearly stated. In addition to the medical record, the therapist also may be required to provide documentation to other sources such as home health or insurance agencies.

Reexamination and Outcomes Assessment

Throughout the course of treatments, therapists routinely perform reexaminations to determine whether patients are progressing. For patients with cardiopulmonary disorders, for example, the therapist may reexamine the patient at every session to determine whether physiological responses to activity are appropriate or whether the patient's lungs are clearing. Results of reexamination are used to modify or redirect interventions. It is important to include documentation of patient progression, including the patient's perception of progression, in each note in order to support the continued justification of skilled services.

As the patient approaches discharge from physical therapy services, the therapist assesses the outcomes of the intervention. The therapist measures the impact of physical therapy services on the patient's impairments, activity limitations, and participation restrictions. Examples of outcome measures often used to assess health-related quality of life in patients with cardiopulmonary disorders include the Chronic Respiratory Questionnaire[30] and Minnesota Living with Heart Failure questionnaire.[31]

The therapist relates the assessment of outcomes to the original goals established by the therapist and patient. As a result of the outcomes assessment, the therapist may refer the patient back to the physician or to another health care professional. A systematic review of medical records from a group of patients with similar diagnoses can be performed to determine program outcomes of selected physical therapy interventions. See Chapter 17 for a discussion of optimizing outcomes.

Purposes of Documentation

To be useful, measurements need to be documented. Measurements that remain in the mind of the evaluator often are forgotten or not remembered accurately. Documentation is important to facilitate and to maximize reimbursement, as well as to ensure efficiency of care through communication among health care professionals. Documentation includes information about results of the examination, assessment of the patient's condition, and the physical therapy diagnosis, prognosis, and plan of care.

Specific reasons for documentation include the following:

- To provide information for other therapists and assistants, who may evaluate and/or treat the patient
- To communicate with the referring physician and other health care professionals
- To provide data to support clinical research, such as treatment effectiveness and efficiency through collection of information on outcomes of various types of care
- To verify and support the skilled nature of physical therapy services provided and to justify reimbursement for those services
- To address legal and risk management issues by documenting the care provided and the individual's response to care

Guidelines for Content and Organization

Writing notes in a clear and concise format is important so that information is conveyed accurately. Examples of unclear notes are those that contain typographical errors, illegible handwriting, or vague statements that can be interpreted in more than one way. Concise notes are more likely to be read by other health care professionals. Most clinicians do not have time in their schedules to read through extensive patient information that may not be relevant. A concise note includes only essential information in a clear communication style free of unnecessary phrases. The APTA's Defensible Documentation Tips include the following[32]:

Use only standard or accepted abbreviations. Facilities have lists of approved abbreviations that are available to those who write, read, and review records.

All notations must include the date and time of service.

Documentation of services rendered must match the billing codes submitted to payers.

Tables, headings, and subheadings can be used to help organize the information in an easy-to-find format. Notes must clearly demonstrate the need for skilled, medically necessary services by the physical therapist and the physical therapist assistant.

Patient progression should be evident, with data and assessments provided to support the individual's achievement of goals or the lack of progression toward set goals.

Communications with the patient, family, health care team, payers, and other related parties involving care should be documented in the chart.

Documentation is essential when an unusual or adverse event occurs. For example, abnormal responses to activity that may appear relatively benign are important to record. Abnormal responses include dizziness, chest pain, or dysrhythmias. An unusually high or low heart rate or blood pressure response also should be noted. Combined with information reported by the patient and findings from other health care professionals, these results may indicate significant changes in the patient's cardiopulmonary status.

HIPAA Guidelines

The Health Insurance Portability and Accountability Act (HIPAA) includes federal guidelines that protect the confidentiality of health information. Personal protected health information (PHI) is to be shared only with persons authorized to view the information (i.e., professionals involved in providing health care). Facilities assume the responsibility of designing systems to ensure that health information is protected and kept confidential. When PHI is stored electronically, controls should be established to ensure only authorized access to information. This may include the use of encryption of laptop computers, memory cards, thumb drives, PDAs, and other portable devices. Therapists must ensure that discussions involving patients' health information occur in private locations. All health care professionals are bound by these guidelines. Further information may be found at the U.S. Department of Health and Human Services website (www.hhs.gov/ocr/hipaa/).

Summary

Measurement and documentation are important components in the process of providing patient care. Therapists select measurements because they reveal information about patient characteristics that is needed to determine appropriate directions for intervention. Performing measurements in a consistent way allows comparison of patient characteristics at varied points in time. The recording, or documentation, of the results of measurements and other information about the patient serves as a legal record. Although documentation formats vary among facilities, information from records can be organized to include the following topics: examination, evaluation, diagnosis, prognosis and plan of care, interventions, and reexamination. Documentation can be viewed as a way to assist therapists to organize their findings, reflect on the significance of the findings, and generate an efficient and comprehensive care plan.

Review Questions

1. Describe and give examples of nominal, ordinal, ratio, and interval measurements.
2. Define sensitivity and specificity of tests.
3. Describe four purposes for documenting the results of patient assessment and responses to interventions.
4. Provide an example of an impairment, activity limitation, and participation restriction that is common in patients with cardiopulmonary disorders.
5. Describe each of the components of patient management: examination, evaluation, diagnosis, prognosis, and plan of care.

References

1. Task Force on Standards for Measurement in Physical Therapy: Standards for tests and measurements in physical therapy practice. *Phys Ther* 71(8):589–622, 1991.
2. Rothstein JM, Echternach JL: *Primer on measurement: An introductory guide to measurement issues*, Alexandria, Va, 1993, American Physical Therapy Association.
3. O'Rourke RA, O'Gara PT, et al: Diagnosis and management of patients with chronic ischemic heart disease. In *Hurst's the heart*. V. Fuster, R. O'Rourke, R. Walsh and P. Poole-Wilson, http://accessmedicine.com/content.aspx?aID=3068873, 2008.
4. Borg G: Rating scales for perceived physical effort and exertion. *International encyclopedia of ergonomics and human factors*. W. Karwowski. New York, 2006, Taylor & Francis Inc, pp 538–541.
5. Price DD, McGrath PA, Rafii A, Buckingham B: The validation of visual analogue scales as ratio scale measures for chronic and experimental pain. *Pain* 17(1):45–56, 1983.
6. Neely G, Ljunggren G, Sylven C, Borg G: Comparison between the Visual Analogue Scale (VAS) and the Category Ratio Scale (CR-10) for the evaluation of leg exertion. *Int J Sports Med* 13(2):133–136, 1992.
7. Shortell SM, Richardson WC: *The evaluation process. Health program evaluation*, St Louis, 1978, Mosby.
8. Brooks D, Interrater TJ: Reliability of Auscultation of Breath Sounds Among Physical Therapists. *Phys Ther* 75(12):1082–1088, 1995.
9. Orchard T, Strandness D, Jr: Assessment of peripheral vascular disease in diabetes. Report and recommendations of an international workshop sponsored by the American Diabetes Association and the American Heart Association September 18-20, 1992 New Orleans, Louisiana. *Circulation* 88(2):819–828, 1993.
10. Yamaya Y, Bogaard HJ, Wagner PD, et al: Validity of pulse oximetry during maximal exercise in normoxia, hypoxia, and pyperoxia. *J Appl Physiol* 92(1):162–168, 2002.
11. Cranley JJ, Canos AJ, Sull WJ: The diagnosis of deep venous thrombosis: Fallibility of clinical symptoms and signs. *Arch Surg* 111(1):34–36, 1976.
12. Kahn SR: The clinical diagnosis of deep venous thrombosis: integrating incidence, risk factors, and symptoms and signs. *Arch Intern Med* 158(21):2315–2323, 1998.
13. Rothstein JM, Echternach JL, et al: The hypothesis-oriented algorithm for clinicians II (HOAC II): A guide for patient management. *Phys Ther* 83(5):455–470, 2003.
14. Wells PS, Hirsh J, Anderson DR, et al: Accuracy of clinical assessment of deep-vein thrombosis. *Lancet* 345(8961):1326–1330, 1995.
15. Jette AM: Toward a common language for function, disability, and health. *Phys Ther* 86(5):726–734, 2006.
16. Pickering TG, Hall JE, Appel LJ, et al: Recommendations for Blood Pressure Measurement in Humans and Experimental Animals: Part 1: Blood Pressure Measurement in Humans: A Statement for Professionals From the Subcommittee of Professional and Public Education of the American Heart Association Council on High Blood Pressure Research. *Hypertension* 45(1):142–161, 2005.
17. American Thoracic Society: ATS Statement: Guidelines for the Six-Minute Walk Test. *Am J Respir Crit Care Med* 166(1):111–117, 2002.
18. World Health Organization: Towards a Common Language of Functioning, Disability and Health. http://www.who.int/classifications/icf/training/icfbeginnersguide.pdf. Accessed on November 29, 2010.
19. APTA: APTA Endorses World health Organization ICF Model. Retrieved March 15, 2011 from http://www.apta.org/Media/Releases/APTA/2008/7/8/, 2008.
20. Jewell DV: *Guide to Evidence-based physical therapy practice*, Sudbury, Mass, 2008, Jones and Bartlett Publishers.

21. Redelmeier DA, Bayoumi AM, Goldstein RS, Guyatt GH: Interpreting small differences in functional status: the six minute walk test in chronic lung disease patients. *Am J Respir Crit Care Med* 155(4):1278–1282, 1997.
22. Puhan MA, Mador MJ, Held U, et al: Interpretation of treatment changes in 6-minute walk distance in patients with COPD. *Eur Respir J* 32(3):637–643, 2008.
23. Bradley J, Howard J, et al: Reliability, repeatability, and sensitivity of the modified shuttle test in adult cystic fibrosis. *Chest* 117(6):1666–1671, 2000.
24. Ries AL: Minimally clinically important difference for the UCSD Shortness of Breath Questionnaire, Borg scale, and visual analog scale. *COPD: Journal of Chronic Obstructive Pulmonary Disease* 2(1):105–110, 2005.
25. APTA: Guide to physical therapist practice, ed 2. *Phys Ther* 81:9–744, 2001.
26. Enright PL, Sherrill DL: Reference equations for the six-minute walk in healthy adults. *Am J Respir Crit Care Med* 158(5):1384–1387, 1998.
27. Cote CG, Pinto-Plata V, et al: The 6-min walk distance, peak oxygen uptake, and mortality in COPD. *Chest* 132(6):1778–1785, 2007.
28. Cahalin LP, Mathier MA, et al: The six-minute walk test predicts peak oxygen uptake and survival in patients with advanced heart failure. *Chest* 110(2):325–332, 1996.
29. Jenkins SC: 6-Minute walk test in patients with COPD: clinical applications in pulmonary rehabilitation. *Physiotherapy* 93(3):175–182, 2007.
30. Williams JEA, Singh SJ, et al: Development of a self-reported Chronic Respiratory Questionnaire (CRQ-SR). *Thorax* 56(12):954–959, 2001.
31. Rector TS, Cohn JN: Assessment of patient outcome with the Minnesota Living with Heart Failure questionnaire: reliability and validity during a randomized, double-blind, placebo-controlled trial of pimobendan. Pimobendan Multicenter Research Group. *Am Heart J* 124(4):1017–1025, 1992.
32. American Physical Therapy Association: Defensible Documentation Tips, www.apta.or/documention. Accessed on March 25, 2011.

Chapter 8

II

History

Willy E. Hammon III and Elizabeth Dean

KEY TERMS

Cough
Dyspnea
History
Pain

CHAPTER OUTLINE

The value of a history depends in large part on the skill of the interviewer. When eliciting the history from a patient, the physical therapist must be alert to recognize the symptoms that are indicative of cardiac and pulmonary disease. This information is then used in the decision-making process to select the most appropriate intervention for the individual. This chapter presents a comprehensive approach to history taking. Physical therapists may find part or all of this information applicable, depending on the particular circumstances.

The Interview

Obtaining a thorough and accurate patient history is truly an art. One important goal of history taking is to establish a good patient-therapist rapport. The patient must be allowed to explain the history in his or her own words and at a comfortable pace.[1] If the therapist appears hurried, distracted, preoccupied, irritated, or uncaring; is often interrupted; or fails to be an attentive listener, the patient-therapist relationship will likely suffer.

The interviewer must be careful not to allow personal feelings about the patient's grooming, appearance, demeanor, or behavior during the interview to unduly question the validity of the chief complaints.[2] By the time the patient is referred for physical therapy, he or she may have seen one or more physicians, have been subjected to a number of noninvasive or invasive studies, or have been prescribed oral or inhaled medications with variable or unsatisfactory alleviation of symptoms. The patient is likely to manifest a degree of anxiety and frustration. Therefore, the therapist's approach, history-taking method, and interviewing style are important for gaining the patient's confidence and cooperation.

The patient history interview can be divided into the data-gathering and interpretative sections.[3] The data-gathering segment begins with asking why the patient has sought medical attention and has been referred for physical therapy services. In other words, what is the patient's chief complaint—the symptom that caused the patient to seek help?

Each chief complaint should be carefully explored. Supplementary questions should be nonleading, using words the patient can easily understand. This allows the interviewer to determine the significance of the complaint. An in-depth knowledge of cardiopulmonary pathophysiology allows the therapist to gather data about the patient's symptoms while also interpreting the likely type of cardiopulmonary dysfunction that exists. This in turn serves as a basis for the therapist to begin to select the appropriate assessment and treatment modalities for the individual.

It is important to remember that patient satisfaction is greatest if the patient is allowed to fully express major concerns without being interrupted. In addition, the chance of missing what is really of greatest concern to the patient is reduced if the patient is allowed sufficient time to describe it in his or her own words. Studies have shown that this usually takes only 1 to 3 minutes.

The patient's view of what the problem is and his or her suggestions for addressing the problem should be included in the interview. Patients are more satisfied when they are allowed and encouraged to participate in the interview. Patient involvement in the process also leads to improvement in the establishment of short- and long-term goals.

The depth of the history taken by the physical therapist can vary according to the following factors:

- Whether the individual is an inpatient or an outpatient. Many inpatients have detailed medical records available for the therapist to review. This reduces the amount of information the physical therapist needs to obtain from the patient during an interview. If the information in the chart is scant, or if the individual is an outpatient with only a treatment referral and few or no medical records available, the physical therapist should obtain a more detailed history.
- Whether the treatment order is narrow or broad in scope
- The acuteness of the patient's illness, level of consciousness, and ability to provide accurate information

Smoking History

The patient should be asked about his or her tobacco-smoking history.[3] The number of pack-years of cigarette smoking may be calculated (average number of packs per day multiplied by the number of years smoked) as a relative risk for lung cancer and COPD. Regular smoking of marijuana is more damaging to lung health in the short term as well as potentially long term.[4]

Family History

The family history is useful in evaluating the possibility of hereditary pulmonary diseases, such as alpha$_1$-antitrypsin deficiency, cystic fibrosis, allergic asthma, hereditary hemorrhagic telangiectasia, and others.[5,6] A family history of diabetes, hypertension, coronary artery disease (CAD), or rheumatic fever raises the possibility that these conditions might exist in the patient as well.[7]

Occupational History

Taking an occupational history is particularly important for pulmonary patients who arrive for physical therapy with little or no accompanying medical information. The internal surface of the lung measures 50 to 100 m^3 and is in constant contact with the environment.[5] Jobs that involve exposure to silica or silicates (e.g., miners, sandblasters, foundry workers, stone cutters, brick layers, and quarry workers) or other inorganic substances place workers at risk for combinations of obstructive and restrictive lung disease (e.g., silicosis). Construction workers, shipyard workers, pipefitters, and other industrial workers exposed to asbestos are at increased risk for developing a restrictive lung disease such as asbestosis.[8] Benign pleural plaques may be found on the diaphragmatic pleurae and bilaterally between the 6th and 10th ribs on the anterolateral or posterolateral chest wall. Progressive pleural thickening rarely occurs. These individuals have an increased incidence of malignant neoplastic diseases such as bronchogenic carcinoma and malignant mesothelioma. Some firefighters, iron workers, and other rescuers working at the World Trade Center disaster site following September 11, 2001, have developed respiratory symptoms and disorders.[9,10]

Coal workers are exposed to coal mine dust. About 10% have simple pneumoconiosis, whereas a smaller proportion develop the complicated form of the condition—progressive massive pulmonary fibrosis.[11]

A history of paroxysmal coughing, chest tightness, or dyspnea that is worse during the work week but remits on weekends (or other regular days off work) strongly suggests occupational asthma.[11] This condition is difficult to diagnose because symptoms commonly occur several hours after exposure to the provoking agent. Causal agents include grain dusts, wood dusts, formalin, enzyme detergents, ethanolamines (in spray paints and soldering flux), nickel, and hard metals (e.g., tungsten carbide). Workers exposed to cotton flax and hemp dusts may develop byssinosis, an obstructive lung disease. In the early stages, this condition is reversible, but long-term exposure over a number of years causes chronic irreversible obstructive lung disease.

A history of fever, cough, shortness of breath, and recurrent pneumonias in farmers in the northern United States suggests farmer's lung.[11] This is the most common hypersensitive pneumonitis; it is caused by inhaling fungal agents such as thermophilic actinomycetes. Long-term exposure can lead to pulmonary fibrosis. Numerous occupations expose workers to factors that cause hypersensitive pneumonitis.

Prior Treatment

It is important to determine what treatment(s) the patient has received for his or her condition. Specifically, has the patient ever received physical therapy for this or any other condition? What types of treatments were done? Were they helpful in improving or resolving the condition? In this way, it is possible to determine what treatment modalities have been used, which of them the patient believes may have merit, and which the patient finds objectionable or lacks confidence in, thus avoiding alienating the patient by repeating what he or she believes to be ineffective therapy.

Questionnaires

Questionnaires can be used in a number of ways. Printed symptom or medical questionnaires can be beneficial or detrimental to the patient-therapist relationship, depending on how they are used. Questionnaires can expedite the data-gathering portion of the initial visit by allowing the patient to note in advance all symptoms, medical conditions, surgeries, occupations, medications, and other factors that may influence physical therapy intervention. They can reduce the amount of nontreatment time therapists may otherwise spend inquiring about irrelevant symptoms and conditions. Printed questionnaires also allow patients sufficient time to recall relevant information and respond more accurately than they often do in an interview setting.[5] Used in this way, a printed questionnaire can be a valuable tool for expediting a comprehensive evaluation of cardiopulmonary patients. However, if questionnaires are used improperly, they can depersonalize the history-taking portion of the initial visit.[1] If the physical therapist allows the printed form to become a substitute for interaction with the patient, patient satisfaction will be low and the patient-therapist relationship will suffer.

In addition, questionnaires are being increasingly used as standardized outcome measures to assess activity and participation capacity, as well as quality of life and life satisfaction (see Chapter 17). Many questionnaires have been validated and are reliable when used in the clinical setting.

Dyspnea

Dyspnea, commonly referred to as breathlessness or shortness of breath, can be defined as the sensation of difficulty in breathing.[12] It is one of the most common reasons for patients to seek medical attention. Dyspnea is difficult to quantitate because it is subjective and at times is normal (i.e., at high altitudes and during or following vigorous exercise). Also, patients of different backgrounds use different descriptors for their breathlessness.[13] Dyspnea is a symptom of cardiac and pulmonary diseases, among other conditions.

When a patient complains of shortness of breath or breathlessness, it should be noted that this complaint is often unrelated to the patient's arterial oxygen level (PaO_2). Many times, it appears that altered mechanical factors during breathing contribute to the sensation of breathlessness.[14] Numerous receptors that have a role in sensing dyspnea have been identified; they include vagal receptors (e.g., irritant, stretch, and J-receptors), chemoreceptors, proprioceptive receptors (e.g., tendon organs, muscle spindles, joint and skin receptors), and upper airway receptors.[3]

Analyzing the oxygen transport system (Figure 8-1) can help the physical therapist to determine the likely cause of each patient's dyspnea and the most appropriate physical therapy intervention. The delivery of oxygen from ambient air to the mitochondrion within the cell depends on the intact interaction of the respiratory, cardiovascular, and muscular systems. Also, carbon dioxide (CO_2) is eliminated in the opposite direction. Dyspnea can be caused by dysfunction in any of the systems.

Dyspnea commonly occurs when the body's requirement for breathing (ventilation) exceeds the body's capacity to provide it.[3] In other words, the symptom varies directly with the body's demand for ventilation and, inversely, with the body's ventilatory capacity.

There are three basic causes of dyspnea: [12]

1. An increased awareness of normal breathing
2. An increase in the work of breathing
3. An abnormality in the ventilatory system itself

An increased awareness of normal breathing is usually related to anxiety.[5] The patient commonly complains of "not getting a deep enough breath," a feeling of "smothering," or "not getting air down in the right places."[15] These sensations have been designated as psychogenic dyspnea. The patient's breathing pattern is irregular, with frequent sighs. When severe, it is associated with tingling of the hands and feet, circumoral numbness, and lightheadedness. Coaching the patient to hyperventilate and to reproduce the symptoms may help the patient better understand the cause of these symptoms and how to control them.[5] The hyperventilation syndrome is properly diagnosed only after organic causes have been excluded and pulmonary function tests indicate normal respiratory mechanics and PaO_2.

The second cause of dyspnea is an increase in the work of breathing. Greater inspiratory pressures must be generated by the respiratory muscles to move air in and out of the lungs when the mechanical properties of the lungs have changed. This may be related to an increase in lung water resulting from cardiac disease or the high cardiac output of anemia. A loss of compliance (increased lung stiffness) because of diffuse inflammatory or fibrotic lung disease often causes shortness of breath. Small or large airway obstruction as a result of bronchoconstriction, sputum, inflammation, and other effects commonly produces dyspnea.

The third cause of dyspnea is an abnormality in the ventilatory apparatus or pump. The ventilatory apparatus consists of the thoracic cage, respiratory muscles, and nerves.

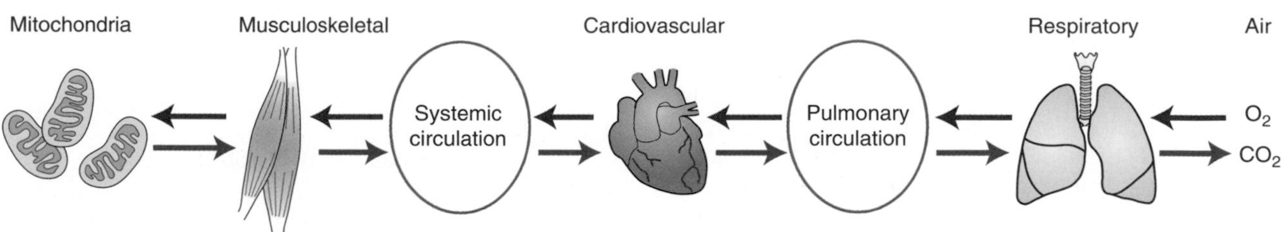

Fig. 8-1 Schematic illustration of the oxygen transport system, which involves the interaction between the respiratory, cardiovascular, and musculoskeletal systems. *(Reprinted with permission from Mahler D: Dyspnea: Diagnosis and management.* Clin Chest Med *8:215-230, 1987.)*

Any of these may become dysfunctional. Thoracic cage abnormalities include kyphoscoliosis, extreme obesity, and large pleural effusions. Diseases of the respiratory muscles include polymyositis and muscular dystrophy. Neurological abnormalities include spinal cord injuries, phrenic nerve injuries, brachial plexus neuropathy, ascending polyneuritis (Guillain-Barré syndrome), myasthenia gravis, amyotrophic lateral sclerosis, poliomyelitis, neurotoxins, and exposure to paralytic agents.

The time course of the appearance and progression of dyspnea should be identified.[6,16] Acute dyspnea is common in pulmonary embolism, pneumothorax, acute asthma, pulmonary congestion related to congestive heart failure (CHF), pneumonia, and upper airway obstruction. Most of these conditions require immediate physician evaluation of the acute problem before physical therapy intervention. Subacute or chronic progression of dyspnea generally presents, over time, as increasingly severe dyspnea with exertion. It occurs with emphysema, restrictive lung disorders such as pulmonary fibrosis, chest wall deformities, respiratory muscle dysfunction, occupational lung diseases, chronic CHF, and large pleural effusions.

Dyspnea may also be related to body position.[16] Therefore, when evaluating dyspnea, the physical therapist should ask whether the patient:

- Has difficulty breathing when reclining horizontally
- Finds it necessary to be propped up on several pillows to sleep at night (orthopnea)
- Has more difficulty breathing when reclining on one side (trepopnea)
- Wakes up at night short of breath and feels the need to sit up or walk around the room to "catch your breath" (paroxysmal nocturnal dyspnea)

Acute Dyspnea

A patient who has acute dyspnea requires a rapid and thorough history and physical assessment. The physical therapist should ask several important questions to address the possible causes of acute dyspnea:[14]

1. Are you short of breath at rest? If the answer is yes, it suggests a severe physiological dysfunction. The patient likely needs prompt evaluation by a physician if this is of recent onset and the patient has not had a medical workup.
2. Do you have chest pain? If so, what part of your chest? Unilateral localized chest pain raises the possibility of spontaneous pneumothorax, pulmonary embolism, or chest trauma.
3. What were you doing immediately before or at the time of the onset of shortness of breath? Approximately 75% of spontaneous pneumothoraces occur during sedentary activity, 20% happen during some strenuous activity, and 5% are related to coughing or sneezing. A history of immobilization of a lower extremity, recent surgery, bed rest, travel requiring prolonged sitting, obesity, CHF, and venous disease of the lower extremities are all risk factors for pulmonary embolism. If the patient's symptoms are related to chest trauma, the fact that a fall, a blow, or an accident occurred can usually be quickly established.
4. Do you have any major medical or surgical conditions? Cystic fibrosis, chronic obstructive pulmonary disease (COPD), interstitial lung disease, and malignancies are important causes of secondary spontaneous pneumothorax.

Acute dyspnea in cardiac patients is difficult to assess because the signs and symptoms are so similar to those caused by pulmonary disease. It is most often due to arrhythmias and acute coronary ischemia with associated left ventricular dysfunction, but it can be caused by any cardiac disorder.[16]

If the therapist strongly suspects pneumothorax, pulmonary emboli, or an acute cardiac disorder on the basis of the history and physical assessment, the patient should be referred for immediate medical evaluation.

Dyspnea on Exertion

Dyspnea on exertion is a common complaint of patients with cardiopulmonary dysfunction. Dyspnea during exercise or exertion usually precedes dyspnea at rest.[17] It most often is a result of chronic pulmonary disease or CHF. Some causes of dyspnea during exertion or exercise are listed in Table 8-1.

It is important to establish the amount of activity required to produce dyspnea. Various scales[18,19] have been developed to categorize the level of dyspnea and impairment present in patients (Figure 8-2 and Table 8-2). The patient should be asked about daily activity and what activities produce breathlessness.[20] Does the patient become short of breath climbing a flight of stairs or walking uphill? Is the patient able to walk and talk simultaneously? Does walking more slowly affect the individual's dyspnea?

In addition, the time at which the patient began to notice an increase in shortness of breath should be noted. A recent onset of dyspnea is more characteristic of heart failure than of chronic lung disease, which has a longer, more insidious onset. Acute pulmonary problems such as pneumothorax, atelectasis, pneumonia, and other conditions superimposed on chronic lung disease can also explain a recent intensification of symptoms.

Fig. 8-2 The visual analogue scale is a vertical line 100 mm in length. The patient is asked to make a mark along this line that represents his or her level of breathlessness. The distance of the patient's mark above zero represents the measurement of dyspnea. *(Reprinted with permission from Mahler D: Dyspnea: Diagnosis and management.* Clin Chest Med *8:215-230, 1987.)*

Table 8-1 Disorders Limiting Exercise Tolerance, Pathophysiology, and Discriminating Measures

Disorders	Pathophysiology	Measures That Deviate From Normal
PULMONARY		
Obstructive lung disease	↓ Ventilatory capacity due to airflow limitation, increased ventilatory requirement due to V/Q mismatching, hypoxic stimulation to breathing	↓ VO_2 max, ↑ VD/VT, ↑ P(a–ET)CO_2, ↑ P(A–a)O_2, ↓ breathing reserve (MVV–VE_2 max), ↓ HR at maximal WR (↑ HR reserve), abnormal (trapezoidal) expiratory flow pattern
Restrictive lung disease	↓ Lung volumes, especially IC and TLC; V/Q mismatching, hypoxemia	↓ VO_2 max, ↑ VT/IC, RR >50 at maximal WR, ↓ breathing reserve, ↑ VD/VT, ↑ P(a–ET)CO_2, progressively ↓ PaO_2 and ↑ P(A–a)O_2 with ↑ WRs
Chest wall defects	Respiratory pump dysfunction due to muscle weakness or ↓ chest wall compliance	↓ VO_2 max, ↑ VT/IC, ↑ RR at low WRs, nl $\Delta VO_2/\Delta WR$, ↓ breathing reserve, ↓ HR at maximal WR, nl PaO_2
Diseases of pulmonary circulation	↓ Pulmonary perfusion leading to V/Q mismatching	↑ V_E at submaximal WRs, ↑ VD/VT, ↑ P(a–ET)CO_2, progressively ↓ PaO_2 and ↑ P(A–a)O_2 with ↑ WRs, ↓ VO_2 max, ↓ AT, more shallow $\Delta VO_2/\Delta WR$ as WR is ↑ toward maximum, ↓ O_2 pulse (VO_2 max/HR)
CARDIAC		
Coronary insufficiency	Relative imbalance between myocardial oxygen supply and demand, causing myocardial ischemia	May have chest pain and ischemic ECG changes, ↓ VO_2 max, ↓ AT, ↓ O_2 pulse, more shallow $\Delta VO_2/\Delta WR$ as WR is ↑ toward maximum, ↑ HR/ VO_2, ↑ breathing reserve, metabolic acidosis at low WRs → ↑ WRs→V_E, abnormal BP responses
Valvular	Cardiac output limitation due to ↓ effective SV	↓ VO_2 max, ↓ AT, ↓ O_2 pulse, more shallow ΔVO_2 max/ΔWR as WR is ↑ toward maximum, ↑ HR/ VO_2, ↑ breathing reserve, metabolic acidosis at low WRs → ↑ V_E, abnormal BP responses
Myocardial	Cardiac output limitation due to ↓ EF and SV	
OTHER		
Obesity	↑ Energy cost to move body; if severe, restrictive lung dysfunction and pulmonary insufficiency	↑ VO_2 per workload, nl O_2 pulse when predicted from ht, ↓ VO_2 max/wt and AT/wt but nl VO_2 max/ht and AT/ht (unless extremely obese), ↑ P(A – a)O_2 at rest that normalizes during exercise, nl VD/VT
Peripheral arterial disease	Impaired ability to ↑ blood flow to working muscles	Leg pain (claudication), ↓ $\Delta VO_2/\Delta WR$, ↓ VO_2 max, ↓ AT, possible hypertensive BP response
Anemia	↓ Oxygen-carrying capacity	↓ Hemoglobin and hematocrit, ↓ VO_2 max, ↓ AT, ↓ O_2 pulse, nl VD/VT, P(a – et)CO_2, and P(A – a)O_2
Musculoskeletal disorders	Musculoskeletal coupling inefficiency; inflammation	↓ Mechanical efficiency (VO_2 per workload), ↓ maximal WR; possible pain and abnormal movement patterns
Chronic metabolic acidosis	Due to poorly controlled DM, CRF, CHF, or ingestion of certain drugs	↓ HCO_3^-, steep / VCO_2 relationship, nl P(a–ET)CO_2 and P(A–a)O_2, nl VD/Vt
Deconditioning	Inactivity or prolonged bed rest leading to loss of ability to effectively redistribute systemic blood flow	↓ VO_2 max, ↓ AT, ↓ O_2 pulse, ↑ breathing reserve, metabolic acidosis at lower WRs → ↑ V_E
Anxiety reaction	Hyperventilation and respiratory alkalosis with precisely regular RR, although possible breath-holding episodes	Abrupt tachypnea that sometimes starts at rest, ↓ $PaCO_2$, respiratory alkalosis
Malingering, poor effort	Very irregular breathing with periods of hyperventilation and hypoventilation	AT not achieved or ↑ compared with VO_2 max, ↑ breathing and HR reserve; often irregular breathing pattern with periods of tachypnea and bradypnea producing wide swings in $PaCO_2$ and $PetCO_2$ unrelated to changes in WR

↓, Decreased; ↑, increased; →, leading to; Δ, change in; AT, anaerobic threshold; BP, blood pressure; CHF, chronic heart failure; CRF, chronic renal failure; DM, diabetes mellitus; ECG, electrocardiogram; EF, ejection fraction; HR, heart rate; ht, height; IC, inspiratory capacity; MVV, maximal voluntary ventilation; nl, normal; P(A–a)O_2, alveolar–arterial oxygen difference; $PaCO_2$, partial pressure of arterial carbon dioxide; P(a–ET)CO_2, arterial–end-tidal carbon dioxide difference; PaO_2, partial pressure of arterial oxygen; $PetCO_2$, partial pressure of end-tidal carbon dioxide; RR, respiratory rate; SV, stroke volume; TLC, total lung capacity; VCO_2, carbon dioxide production; VD/VT, ratio of dead space volume to tidal volume; V_E, minute ventilation; V_E max, maximal minute ventilation; VO_2, oxygen consumption; VO_2 max, maximal oxygen consumption; V/Q, ventilation–perfusion; WR, work rate; wt, body weight. Data from American Thoracic Society/American College of Chest Physicians ATS/ACCP statement on cardiopulmonary exercise testing. *Am J Respir Crit Care Med* 167:211–277, 2003; Wasserman K: Dyspnea on exertion. Is it the heart or the lungs? *JAMA* 248:2039–2043, 1982; Wasserman K, Hansen JE, Sue DY, et al: *Principles of Exercise Testing and Interpretation*. Philadelphia, 1987, Lea & Febiger; and Weisman IM, Zeballos RJ: An integrative approach to the interpretation of cardiopulmonary exercise testing. *Prog Respir Res* 32:300–322, 2002. In Watchie J. *Cardiovascular and Pulmonary Physical Therapy: A Clinical Manual*, ed 2. St. Louis, 2010, Saunders.

Table 8-2 American Thoracic Society Dyspnea Scale

Grade	Degree	Description
0	None	Not troubled with breathlessness except with strenuous exercise
1	Slight	Troubled by shortness of breath when hurrying on level ground or walking up a slight hill
2	Moderate	Walks slower than people of the same age on level ground because of breathlessness or has to stop for breath when walking at own pace on level ground
3	Severe	Stops for breath after walking about 100 yards or after a few minutes on level ground
4	Very severe	Too breathless to leave the house or breathless when dressing or undressing

Reprinted with permission from Brooks SM: Surveillance for respiratory hazards, *ATS News* 8:12-16, 1982.

Is wheezing present with the dyspnea on exertion? Has there been an associated weight gain? Does the patient have a positive smoking history and sputum production? If a positive response is received, these suggest that COPD is the primary cause of symptoms.[20]

The basic defect that cardiac diseases produce during exertion is a limited cardiac output, which is caused primarily by a reduced stroke volume.[17] To compensate for the relatively low stroke volume, the patient develops a rapid heart rate and a wide arteriovenous O_2 difference (decreased capillary PO_2) at an inappropriately low work rate. Therefore the exercising muscles (both skeletal and myocardial) have increased difficulty getting an adequate oxygen supply to perform the necessary work: this results in dyspnea, fatigue, or pain. The lactic acidosis that results from the low level of oxygen delivery to the muscles can be measured by either invasive or noninvasive gas-exchange methods during exercise testing. The functional and therapeutic capacity of the patient with heart disease can be estimated on the basis of the history and symptoms (Table 8-3).

Dyspnea in patients with cardiac disorders is usually related to metabolic acidosis-induced hydrogen ion stimulus. Also, increased pressure in the right side of the heart and pulmonary circulation during exertion may stimulate mechanoreceptors that increase ventilation and induce dyspnea.

Diseases that involve the lungs or thoracic cage generally prevent external respiration (ventilation) from keeping pace with internal respiration (in the cells).[17] In other words, patients outwalk or outrun their lungs during activities or exertion. The primary symptom that limits exercise in patients with pulmonary disorders is dyspnea, which occurs because of the difficulty they have eliminating the CO_2 produced by metabolism. Some individuals, such as those with pulmonary fibrosis and some of those with COPD, do experience a decrease in PO_2 with exercise. Hence dyspnea on exertion in pulmonary patients is usually related to hypoxic or hypercapnic stimuli.

Table 8-3 Functional and Therapeutic Classification of Patients with Heart Disease

Classification	Parameters
FUNCTIONAL CLASSIFICATION	
Class I	Patients with cardiac disease but without resulting limitations of physical activity; ordinary physical activity does not cause undue fatigue, palpitation, dyspnea, or anginal pain.
Class II	Patients with cardiac disease resulting in slight limitation of physical activity; they are comfortable at rest. Ordinary physical activity results in fatigue, palpitation, dyspnea, or anginal pain.
Class III	Patients with cardiac disease resulting in marked limitation of physical activity; they are comfortable at rest. Less than ordinary physical activity causes fatigue, palpitation, dyspnea, or anginal pain.
Class IV	Patients with cardiac disease resulting in inability to carry on any physical activity without discomfort; symptoms of cardiac insufficiency or of the anginal syndrome may be present even at rest. If any physical activity is undertaken, discomfort increases.
THERAPEUTIC CLASSIFICATION	
Class A	Patients with cardiac disease whose physical activity need not be restricted in any way.
Class B	Patients with cardiac disease whose ordinary physical activity need not be restricted but who should be advised against severe or competitive efforts.
Class C	Patients with cardiac disease whose ordinary activity should be moderately restricted and whose more strenuous efforts should be discontinued.
Class D	Patients with cardiac disease whose ordinary activity should be markedly restricted.
Class E	Patients with cardiac disease who should be at complete rest, confined to bed or chair.

Reprinted with permission from the New York Heart Association: *Diseases of the heart and blood vessels: Nomenclature and criteria for diagnosis*, ed 6, Boston, 1964, Little, Brown.

Dyspnea in Cardiac Patients

The cause of dyspnea in cardiac patients is determined by whether an associated stiffness of the lungs (a loss of compliance) is also present.[15] Dyspnea is the primary symptom of a decompensating left ventricle.[7,16] As the ventricle fails to eject the normal volume of blood, it produces chronic pulmonary venous hypertension, congestion, and pulmonary edema, resulting in stiff or less compliant lungs. This, along with modest hypoxemia that augments the respiratory drive, increases ventilation and the work of breathing. Tachypnea is often seen at rest. Exercise exaggerates the pulmonary congestion and edema and promotes arterial and mixed venous hypoxemia, which also increases the amount of dyspnea and tachypnea manifested. Fatigue, resulting from low cardiac output, also affects the respiratory muscles, further increasing the sensation of breathlessness.

Dyspnea in cardiac patients without stiff lungs is seen primarily during exertion or exercise.[15] In uncomplicated pulmonic stenosis, it is probably related to an inadequate cardiac output during exercise. Patients with tetralogy of Fallot and other forms of cyanotic heart disease experience both dyspnea and fatigue during exercise when the arterial oxyhemoglobin saturation has fallen appreciably below the resting level.

Orthopnea

Orthopnea is dyspnea that occurs when the patient is in the recumbent position.[1] The patient may state the need for two or three pillows under the head to rest at night. This symptom is commonly associated with CHF but may also be associated with severe chronic pulmonary disease.

Paroxysmal Nocturnal Dyspnea

Paroxysmal nocturnal dyspnea (PND) is an important type of shortness of breath. This symptom has strong predictive value as a sign of CHF.[1] The patient usually falls asleep in the recumbent position, and 1 or 2 hours later, awakens from sleep with acute shortness of breath. The patient sits upright on the side of the bed or goes to an open window to breathe "fresh air" and get relief from shortness of breath.

The mechanism of PND is the transfer of fluid from extravascular tissues into the blood stream (or intravascularly) during sleep.[20] The intravascular volume of fluid gradually increases until the compromised left ventricle can no longer manage it. The left atrial pressure rises when the rate of lymphatic drainage from the lungs is unable to keep up with the increased volume of fluid. The increased atrial pressure leads to a sufficiently elevated pulmonary capillary pressure to produce interstitial edema. Patients who are light sleepers awaken early with dyspnea. Deep sleepers may not awaken until they develop alveolar edema.

Classic PND cannot usually be eliminated by only elevating the trunk without lowering the legs. The patient must pool blood in the extravascular tissues of the legs to get adequate relief, which usually takes at least 30 minutes. This is why the patient must sit up or stand up and ambulate.

The patient should be asked about the amount of exercise or work performed during the day before an attack of PND. A true episode of left ventricular failure in PND is more likely to occur after a day of unusual exertion, which causes an increased amount of extravascular fluid to accumulate in the legs. If the patient is participating in an exercise or rehabilitation program, the level of exercise may have to be reduced to prevent PND.

Platypnea

Platypnea is the onset of dyspnea when the patient assumes the sitting position from the supine position.[6,16] This unusual phenomenon is commonly found in patients with basilar pulmonary fibrosis or basilar arteriovenous malformation. It can be related to the redistribution of blood flow to the lung bases when assuming the sitting position and the resultant ventilation-perfusion mismatching and hypoxemia.

Trepopnea

Trepopnea refers to dyspnea in one lateral position but not the other.[3] It is caused by the positional mismatching of ventilation to perfusion in unilateral respiratory system pathology such as lung disease, pleural effusion, or airway obstruction.[16,21,22] It also is commonly seen in patients with mitral stenosis.[20] Occasionally, it may be the result of a fall in blood pressure when the patient is in the left lateral decubitus position. If the patient has ischemic heart disease, the reduction in coronary perfusion can cause either angina or dyspnea.

Functional Dyspnea

Functional dyspnea is defined as shortness of breath at rest but not during exertion.[6] It is most commonly seen in young women who complain of the need to take a deep breath or to sigh, and they interpret this sensation as shortness of breath. The physical examination and pulmonary function tests are negative. Reassurance is usually all that is necessary.

Wheezing

Patients who complain of wheezing associated with dyspnea may have pulmonary or cardiac disease. This symptom, if first reported in patients over the age of 40, is often related to heart failure.[1] When it has been confirmed that the wheezing results from heart disease, the patient is said to have cardiac asthma. Wheezing in cardiac patients is a manifestation of narrowed airways and thickened bronchial walls as a result of pulmonary edema.[15] However, if patients have a history of episodes of wheezing and dyspnea since childhood, COPD or asthma is the likely cause. Other pulmonary conditions, such as eosinophilic pneumonia, bronchopulmonary aspergillosis, allergic granulomatosis, and others can cause wheezing.[5] Wheezing must be differentiated from stridor, which is commonly caused by laryngotracheal narrowing due to a tracheostomy scar, trauma of intubation, laryngeal paralysis, epiglottitis, or tumors. Chronic pulmonary patients may also develop heart conditions, so it is good to remember that patients who complain of wheezing may have both cardiac and pulmonary disease.

Cough

Cough is a common symptom of pulmonary disease. The cough mechanism consists of three phases:[23]

1. Inspiratory phase
2. Compressive phase
3. Expiratory phase

Numerous cough-irritant receptors are located on the mucosa of the larynx, trachea, bronchi, pleura, and external auditory canal. These receptors are most sensitive at the glottis and carina and diminish rapidly beyond the fourth-generation bronchi. A cough follows stimulation of these mucosal receptors by any of a number of factors including inflammation, sputum, foreign bodies, noxious gases or odors, chemical substances, endobronchial tumors, and extrabronchial pressure on the trachea or bronchi.[6]

A productive cough is beneficial for clearing the airways of sputum and foreign material and generally should not be inhibited. However, a dry, hacking cough is usually of no value and can have a self-perpetuating irritant effect on the respiratory mucosa. A dry cough may be the initial symptom of certain interstitial lung diseases such as allergic alveolitis, sarcoidosis, and pulmonary fibrosis. Some causes and characteristics of coughs are listed in Table 8-4.

Cough may be the only presenting symptom of asthma and is a common cause of chronic cough.[24,25] In individuals with asthma, cough is precipitated by inhaling cold air and by exercising, and the cough is dry. Cough can precipitate an asthma attack in sensitive patients; in that instance, it is known as cough-induced bronchospasm.

It is important to determine the length of time cough has been present.[6] The most common cause of an acute cough is a viral respiratory infection, which generally resolves within a few days or 2 to 3 weeks. Exposure to noxious gases also precipitates acute coughing.

A cough that has persisted for more than 3 weeks can be termed chronic.[3] The most common cause of chronic cough is chronic bronchitis, which is present in up to 30% of cigarette smokers. The next most common cause is the postnasal

Table 8-4 Some Causes and Characteristics of Coughs

Cause	Characteristics
ACUTE INFECTIONS OF LUNGS	
Tracheobronchitis	Cough associated with sore throat, running nose and eyes
Lobar pneumonia	Cough often preceded by symptoms of upper respiratory infection; cough dry, painful at first; later becomes productive
Bronchopneumonia	Usually begins as acute bronchitis; dry or productive cough
Mycoplasma and viral pneumonia	Paroxysmal cough, productive of mucoid or blood-stained sputum associated with influenza-like syndrome
Exacerbation of chronic bronchitis	Cough productive of mucoid sputum becomes purulent
CHRONIC INFECTIONS OF LUNGS	
Bronchitis	Cough productive of sputum on most days for more than 3 consecutive months and for more than 2 successive years; sputum mucoid until acute exacerbation, when it becomes mucopurulent
Bronchiectasis	Cough copious, foul, purulent, often since childhood
Tuberculosis or fungus	Persistent cough for weeks to months, often with blood-tinged sputum
PARENCHYMAL INFLAMMATORY PROCESSES	
Interstitial fibrosis and infiltrations	Cough nonproductive, persistent; depends on causes
Smoking	Cough usually associated with injected pharynx; persistent, most marked in morning, usually only slightly productive unless succeeded by chronic bronchitis
TUMORS	
Bronchogenic carcinoma	Nonproductive to productive cough for weeks to months; recurrent small hemoptysis common
Alveolar cell carcinoma	Cough similar to bronchogenic carcinoma, except in occasional instances when large quantities of watery, mucoid sputum are produced
Benign tumor in airways	Cough nonproductive, occasionally hemoptysis
Mediastinal tumor	Cough, often with breathlessness, caused by compression of trachea and bronchi
Aortic aneurysm	Brassy cough
FOREIGN BODIES	
Immediate, while still in upper airway	Cough associated with progressive evidence of asphyxiation
Later, when lodged in lower airway	Nonproductive cough, persistent, associated with localizing wheeze
Left ventricular failure	Cough intensifies while body is supine; aggravation of dyspnea
Pulmonary infarction	Cough associated with hemoptysis, usually with pleural effusion

Reprinted with permission from Szidon J, Fishman A: Approach to the pulmonary patient with respiratory signs and symptoms. In Fishman A, editor: *Pulmonary diseases and disorders.* New York, 1988, McGraw-Hill.

discharge syndrome. Patients describe a sensation of secretions dripping from the back of the nose into the throat, prompting throat clearing or coughing. Gastroesophageal disorders are present in 10% to 40% of patients with chronic cough and may contribute to coughing due to microaspiration or irritation of cough receptors in the lower esophagus.[25-27]

Various cardiac conditions may stimulate receptors in the bronchi and provoke coughing.[28] Because the bronchial veins empty into the pulmonary veins (leading to the left side of the heart), the systemic veins, and the superior vena cava (leading to the right side of the heart), venous congestion and coughing may occur with either right- or left-side CHF. It is more common, however, in left-sided CHF. The onset of a cough in a patient with paroxysmal tachycardia or acute myocardial infarction (MI) is often an early symptom of acute left-side heart failure.

Coughing may be caused by other cardiovascular conditions, such as a large left atrium displacing the left main stem bronchus upward, aortic aneurysms placing pressure on the bronchi, and a double aortic arch compressing the trachea.

A specific diagnosis can be made in 80% of cases of chronic cough by an appropriate history alone.[29] Determining the precipitating causes or the time of onset points the clinician to a probable diagnosis. For example, does the patient cough primarily at night? If so, it points to heart failure, esophageal problems, bronchiectasis, or asthma as the potential cause. An early-morning cough is more common in bronchitis and in individuals with postnasal drip. Cough following meals suggests esophageal disease. Cough precipitated by exertion or deep breathing suggests asthma or interstitial lung disease. Allergens or irritant fumes at home or at work may be a cause of cough. Postviral cough may be present for weeks following a viral illness.

Some medications can elicit coughing. Beta blockers prescribed to treat hypertension, migraine headaches, cardiovascular disease (CVD), or glaucoma may precipitate asthma.

Many drugs, including chemotherapeutic agents, can cause interstitial lung disease and coughing.

Cough and wheezing may result from COPD, asthma, or early left heart failure. Early left heart failure predisposes the patient to respiratory infections and may be responsible for chronic bronchitis.

Cough Complications

One of the more common complications of cough is syncope. Tussive, or cough-induced, syncope, which is more common in men than in women, can be recognized through accurate history taking.[5] It is typically reported by middle-aged men who "smoke hard, eat hard, drink hard, and cough hard." They experience fainting or near-fainting following cough paroxysms. The cause is obscure but may be related to vagus-induced cardiac slowing or vasodilation or to high intrathoracic pressures that impair venous return, decrease cardiac output, increase intracranial pressure, and result in a reduced cerebral blood flow. Cough syncope is often resolved by smoking cessation.

Complications of cough include headache, back pain, muscular tears, hematomas, and rib fractures (along the posterior axillary line). Occasionally, vertebral compression fractures (in osteopenic patients), urinary incontinence (UI) (in women), and inguinal hernias (in men) may occur.[30]

Chest Pain

Taking an accurate history is crucial to the proper evaluation of chest pain.[3] Although the definitive cause of chest pain cannot be fully established without diagnostic medical tests, it is usually possible to determine whether the pain originates in the pleurae, chest wall, or thoracic organs by means of careful history taking.

Pleuritic Chest Pain

Pleuritic chest pain originates from the parietal pleura or endothoracic fascia but not the visceral pleura, which have no pain receptors. The patient can usually identify it as being close to the thoracic cage.[15] Pleuritic chest pain worsens sharply with inspiration as the inflamed parietal pleura are stretched with chest wall motion. Deep breathing, coughing, and laughing are extremely painful, requiring the patient to apply pressure over the involved area to control the pain.

Pleuritic chest pain is ordinarily found in patients who have other signs of respiratory illness, such as cough, fever, chills, and malaise. Inflammation of the central portion of the diaphragmatic pleura produces ipsilateral shoulder pain by way of the phrenic nerve.[5] Outer portions of the diaphragmatic pleura are innervated by the 7th through 12th intercostal nerves. Irritation of these pleura causes referred pain in the lower thorax or upper abdomen.[31]

The onset of pleuritic chest pain varies according to its cause.[3] Sudden severe pleuritic chest pain suggests a spontaneous pneumothorax, pulmonary embolism, or infarct. Pulmonary embolism is usually accompanied by sudden dyspnea, hemoptysis, tachycardia, cyanosis, hypotension, anxiety, and agitation.[7]

Cardiac Chest Pain

Three cardinal features are characteristic of cardiac chest pain. The patient should be asked the following questions:[7]

1. Does the pain have maximal intensity from the onset or does it build up for several seconds? Ischemic cardiac pain, or angina, is caused by the myocardium contracting in the absence of an adequate oxygen supply. The same type of pain can be produced by placing a blood pressure cuff around the upper arm and inflating it until the brachial pulse can no longer be palpated at the wrist. If a patient opens and closes a fist, pain will gradually appear and escalate in the forearm. The causal mechanism of this pain is the same as that of myocardial pain: continuing muscular contraction in the absence of an adequate oxygen supply. This type of pain requires several contractions of the myocardium to reach its maximal intensity. In other words, there is a characteristic buildup, or escalation, of angina pain.
2. Can you point to the area of pain with one finger? Anginal pain is characteristically demonstrated by patients' using their entire hand or closed fist against the anterior chest wall. It is described as a sign of angina because it is so typical.[7] By contrast, any pain that can be localized by pointing with a fingertip is unlikely to be angina.
3. Is the pain deep inside your chest, or does it seem as though it is close to the surface? Anginal pain is visceral pain that may be referred superficially but always has a deep internal component.

Myocardial ischemia may be completely painless (silent ischemia). Angina may, in fact, not be painful but rather may be described as discomfort, pressure, squeezing, a tight band, heaviness, burning, or indigestion. It usually is located substernally and radiates into one or both arms, the neck, the jaw, or the back.

Angina is not limited to patients with CAD.[7] Individuals who have normal coronary arteries but an insufficient oxygen supply for a given cardiac workload can also experience angina. These include individuals with anemia, hypertension, tachycardia, and thyrotoxicosis. Hypertrophic and dilated cardiomyopathy can produce typical angina pain, although the latter tends to be intermittent, usually occurring with episodes of CHF. Aortic valve disease can cause angina as a result of impairment of adequate coronary artery blood flow.

Angina is usually precipitated by exertion, such as walking uphill, against the wind, or in cold weather.[7] It is more likely to be brought on after a meal or by emotional stress. The rapid resolution of chest pain by rest or sublingual nitroglycerin strongly suggests a cardiac origin. The pain produced by MI is longer, persisting more than 20 minutes; it occurs at rest and is accompanied by nausea, diaphoresis, hypotension, and dyspnea.

Pulmonary Hypertension

Chest pain related to pulmonary hypertension may mimic angina pectoris. It is usually found in patients with mitral stenosis or Eisenmenger syndrome (pulmonary hypertension related to an interventricular septal defect, a patent ductus arteriosus, or an atrial septal defect). This type of chest pain usually is absent at rest, occurs during exertion, and is invariably associated with dyspnea.[1] It is believed to result from dilation of the pulmonary artery or from right ventricular ischemia. The pain is not relieved by nitrates. Primary pulmonary hypertension may be accompanied by syncope and the Raynaud phenomenon.[6]

Pericardial Chest Pain

Pericardial chest pain is also midline, but because of its anatomic relationship with the mediastinal pleura, it has features that suggest pleural involvement.[3] Deep breathing, coughing, swallowing, movement, and lying down may make it worse. If the central tendon of the diaphragm is involved, the pain may be referred to the left shoulder or scapular area.[7] The patient may report that each heartbeat affects the pain. Sitting up and leaning forward or lying on the right side often relieves the pain.

Esophageal Chest Pain

Diffuse esophageal spasm or esophageal colic is a common cause of chest pain. It is often confused with cardiac pain because it is located substernally, has a squeezing or aching quality, and may radiate into one or both arms.[12] Furthermore, diffuse esophageal spasm may be relieved by sublingual nitroglycerin as a result of its generalized function as a smooth-muscle relaxant.

Pain that radiates through the chest to the back, pain that decreases with a change in position from supine to upright, or relief induced by ingesting antacids all suggest an esophageal origin.[3] Also, diffuse esophageal spasm is often associated with pain on swallowing (odynophagia), dysphagia, and regurgitation of stomach contents. Swallowing hot or cold liquids and emotional stress tend to precipitate this type of chest pain.

Chest Wall Pain

Chest wall pain is the most common type of chest pain. Clues in the patient's history to this type of pain include intermittent occurrence, variable intensity, and local tenderness.[5] Because it is commonly located on the anterior chest wall, many patients believe it is heart pain. However, an important differentiation from cardiac pain is that it does not occur during, but rather following, exertion. It may worsen with inspiration, but its association with trunk motions (flexion, extension, rotation) distinguish it from pleuritic chest pain.

Localized anterior chest pain as a result of costochondritis of the second to fourth costosternal articulations (Tietze syndrome) is described as tender to touch.[12] A complaint of rib tenderness, together with a history of trauma, fall, long-term steroid use, coughing, or upper extremity exertion, suggests rib fracture.

Degenerative disk disease and arthritis of the cervical or thoracic spine, thoracic outlet syndrome, spondylitis, fibromyalgia, kyphoscoliosis, and herpes zoster can all produce chest wall pain.[3,5,32-34] Primary lung cancer that invades the adjoining chest wall, ribs, or spine produces severe, persistent, localized pain.[3] Another possible cause of chest wall pain is the Pancoast syndrome (superior sulcus tumor), in which a primary lung tumor located in the extreme apex of the lung invades the brachial plexus and produces pain in the shoulder, scapular region, or medial aspect of the arm and hand.

Chest wall pain may be caused, rarely, by thrombosis of a superficial vein on the chest wall (Mondor's disease). It is a self-limited condition of unknown origin and can last several weeks.[3] The only physical finding is a subcutaneous cord that can be palpated along the lateral chest wall.

Hemoptysis

Hemoptysis is defined as coughing up blood. It can vary in amount from being blood-streaked sputum to being virtually all blood. The bleeding site may be anywhere in the upper or lower respiratory tract.

The timing and frequency of hemoptysis, as determined in the history, can offer clues about its cause. A history of nosebleeds is significant because blood may be aspirated during sleep at night and expectorated the following morning. Intermittent bouts of hemoptysis are characteristic of respiratory infections such as bronchiectasis, tuberculosis, fungus infections, or broncholithiasis.[5] Persistent expectoration of blood-streaked sputum on a daily basis is highly suggestive of bronchogenic neoplasm.

The lung receives its blood supply in two ways: the pulmonary arteries (a low-pressure system) and the bronchial arteries (a high-pressure system) off the aorta.[6] The appearance of hemoptysis may vary according to which blood supply is involved. If the bronchial vessels are the source, there tend to be large amounts of bright-red blood. This is often the site of bleeding in bronchiectasis, because bronchial arteries undergo enlargement and extensive anastomosis with the pulmonary artery system. In mitral stenosis, where there is increased pulmonary vascular resistance, hemoptysis arises from passively engorged submucosal bronchial veins.[15]

Hemoptysis sourced in the low-pressure pulmonary artery system tends to occur in small amounts and is composed of dark or clotted venous blood.[3] It may arise from the pulmonary parenchyma, as in the case of the highly vascular granulation tissue found in the walls of lung abscesses. These abscesses may be caused by infections, such as tuberculosis, anaerobic bacteria, staphylococci, or chronic irritation by a fungus ball in an abscess cavity. If a blood vessel ruptures in an abscess cavity, hemorrhage tends to be massive, even exsanguinating.

Cardiovascular conditions, such as mitral stenosis, pulmonary infarction, Eisenmenger physiology, and aortic aneurysm, are also associated with hemoptysis.[1] Pink frothy sputum is commonly found with acute pulmonary edema. Physical therapists should carefully evaluate complaints of hemoptysis and be certain of its cause before cautiously conducting treatment.

Fatigue and Weakness

There are multiple causes of fatigue and weakness.[1] Physical therapists should not conclude too quickly that they are related to physical inactivity and decreased muscular strength in sedentary cardiopulmonary patients. The most common causes of complaint of fatigue and weakness are depression, anxiety, and emotional stress. They often accompany anemia, hypothyroidism, and chronic disease states.

Fatigue is commonly associated with CHF. In this condition, it is probably related to cardiac output insufficient to perfuse the entire body adequately, including the skeletal muscles. Generally, fatigue caused by cardiac disease is related to exertion, but fatigue related to anxiety tends to be continuous.[1]

Diuretics used to treat CHF can cause potassium depletion and hypokalemia with resultant weakness. Antihypertensive medications can produce weakness through postural hypotension.

Pedal Edema

CHF is a common cause of bilateral pedal edema.[7] However, 10 to 20 pounds of fluid generally accumulate in the body before foot and ankle swelling is evident. Therefore weight gain is an even earlier indication of fluid retention due to CHF. Occasionally, patients may complain only about an increase in abdominal girth, which results from ascites. When caused by CHF, the onset of ascites virtually always occurs after pedal edema is present. If the amount of ascites is disproportionate to that of pedal edema, restrictive cardiomyopathy or constrictive pericarditis should be a consideration.

It is important to determine whether the patient had dyspnea on exertion before the onset of lower-extremity edema. If the edema is a result of a poorly functioning left ventricle, mitral stenosis, or cor pulmonale, it usually follows dyspnea on exertion.

Patients with CHF and altered renal function commonly report edema of the ankle and lower legs while upright during the day, but indicate a decrease during the night.[1] This is a result of local hydrostatic factors related to the upright position.

Edema may be present in nephrosis or starvation, when the total blood protein falls below 5 g/100 mL (hypoproteinemia). Other causes of pedal edema include liver disease, kidney disease, and anemia. Edema of one leg ordinarily occurs because of local factors such as thrombophlebitis or varicose veins.

Hoarseness

Hoarseness (abnormal vocal cord motion during phonation) is a symptom of laryngeal dysfunction.[5] It is usually associated with upper respiratory tract infections or allergies and resolves in 1 to 2 weeks.[6] Trauma following intubation, laryngeal polyps, or tumors are other common causes of hoarseness. However, this symptom is also related to cardiopulmonary conditions. Because the recurrent laryngeal nerves pass through the upper thorax, intrathoracic pathology that involves one of these nerves can cause unilateral vocal cord paralysis, resulting in hoarseness.[6] These include lung or mediastinal tumors, granulomatous disease, enlarged mediastinal lymph nodes, and pericardial or mediastinal adhesions.

Several cardiovascular conditions can produce hoarseness because the left recurrent laryngeal nerve loops under the arch of the aorta and above the pulmonary artery as it returns to the neck.[1] Therefore an aneurysm of the arch of the aorta, a dilated pulmonary artery or atrium resulting from an atrial septal defect, or mitral stenosis can cause hoarseness.[28]

Hence, if a patient manifests hoarseness, it is necessary to inquire about the length of time it has been present, the patient's smoking history, and any history of cardiac or pulmonary diseases.

Summary

Obtaining an accurate and thorough history is the cornerstone of the physical therapy evaluation process. The probable cause and severity of many cardiopulmonary symptoms can be determined by careful history taking. This information enables therapists to select the most appropriate evaluation and treatment techniques. When properly performed, accurate history taking gains the patient's confidence and cooperation and provides the basis for a good patient-therapist relationship.

Review Questions

1. What are the basic causes of dyspnea?
2. What questions can be asked of a patient with dyspnea in order to determine the likely cause?
3. What scales have been developed to quantitate dyspnea?
4. What are the principal features of chest pain that originates in the pleurae? In the chest wall? In the thoracic organs?
5. What are the cardinal features of cardiac chest pain?
6. What occupations can place workers at risk for respiratory disease?

References

1. Hurst J, Morris DC, Crawley IS, et al: The history: past events and symptoms related to cardiovascular disease. In Hurst J, Schlant RC, Rackley CE, et al, editors: *The heart,* New York, 1990, McGraw–Hill.
2. Birdwell B, Herbers J, Kroenke K: Evaluating chest pain: the patient's presentation style alters the physician's diagnostic approach. *Archives of Internal Medicine* 153:1991–1995, 1993.
3. Snider G: History and physical examination. In Baum G, Wolinski E, editors: *Textbook of pulmonary diseases,* ed 5, Boston, 1994, Little, Brown.
4. Tetrault JM, Crothers K, Moore BA, et al: Effects of marijuana smoking on pulmonary function and respiratory complications. *Archives of Internal Medicine* 167:221–228, 2007.
5. Miller D: The medical history. In Sackner M, editor: *Diagnostic techniques in pulmonary disease,* New York, 1980, Marcel Dekker.
6. Sharf S: History and physical examination. In Baum G, Wolinski E, editor: *Textbook of pulmonary diseases,* ed 4, Boston, 1989, Little, Brown.
7. Marriott H: Taking the history. In Marriott H, editor: *Bedside cardiac diagnosis,* Philadelphia, 1993, JB Lippincott.
8. Varkey B: Asbestos exposure: an update on pleuropulmonary hazards. *Postgraduate Medicine* 74:93–103, 1983.
9. Feldman DM, Baron SL, Bernard BP, et al: Symptoms, respirator use, and pulmonary function changes among New York City firefighters responding to the World Trade Center disaster. *Chest* 125:1256–1264, 2004.
10. Skloot G, Goldman M, Fischler D, et al: Respiratory symptoms and physiologic assessment of ironworkers at the World Trade Center disaster site. *Chest* 125:1248–1255, 2004.
11. Brandstetter R, Sprince N: Occupational lung disease. *Medical Times* 110:56–63, 1982.
12. George R: History and physical examination. In: George R, editor: *Chest medicine: essentials of pulmonary and critical care medicine,* Baltimore, 1990, Williams and Wilkins.
13. Mahler D, Harver A: Clinical measurements of dyspnea. In Mahler D, editor: *Dyspnea,* Mount Kisco, NY, 1990, Futura.
14. Mahler D: Dyspnea: diagnosis and management. *Clinical Chest Medicine* 8:215–230, 1987.
15. Szidan P, Fishman A: Approach to the pulmonary patient with respiratory signs and symptoms. In Fishman A, editor: *Pulmonary diseases and disorders,* ed 2, New York, 1988, McGraw–Hill.

16. Mahler D: Diagnosis of dyspnea. In Mahler D, editor. *Dyspnea*, New York, 1998, Marcel Dekker.
17. Wasserman K: Dyspnea on exertion: is it the heart or the lungs? *JAMA* 248:2039–2043, 1982.
18. Borg G: Psychophysical bases of perceived exertion. *Medical Science of Sports and Exercise* 14:377–381, 1982.
19. Mahler D, Harver A: Do you speak the language of dyspnea? *Chest* 117:928–929, 2000.
20. Constant J: The evolving checklist in history-taking. In *Bedside cardiology*, Boston, 1993, Little, Brown.
21. Remolina C, Khan AU, Santiago TV, Edelman NH: Positional hypoxemia in unilateral lung disease. *New England Journal of Medicine* 304:523–525, 1981.
22. Zack MB, Pontoppidan H, Kazemi H: The effect of lateral positions on gas exchange in pulmonary disease. *American Review of Respiratory Diseases* 110:49–55, 1974.
23. Irwin R, Rosen M, Braman S: Cough: a comprehensive review. *Archives of Internal Medicine* 137:1186–1191, 1977.
24. Dicpinigaitis DV: Cough in asthma and eosiniphilic bronchitis. *Thorax* 59:71, 2004.
25. Morice AH, Kastelik JA: Chronic cough in adults. *Thorax* 58:901–907, 2003.
26. Fontana GA, Pistolesi M: Chronic cough and gastro-esophageal reflux. *Thorax* 58:1092–1095, 2003.
27. Irwin RS, Madison M: The diagnosis and treatment of cough. *New England Journal of Medicine* 343:1715–1721, 2000.
28. Goldberger E: Symptoms referable to the cardiovascular system. In Goldberger E, editor: *Essentials of clinical cardiology*, Philadelphia, 1990, JB Lippincott.
29. Stulberg M: Evaluating and treating intractable cough—Medical Staff Conference, University of California, San Francisco. *Western Journal of Medicine* 143:223–228, 1985.
30. Braman S, Corrao W: Cough: differential diagnosis and treatment. *Clinical Chest Medicine* 8:177–188, 1987.
31. Fraser RS, Muller NL, Colman NC: The clinical history and physical examination. In Fraser RS, Muller NL, Colman NC, et al, editors: *Diagnosis and diseases of the chest*, Philadelphia, 1999, WB Saunders.
32. Epstein S, Gerber L, Borer J: Chest wall syndrome: a common cause of unexplained cardiac pain. *JAMA* 241:2793–2797, 1979.
33. Pellegrino M: Atypical chest pain as an initial presentation of primary fibromyalgia. *Archives of Physical Medicine Rehabilitation* 71:526–528, 1990.
34. Wise C, Semble E, Dalton C: Musculoskeletal chest wall syndromes in patients with noncardiac chest pain: a study of 100 patients. *Archives of Physical Medicine Rehabilitation* 73:147–149, 1992.

Pulmonary Function Tests

Donna Frownfelter

KEY TERMS

Dead space
Expiratory reserve volume
Functional residual capacity
Inspiratory capacity
Inspiratory reserve volume
Lung capacities
Lung volume
Obstructive component
Predicted values
Restrictive component
Residual volume
Tidal volume
Total lung capacity
Vital capacity

CHAPTER OUTLINE

Pulmonary function tests are usually ordered when patients go to their primary physician or a pulmonary specialist with complaints of shortness of breath, cough, decreased activity, and dyspnea. When the history is taken, patients' complaints are due to their breathing problem, for example they are short of breath walking up stairs or dressing. As dyspnea begins to affect their daily life more and more, people will often make lifestyle changes, such as selling a two-story house and moving to a ranch house with no stairs or altering the way they dress (e.g., wearing housecoats or jogging pants that are easier to put on and take off). Often, people think that their breathing problems are just part of getting older, and they try to change their lifestyle to accommodate their limitations and avoid doing things that make them short of breath. In many cases, by the time a patient comes to the care provider with these complaints, he or she is already showing signs of moderate to severe chronic obstructive pulmonary disease (COPD). As will be discussed in this chapter, this is a very good reason for considering office spirometry to be a "fifth vital sign." Suggestions have been made that all smokers and any nonsmoker over 40 years of age should have office spirometry. If the values are abnormal, even though patients may not be experiencing noticeable lifestyle changes, the appropriate drug therapy regimen can be implemented and patients who are smokers will have a definite motivation to quit smoking.

Pulmonary function tests (PFTs) help in the evaluation of the mechanical function of the lungs.[1] They are based on researched norms, taking into account sex, height, and age. For example, there are predicted values for a male, age 65, who is 6 feet tall.[2,3] Race and ethnic differences also play roles in the reference values and need to be taken into account for diagnostic and research purposes.[4–6]

When the patient performs the test, actual results (observed) are compared with the predicted value expected of a person of that gender, height, and age to see whether he or she falls within the "normal" range or has a restrictive, obstructive, or a mixed component, based on the tests. If the patient is not within the normal range, a bronchodilator is given, and the test is repeated to see whether there is significant improvement with medication. Basically, the pulmonary function tests are categorized as volume, flow, or diffusion studies. Diagnosis of pulmonary disease or dysfunction and improvement with treatment are evaluated after interpreting a patient's pulmonary function tests.

Spirometry is the most useful and commonly available test of pulmonary function. Both pulmonologists and primary care physicians commonly use screening spirometry in their offices in order to assess patients and to evaluate the effectiveness of treatment being given to the patient.[7]

Patients with asthma and COPD make up a large portion of the primary care physician's caseload. COPD is often diagnosed in the moderate to severe stage of the disease. The diagnosis of COPD can be made quite easily with spirometry, taking the patient's symptoms and history into account. Smokers can be evaluated for early lung disease, and this can serve as a "teachable moment" for them to quit smoking.[8]

Yawn and colleagues (2007)[9] compared the office spirometry interpretations of pulmonary experts with those of family physicians. They found agreement in 78% of the completed tests. In addition, following spirometry, changes were implemented in the management of 48% of patients. Of interest, there was closer correct interpretation of pulmonary functions between family physicians and pulmonologists in patients who had asthma, versus those with COPD.

Preoperative Pulmonary Evaluation

Preoperative pulmonary evaluation can predict postoperative pulmonary complications.[10–12] As people are living longer lives, more older adults will be candidates for surgery. From 1980 to 1995 the rates of cardiovascular surgical procedures in patients over 65 tripled.[13] In 1997 the performance of 10 of the most common surgical procedures in the United States totaled 1 in 350,0000 operations in the 65- to 84-year-old age group.[14] Considering the comorbidities of an aging population and the concern about complications in older adults, a thorough preoperative pulmonary screening is recommended.[11]

Risk factors that contribute to postoperative complications include smoking, older age, obesity, poor health, and chronic obstructive pulmonary disease.[11] Additional procedure-related risk factors include the site of surgery (abdominal, chest wall versus extremity, duration of surgery, and type of anesthesia or neuromuscular blockage).[15]

Office Spirometry to Improve Early Detection of Chronic Obstructive Pulmonary Disease

The National Lung Health Education Program has recommended that office spirometry be used to screen for subclinical lung disease in adult smokers. For patients who are smokers or for any patients over 40 who have unexplained dyspnea, cough, wheezing, or excessive mucus, spirometric measurements can be considered another vital sign to measure during the routine physical examination, along with blood pressure and cholesterol levels.[16,17]

In a study of 35- to 70-year-old individuals visiting their general practitioners, patients were given a questionnaire on symptoms of obstructive lung disease.[18] Spirometry was performed in patients with positive answers to the questions and in a random sample of 10% of the group. It was found that 42% of the newly diagnosed cases of obstructive disease would not have been detected without spirometry. The researchers concluded that office spirometry is essential in general practice and can be done by general practitioners who have training in the performance and interpretation of the pulmonary function tests. It is essential that there be good quality assurance and good training when these tests are performed in a general practitioner's office. Studies have shown variability between the results of pulmonary function tests done in the office versus those done in a lab, so the results should not be considered interchangeable.[19,20]

Respiration: Effect of Anatomical and Physiological Dead Space

The most important function of the lungs is to supply the body with oxygen and to the remove carbon dioxide (CO_2) that is produced as a waste product of metabolism. As this continuous gas exchange takes place, sufficient ventilation is needed to move the gases to the alveoli. A number of conducting airways in the lungs, from the trachea down to the terminal bronchi, do not participate in respiration but only move the gases to the alveoli. The volume of this series of airways is known as anatomical dead space. Generally, the anatomical dead space is proportional to the adult body weight. For example, in a 150-pound person, there is an anatomical dead space of approximately 150 mL. A normal tidal volume (TV), the breath normally taken, has to be large enough to reach the alveoli well past the anatomical dead space. In a normal adult, the TV is generally 450 to 600 mL. The anatomical dead space would thus represent about one-third of the TV. The rest of the breath would reach the alveoli and be considered "alveolar ventilation." In many neurologically impaired patients who have limited TVs, it is important to note that little alveolar ventilation may be taking place when the patient is breathing in a rapid and shallow pattern. For example, if a patient's TV is 200 mL, 150 mL would be anatomical dead space, and only 50 mL of each breath would be effective alveolar ventilation.

Many diseases and conditions can alter the volume of dead space that requires ventilation. In some cases the dead space decreases—for instance, in a pneumonectomy, when it is physically removed, or in asthma, when bronchospasm may narrow the airways. In other conditions such as pulmonary embolism, dead space increases when ventilated areas of lung cease to be perfused. The alveoli continue to receive fresh gas, but there is no blood available for gas exchange. This type of dead space is known as physiological dead space.

When dead space is increased, a larger percentage of the tidal volume is ventilating the dead space, leaving a smaller percentage for alveolar ventilation. The patient must work harder to get enough air to the functioning alveoli. This causes increased work of breathing and may result in patient fatigue. Work of breathing, or minute ventilation (MV), is defined as the TV times the respiratory rate (RR). The formula for minute ventilation is: $MV = TV \times RR$. For example, an MV of 8 L per minute = 500 mL × 16 breaths per minute. When the ventilatory rate increases, the TV decreases; thus the effective alveolar ventilation decreases.

Neurological and neuromuscular weakness may result in the inability to reach a normal TV. Similarly, surgical procedures or pain caused by fractured ribs can also compromise a patient's ability to take a breath. Patients given a thoracolumbosacral orthosis (TLSO), or a corset for low back pain, may find their pulmonary function compromised by the restriction of the rib cage and abdomen. As the TV drops, a large percentage of the breath is anatomical dead space. This results in increased work of breathing for the patient and may ultimately result in respiratory failure if the patient is unable to provide effective alveolar ventilation.

Lung Volumes

The lung has four volumes: TV, inspiratory reserve volume (IRV), expiratory reserve volume (ERV), and residual volume (RV) (Figure 9-1).

- TV is the normal breath.
- IRV is the maximum amount of air that can be inhaled above a normal inspiration.
- ERV is the maximum amount of air that can be expired after a normal exhalation.
- RV is the volume of gas that remains in the lungs at the end of a maximum expiration.

Changes in RV can help in the diagnosis of certain medical conditions. An increase in RV means that even with maximum effort, the patient cannot exhale excess air from the lungs. This results in hyperinflated lungs and indicates that certain changes have occurred in the pulmonary tissue, which in time may cause mechanical changes in the chest wall (e.g., increased [AP] diameter, flattened diaphragm). These changes may be reversible in patients with partial bronchial obstruction, such as young patients with asthma, or irreversible, as in patients with advanced emphysema. Restrictive lung disease can cause a decrease in residual volume, as can cancer of the lung, microatelectasis, or musculoskeletal impairment.[21]

Lung Capacities

A lung capacity is two or more volumes added together (see Fig. 9-1). The capacities include total lung capacity (TLC), vital capacity (VC), inspiratory capacity (IC), and functional residual capacity (FRC).

TLC is the amount of gas the lung contains at the end of a maximum inspiration. It is made up of all four lung volumes. An increased TLC is seen with hyperinflation, such as in emphysema. A decrease in TLC may be seen in restrictive lung disease, such as pulmonary fibrosis, atelectasis, neoplasms, pleural effusions, and hemothorax, as well as in restrictive musculoskeletal problems, such as spinal cord injury and kyphoscoliosis. Decreased TLC can also be secondary to morbid obesity or pregnancy.

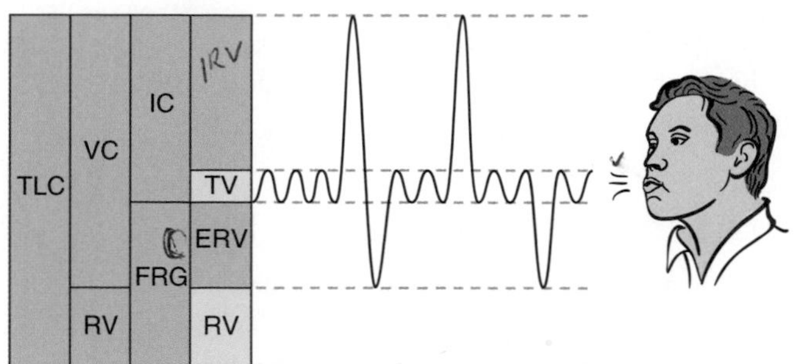

Fig. 9-1 A spirogram (pulmonary function testing).

VC is the maximum amount of gas that can be expelled from the lungs by forceful effort after a maximum inspiration. It contains the IRV, TV, and ERV. A decrease in VC can occur as a result of absolute reduction in distensible lung tissue. This is seen in pneumonectomy, atelectasis, pneumonia, pulmonary congestion, occlusion of a major bronchus by a tumor or foreign object, and restrictive lung disease, due to either a primary cause such as pulmonary fibrosis or a secondary cause such as the application of a TLSO.

A decrease in VC may also be seen without primary lung disease or airway obstruction. In neuromuscular or musculoskeletal dysfunction, VC can be compromised (as in Guillain-Barré syndrome, spinal cord injury, drug overdose, motor vehicle accident with fractured ribs, severe scoliosis, pectus excavatum, and kyphoscoliosis). Additional contributing factors, such as morbid obesity, pregnancy, enlarged heart, and pulmonary effusion, may involve limitation of expansion of the lungs.

IC is the maximum amount of air that can be inspired when starting at the resting expiratory level. It contains the IRV and the TV.

FRC is the volume of air remaining in the lungs at the resting expiratory level. It contains the ERV and the RV. The FRC prevents large fluctuations in PaO_2 with each breath. An increase in FRC represents hyperinflation of the lungs. It causes the thorax to be larger than normal, which results in muscular inefficiency and some mechanical disadvantage. Patients on mechanical ventilators may increase their FRC with positive pressure and by additional modes such as positive end-expiratory pressure (PEEP). Spontaneously breathing patients can also be on continuous positive airway pressures (CPAP and BIPAP), which keep the lungs at a positive airway pressure to improve ventilation and oxygenation.

Air Flow Measurements

Forced Expiration

When a patient performs a VC maneuver, it can either be slow or fast. During exhalation, the amount of air exhaled over time can be measured. In a slow VC, a patient with emphysema can take a great deal of time to empty his or her lungs. In a forced VC, a normal individual can exhale 75% of the VC in the first second of exhalation (FEV_1). Patients with emphysema often have greatly decreased VCs, only 40% of which are predicted. Some pulmonary function laboratories also offer an FEV_6, which measures the flow at six seconds rather than just at 1 second.

Flow Volume Curve

The flow volume curve is helpful in diagnosing lung disease because it is independent of effort. The curve in Figure 9-2 demonstrates that flow rises to a high value and then declines over most of expiration.[22] In restrictive lung disease, the maximum flow rate is reduced, as is the total volume exhaled. In obstructive lung disease, the flow rate is low in relation to

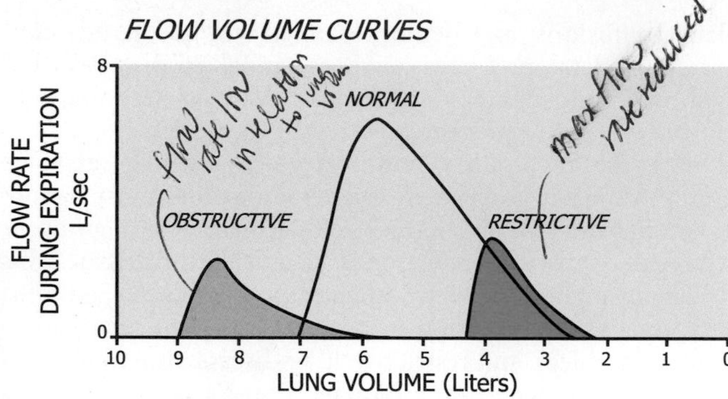

Fig. 9-2 Comparison of flow volume curves in the normal patient and in the patient with obstructive and restrictive lung disease.

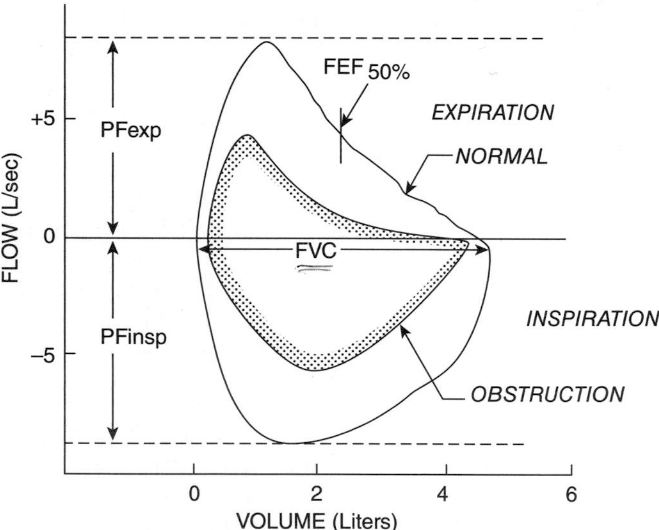

Fig. 9-3 Comparison of flow volume loops in the normal patient and in the patient with obstructive lung disease.

lung volume, and a scooped-out appearance is often seen (see Figure 9-2).

Another diagnostic test that uses forced expiration is the flow volume loop. It is a graphic analysis of the flow generated during a forced expiratory volume maneuver followed by a forced inspiratory volume maneuver (Figure 9-3). This graph offers a pictorial representation of data from many individual tests (e.g., peak inspiratory and expiratory flow rates, FVC, and FEV). The shape of the graph may also be helpful in diagnosing disease, because again there is a more scooped-out appearance in cases of obstructive disease.

Closing Volume and Airway Closure

The assessment of closing volume is used to help diagnose small-airway disease. A test called the single-breath nitrogen (N_2) washout is used for assessing closing volume and closing capacity of the small airways. In this test, the patient takes a single VC breath of 100% oxygen. During complete exhalation, the N_2 concentration can be measured. The characteristic tracing of N_2 concentration can be measured. The characteristic tracing of N_2 concentration versus lung volume reflects the sequential emptying of differentially ventilated lung units,

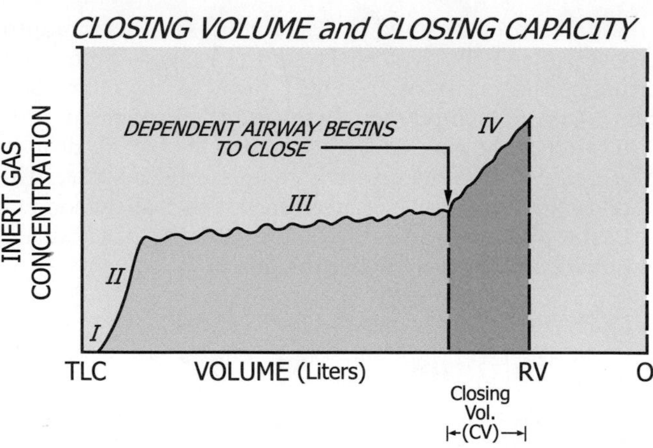

Fig. 9-4 The single-breath nitrogen washout test to assess airway closure.

resulting in different expiratory concentrations of N_2. Four phases can be identified (Figure 9-4). Phase I contains pure dead space and virtually none of the potential N_2 from the RV. Phase II is associated with an increasing N_2 concentration of a mixture of gas from the dead space and alveoli. The plateau in N_2 concentration observed in phase III reflects pure alveolar gas emanating from the base and middle lung zones. Phase IV occurs toward the end of expiration and is characterized by an abrupt increase in N_2 concentration. This high N_2 concentration reflects the closure of airways at the base of the lungs and the expiration of gas from the upper lung zones, because in the single breath of 100% oxygen, less oxygen was initially directed to this area.

Closing volume is the lung volume at which the inflection of phase IV, the marked increase in N_2 concentration after the plateau, is observed. Closing capacity refers to closing volume and RV. The same characteristic tracing of the single-breath nitrogen washout test can be obtained by the inhalation of a bolus of tracer gas (e.g., argon, helium, xenon 133).

The closing volume is 10% of the vital capacity in young, healthy individuals. It increases with age and is 40% of the vital capacity at age 65. Closing volume is used as an aid in the diagnosis of small-airway disease and as a means of evaluating treatment and drug response.

Maximum Voluntary Ventilation

Maximum voluntary ventilation measures the maximum breathing capacity of the patient. It reflects strength and endurance of the respiratory muscles. The patient is asked to pant for 15 seconds into the spirometer tubing. The results are commonly examined preoperatively with the other results to determine a patient's prognosis for success after surgery, such as his or her ability to cough, to take deep breaths, and to enhance airway clearance.

Diagnosis of Restrictive and Obstructive Lung Disease

Physicians use the results of pulmonary function tests to diagnose lung disease or characteristic components of lung disease such as bronchospasm. A restrictive component describes

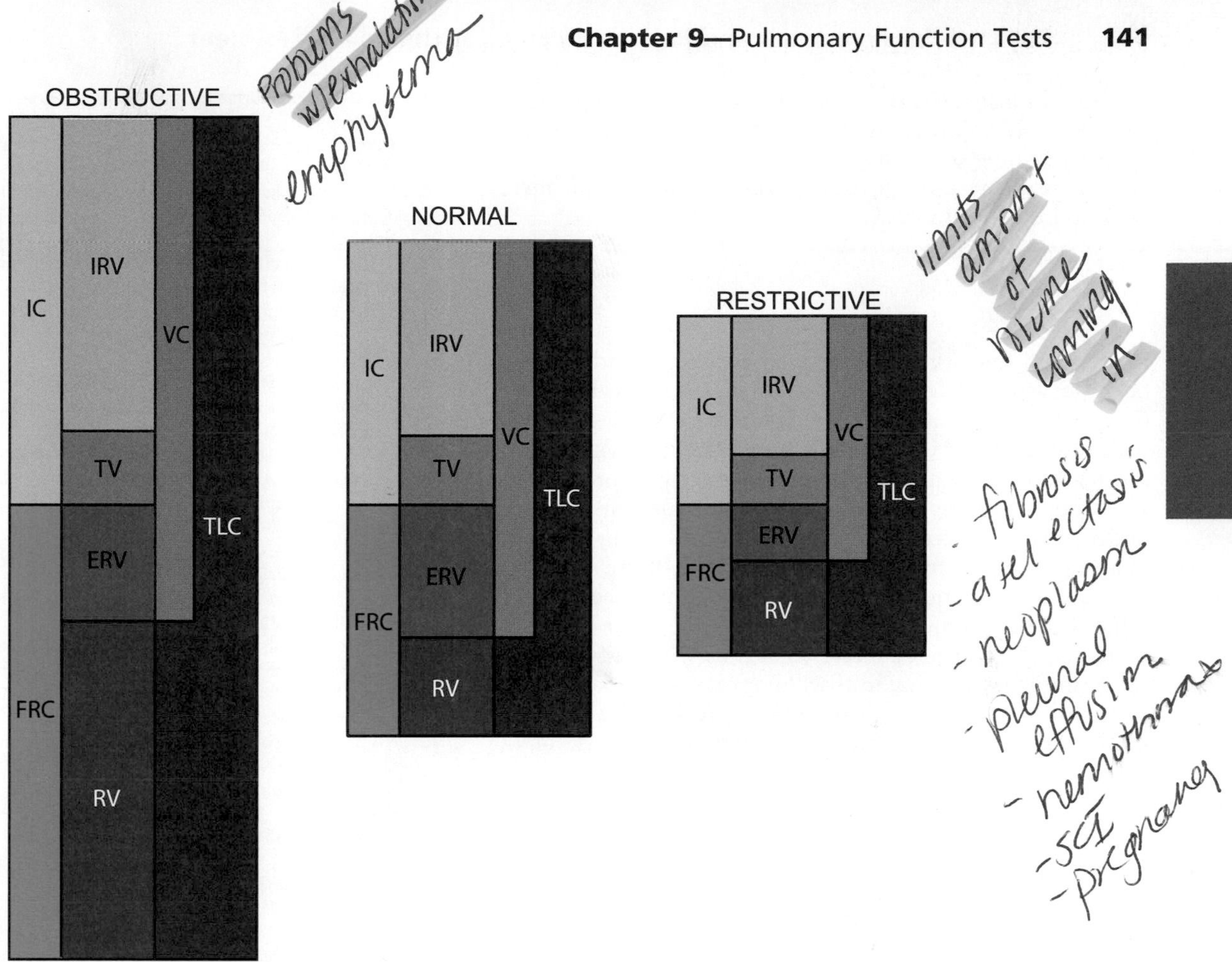

Fig. 9-5 Examples of proportional changes in lung volumes and capacities characteristic of obstructive and restrictive lung diseases.

conditions that limit the amount of volume coming into the lungs (restriction to inspiration). An obstructive component generally relates to problems in exhalation air flows and characteristic patterns of obstruction, such as in the first second of expiration FEV_1 measurement. Patients do not commonly have only one primary disease process but may have overlapping lung conditions.[23] A diagnosis may read, "PFTs consistent with moderate emphysema with bronchospastic component; good response to bronchodilators." A patient with an abnormal PFT is given a bronchodilator and retested. If there is a 15% to 20% increase in the PFT after bronchodilators are administered, they will be a recommended part of the patient's medications. However, some patients are given a trial of bronchodilators, even if there is not such a dramatic response on PFTs.

A pictorial demonstration of the differences in obstructive and restrictive lung disease is shown in Figure 9-5. Disease has a marked effect on pulmonary function; yet TV usually remains 10% of total lung capacity until the disease is relatively severe. Physiological pulmonary reserves in both disease processes are limited and generally affect a patient's response to exercise. Exercise is limited by the ventilatory status rather than by a cardiac end point. As obstructive lung disease progresses, TLC, FRC, and RV are markedly increased. In severe COPD, the increased FRC can compromise the VC. More energy is expended to breathe than that expended by a normal individual. This effect can be disproportionally increased with minimal amounts of activity. In restrictive lung disease, restriction of the chest wall or lung tissue can produce a decrease in TLC. A VC of 80% or less of predicted values for a patient is considered a diagnostic feature. A residual decline in FRC potentiates airway closure.

The phenomenon of closing volume in the lungs is particularly significant to physical therapists who prescribe breathing exercises and body positioning and can thereby alter pulmonary mechanics and gas exchange. These treatment interventions may have pronounced effects on lung volumes and airway closure.[24] At low lung volumes (e.g., breathing at FRC, in the Trendelenberg position, and in lung disease) intrapleural pressures are generally less negative, and the pressure of dependent lung regions may equal or exceed atmospheric pressure. Intrapleural pressure is less negative because the lungs are less expanded and elastic recoil is decreased. As a result, airway closure is potentiated. In young individuals, closure is evident at RV; however, in older individuals, closure is observed at higher lung volumes, such as at FRC. Premature closure of the small airways results in uneven ventilation and impaired gas exchange with a given lung unit. Airway closure occurs more readily in chronic smokers and in patients with lung disease.

Aging has a significant effect on airway closure. With aging, a loss of pulmonary elastic recoil results in a loss of intrapleural negative pressure. In older individuals, therefore, airway closure occurs at higher lung volumes. For example, closure has been reported to occur at the age of 65 in the upright lung during normal breathing. In the supine position, where FRC is reduced, closure occurs at a significantly younger age (about age 44). In addition to the often compounding effect of age, the lung volume at which airway closure occurs increases with chronic smoking and lung disease and is changed with alterations in body position.[25,26]

Summary

Pulmonary functions change as a patient's condition gets better or worse.[27,28] There are normal declines in volumes and flows with aging, as well as with disease processes. Basic bedside spirometry is often done to assess a patient's breathing mechanical ability and screen preoperatively to predict possible postoperative complications, especially in high-risk patients. Bedside screening can detect improvement or decline in a clinical status. In a patient with Guillain-Barré syndrome, as breathing becomes labored, the VC is monitored to determine whether a ventilator is needed. On the other hand, in a patient with obstructed airways, such as with cystic fibrosis, the pulmonary function tests will improve.[29] In a patient with spinal cord injury or neuromuscular weakness, as strength improves, vital capacity increases. However, because of the lack of abdominal muscles, the flows may be reduced.

Review Questions

1. What effect will an obstructive or restrictive component have on exercise performance?
2. Why is it important to compare the patient's predicted values with the actual observed values in a pulmonary function test?
3. What response should you assess to determine whether bronchodilators have a positive effect on pulmonary function?
4. How can pulmonary function tests be used to assess patient improvement or decline over a period of time?
5. What is the value of using pulmonary function tests as another vital sign?

References

1. Cherniak RM: Evaluation of respiratory function in health and disease. *Disease-a-Month* 38:505–576, 1992.
2. Morris J, Koski A, Johnson L: Prediction nomograms (BTPS) spirometric values in normal males and females. *American Review of Respiratory Diseases* 163:57–67, 1971.
3. Zelenik J: Normative aging of the respiratory system. *Clinical Geriatric Medicine*19:1–18, 2003.
4. Aelony Y: Ethnic norms for pulmonary function tests. *Chest* 99:1051, 1991.
5. Cruz-Merida AJ, Soto-de la Fuente AE, Mendez-Vargas MM, et al: Prediction equations for spirometric parameters in Mexican adult population. *Archives of Medical Research* 35:446–449, 2004.
6. Hankinson J, Odencrantz J, Fedan K: Spirometrical reference values from a sample of the general U.S. population. *American Journal of Respiratory Critical Care Medicine* 159:179–187, 1999.
7. Hayes D, Kraman S: The physiologic basis of spirometry. *Respiratory Care Dec* 54(12):1717–1726, 2009.
8. Price D, Yawn B, Jones R: Improving the differential diagnosis of chronic obstructive lung disease in primary care. *Mayo Clinic Proceedings* 85(12):1122–1129, 2010.
9. Yawn B, Enright P, Lemanske R, Jr, et al: Spirometry can be done in family physicians' offices and alters clinical decisions in management of asthma and COPD, *Chest* 132(4):1162–1168, 2007, doi:10.4065/mcp.2010.0389.
10. Kocabas, A, Kara, K, Ozgur, G, et al: Value of preoperative spirometry to predict postoperative complications. *Respiratory Medicine* 90:25–33, 1996.
11. Smetana G: Preoperative pulmonary evaluation. *New England Journal of Medicine* 340:937–944, 1999.
12. Wang JS: Pulmonary function test in preoperative pulmonary evaluations. *Respiration Medicine* 98:598–605, 2004.
13. Kozak LJ, McCarthy E, Pokras R: Changing patterns of surgical care in the United States 1980–1995. *Health Care Finance Review* 21:31–49, 1999.
14. Agency for Healthcare Research and Quality: *HCUPnet. Healthcare cost and utilization project*, Rockville, Md, 2001, AHRQ. http://hcupnet.ahrq.gov/.
15. Trayner E, Celli B: Postoperative pulmonary complications. *Medical Clinics of North America* 85:1129–1139, 2001.
16. Petty T: Testing patients' lungs: spirometry as part of the physical examination. *Clinical Therapy* 21:1908–1922, 1999.
17. Petty T: Simple office spirometry. *Clinical Chest Medicine* 22:845–859, 2001.
18. Buffels J, Degryse J, Hetman J, et al: Office spirometry significantly improves early detection of COPD in general practice. *Chest* 125:1394–1399, 2004.
19. Eaton T, Withy S, Garrett JE, et al: Spirometry in primary care practice: the importance of quality assurance and the impact of spirometry workshops. *Chest* 116:416–423, 1999.
20. Schermer T, Jacobs JE, Chavannes NH, et al: Validity of spirometric testing in a general population of patients with COPD. *Thorax* 58:861–866, 2003.
21. Smith RM, Dickson RA: Changes in residual volume relative to vital capacity and total lung capacity after arthrodesis of the spine in patients who have idiopathic scoliosis. *Bone and Joint Surgery of America* 76:153, 1994.
22. Rahn H: The pressure-volume diagram of the thorax and lung. *American Journal of Physiology* 146:161, 1946.
23. Clausen JL: *Pulmonary function testing guidelines and controversies*. London, 1984, Grune and Stratton.
24. Dean E: The effect of body position on pulmonary function. *Physical Therapy* 65:613–618, 1985.
25. Berry R, Pai U, Fairshter R: Effect of age on changes in flow rates and airway conductance after a deep breath. *Journal of Applied Physiology* 68:635–643, 1990.
26. Zadai C: Pulmonary physiology of aging: the role of rehabilitation. *Topics in Geriatric Rehabilitation* 1:49–56, 1985.
27. Emery CE: Psychological outcome of a pulmonary rehab program. *Chest* 100:613–617, 1991.
28. Emerson CL, Lukens TW, Effron D: Physician estimation of FEV_1 in acute exacerbation of COPD. *Chest* 105:1709–1712, 1994.
29. Versteegh FGA, Neijens HJ, Bogaard JM, et al: Relationship between pulmonary function, O_2 saturation during sleep and exercise with cystic fibrosis. *Advanced Cardiology* 35:151–155, 1986.

Arterial Blood Gases

Donna Frownfelter

KEY TERMS

Acid-base balance
Alveolar ventilation
Arterial blood gas
Hypoxemia
Oximetry
Oxygen saturation
Partial pressure of gases
Pet CO_2
Transcutaneous CO_2
Henderson-Hasselbach equation
Arterial blood gas interpretation

CHAPTER OUTLINE

An arterial blood gas is a physiological assessment tool that measures a patient's acid-base balance, alveolar ventilation, and oxygenation status.[1] It is a valuable resource for obtaining information from respiratory monitoring in the intensive care unit, for conducting follow-up of outpatients, and for evaluating the treatment and the progress of their diseases. There has been a trend toward finding more noninvasive techniques to serve these purposes. This trend has been motivated by the desire to spare patients from being "stuck" so frequently and to avoid the risk for infection posed by indwelling cannulas in patients who already are ill and have weakened immune systems. Physical therapists frequently use oxygen saturation for assessment, but this is insufficient in many patients. When a patient has been thoroughly examined and it is determined that the arterial blood gas values are relatively stable, the physical therapist should compare those values to subsequent readings on the oximeter. Therapists need to consider the blood gas trends, acid/base status, and alveolar ventilation and then correlate those findings to the patient's signs and symptoms, the physiological monitoring of HR, BP, and RR, and the perceived exertion with exercise. In many cases we need to consider a multisystem approach without examination and evaluation. Oximetry readings are important but must be evaluated in light of all body systems, not just the oximetry readings.

Arterial blood gas evaluation and interpretation can be confusing. The purpose of this chapter is to provide the background needed to understand what the arterial blood gas measures and how it can be applied clinically to improve the evaluation and assessment of patients. It cannot be overemphasized that the arterial blood gas is an essential part of the total examination and evaluation. In the case of a complex patient who has both respiratory and metabolic issues and there is no straightforward or "easy" interpretation, interdisciplinary team members often collaborate to evaluate the patient's arterial blood gases. It is extremely valuable for a new physical therapist to make ward rounds with the pulmonary physicians, nurses, and respiratory care practitioners, learning about physiological assessment through discussions and questioning during these rounds.

A further goal of this chapter is to help the clinician evaluate and interpret arterial blood gases more effectively and to integrate the information into treatment planning and the patient's overall progress. However, it is important to remember that blood gases provide a single, static picture of a patient's condition at a given time; as such, they are important in the management of acutely ill, unstable patients. As a patient's condition changes, new arterial blood gas results must be obtained and evaluated to determine whether the patient is improving or declining.

Noninvasive Monitoring

Noninvasive monitoring has become more readily available and is used to measure expired carbon dioxide (Pet CO_2) and transcutaneous CO_2 (T CO_2) in neonatal and pediatric patients. New studies are showing that a universal pulse oximetry screening of all neonates before they are discharged would improve the detection rate of congenital heart disease. In a survey conducted in the United Kingdom by Kang and colleagues, it was found that 209 (93%) of the 224 units contacted did not use pulse oximetry routinely. In the neonatal units that did use pulse oximetry, if the saturation was abnormal, they also did echocardiography. Two other units obtained not only echocardiogram, but also x-rays and ECG. The conclusion was that this should be used with national guidelines to supplement the postnatal examination.[2]

A similar study was conducted by Arlettaz and colleagues to determine whether pulse oximetry could detect congenital heart disease in newborns. It was noted that about half of all newborns who had congenital heart disease were asymptomatic in the first few days of their life. However, early detection of this condition is important because treatment outcomes are related to the time of the diagnosis, and early identification leads to best outcomes. The authors studied the effectiveness of oximetry on the first day of life for early detection of congenital heart disease in neonates who appeared normal. They also examined whether pulse oximeter screening in addition to the clinical examination of the patient would yield more results in the diagnosis of congenital heart disease than would examination alone. If pulse oximetry was less than 95%, echocardiography was done. Of the 3262 newborns screened, 24 infants had repeated oxygen saturations of less than 95%. Of these neonates, 17 had congenital heart disease and the other 5 had persistent pulmonary hypertension. Arlettaz and colleagues concluded that pulse oximetry screening in the first few days of life is an effective tool to identify cyanotic congenital heart disease in otherwise healthy newborns.[3]

Pulse oximetry has also been used to measure trends in oxygen saturation in patients before, during, and after exercise. For patients who are nervous about exercising, the oximeter can be used to check their saturation level and assure them that they are safe as they exercise. If they are feeling short of breath during exercise, they can stop to look at the value on the oximeter, which will usually return to baseline within a couple of minutes. This gives patients more confidence to exercise. These measures have resulted in fewer invasive arterial sticks and in the ability to monitor patients in an ongoing manner; in addition, they have made it possible to improve the care of patients with cardiovascular and pulmonary illness and to administer the most appropriate ventilation and oxygenation support. Many pulmonary physicians are encouraging patients to obtain a less expensive model that they can carry with them. Such a device will let patients follow their trends and help them to be safer. If more desaturation than normal is measured or anything out of the ordinary occurs, patients are instructed to call their doctor. An early visit may help to prevent exacerbations of their disease.

Partial Pressure of Gases

To better understand blood gases, it is important to remember the properties of gases. The earth's atmosphere consists of gas molecules that have mass and are attracted to the earth's center of gravity. At the surface, this atmospheric weight exerts a pressure that can support a column of mercury 760 mm high.

Dalton's law states that in a mixture of gases, the total pressure is equal to the sum of the partial pressures of the separate gases. Oxygen is 20.9% of the atmosphere, so it has a partial pressure of 159 ($760 \times 20.9\% = 159$). Nitrogen is 79% of the atmosphere; thus it has a partial pressure of 600 ($760 \times 79\% = 600$). Other gases make up 0.1% of the atmosphere.

The diffusion of gases across semipermeable membranes shows gradients from higher concentrations to lower concentrations. Each gas moves independently from the others.

During respiration, oxygen and CO_2 exchange across the alveolar capillary membrane. Special situations may affect the normal progress of respiration and gas exchange.

Normally, alveolar units ventilate and capillary units bring oxygenated blood to the tissues, excreting CO_2 back into the alveoli to be removed through the lungs. Some abnormal situations may occur, however, such as shunts and dead-space units. In a shunt unit, the alveoli have collapsed, but blood flow continues and is unable to pick up oxygen. An example of this is atelectasis, in which a lung segment or part of a segment has retained secretions and lung tissue distal to the mucous plug collapses. Circulation continues but oxygenation does not occur, and the PO_2 decreases. On the other hand, a dead-space unit can have ventilation but not perfusion. This occurs with pulmonary embolism, when a blood clot obstructs the circulation. The oxygen is available in the ventilated alveoli, but with no circulation, a dead unit is credited. Figure 10-1 demonstrates the regional differences seen in respiratory units.

Normal Blood Gas Values

The acid-base balance is denoted by the pH scale; it ranges from 1 to 14, where 1 is the most acidic and 14 the most basic. The arterial pH values are normally 7.35 to 7.45. If the pH is below 7.35, the patient is considered to be in a more acidotic state. If the pH is above 7.45, the patient is considered to be in a more alkalotic state.

Alveolar ventilation is reflected in the partial pressure of carbon dioxide (PCO_2). Normal PCO_2 values are 35 to 45 mm Hg. If the PCO_2 is below 35 mm Hg, the patient is said to be hyperventilating (having increased ventilation, blowing off more CO_2 than normal). If the PCO_2 is above 45 mm Hg, the patient is hypoventilating (having decreased alveolar ventilation, not blowing off enough CO_2 to maintain normal alveolar ventilation).

Arterial oxygen is measured as PO_2, the partial pressure of oxygen. Normal values are 80 to 100 mm Hg. If the PO_2 is below 80 mm Hg in someone younger than 60 years of age, the patient is hypoxemic. A value of 60 to 80 mm Hg is considered mild hypoxemia; 40 to 60 mm Hg is considered

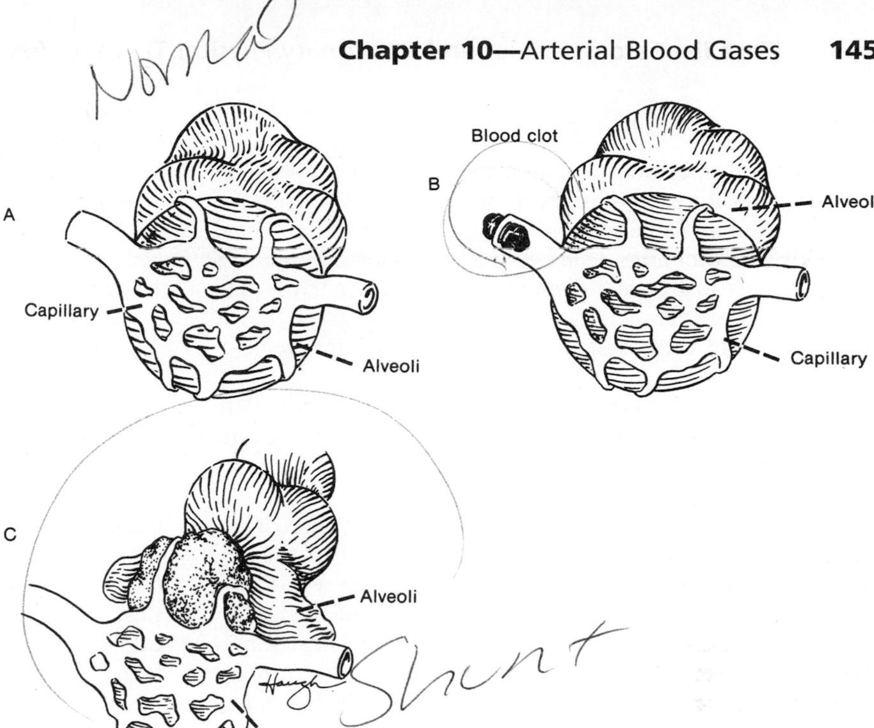

Fig. 10-1 **A,** Normal alveolus. **B,** Dead space. **C,** Shunt.

moderate hypoxemia, and less than 40 mm Hg is severe hypoxemia.[1]

Base Excess/Base Deficit

The blood normally has the capacity to buffer acid metabolites. The normal level of base HCO_3^- in the blood is 22 to 26 millimoles per liter (mmol/L). This buffering capacity diminishes in the presence of acidemia or alkalemia. Acidosis is an abnormal acid-base balance in which the acids dominate. Alkalemia is an abnormal acid-base balance in which the bases dominate. When there is a decrease in HCO_3^-, it is seen in a negative base excess and referred to as a base deficit, which is usually seen as a negative number on the blood gas report, such as −3.

As one looks at the base excess and the base deficit (BE/BD), it is helpful to determine whether the patient's condition is acute or chronic. This state can also be thought of as uncompensated (acute); partially compensated; or completely compensated (chronic). The pH is the key to making this determination. If the pH is not in the normal 7.35 to 7.45 range, the patient is in an acute state. As the balance progresses back toward normal, it may be partially compensated. When a normal pH exists, it is compensated, or chronic. The interpretation comes from looking at the BE/BD and then at the pH. Having a series of arterial blood gases for comparison is helpful, for example, in a patient with respiratory failure and on a ventilator; the patient's improvement can be documented.

Another example is that of a patient in the chronic state who has chronic obstructive pulmonary disease (COPD) and is retaining CO_2 at a level of 55 mm Hg. If the pH reads 7.25, this would be considered an acute state. As the body retains base, the pH will rise back toward normal. If the pH is 7.32 with a PCO_2 of 55 and +3 base excess, the status would be partially compensated. If the pH is within normal limits, with a PCO_2 of 55 and a pH of 7.35, the status would be compensated or chronic. This is a means of identifying people who are chronic CO_2 retainers.

Hemoglobin

Hemoglobin (Hgb) is the main component of the red blood cell. It is crucial for oxygen transport. The normal Hgb range is 12 to 16 g/100 mL blood. In patients who have lost blood through surgical procedures or disease, the decreased hemoglobin can account for their extreme weakness as a result of decreased total oxygen transport capacity. Some of the patients at highest risk are those who have just undergone joint replacement in which there has been much blood loss. Often their Hgb levels are only 8, and because they are considered "orthopedic" patients, it is thought that the low levels can be overlooked. In addition, patients with advanced COPD can at times desaturate (pulse oximetry below 90%) with exercise when the PO_2 is low (i.e., PO_2 55-60). Pulse oximetry is essential for monitoring the exercise of patients with low PO_2, low Hgb, or both.

Cyanosis, the presence of a bluish color to the skin, mucous membranes, and nail beds, is indicative of an abnormal amount of reduced Hgb concentration, usually greater than 5 g of reduced Hgb. The presence of cyanosis suggests a high probability of hypoxemia; however, hypoxemia can occur without cyanosis. Two examples may be cited, one in which an anemic patient with hypoxemia can have little cyanosis, and the other in which a patient with polycythemia can have cyanosis with minimal hypoxemia.

There is a predictable relationship between the arterial oxygen saturation of the Hgb and the PO_2. It is represented in the oxyhemoglobin dissociation curve as follows. When oxygen saturation is monitored during exercise, saturation is kept at or above 90%. As the curve denotes at a level of approximately 60 mm Hg, the saturation is about 90%. As the PO_2 drops at the sharp part of the curve, there is a marked decrease in oxygen saturation for every mm Hg PO_2.[4]

Acid-Base Balance

Normal body metabolism consists of the consumption of nutrients and the excretion of acid metabolites. Acid metabolites must be kept from accumulating in large amounts because the body's cardiovascular and nervous systems operate in a relatively narrow free hydrogen ion (H^+) range (narrow pH). Free H^+ concentration is discussed as pH ($-\log[H^+]$). The maintenance of body systems requires an appropriate acid-base balance.[5]

Approximately 98% of normal metabolites exist in the form of CO_2, which reacts readily with water to form carbonic acid.

$$CO_2 + H_2O\ Ø''\ H_2CO_3$$

Carbonic acid (H_2CO_3) can exist as either a liquid or a gas. Because carbonic acid can change to CO_2, much of the acid content can be excreted through the lungs during respiration. In this way, the lungs can help regulate the pH of the body.

The Henderson-Hasselbach equation demonstrates how the H^+ concentration results from the dissociation of carbonic acid and the interrelationship of the blood acids, bases, and buffers.

$$H_2O + CO_2\ Ø''\ H_2CO_3H^+ + HCO_3^-$$

Renal Buffering Mechanisms

The kidneys are the main route of excretion of the normal metabolic acids. H^+ is excreted in the urine and also resorbed by bicarbonate into the blood. In this manner, the kidneys can respond when there is an acid-base imbalance and return the body to normal homeostasis. Buffering the acid component and holding on to HCO_3^- can bring the pH to a more alkalotic range. The arterial blood gas result includes a comment about base excess/base deficit. Following that number and watching the change in pH is very helpful in monitoring patients to see whether they are improving or declining.

Chemoreceptor Response to Hypoxemia

The peripheral chemoreceptors, the carotid bodies, and the aortic bodies are located at the bifurcation of the internal and external carotid arteries and the arch of the aorta. These receptors are nervous tissue with a high metabolic rate and an abundant oxygen supply. When tissue PO_2 decreases, the response of these receptors to the brain is to increase ventilation and cardiac output. When that is not sufficient to effect a normal PO_2, supplemental oxygen or increased mechanical assistance such as continuous positive airway pressure (CPAP) is administered.[6]

Blood Gas Interpretation

Consider the normal values for the arterial blood gas: pH, PCO_2, PO_2, O_2 saturation, and base. With any given patient, there may be a range used (see below) that will be considered in light of the patient's disease, current acute or chronic status, and signs and symptoms. At times, these values will be considered "acceptable ranges," rather than ideal.

Once the norms for the pH, PCO_2, PO_2, and base have been established for a given patient, they should be considered first in the interpretation. Is the current value normal or not? Is the patient acute (uncompensated), partially compensated, or fully compensated (chronic)?

A stepwise interpretation can be helpful. Performing the assessment in the same order each time provides a comprehensive and standard overview.

1. Look at the PCO_2 to determine whether there is normal alveolar ventilation.
2. Look at the pH to see whether there is a normal acid-base balance or whether it is acute or chronic.
3. Look at the PO_2 to see whether there is normal oxygenation or whether there is hypoxemia and to what degree.
4. Look at the base excess/base deficit BE/BD.

It is important to note additional clinical considerations. Is the patient receiving oxygen or mechanical ventilation? If the patient is on increased inspiratory oxygen (FIO_2) of 40% and the PO_2 is not close to acceptable levels, it is more of a concern than if the patient is on a low FIO_2 and the PO_2 is within normal limits. Similarly, if the patient is on mechanical ventilation, the blood gases should be close to normal. The exception would be a patient who is a chronic CO_2 retainer; that patient would be ventilated to his or her normal level (i.e., at the PCO_2 level where the pH becomes closer to normal).

Acceptable Ranges of Arterial Blood Gases

At times, for various medical reasons, an acceptable range of blood gases will be used, rather than trying to get an ideal reading. The following ranges may be acceptable, depending on the physician and the patient's particular circumstances.

- pH 7.30 to 7.50
- PCO_2 30 to 50 mm Hg
- pH 7.45 and above alkalemia
- pH 7.35 and below acidemia

The relationship between the pH and the PCO_2 should be noted. In general, as the PCO_2 rises, the pH will decrease. There is also predictable change caused by variation in carbonic acid. Some general rules of thumb include:

- For every 20 mm Hg increase in PCO_2, the pH decreases by 0.10 (PCO_2 60, pH 7.25)
- For every 10 mm Hg decrease in PCO_2, the pH increases by 0.10 (PCO_2 25, pH 7.50)

There is also a relationship between the PCO_2 and the plasma bicarbonate.

- For every increase of 10 mm Hg in the PCO_2, there is a decrease of 1 mmol/L of plasma bicarbonate
- For every 10 mm Hg PCO_2, there is a decrease in plasma bicarbonate of 2 mmol/L

By knowing these guidelines, the therapist can determine whether the changes in the arterial blood gases are in line with respiratory problems as opposed to metabolic problems such as acidosis due to diabetic ketoacidosis, in which the base deficit can be very low and the pH can be low (acidemic), but the PCO_2 can be within normal limits.[5,7]

Potential Causes of Error in Arterial Blood Gas Sampling

The accuracy of arterial blood gas results depends on many factors: proper collection of the arterial sample, the handling of the sample from the patient to the laboratory, and the method by which the sample was analyzed. Possibilities for error exist all along the pathway. Great care must be taken to create proper protocol for all steps, and laboratories need to remain vigilant to decrease errors. Some of the common problems are nonarterial samples (venous blood versus arterial blood), air bubbles in the syringe, inadequate anticoagulant in the sample, and delayed analysis of a noncooled sample.[8]

Respiratory Failure

Respiratory failure is defined as the inability of the pulmonary system to meet the metabolic demands of the body (i.e., ventilation and oxygenation).[5] The blood gases usually show a pH below 7.30 and a PCO_2 above 50. Generally, the patient is also hypoxemic.

During the acute phase, the kidneys have not started to compensate, and the base HCO_3^- is within normal limits. Later, a base excess can be noted as the kidneys try to compensate for the acidotic pH. Chronic respiratory failure can be noted by an increased PCO_2, a pH within normal limits, and a low PO_2.

In assessing the PO_2, the following ranges are used: mild hypoxemia, less than 80 mm Hg; moderate hypoxemia, 60 to 80 mm Hg; and severe hypoxemia, below 40 mm Hg.

Positional changes can affect the oxygenation status. For example, unilateral right lower lobe atelectasis with the patient lying on the right side causes increased blood flow to the right lung, which is collapsed. This causes increased shunting and a decrease in oxygenation (differential shunting). If the patient lies on the left side, the oxygenation will improve. When the patient lies in a supine position, a mixed PO_2 can be observed.

When hypoxemia is noted, treatment consists of oxygen therapy, CPAP or biphasic positive airway pressure, and alleviation of the cause of hypoxemia, if possible. This may be achieved by means of airway-clearance techniques or medication, in addition to the oxygen therapy or mechanical ventilation. Oxygen therapy treats the hypoxemia, decreases the patient's work of breathing, and decreases myocardial work.

Factors Affecting Arterial Blood Gases

Many normal causes affect arterial blood gases, such as extremes of age, from neonates to older adults. The neonate has many changes going on in the initial life process; fetal circulation changes dramatically in the first hours and days of life. In the older adult patient, decreases in cardiac output (CO), residual volume (RV) of the lungs, and maximal breathing capacity gradually lower PO_2 over the course of the life cycle. It is estimated that after 60 years of age, the PO_2 decreases by 1 mm Hg per year of age from 60 to 90 years.

Exercise or any increase in activity above rest may result in significantly increased oxygen consumption in patients with cardiopulmonary dysfunction. In the normal population, the human body compensates by increasing oxygen consumption to meet the workload. Usually, a plateau is reached and a constant oxygen consumption for that activity is achieved. In patients with cardiopulmonary dysfunction, oxygen consumption continues to increase, even at the same workload in untrained patients. It is important to monitor oxygen saturation to prevent desaturation in these patients.[4] During pregnancy, hormonal and mechanical factors may have negative effects on cardiopulmonary function. In the last trimester, women commonly observe shortness of breath and difficulty in taking a deep breath because of hormonal issues and diaphragmatic encroachment.

In a small study by Sunyal and colleagues assessing oxygen saturation in pregnant women to try to evaluate the lung function in pregnancy, 32 women (25 to 35 years old) without any recent respiratory disease were monitored during each trimester. The study compared eight healthy nonpregnant women as an age-matched control group. In the pregnant women, the oxygen saturation levels increased progressively each trimester: first trimester (97.73% ± 0.30), second trimester (98.05% ± 0.54), and third trimester (98.40% ± .30). The oxygen saturation readings were higher in the pregnant women than in the nonpregnant women. The study conclusion was that the increased oxygen saturation during pregnancy was related to increased ventilation and a rising progesterone level, which reaches a peak in the later phases of pregnancy.[9]

During sleep there is a decrease in minute ventilation and a decreased responsiveness to CO_2 and hypoxemia. Many patients who have undergone spinal cord injuries or cerebrovascular accidents, who have COPD, who have significant neuromuscular changes such as kyphoscoliosis, or who are morbidly obese have been noted to have apnea and hypoxemia during sleep. The possibility of these conditions should be considered in any patient with daytime somnolence who complains of difficulty sleeping or staying awake during the day or who has trouble following directions or is mentally confused. Often the patient's spouse or partner will report that the patient is restless in bed and snoring increasingly. Some may actually notice that the patient stops breathing at times during sleep. These patients need to be referred for a sleep study to evaluate their breathing, oxygenation, and oxygen saturation at night. Physical therapists can help by monitoring these patient populations, by understanding and watching for the signs and symptoms listed above, and by communicating with the patient's partner (if the patient has one) to ask about specific details in the patient's sleeping patterns and whether there have been any noticeable changes in function.

Barometric Pressure Can Affect Oxygenation

Low barometric pressure associated with high altitude significantly decreases the amount of oxygen available to an individual. As noted before, the partial pressure of oxygen is dependent on the total atmospheric pressure. When the total pressure is reduced, less O_2 is available. This is particularly important if a patient already has a decreased PO_2 and is traveling to an area with lower barometric pressure. Patients on oxygen need an oxygen prescription that is based on the area in which they are living. Dr. Petty, who practiced in Colorado, urged his patients to buy an oximeter to carry with them. His motto was "titrate where you migrate."

Barometric pressure increases, such as in a hyperbaric oxygen chamber with higher barometric pressure, can help deliver increased oxygen for a select group of patients. Wound-healing needs and carbon monoxide poisoning are two such indications. Hyperbaric chambers are not found in all hospitals, but when the need arises, a search can find the one closest for treatment.

Other Factors That Can Influence the Arterial Blood Gas

Increased temperature (a febrile state) can increase metabolism and therefore increase oxygen consumption, decrease PO_2, and consequently, increase alveolar ventilation, which will decrease PCO_2. Decreased temperatures can decrease oxygen consumption, as is seen in patients who have survived for several minutes in cold water and are then resuscitated or in patients who are kept in a state of hypothermia to decrease body functions and preserve oxygen while medical staff members do their best to stabilize the patient.

On the arterial blood gas report it is important to note the status of the patient at the time the blood gas is drawn. Usually, patients are at rest when the blood gas is drawn. If the PO_2 is low at rest (60 mm Hg), it is close to the sharp part of the oxyhemoglobin dissociation curve, and the patient may desaturate quickly with an increase in exercise.

If the patient is on supplemental oxygen and the PO_2 is only 55 mm Hg, the PO_2 is still inadequate because of the additional O_2.[10-12] Any patient on oxygen at rest should be evaluated for appropriate oxygenation with exercise. Most patients' blood gases are drawn at rest, not with exercise. Similarly, if a patient is on mechanical ventilation, the blood gases should be within or near normal limits.

Noninvasive Monitoring

Noninvasive monitoring of respiratory function is convenient, is accurate in showing trends, involves minimal complications, and causes little discomfort for the patient. The modalities are used as part of an ongoing examination, along with clinical monitoring. Noninvasive monitoring tools include pulse oximetry, transcutaneous oxygen (Ptc O_2), transcutaneous PCO_2 (Ptc CO_2), and end-tidal CO_2 using capnography.

Pulse Oximetry

Pulse oximetry provides estimates of arterial oxyhemoglobin saturation (SaO_2) by utilizing selected wavelengths of light to noninvasively determine the saturation of oxyhemoglobin (SpO_2).[13]

INDICATIONS FOR PULSE OXIMETRY

There are several reasons to perform pulse oximetry.

1. To monitor the adequacy of arterial oxyhemoglobin saturation
2. To evaluate the patient's response to interventions and exercise
3. To meet third-party payers' need to document desaturation and prescribe oxygen in order to meet regulations[14]

PRECAUTIONS FOR PULSE OXIMETRY

If a patient needs ongoing measurement of pH, PCO_2, and total Hgb, the presence of abnormal Hgb may be a "relative" contraindication for pulse oximetry.[13] If the Hgb is low (i.e., 7-8, or virtually half the normal Hgb), the oxygen saturation may be above 90% at rest but as soon as exercise begins, the patient will usually desaturate very quickly. Thus pulse oximeter reading needs to be monitored before, during, and after exercise/activity to have a better overall view of the physiological response to the intervention. The other vital signs need to be evaluated as well.

A probe is attached to the patient's finger, toe, or earlobe, and a measurement is made of the amount of light that is absorbed (i.e., relayed to a microprocessor that calculates SaO_2). It can be read intermittently or displayed continuously. In addition, a pulse reading is given.

A reading taken at rest as an additional vital sign, along with HR, BP, and RR, provides a baseline before exercise. When an exercise workload is given, the parameters can be compared to see whether the patient has a normal or abnormal response to exercise. The recommendation is to keep the O_2 saturation above 90% during exercise. Supplemental oxygen can be titrated to keep the O_2 saturation within the appropriate range. This is done in conjunction with the physician because it is not in the scope of practice for physical therapists to change FIO_2 levels without a consultation and physician's order. Many hospitals that deal with critically ill patients as an interdisciplinary team will have standing orders to cover this situation. The orders may read, for instance, "titrate oxygen to keep the O_2 sats above 90% with exercise." In this case, limits to how high the FIO_2 may be raised need to be considered, as well as changing the oxygen delivery system to get a more consistent level of oxygenation, especially during activity.

Situations exist in which pulse oximetry may not yield accurate results: abnormal Hgb, jaundice, anemia, low perfusion (i.e., diabetes), the use of intravascular dye such as methylene blue, deeply pigmented skin, and dark nail polish.[15] In addition, movement artifacts and highly lit fluorescent lights can have an effect on the readings. These concerns must be appreciated by therapists, especially during exercise, to ensure proper readings and correct evaluation of responses to exercise.

Documentation of patients' responses to exercise can be included with vital sign notations: ECG, HR, BP, RR, and SpO_2 may be recorded. The readings taken at rest, during exercise, and at the end point of exercise are important, as well as the time it takes for the patient to recover (to return to baseline). This information documents the physiological response to exercise.

Transcutaneous Oxygenation

To test for transcutaneous oxygenation (Ptc CO_2), a sensor is applied to the skin on the anterior chest or abdomen. The sensor is heated to produce localized erythema. This method is used primarily in the neonatal and pediatric intensive care units. There is an equilibration time of about 10 to 15 minutes, and the sensor must be calibrated to ensure accurate results. Inaccurate measurements may be caused by hypothermia, shock, severe anemia, edema, severe acidosis, and dislodgement of the sensor. Cases of thermal injury have occurred.

Transcutaneous Carbon Dioxide

Transcutaneous carbon dioxide (Tc CO_2) measurements are used in the neonatal ICU, where continuous monitoring is indicated, especially if the baby is not intubated or being mechanically ventilated. The Tc CO_2 has a skin sensor and is most effective in monitoring hemodynamically stable patients. The sensor must be calibrated and must be rotated frequently to prevent burns. A relatively close correlation exists between arterial PCO_2 and Pt CO_2, and the latter has the additional benefit of requiring fewer needle sticks.

A study by Sandberg and colleagues performed in the neonatal intensive care unit (NICU) evaluated the accuracy of transcutaneous (Tc) blood gas monitoring in newborn infants, including infants with extremely low birth weights. The measurements were taken under "stable conditions." Some differences were found in arterial measurements versus Tc measurements, related to body weight, postnatal age, and the amount of oxygen each neonate required. Overall, Sandberg and colleagues concluded that there was good agreement between the two methods and that it was clinically acceptable to use Tc in their NICU. They added that although it would not replace the need for doing arterial blood gases, Tc monitoring would be a good supplement to use in assessing neonates.[16]

End Tidal Carbon Dioxide

Capnography uses infrared spectroscopy or mass spectrometry reading of expired CO_2 to analyze CO_2 content in a continuous reading. There is also a wave display of the breath-to-breath readings. The waveform can be divided into segments that represent various phases of the respiratory cycle. In the beginning of a normal exhalation, gas is expelled from the anatomical dead space and has a low CO_2 reading. As more alveoli empty, there is an increasing proportion of alveolar gas in relationship to dead space gas and thus a greater concentration of CO_2. A plateau level is reached when there is a nearly constant CO_2 concentration (alveolar plateau). At the alveolar plateau, the end tidal CO_2 concentrations closely approximate the arterial PCO_2. Then with inspiration, the CO_2 concentration decreases rapidly to baseline.

The end tidal CO_2 readings help monitor changes in the ventilatory status and assist in determining the need for changes in the ventilator settings to improve alveolar ventilation.[17] Most notable is the ability to see trends in these readings and maintain an ongoing monitoring system that can allow for early detection of complications, such as pneumothorax, hypoventilation, pulmonary embolism, or fat embolism (any increase in dead space). The end tidal CO_2 readings have also been used to determine the proper positioning of feeding tubes and endotracheal tubes.[18,19]

Summary

This chapter discusses the normal arterial blood gases and the significance of their values. A guide to the interpretation of blood gases is proposed. The relationships between pH and PCO_2, between PCO_2 and HCO_3^-, and between O_2 saturation and PO_2 are examined. Predictable changes that are caused by respiratory changes are described. In addition, it is noted that metabolic changes can have marked effects on blood gases. Oxygen therapy and airway-clearance techniques can improve hypoxemia.

Position changes can be detrimental, causing differential shunting, or can improve the PO_2 by means of better ventilation-perfusion matching. For example, if the affected lung that has pneumonia is placed down (i.e., lying on the side of the pneumonia), there will be more perfusion passing by the poorly ventilated lung and the PO_2 will decrease. If the well ventilating lung is placed down the PO_2 will improve.

Noninvasive monitoring has been a great advance; it is now possible to see ongoing trends in a patient and assess complications early so that patients can be moved forward more safely and efficiently. Noninvasive monitoring can also be an adjunct to exercise, as will be discussed in Chapter 43.

Physical therapists must have a thorough understanding of the various respiratory monitors so that they are better equipped to provide comprehensive evaluation and assessment, thus allowing them to safely encourage patients to progress to their optimal rehabilitation outcomes.

Review Questions

1. Which factors may affect arterial blood gases?
2. What effect does an increased temperature in a patient have on the blood gases, and how does this relate clinically to treating a patient with an elevated temperature?
3. How has noninvasive monitoring improved the ability to monitor patients?
4. What parameters of the blood gas reading will guide you in determining whether the patient is a chronic CO_2 retainer?
5. What effect can body position have on blood gases, and how can this knowledge be used therapeutically?
6. What precautions need to be considered for effective reading of arterial blood gases?
7. Which patient diagnoses may pose more chances for error in oxygen saturation readings?
8. What arterial blood gas reading would prompt you to hold physical therapy treatment?
9. What would you follow on the arterial blood gas reading to determine improvement in alveolar ventilation or oxygenation status before increasing activity or exercise?

References

1. Cherniak RM: Evaluation of respiratory function in health and disease. *Disease Monitor* 38:505–576, 1992.
2. Kang S, Tobin S, Kelsall W: Neonatal Pulse oximetry screening: A National Survey. *Acta Paediatr* 101111:1651–2227, 2011, Feb 15, EPub ahead of print.
3. Arlettaz R, Bauschatz AS, Mönkhoff M, et al: The contribution of pulse oximetry to the early detection of congenital heart disease in newborns. *Eur J Pediatr* 165(2):94–98, 2006 Feb.
4. Guyton A: *Textbook of medical physiology*, ed 7, Philadelphia, 1986, WB Saunders.
5. Shapiro BA: Evaluation of blood gas monitors: Performance criteria, clinical impact, and cost/benefit (editorial comment). *Critical Care Medicine* 22:546–548, 1994.
6. Tarpy SP, Farber HW: Chronic lung disease: When to prescribe home oxygen. *Geriatrics* 49:27–28, 31–33, 1994.
7. Shapiro BA, Peruzzi W, Templin R: *Clinical application of blood gases*, ed 5, St Louis, 1994, Mosby.
8. Pramad S, Gunchan P, Sandeep P: Interpretation of arterial blood gas. *Indian J Crit Care Med* 14(2):57–64, 2010, Apr-Jun.
9. Sunyal D, Amin MR, Molla MH, et al: Assessment of percentage saturation of hemoglobin with oxygen in arterial blood of pregnant women. *J Bangladesh Soc Phsiol* Dec(1):10–13, 2006.
10. Brunelli A, Al Refai M, Monteverde M, et al: Predictors of exercise oxygen desaturation following major lung resection. *European Journal of Cardiothoracic Surgery* 24:145–148, 2003.
11. Carpenter KD: Oxygen transport in the blood. *Critical Care Nurse* 11:20–33, 1991.

12. Emtner M, Porszasz J, Burns M, et al: Benefits of supplemental oxygen in exercise training in nonhypoxemic chronic obstructive pulmonary disease patients. *American Journal of Respiratory Critical Care Medicine* 168:1034–1042, 2003.
13. American Association for Respiratory Care: Clinical practice guidelines. *Respiratory Care* 36:1406–1409, 1991.
14. Welch JP, DeCesare MS, Hess D: Pulse oximetry: Instrumentation and clinical applications. *Respiratory Care* 35:584–601, 1990.
15. Schnapp LM, Cohen NH: Pulse oximetry: Uses and abuses. *Chest* 98:1244–1250, 1990.
16. Sandberg KL, Brynjarsson H, Hjalmarson O: Transcutaneous blood gas monitoring during neonatal intensive care. *Acta Paediatr* 1651–2227, 2011, Jan 18.
17. Healey CJ, Fedullo AJ, Swinburne AJ, et al: Comparison of noninvasive measurements of carbon dioxide tension during withdrawal from mechanical ventilation. *Critical Care Medicine* 15:764–768, 1987.
18. Ahrens T, Wijeweera H, Ray S: Capnography: A key underutilized technology. *Critical Care Nursing Clinics of North America* 11:49–62, 1999.
19. Burns SB, Carpenter R, Truwit JD: Report on the development of a procedure to prevent placement of feeding tubes into the lungs using end-tidal CO_2 measurements. *Critical Care Medicine* 29:936–939, 2001.

Imaging of the Chest

Myriam Riboh and Patrick Knott

KEY TERMS

Aortic aneurism
Cardiac hypertrophy
Cardiac silhouette
Computed tomography
Consolidation
Hemothorax
Inspiratory effort
Ionizing radiation
Magnetic resonance imaging
Mediastinal widening
Nonionizing radiation
Pleural effusion
Pneumonia
Pneumothorax
Positron emission tomography
Radiolucent
Radionuclide imaging
Radiopaque
Ventilation-perfusion scan

CHAPTER OUTLINE

Wilhelm Roentgen discovered the x-ray in 1895 and won the very first Nobel Prize in physics (1901) for this discovery.[1] Since that time, radiography has been used in medicine to image the chest structures. Ionizing radiation has its disadvantages, however, as Thomas Edison learned when his laboratory assistant, Clarence Daley, became the first scientist to die of radiation exposure in the United States.[1] By the 1940s, ultrasound was being used as a way to image the body using nonionizing radiation.[1] Computed tomography (CT) was developed in the 1970s, and magnetic resonance imaging (MRI) in the 1980s.[1] All these methods have been used to image the chest, and each offers distinct advantages and disadvantages for the patient and the clinician.

Most imaging machines still use film to capture the image, but newer systems are using digital formats. In either case, the basic methods are similar: x-rays are generated when the anode of an x-ray tube is bombarded with electrons from the cathode of the tube. The collision gives off energy in the form of x-radiation, which travels out of the tube and through the patient, then hitting the imaging cassette. The cassette contains film or a digital imaging sensor. The image is then processed by a digital processor or a film developer (Figure 11-1).

The film turns black (is exposed) if the x-rays pass through the patient and reach the film surface. If the x-rays are reflected or absorbed by the patient, they do not reach the film, and the resulting image stays white (unexposed). The patterns and shades of light and dark on the film reflect the differing densities present in the part of the human body being imaged.

The darkest images on a film (also called radiolucent areas) represent pockets of air within the body. Fat is denser than air, and it produces a dark-gray image. Muscle and other soft tissues are more dense and produce a much lighter gray image. Finally, bone is the most dense natural substance in the body and produces a white image. Metallic objects are even more dense (also called radiopaque) than bone and produce a pure white image (Figure 11-2).

Figure 11-2, *A*, demonstrates all the different densities. This lateral view of the knee shows metal from a total knee replacement, along with bone, muscle, fat, and on either side of the patient's knee, air.[2]

The x-ray image is a summation of all the densities that the x-rays have passed through. The different layers of tissue that are on top of one another are flattened into a single two-dimensional image. Sometimes the various densities lie next to one another and are easily distinguished in the image. Other times the two densities overlap one another and are blurred together in the image. For this reason, the patient is usually positioned so that two or more images can be taken at a right angle to one another. This allows structures that are overlapping in one orientation to be seen side-by-side with the other orientation.[1,3]

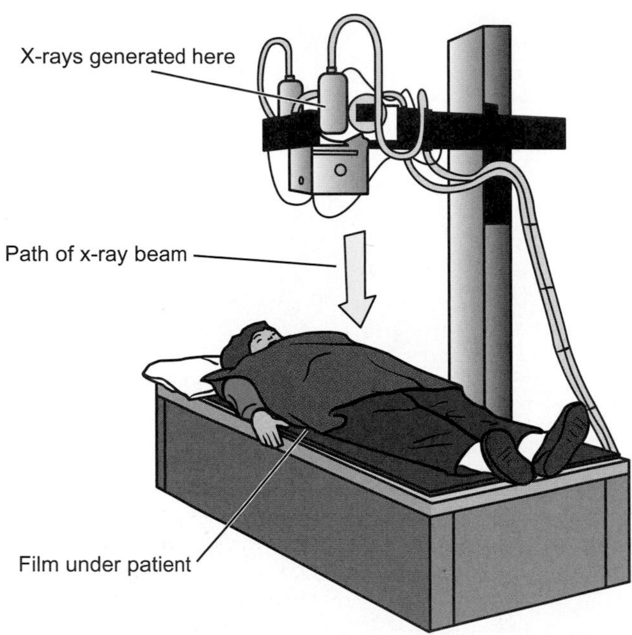

Fig. 11-1 A typical x-ray machine.

The Radiograph and Its Evaluation

The process for evaluating a radiograph can be broken down into several stages. The initial evaluation should verify all of the technical details of the scan; subsequent stages look at various aspects of the anatomy imaged.

Initial Evaluation

The initial stage is when the technical details of the images are noted:

- Correct patient identifying information
- Correct body part imaged
- Body part imaged with two projections
- Quality of the exposure of the film

Before proceeding with any further evaluation, the first step is to check that the information identifying the patient has been properly provided on the image and that the image is indeed of the patient in question. Identifying information usually consists of the patient's full name, date of birth, and if possible, their sex and social security number. Failing to verify this basic information can lead to medical errors in one or multiple patients.

Next, check that the part of the body in question is indeed the part that was imaged and that it was done in at least two projections oriented 90 degrees apart (for example, one view from the front and one from the side). The left and right sides of the patient should be indicated on the films so that they can be viewed in proper orientation. A marker should also indicate the patient's position at the time of the radiograph. For instance, a frontal chest radiograph can be taken with the patient standing, sitting, or lying down.

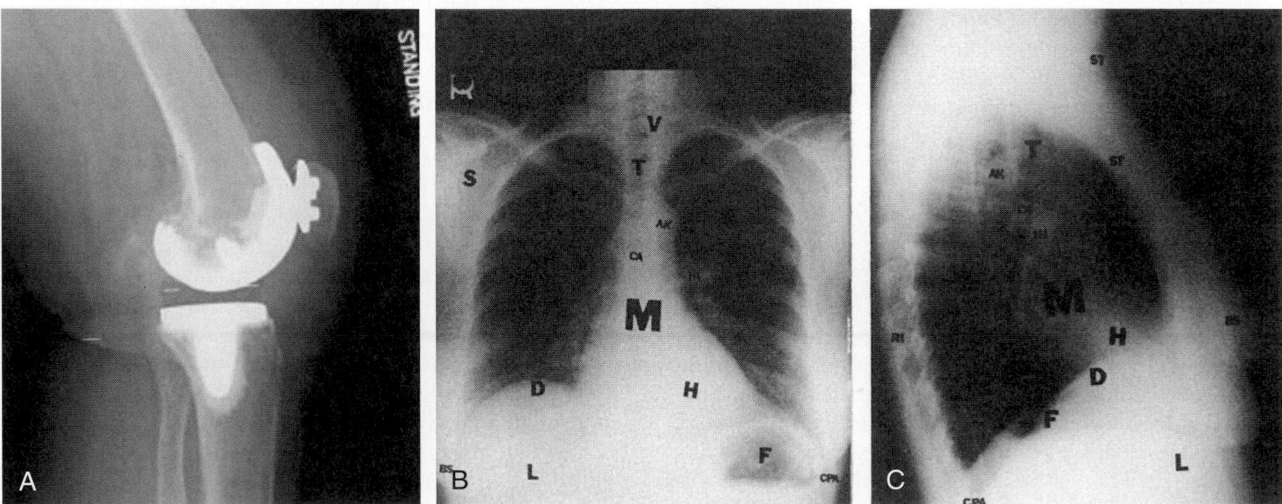

Fig. 11-2 A, This radiograph of a knee with a total joint replacement shows the differences in density among air, fat, muscle, bone, cement, and titanium. **B,** PA radiograph, and **C,** lateral radiograph; these two views anatomically localize the basic structures that must be reviewed during the evaluation of chest radiographs. Some of the structures are seen in both views, whereas others are seen in only one view. During evaluation, the therapist should be able to see and identify the following basic anatomical structures:

Soft tissues and extrathoracic structures: soft tissues (*ST*), breast shadows, (*BS*), diaphragm (*D*), liver (*L*), and fundus of stomach (*F*)

Bony thorax: ribs (*RI*), vertebrae (*V*), scapulae (*S*, seen best on PA), clavicles (*C*, seen best on PA), and sternum (*S*, seen best on lateral)

Mediastinal structures: mediastinum (*M*), trachea (*T*), carina (*CA*), aortic knob (*AK*), heart (*H*), anterior clear space (*ACS*, seen best on lateral), and hilus of lungs (*HI*)

Lung fields: hilus of lungs (*HI*), pulmonary vessels (arise from hilus and branch outward), costophrenic angles (*CPA*), and lung apices (*LA*, seen best on PA) (***A*** *from GE Healthcare.)*

Table 11-1 **Standard Radiograph Projections**

View	Description
AP (anteroposterior)	Frontal view, taken with the patient facing the x-ray tube, with the back toward the film
PA (posteroanterior)	Looks the same as the AP, but the patient is positioned facing the film
Right lateral	Side view, with the right side against the film
Left lateral	Side view, with the left side against the film
Oblique	A view taken at a 45-degree angle, between the AP and the lateral views

Finally, check the overall exposure of the film. If all the structures are too dark, the film has been overpenetrated. It should be retaken using less radiation. If all the structures are too light, the film has been underpenetrated and should be retaken using more radiation.

Evaluation for Pathology

Overview

After verifying the technical aspects of the images, the diagnostic evaluation can begin. It will help to first review the different projections that have been taken (Table 11-1). There are special views that position the patient in such a way that a particular area of interest is oriented for optimal visualization.

The standard chest radiograph is taken as a posteroanterior (PA) and a left lateral view, with the patient standing. These two views position the heart closest to the film; clinicians use the radiograph to judge the size of the heart, and the farther away from the film the heart is, the more it will appear magnified. This concept is easy to understand if you shine a light on your hand and view the resulting shadow on the wall. The closer your hand is to the wall, the more its shadow's size is true to life. The farther away the hand gets from the wall, the larger and fuzzier the shadow appears. The evaluation of the heart and lungs is most accurate when these structures are positioned close to the film during imaging.

The next step in evaluating a chest radiograph is to do a quick scan of the entire image to look for obvious or life-threatening abnormalities. General anatomy should be identified, including:

- Spine
- Sternum
- Clavicles and ribs
- Right and left diaphragms
- Abdominal organs
- Heart
- Mediastinum and great vessels
- Trachea
- Main bronchi
- Lungs

At this point it is also important to assess the position of the patient by looking at the clavicles to ensure they are aligned. If they are rotated, this could distort images of the lungs, heart, and other important structures. The image should also be scanned for any nonanatomical findings such as pacemakers, tubes, electrical leads, staples, etc. If old films exist in the patient record, it is helpful to compare the current findings with the old. Once this is done, a more thorough evaluation is begun (Table 11-2).

Table 11-2 **Summary of Chest X-Ray Evaluation**

Focus	Findings
Patient information	Name, date of birth, social security number, sex, existence of any old films.
Nonanatomical findings	Pacemakers, ECG leads, buttons, surgical remnants (e.g., staples), foreign bodies.
General inspection	Check rotation of chest by evaluation of the clavicles. Does anything "jump out" at you? Is everything present that should be there?
Bones	Are the appropriate number present? Are they in normal anatomical position? Any fractures, lesions?
Trachea	Is it midline? Is it narrowed? Are there any foreign bodies?
Lungs	Assess inspiratory effort, diaphragms, lung tissue, full expansion of lungs, opacities, infiltrates.
Heart	Size, borders, shape.
Mediastinum	Is it widened?

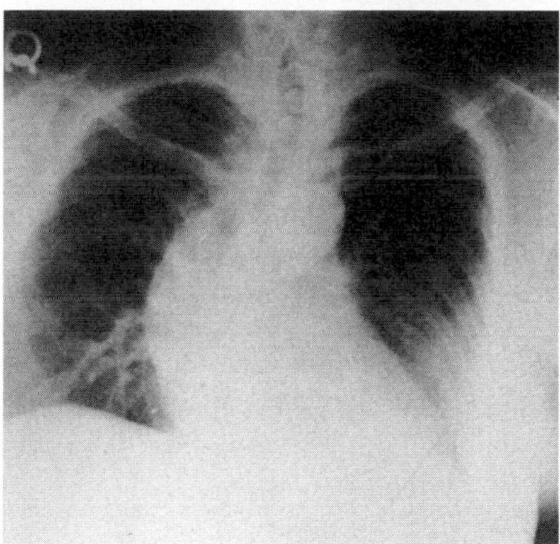

Fig. 11-3 This chest radiograph of a patient with kyphoscoliosis reveals a markedly abnormal, reverse-S–shaped curve of the thoracic spine that is deforming the mediastinal structures and the ribs. This patient is breathing primarily with the diaphragm.

Bony Skeleton

The bony skeleton (Figure 11-3) should be checked for signs of fracture, especially along the margins of the ribs. Fractures are seen as radiolucent lines within the bone or as disruptions of the smooth cortical line at the edges of the bone. Unexplained fragments of bone that are not in a normal anatomical position are another sign of fracture.

Inspiratory Effort

The inspiratory effort should be evaluated. Patients are asked to take a deep breath at the time of the radiograph, and this deep inspiration should make it possible to visualize 10 to 12 ribs within the thoracic cavity. If a radiograph is taken during expiration or during a poor inspiratory effort, the ribs will appear very close together and the lower ribs will be seen below the level of the diaphragm. It is important to take notice of this, as poor inspiratory effort can mask findings in the lungs, or make some findings appear more pronounced than they really are. Inspiratory effort is also important to note because it can provide a quick guide to your patient's respiratory ability.

Position of the Diaphragm

The position of the diaphragm should be noted. Its position, shape, clarity, and the appearance of the costophrenic angles are important, remembering that anatomically, the left (L) diaphragm is usually lower than the right (R) diaphragm. The costophrenic angles are where the diaphragm meets the chest wall. In these thin, pointy areas at the base of the chest cavity, blood or fluid accumulations inside the chest can be seen on an upright film. Such accumulations can affect patient lung capacity and thus oxygenation.

Trachea

Another important structure to evaluate is the trachea, which should be visible at the upper portion of the CXR, with a more radiolucent density, similar to the lung fields. The trachea should be in the midline on the PA view, and the carina (where the trachea branches into the two main stem bronchi) should also be visible. A shift from midline can indicate tension in the chest wall such as that found with some pneumothoraces. Narrowing and/or any foreign objects in the trachea can indicate respiratory distress and must be evaluated immediately.

Lung Fields

Next, the lung fields should be evaluated for uniform density and vascular markings throughout. The hilar area, where the vascular and airway structures converge, is normally more dense and can be an area of importance when looking for masses or tumors. The peripheral lung fields, where the smallest vascular and airway structures are, appear the smoothest and least dense. Comparing them side by side for symmetry helps in the recognition of abnormal areas. Conditions such as pneumonia, tumor, effusion, or other disease processes lead to consolidation of lung tissue, making it more dense than tissue in the rest of the lung fields (Figure 11-4).

Full expansion of the lung fields is also important to evaluate. A pneumothorax causes part of the lung to collapse, creating a less dense empty space in the chest cavity that is devoid of any pulmonary or vascular markings (Figure 11-5). Conversely, a hemothorax or pleural effusion fills the chest cavity with fluid that is denser than normal lung tissue (Figure 11-6). Both of these abnormalities are evident on chest radiographs and can affect oxygenation, as discussed above.

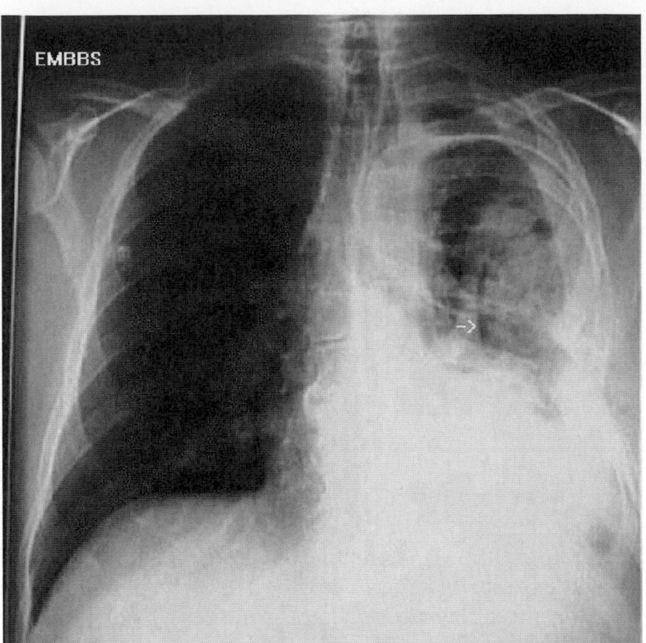

Fig. 11-4 Left-sided empyema with consolidation of lung tissue. *(From EMBBS. Emergency Medicine and Primary Care Home Page. www.embbs.com.)*

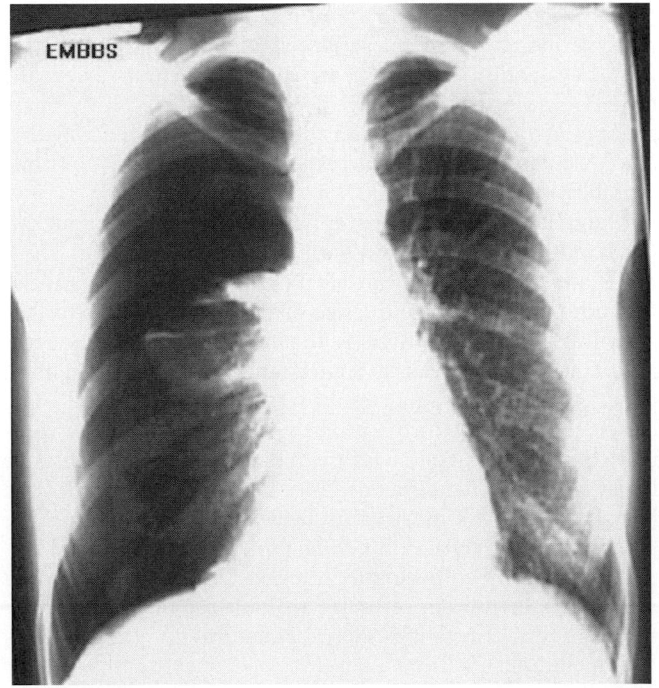

Fig. 11-5 Right-sided pneumothorax. *(From EMBBS. Emergency Medicine and Primary Care Home Page. www.embbs.com.)*

Heart Size

Normally, the heart is about as wide as one-half of the chest cavity. Measuring the cardiac silhouette and then measuring the width of the hemithorax (from the center of the sternum to the outer edge of the ribs) for comparison helps to identify conditions such as cardiac hypertrophy due to chronic or acute heart failure. Next, the shape and the borders of the heart should be examined. For example a "boot shaped" heart

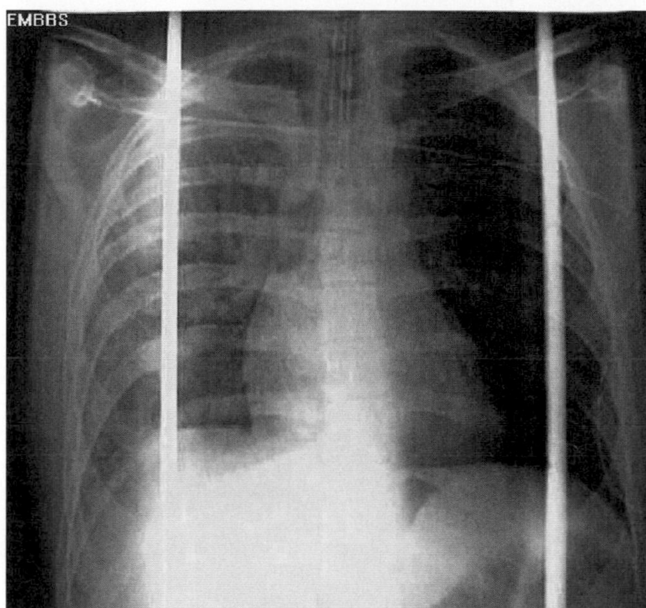

Fig. 11-6 Right rib fractures with right hemothorax. *(From EMBBS. Emergency Medicine and Primary Care Home Page. www.embbs.com.)*

can indicate congenital heart deformities in children, and the loss of a distinct heart border could indicate an infiltrate in the adjacent lung tissue.

Mediastinum

The width of the mediastinum is also important to evaluate. The mediastinal structures should be just wider than the thoracic spine. When the dense structures in this area are much wider than expected, a life-threatening aortic aneurism should be suspected. As the aortic arch widens, it projects a higher-density shadow over the upper left chest cavity that is visible on the radiograph (Figure 11-7).

Other Disease States

Other common disease states can have typical findings on chest radiographs. The hyperinflation caused by an acute asthma attack may present as increased bronchial markings throughout the lung fields, a flattened diaphragm, and a maximally expanded chest cavity. Chronic obstructive pulmonary disease (COPD) causes similar effects, including a barrel-shaped chest (increased anteroposterior [AP] diameter), a flattened diaphragm, and an overall decreased density of the pulmonary markings.

Other Imaging Methods

Computed Tomography

CT scans of the chest can be a useful diagnostic tool for certain diseases (Figure 11-8). Like standard radiographs, CT uses ionizing radiation, but it allows for rapid scanning in much more detail. The CT scan generates pictures that are "slices" through the patient in the axial plane (Figure 11-9). Although bone is visualized much better than soft tissues, a CT scan can still provide excellent images of the lungs, vascular structures,

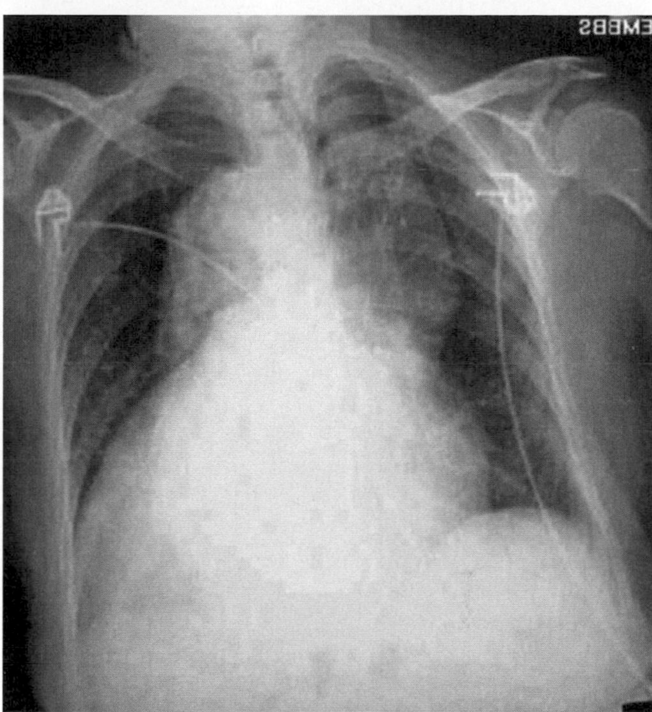

Fig. 11-7 Thoracic aortic aneurism with widened mediastinum. *(From EMBBS. Emergency Medicine and Primary Care Home Page. www.embbs.com.)*

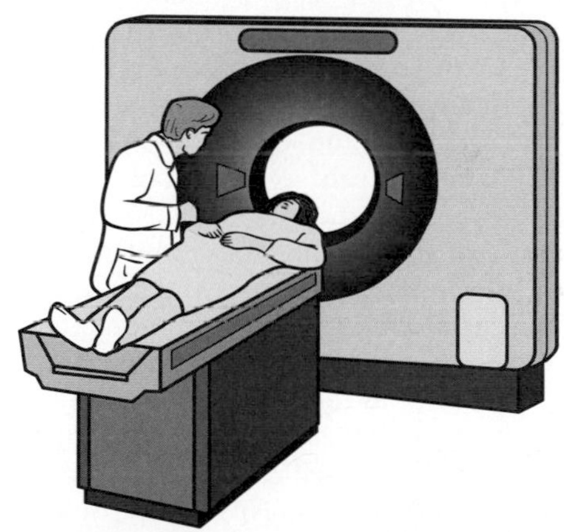

Fig. 11-8 Computed tomography (CT) scanner.

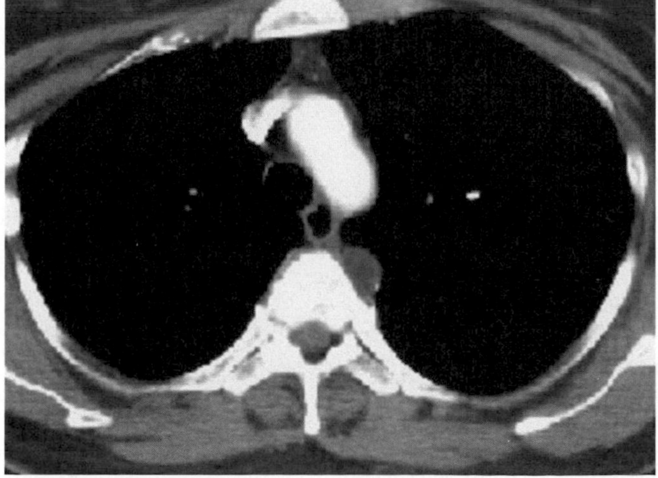

Fig. 11-9 Chest CT showing spine, pulmonary spaces, and aortic arch. *(From GE Healthcare.)*

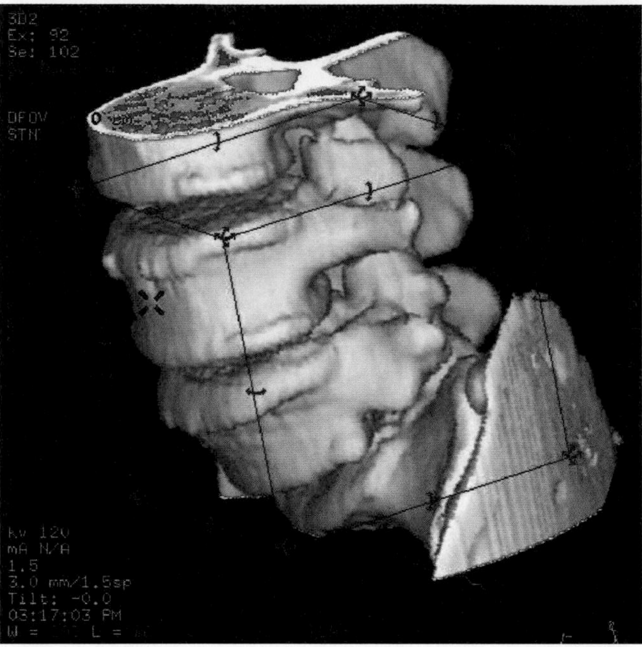

Fig. 11-10 Three-dimensional reconstruction generated by a CT scanner. *(From GE Healthcare.)*

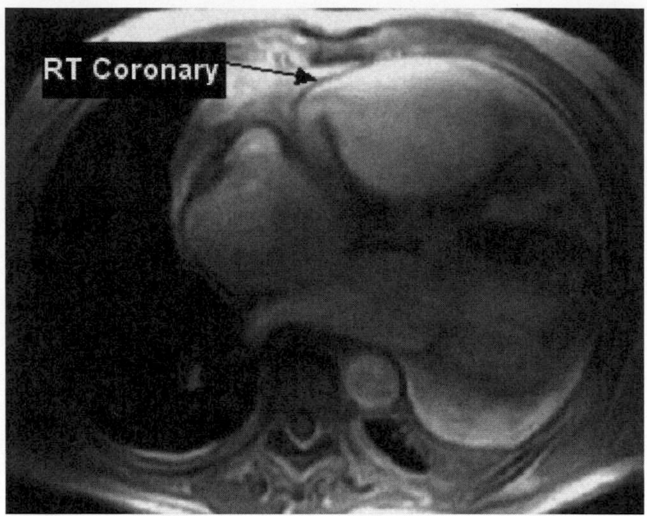

Fig. 11-11 Cardiac MRI evaluating the coronary arteries. *(From GE Healthcare.)*

and heart. New software can produce three-dimensional images that show the anatomy beautifully (Figure 11-10), and the sensitivity of these machines can allow for the detection of very small amounts of calcification in the coronary arteries, which can be an indication of early heart disease. Newer "ultrafast" CT scanners can see more subtle changes in the coronary arteries because they take images so quickly that they seem to "stop" or "freeze" the action and movement of the heart. This results in clearer pictures and the ability to discern small details more accurately.[4] Another modality, called spiral CT scan, provides higher resolution and more rapid images, making it very helpful in the diagnosis of pulmonary embolism, because it can visualize vessels with great precision. In certain cases, an iodine-based dye must be injected intravenously to enhance CT images. This dye can exacerbate renal disorders, and should thus be used with caution.

As CT scans become more and more precise, they are also used more frequently. This increased use raises a concern regarding the radiation exposure of patients undergoing these studies. Although radiation exposure is also a factor with conventional radiography of the chest, the level of exposure with computed tomography has been documented to be much higher. A typical chest CT will expose a patient to the radiation equivalent of 50 to 450 chest x-rays. This increase in radiation exposure had been linked to cancer development later in life, most notably in the pediatric population. Because of this risk, other chest imaging techniques may be considered if appropriate.[5,6]

Magnetic Resonance Imaging

Magnetic resonance imaging of the chest can be performed to evaluate the soft tissues of the chest cavity.[7] MRI has the advantage of using magnetic energy rather than ionizing radiation, so there is no harmful exposure for the patient. MRI scans also provide much higher-quality views of soft tissues than can be achieved by CT scans, but MRI is more expensive and takes nearly an hour to complete. A chest CT can be done in less than a minute, making it a better choice for evaluation of trauma (Figure 11-11). MRI is most useful when evaluating heart function/wall movement, vasculature of the heart and lungs, tumor size and staging, and respiratory movement of the muscles and diaphragm.[4,8]

Radionuclide Ventilation-Perfusion Scan

A radionuclide ventilation-perfusion (VQ) scan can be used to detect conditions that affect blood flow in the lung parenchyma. Radioactive isotopes are injected into the blood stream and are also inhaled into the lungs. Scanning for the location of these isotopes can then determine the extent to which the lungs have been ventilated and perfused. A mismatch (for instance, an area that was perfused with gas but not perfused with blood) would indicate that a blood clot had become caught in the pulmonary vasculature. Research has found, however, that VQ scans produce a high number of indeterminate results, and newer CT images have been found to be more accurate. A pulmonary angiogram is still the definitive test for a pulmonary embolism, but it is an invasive test that must be administered in the cardiac catheterization laboratory and involves injection of dye into the arterial vasculature; thus other imaging methods should be considered when appropriate.

Positron Emission Tomography Scan

Positron emission tomography (PET) scanning is a newer form of radionuclide imaging that helps show the function of organs rather than just their structure. For instance, the amount of radio-labeled glucose taken up by heart muscle cells can help clinicians determine whether the muscles have died after a myocardial infarction or whether they are still alive. This makes the PET scan a crucial decision-making tool: if the post-MI heart muscle cells are alive, they would benefit from bypass surgery, whereas if they are dead, bypass surgery would not be worthwhile. This modality is also very helpful in the localization of tumors in the chest cavity; these tumors are highly metabolic and have high uptake of the radionuclide, thus "lighting up" on a PET scan.[9]

Ultrasound

Ultrasound is an imaging modality commonly used in the abdomen, but because the sound waves bounce off bone, it is much less useful in the chest cavity. Ultrasound is sometimes used to identify pockets of fluid during thoracocentesis, but a CT scan is more commonly used whenever the precise placement of a needle in the chest is necessary. Ultrasound can also be useful to assess cardiac function via a modality known as transesophageal ultrasound.[10]

Summary

There are a variety of ways to image the chest. The standard chest radiograph is still an important way to gather information quickly, inexpensively, and at low risk for the patient. A physical therapist should be familiar with the basic techniques of reading a chest radiograph and should be able to identify common abnormalities viewable by x-ray, as well as other imaging methods, in order to better adapt their therapy regimen to fit the patient's needs and oxygen demands.

Review Questions

1. What do the differing densities seen on a standard chest radiograph represent?
2. What are the basic steps in reading a chest radiograph?
3. What are the signs, visible on a chest radiograph, of the following disorders: pneumothorax, hemothorax, consolidation, and thoracic aneurism?
4. How does nuclear imaging give the clinician physiological and anatomical information about the patient?

References

1. Novelline RA: *Squire's fundamentals of radiology*, ed 5, Cambridge, Mass, 1999, Harvard University Press.
2. Johnson TR, Steinbach LS: *Essentials of musculoskeletal imaging*, Rosemont, Ill, 2004, American Academy of Orthopaedic Surgeons.
3. Rothenberg MA: *Understanding x-rays: A plain English approach*. Eau Claire, Wisc, 1998, Professional Education Systems.
4. Nagel E, Lehmkuhl HB, Bocksch W, et al: Noninvasive diagnosis of ischemia-induced wall motion abnormalities with the use of high-dose dobutamine stress MRI: Comparison with dobutamine stress echocardiography. *Circulation* 16;99(6):763–770, 1999.
5. Brenner, DJ, Hall, EJ (2007). Computed Tomography—An increasing Source of Radiation Exposure. *New England Journal of Medicine* 22(357):2277–2284, 2007.
6. Kalra MK, Maher MM, Rizzo S, et al: Radiation exposure from chest CT: Issues and strategies. *J Korean Med Sci* 19:159–166, 2004.
7. Hierholzer J, Luo L, Bittner RC, et al: MRI and CT in the differential diagnosis of pleural disease. *Chest* 118:604–609, 2000.
8. Kotani T, Minami S, Takahashi K, et al: An Analysis of chest wall and diaphragm motions in patients with idiopathic scoliosis using dynamic breathing MRI. *Spine* 29(3):298–302, 2004.
9. Wilkie SWA, Gomersall LN, Denison AR, et al: Current imaging practice in lung cancer. *Imaging* 20:278–288, 2008.
10. Beckh S, Lessnau B, Lessnau KD: Real-time chest ultrasonography: A comprehensive review for the pulmonologist. *Chest* 122:1759–1773, 2002.

II

Chapter 12

Electrocardiogram Identification

Christian Evans and Gary Brooks

KEY TERMS

Artifact
Bradycardia
Depolarization
Dysrhythmia
Ectopic focus
Electrocardiogram
Supraventricular
Syncytium
Tachycardia

CHAPTER OUTLINE

Electrical signaling is a primary method of communication, control, and regulation in the human body, and nowhere is this method employed with greater precision and elegance than in the heart. The rate, rhythm, and conduction of electrical signals are critical to cardiac function; these are the rhythmic electrical impulses that cause the mechanical contraction, or pumping, of the heart muscle. This electrical current is detectable by electrodes that are placed on the surface of the skin. The flow of current during the cardiac cycle is then recorded as the characteristic waveforms of the electrocardiogram (ECG; sometimes also called EKG). Mechanical events such as the contraction and relaxation of the myocardium are inferred from the waveforms produced by the ECG.

The ECG is an essential tool for the diagnosis and medical management of patients with cardiac disease. Information provided by the ECG may also assist the physical therapist in the assessment of a patient's readiness for and response to physical activity. Physical therapists in many different practice environments have access to information afforded by the ECG. For example, in the intensive care unit or acute care setting or during cardiac rehabilitation, a patient's ECG may be continuously monitored via telemetry (a remote monitoring system in which ECG signals are sent via radio waves to a distant receiver) or by a bedside unit. In both the acute and outpatient settings, past significant ECG recordings, as well as an interpretation, may be available in the medical record. Documentation accompanying a referral for outpatient physical therapy may also include a reference to the patient's ECG. It is therefore crucial that all physical therapists have a basic understanding of the uses and limitations of the ECG in their practices.

As an example of how an understanding of ECG interpretation may be useful for physical therapists, consider the following scenario. A physical therapist in a cardiac intensive care unit (CCU) initiates exercise for a patient recovering from open-heart surgery. The patient's ECG has been stable throughout the postoperative recovery phase, but the patient has not yet been challenged with moderate intensity activity or exercise. The therapist gets the patient up and begins an appropriate level of exercise; however, with this greater demand on the heart, the patient develops an exercise-induced dysrhythmia. This abnormal rhythm may be mild and fairly benign, or it could be malignant or life-threatening. If the physical therapist is able to interpret the ECG accurately in this situation, this dysrhythmia may be caught and then referred to and treated by the physician. If the dysrhythmia is not recognized, a less favorable outcome may occur.

This chapter briefly reviews the basic anatomy and physiology of the myocardial conduction system as it relates to the ECG. The configuration of the normal ECG is presented and discussed, along with several methods of quickly determining heart rate and rhythm from an electrocardiographic record, or ECG "strip." Some of the more common dysrhythmias are examined, as are some other pathological features. Throughout the chapter, the uses and limitations of the ECG in physical therapy practice are highlighted.

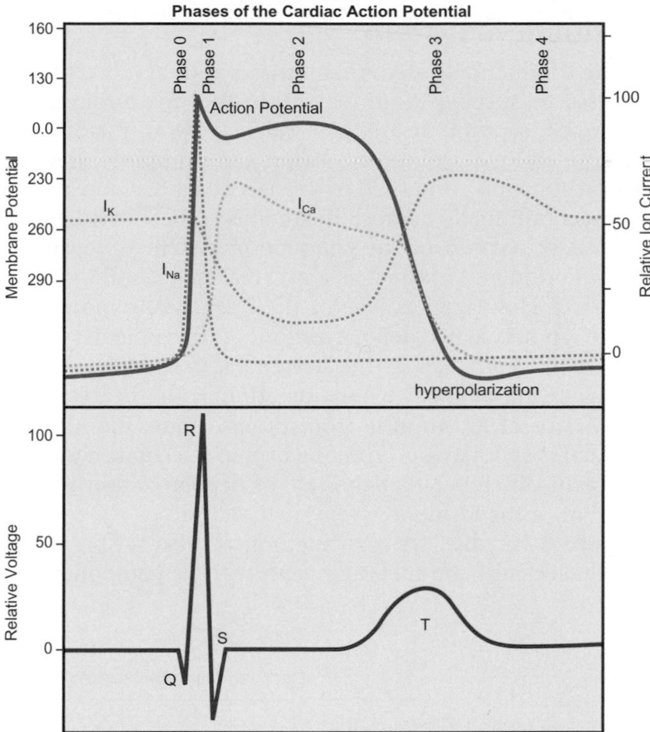

Fig. 12-1 Relationship of an individual ventricular cardiomyocyte action potential to the ECG. **A,** The time-dependent ionic currents (I_K, I_{Na}, and I_{Ca},) of an individual ventricular cardiac cell that determine the shape, amplitude, and duration of the cell's action potential (shown in red). The action potential can be broken down into five distinct phases (0-4). **B,** The QRS complex and T wave of the ECG are temporally related to the cardiac action potential and the phases. However, the ECG also reflects the anatomical orientation of the wave of depolarization through the heart and the location of the recording electrodes.

Physiology and Anatomy of the Conduction System

Cardiac Action Potential

The cardiac action potential is generated by the flow of ions across myocardial cell membranes; it has a distinctive shape and five phases (phases 0 to 4).[1] In the cell's resting state, a negative membrane potential exists, based on the selective permeability of the cardiac cell membrane and the relative concentrations of sodium (Na^+), calcium (Ca^{2+}), and potassium (K^+) ions in the internal and external cellular environments. The relative time-sensitive ionic currents for each species are color-coded and labeled in Figure 12-1, and the cardiac action potential is superimposed over the individual currents that compose it. At rest, a typical ventricular cardiomyocyte membrane is primarily permeable only to K^+ ions, allowing the movement of K^+ out of the cell until the charge inside is approximately −90 mV, relative to the charge outside. This is the resting membrane potential of the cardiomyocyte and is close to the equilibrium potential for K^+. The membrane potential changes rapidly at the onset of depolarization, with the opening of Na^+ and Ca^{2+} channels, allowing these ions to cross the membrane and enter the cell. Calcium then becomes available for contraction of cardiac muscle myofibrils.

During depolarization, the membrane's potential becomes positive and the cell contracts. As in skeletal muscle, the Na+ channels are fast-opening and fast-closing mechanisms, allowing Na+ to rapidly enter the myocardial cell on depolarization (referred to as phase 0 of the cardiac action potential in Figure 12-1). Unlike skeletal muscle, however, cardiac muscle has a prolonged action potential as a result of the slower and extended opening of the Ca^{2+} channels. After initial depolarization, some K^+ channels remain open while others close, and repolarization begins (phase 1) as a result of outward K^+ current flowing through the open K^+ channels. A plateau phase (phase 2) of the action potential exists, during which the outward flow of K^+ ions is balanced by an inward flow of Ca^{2+} ions. This prolongs depolarization and delays return to the resting membrane potential. Closure of the slow Ca^{2+} channels at onset of repolarization is accompanied by the opening of additional K^+ channels, causing a rapid outflow of K^+, which completes repolarization (phase 3 in Figure 12-1), restoring resting negative membrane potential. During the cell's resting phase (phase 4 of Figure 12-1), Na^+ and Ca^{2+} are actively pumped out of the cell, and K^+ is pumped into the cell, restoring the ionic gradients needed for repolarization.[1,2,3]

Each cell has an absolute refractory period during depolarization, meaning that an additional stimulus will not cause an additional depolarization. A brief but important relative refractory period follows depolarization, during which a stimulus of greater than normal intensity is necessary to depolarize the cell again. The refractory period of atrial cells is significantly shorter than that of ventricular cells, allowing a more rapid intrinsic atrial rhythm than intrinsic ventricular rhythm. Therefore atrial rhythms pace the heart, including the ventricles, given intact atrioventricular (AV) conduction.

From Figure 12-1 it can be seen that certain ionic currents contribute to particular phases of the cardiac action potential. The Na^+ current is the predominant factor in the initial depolarization, whereas the Ca^{2+} current is important in the plateau phase, and the K^+ currents are important in the duration of the action potential and in repolarization. Many of the drugs used to treat dysrhythmias work on the channels for one or more of these three ions and affect their permeability. Furthermore, the electrical current produced by these ionic currents is transmitted through the conductive tissues surrounding the heart. The "wave" of depolarization that is propagated through the conduction system and contractile tissue of the heart, as well as repolarization, which takes place in a particular spatial manner, are detectable by the surface electrodes of the ECG.

Conduction System

It is the conduction system that initiates and rapidly transmits impulses to specific locations within the myocardium (the atria, apex, septum, and lateral wall), allowing for effective, coordinated myocardial contraction and pumping. The conduction system is composed of specialized cardiac muscle that contracts minimally because it contains few contractile myofibrils. Any portion of the conduction system is capable of self-excitation and may act as a pacemaker, generating action potentials. However, because of the intrinsically more rapid rate of spontaneous depolarization of the sinoatrial (SA) node, it normally acts as the heart's pacemaker. The rate of depolarization of the SA node determines the heart rate. In the absence of an impulse from the SA node, the AV node depolarizes spontaneously, taking over as pacemaker, with the important difference that the rate of depolarization is lower than that of the SA node.

Figure 12-2 displays the anatomical association of the cardiac electrical conduction system with its components on the ECG. Atrial depolarization is initiated by a spontaneously generated impulse that originates in the SA node. The impulse is then transmitted throughout the atrial muscle, resulting in atrial contraction. The event is recorded as the P wave of the ECG. The impulse is also transmitted, via rapidly conducting internodal pathways, to the AV node. Atrial repolarization is not recorded by the ECG because it occurs during ventricular depolarization.

Impulse conduction slows within the AV node considerably, resulting in a delaying of the impulse before it reaches the ventricular conduction system. The pause in impulse propagation allows the atria to contract and fill the ventricles with blood. The P-R interval of the ECG represents this period between the onset of atrial depolarization and the onset of ventricular depolarization. Normally the P-R interval lasts between 0.12 and 0.20 second.[4]

Following passage through the AV node, the impulse continues to the AV bundle (bundle of His) and then to Purkinje fibers, which transmit the impulse rapidly to the ventricular endocardium. Ventricular depolarization corresponds to

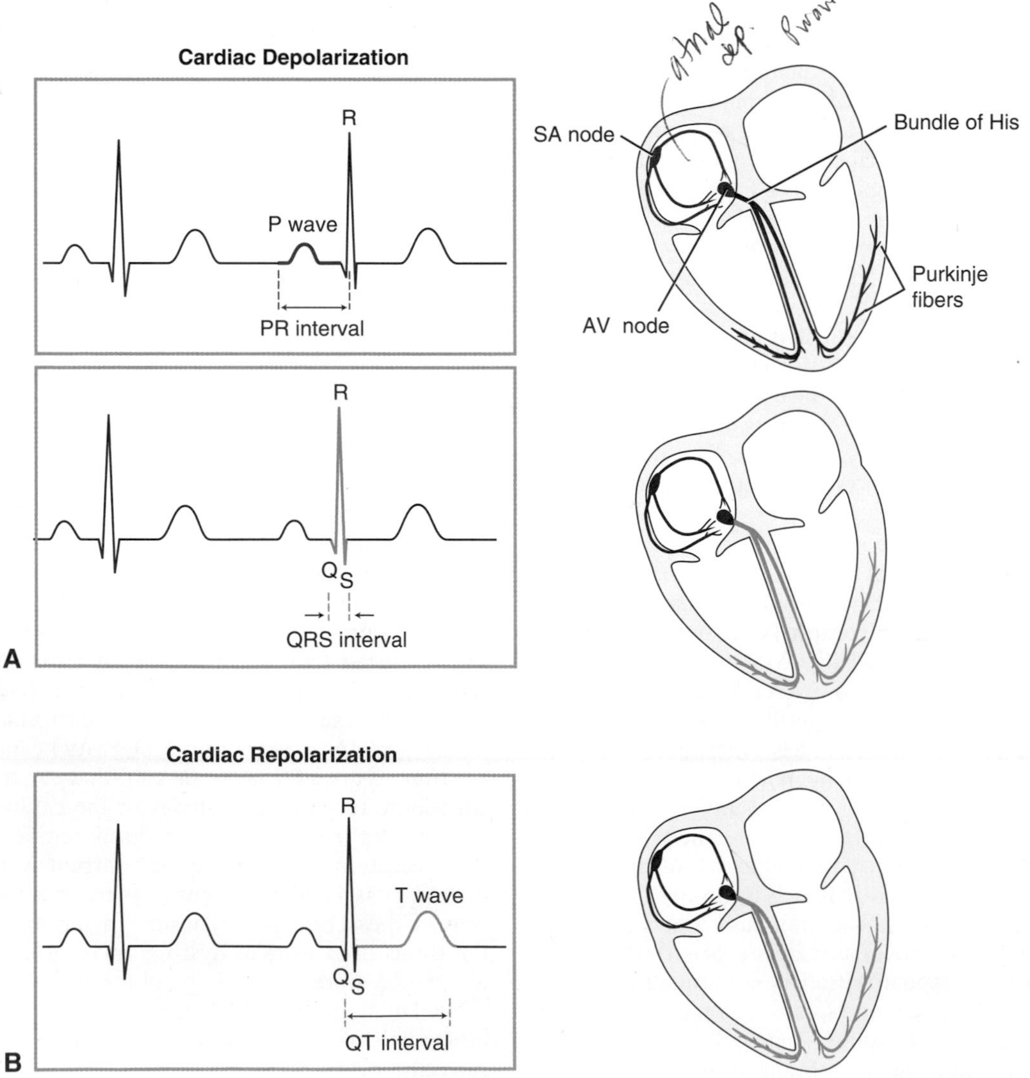

Fig. 12-2 Relationship of ECG complex to conduction pathway. **A,** The sequence of events in depolarization: the wave of depolarization spreads from the SA node through the atria to the AV node. After a delay in the AV node, it travels through the bundle of His to the Purkinje fibers to the ventricular myocardium. The delay at the AV node accounts for the duration of the P-R interval. QRS duration is dependent on normal propagation from the atria and an intact ventricular conduction system. **B,** Ventricular repolarization.

phase 0 of the cardiac action potential (see Figure 12-1) and is represented in the ECG by the QRS complex. The depolarization wave propagates relatively slowly throughout the ventricular myocardium. The span of time elapsing during ventricular depolarization is reflected by the QRS interval, which normally ranges between 0.06 and 0.1 seconds. Ventricular depolarization originates in the interventricular septum, creating the Q wave, which is normally small or absent, depending on the lead. The depolarization wave next spreads to the apex and then to the right and left ventricles, causing the R and S waves. Depolarization also propagates in an endocardial to epicardial direction within the ventricles.[2,3] A normal QRS duration indicates that the impulse originated in the SA node or a region above the AV node (supraventricular). A long QRS interval (≥0.1 second) suggests that the impulse arose from the ventricle or originated abnormally in supraventricular tissue. The normal sequence of depolarization is as follows: SA node to AV node to bundle of His to Purkinje fibers to the ventricular myocardium. When this sequence is followed, the ECG correlates with the mechanical events of the cardiac cycle as shown in Figure 4-13.

After ventricular depolarization, the ECG deflection returns to baseline, and this pause in electrical activity corresponds with the plateau phase (phase 2) of the cardiac action potential. Ventricular repolarization is represented by the T wave and corresponds to phase 3 of the cardiac action potential. The configuration of the S-T segment is an important marker of myocardial ischemia or infarction. Following the T wave, a U wave may also be present. The source of the U wave is not well understood.[5] Although U wave inversion may indicate ischemia involving the left ventricular wall,[6] it is not a unique marker and is not as sensitive as S-T segment changes in predicting ischemia; therefore it is not a useful clinical marker.[7]

Within the ventricle, individual cardiomyocytes are in direct communication with each other via gap junctions. This facilitates rapid spread of the wave of depolarization from cell to cell, allowing the right and left ventricular heart muscle to function as a syncytium, or a single pumping unit.[8] Note that the ventricles remain in a state of contraction until slightly after repolarization. This period of contraction corresponds to the Q-T interval on the ECG. Diastole, therefore, begins subsequent to the end of the T wave and continues until the next ventricular depolarization. Note also that atrial depolarization and contraction occur during diastole.

Electrocardiogram

Recording the Electrocardiogram

Before examining the timing of the wave forms and the rhythms of the ECG, a basic understanding of the principles of electrocardiography is needed. A standard 12-lead configuration is used for the diagnosis and medical management of cardiac conditions (Figure 12-3): six leads record the electrical signals in the frontal plane, and six leads record signals in the transverse plane. The placements of the 10 electrodes for a 12-lead ECG are shown in Figure 12-4 (note that 12 electrodes are not necessary because some leads serve a dual purpose).

The frontal-plane leads include three standard bipolar limb leads, referred to as leads I, II, and III, and three augmented unipolar limb leads, referred to as aVR (right arm), aVL (left arm), and aVF (left leg). These two sets of leads share the same electrodes but view the electrical activity of the heart from different perspectives. The bipolar leads have a single positive and a single negative electrode and record the difference in electrical potential between them. The augmented limb leads have a single positive electrode and derive the negative electrode from the combination of the other electrodes. The standard limb leads form a triangle, known as the Einthoven's triangle, around the heart that allows for advanced calculations related to the net vector of depolarization, or the axis of the heart (an index of the cardiac mass and position). If only a single lead is recorded, standard limb lead II is often chosen because all of the deflections are typically upright.[4]

The transverse-plane leads are referred to as the precordial, or chest, leads. These six leads form a semicircle around the anterior aspect of the heart; their placement is described in Figure 12-4. In addition to the three electrodes for the limb leads and the six electrodes for the chest leads, a 10th electrode that serves as a neutral ground must be used to reduce artifacts and stabilize the baseline. Imagine that each of the 12 leads "views" the heart from a different angle, therefore recording events in different locations of the heart in different ways. By convention, the waveform on the ECG is positive (upward) as current travels toward a positive electrode or lead and is negative (downward) when current travels away from a lead. Other lead configurations may be used for exercise testing.[9] Single-lead monitoring is commonly used during exercise training or in the acute care settings.

Evaluating the ECG Strip

The evaluation of an ECG should be approached in a systematic fashion. The following questions are useful for appreciating the information that is relevant to current clinical practice.[10]

What is the rate and pattern (regularity) of the rhythm? Is the R-R interval (the distance between successive R waves) equal for each beat? This indicates regularity of the beats.

Does a P wave precede every QRS complex? This indicates that the rhythm is atrial.

Is there a QRS complex after every P wave? This indicates conduction of impulses from the atria to the ventricles.

What is the P-R interval? A P-R interval of 0.12 to 0.20 second indicates normal conduction from atria to ventricles. A P-R interval >0.2 seconds indicates a conduction delay or block.

Is the QRS complex of normal duration and morphology (shape)? A QRS complex greater than 0.1 second indicates either that an impulse arose within a ventricle or was conducted abnormally through the ventricular conduction system.

By answering each of these questions, the tendency to "eyeball" the rhythm and make a quick, but inaccurate assessment is avoided.

Determination of Heart Rate

Several quick methods can be used to estimate heart rate. Most printed and displayed ECG recordings indicate a heart rate. This must be interpreted with caution, however, because the presence of artifact (extraneous deflections of the waveform caused by movement or electrical interference) may render an automated heart rate calculation inaccurate. This is a common

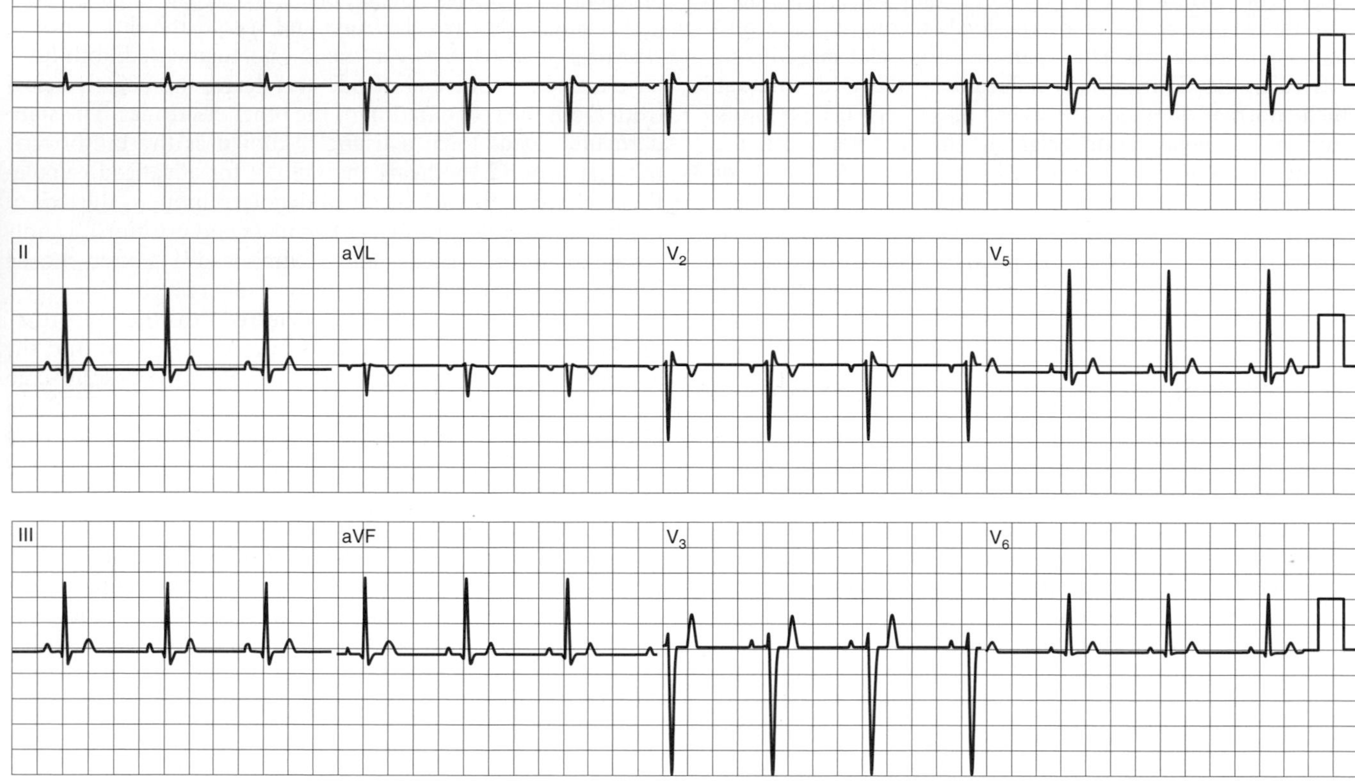

Fig. 12-3 A normal 12-lead ECG.

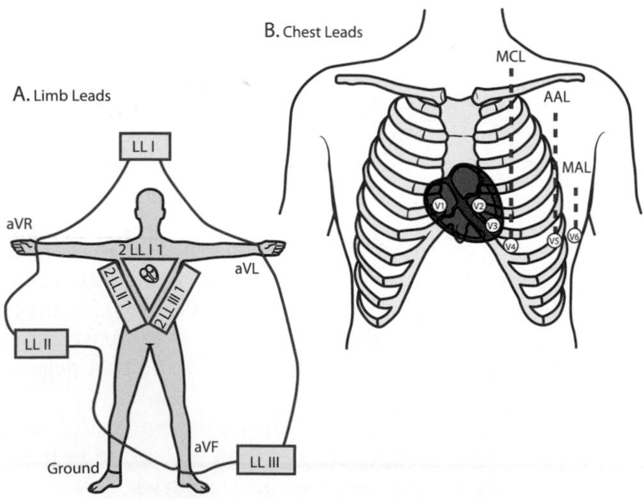

Fig. 12-4 Anatomical placement of the 12-lead electrocardiogram electrodes. **A,** The placement of the electrodes for the three standard limb leads (LL), LL I, LL II, and LL III; and the placement for the augmented limb leads, aVR (right arm), aVL (left arm), and aVF (left leg). The standard limb leads are bipolar leads, whereas the augmented limb leads are unipolar. **B,** The placement of the six chest leads, or precordial leads, V1 to V6. Leads V1 and V2 are placed over the fourth intercostals spaces, on the left and right of the sternum, respectively. Typically, V4 is placed next on the midclavicular line (MCL) at the fifth intercostals space. V3 is placed midway between V2 and V4. V6 is placed next on the midaxillary line (MAL) on the same plane as V4. The V5 lead is placed at a point midway between V4 and V6, at the anterior axillary line (AAL). A 10th electrode must be attached (shown here attached to the right leg) to minimize artifact. Abbreviations: *AAL,* anterior axillary line; *LL,* standard limb lead; *MAL,* midaxillary line; *MCL,* midclavicular line.

problem during activity or exercise, the circumstances during which many physical therapists monitor patients. It is possible to calculate or to estimate a heart rate on the basis of a printed ECG strip because, by convention, the recording paper is divided into 1-mm squares and larger 5-mm squares, which are defined by heavier lines (Figure 12-5). Also by convention, the standard paper speed for an ECG recording is a rate of 25 mm per second, and most recorders mark each 3-second interval. Each millimeter of length then represents $\frac{1}{25}$, or 0.04 second, and each 5-mm block represents $\frac{1}{5}$, or 0.20 second. Some monitor systems, however, place a mark on the recording paper at 25-mm, or 1-second intervals.

There are several methods of estimating heart rate from a printed ECG strip (Figure 12-6). On the strip, find an R wave located on or near a heavy vertical line. Proceeding to the right of that R wave, for each subsequent heavy vertical line, assign the following numbers: 300 for the first heavy line encountered, 150 for the next, followed by 100, 75, 60, 50, and 42 (Figure 12-6, *A*). Stop at the first heavy vertical line following the next R wave that is encountered. The heart rate may be estimated as falling between values to the left and right. In Figure 12-6, the rate would be estimated as falling between 100 and 75, or close to 80 beats per minute.

In many clinics, rulers are available that are calibrated so that heart rate may be estimated quickly by aligning markings on the ruler with features of the ECG strip. For example, after the arrow on the ruler is placed on an R wave, count two R waves to the right and read the number at that position on the ruler. In Figure 12-6, *B,* this method approximates the heart rate as 74 beats per minute. It is important to note that the

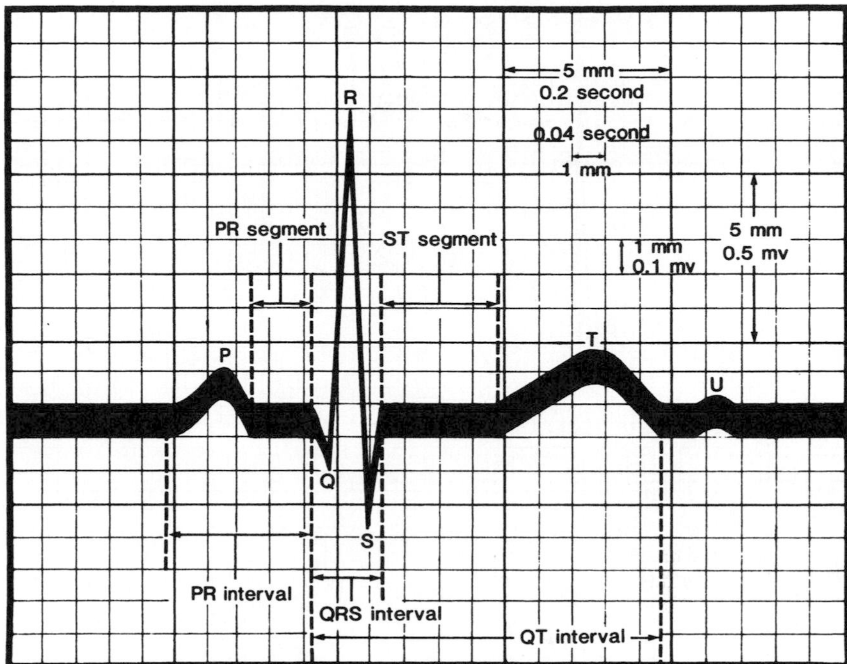

Fig. 12-5 A normal ECG showing characteristic waves, intervals, and segments, and some of the features of the tracing paper.

preceding two methods are useful only if the rhythm of the ECG strip is regular (i.e., the R waves are equally spaced, occurring at consistent intervals). Should the rhythm be irregular, with R waves appearing at varying intervals, another method must be employed to estimate the heart rate.

A common and easy method for estimating the heart rate is to count off the number of R waves in a 6-second strip. Depending on whether the ECG recorder makes a mark every 1, 3, or 6 seconds, count off the appropriate number of seconds to obtain a 6-second strip. The procedure is as follows: Start at the mark corresponding to the beginning of the 6-second period and proceeding from left to right, count the number of R waves within the 6-second recording. Now multiply by 10. That is the estimated heart rate, rounded down to the nearest 10 beats per minute. Several 6-second strips may be analyzed to document the heart rate range of an irregular rhythm. The rate of the irregular rhythm in Figure 12-6, *C*, is estimated at approximately 60 beats per minute.

Evaluation of Rhythms

Electrocardiographic monitoring is an important evaluation tool during the treatment of individuals with a history of, or potential for, acute myocardial infarction (MI) or myocardial ischemia. Most cardiac deaths are a result of lethal dysrhythmias, for which there is increased risk in the presence of infarction or ischemia. Rapid recognition of lethal dysrhythmias, or dysrhythmias that may deteriorate into lethal dysrhythmias, is essential for all health professionals involved in the care of individuals with cardiac disease. The dysrhythmias described in this chapter are those that are either common or dangerous in terms of mortality and morbidity.

Normally, a cardiac impulse is generated by the SA node, causing atrial depolarization. This is followed by a slight delay in the AV node, after which the impulse is conducted to the ventricles, causing ventricular depolarization. These events are shown in Figure 12-7 in their normal spatial and temporal sequence and in normal sinus rhythm. A P wave precedes every QRS complex and every P wave is, in turn, succeeded by a QRS complex. This occurs within an interval of 0.12 to 0.20 second (one large box), as determined by the P-R interval. The QRS complexes occur within a range of 0.04 to 0.12 second, indicating that ventricular impulse conduction and depolarization is occurring in a normal interval. The positively deflected T wave indicates normal ventricular repolarization. Because the SA node spontaneously depolarizes at a rate of between 60 and 100 beats per minute, the rate of normal sinus rhythm must fall within these limits.

The identification of dysrhythmias affects clinical decision making, particularly with regard to a patient's readiness for or response to activity. The clinical significance of dysrhythmias ranges from benign to lethal. The clinical significance of a given dysrhythmia is determined by a number of considerations. Some of these considerations include the following: Is there evidence of hemodynamic compromise? Is the dysrhythmia a new or unusual finding? Might the dysrhythmia be a precursor to a more serious or perhaps lethal dysrhythmia? Is this an acute occurrence or a chronic dysrhythmia pattern? The clinical response to a patient with a dysrhythmia depends on the answers to these questions and the treatment setting.

Dysrhythmia Identification

Supraventricular Dysrhythmias

Supraventricular dysrhythmias arise from an abnormality in impulse generation or conduction "above" the level of the ventricles. A sinus rhythm is any rhythm established by impulses from the SA node. Thus, depending on where the abnormality occurs—in the atria or at the level of the AV junction—a supraventricular dysrhythmia may be categorized as sinus, atrial, or junctional.

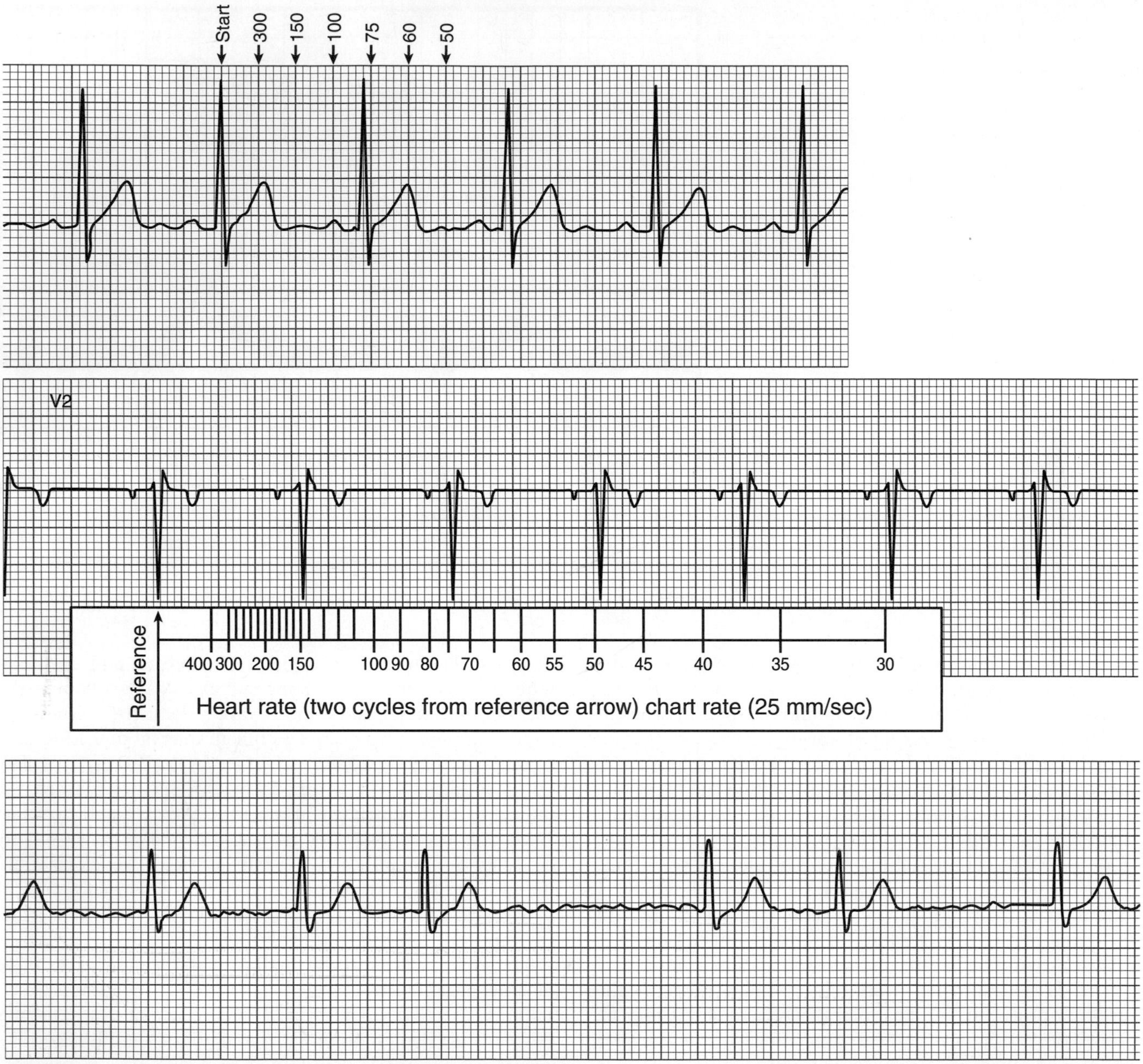

Start 300 150 100 75 60 50

V2

Reference

400 300 200 150 100 90 80 70 60 55 50 45 40 35 30

Heart rate (two cycles from reference arrow) chart rate (25 mm/sec)

Fig. 12-6 Estimating heart rate. **A,** Count-off method. **B,** Using a rate-ruler. **C,** Heart rate estimation in an irregular rhythm (atrial fibrillation).

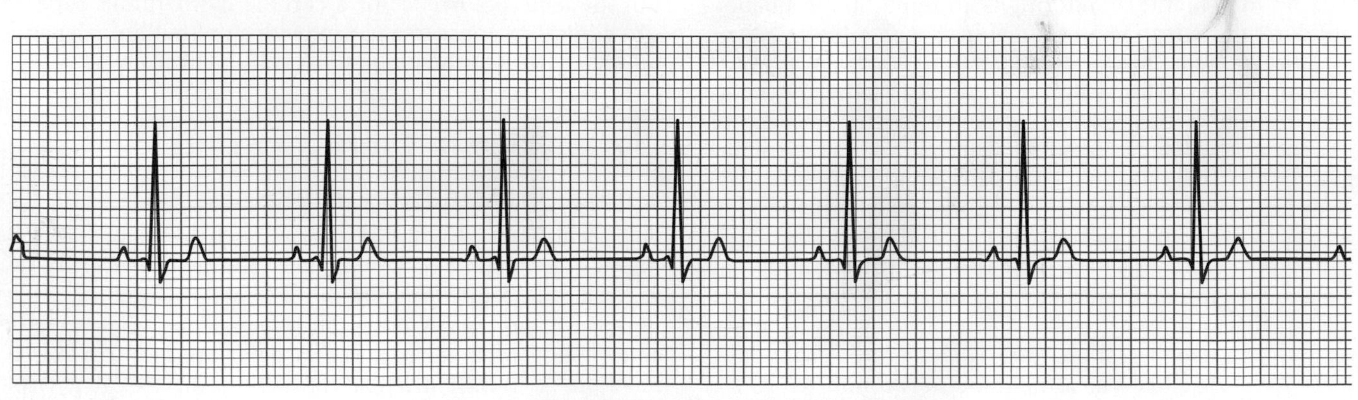

Fig. 12-7 Normal sinus rhythm.

A cardiac dysrhythmia may be a sinus rhythm but with an irregular or abnormally rapid or slow rate (Figure 12-8). Sinus dysrhythmia is an irregular sinus rhythm with varying R-R intervals (Figure 12-8, *A*). This is a normal variant that is associated with the individual's respiratory pattern. Sinus bradycardia is a sinus rhythm occurring at a rate of less than 60 beats per minute (Figure 12-8, *B*). This rhythm may significantly reduce cardiac output, causing hemodynamic compromise, manifested by hypotension or symptoms such as dizziness, lightheadedness, or syncope. On the other hand, individuals taking beta blockers, a group of medications that slow the heart, may exhibit this as their normal rhythm, as might individuals who achieve a high level of physical conditioning. Sinus tachycardia is a sinus rhythm occurring at a rate of greater than 100 beats per minute (Figure 12-8, *C*). Sinus tachycardia, or any other form of tachycardia, increases myocardial oxygen demand, or the workload on the heart. This may initiate or exacerbate ischemia in the presence of coronary artery disease (CAD).

A beat or rhythm that does not originate in the SA node is considered to represent an ectopic focus or pacemaker. One common form of dysrhythmia is a "premature" complex (i.e., a beat that occurs sooner than expected given the established rhythm). A premature atrial complex, or PAC, is an early beat that has an ectopic atrial origin (Figure 12-9). An R wave appears closer to its preceding R wave than the other R waves in the established rhythm. The P wave of the odd beat may have a different shape or may be inverted relative to the normal P waves, indicating that it came from a focus other than the SA node, but the associated QRS complex is always preceded by a P wave, meaning that the impulse first depolarized the atria before being conducted to the ventricles. Sometimes the AV junction may initiate an early beat, causing a premature junctional complex, or PJC. When this occurs, the R wave appears earlier; however, there may be no associated P wave, or there may be an unusual P wave, one that is inverted or follows the QRS complex. An inverted or late P wave indicates that the impulse was conducted in a retrograde

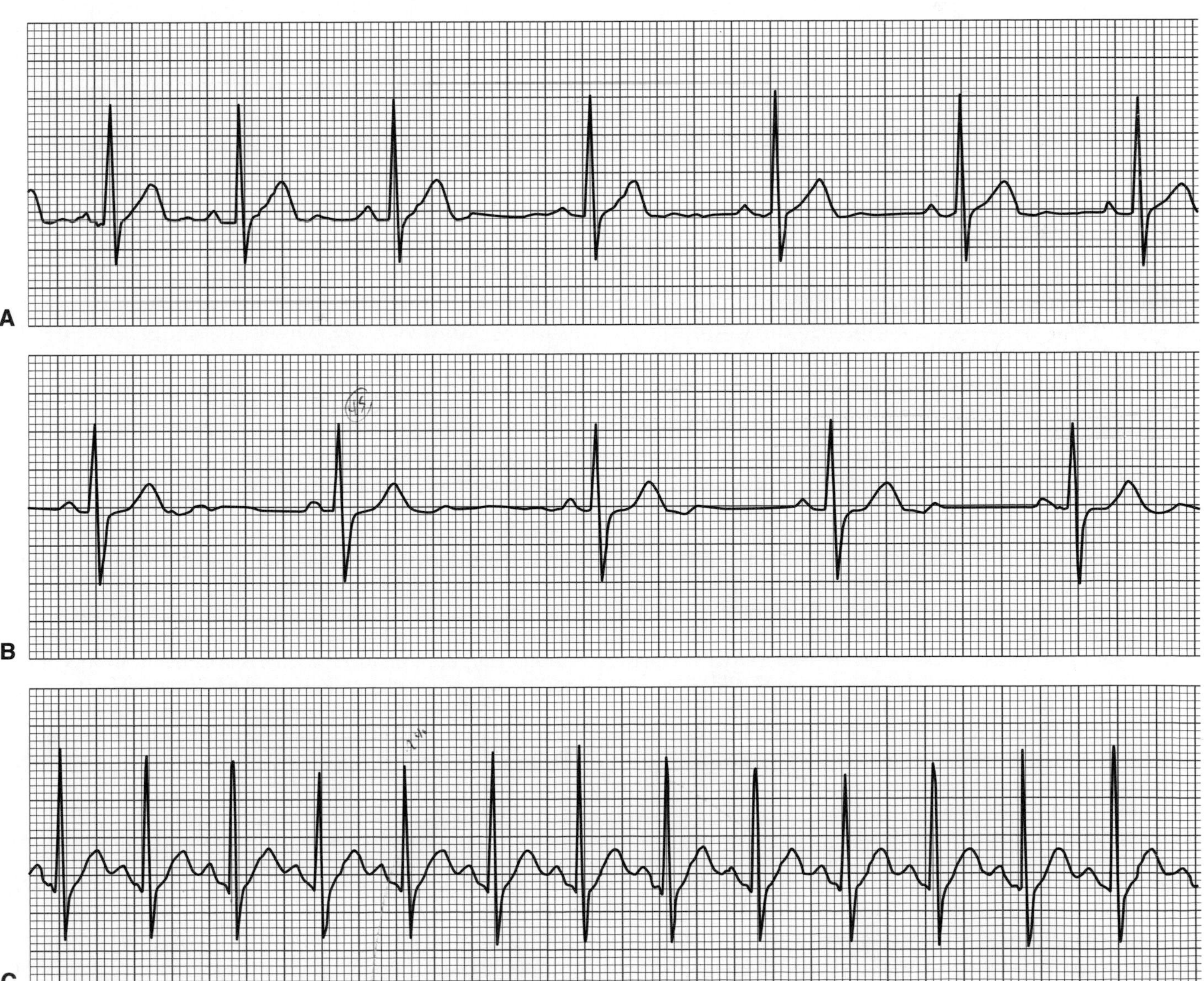

Fig. 12-8 Sinus rhythm but with an irregular or abnormally slow or rapid rate. **A,** Sinus dysrhythmia. **B,** Sinus bradycardia. **C,** Sinus tachycardia.

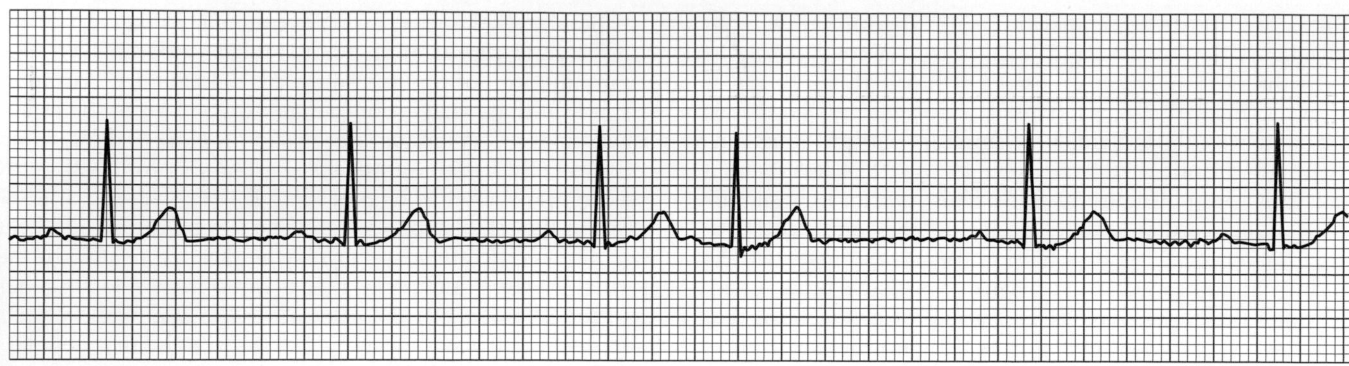

Fig. 12-9 Premature atrial complex.

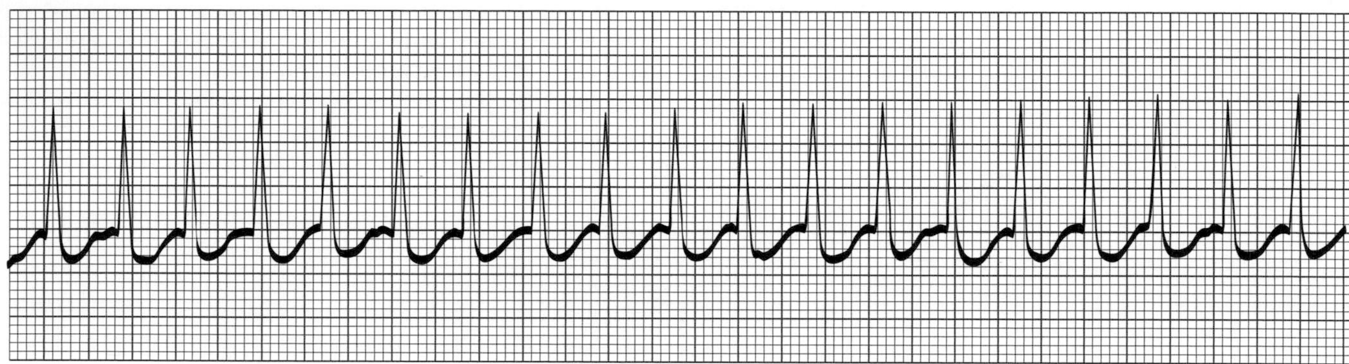

Fig. 12-10 Supraventricular tachycardia.

(backward) fashion. Clinically, a premature atrial or junctional complex may be palpated as a "skipped" or early beat during pulse taking, or the patient may perceive a palpitation or skipped beat. Otherwise, these dysrhythmias are usually of little clinical significance.[4,11]

A more serious supraventricular dysrhythmia is supraventricular tachycardia, or SVT. In this dysrhythmia, the heart rate is rapid, exceeding 150 beats per minute. The tachycardia may be sustained, lasting hours or even days, or it may be "paroxysmal" (PSVT), appearing abruptly and spontaneously reconverting to the previous rhythm within seconds or minutes. The P wave is often not visible, making assessment of atrial or junctional origin difficult. According to the 2005 American Heart Association guidelines, tachycardia is classified on the basis of the width of the QRS complex. So called "narrow-complex tachycardia" refers to a rapid rhythm with a QRS <0.12 seconds. These types of tachycardia originate above the ventricle and are "supraventricular." Wide complex tachycardia (QRS >0.12 seconds) is usually ventricular in origin and is discussed below. Distinguishing between these two types of tachycardia is important since the ventricular form is more serious and a life-threatening condition. The R-R interval in supraventricular tachycardia is markedly shortened. Figure 12-10 demonstrates supraventricular tachycardia at a rate of 190 beats per minute. Other related forms of SVT include paroxysmal atrial tachycardia (PAT) and multifocal atrial tachycardia (MAT). Clinically, patients with SVT may perceive a "racing" heart rate, which may be quite distressing. At very rapid heart rates, for example, greater than 170 beats per minute, diastolic ventricular filling time is markedly reduced, which may cause hemodynamic compromise. Symptoms associated with inadequate cardiac output, such as dizziness, lightheadedness, and syncope may ensue. Some individuals with SVT remain asymptomatic, the rhythm being detected incidentally, for example, during routine pulse or telemetry monitoring.

Atrial fibrillation is the most common clinically encountered dysrhythmia; it is seen in approximately 0.4% of the general population, but in more than 6% of patients over age 80.[12] Atrial fibrillation is characterized by inconsistent, irregular R-R intervals with an absence of true P waves (see Figure 12-6, *C*). P waves may be replaced by multiple, fibrillatory F waves of varying configurations. This dysrhythmia is characterized by the presence of many impulses simultaneously, generated from multiple locations within the atria. The atria, therefore, are not pumping effectively which, in turn, may impair ventricular contraction, resulting in a reduction in cardiac output of up to 25%. This is because of the loss of the additional ventricular filling supplied by atrial contraction. Impulses do conduct through the AV junction to the ventricles; however, this occurs inconsistently and results in the irregular R-R interval. The ventricular response to atrial fibrillation is important. A rapid ventricular response, resulting in tachycardia, may cause hemodynamic compromise with associated symptoms or poor activity tolerance. Of additional clinical significance is the association between atrial fibrillation and embolic cerebrovascular accidents. Stasis of blood within the noncontracting atria may allow for thrombus formation. Figure 12-6, *C* illustrates atrial fibrillation with a "controlled" (i.e., fewer than 100 beats per minute) ventricular response. Pulse monitoring of an individual in atrial fibrillation reveals an irregular pattern.

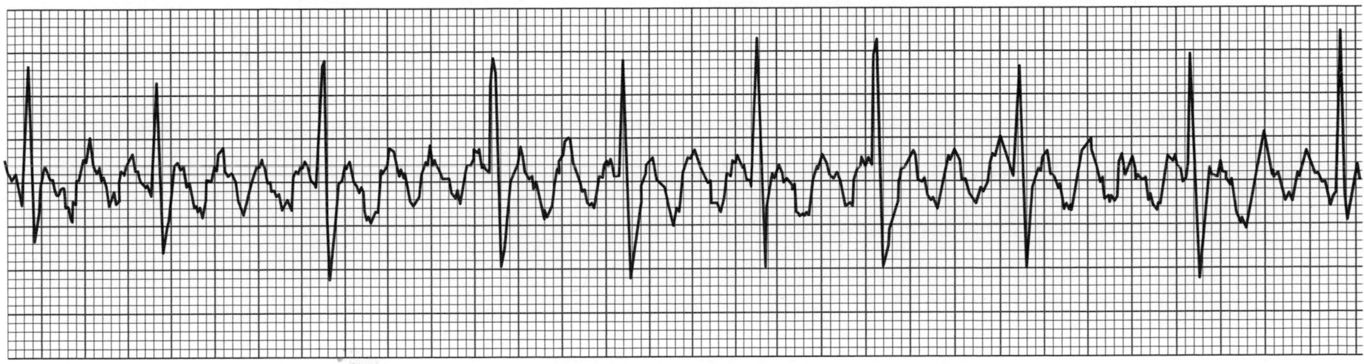

Fig. 12-11 Atrial flutter.

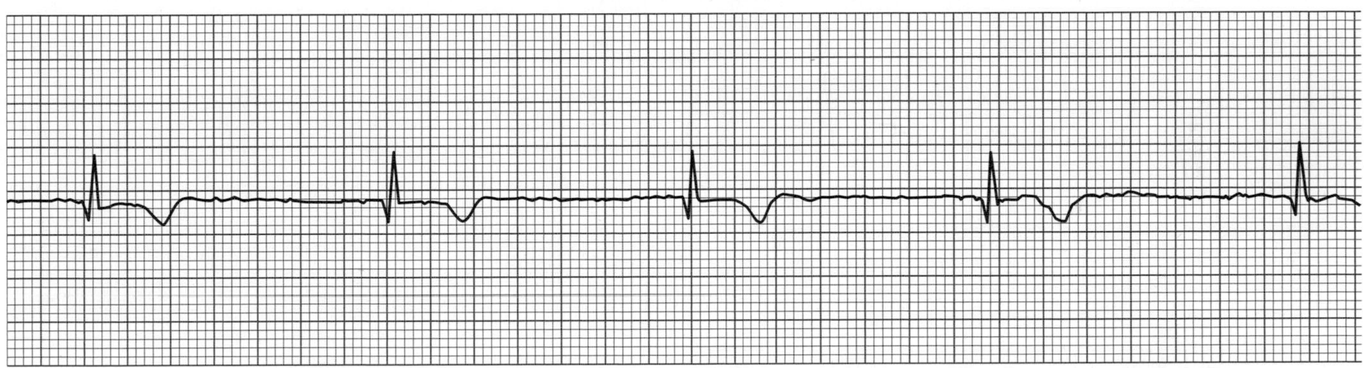

Fig. 12-12 Junctional rhythm.

Another dysrhythmia that is characterized by abnormal atrial activity is atrial flutter (Figure 12-11). In this rhythm, P waves are replaced by F waves that have a distinctive morphology often referred to as a saw-tooth or picket-fence appearance. Of clinical importance is the ratio of atrial to ventricular conduction and whether or not the patient is hemodynamically stable.[4,11]

Because the intrinsic rate of spontaneous depolarization of the AV node is less than that of the SA node, spontaneous AV node depolarization is normally prevented. However, in the absence of an atrial impulse, the AV node depolarizes spontaneously and generates an impulse that then is conducted to the ventricles. Thus in junctional rhythm or nodal rhythm (Figure 12-12), the QRS complex is not preceded by a P wave. The AV node may generate an isolated "escape" beat, or it may take over as the heart's pacemaker. Sustained nodal or junctional rhythm is usually between 40 and 60 beats per minute, corresponding with the inherent rate of spontaneous AV node depolarization.

Ventricular Dysrhythmias

An ectopic pacemaker below the atria and outside the normal conduction system, such as a region in the ventricular myocardium, may give rise to a ventricular dysrhythmia. Ventricular dysrhythmias may be distinguished from supraventricular dysrhythmias in that the QRS duration of a ventricular dysrhythmia is longer than the normal 0.12 second. The appearance of ventricular dysrhythmias may be characterized as being "wide and weird." It is important to point out that not all rhythms with a long QRS result from impulse generation within the ventricles. A disturbance in impulse conduction through the ventricles can also lead to a long QRS.

The reason for the widening of the QRS complex resulting from ventricular impulse conduction disturbance or impulse generation is apparent when one considers the normal conduction of a sinus impulse within the ventricles. An impulse normally is rapidly conducted to ventricular myocardium via the Purkinje fibers. This ensures that the impulse reaches all regions of the ventricular myocardium in a timely fashion, with subsequent coordinated depolarization and contraction. Within the ventricular myocardium itself, however, propagation of the depolarization wave proceeds more slowly as a result of the syncytial arrangement of myocardial cells.

An impulse generated within the ventricles, outside the normal conduction pathways, initially depolarizes surrounding local myocardium. The depolarization wave then spreads outward from that focus, but it is propagated at a slower velocity. Ventricular contraction, in this case, is not coordinated; some regions contract well before the depolarization wave reaches regions remote from the ectopic focus. It follows that the ventricular ejection of blood is reduced during an ectopic beat (Figure 12-13). An ECG rhythm (Figure 12-13, bottom) is recorded simultaneously with the record of arterial blood pressure monitoring (top). The appearance of the wide and weird complex results in significant diminution of the corresponding arterial pressure wave. Ventricular dysrhythmias are strongly associated with serious heart disease, but it is often not clear whether the dysrhythmia is the cause or the result of the heart condition.[13]

The most common form of ventricular dysrhythmia is a premature ventricular complex (PVC). In Figure 12-13 the

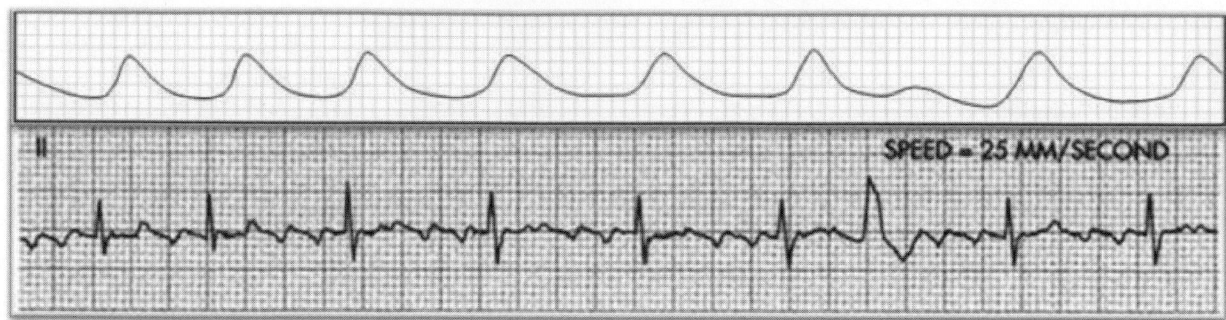

Fig. 12-13 Diminished arterial pressure wave following a PVC.

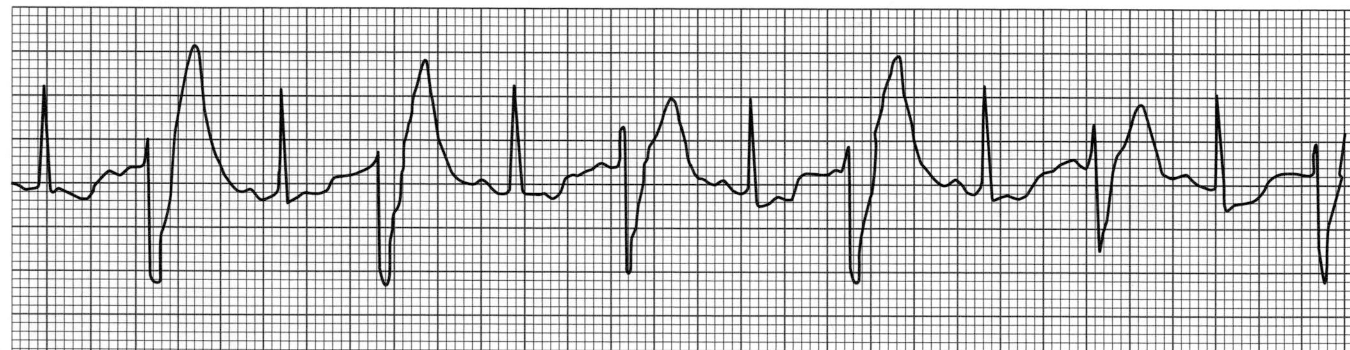

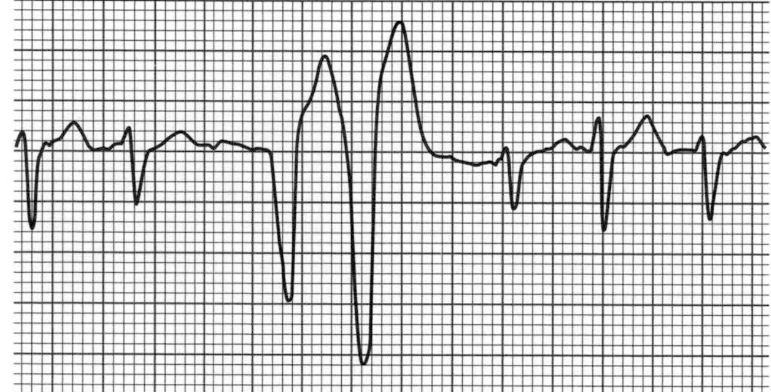

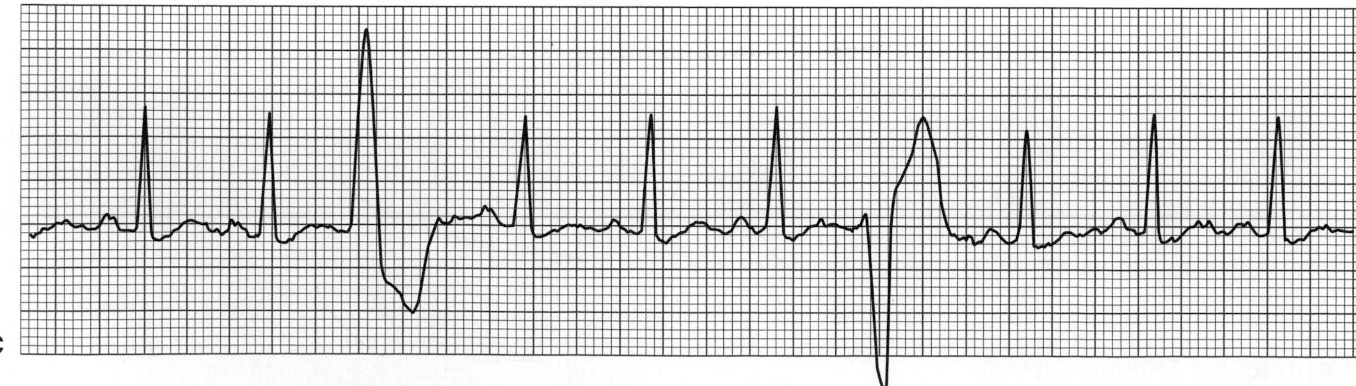

Fig. 12-14 PVC patterns. **A,** Ventricular bigeminy. **B,** Ventricular couplet. **C,** Multifocal PVCs.

QRS complex appears early, interrupting the established rhythm. An electrical pause often follows a PVC, after which the established rhythm resumes. Clinically, a PVC may be perceived by a patient as a skipped beat or a palpitation. If a PVC occurs during pulse monitoring, the examiner will likely sense a skipped, or irregular, beat.

PVCs sometimes happen in patterns, occurring at regular intervals (Figure 12-14). A PVC occurs in ventricular bigeminy on every second beat (Figure 12-14, *A*), in ventricular trigeminy on every third beat, and in ventricular quadrigeminy on every fourth beat. With these rhythms, a regularly irregular pattern may be noted during pulse monitoring.

PVCs may also occur twice in succession as a ventricular couplet, as seen in Figure 12-14, *B*.

PVCs that originate from more than one ectopic focus are termed multifocal PVCs. In this circumstance, the waveforms will have different morphologies according to the locations of the ectopic foci. Remember that the positive or negative deflection of the waveform depends on the direction of depolarization, as viewed by the lead used for monitoring. In Figure 12-14, *C*, the first PVC shown has an initial positive deflection, whereas the second PVC seen has an initial negative deflection. Each of these PVCs comes from a different ectopic focus.

The physical therapist's decision-making process in response to observation of ventricular ectopic beats is complex and may not be grasped easily by the entry-level practitioner. Factors such as the presence or absence of symptoms, the acuity of the patient, and whether the rhythm is a new finding all influence a clinical response. The presence of a pattern such as bigeminy, couplets, or a multifocal pattern is also considered. Further elucidation of clinical responses to most dysrhythmias is beyond the scope of this chapter; however, some dysrhythmias demand an immediate response once they have been observed.

Ventricular tachycardia (V-tach, or VT) (Figure 12-15) is defined as three or more consecutive PVCs at a rate greater than 100 beats per minute.[14,15] This is a serious and potentially lethal dysrhythmia that requires that emergency measures be undertaken. During V-tach all complexes are ventricular in origin. V-tach sometimes occurs in runs of three or more ectopic complexes followed by reversion to the baseline rhythm, or it may be sustained. Effective circulation may be preserved, or it may be seriously compromised or absent in sustained V-tach. A patient may be asymptomatic, particularly if only a brief run of V-tach was experienced. If VT is sustained, the patient may be asymptomatic, symptomatic, or unconscious and pulseless. The physical therapist's response depends on the rhythm (regardless of whether it is sustained) and on whether the patient is symptomatic or conscious. Clinical responses range from cessation of activity, ongoing patient monitoring, and immediate notification of a physician to a full code.

Ventricular fibrillation (V-fib) is a lethal dysrhythmia accompanied by immediate loss of consciousness and loss of circulation (i.e., cardiac arrest). It is characterized by disorganized, simultaneous firing of multiple, ectopic ventricular foci and there is no organized rhythm (Figure 12-16). Effective ventricular contraction ceases and cardiopulmonary resuscitation is indicated until defibrillation is available. Death follows unless defibrillation with an automated external defibrillator (AED) or other device successfully restores an effective rhythm. Conditions that render the myocardium vulnerable to ventricular fibrillation include V-tach, myocardial ischemia or infarction, dilation of the heart, hyperkalemia, and electric shock.[3]

If not successfully treated, V-fib may further degenerate into asystole, which indicates complete absence of ventricular electrical activity (see Figure 12-16). Asystole may also occur as a primary event. This is known colloquially as flat-line rhythm. Like ventricular fibrillation, asystole requires that cardiopulmonary resuscitation begin immediately to save the patient's life.

Care must be taken to distinguish an apparent lethal dysrhythmia from lead disconnection or movement artifact. Unwary therapists have hastily summoned help upon

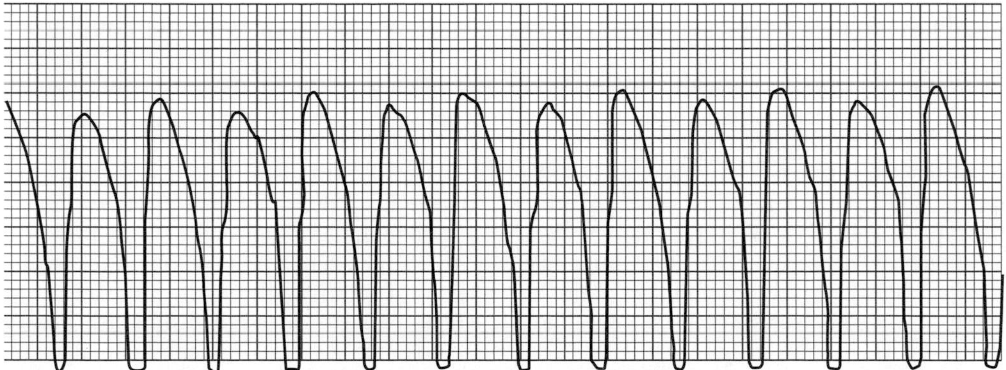

Fig. 12-15 Ventricular tachycardia.

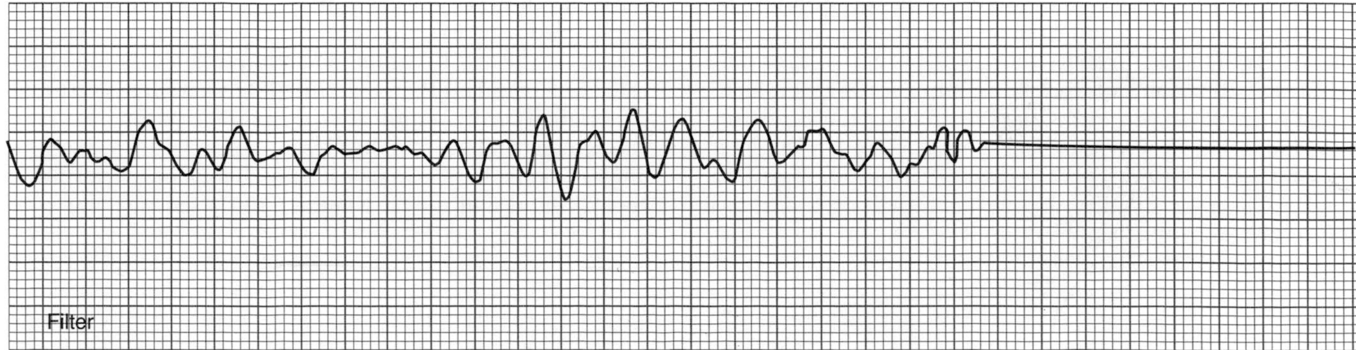

Fig. 12-16 Ventricular fibrillation degenerating into asystole.

observing V-fib or asystole, only to feel foolish when a lead is reattached to the patient and normal rhythm is restored. These dysrhythmias are always accompanied by loss of consciousness and pulse; therefore, a clinician should assess the patient before taking action. Similarly, during activity or exercise, movement artifact may easily be mistaken for V-tach. By assessing the patient and asking him or her to hold still, the issue may be quickly resolved.

Conduction Blocks

Conduction blocks are another type of ECG abnormality with which physical therapists should be familiar. The propagation of a cardiac impulse may be inhibited or terminated along the conduction pathway. Blockage can occur at the sinus node, between the atria and ventricles, or within the ventricular conduction system. Sinus block occurs if the impulse cannot propagate beyond the sinus node. In this case, the AV junction usually takes over as the pacemaker, and a junctional rhythm is seen with the absence of P waves.

More common are the AV blocks (Figure 12-17). They are ranked as first-, second-, or third-degree, depending on the extent of delay or obstruction of the cardiac impulse between the atria and ventricles. First-degree AV block is characterized by a prolongation of the P-R interval beyond its normal 0.2 second (Figure 12-17, *A*). Remember that the P-R interval is measured from the *beginning* of the P wave to the *beginning* of the QRS complex. Each impulse is delayed between the atria and ventricles, but each eventually reaches the ventricular conduction system, resulting in a normal QRS complex. Thus for each P wave, there is a QRS complex; therefore the conduction ratio is 1 : 1.

Second-degree AV block takes two forms, although in each form there are some sinus impulses that are not conducted to the ventricles. In second-degree block Mobitz type 1, also known as Wenckebach periodicity or block, the P-R interval lengthens progressively until a P wave fails to conduct to the ventricles (Figure 12-17, *B1*). Notice how the first three P-R intervals lengthen until, after the fourth P wave, a QRS complex fails to appear. The cycle then repeats itself. Second-degree block Mobitz type 2 (Figure 12-17, *B2*) is characterized by a fixed P-R interval with a "dropped" QRS following every second, third, or fourth P wave. The conduction ratio in Figure 12-17, *B2* is 3 : 1, or three P waves for each QRS complex. Both first- and second-degree AV blocks are considered to be incomplete heart blocks.

Third-degree AV block, or complete heart block, is also known as AV dissociation. In this rhythm, P waves are present, but there is no relationship between P waves and QRS complexes. Typically, a longer strip of rhythm is required to make this diagnosis. P waves may be superimposed on QRS complexes, but none of the sinus impulses are conducted to the ventricles; the atria and ventricles are contracting independently of each other. In the absence of clinical intervention such as artificial pacing (Figure 12-17, *C*), ventricular depolarization is initiated by a junctional or ventricular pacemaker.

Clinically, AV blocks range in severity from benign, as is usually the case with first-degree AV block, to potentially lethal. Whether hemodynamic compromise occurs depends on the extent of impairment of cardiac output caused by too slow a rate of ventricular contraction.[4] Slow rates of ventricular contraction may cause lightheadedness or syncope. In most cases of third-degree block, treatment now includes the implantation of an artificial pacemaker. In Figure 12-17, C, the needle-like spikes indicate that an artificial pacemaker is depolarizing the ventricles at a rate of 60 beats per minute.

Myocardial Ischemia or Infarction

The ECG provides much more information than that gleaned from dysrhythmia analysis. Because physical therapists often treat patients with coronary heart disease, information regarding myocardial ischemia or infarction (MI) is also of interest. Although physical therapists do not medically diagnose myocardial ischemia or MI, they should have a working knowledge of its electrocardiographic evidence and the consequences of ischemia. During myocardial ischemia, blood flow to a portion of myocardium is compromised, resulting in alteration of myocardial metabolism. In MI, a portion of myocardium has died, but an adjacent zone of ischemic myocardial cells endures. These ischemic cells may remain leaky and partially depolarized. A persistent current flows from the injured regions to the healthy regions (that are fully polarized), resulting in a current of injury, which is seen as a shift in the S-T segment above or below the isoelectric line (Figure 12-18).[3,8] S-T segment shifts have significant diagnostic value. For example, S-T segment elevation (Figure 12-18, *A*) is associated with transmural MI, whereas S-T segment depression (Figure 12-18, *B*) is associated with nontransmural or subendocardial MI. Also, the onset of S-T segment depression during activity is often considered diagnostic of myocardial ischemia.[12,16] Figure 12-18, *B* is an example of exercise-induced S-T segment depression observed in one lead during exercise.

The following is a brief discussion of other abnormalities of the ECG observed in coronary artery disease (CAD). A prominent, pathological Q wave is indicative of a transmural MI.[8,12] Indeed, non-Q is synonymous with nontransmural, in terms of MI. In addition, the presence of a prominent Q wave (Figure 12-19) does not distinguish between an old and an acute event. Figure 12-20 shows an algorithm for the classification of ischemia and MI based on the ECG.[16]

The T wave itself may also undergo changes during myocardial ischemia or MI. During ischemia, for example, the T wave may invert as a result of prolongation of repolarization.[3] Similarly, during MI, changes in the T wave may evolve with the infarct, at first becoming indistinguishable within an elevated S-T segment, then inverting, then perhaps reverting to the original configuration after the passage of time. Although ST segment changes and the presence of a Q wave are compelling indicators for the diagnosis of ischemia or MI, it must be kept in mind that they are neither 100% sensitive nor 100% specific.

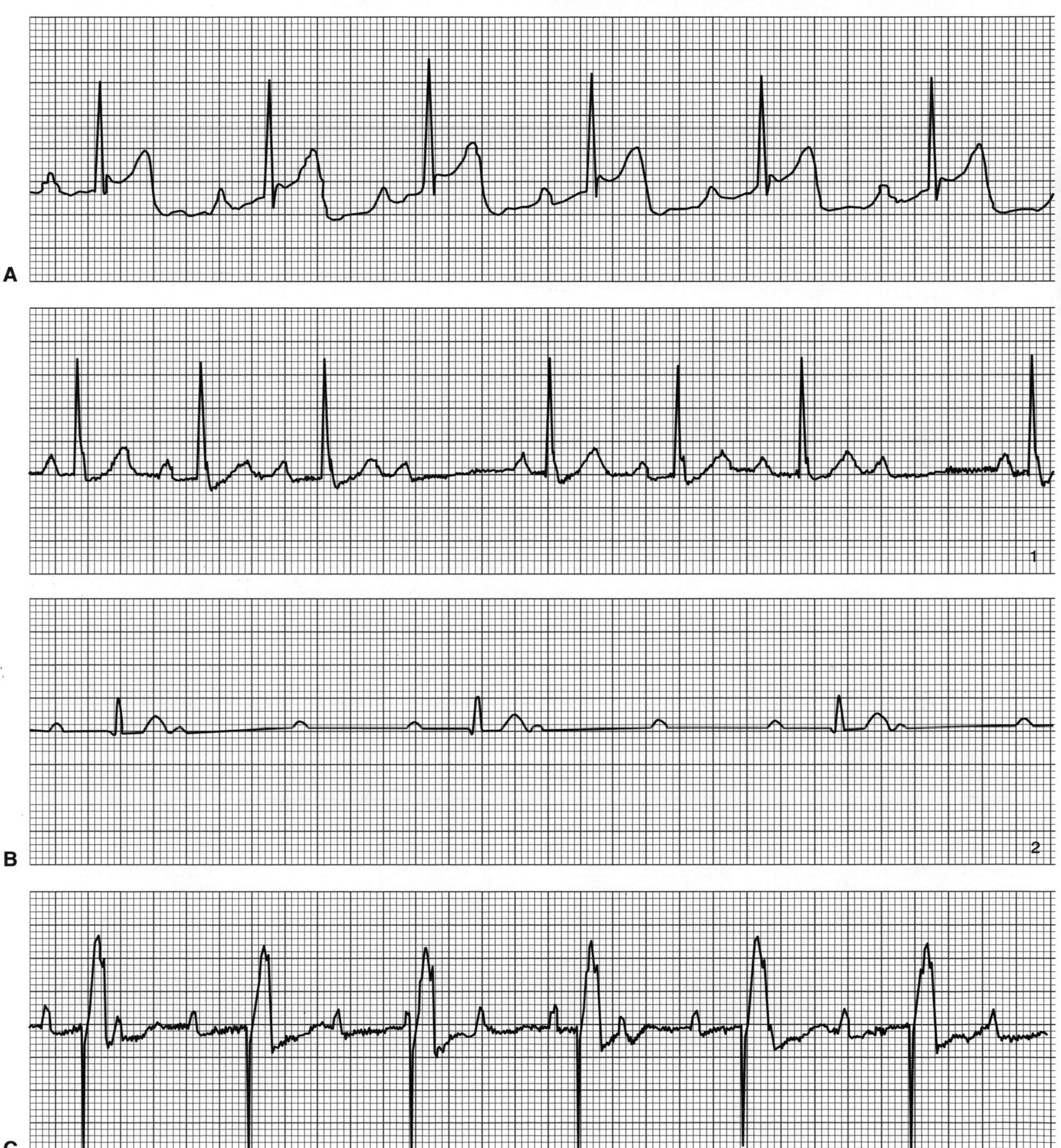

Fig. 12-17 AV blocks. **A,** First-degree AV block. **B,** Second-degree AV block: *1,* Mobitz type 1; *2,* Mobitz type 2. **C,** Third-degree AV block with ventricular pacing.

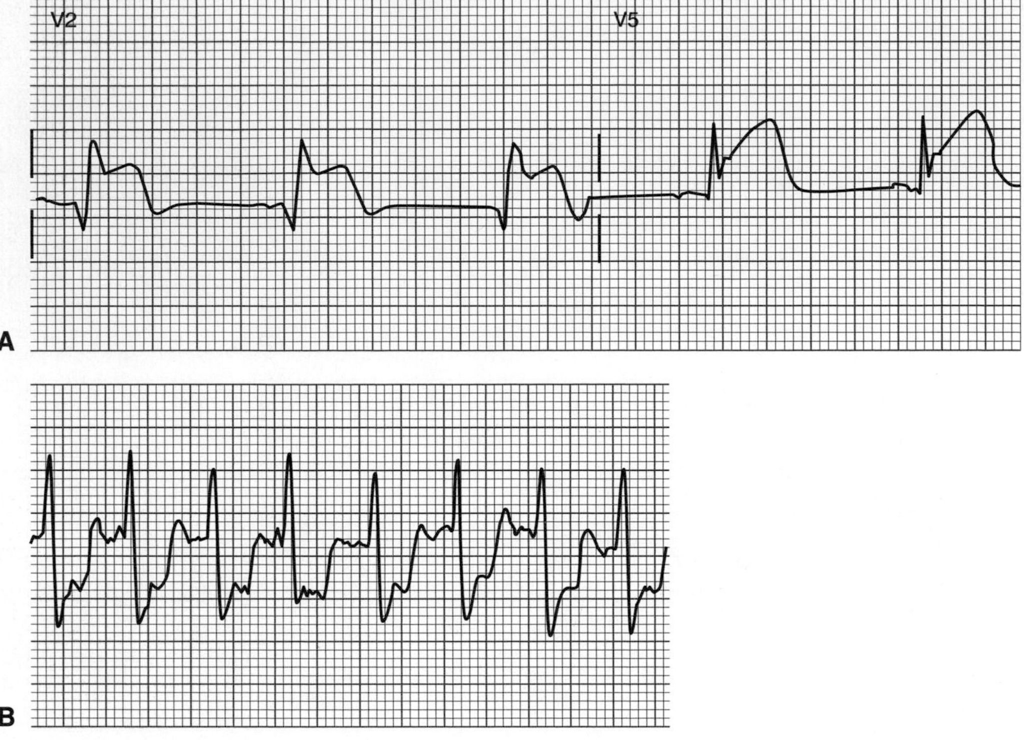

Fig. 12-18 S-T segments. **A,** Elevation during myocardial infarction. **B,** Depression during exercise.

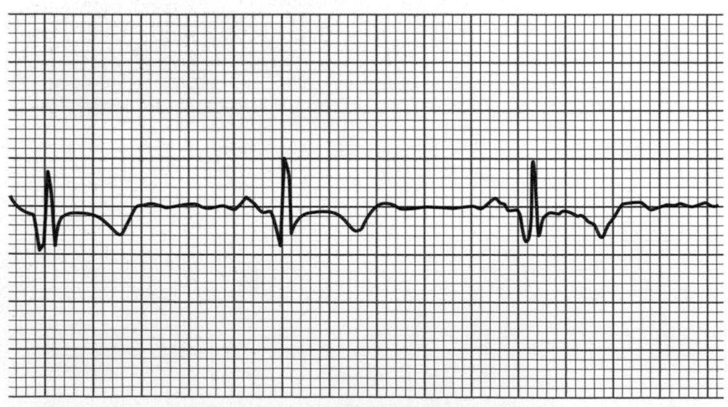

Fig. 12-19 Significant Q wave.

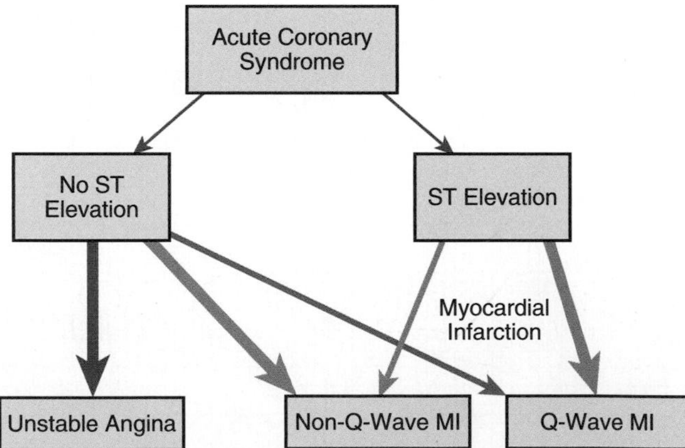

Fig. 12-20 Algorithm for ECG diagnosis of ischemia or acute myocardial infarction. *(From Antman EM, Anbe DT, Armstrong PW, et al. ACC/AHA guidelines for the management of patients with ST-elevation myocardial infarction; A report of the American College of Cardiology/American Heart Association Task Force on Practice Guidelines [Committee to Revise the 1999 Guidelines for the Management of patients with acute myocardial infarction].* Circulation *110(5):588-636, 2004.)*

Summary

Understanding the significance of a normal ECG and abnormal tracing is fundamental to contemporary physical therapy practice. Changes in cardiac rhythm can occur during activity and exercise, as well as at rest. The physical therapist needs to understand the factors that alter ECG rhythm (pathological, such as ischemia and/or impaired cardiac neural conduction system, and nonpathological, such as stress and coffee) and how the capacity to respond to physical activity and exercise can be altered. Optimal electromechanical coupling within the myocardium helps ensure that cardiac output is appropriate to supply the working muscles and tissues with the oxygen they require. Also, such knowledge informs the physical therapist about monitoring precautions and the level of safety that needs to be observed.

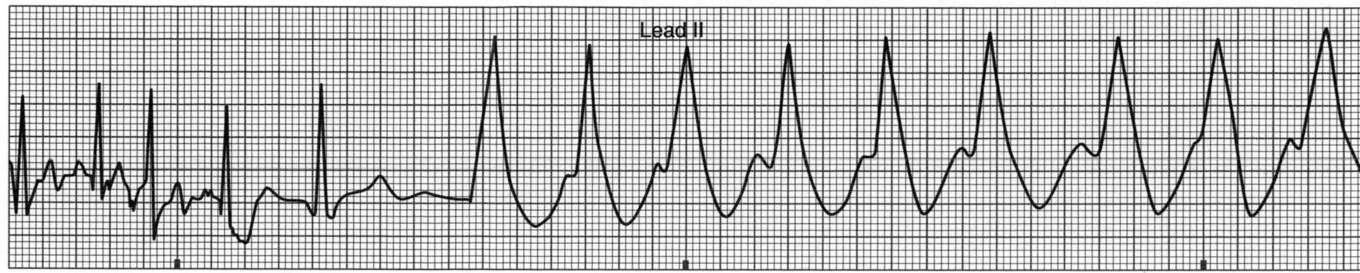

Fig. 12-21 ECG tracing for Case Study 1.

Cases Studies

Case Study 1

An 81-year-old man is referred to physical therapy 2 days after angioplasty for treatment of coronary heart disease and blockages in the left circumflex and diagonal arteries. The patient has had an uncomplicated course and no cardiac arrhythmias since surgery. He is evaluated in the physical therapy gym and given a submaximal predictive treadmill test with electrocardiogram monitoring. The test consists of walking a 5% grade at 3 mph for 5 minutes. His ECG is normal at rest, but at 4 minutes of ambulation he complains of shortness of breath and requests that the test be stopped. The ECG in the last 6 seconds of ambulation is shown below (Figure 12-21). Answer the questions related to these findings. The answers can be found after the Review Questions.

1. Identify this dysrhythmia.
2. What are the hemodynamic and functional consequences of this dysrhythmia?
3. What action should be taken by the evaluating physical therapist?

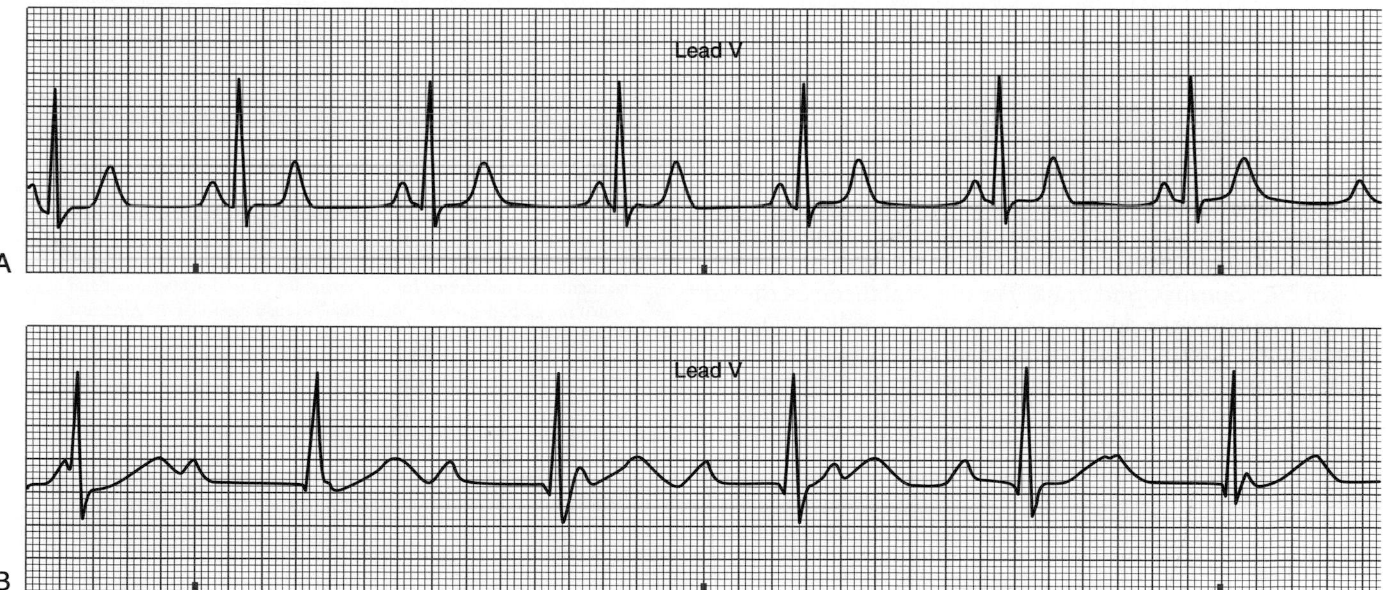

Fig. 12-22 ECG tracing for Case Study 2. **A,** Normal ECG. **B,** Typical dysrhythmia during 24-hour Holter monitoring.

Case Study 2

A 20-year-old basketball player is referred to a sports medicine clinic for a medical examination because of a knee injury. The physical examination shows mild tenderness and edema of the right knee but no other medical problems. During the examination by the physician, the athlete confides that he often experiences dizziness throughout the day. The physician performs a single-lead electrocardiogram and exercise test at that time. The test shows sinus bradycardia at rest and a normal response to exercise (Figure 12-22, *A*). The patient is sent home with a Holter monitor (a device that records an ECG continuously over a 24-hour period). Analysis of the recording reveals that the pattern in Figure 12-22, *B*, is occurring sporadically approximately 25% of the time.

1. Identify this dysrhythmia and determine the patient's heart rate (3-second intervals are marked on the strip).
2. What are the possible hemodynamic consequences when this dysrhythmia occurs, and how could it lead to the patient's complaint of dizziness?

Review Questions

1. How may the following dysrhythmias be perceived by a clinician without the benefit of ECG monitoring? How may they be perceived by a patient?
   Atrial fibrillation
   Supraventricular tachycardia
   Premature ventricular contractions
   Third-degree AV block
   Ventricular fibrillation
2. What determines the clinical significance of a dysrhythmia?
3. What property of the SA node allows it to pace the heart? Under what conditions do other portions of the conduction system act as pacemakers?
4. Does an impulse originating within the ventricular myocardium generate an effective myocardial contraction? If not, why not?
5. Why is ECG monitoring indicated after myocardial infarction?
6. What event is represented by each of the following:
   P wave
   QRS complex
   T wave
   U wave
7. What is the possible clinical significance of S-T segment depression? Of S-T segment elevation? What symptoms might be anticipated in the presence of those conditions?

Answers to Case Study 1:

The ECG shows the beginning of a run of ventricular tachycardia with a rate of approximately 100 beats per minute. The consequences of this dysrhythmia range from asymptomatic to signs and symptoms of angina and acute heart failure to loss of consciousness and death. The physical therapist should help the patient to lie down as quickly, but as safely, as possible in a supine position and continue to observe and monitor him. Depending on the patient's symptoms and whether the V-tach is sustained, the therapist should either notify the physician immediately and discuss the course of action or call a code.

Answers to Case Study 2:

Careful inspection of panel B in Figure 12-22 reveals that there is complete dissociation of the ventricular rhythm from the atrial rhythm, indicating third-degree or complete heart block. The rhythm strip shows that a regular atrial pattern (P waves) is superimposed on a regular ventricular rhythm (QRS complexes), but the QRS complexes do not follow the P waves. The heart rate is the ventricular rate and therefore approximately 40 beats per minute. Third-degree heart block results in asynchrony between the atrial ejection and the ventricular filling. In addition, the ventricular rate is typically very low and the combined effects of decreased filling and low heart rate may cause decreased blood pressure. The resulting hypotension, particularly during changes in position or movement, may lead to dizziness.

References

1. Roden DM, Balser JR, George AL, Anderson ME: Cardiac ion channels. *Annual Reviews in Physiology* 64:431–475, 2002.
2. Koeppen BM, Stanton BA, editors: *Berne & Levy physiology*, ed 6, Philadelphia, 2010, Mosby Inc.
3. Guyton AC, Hall JE: *Textbook of medical physiology*, Philadelphia, 2006, WB Saunders.
4. Huszar RJ: *Basic dysrhythmias, interpretation and management*, ed 3, St. Louis, 2002, Mosby.
5. Surawicz B: U wave: facts, hypotheses, misconceptions, and misnomers. *Journal of Cardiovascular Electrophysiology* 9:1217–1228, 1998.
6. Kodma K, Hiasa G, Ohtsuka T, et al: Transient U wave inversion during treadmill exercise testing in patients with left anterior descending coronary artery disease. *Angiology* 51:581–589, 2000.
7. Ritsema van Eck HJ, Kors JA, Herpen G: The elusive U wave: a simple explanation of its genesis. *Journal of Electrocardiology* 36:133–137, 2003.
8. Opie LH: *Heart physiology, from cell to circulation*, ed 4, Philadelphia, 2004, Lippincott Williams and Wilkins.
9. American College of Sports Medicine: *Guidelines for exercise testing and prescription*, Baltimore, Md, ed 8, 2009, Lippincott Williams & Wilkins.
10. Cummins RO, editor: *Advanced cardiac life support: principles and practice (ACLS: the reference textbook)*, Dallas, 2003, American Heart Association.
11. Brown KR, Jacobson S: *Mastering dysrhythmias: a problem-solving guide*, Philadelphia, 1988, FA Davis.
12. American College of Cardiology, American Heart Association: Key data elements and definitions for measuring the clinical management and outcomes of patients with atrial fibrillation: a report of the American College of Cardiology. ACC/AHA, 204. doi:10.1016/j.jacc.2004.06.04, 2004.
13. Bhushan M, Asirvatham SJ: The conundrum of ventricular arrhythmia and cardiomyopathy: which abnormality came first? *Curr Heart Fail Rep* 6(1):7–13, 2009.
14. Akhtar M: Clinical spectrum of ventricular tachycardia. *Circulation* 82:1561–1573, 1990.
15. Samie FH, Jalife J: Mechanisms underlying ventricular tachycardia and its transition to ventricular fibrillation in the structurally normal heart. *Cardiovascular Research* 50:242–250, 2001.
16. American College of Cardiology, European Society of Cardiology: Myocardial infarction redefined—a consensus document of the Joint European Society of Cardiology/American College of Cardiology. http://www.acc.org/clinical/consensus/mi%5Fredefined/redefined.pdf; retrieved January 7, 2005, 2000.

Chapter 13 II

Multisystem Assessment and Laboratory Investigations

Elizabeth Dean

KEY TERMS

Blood
Endocrine function
Heart
Immune function
Kidneys
Liver
Lungs
Multisystem assessment
Peripheral vascular circulation

CHAPTER OUTLINE

The purpose of this chapter is to describe the rationale for multisystem assessment in the patient managed for cardiovascular and pulmonary dysfunction and to discuss some common laboratory tests related to multisystem assessment. The bases of tests that assess the function of the following organ systems are presented: blood, pulmonary, cardiac, peripheral vascular, kidney, endocrine, liver, and immune systems. The normal ranges are given for common laboratory tests and investigations. The information in this chapter is supplemental to the elements of the cardiovascular and pulmonary assessments and related laboratory investigations described in other chapters of Part II.

The oxygen transport system affects and is affected by virtually every organ system in the body. The signs and symptoms of systemic disease can mimic other conditions, including cardiovascular and pulmonary dysfunction, which is treated by physical therapists. Therefore the physical therapist must be able to differentiate among these presentations to determine what treatment, if any, is indicated, and what treatments may be contraindicated. Knowledge of multisystem function helps to confirm a diagnosis, as well as to predict a patient's response to treatment and his or her recovery and prognosis. In addition, this information is crucial in guiding clinical decision making, that is, refining and modifying treatment prescription. These abilities have become increasingly important in this era of professional accountability and with the advent of direct patient access.

Rationale for Multisystem Assessment

The cardiovascular and pulmonary systems support cellular respiration and life. Thus every system and every cell in the body is affected by the adequacy of oxygen transport, which is dependent on cardiovascular and pulmonary function. In addition, these systems are affected by virtually every other system in the body. The cardiovascular and pulmonary physical therapist, therefore, needs thorough knowledge of multisystem function and of the interdependence of the organ systems, as well as the ability to assess multisystem function and to integrate this information into a comprehensive and progressive treatment plan.

The lungs and heart are anatomically and physiologically interdependent, and they function as a unit to transport oxygen via the peripheral circulation so as to perfuse and nourish tissues. Tissue homeostasis is dependent on the adequacy of the anatomy and physiology of the blood. The adequacy of peripheral perfusion determines the adequacy of the function of all organ systems in the body. Therefore knowledge of the failure of the various organ systems can reflect impaired oxygen transport or may identify a threat to oxygen transport.

The elements of laboratory evaluation and testing, as well as the normal values, have been compiled from the following sources: Dean (1999)[1]; Fischbach (2004)[2]; Hall (2010)[3]; Jacobs et al (2001)[4]; Le Fever Kee (2000)[5]; Pagana and Pagana (2002)[6]; and Wallach (2000)[7].

Elements of Multisystem Assessment

Blood

Some common blood tests are listed in Table 13-1, along with their normal values.

The average blood volume consists of 5 L of blood—3 L of plasma and 2 L of cells. Plasma is the medium that suspends and transports blood cells. The complete blood count (CBC) is one of the most commonly ordered laboratory procedures. This basic screening test helps to establish the patient's diagnosis, treatment response, recovery, and prognosis. The CBC includes the red blood cell count (RBC), a variety of red blood cell indices, differential white blood cell count (WBC), hematocrit (Hct), hemoglobin (Hgb), and platelet count.

Tests of coagulation and hemostasis reflect bleeding pathology, which often involves injury of blood vessels and cells. Damage to the blood vessel wall leads to constriction, a primary mechanism of hemostasis. Circulating platelets adhere to exposed subendothelial tissues, which can predispose thrombus formation.

The fluidity of the blood is regulated by the facilitation and the inhibition of thrombin formation. When these two processes are in balance, the blood has an optimal consistency; it is neither too thick nor too thin. This allows blood to flow optimally through the circulation without unduly affecting the work of the heart. Blood vessel injury can disrupt this balance and can promote coagulation.

Disseminated intravascular coagulation (DIC) results from an imbalance between the formation and deposition of fibrin, which leads to the formation of thrombi. The continuous production of thrombin causes depletion of the coagulation factors, and bleeding results. Tests used to assess bleeding capacity include thrombin time and fibrin clotting time (partial thromboplastin time [PTT]).

Proteins (amino acids) serve as regulators of metabolism. Examining and measuring proteins provides much useful clinical information because proteins regulate many important physiological functions in the body. Plasma proteins serve as a source of nutrition for the body tissues and function as buffers when combined with hemoglobin.

Albumin, a protein formed in the liver, maintains normal water distribution in the body (colloid osmotic pressure). It transports blood constituents such as ions, pigments, bilirubin, hormones, fatty acids, enzymes, and certain drugs. Approximately 55% of total protein is albumin. The remainder is globulin, which functions in antibody formation, and other plasma proteins (fibrinogen and prothrombin) involved with coagulation.

Two other blood proteins are noteworthy. Hemoglobin A1c or glycated hemoglobin provides a measure of plasma glucose concentration over time, and values over 6% has become a marker for type 2 diabetes mellitus. High values of hemoglobin A1c are associated with complications of diabetes. The C reactive protein is a marker of inflammation. In acute infection it rises markedly. However, perhaps more importantly, this protein is elevated in people with risk factors of or manifestations of chronic lifestyle-related conditions such as ischemic heart disease. The western lifestyle has been described as pro-inflammatory in that lifestyle behaviors such as smoking, high fat diet, inactivity, and stress common in high-income countries such as western countries, contribute to a systemic low-grade inflammatory state. Measures of these proteins are important to the physical therapist to evaluate outcomes of health education and exercise.

Lactic acid, a product of carbohydrate metabolism, is produced when cells receive inadequate oxygen in relation to oxygen demand (anaerobic metabolism). When the production of lactic acid exceeds its removal from the blood by the liver, lactic acid accumulates in the blood.

Cholesterol is used in the production of steroid hormones, bile acids, and cell membranes. Cholesterol is found in muscles, red blood cells, and cell membranes. Low-density and high-density lipoproteins (LDLs and HDLs) transport cholesterol in the blood. High levels of LDLs and low levels of HDLs are associated with atherosclerosis and increased risk for coronary artery disease (CAD).

Electrolyte assessment is based on the electrolyte constituents of a blood or urine sample. Although present in minute quantities, electrolytes are essential in maintaining normal cellular function and homeostasis. The electrolytes that are routinely studied are sodium, potassium, chloride, calcium, phosphorus, and magnesium.

Pulmonary Function

See Chapters 9 and 15 for a detailed description of the assessment of the pulmonary system and its function.

Cardiac Function

A detailed description of the assessment of the cardiac system and its function appears in Chapters 11, 12, and 15.

Peripheral Vascular Function

Assessment of the peripheral vascular circulation is essential to provide information regarding central and peripheral hemodynamic status as well as peripheral tissue perfusion. This assessment is crucial in establishing the integrity of the patient's hemodynamic status at rest and during the physical and exercise stress that is associated with most physical therapy treatments. Laboratory tests include segmental blood pressure studies, skin temperature studies, pulse wave analysis, Doppler ultrasound studies, and arteriography. The physical examination corroborates the results of the laboratory investigations and includes the patient's history; inspection of the integrity of the peripheral circulation, particularly to the extremities; palpation to assess peripheral pulses; and auscultation, which can be helpful in detecting bruits or areas of turbulent blood flow associated with arterial stenoses.

Table 13-1 Common Tests of Multisystem Function and Their Normal Values: Blood Tests

Test	US Unit	SI Unit
Red blood cell count (RBC)		
Men	4.4-6.2 million/µL	4.5-6.2 × 10^{12}/L
Women	4.0-5.5 million/µL	4.0-5.5 × 10^{12}/L
Hemoglobin (Hgb)		
Men	13.6-18 g/dL	8.44-11.17 mmol/L
Women	12-16 g/dL	7.45-9.9 mmol/L
Hemoglobin A1c	<6%	
Hematocrit (Hct)		
Men	39%-51%	0.39-0.59
Women	35%-47%	0.35-0.47
Platelet count	150,000-400,000/mm^3	150-400 × 10^9/L
Prothrombin time (PT)	10-15 seconds	10-15 seconds
Partial thromboplastin time (PTT)	<70 seconds	<70 seconds
White blood cell count (WBCC)*		
Men	4500-11,000/µL	4.5 × 11.0 × 10^9/L
Women	4500-11,000/µL	4.5 × 11.0 × 10^9/L
Erythrocyte sedimentation rate (ESR)		
Men	15-20 mm/hr	
Women	20-30 mm/hr	
Proteins		
Albumin	3.5-5.0 g/dL	35-50 g/L
Alpha$_1$ globulin	0.1-0.4 g/dL	1.0-4.0 g/L
Alpha$_2$ globulin	5.0-10 g/dL	0.5-1.0 g/L
Beta globulin	7.0-12 g/dL	0.7-1-2 g/L
Gamma globulin	8.0-16 g/dL	0.8-1.6 g/L
Fibrinogen	200-400 mg/dL	2.2-4.0 g/L
Lactate		
Venous	0.5-2.2 mEq/L	0.5-2.2 mmol/L
Arterial	0.5-1.6 mEq/L	0.5-1.6 mmol/L
Electrolytes (blood)		
Sodium (Na^+)	136-145 mEq/L	136-145 mmol/L
Potassium (K^+)	3.5-5.3 mEq/L	3.5-5.0 mmol/L
Calcium (Ca^{2+})[†]		
Total	8.2-10.7 mg/dL	2.10-2.70 mmol/L
Ionized	4.45-5.30 mg /dL	1.10-1.30 mmol/L
Chloride (Cl^-)	95-108 mEq/L	95-108 mmol/L
Cholesterol total		
Men ≤40 years	124-270 mg/dL	3.21-699 mmol/L
Men >40 years	151-277 mg/dL	3.91-7.17 mmol/L
Women ≤40 years	122-242 mg/dL	3.16-6.27 mmol/L
Women >40 years	147-303 mg/dL	3.81-7.85 mmol/L
Creatine kinase (total)		
Men	20-200 international units/L	20-200 international units/L
Women	20-180 international units/L	20-180 international units/L
C reactive protein	Normal: <0.8 mg/L Low risk: <1.00 mg/L Average risk: 1.00-3.00 mg/L High risk: >3.00 mg/L	

*Differential WBCC includes counts of neutrophils, eosinophils, basophils, lymphocytes, and monocytes.

[†]Norm 46%-56% of total serum.

Normal values may vary depending on the laboratory performing the measurement. Within-subject variation occurs as a result of age and variations in the pretest standardization procedures.

Some common tests of peripheral vascular function are listed in Table 13-2, along with their normal values.

Kidney Function

Urine consists of the end products of cellular metabolism and is produced by the large volumes of blood (approximately 25% of the cardiac output [CO]) that flow through the kidneys. When the kidneys are compromised, death can ensue within a few days. Although fluid is lost through several routes, the kidneys are primarily responsible for processing and regulating fluid balance in the body.

Urea, the major nonprotein nitrogenous end product of protein catabolism, is measured in the blood as blood urea nitrogen (BUN). The urea is then carried to the kidneys by the blood to be excreted in the urine.

Creatinine is a byproduct in the breakdown of muscle creatine phosphate resulting from energy metabolism. The production of creatinine is constant as long as muscle mass is constant. Kidney dysfunction reduces the excretion of creatinine, resulting in increased levels of blood creatinine. Analysis of urine for creatinine provides an index of kidney function.

Increased osmolality stimulates the secretion of antidiuretic hormone (ADH) that acts on renal tubules. This results in the reabsorption of water, more concentrated urine, and less concentrated serum.

Some common tests of kidney function are listed in Table 13-3, along with their normal values.

Endocrine Function

Endocrine glands are responsible for producing the substances and neuromediators responsible for maintaining homeostasis and enabling the body to adapt when physically and psychologically challenged or perturbed from a resting state. The key endocrine glands are the pancreas, the thyroid gland, and the adrenal glands. Endocrine glands regulate metabolism and are responsible for increasing blood flow and pressure and for reducing vascular resistance when metabolic demands increase.

Some common tests of endocrine function are listed in Table 13-4, along with their normal values.

Pancreatic Function and Insulin Production

Insulin, a hormone produced in the pancreas by the beta cells of the islets of Langerhans, regulates the metabolism of carbohydrates (as do the liver, adipose tissues, muscles, and other target cells) and is responsible for maintaining a constant level of blood glucose. The rate of insulin secretion is determined primarily by the level of blood glucose perfusing the pancreas and also by hormonal status, the autonomic nervous system, nutritional status, smoking, restricted mobility, physical stress such as traumatic insult to the body during illness and injury, and pharmacological agents.

Table 13-2 Common Tests of Multisystem Function and Their Normal Values: Tests of Peripheral Vascular Function

Test	Normal Values
Skin temperature	Ranges from ambient temperature to 30° C (86° F)
Ankle systolic pressures	97% of brachial pressure
Peripheral pulses	Apex heart rate
Capillary filling after quick pressure over the nail bed	Instantaneous filling

Table 13-3 Common Tests of Multisystem Function and Their Normal Values: Tests of Kidney Function

Test	US Unit	SI Unit
Blood urea nitrogen (BUN)	5-20 mg/dL	1.8-7.1 mmol/L
Creatinine (urine)		
Men	<40 mg/24 hr	0-307 μmol/day
Women	<80 mg/24 hr	0-615 μmol/day

Normal values may vary depending on the laboratory performing the measurement. Within-subject variation occurs because of age and variations in the pretest standardization procedures.

Table 13-4 Common Tests of Multisystem Functions and Their Normal Values: Tests of Endocrine Function

Test	US Unit	SI Unit
PANCREATIC FUNCTION		
Glucose tolerance test		
Fasting glucose	<110 mg/dL	<6.1 mmol/L
At 2 hr glucose	<140 mg/dL	<7.8 mmol/L
Insulin		
12 hr fasting	<17 international units/mL or 110 mg/L	117 pmol/L
Amylase		
Blood level	30-110 units/L	30-110 units/L
THYROID FUNCTION		
Total thyroxine (T_4)	4.5-12.0 mcg/dL	58.5-155 nmol/L
Total triiodothyronine (T_3)	80-230 mcg/dL	1.2-3.5 nmol/L
ADRENAL FUNCTION		
Epinephrine	0-140 pg/mL	0-762 pmol/L
Norepinephrine	200-1700 pg/mL	1088-9256 pmol/L
Cortisol		
Morning	5-28 mcg/dL	138-773 nmol/L
Evening	2-14 mcg/dL	55-386 nmol/L

Normal values may vary depending on the laboratory performing the measurement. Within-subject variation is dependent on age and variations in the pretest standardization procedures.

Amylase is an enzyme produced in the salivary glands, pancreas, and liver; it converts starch to sugar. Inflammation of the pancreas or salivary glands results in more of the enzyme entering the blood. The amylase test is used to diagnose and monitor the treatment of acute pancreatitis.

Thyroid

The function of the thyroid gland is to take iodine from the circulating blood, combine it with amino acid tyrosine, and convert it into the thyroid hormones thyroxine (T_4) and triiodothyronine (T_3). Thyroid hormones have a profound effect on metabolic rate. Increased metabolism causes more rapid use of oxygen than normal and causes greater quantities of metabolic end products to be released from the tissues. These effects cause vasodilation in most of the body tissues, thus increasing blood flow. An increase in the thyroid hormones increases cardiac output, heart rate, force of cardiac contraction, blood volume, arterial blood pressure, oxygen consumption, and carbon dioxide (CO_2) production; hence there is an increase in the rate and depth of breathing and increased appetite, food intake, and gastrointestinal motility. The thyroid gland also stores T_3 and T_4 until they are released into the blood stream under the influence of thyroid-stimulating hormone (TSH) from the pituitary gland.

Adrenal Function

Catecholamines, epinephrine, and norepinephrine are produced by the adrenal medulla of the adrenal glands. Urine samples are used to test for these important vasoactive neurotransmitters in the investigation of various disorders. In addition to their vasoactive properties, the catecholamines are essential in stimulating the sympathetic response in the fight-or-flight mechanism.

Cortisol is produced by the adrenal cortex of the adrenal glands and is involved with metabolism of carbohydrate, protein, and fat. In addition, it inhibits the action of insulin and thus the uptake of glucose by the cells. The normal secretion of cortisol varies diurnally (i.e., it is high in the morning and low in the evening). In addition, cortisol is a stress hormone.

Liver Function

Liver function is especially important in that dysfunction of this organ can be life-threatening. The liver has a primary role in carbohydrate and protein metabolism; it produces bile and is responsible for detoxification of the blood. Its function is assessed by tests of liver enzymes such as amylase and alkaline phosphatase.

Some common tests of liver function are listed in Table 13-5, along with their normal values.

Table 13-5 Common Tests of Multisystem Function and Their Normal Values: Tests of Liver Function

Test	US Units	SI Units
Alkaline phosphatase	44-147 units/L	44-147 units/L
Bilirubin		
Direct	0.0-0.3 mg/dL	1.7-5.1 μmol/L
Indirect	0.1-1-0 mg/dL	1.7-17.1 μmol/L

Normal values may vary depending on the laboratory performing the measurement. Within-subject variation occurs as a result of age and variations in the pretest standardization procedures.

Immunological Function

Immunological function is dependent on the adequacy of the function of several tissues and organs—namely, bone marrow, the thymus gland, the lymph nodes, and the vessels of the lymphatic system, spleen, tonsils, and intestinal lymphoid tissue. Immunological function can break down if insufficient protective immune factors are produced, or if the system is overwhelmed by an invading organism for which the body has inappropriate or insufficient resistance.

Some common tests of immunological function are listed in Table 13-6, along with their normal values. Specific detailed accounts of immmunodiagnostic studies and tests for autoimmune deficiencies are beyond the scope of this chapter but can be reviewed in Fischbach (2004)[2] and Le Fever Kee (2000)[5].

Table 13-6 Common Tests of Multisystem Function and Their Normal Values: Tests of Immunological Function

	Differential White Blood Cell Count	
	Absolute Value (cells/μL)	**Relative Value (by %)**
Neutrophils	2500-8000	55-70
Lymphocytes	1000-4000	20-40
Monocytes	100-700	2-8
Eosinophils	50-500	1-4
Basophils	25-100	0.5-1

Normal values may vary depending on the laboratory performing the measurement. Within-subject variation occurs from age and variations in the pretest standardization procedures.

Summary

This chapter describes the rationale for multisystem assessment in the patient being managed for cardiovascular and pulmonary dysfunction and discusses some common tests of multisystem function. The cardiovascular and pulmonary systems affect, and are affected by, virtually every other organ system in the body. Thus primary cardiovascular and pulmonary dysfunction can lead to complications in many organ systems and vice versa; dysfunction of other organ systems can have cardiovascular and pulmonary manifestations. In addition, the signs and symptoms of systemic conditions can mimic other conditions treated by physical therapists. Therefore the physical therapist must be able to differentiate among these presentations in order to determine whether a pathology will respond to management by physical therapy, what treatments are not indicated, and what treatments may be contraindicated. Multisystem monitoring provides the fundamental information needed to guide clinical decision making, that is, to refine and progress the treatment prescription. These abilities are essential in contemporary physical therapy practice.

Review Questions

For each of the following types of tests assessing organ system function, (a) describe the test(s) and (b) explain the clinical implications of high or low values for the physical therapist.

1. Describe blood composition tests.
2. Describe pulmonary function tests.
3. Describe tests of heart function.
4. Describe tests of peripheral vascular function.
5. Describe tests of kidney function.
6. Describe tests of endocrine function.
7. Describe tests of liver function.
8. Describe tests of immune function.

References

1. Dean E: Preferred practice patterns in cardiopulmonary physical therapy: a guide to physiologic measures. *Cardiopulmonary Physical Therapy Journal* 10:124–134, 1999.
2. Fischbach F, Dunning MB: *A manual of laboratory diagnostic tests*, ed 8, Philadelphia, 2008, Lippincott Williams & Wilkins.
3. Guyton AC, Hall JE: *Textbook of medical physiology*, ed 12, Philadelphia, 2010, Elsevier.
4. Jacobs DS, Kasten BL, Demott WR: *Laboratory test handbook*, ed 5, Cleveland, Ohio, 2001, Lexi-Comp.
5. Le Fever Kee J: *Handbook of laboratory and diagnostic tests with nursing implications*, ed 6, Paramus, NJ, 2001, Prentice Hall.
6. Pagana KD, Pagana TJ: *Mosby's diagnostic and laboratory test reference*, ed 8, Philadelphia, 2006, Elsevier.
7. Wallach J: Interpretation of diagnostic tests: a synopsis of laboratory medicine, ed 8, Philadelphia, 2006, Lippincott Williams & Wilkins.

Chapter 14

II

Special Tests

Gail M. Huber

KEY TERMS

Computed tomography
Echocardiography
Ejection fraction
Hibernating myocardium
Magnetic resonance imaging
Myocardial viability
Radionuclide angiography
Radionuclide imaging
Stunned myocardium
Ventilation-perfusion scan

CHAPTER OUTLINE

The medical workup of a patient with cardiac or pulmonary disease uses many tools. The patient interview, physical examination, chest x-ray, and electrocardiogram (ECG) can provide adequate information to make a diagnosis. However, when the diagnosis remains unclear, special tests that use more complex technology are required. These special tests may be invasive or noninvasive. Current clinical practice guidelines recommend that noninvasive tests be performed before invasive tests such as angiography.[1] Nuclear medicine offers a variety of noninvasive tests for evaluation of cardiac and pulmonary function. Echocardiography, which is particularly useful in children, is another noninvasive method that provides information about the cardiovascular system, including valve function, ventricular performance, and estimation of filling pressures. In comparison with cardiovascular tests, special tests of the respiratory system are less commonly required in the initial diagnosis and treatment of disease. The generally high-quality information obtained from standard x-ray examination in combination with the patient's respiratory symptoms, pulmonary function tests, and the results of the physical examination is usually sufficient, making special tests unnecessary.[2-4]

However, in some cases, an invasive test is still the best choice. Pulmonary and cardiac angiography is not without risk; however, for evaluating blood flow in the heart and lungs, as well as determining cardiac anatomy and direct volume and pressure measures, it is without equal. Another invasive test that is often warranted is transesophageal echocardiography.

Following the initial assessment of the problem, these same special tests may be used to assist in the determination of appropriate therapy and to evaluate prognosis and response to treatment. The noninvasive tests, in particular, are important in determining ongoing surgical, interventional, or medical therapy. Physical therapists must have a strong understanding of all special tests (invasive and noninvasive) and

Table 14-1 **Tests Used for Diagnosis and Prognosis in Ischemic Heart Disease**

Test Type	Sensitivity*	Specificity*	Predictive Accuracy*
Exercise ECG	68%	77%	73%
Duke treadmill score	–	–	80%
Thallium-201 perfusion scan	85%	85%	85%
Technetium-99m sestamibi/SPECT	88%	72%	80%
Adenosine SPECT	90%	82%	85%
Exercise echocardiography	85%	81%	80%
Dobutamine echocardiography	88%	84%	86%
Computed tomography: electron beam computed tomography (EBCT) calcium score	60%	70%	65%

*Data vary according to studies included and characteristics of patient group studied (e.g., number of coronary vessels involved). From Kones R: Recent advances in the management of chronic stable angina. I: Approach to the patient, diagnosis, pathophysiology, risk stratification, and gender disparities. *Vascular Health and Risk Management* 6:635-656, 2010.

how they are used in making a differential diagnosis and determining treatment.

Various factors are involved in the decision of which special tests may be beneficial for a patient. These tests afford different benefits to patients in terms of diagnostic and prognostic accuracy (Table 14-1). Radiation exposure is an additional factor in selection of tests. These tests have helped to clarify our understanding of the physiology and pathophysiology of the cardiovascular and pulmonary system. Therapists need to understand the pathophysiological basis for a patient's movement dysfunctions to select the most appropriate treatment strategies. Many special tests can and are being used in research to evaluate treatment interventions. For example, radiolabeled aerosols are used to evaluate mucociliary clearance, providing a method to evaluate the effectiveness of pulmonary hygiene techniques.[5] Clinically, physical therapists need to use information from the tests to develop a framework for predicting how the patient may respond to a physical therapy intervention. For example, nuclear imaging can provide information about left ventricular ejection fraction. This information helps the therapist determine whether the patient should be stratified into high-risk or low-risk categories. Monitoring of an exercise session may depend on the risk level, and the therapist's interpretation of the patient's response to treatment may be affected by this information.

This chapter will review some of the special technology used to examine the cardiac and pulmonary systems. First, the general method used to acquire data will be described. Next, the type of data available from the technology will be defined, and finally, specific application to the cardiac or pulmonary system will be discussed.

Nuclear Imaging Systems

Physics of Nuclear Imaging

A general view of how nuclear imaging systems work should help the physical therapist understand some of the differences between the wide variety of tests used today. This area of medicine continues to experience rapid growth and change as technology changes the equipment used to perform the test, the radiopharmaceuticals available, and the speed at which data can be acquired and analyzed.

Radionuclide imaging allows for the noninvasive acquisition of images from a variety of body tissues. An imaging system requires three basic parts. The first requirement is a radiopharmaceutical that emits gamma radiation and is taken up by the body tissue of interest. Next, a radiation detector or camera is needed. Finally, computers are required to collect and analyze the data. Thus an image is formed based on the brightness of the tissue, which is proportional to the radiation the tissue has absorbed.[6]

Radionuclides are elements that are unstable; they gain stability by emitting particles or photons. This is called radioactive decay, and gamma radiation is released. Radionuclides are either cyclotron- or generator-produced. The cyclotron accelerates alpha-particles, deuterons, and protons to energies suitable for the production of the required radionuclide.[7] A radionuclide generator is a system of a long-lived parent radionuclide which decays to produce a daughter radionuclide. The system is constructed so that the daughter can be removed (called "milking" the generator) for patient use.[8] A generator system produces short-lived radionuclides.[7]

These elements are often attached to other substrates for transport in the body to the particular tissue of interest. The radionuclide is administered via an intravenous infusion. The elements have differing characteristics, such as energy output and half-life. Because of their varied distribution in the body tissues, they provide different information.

Detection of the radioactive energy emitted by a specific radiopharmaceutical requires a camera. When certain materials are struck by ionizing radiation, light is emitted. A scintillation detector detects this light (Figure 14-1). A gamma camera (a scintillation detector) is able to detect photons exiting the body. It uses a large, collimated crystal monitored by an array of photomultiplier tubes.[9] A collimator is a device that allows only those photons traveling in an appropriate direction to reach the crystal. There are several types of collimators: parallel-hole collimators (most common), pinhole collimators, and converging and diverging collimators. The photomultiplier tube records the amount of light from the

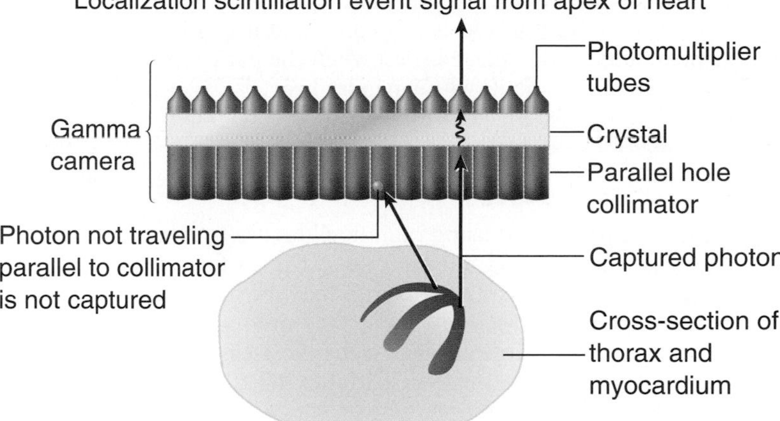

Fig. 14-1 Diagrammatic illustration of a multi-hole collimator where gamma rays admitted in line with the collimator holes are transmitted to the crystal, whereas gamma rays emitted obliquely are absorbed by the collimator septa. *(From Hendee WR, Ritenour R, editors:* Medical imaging physics, *ed 3. St. Louis, 1992, CV Mosby.)*

crystal and converts it into a voltage that is proportional to the intensity of the light.[9] The camera system is connected to a computer that stores the light images. The computer is able to derive two-dimensional images from the data. The newer software algorithms that construct the images have improved, allowing for better spatial resolution, contrast, and overall image quality.[10]

Planar Imaging

A single crystal camera produces a two dimensional or planar image. Multicrystal cameras also produce planar images but are also able to perform fast, dynamic imaging used in first pass and gated studies. Planar images are unable to reflect the depth of an image.[6] Planar imaging may be the only option available for obese patients who do not "fit" the single-photon emission computed tomography (SPECT) camera or for those who cannot remain immobile.[11]

Single-Photon Emission Computed Tomography Imaging

The most common nuclear study of myocardial perfusion is SPECT imaging.[12] Planar images or tomographs are collected by rotating the scintillation detectors (single-, dual-, or triple-head scintillation cameras) around the patient, taking images at 3-degree increments.[10] SPECT images allow for quantification of radioactivity.[6] However, attenuation artifacts (absorption of the radioactive energy by other body tissues, preventing the camera from detecting it) are greater than with planar images, particularly those images involving the inferior wall of the heart in men and the anterior wall in women, and may produce false-positive scans.[13] Quality of the images is dependent on the use of stringent quality control measures and experience of the staff. The most commonly used radionuclides are thallium-201, technetium-99m-sestamibi, and technetium-99m-tetrofosmin.[14] Image quality is also patient-dependent. Patients must be able to lie perfectly still for 15 to 20 minutes, with their hands over their heads, while data are collected. Newer systems allow for a 50% reduction in duration of the scan as well as reduced processing time.[10] Currently available systems also allow for seated positioning.[10]

Therapists should identify patients who would have difficulty with arm movements or with remaining still. For these patients, other imaging modalities such as echocardiography may be appropriate.

Positron Emission Tomography

Positron emission tomography (PET) uses positron-emitting radionuclides. The images obtained by PET can provide information regarding cellular processes in living tissue. Both cardiac and lung tissue can be quantitatively examined to obtain information on metabolism, blood perfusion, tissue viability, autonomic regulation, and other processes.[15,16] PET is valuable in delineating myocardial areas with reversible and irreversible injury, thus assessing the feasibility of revascularization, in patients with CAD or left ventricular dysfunction.[17] PET studies use short scanning times (5-35 minutes) and because of the short half-life of PET tracers, multiple scans can be repeated in a relatively short period of time.[18] Although PET scans offer superior imaging, in part due to greater correction for attenuation artifact,[18] PET's technological complexity, short-lived radio tracers, and specialized equipment have resulted in high costs and more limited clinical application.[15] However, because of increased PET use in oncology imaging, opportunities for imaging of the cardiorespiratory system are now increasing.[15,19] Current FDA-approved PET nuclides are rubidium-82 (82-Rb), 13N-ammonia (13-NH3), and fluorine-18-fluorodeoxyglucose (18F-FDG).[15]

Nuclear Tests of the Cardiovascular System

First-Pass and Gated Equilibrium Scans

In a first-pass study, data are collected on a radiolabeled bolus of blood as it passes through the cardiac chambers, which is one method of radionuclide angiography. A first-pass scan allows for clear identification of the four cardiac chambers. During first-pass studies, data are collected over several cardiac cycles. Gated equilibrium studies or multiple-uptake gated acquisition (MUGA) scans average several hundred cardiac cycles. Each R wave of the ECG triggers the acquisition of data; thus the average cycle observed is the compilation of many cycles.[20] The quality of the image is best when the patient has a stable sinus rhythm. Patients with irregular heart rates, such as atrial fibrillation, have images of poorer quality.

Exercise Stress Studies

Many of the tests performed using radionuclides are coupled with an exercise test. A treadmill exercise test is performed, and at the peak of exercise, a tracer is injected. Shortly afterward, depending on the tracer, images are acquired. Exercise imaging enhances the identification of ischemic areas. These tests are then often compared with rest studies. Rest/stress or stress/rest protocols can be used.[14]

Pharmacological Stress Studies

Some patients are unable to exercise to an intensity sufficient to produce stress on the cardiovascular system. When patients are unable to exercise, pharmacological agents can be administered instead. For example, dipyridamole (Persantine) can be used to dilate the patient's coronary arteries; or to increase the metabolic demand of the heart, beta-agonists such as adenosine and dobutamine are most commonly used. The newest approved agent is regadenoson, a selective A2A adenosine receptor agonist. Pharmacological stress tests can be coupled with SPECT and PET nuclear imaging techniques or with echocardiography to determine regions of ischemic myocardium suggesting functionally significant blockage in the coronary artery supplying that area.

Nuclear-Derived Measurements

Data derived from radionuclide images provide information about perfusion, function, and viability. Radionuclides taken up by the myocardium provide a picture of the heart that includes wall thickness and an outline of the chamber. In radionuclide angiography, which includes first-pass and gated studies, the blood is highlighted as it passes through the chambers. Qualitative and quantitative measurements can be taken.

The most important of these measurements, the ejection fraction (right and left ventricle) is a measure of myocardial function. It is derived from quantitative counts of the ventricular area during diastole and systole:[20]

$$([\text{end-diastolic counts} - \text{end-systolic counts}] \times 100) / \text{end-diastolic counts}$$

Left ventricular ejection fraction (LVEF) has been shown to be predictive of mortality. LVEF normally ranges from 50% to 85%, whereas LVEF below 40% indicates moderate-severe congestive heart failure.[21,22] LVEF is linearly related to mortality up to 45% EF[23] and inversely related to moderate- to large-sized infarcts.[24] Right ventricular ejection fraction (RVEF) has been found to have a wide range of normal values (35% to 75%)[25] but is not as predictive of function without data about wall motion abnormalities. The strongest radionuclide predictor of outcome is the exercise LVEF. In terms of predicting outcome, multivariate analysis of clinical data, catheterization data, and radionuclide measurements have shown that the radionuclide results (exercise LVEF, resting end-diastolic volume, and change in heart rate [HR]) have the same prognostic power as the catheterization data.[26]

Another important measurement is wall motion. Quantitative and qualitative evaluation of the movement of the myocardium can be made. Wall thickness and wall movement are compared during systole and diastole. Assessments are made about akinesia (absence of wall motion), global or regional hypokinesia (reduction of wall motion), and dyskinesia (outward bulging of the wall during systole).[27] Global left ventricular function is a strong predictor of survival. It can help clinicians differentiate a weak heart from one that is stiff, thus allowing the appropriate treatment. Regional wall function, when correlated with knowledge of coronary artery anatomy, allows for the identification of potential blockages or areas of infarct. Assessing wall thickness can provide information about hypertrophy or aneurysm but is done more reliably by echocardiography.

Infarct size is an important measurement because it predicts short-term mortality. It is also important as a clinical endpoint in determining the effectiveness of reperfusion strategies and pharmacological interventions, which should result in a decrease of infarct size.[28] The size of a myocardial infarct can be estimated by using the measurements previously described (i.e., ejection fraction, end-systolic volume, and global or regional wall motion).[28] Perfusion defects of the myocardium can be measured acutely, after intervention, or during recovery.

Anatomical measurements of chamber size can be made. From these data, chamber volume can be calculated, as well as stroke volume and cardiac output (Table 14-2).

Myocardial Perfusion Imaging

Perfusion of the myocardium is a vital factor in the viability and function of the heart. Information about myocardial perfusion is used for diagnostic decisions, treatment decisions, and prognosis. Perfusion of the myocardium under rest and exercise conditions is important in the diagnosis of CAD. For those patients with left ventricular dysfunction, identifying tissue that is viable but still at risk is critical for improving long-term outcomes. The efficacy of reperfusion strategies, such as angioplasty and thrombolytic therapy, must be evaluated. Information gained from combined perfusion and metabolic studies has helped to increase the understanding of ischemic myocardium. Two types of contractile dysfunction have been delineated. Hibernating myocardium is the result of prolonged ischemia. In this case, the contractility of the muscle fiber is affected so that there may appear to be regional wall motion abnormalities. The tissue is alive but not contracting. It is theorized that this is a measure to reduce energy expenditure and ensure myocyte survival. The second condition, myocardial stunning, occurs under conditions of acute ischemia. In this case, contractile dysfunction that initially occurs during the acute ischemic episode persists for some time after perfusion has returned to normal. Both conditions are reversible. Patients demonstrating hibernating myocardium may benefit from revascularization procedures. Patients with stunned myocardium may only require supportive care until contractile function returns.[29] The type of imaging performed and the specific radiopharmaceutical used provides similar but not necessarily interchangeable imaging results and measurements.[14]

Table 14-2 **Summary of Special Tests of the Cardiopulmonary System**

	Specific Tests	Clinical Findings
Cardiac Tests		
Nuclear imaging	**Planar, SPECT, MUGA, First pass** Common isotopes: 201-Thallium, 99m-Technitium sestamibi, 99 Technitium-tetrofosmin **PET Scans** Common isotopes: 82-rubidium 13-N-ammonia,15-O labeled water, and 18-fluorine-fluorodeoxyglucose (18F-FDG)	Evaluates myocardial perfusion, used in exercise stress studies and to assess reversibility of defects. Quantitatively can be used to determine: ejection fraction (EF), stroke volume (SV), cardiac output (CO), regional function, ventricular volumes, intracardiac shunt, valvular regurgitation. Quantitatively assesses cell activity of living tissue. Has ability to assess glucose (18F-FDG) and oxidative metabolism, perfusion and potential for revascularization.
Echocardiography	**M-mode; 2-D; transespophageal (TEE); Doppler; myocardial contrast echo (MCE)**	Evaluates myocardial structure. 2-D used in exercise stress studies. 2-D Quantitatively measures: chamber size, wall thickness, valve structure TEE and function, pressure and flow through valve, valve area, EF.
Computed tomography (CT)	Electron-based CT (EBCT)	Identifies calcium concentration in tissues, which is related to the amount of atherosclerotic plaque.
Magnetic resonance imaging (MRI)	MRI with contrast (Gandolium-DTPA)	Identifies ventricular volumes, EF, CO. Contrast imaging can be used to identify perfusion defects, flow, areas of infarction.
Angiography		Quantitative measures of pressure, resistance, flow, oxygen consumption, arteriovenous oxygen difference EF, CO
Pulmonary Tests		
	Specific Tests	**Clinical Findings**
Pulmonary scans	**Perfusion scan** Common isotopes: MAB **Ventilation scan** Common isotopes: 99m-Tc -DTPA **Gallium scan** **PET Scans** Common isotopes: 18F-FDG	Identifies regions of decreased pulmonary perfusion, used to identify pulmonary embolism. Identifies regions of decreased ventilation. Used in conjunction with 133-Xe perfusion scan to identify patients with pulmonary embolism. Identification of neoplastic or inflammatory pulmonary lesions Aids in differential diagnosis of solitary pulmonary nodules, inflammation and malignant lesions.
Computed tomography	High-resolution CT; spiral CT	HRCT used in the diagnosis of bronchiectasis; spiral CT can be used to diagnose PE.
Magnetic resonance imaging	Dynamic MRI Gd-DTPA contrast	MRI with contrast used for MR angiography; dynamic MRI used in workup of lung transplant to examine ventilation, pulmonary mechanics
Angiography		For diagnosis of PE

Thallium-201

Thallium-201 (201-TL) is the oldest radioactive isotope used in myocardial perfusion studies.[14] It is a cyclotron-produced isotope that emits low-energy radiation (68 to 80 kiloelectron volts [keV]). Thallium concentrations in the myocardium depend on 201-TL properties, uptake, and redistribution. Administered intravenously, its distribution throughout the body depends on blood flow, and within 5 minutes, myocardial uptake represents myocardial blood flow.[30] The first-pass myocardial uptake coefficient is 85%.[14] Extraction from the blood and transport across the cell membrane depend on active and passive transport mechanisms. Thallium is transported across the cell membrane through the sodium-potassium ATPase pump and facilitative diffusion.[30] Normally perfused and functioning myocardium will take up the thallium tracer, while damaged cells will demonstrate weaker uptake. Within 15 minutes thallium begins washout (also called redistribution) in normal myocardium. Images taken 4-24 hours later show clearance of the 201-Tl, again as a result of normal blood flow, while abnormal cells have more tracer as it has not been washed out.[30]

Thallium-201 images can be qualitatively and quantitatively evaluated. Normally perfused myocardium demonstrates uniform uptake of the tracer. Uniform uptake can occur as long as blockages are less than 50% of the artery. Ischemic but viable myocardium initially appears as areas of decreased uptake; these areas fill in over time, a function of redistribution. Because blood flow is decreased, clearance of thallium-201 from the defect region is slower.[30] In infarcted areas, these defects remain unchanged over time. Thus perfusion and tissue viability can be assessed with 201-TL. Qualitative evaluation requires visual inspection of the images. Quantitative evaluation is performed by specialized software individual to the imaging system used. The computer analyzes the amount of radioactivity taken up in a particular region of interest (ROI). It then quantifies this count so that regions can be compared with each other and with normalized data. In this way, unperfused or hypoperfused areas can be identified (Figure 14-2).

Thallium-201 is used to acquire planar and SPECT images for rest studies, exercise stress studies, and pharmacological stress studies. The traditional thallium-201 stress study calls for injection of the tracer at the peak of exercise with collection of the stress data within 10 to 15 minutes. The redistribution study is completed at a minimum of 4 hours later. Alternative study protocols include reinjection of thallium before the 4-hour redistribution study and use in dual-isotope studies.[30] Reinjection of thallium and repeat imaging 24 hours after initial study can help identify severely ischemic (greater than 90% blockage) areas, which may take much longer to demonstrate redistribution.

Technetium-99m-Sestamibi or Technetium-99m-Tetrofosmin

The technetium (Tc)-99m–based radionuclides were developed because of a number of advantages they have over thallium imaging. Sestamibi and tetrofosmin provide improved SPECT image quality as a result of higher count rates and higher energy, in the 140 keV range. Tc-99m is generator-produced. These isotopes have a 6-hour half-life and are excreted via the hepatobiliary system.[14] Because of the short half-life, higher doses can be injected, and although the percentage of extraction is lower (65% for sestamibi and 54% for tetrofosmin), uptake in relation to flow is similar to that of thallium.[14] These factors result in higher count rates, which thus allow the use of gated images and first-pass acquisition studies. Higher count rates are preferred when evaluating obese patients. One of the greatest limitations of Tc-99m is that it does not readily redistribute; therefore reversibility of defects cannot be ascertained as well as with thallium. This factor is one reason thallium is much more popular. Two-day protocols or dual isotope protocols can be used to overcome this limitation.[31] Lack of redistribution has been exploited in evaluating the impact of thrombolytic therapy in acute situations. A patient with an acute myocardial infarction (MI) can be injected with tracer, given thrombolytics, stabilized, and scanned 4 hours later. The scan results show myocardial perfusion at the time of injection when the myocardium was ischemic. Later scans demonstrate the new perfusion situation.

Protocols using this isotope are designed to take advantage of the rapid uptake and washout. When used with pharmacological stress studies, a rest-stress study can be completed within minutes.[32] This may have future application in studying reperfusion following balloon angioplasty or reperfusion therapy with thrombolytic agents.[32]

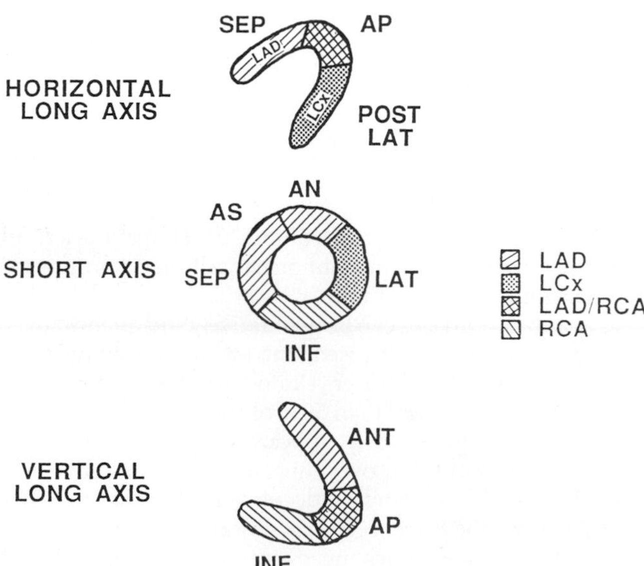

Fig. 14-2 Illustration of the SPECT series. Representative mid-ventricular slices of the three projections most frequently used for SPECT thallium display. *LAD,* left anterior descending; *LCx,* left circumflex; *RCA,* right coronary artery; *SEP,* septum; *AP,* apical; *LAT,* lateral; *POST LAT,* posterior lateral; *INF,* inferior. *(From Fisher KC: Qualitative SPECT thallium imaging: Technical considerations and clinical applications. In Guiberteau MJ, editor:* Nuclear cardiovascular imaging, *New York, 1990, Churchill Livingstone.)*

Positron Emission Tomography Tracers

PET tracers are also used to evaluate perfusion. The most commonly used tracers are 13N-ammonia, rubidium-82, and 15-O-labeled water.[33,34] The benefit of using PET tracers is that it is possible to quantify myocardial blood flow in mL/g/min.

13N-Ammonia

13N-Ammonia (13-NH3) provides high-quality images of myocardial perfusion because of its high first-pass extraction fraction (80%).[34] The tracer diffuses into myocardial cells and becomes trapped.[15]

Rubidium-82

One of the oldest approved tracers, rubidium-82 (82-Rb) is taken up by the myocardium via the Na/K-ATPase mechanism. Imaging myocardial blood flow is not optimal, because first-pass extraction is only 60% and uptake becomes nonlinear with increased blood flow.[34] However, it is easily produced via generator. The very short half-life of 82-Rb is useful in the clinical setting. It is most often used with pharmacological stress studies.[34]

15-O-Labeled Water

The PET tracer 15-O-labeled water (H2-15O) can be delivered by a variety of methods. It can be administered by bolus injection (the same method used for 82Rb and 13-NH3), but it can also be inhaled or given as an infusion. Myocardial uptake is uniform over a wide range of flow rates and is modeled as an inert freely diffusible tracer, which easily crosses capillary and sarcolemmal membranes.[33] However, the short half-life and reduced count density of H2-15O result in less-than-optimal image quality, making visual analyses problematic.[34] H2-15O is not currently an FDA-approved tracer.

Myocardial Metabolism

Fluorine-18-Fluorodeoxyglucose

Fluorine-18-fluorodeoxyglucose (18F-FDG) is a glucose analogue that crosses the capillary and sarcolemmal membrane at a rate proportional to that of glucose. 18F-FDG becomes trapped in the myocardium, because it is not a useful substrate in metabolic pathways. The distribution of 18F-FDG is relative to uptake of unlabeled glucose.[35] Glucose utilization is therefore used as a marker of tissue viability.

Identification of areas with normal metabolism, altered metabolism, or no metabolism is based on the use of glucose as an energy substrate. Normally perfused myocardial cells use a combination of fatty acids and carbohydrates for adenosine triphosphate (ATP) production when in a fasting state and use glucose as the primary energy source in the postprandial state. Ischemic myocardium uses glucose in the fasting state and the postprandial state. Infarcted or scarred areas show no metabolic activity. Therefore increased uptake of 18F-FDG in the postprandial state occurs in both hibernating and normal myocardium, but in the fasting state, it occurs only in the hibernating myocardium. Clinical studies in patients with infarct showed that areas with persistent thallium-201 perfusion defects have evidence of remaining metabolic activity in 47% of regions when studied with a PET scan, indicating overestimation of irreversible injury. Use of reinjection and late redistribution imaging has significantly lowered this number.[36] The implication derived from this finding is that in areas with perfusion defects, if glucose activity remains, the region is viable (mismatch pattern); conversely, if such activity is absent, the area is likely to be infarcted or necrotic (match pattern).[37] Viewed in functional terms, mismatch simply implies the potential for improvement; match implies no potential for improvement in contractility after successful revascularization.[38]

11C-Acetate

Another way to evaluate myocardial viability is to use an isotope that is incorporated into the metabolic pathways related to myocardial oxygen consumption. 11C-acetate in its activated form, acetyl-CoA, represents the entry point for all metabolic pathways into the tricarboxylic acid cycle, which is tightly coupled to oxidative metabolism. Its advantage over 18F-FDG is that it does not rely on substrate use (i.e., glucose versus fat metabolism). 11C-acetate accurately reflects oxidative metabolism and can distinguish viable from nonviable myocardium in both acute and chronic ischemic conditions.[39]

Nuclear Tests of the Pulmonary System

Ventilation-Perfusion Lung Scan

The ventilation-perfusion (VQ) lung scan is a combination of two separate imaging procedures. It is primarily used in the diagnosis of pulmonary embolism (PE), with limited use for other clinical problems.[40] The perfusion portion requires the injection of radioactive tracer. Technetium-99m- macroaggregated albumin is accepted (almost universally) as the perfusion tracer of choice.[41] The ventilation scan requires the inhalation of radioactive gas, usually 133-XE gas or Tc-99m-diethylenetriamine pentaacetic acid (DTPA) aerosol. Other isotopes can be used for ventilation scanning (e.g., Kr-81M, Xenon-127), but they are more difficult to obtain (Figure 14-3).

A normal perfusion scan essentially rules out recent pulmonary embolus. If the perfusion scan is abnormal, it is compared with the ventilation scan for match or mismatch of defects. An interpretation scheme is used, such as Pioped, which classifies the probability of PE as present (high probability), absent (normal or very low probability), and nondiagnostic (low probability or indeterminate).[5,41] Patients with high-probability scans should begin anticoagulation therapy.[41] The D-dimer test and pretest probability of a PE also help to determine if the patient is high probability and thus requires anticoagulation.

Since the PIOPED II conclusion that computed tomography pulmonary angiogram (CTPA) has superior diagnostic accuracy for pulmonary emboli, the VQ scan is used less frequently.[41-44] However, VQ scans remain valuable for patients concerned with radiation exposure, intolerance to intravenous contrast agents or during pregnancy.[45]

Miller and O'Doherty[5] note other applications of ventilation/perfusion scanning, including monitoring of response to radiotherapy and assessment of resectability of bullae. The scan is used to predict whether someone can tolerate a pneumonectomy based on percent flow to the opposite lung and extent of disease present.

Positron Emission Tomography

PET scans using 18F-FDG isotopes are being used to identify metabolically active tissue (glucose metabolism) in the lungs. It has found application in the differential diagnosis of pulmonary nodules, inflammation, and potential malignant lesions.[46] PET with 18F-FDG is used as a diagnostic tool for pulmonary nodules and mass lesions.[46] Solitary pulmonary nodules (SPN) are often found during screening tests. They are of significant concern because of the risk for malignancy. Gould and colleagues[46] performed a meta-analysis and concluded that sensitivity is 96.8% and specificity is 77.8% for detecting malignancy in SPNs. PET 18F-FDG is not recommended for nodules less than 1 cm in size.[47] In addition to difficulty accessing PET scanners, cost may be a limiting factor—based on Medicare reimbursement figures, PET scans using 18F-FDG can cost six times more than conventional CT scans of the chest.[47]

Gallium Scintigraphy

PET or SPECT imaging has largely replaced gallium scanning for lung disease.[48] However, this isotope is still used in some centers and in specific clinical situations. Gallium-67-citrate binds with transferrin. This complex binds with transferrin-receptors in neoplastic cells while in areas of inflammation and infection gallium binds to lactoferrin and siderophores.[48] The radioisotope is injected intravenously, but it takes 48 to 72 hours before imaging can be performed; this delay is one reason it is out of favor.

Gallium is used in the evaluation of patients with inflammation and infection. Non-infectious inflammatory processes include: sarcoidosis, amiodarone toxicity, following cytotoxic therapy with bleomycin, and interstitial pulmonary fibrosis, as well as many other entities.[48] Gallium scanning is used to monitor response to treatment in lymphoma and where PET scans are not available can be useful in the diagnosis of lung cancer.[48] Gallium continues to be useful in infections (e.g., TB) as it helps discriminate active infection from fibrosis. Similarly, discriminating active disease from scarring is useful in

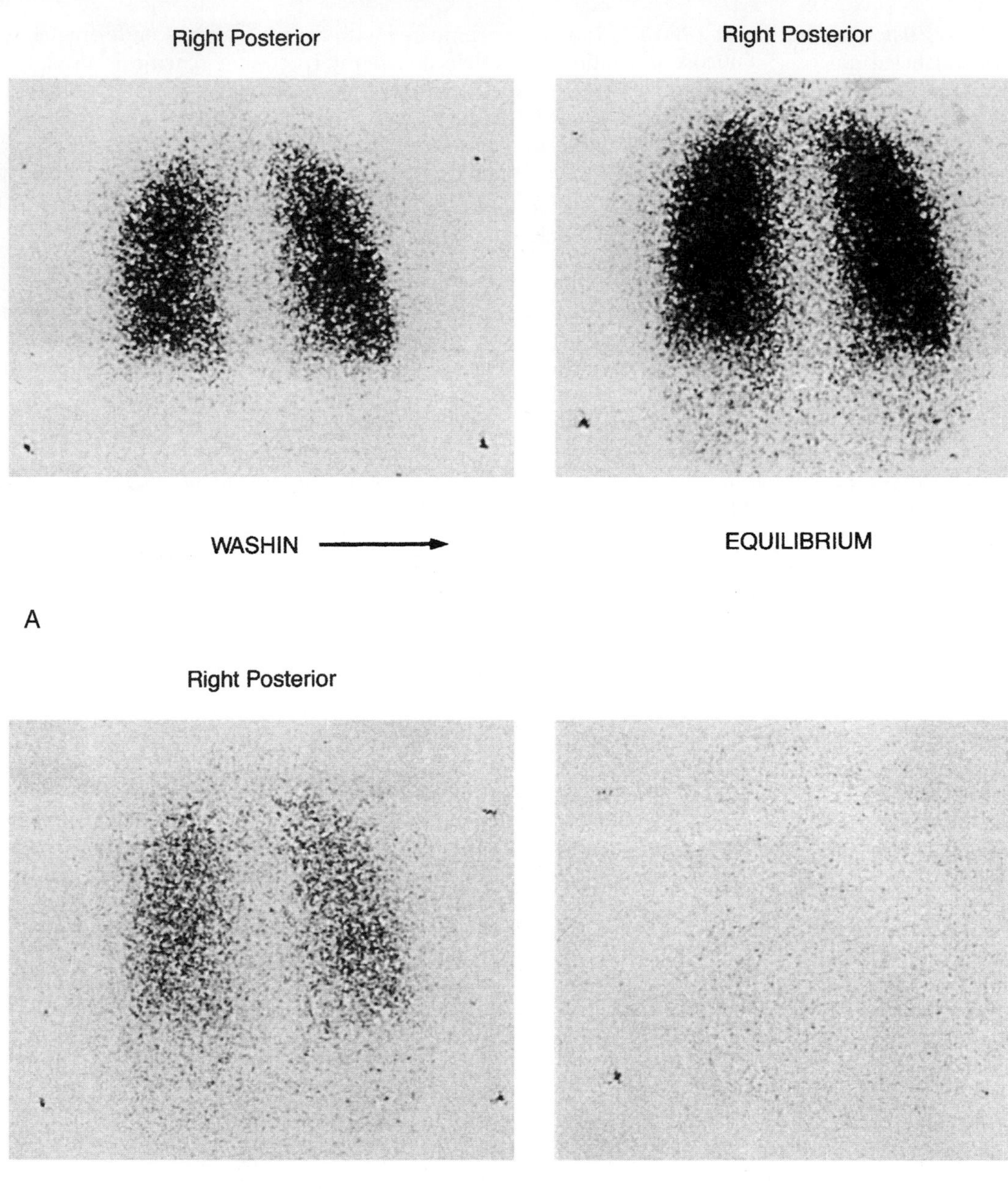

Fig. 14-3 The value of ventilation/perfusion lung scans in the diagnosis of thromboembolism. A xenon inhalation lung scan **(A)** discloses normal ventilation parameters during the washin, equilibrium, and washout phases.

evaluating AIDS patients with *Pneumocystis carinii* pneumonia (PCP).[48] The sensitivity of gallium scanning for *PCP in patients with AIDS* approaches 94% to 96%.[43]

Angiography

Angiography is the radiographic examination of the arterial system using an opaque contrast dye injected into the arterial segment to characterize flow. Angiography provides information about the detailed structural anatomy of the vascular system under study. Angiography requires an x-ray generator tube and image intensifier/cine camera.[49] The radiopaque dye is injected into the vascular supply of the region of interest. Radiographic images can then monitor the contrast material as it moves through the circulation. The development of coronary angiography via cardiac catheterization techniques allowed for the development of many of the catheter-based interventions now used today.[50]

Cardiac Imaging

The gold standard with which many of the cardiac noninvasive tests are compared is that of cardiac catheterization. It is an invasive test, with a small but serious risk to the patient.

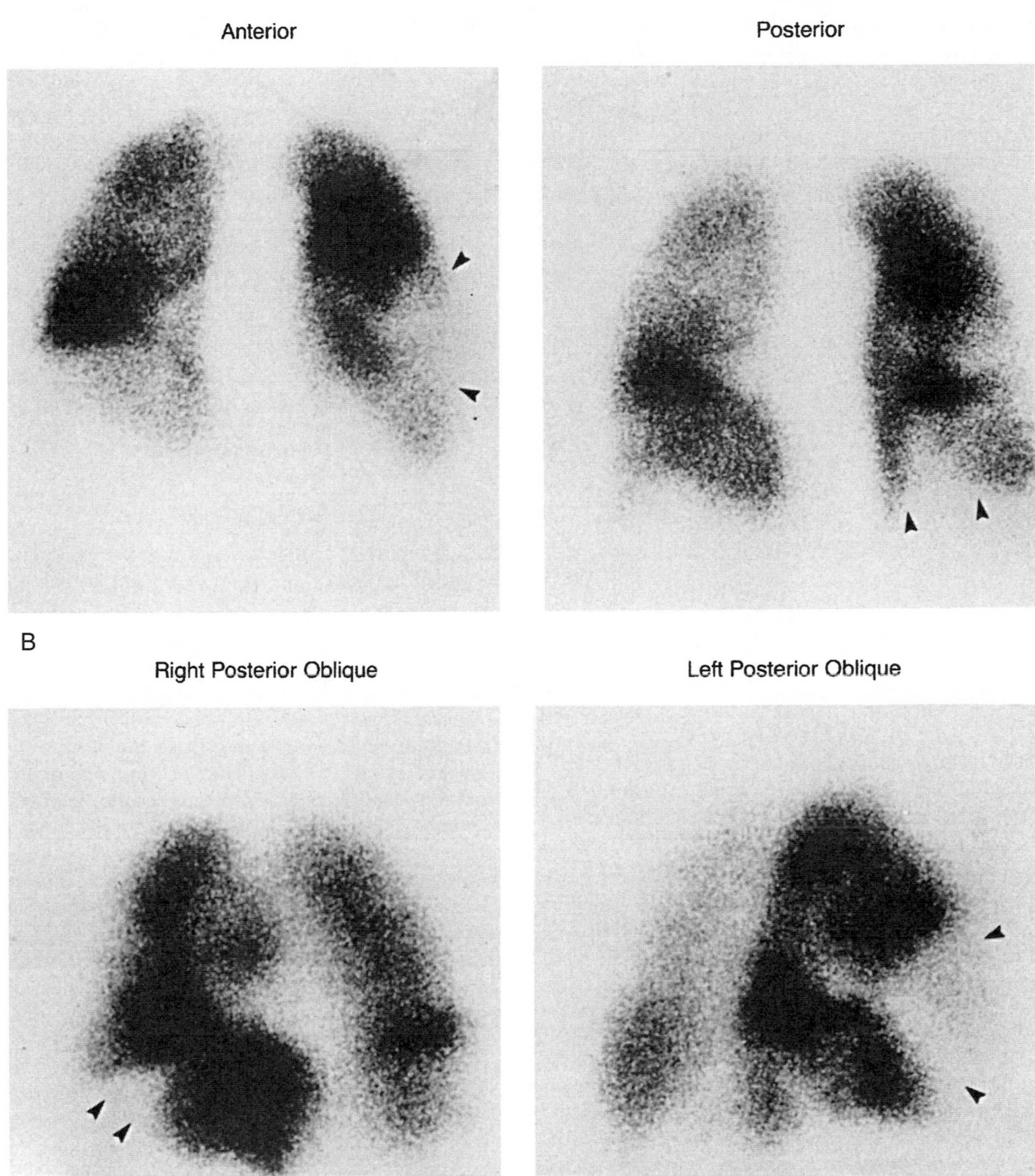

Fig. 14-3, cont'd Corresponding technetium-99m–labeled macroaggregated albumin perfusion lung scans **(B)** in anterior, posterior, and right and left posterior oblique projections identify multiple segmental filling defects throughout both lungs (*arrowheads*). These findings, in concert with the ventilation study are virtually diagnostic (high probability) of pulmonary thromboembolism. The patient was a 65-year-old man with acute dyspnea. *(From Fraser RS, Paré PD, Coman N, et al:* Diagnosis of diseases of the chest, *ed 4, Philadelphia, 1999, WB Saunders.)*

Complications include death, stroke, MI, bleeding, arterial trauma or thrombus, renal dysfunction, and arrhythmias.[49] The test is indicated in patients presenting with ST elevated MI (STEMI) who are candidates for reperfusion as well as those presenting with chest pain and non-STEMI who are at risk for further cardiac events.[51] There is some debate as to whether the NSTEMI population should undergo a coronary angiogram with potential for revascularization within 24 hours or should wait. Current guidelines recommend the early procedure.[52] Patients who have CAD with angina that is unresponsive to medical therapy may also need catheterization.

The procedure for cardiac catheterization of the left side of the heart requires the threading of a catheter, guided by fluoroscopy, through the femoral artery or brachial artery to the aorta. Direct measurements of chamber pressures, blood flow, and oxygen saturation can be obtained. When selective coronary arteriography is performed, radiopaque contrast material is injected from the catheter into the left main or right coronary artery. Cine recordings are made after the injection, and injections are repeated until the entire coronary tree is visualized. The location of an arterial obstruction can be identified, as well as the percentage of blockage (stenosis) (Figure 14-4).

More recently, additional physiological measures can be obtained that provide flow and pressure data at the site of the lesion within the coronary artery.[53] These measures have become particularly important for monitoring outcomes after the administration of reperfusion therapy (e.g. thrombolytics, angioplasty, stenting).[54,55] Coronary artery flow grades—for example, thrombolysis in myocardial infarction (TIMI) grades 0-3—are based on the visual analysis of the rate of opacification of the artery of interest, typically 90 minutes after intervention.[54] TIMI myocardial perfusion grades (TMPG 0-3), or myocardial blush, grade the reperfusion of the myocardium by the contrast medium.[55] Higher TIMI and TMPG grades have been associated with reduced mortality over 2 years.[55]

Cardiac ventriculography is a procedure in which dye is injected into the ventricle and the entire chamber becomes outlined. Several cardiac cycles are recorded on cine. This provides valuable information about global and segmental wall motion, valve motion, and the presence of abnormal anatomy.

Pulmonary Imaging

Pulmonary angiography is used primarily for the diagnosis of PE. It is the gold standard with which ventilation/perfusion scans are compared.[41] Contrast dye is injected into the pulmonary circulation through the pulmonary artery. Additional techniques such as balloon occlusion, segmental injections, or increased magnification improve the sensitivity of the test.[40] Interobserver reliability studies performed on the interpretation of pulmonary angiograms are 83% to 86%.[41]

Echocardiography

Another noninvasive method of evaluating the heart uses the physical properties of sound. Echocardiography (sometimes simply called "echo") provides information about blood flow, structure, and function of the heart. Motion mode (M-mode) and two-dimensional (2-D) images are highly reliable methods of evaluation. Recent developments of technique and technology include color flow Doppler echo, transesophageal echo, and intravascular echo. These techniques, when used in combination, can provide much of the information previously available only by cardiac catheterization.[56,57] Echocardiography is an important tool in the assessment and management of patients with thoracic trauma.[58]

Physics of Echocardiography

Imaging systems that use ultrasound require a source for generation of the sound wave, a transducer, and a receiver to pick up the reflected sound waves. Sound is absorbed or reflected differentially by specific tissues. Therefore the sound wave reflected from muscle differs from that reflected from vascular space, or valvular structures. Returning signals are converted into electrical signals that generate an image. This is the basis for M-mode and 2-D echo. In M-mode echocardiography, the transducer transmits a single sound wave through the chest wall (transthoracic echocardiography, or TTE). A thin slice of the heart, an "ice pick" view, directly under the sound wave, reflects the wave back to the transducer. M-mode, though useful when a high-resolution image is required, is rarely used.[59] The primary diagnostic mode is 2-D. In 2-D echocardiography, the transducer is able to pick up a wedge section of the heart. In 2-D mode, the transducer acts as the transmitter and receiver. A "real time" two-dimensional picture of the heart is recorded on videotape. The heart can be viewed in motion, and wall motion can be evaluated (Figure 14-5).

Doppler Echocardiography

Doppler echocardiography relies on the Doppler effect to determine velocity. When a sound wave is aimed at moving objects, such as red blood cells, the known transmitted frequency from the soundhead and the reflected frequency differ, a phenomenon known as a frequency shift. The greater the frequency shift, the greater the speed of the targeted object.[57] *Velocity of flow* is the term used to express Doppler frequency shifts. Both continuous-wave and pulsed-wave Doppler modes are used.

Color flow Doppler echocardiography was introduced in the mid-1980s. It is usually superimposed on a two-dimensional image in real time but can be used with M-mode. It is a method that displays anatomical and spatial blood flow velocity estimates with indication of flow direction in real time.[60] Color is matched based on the direction of flow, and shading is indicative of intensity based on the mean velocity flow estimates.[60] It is primarily used to assess the extent of regurgitant jets across "leaky valves," as well as to indicate areas of abnormal shunts such as atrial septal defects. Turbulence created by narrowed valves creates wide color shading.

Measurements Derived from Echocardiography

Echocardiographic results can be viewed qualitatively and quantitatively. An experienced viewer can analyze the anatomical relationships and structure of the heart, wall motion, valve movement and configuration, and chamber size.

Quantitative measures are calculated from the Doppler frequency shifts. Velocity measures can be used in other equations to estimate pressure and valve area. The modified Bernoulli equation is used to calculate pressure changes around the valve:

$$\Delta P \text{ (mm Hg)} = 4 \times V_{max}^{2} \text{ (m/sec)}$$

where P is the pressure gradient across the valve and V is the velocity of blood flow through the valve.

These measurements allow calculation of stenotic valve gradients and right-sided filling pressures, valve regurgitation, and shunt volumes.[57] Valve regurgitation and shunt calculations are more complicated than the Bernoulli equation alone.

Another important quantitative measure is the estimated area of the valve. The continuity equation is used to estimate valve area. It is based on the principle of conservation of mass;

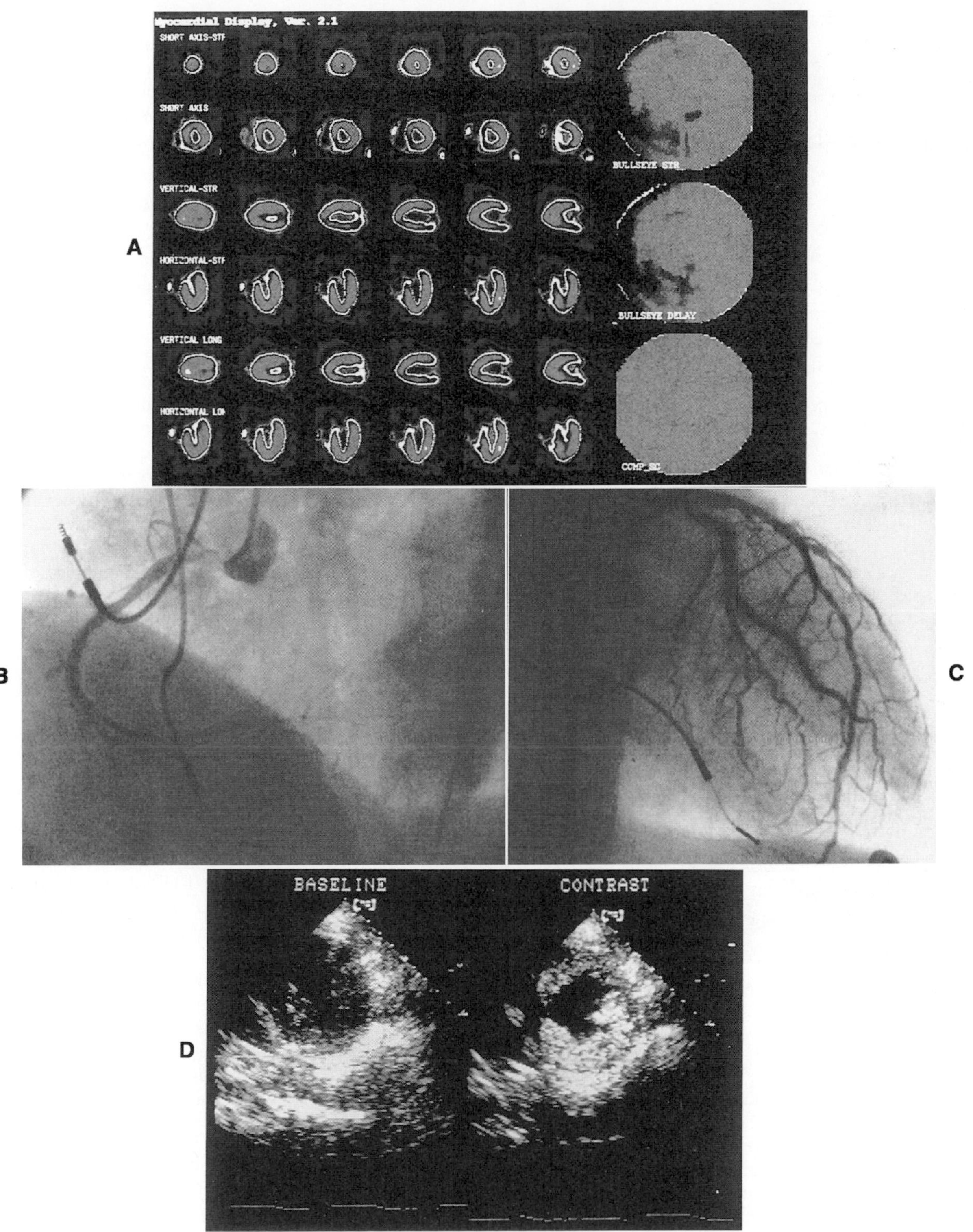

Fig. 14-4 Stress single-photon emission computed tomography reoriented and polar plot images. **A,** Right coronary artery arteriogram; **B,** left anterior descending coronary artery arteriogram; **C,** circumflex coronary arteriogram; and the short-axis two-dimensional echocardiographic images **(D)** at baseline (*left*) and after contrast injection down the LAD coronary artery (*right*). Although this patient had a normal dobutamine thallium-201 SPECT with no discernible perfusion defect after comparison to the normal databank (COMPSC) **(A),** the right coronary artery is noted to have a subtotal ostial stenosis **(B)**. No collaterals are observed to the right coronary artery after left main contrast injection **(C)**. However, on echocardiography **(D),** intense contrast enhancement is noted in the inferior wall after injection of sonicated microbubbles down the LAD, verifying the presence of coronary collaterals to the right coronary artery. Despite a severe right coronary artery stenosis, this patient did not develop a stress perfusion defect because of the well-developed collateral circulation, which was apparent on echocardiography but not arteriography. *(From Malunarian JJ: State of the art for CAD detection: Thallium 201. In Zarit BL, Beller GA, editors:* Nuclear cardiology, *ed 2, St. Louis, 1999, CV Mosby.)*

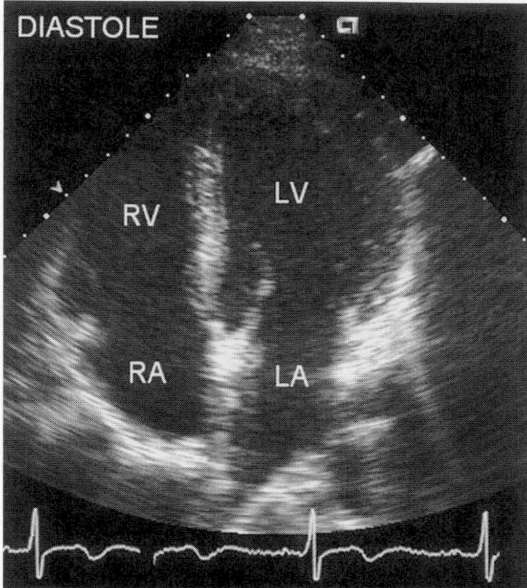

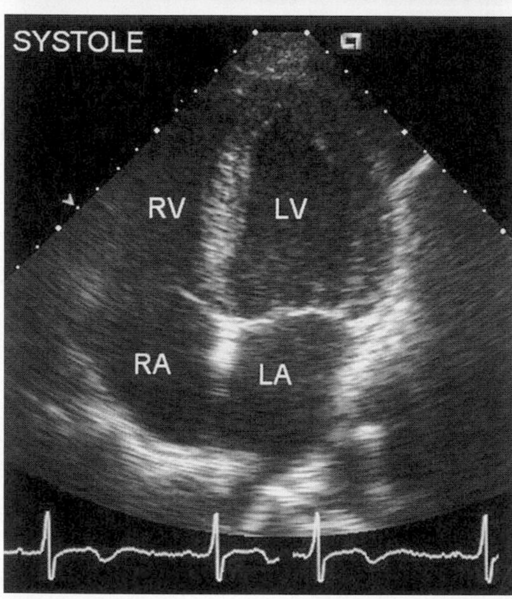

Fig. 14-5 Normal 2-D echo images at end-diastole (*above*) and end-systole (*below*). *(From Otto CM:* Textbook of clinical echocardiography, *ed 2, Philadelphia, 2000. WB Saunders.)*

that is, in a normal heart, the volume of blood that enters the right atrium should be conserved as it passes through the other chambers (stroke $volume_1$ = stroke $volume_2$). Since the volume before the valve must be equal to the volume after the valve, it is possible to measure flow velocity before and after the valve and then solve for the area of the valve:

$$A_1 \times V_1 = A_2 \times V_2, \text{therefore } A_2 = (A_1 \times V_1)/V_2$$

where V_1 is the velocity of flow at one side of the valve, V_2 is the flow velocity at the other side of the valve, and A is the cross-sectional area.[57]

Exercise Studies

Exercise echocardiography can be done immediately following physiological stress (treadmill or bicycle exercise) or pharmacological stress (dipyridamole, adenosine, or dobutamine). Pharmacological stress offers the advantage of the patient being in a stable position throughout the test. If monitoring during physiological stress conditions is desired, the bicycle test, in the semirecumbent or supine position, is preferred because imaging cannot be performed during a treadmill test.[61]

Transesophageal Echocardiography

Because of consistent technical difficulties with TTE, the technique of transesophageal echocardiography (TEE) was developed to improve spatial resolution. TEE can obtain M-mode, 2-D, 3-D, and color flow Doppler images by using a small probe mounted on the tip of a modified gastroscope. TEE is considered minimally invasive. The probe is advanced into the esophagus, similar to placement of a gastric tube by nasal or oral route, and positioned so that multiple views of the heart are available.[62] For cardiac output measures, it is advanced to the midthoracic level.[63] The technique can be performed on anesthetized patients during surgery and monitored postoperatively; on mildly sedated patients (e.g., those on mechanical ventilation or trauma patients in the intensive care unit); and on those suspected of having aortic dissection or aortic injury.[58] TEE is frequently used for diagnosis of congenital heart disease, evaluation of valve function, and determination of thromboembolic risk. It has become an important monitoring tool during cardiac catheterization procedures and surgery.[64]

TEE is used to assess cardiac valve function as well as to monitor treatment. Image quality of TEE is better than that of TTE. This is especially true when visualizing the mitral valve, because of the proximity to the transducer (valves positioned farther from the transducer afford lower-quality images).[65] It is used to monitor prosthetic valve function, as well as to diagnose and monitor infective endocarditis, particularly the status of valve vegetation. TEE provides superior visualization (compared with TTE) of the left atrium and left atrial appendage, which are often the source of thrombi causing transient ischemic attack (TIA) or stroke. TEE Doppler studies can examine left atrial flow velocities, which also indicate increased stroke risk. TEE Doppler has been successfully used to decrease morbidity and length of stay when hemodynamic management of the patient is critical.[63] TEE has now progressed to 3-D real-time imaging, which allows for improved imaging and quantification of LV function, including preload, afterload, and contractility.[65]

Myocardial Contrast Echocardiography

The ability of echocardiography to evaluate myocardial perfusion was historically based on observation of wall motion abnormalities. The development of a contrast agent that can be used with echocardiography has ushered in noninvasive techniques that do not rely on radioactive agents (see Figure 14-3). In myocardial contrast echocardiography (MCE), microbubbles of air encapsulated in a thin shell are introduced by IV infusion or bolus injection into the venous system as the contrast agent.[66] These small bubbles (<6-10 μm) oscillate when exposed to ultrasound energy and produce harmonic signals (a multiple of the ultrasound frequency) that are then used to produce the images.[67] Although numerous studies have shown the potential benefit of MCE for bedside and stress perfusion imaging, the FDA has not approved it for this use.[68]

Computed Tomography

Computed tomography (CT) was first developed in the 1970s, allowing the visualization of cross-sectional views of body organs, as opposed to the planar views possible with standard radiographs.[69] Further technological developments in CT have made possible such rapid scan times that CT of the respiratory system can be completed in a single breath-hold, resulting in scans of improved spatial resolution and diagnostic utility.[70] Electron beam CT has found application in the examination of the cardiac system and is currently used as part of risk stratification for asymptomatic patients.[71]

Physics of Computed Tomography

A computed tomographic scan (CT scan) acquires images of a fixed thickness (a cross-sectional slice), which allows examination of a specific part of the body. CT scanners use an x-ray source, collimators, x-ray detectors, and computers to reconstruct the cross-sectional images from the acquired data.[69] The x-ray source rotates around the patient, the speed of rotation dictating how long it takes to acquire a single slice (about 1 second). Slice thickness and the space between slices determine the quality of the spatial resolution of the images. The spatial resolution required depends on the type of tissue being examined and the suspected diagnosis. Imaging can be done with a single-detector or newer multiple-detector row scanners (4, 8, or 16 rows).[72] Multidetector CT (MDCT) scanners allow for faster acquisition of images. Spiral CT scanners simultaneously rotate the source and move the table and patient for continuous data acquisition and improved resolution.[73] The most rapid scanning times are achieved by electron beam computed tomography (EBCT), also called ultrafast CT. EBCT uses an electron gun to generate x-rays to a fixed tungsten "target."[71] The electron beam is electronically moved, rather than mechanically rotated, resulting in images that can be made in milliseconds. The cost and the limited number of available EBCT scanners are factors that limit their routine use.[72]

Cardiac Imaging

Electron-beam tomography is currently used to identify calcium in atherosclerotic plaques within the coronary arteries.[71] A scoring system developed to quantify the amount of calcium in the coronary arteries is used to identify future risk of cardiac events.[71] Scores are based on Housenfeld units (HU), which are based on the tissue attenuation factor. Calcified areas are identified in the coronary tree and given scores based on HU > 130. Scores are summed across all identified lesions (Agatston method) to provide a total coronary calcium score.[74] In general, the greater the amount of calcium detected, the greater the amount of atherosclerotic plaque in the coronary arteries. A limitation of EBCT is that it cannot localize the plaque anatomically. Sensitivity and specificity for EBCT for CAD is 91% and 49%, respectively.[71] Research is currently being done to determine whether EBCT tests adds valuable data to cardiac risk assessment.[75] In a sample of nearly 9000 asymptomatic low- to intermediate-risk middle-aged adults, the relative risk for a cardiac event significantly increased at higher quartiles of calcium scores.[75] However, it is not recommended for screening in asymptomatic patients or for patients at high pretest probability for CAD.[76,77] Cardiac CT has been deemed appropriate for symptomatic individuals with low to intermediate pretest probability of significant coronary stenosis or pre-operative evaluation in low-risk patients.[77] A particular strength of CT is its ability to image cardiac structure and ventricular function.[77]

Pulmonary Imaging

Compared with standard radiography, CT is not commonly used in the initial diagnosis of pulmonary disease. However, the CT scan has been found to be a useful first-line diagnostic tool in the evaluation of mediastinal disease, including mediastinal masses, staging of mediastinal cancers, and identification of cysts.[40]

High-resolution computed tomography (HRCT) has improved the documentation of morphological changes associated with chronic airflow obstruction. Webb's 1994 review[78] of the application of this new technology identified the utility of this test in a variety of obstructive diseases. HRCT is sensitive in the diagnosis of early emphysema, although it is rarely used clinically. In cystic disease, such as histiocytosis X and lymphangiomyomatosis, HRCT is able to demonstrate cysts less than 10 mm in diameter and can also visualize wall thickness.

In the diagnosis of bronchiectasis, HRCT demonstrates a high specificity (Figure 14-6) and is the procedure of choice after standard chest radiography. It can discriminate among the three different types of abnormal bronchi seen in bronchiectasis (cylindrical, varicose, and cystic); however, there is little clinical significance in this distinction.[78] HRCT can be used to differentiate lymphangitic spread of cancer versus heart failure when that distinction is clinically unclear. It also can be used to evaluate clearing of persistent pneumonias. Overall, HRCT has helped clarify disease morphology, but its clinical significance for diagnosis and for patient pulmonary function is less clear.

Spiral CT, with and without a contrast agent, has become the test of choice in the diagnosis of acute pulmonary embolism.[79] Multidetector scans (>4 detectors) provide sensitivity and specificity >83% and 89% respectively.[79] The combination of CT and V/Q scans provide examination of lung function (V/Q) and structure (CT) which may surpass CT alone for diagnosis of PE.[80] Hybrid cameras that can perform both V/Q SPECT and CT will increase utilization of these scans. Future applications may be seen in planning radiation therapy of the lung and lung volume reduction surgery.[81]

Magnetic Resonance Imaging

Technically, MRI, which was adopted clinically in the 1970s, uses nuclear magnetic resonance to build tissue images—that is, nuclei are made to resonate in a magnetic field.[82] However, since MRI is a technique that does not use radiopharmaceuticals or ionizing radiation, it was thought to be less confusing to leave "nuclear" out of the name. Thus MRI is a noninvasive, test that involves no exposure to radiation and is able to

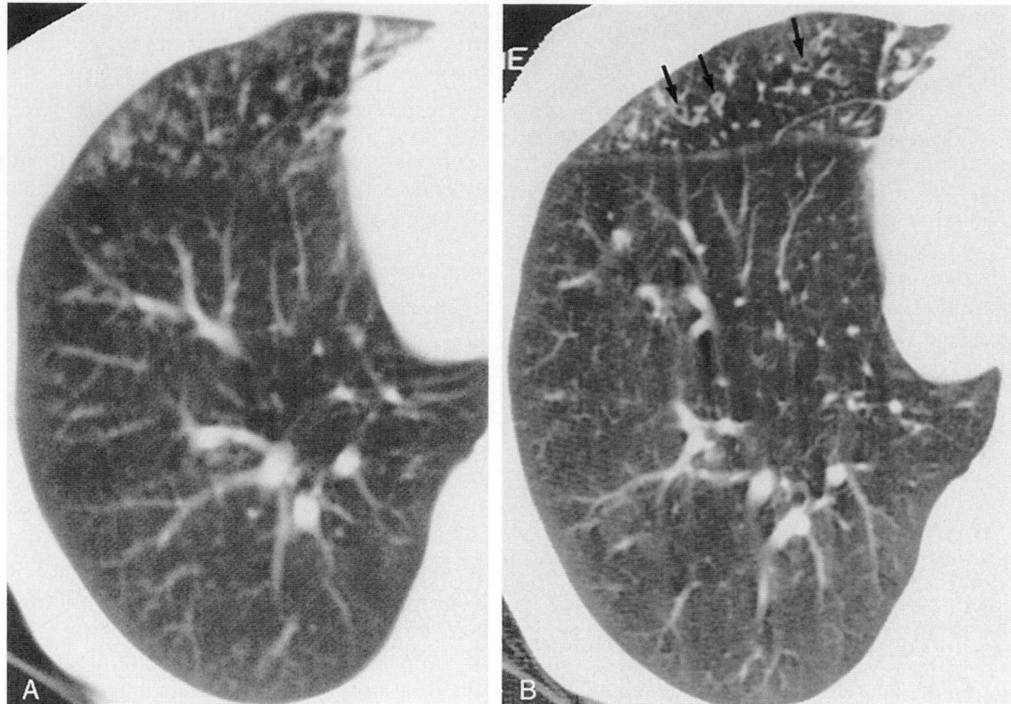

Fig. 14-6 HRCT versus conventional CT for bronchiectasis. A conventional 10-mm-collimation CT scan **(A)** in a 65-year-old woman demonstrates small focal areas of ground-glass attenuation and consolidation in the right middle lobe. An HRCT scan (1.5-mm collimation) **(B)** performed immediately after the conventional CT scan demonstrates right middle lobe bronchiectasis (*arrows*). *(From Fraser RS, Paré PD, Coman N, et al:* Diagnosis of diseases of the chest, *ed 4, Philadelphia, 1999, WB Saunders.)*

provide high quality imaging without the use of contrast dyes. Furthermore, with the development of ultrafast imaging, MRI has found utility for the examination of the cardiovascular and pulmonary systems.

Physics of Magnetic Resonance Imaging

MRI relies on the creation of a stable, powerful magnetic field that causes hydrogen (also carbon-13, fluorine-19, and sodium-23) nuclei to align with the field. A radiofrequency pulse specific to the hydrogen (or other) nuclei causes the nuclei to resonate.[82,83] Additional magnets that apply magnetic fields of different gradients are used to locate the image. When the radiofrequency is turned off, the nuclei release the stored energy. This energy is analyzed via Fourier transformation, which results in the image. The images are highly dependent on the timing and magnitude of the radiofrequency.[84] Data acquisition can take 20 to 90 minutes, during which the patient must remain immobile. Application of MRI to the cardiac and pulmonary system was initially limited by the continuous movement of the heart and lungs, but the development of ultrafast imaging has overcome some of these problems.[85] Contrast materials such as gadolinium diethylenetriamine pentaacetate (Gd-DTPA) can be used to enhance signal intensity.

Cardiac Imaging

MRI is a useful technique in evaluating cardiac structures. It can identify cardiac masses and is the modality of choice for evaluating the pericardium. MRI is still secondary to CT in evaluating the mediastinum and detecting CAD.[84,86] Coronary artery imaging is still problematic due to cardiac motion.[87] Cardiac images from MRI do allow the measurement of right and left ventricular volumes, ejection fraction, and cardiac output.[82, 87] MRI is able to detect tissue composition such as myocardial fat infiltration and identification of myocardial edema caused by inflammation or ischemia.[87] Data collection of the heart requires the use of different testing sequences and specialized equipment to capture the beating heart.[87]

Tests to Evaluate Myocardial Perfusion

Contrast agents such as Gd-DPTA can be used in stress MRI studies to examine perfusion defects in the myocardium.[72] Cardiac MRI is able to characterize blood flow, as well as uptake and washout of the contrast agent. Unlike other modalities, cardiac MRI can distinguish tissue layers, enabling identification of areas of subendocardial or transmural defects.[72] MRI can also identify areas of myocardial edema, which is the result of ischemia. This allows identification of at risk areas which will benefit from reperfusion interventions. [87]

Tests to Evaluate Myocardial Viability

The viability of cardiac tissue can be examined with MRI, using delayed contrast enhancement Gd-DPTA as the contrast agent.[82] Images are taken 10 minutes after the intravenous administration of the agent. An inversion time pulse sequence allows the normal myocardial tissue to fade and the infarcted or scar tissue to be enhanced.

Pulmonary Imaging

Evaluation of the lung parenchyma presents unique problems because of respiratory movement, low proton density, and the air-tissue interface.[85] The development of ultrafast imaging pulse sequences, called dynamic MRI, has improved the utility of this noninvasive test for evaluation of the pulmonary system. Contrast agents such as Gd-DTPA are used to perform MR angiography to diagnose pulmonary embolism.[88] The use of MRI to provide noninvasive evaluation of PE has application in special cases, where typical tests are inconclusive.[88] Without contrast, dynamic MRI is being used to study biomechanical function of the diaphragm and chest wall in patients with and without pulmonary disease. These studies are important for patients undergoing lung volume reduction surgery.[89]

The use of gaseous contrast agents such as hyperpolarized helium-3 (HHe-3), with dynamic MRI and lung motion correction, is a promising new development that allows examination of gas distribution in the lungs.[85, 90] These studies have shown that dynamic MRI with contrast HHe-3 contrast can discriminate healthy lung grafts from native diseased lung in transplant patients[85] and identify ventilation defects that correlate with decreased FEV_1 in patients with asthma.[90]

Bronchoscopy

Bronchoscopy is often used as both a diagnostic and a therapeutic treatment modality.[91] It allows direct visualization of the trachea and its major subdivisions. Fiberoptic bronchoscopy has virtually replaced bronchography.[40] In fiberoptic bronchoscopy, a flexible tube is inserted into the trachea of mildly sedated patients. This tube is able to enter small bronchial subdivisions. Secretions can be removed for evaluation or as a treatment. It is also possible to obtain biopsy samples using tiny forceps or cell brushings. Bronchoscopy is particularly important in the diagnosis of bronchogenic carcinoma.[92]

Summary

Many tests are available to identify cardiopulmonary dysfunction. The attending physician determines which tests are appropriate for the patient's particular medical condition. When the tests are completed, results are given, and an evaluation of the results is documented. Physical therapists need to understand the results of the tests and how they will apply to patient function and response to exercise. This understanding applies to the selection of exercise and work loads the therapist prescribes for the patient. Until a physical therapist reaches a certain maturity level (in terms of experience), as well as a level of understanding and application of the test results to patient treatment, it is highly encouraged that the therapist discuss the tests and the results with the patient's physician. These discussions are excellent learning opportunities, both for the physical therapist and for the physician, who may gain a better understanding of what physical therapy has to offer the patient with cardiopulmonary dysfunction.

Review Questions

1. Why is the ejection fraction an important measure of myocardial function?
2. What is the difference between stunned myocardium and hibernating myocardium?
3. How does EBCT identify CAD risk?
4. Which tests can be used to evaluate myocardial viability?
5. Which test provides the best anatomical information?

References

1. Kones R: Recent advances in the management of chronic stable angina I: Approach to the patient, diagnosis, pathophysiology, risk stratification, and gender disparities. *Vascular Health and Risk Management* 6:635–656, 2010.
2. Dyer DS, Khan AR, Mohammed T-L, et al: ACR appropriateness criteria on chronic dyspnea, suspected pulmonary origin. *J Thorac Imaging* 25:W21–W23, 2010.
3. Lynch T, Bialy L, Kellner JD, et al: A systematic review on the diagnosis of pediatric bacterial pneumonia: When gold is bronze. *PLoS ONE* 2010 Aug 6;5(8):e11989, 2010.
4. Rogers TK: Primary care radiography in the early diagnosis of lung cancer. *Cancer Imaging* 10:73–76, 2010.
5. Miller RF, O'Doherty MJ: Pulmonary nuclear medicine. *European Journal of Nuclear Medicine* 19:355–368, 1992.
6. Maass-Moreno R, Bachrach SL: Imaging instrumentation. In Iskandrian AE, Verani MS, editors: *Nuclear Cardiac Imaging*, ed 3, Oxford, 2003, University Press.
7. Murphy PH: Radiation physics and radiation safety. In Iskandrian AE, Verani MS, editors: *Nuclear Cardiac Imaging*, ed 3, Oxford, 2003, University Press.
8. Fernandez R: Radionuclides in Nuclear Cardiology: Current Status and Limitations.
9. Beller G: *Clinical Nuclear Cardiology*. Philadelphia, 1995, W.B. Saunders.
10. Patton JA, Slomka PJ, Germano G, et al: Recent technologic advances in nuclear cardiology. *J Nucl Cardiol* 14:501–513, 2007.
11. Watson DD: Acquisition, processing, and quantification of nuclear cardiac images. In Iskandrian AE, Verani MS, editors: *Nuclear Cardiac Imaging*, ed 3, Oxford, 2003, University Press.
12. Patton JA, Turkington TG: SPECT/CT physical principles and attenuation correction. *J Nucl Med Technol* 36:1–10, 2008.
13. Schwaiger M: Myocardial perfusion imaging with PET. *Journal of Nuclear Medicine* 35:693–698, 1994.
14. Baggish AL, Boucher CA: Radiopharmaceutical agents for myocardial perfusion imaging. *Circulation* 118:1668–1674, 2008.
15. Bengel FM, Higuchi T, Javad MS, et al: Cardiac positron emission tomography. *J Am Coll Cardiol* 54:1–15, 2009.
16. Chen DL, Kinahan PE: Multimodality molecular imaging of the lung. *J Magn Reson Imaging* 32:1409–1420, 2010.
17. Klocke FJ, Baird MG, Lorell BH, et al: American College of Cardiology; American Heart Association; American Society for Nuclear Cardiology. ACC/AHA/ASNC guidelines for the clinical use of cardiac radionuclide imaging–executive summary: a report of the American College of Cardiology/American Heart Association Task Force on Practice Guidelines (ACC/AHA/ASNC Committee to Revise the 1995 Guidelines for the Clinical Use of Cardiac Radionuclide Imaging). *J Am Coll Cardiol* 42(7):1318–1333, 2003.
18. Rahmim A, Zaidi H: PET versus SPECT: strengths, limitations and challenges. *Nucl Med Commun* 29(3):193–207, 2008.
19. Schwaiger M, Ziegler S, Nekolla SG: PET/CT: Challenge for nuclear cardiology. *J Nucl Med* 46:1664–1678, 2006.
20. Williams KA, Borer JS, Supino D: Radio nuclide angiography. In Iskandrian AE, Verani MS, editors: *Nuclear Cardiac Imaging*, ed 3, Oxford, 2003, University Press.
21. Dyer GSM, Tifer MA: Heart Failure. In Lilly LS, editor: *Pathophysiology of Heart Diseases*, ed 3, Philadelphia, 2003, Lippincott Williams & Wilkins.
22. Jessup M, Brozena S: Heart Failure. *New England Journal of Medicine* 348:2007–2018, 2003.
23. Curtis JP, Sokol, SI, Wang Y, et al: The association of left ventricular ejection fraction, mortality, and cause of death in stable outpatients with heart failure. *J Am Coll Cardiol* 42:736–742, 2003.
24. Pride YB, Giuseffi JL, Mohanavelu S, et al: Relation between infarct size in ST-segment elevation myocardial infarction treated successfully by

percutaneous coronary intervention and left ventricular ejection fraction three months after the infarct. *Am J Cardiol* 106(5):635–640, 2010.
25. Kinch J, Ryan T: Right ventricular infarction. *N Engl J Med* 330(17):1211–1217, 1994.
26. Port S: The role of radionuclide ventriculography in the assessment of prognosis in patients with CAD. *Journal of Nuclear Medicine* 35:721–725, 1994.
27. Otto CM: *Textbook of Clinical Echocardiography*. Philadelphia, 2000, W.B. Saunders.
28. Gibbons RJ, Valeti US, Aaroz PA, et al: The quantification of infarct size. *J Am Coll Cardiol* 44:1533–1542, 2004.
29. Schinkel AFL, Bax JJ, Delgado V, et al: Clinical relevance of hibernating myocardium in ischemic left ventricular dysfunction. *The American Journal of Medicine* 123:978–986, 2010.
30. Pagnanelli RA, Basso DA: Myocardial perfusion imaging with 201Tl. *J Nucl Med Technol* 38:1–3, 2010.
31. Berman D, Hosen S, Van Train K, et al: Myocardial perfusion imaging with technitium-99M-sestamibi comparative analysis of available imaging protocols. *Journal of Nuclear Medicine* 35:681–688, 1994.
32. Johnson L: Myocardial perfusion imaging with technetium-99m-teboroxime. *Journal of Nuclear Medicine* 35:689–692, 1994.
33. Kaufmann PA, Camici PG: Myocardial blood flow measurements by PET: Technical aspects and clinical applications. *J Nucl Med* 46:75–88, 2005.
34. Schindler TH, Schelbert HR, Quercioli A, et al: Cardiac PET imaging for the detection and monitoring of coronary artery disease and microvascular health. *JACC: Cardiovascular Imaging* 3:623–640, 2010.
35. Maddahi J, Schelbert H, Brunken R, et al: Role of thallium-201 and PET imaging in evaluation of myocardial viability and management of patients with coronary artery disease and left ventricular dysfunction. *Journal of Nuclear Medicine* 35:707–715, 1994.
36. Hendel R: Single-photon imaging for the assessment of myocardial viability. *Journal of Nuclear Medicine* 35(4 suppl):23s–31s, 1994.
37. Niemeyer MG, Van der Wall EE, Pauwels EKJ, et al: Assessment of acute myocardial infarction by nuclear imaging techniques. *Angiology* 43:720–733, 1992.
38. Schelbert H: Metabolic imaging to assess myocardial viability. *Journal of Nuclear Medicine* 35(4 suppl):8s–14s, 1994.
39. Bergman S: Use and limitations of metabolic tracers labeled with positron-emitting radionuclides in the identification of viable myocardium. *Journal of Nuclear Medicine* 35(4 suppl):15s–22s, 1994.
40. Lillington G: *A diagnostic approach to chest disease*. Baltimore, 1987, Williams and Wilkins.
41. Sostman HD, Stein PD, Gottschalk A, et al: Acute pulmonary embolism: sensitivity and specificity of ventilation-perfusion scintigraphy in PIOPED II study. *Radiology* 246(3):941–946, 2008.
42. Douma RA, Kamphuisen PW, Buller HR: Acute pulmonary embolism. Part 1: epidemiology and diagnosis. *Nat. Rev. Cardiol* 7:585–596, 2010.
43. Kramer E, Divgi C: Pulmonary applications of nuclear medicine. *Clinics in Chest Medicine* 12(1):55–75, 1991.
44. Weiss CR, Scatarige JC, Diette GB, et al: CT pulmonary angiography is the first-line imaging test for acute pulmonary embolism: a survey of US clinicians. *Acad Radiol* 13:434–446, 2006.
45. Hope WW, Demeter BL, Newcomb WL, et al: Postoperative pulmonary embolism: timing, diagnosis, treatment, and outcomes. *American Journal of Surgery* 194:814–819, 2007.
46. Gould MK, Maclean CC, Kuschner WG, et al: Accuracy of positron emission tomography for diagnosis of pulmonary nodules and mass lesions. *JAMA* 285:914–924, 2001.
47. Tan BB, Flaherty KR, Kazerooni EA, et al: The solitary pulmonary nodule. *Chest* 123:89S–96S, 2003.
48. Schuster DM, Alazraki N: Gallium and other agents in diseases of the lung. *Seminars in Nuclear Medicine* 32:193–211, 2002.
49. Reagan K, Boxt L, Katz J: Introduction to coronary arteriography. *Radiologic Clinics of North America* 32:419–433, 1994.
50. Ryan TJ: The coronary angiogram and its seminal contributions to cardiovascular medicine over five decades. *Circulation* 106:752–756, 2002.
51. Kushner FG, Hand M, Smith DE, et al: 2009 Focused Updates: ACC/AHA Guidelines for the management of patients with ST-elevation myocardial infarction. *J Am Coll Cardiol* 54:2205–2241, 2009.
52. Wright RS, Anderson JL, Adams CD, Bridges CR, et al: 2011 ACCF/AHA focused update of the guidelines for the management of patients with unstable angina/non-ST-elevation myocardial infarction. *J Am Coll Cardiol* 57:1920–1959, 2011.
53. Kern MJ: Coronary physiology revisited: Practical insights from the cardiac catheterization laboratory. *Circulation* 101:1344–1351, 2000.
54. Kern MJ, Moore JA, Aguirre FV, et al: Determination of Angiographic (TIMI Grade) Blood Flow by Intracoronary Doppler Flow Velocity During Acute Myocardial Infarction. *Circulation*. 94:1545–1552, 1996.
55. Gibson CM, Cannon CP, Murphy SA, et al: Relationship of the TIMI myocardial perfusion grades, flow grades, frame count, and percutaneous coronary intervention to long-term outcomes after thrombolytic administration in acute myocardial infarction. *Circulation* 105:1909–1913, 2002.
56. Grossman W: *Cardiac Catheterization and Angiography*, ed 3, Philadelphia, 1986, Lea & Febiger.
57. Anavekar NS, Oh JK: Doppler echocardiography: a contemporary review. *J Cardiology* 54:347–358, 2009.
58. Kohli-Seth R, Neuman T, Sinha R, et al: Use of echocardiography and modalities of patient monitoring of trauma patients. *Current Opinion in Anaesthesiology* 23:239–245, 2010.
59. Feigenbaum H: Role of M-mode Technique in Today's Echocardiography. *Journal of the American Society of Echocardiography* 23:240–257, 2010.
60. Waggoner AD, Perez J: Principles and physics of Doppler. *Cardiology Clinics* 12:385–389, 1990.
61. Armstrong GP, Griffin BP: Exercise echocardiographic assessment in severe mitral regurgitation. *Coronary Artery Disease* 11:23–30, 2000.
62. Kerber R: *Echocardiography in coronary artery disease*. Mount Kisco, NY, 1988, Futura Publishing.
63. Schober P, Loer SA, Schwarte LA: Perioperative hemodynamic monitoring with transesophageal Doppler technology. *Anesth Analg* 109:340–353, 2009.
64. Peterson GE, Brickner E, Reimold SC: Transesophageal echocardiography. *Circulation* 107:2398–2402, 2003.
65. Kwak J, Andrawes M, Garvin S, et al: 3-D Transesophageal echocardiography: A review of recent literature 2007-2009. *Curr Opin Anaesthesiol* 23:80–88, 2010.
66. Rocchi G, Fallani F, Bracchetti G, et al: Non-invasive detection of coronary artery stenosis: a comparison among power-Doppler contrast echo, 99Tc-Sestamibi SPECT and echo wall-motion analysis. *Coronary Artery Disease* 14:239–245, 2003.
67. Mulvagh SL: Myocardial perfusion by contrast echocardiography: diagnosis of coronary artery disease using contrast-enhanced stress echocardiography and assessment of coronary anatomy and flow reserve. *Coronary Artery Disease* 11:243–251, 2000.
68. Porter TR, Xie F: Myocardial perfusion imaging with contrast ultrasound. *JACC Cardiovasc Imaging* 3(2):176–187, 2010.
69. Fraser RS, Paré PD, Coman N et al: *Diagnosis of Diseases of the Chest, Vol. I*, ed 4, Philadelphia, 1999, W.B. Saunders Co.
70. Bakal CW: Advances in imaging technology and the growth of vascular and interventional radiology: A brief history. *J Vasc Interv Radiol* 2003 Jul;14(7):855–860, 2003.
71. O'Rourke RA, Brundage BH, Froelicher VF: American College of Cardiology/American Heart Association expert consensus document on electron-beam computed tomography for the diagnosis and prognosis of coronary artery disease. *Journal of American College Cardiology* 36:326–340, 2000.
72. Nikolaou K, Poon M, Sirol M, et al: Complementary results of computed tomography and magnetic resonance imaging of the heart and coronary arteries: a review and future outlook. *Cardiology Clinics* 21:639–655, 2003.
73. Dawn SK, Gotway MB, Webb WR: Multidetector-row spiral computed tomography in the diagnosis of thoracic diseases. *Respiratory Care* 46(9):912–921, 2001.
74. Berman DS, Hachamovitch R, Shaw LJ, et al: Roles of nuclear cardiology, cardiac computed tomography, and cardiac magnetic resonance: assessment of patients with suspected coronary artery disease. *J Nucl Med* 47:74–82, 2006.
75. Kondos GT, Hoff JA, Serukov A, et al: Electron-beam tomography coronary artery calcium and cardiac events. *Circulation* 107:2571–2576, 2003.
76. Chow BJW, Larose E, Bilodeau S, et al: The "what, when, where, who and how?" of cardiac computed tomography in 2009: guidelines for the clinician. *Can J Cardiol* 25:136–140, 2009.
77. Taylor AJ, Cerqueira M, Hodgson J McB, et al: ACCF/SCCT/ACR/AHA/ASE/ASNC/NASCI/SCAI/SCMR 2010 appropriate use criteria for cardiac computed tomography. *J Am Coll Cardiol* 56:1864–1894, 2010.
78. Webb WR: High-resolution computed tomography of obstructive lung disease. *Radiologic Clinics of North America* 32:745–757, 1994.
79. Henzler T, Barraza JM, Nance JW, et al: CT imaging of acute pulmonary embolism. *J Cardiovascular Computed Tomography* 5:3–11, 2011.
80. Gutte H, Mortensen J, Jensen CV, et al: Detection of pulmonary embolism with combined ventilation-perfusion SPECT and low-dose CT: head-to-head

comparison with multidetector CT angiography. *J Nucl Med* 50:1987–1992, 2009.
81. Roach PJ, Gradinscak DJ, Schembri GP, et al: SPECT/CT in V/Q scanning. *Semin Nucl Med* 40:455–466, 2010.
82. Forder JR, Pohost GM: Cardiovascular nuclear magnetic resonance: Basic and clinical applications. *Journal of Clinical Investigation* 111:1630–1639, 2003.
83. Gould TA: How MRI works. How Stuff Works. Accessed August 19, 2004. www.howstuffowrks.com.
84. Mayo J: Magnetic resonance imaging of the chest. *Radiol Clin North Am* 32(4):795–809,1994 Jul.
85. Gast KK, Puderbach MU, Rodriguez I, et al: Distribution of ventilation in lung transplant recipients: evaluation by dynamic 3He-MRI with lung motion correction. *Investigative Radiology* 38:341–348, 2003.
86. Schuijf JD, Bax JJ, Shaw LJ, de Roos A, et al: Meta-analysis of comparative diagnostic performance magnetic resonance imaging and multislice computed tomography for noninvasive coronary angiography. *Am Heart J* 151:404–411, 2006.
87. Figtree GA, Lonborg J, Grieve SM, et al: Cardiac magnetic resonance imaging for the interventional cardiologist. *J Am Coll Cardio Intv* 4:137–148, 2011.
88. Meaney JF, Weg JG, Chenevert TL, et al: Diagnosis of pulmonary embolism with magnetic resonance angiography. *New England Journal of Medicine* 336:1422–1427, 1997.
89. Suga K, Tsukuda T, Awaya H, et al: Interactions of regional respiratory mechanics and pulmonary ventilatory impairment in pulmonary emphysema: assessment with dynamic MRI and Xenon-133 single-photon emission CT *CHEST* 117:1646–1655, 2000.
90. Samee S, Altes T, Powers P, et al: Imaging the lungs in asthmatic patients by using hyperpolarized helium-3 magnetic resonance: assessment of response to methacholine and exercise challenge. *J Allergy Clin Immunol* 111:1205–1211, 2003.
91. Mars M, Ciesla N: Chest physical therapy may have prevented bronchoscopy and exploratory laparotomy: A case report. *Cardiopulmonary Physical Therapy Journal* 4(1):4–6, 1993.
92. Price S, Wilson L: Pathophysiology: Clinical concepts of disease processes. New York, 1986, McGraw-Hill.

II

Chapter 15

Clinical Evaluation and Assessment of the Cardiovascular and Pulmonary System

Donna Frownfelter and Susan M. Butler McNamara

KEY TERMS

Patent examination and assessment
Identification of CVP impairments
Patient/family history
Physical examination
Chest wall symmetry
Congenital chest wall anomalies
Dyspnea
Fremitus
Auscultation of breath sounds
Normal
Adventitious breath sounds
Crackles
Hyperresonant
Egophony ("e to a changes")
Auscultation of breath sounds
Rhonchi
Chest wall mobility
Symmetry
Causes for asymmetry
"Red flag"

CHAPTER OUTLINE

The Guide to Physical Therapist Practice provides a thorough patient management model.[1] It identifies the key components necessary for a thorough examination and evaluation of the patient, tests and measures, identification of impairments, and interventions and outcomes that help the therapist in providing a multisystem examination and evaluation that will lead to appropriate treatment and achievement of optimal function and goals (see Figure 17-2).

This chapter will follow and focus on the flow of the examination, which includes patient and family history, systems review, tests and measures overview, evaluation leading to interventions, and identifying and reaching appropriate outcomes. This flow may continue in a forward, circular manner, or it may go back and forth as a patient's condition either improves or declines. It is an active process, which may lead to achieving expected outcomes, discharge, or discontinuation of therapy based on many factors. A given patient may have more than one impairment, so all conditions or a multisystem examination should be done to identify all impairments. In addition, prevention and risk factor assessment must be done. For example, if an orthopedic patient is referred for treatment following a total knee replacement (TKR), the therapist may find that he is also prehypertensive with elevated BP and HR, has a family history of heart disease, and is a smoker. Thus, in addition to treating for the primary referral diagnosis of TKR, the therapist may also use the 6A Prevention Pattern to try to decrease the patient's risk factors for cardiovascular and pulmonary (CVP) disease and to promote wellness.

It is important to remember that although patients may be referred to the physical therapist for a primary cardiovascular and/or pulmonary impairment, they may also have a secondary cardiovascular and/or pulmonary impairment that may or may not have been diagnosed or identified. Another example would be a patient referred to physical therapy after having a cardiovascular accident (CVA). This patient may have right-sided weakness, be slumped to the right side, and have decreasing ventilation on the right lung. Weak pharyngeal muscles may be increasing the patient's risk for aspiration. In addition, a decreased vital capacity and weakened abdominal muscles may reduce the patient's ability to keep the airway clear, and poor breath support may make it difficult for the patient to speak clearly, if at all. If the therapist only considers the primary diagnosis of CVA, the potentially life-threatening secondary cardiovascular and pulmonary impairments would be missed, which would limit optimal outcomes.

Screening for risk factors for cardiovascular and pulmonary issues is essential in all patients, including a thorough family history and assessment of other risk factors. A patient may come to the physical therapist after having a "simple" orthopedic procedure such as an ACL repair, but after discussing family history it is discovered that the 30-year-old patient's father died at age 32 after a massive heart attack. If the therapist checks the patient's BP on screening, finds that it is 180/100, and discovers that the patient hasn't been to a doctor in years, the therapist can identify risk factors and help to provide secondary prevention, as well as the primary treatment.

The examination and evaluation provide the therapist with a baseline, against which future visits or sessions will be compared. Depending on the site of practice (e.g., acute care versus long-term care or outpatient, school, or home care), this may occur each time the therapist sees the patient or once a week; regardless, the baseline data are essential as a place to start.

History: Review and Interview

Medical Chart Review

The first component in the examination is obtaining a history. Initially, this can be a review of the medical chart, paying close attention to the notes of the physician, the nurse, and the physician assistant and looking through lab values, tests that were ordered and their results, vital signs, and summary notes. Each practice setting has a variety of available information; as a rule, the more acute the patient's condition is, the more notes, tests, and results there are to review. It is helpful to learn to screen the chart quickly but also thoroughly in order not to miss information. After the chart review, the therapist should discuss the patient's case with the nurse, physician, physician's assistant, and/or other members of the interprofessional team to help develop an understanding of the patient's condition before beginning the examination.

Patient/Family Interview

If a direct patient interview is possible, asking specific open-ended questions is most valuable. It is optimal to interview the patient directly, and even if the person has some limitations, the initial questions should be directed to the patient. If the patient is very ill or cognitively impaired and unable to provide information, the family and significant others in his or her life may be able to give important information not found directly on the medical chart. It is important for the physical therapist to take the time to listen carefully to what is expressed and relate it to what was found in the chart before performing the examination and evaluation.

In outpatient settings, rehabilitation facilities, or schools, very little information may be available other than a physician's referral and/or notes. In these cases, the therapist needs to be effective at drawing out important information from the patient during the interview. It is important to be thorough and yet be aware of appropriate time management and efficiency. Interviewing is a skill that improves with practice as the therapist gains more knowledge of diagnoses and patient presentations and becomes better able to obtain information in an organized efficient manner.

A sequencing strategy is helpful in reviewing charts. With experience most therapists develop a specific system that works well for them. Here is just one example of a strategy for reviewing charts:

1. Read the history and the physical and admission medical notes (i.e., the preadmission symptoms, past medical history)—this includes the physician's notes and the nurse's notes.
2. Read the most recent medical notes.
3. Scan the remainder of the chart.
4. Read any reports from medical specialists and consultants, such as pulmonologists, neurologists, or oncologists.
5. Review any pertinent lab tests, such as chest radiograph, arterial blood gases (ABGs), complete blood count (CBC), cardiac tests, CAT scans, and MRIs.
6. Review medications—in particular, pulmonary and cardiac drugs.
7. Review any procedures performed (e.g., surgery, intubation, chest tubes, NG tubes).
8. Review the psychosocial information (e.g., family, support systems, education, financial concerns, psychological issues, architectural barriers).

In acute care, discharge planning begins with the first time a therapist sees a patient. Patients are often in the hospital only a brief time, and the physical therapist will be asked to make recommendations for discharge. Any detail of a patient's background that would affect discharge planning is crucial to know, even on the first day of treatment. Additional information that may be helpful to review (and falls into the category of "as time allows") includes any documentation recorded by other health professionals, such as nurses, occupational therapists, or speech pathologists. Finally, when the initial chart review is finished, a mental picture of the patient should exist, even before the physical therapist steps into the patient's hospital room.

Details regarding the patient interview have been covered in Chapter 7. However, there are questions that should be posed to any patient, even if his or her primary condition is not cardiovascular and/or pulmonary. The patient whose primary referring impairment is musculoskeletal or neurological needs to have a screening of the cardiovascular and pulmonary system. The therapist should consider the following questions: What is the patient's smoking history? Does the patient have a family history of premature coronary artery disease (i.e., a parent or sibling who had a myocardial infarction)? Can the symptoms presented also be signs of a cardiovascular or pulmonary illness? Does the patient have an active or a sedentary lifestyle? What activities precipitate the patient's symptoms? Do these symptoms include breathlessness? Are there problems with airway clearance, congestion, etc.?

Every patient should be seen as a human being with multiple organ systems. The patient's problem, whether orthopedic or cardiovascular and pulmonary, should not be viewed in isolation. Another example is the outpatient with a physical therapy diagnosis of low back pain. When questioned about limiting symptoms, the patient might describe cramping leg pain, which is suggestive of peripheral vascular disease (PVD). This should be considered a "red flag" that would lead the therapist to look further into cardiovascular and pulmonary issues or impairments. If this is not taken into consideration and the patient is treated only for low back pain, optimal outcomes and function cannot occur.

System Review and Tests and Measures

Physical Examination of the Chest

After the general physical therapy examination of muscle strength, ROM, activity, and function, the physical examination of the chest comes next. The therapist begins by obtaining vital signs (BP, HR, T, etc.) and then progresses to the examination of the chest wall and auscultation of the heart and lungs. When the information provided by each of these techniques is integrated with the patient's history, interview, and chart review, the physical therapist can then do the assessment and identify the impairment, prognosis, and appropriate interventions that will lead to optimal outcomes for the patient. It is important to include all of these assessments in an appropriate sequence. For instance, auscultating breath sounds without evaluating the patient's posture or asymmetry of the chest wall would fail to provide needed clues to the total patient picture and would not facilitate the development of an appropriate plan of care for the patient. All components of the examination must be considered before deciding which interventions should be implemented and which goals and/or outcomes can be developed.

Before we discuss the individual aspects of the chest assessment, a review of the pertinent anatomic landmarks and topographic lines is warranted. Knowledge of the superficial anatomy and its relationship to the underlying heart and lungs aids the therapist in making crucial decisions. The topographical lines allow for more accurate descriptions of the physical findings.

Topographic Anatomic Landmarks

Key anatomic structures include the following:

- Sternum
- Clavicles
- Suprasternal notch
- Sternomanubrial angle (angle of Louis for identification of the second rib)
- Costal angle
- Vertebra prominens

See Box 15-1 and Figure 15-1 for specific definitions and anterior and lateral views of the thorax. Imaginary topographic lines are used to more clearly describe any physical findings (e.g., location of surgical incisions, abnormal breath sounds, etc.; Figure 15-2).

The anterior view of the thorax has three vertical lines:

- Midsternal line (MSL)—a vertical line bisecting the sternum
- 2 Midclavicular lines (MCLs)—parallel to the MSL, bisecting each clavicle; the borders of the lower lung cross the sixth ribs at the MCLs

Laterally, there are also three vertical lines, originating in their respective axillary folds:

- Anterior axillary line (AAL)
- Midaxillary line (MAL)
- Posterior axillary line (PAL)—like the MCLs, these lines are bilateral

The posterior chest has the following three lines:

- Vertebral or midspinal line—runs through the spinous processes of the vertebrae
- 2 Midscapular lines (MSLs)—parallel to the midspinal line, bisecting the inferior angles of the scapulae

Box 15-1 Anatomic Structures

- Suprasternal notch: A depression palpable at the top of the sternum
- Sternomanubrial angle: A bony bump where the manubrium meets the body of the sternum; about 5 cm distal to suprasternal notch; also known as the angle of Louis; palpating lateral to this junction, the second ribs are found; they are reference points for identifying intercostal spaces and successive ribs; also, a superficial marking for where the underlying trachea divides into right and left main stem bronchi
- Costal angle: The angle formed by the joining of the costal margins with the sternum; normally, no greater than 90 degrees
- Vertebra prominens: The spinous process of the seventh cervical vertebra (C7); allows numbering of thoracic vertebra

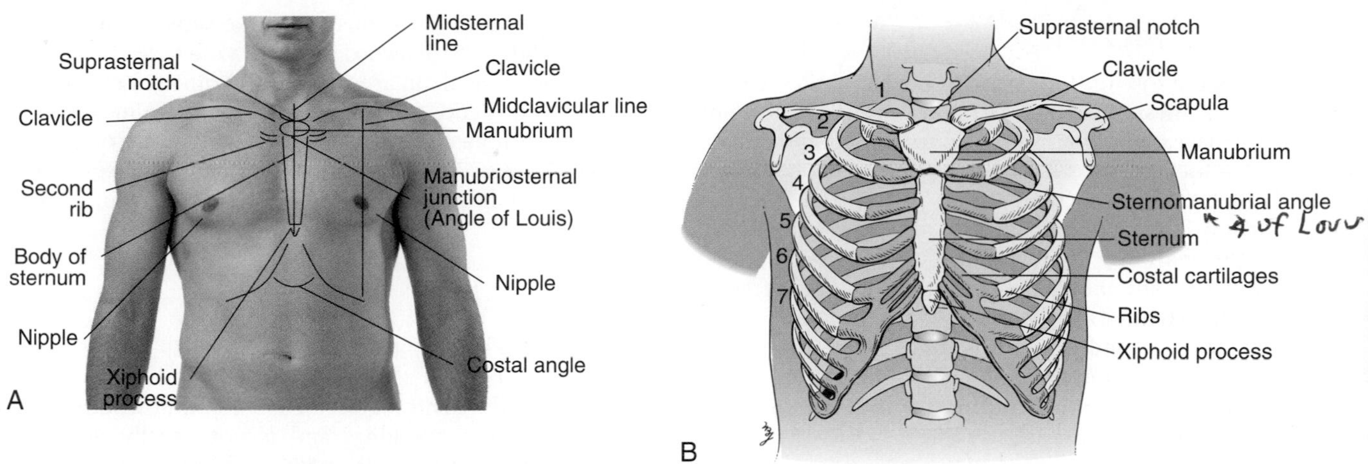

Fig. 15-1 Anatomy of the chest. **A,** Topographic landmarks of the chest. **B,** Bony chest skeleton. *(**A** from Thompson JM, Wilson SF:* Health assessment for nursing practice, *St Louis, 1996, Mosby.* ***B*** *from Schwartz MH:* Textbook of physical diagnosis: History and examination, *ed 6, St Louis, 2010, Saunders.)*

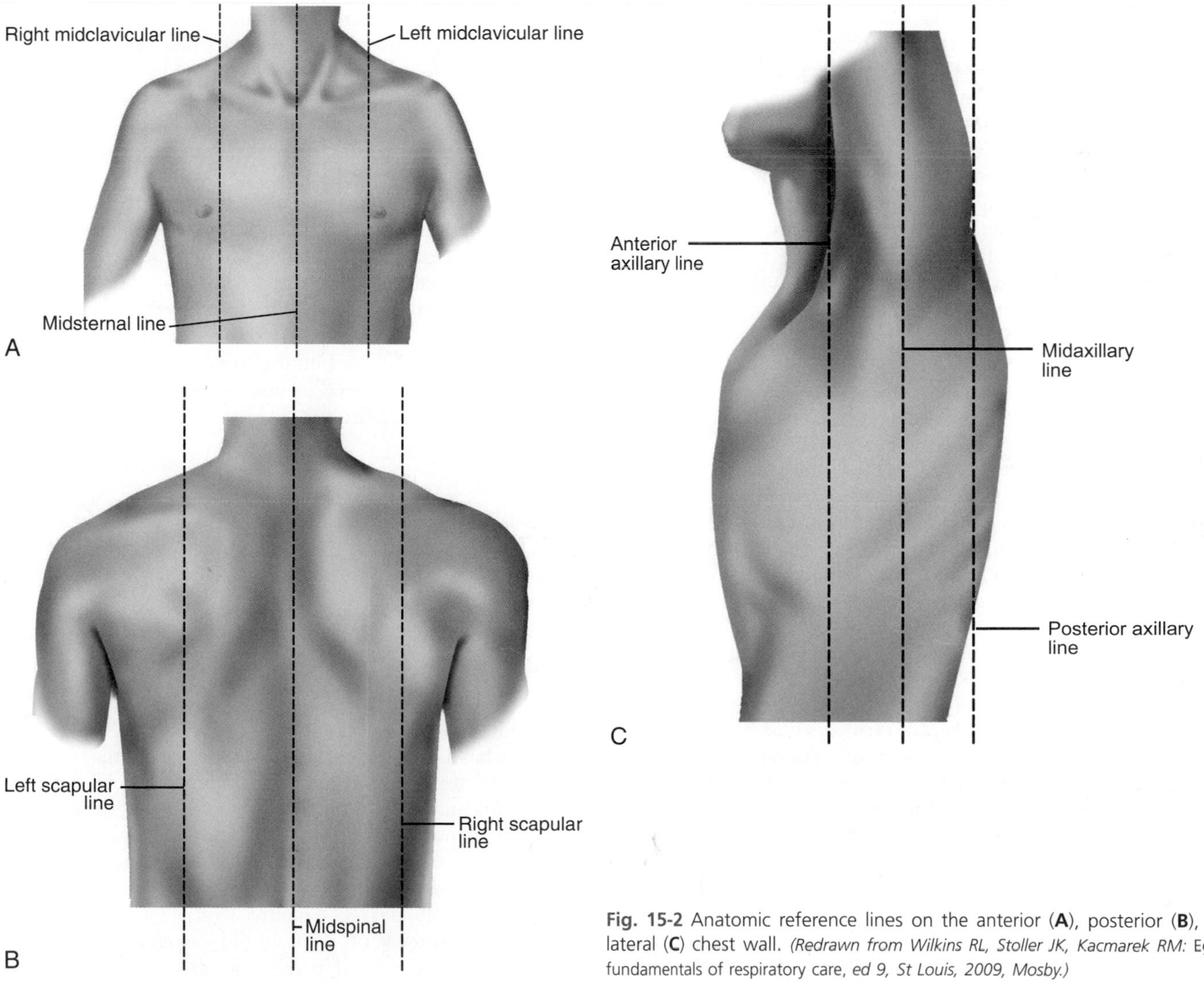

Fig. 15-2 Anatomic reference lines on the anterior (**A**), posterior (**B**), and lateral (**C**) chest wall. *(Redrawn from Wilkins RL, Stoller JK, Kacmarek RM:* Egan's fundamentals of respiratory care, *ed 9, St Louis, 2009, Mosby.)*

Visual Inspection

Inspection is the foremost element of a systematic review of the chest. The physical therapist should not only observe the features of the patient, but also consider the equipment and any aspect of the patient's surroundings that would contribute to delineating the true picture of that patient. The therapist should already have a preliminary idea of the patient based on review of the chart and discussion with the physician, nurse, or physician assistant. Interacting with the patient is necessary to determine whether the initial assessment was realistic. Other clinical signs and symptoms the patient exhibits will also be taken into account during the first interaction. Examination and evaluation should continue during any subsequent interventions and patient visits.

General Appearance

The examination should begin as soon as the therapist walks into the patient's room. Many questions about the appearance of the patient, as well as his or her surroundings, must be considered in order to help determine the patient's status. The following are some examples of questions typical for the acute care setting:

Does the patient appear comfortable? Is there any facial grimacing? Is the patient awake and alert or somnolent or disoriented? Is there any nasal flaring, wheezing, or pursed-lip breathing? (These are signs of respiratory distress. Nasal flaring can be defined as the outward movement of the nares with inspiration.[2]) Are the accessory muscles of respiration (i.e., sternocleidomastoid and trapezius) hypertrophied? How is the patient positioned? Is the patient resting comfortably or leaning forward over the bedside table and struggling for breath? What is the patient's build—stocky, thin, or cachectic? Is the patient's mobility limited? Can the patient sit unsupported? Should the assessment be performed in stages, allowing the patient to be supine and then to lie on each side? Is there any extra equipment in the patient's surroundings? Is the patient using supplemental oxygen? Is the oxygen delivered through a nasal cannula or other device? What is the fraction of inspired oxygen (FiO_2)? Are there any monitoring lines, and where are they located? For instance, if an arterial line is present, is it placed in the radial or the femoral artery? Are there electrocardiogram (ECG) leads? Is it a hard line (directly connected to a monitor) or a telemetry line (communicating through radio transmitter)? Are there intravenous (IV) sites? Are they peripheral (antecubital) or central (subclavian or jugular)? Is there a urinary catheter? Are there chest tubes?

These are just a few examples. In other settings, different questions will apply (such as posture and breathing considerations related to functional activities). However, many of these same questions will apply, regardless of the setting. Remember that a visual inspection of general appearance does not apply only to the patient but also to the immediate surroundings, including any equipment or devices that may be attached to the patient. It is extremely important to know what equipment is being used, to understand the purpose of each medical devices, and to be aware of how movement may affect these devices. All tubes and lines attached to the patient must be identified and thought must be given to what may happen to each of these before any physical therapy activity or intervention is performed. In certain cases, a line or tube being dislodged or detached could be a life-threatening occurrence (such as with an arterial line). In other cases, a dislodging or disturbance of lines may only cause inconvenience (such as with an IV) or discomfort (in the case of a urinary catheter). Regardless of the potential consequences, extreme care and planning must precede any movement of or by patients.

Skin

Does the skin have a pink, healthy color or a pallor? Is cyanosis present? Cyanosis is a bluish tinge that can be seen centrally or peripherally. Central cyanosis is a result of insufficient gas exchange within the lungs and is not usually seen unless oxygen saturation is less than 80%. A bluish tint may be seen at the mucous membranes (e.g., tongue and lips). Peripheral cyanosis, on the other hand, occurs when oxygen extraction at the periphery is excessive. This type is more closely associated with states of low cardiac output. Areas to observe for peripheral cyanosis include fingertips, toes, nose, and nail beds. A differentiating feature between central and peripheral cyanosis is that peripheral cyanosis normally occurs in the cooler body parts, such as the nail beds, and usually vanishes when the part is warmed. In contrast, central cyanosis does not disappear when the area is warmed.

Are any scars, bruises, or ecchymoses observed? Are there reddened areas suggestive of prolonged pressure? Do the bony landmarks appear more prominent than usual? Are there any signs of trauma to the thorax or any other body parts? Does the skin appear edematous? Does this edema appear to limit joint motion? Are there any surgical incisions, new or old? Do these incisions appear to be healed or seem reddened and swollen? Is there evidence of clubbing of the digits? Digital clubbing can be defined as the loss of angle between the nail bed and the distal interphalangeal joint (Figure 15-3). The cause of clubbing is explained by a variety of theories, including increased perfusion secondary to hypoxemia with arterial desaturation, but this is not an exclusive phenomenon; clubbing has also been observed in nonpulmonary diseases such as hepatic fibrosis and Crohn's disease.[2-4]

Neck

Are the accessory muscles of respiration being recruited for a resting breathing pattern? Do the sternocleidomastoid or trapezius muscles appear prominent? This is an early sign of obstructive lung disease.[2]

Jugular Venous Distention

The jugular veins empty into the superior vena cava and reflect right-sided heart function. Right atrial pressure (RAP) is evident based on the extent to which the jugular venous pulse (JVP) can be visualized. The more superficial external jugular veins may be seen superior to the clavicles; the internal jugular veins, though larger, lie deep beneath the sternocleidomastoids and are less visible. Jugular venous distention (JVD) can be best seen when the patient lies with the head and neck at an angle of 45 degrees (Figure 15-4). The presence or absence of symmetry of JVD should be noted. The veins are distended bilaterally if there is a cardiac cause such as

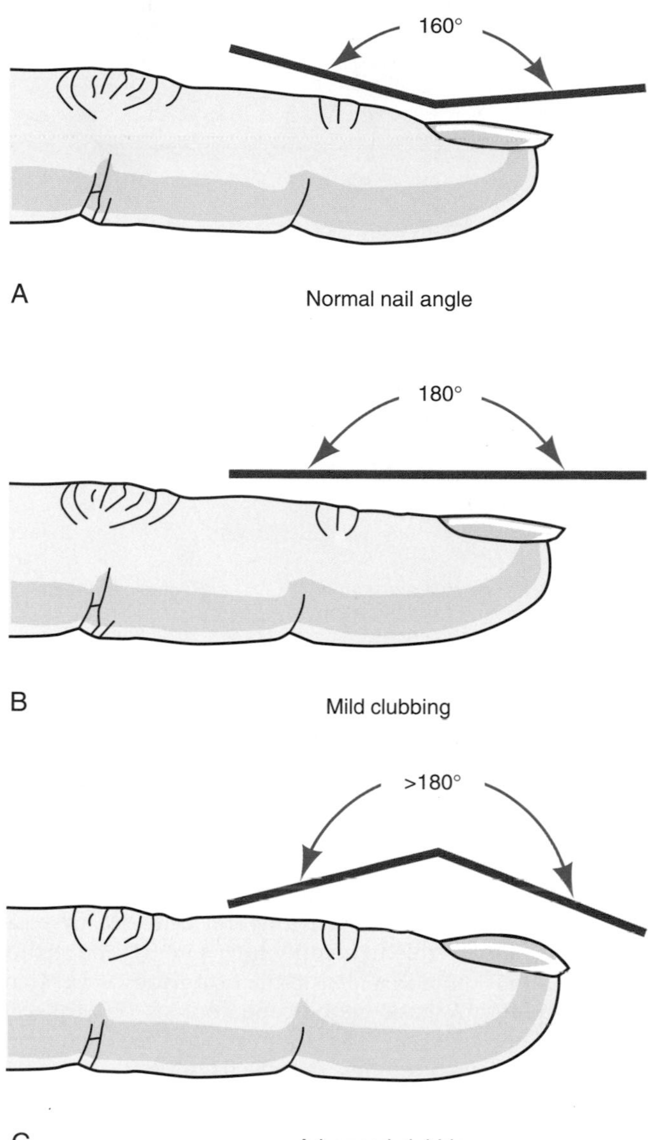

Fig. 15-3 A, Clubbing of the fingers is best assessed by determining the ratio of the diameter at the base of the nail, **B** and **C,** to the diameter at the distal interphalangeal joint. This ratio is normally less than 1. *(From George RB:* Chest medicine, *ed 2, Baltimore, 1990, Williams and Wilkins.)*

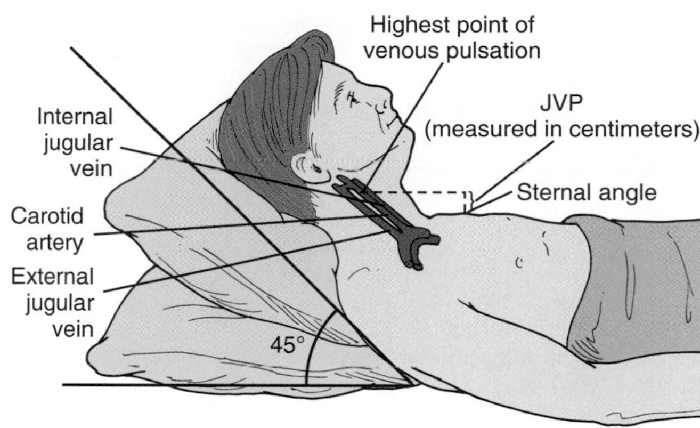

Fig. 15-4 Proper positioning to observe jugular venous distention. *(From Seidel HM:* Mosby's guide to physical examination, *ed 5, Philadelphia, 2003, Mosby.)*

congestive heart failure (CHF). A unilateral distention is an indication of a localized problem.[4]

Chest Wall Configuration

The normal thoracic cage is elliptically shaped when free of disease. The anteroposterior (AP)-to-lateral diameter is 1:2 or 5:7. The angle of the ribs is less than 90 degrees. The ribs articulate with the vertebra posteriorly, at a 45-degree angle. The thorax should be observed anteriorly, laterally, and posteriorly. In patients with COPD, the ribs become more horizontal and the AP diameter increases; thus the term *barrel chest* is used. In infants, the chest is round, with the anteroposterior and transverse or lateral diameters of about equal dimensions. As a child grows to adulthood, the chest becomes more elliptical. With the aging process, the chest returns to a more rounded appearance. The increased anteroposterior diameter in this population is a result of the multiple factors of decreasing lung compliance, decreased strength of the thoracic and diaphragmatic muscles, and skeletal changes in the thoracic spine. The symmetry or absence thereof of the thoracic cage should also be noted. Asymmetry can be the result of structural defects or an underlying intrathoracic pathology or neurological weakness. Various impairments will be seen in different views, as mentioned above, anteriorly, laterally or posteriorly.

Structural defects of the anterior chest may include the following: pectus excavatum, or funnel chest—a depressed lower sternum that usually causes restriction only when it is severe; pectus carinatum, or pigeon chest—a prominent upper sternum that does not restrict chest wall movement; and flail chest—an inward movement of the chest wall with inspiration, such as with multiple rib fractures.

Other structural defects are spinal deformities. These are best viewed posteriorly. Kyphoscoliosis is one example of how a posterior and lateral spinal deviation can limit chest wall and lung expansion. Another example is a patient with COPD, who usually has a forwardly tilted head and thoracic kyphosis (Figure 15-5).

Breathing Patterns

Respiratory rates normally range between 14 and 20 breaths per minute in adults (ages 15 and older). In children, the following ranges are normal: newborn, 30 to 60 breaths per minute; early childhood, 20 to 40 breaths per minute; late childhood, 15 to 25 breaths per minute.[5]

Eupnea is a normal breathing cycle. Apnea is a temporary halt in breathing. Tachypnea is a rapid, shallow breathing pattern; this is an indicator of respiratory distress. Bradypnea exists when respiration is slowed to less than 12 breaths per minute. Causes could be neurologic or metabolic. Kussmaul breathing is an increased rate and depth of respirations and is associated with metabolic acidosis.

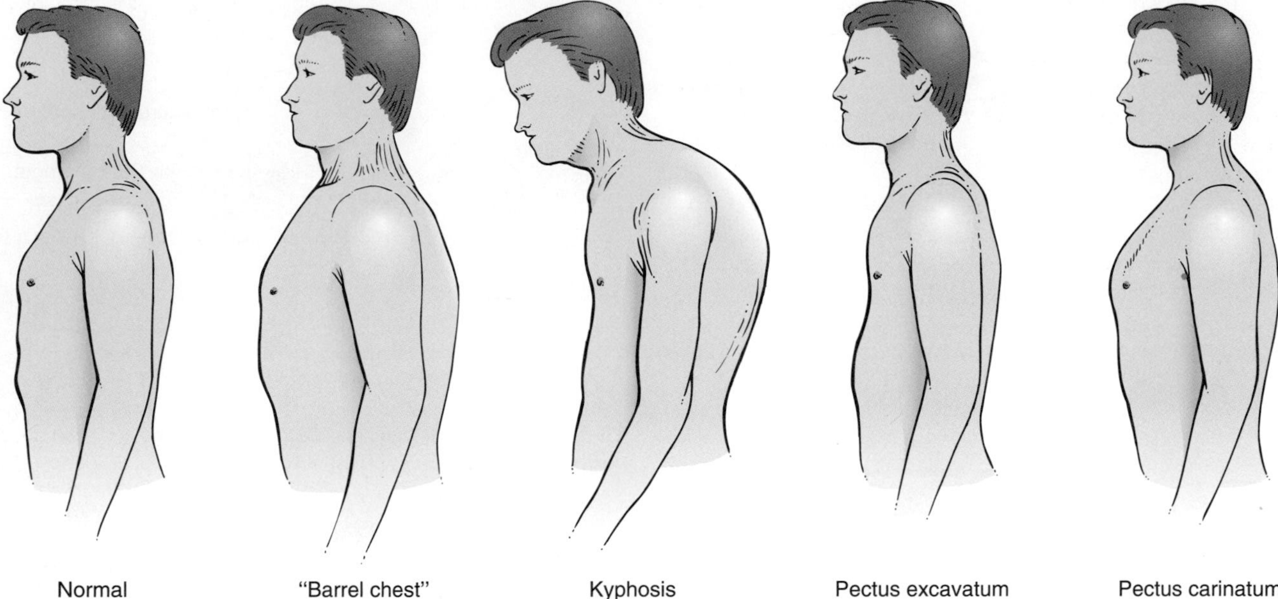

Fig. 15-5 Chest wall configurations. *(From Schwartz MH:* Textbook of physical diagnosis: History and examination, *ed 6, St Louis, 2010, Saunders.)*

Dyspnea is the patient's subjective feeling of shortness of breath. Dyspnea worsens as the severity of the disease increases. An easy method for documenting the level of dyspnea is to count the numbers of words that the patient is able to speak per breath. For instance, six-word dyspnea is not as significant as one-word dyspnea. The type of activities that elicit shortness of breath should also be ascertained. For example, is breathlessness precipitated by stair climbing, taking a shower, and so forth? The normal ratio of inspiratory time to expiratory time is 1:2. As the respiratory rate increases, the inspiration-to-expiration (I:E) ratio decreases to 1:1. This is seen in respiratory distress; as the patient struggles to breathe in, the expiratory phase is shortened, and a vicious circle continues. With pursed-lip breathing, the idea is to prolong the expiratory phase and slow the breathing pattern.

Other objective ways of measuring dyspnea (e.g., the Borg scale, the ventilator response index [VRI], the American Thoracic Society Dyspnea Scale, the Bog Scale of Perceived Exertion) are discussed in Chapter 8. Choosing a scale that the patient understands and can easily use will work best for identifying activities and interventions that cause more or less dyspnea. Later, patients can use the scale to self-monitor their dyspnea in relation to their activities and know when to increase or decrease activity secondary to dyspnea.

Auscultation

Auscultation is the art of listening to sounds produced by the body. Lung and heart sounds are the focus of this chapter. Skill in auscultation is dependent on the following four factors.

1. A functional stethoscope
2. Proper technique
3. Knowledge of the different categories of lung sounds: normal, abnormal, adventitious breath sounds, and voice sounds
4. Knowledge of the various categories of heart sounds and murmurs

Stethoscope

A stethoscope need not be sophisticated to be effective. A physical therapist skilled in auscultation can use any basic stethoscope and be able to identify lung sounds. The stethoscope functions more as a filter to the extraneous noises than as an amplifier. A basic stethoscope consists of earpieces, tubing, and a chest piece. The bell portion of the chest piece assesses low-pitched sounds (i.e., heart sounds). The diaphragm portion discerns high-pitched sounds (Figure 15-6). The tubing should not be so long that sound transmission is dampened. An appropriate length is between 30 cm (12 inches) and 55 cm (21 to 22 inches). The earpieces should fit the physical therapist's ears comfortably and allow the tuning out of external sounds. Another consideration is to position the earpieces anteriorly, or forward toward the ear canals. Warming the diaphragm before placing it on the patient's skin is appreciated by the patient.

A study by Gurunga and colleagues evaluated the use of computer lung sound analysis as a diagnostic aid for auscultation. Their conclusion was that the interlistener automated variability was limited by the acuity of the individual listeners and that the use of the automated identification of lungs sounds may improve the overall sensitivity to more accurately pick up wheezes and crackles. The computerized lung sound analysis was 80% more specific and 85% more sensitive to wheezes and crackles. The authors concluded that their data are limited but may prove clinically promising in the future.[6]

Technique

Environment is another element in the correct performance of auscultation. The room or cubicle should be as quiet as possible. Television and radio should be turned off, and any extraneous noises should be minimized or eliminated. This is especially important when auscultation is a new technique for the therapist. Clothing should be removed or draped so that it does not interfere in the assessment of the breath sounds. The patient should be in a sitting position, if possible, for lung sounds. The anterior, lateral, and posterior aspects of the chest should be auscultated both craniocaudally (apices to bases) and side to side (Figure 15-7). The physical therapist places the diaphragm on the patient's skin so that it lies flat. The patient is instructed to breathe in and out through the mouth. A slightly deeper breath than tidal breathing is suggested. A minimum of one breath per bronchopulmonary segment allows for a comparison of the intensity, pitch, and quality of the breath sounds. Moving the diaphragm from one side to the other side while simultaneously moving it craniocaudally enables the therapist to compare the right side of the chest with the left side of the chest.

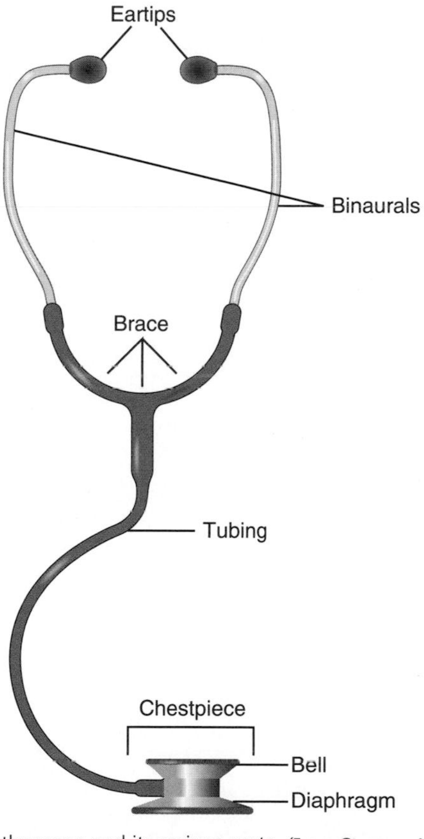

Fig. 15-6 Stethoscope and its various parts. *(From Cameron MH, Monroe L:* Physical rehabilitation: Evidence-based examination, evaluation, and intervention, *Philadelphia, 2007, WB Saunders.)*

Chest Sounds

Chest sounds may be divided into the following categories.

1. Breath sounds—normal, abnormal, adventitious
2. Extrapulmonary sounds—pleural or friction rubs
3. Voice sounds—egophony, bronchophony, whispered pectoriloquy
4. Heart sounds

Breath Sounds

The terminology of breath sounds provided in this chapter is a compilation of multiple resources and clinical experience. Recognition of normal breath sounds is the key to the identification of abnormal and adventitious sounds because it offers the listener a point of reference. Normal breath sounds can be broken down into bronchial, bronchovesicular, and vesicular. The American Thoracic Society (ATS) and the American College of Chest Physicians (ACCP) have attempted to provide standardization of the nomenclature and continue to conduct surveys of health care professionals for use of this terminology in clinical practice.

Bronchial sounds can be described as high-pitched and are heard in both the inspiratory and the expiratory phase. A distinguishing feature is the pause that exists between the inspiratory and expiratory phases (Figure 15-8). These sounds are also described as tracheal because their normal location is over the trachea. Bronchovesicular sounds are similar in that they are also high-pitched and have equal inspiratory and expiratory cycles. However, a differentiating feature is the lack of a pause (see Figure 15-8). Bronchovesicular sounds are heard best wherever the bronchi, or central lung tissue, are close to the surface. These areas are supraclavicular and suprascapular (the apices), as well as parasternal and interscapular (the bronchi). The ATS and ACCP, in their 1977 recommendations for pulmonary nomenclature, used the term *bronchial* to include both bronchial and bronchovesicular sounds. The difference is minor (the pause between the inspiratory and expiratory phases). This recommendation is meant to provide uniformity to lung-sound terminology. Vesicular breath sounds are heard over the remaining peripheral lung fields. These sounds have primarily an inspiratory component, with only the initial one-third of the expiratory phase audible. Their intensity is also softer because of the dampening effect of the spongy lung tissue and the cumulative effect of the air entry from numerous terminal bronchioles. The idea that

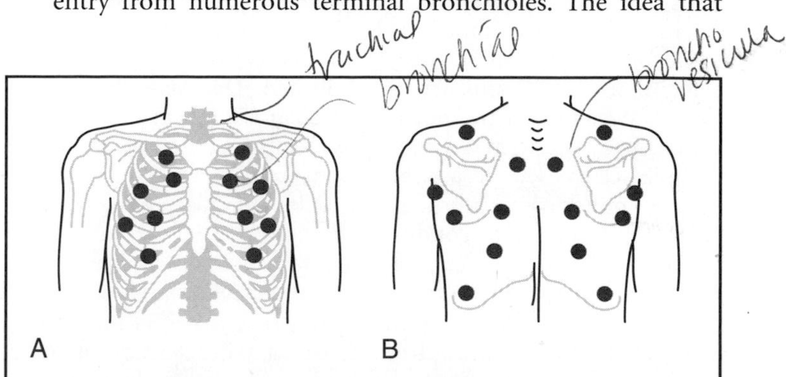

Fig. 15-7 One method of auscultating the chest. **A,** The chest. **B,** The back. *(Redrawn from Buckingham EB:* A primer of clinical diagnosis, *ed 2, New York, 1979, Harper & Row. In Hillegass E:* Essentials in cardiopulmonary physical therapy, *ed 3, St Louis, 2011, Saunders.)*

BRONCHIAL
loud, high-pitched; hollow quality; heard over manubrium; louder on expiration; distinct pause between inspiration (I) and expiration (E)

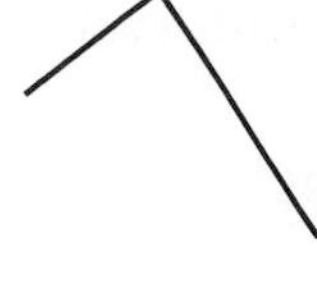

BRONCHOVESICULAR
mixture of bronchial and vesicular; I: E is 1:1; heard over main-stem bronchi anteriorly, ICS #1 and #2; posteriorly, between scapulae

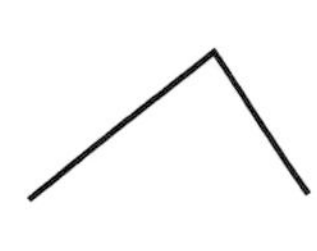

VESICULAR
soft, low-pitched; heard over peripheral lung tissue; no pause between I and E; ratio is 3:1

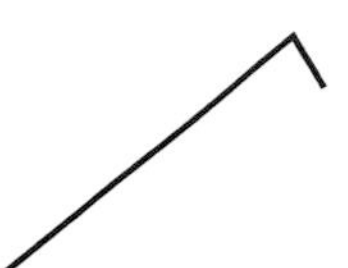

Fig. 15-8 Normal breath sounds.

vesicular sounds reflect air entry in the alveoli has been disproved. Thus, as the therapist auscultates from top to bottom, the breath sounds are quieter at the bases than at the apices. Infants and small children have louder, harsher breath sounds. This is as result of the thinness of the chest wall and the airways' being closer to the surface.

ABNORMAL BREATH SOUNDS

Abnormal breath sounds can be described as changes in the sound transmission as a result of an underlying pathologic process. Sound is filtered by the lung tissues because these organs are air-filled; thus sound transmission is dampened over the bases more than over the apices. On the other hand, sound transmission is enhanced when a liquid or solid is the medium. Certain lung pathologies produce abnormal lung sounds. Abnormal sounds can be divided into three types: bronchial, decreased, and absent. Bronchial sounds occur in peripheral lung tissue when it becomes airless—either partially or completely. In a consolidating type of pneumonia, the lung tissue is "airless" because of the complete obstruction of segmental or lobar bronchi by secretions. Sound from the adjacent bronchi is enhanced and becomes higher pitched, and the expiratory component is louder and more pronounced. Compression of lung tissue from an extrapulmonary source also produces bronchial sounds. Examples include compression secondary to increased pleural fluid (pleural effusion) or tumor. *Tubular breath sounds* is a term used synonymously to mean abnormal bronchial breath sounds.

Decreased or absent breath sounds occur when sound transmission is diminished or abolished. Decreased breath sounds occur when the normal vesicular sounds are further diminished. The term *absent sounds* means that no sounds are audible. Decreased or absent sounds can be caused by an internal pulmonary pathology or can be secondary to an initially nonpulmonary condition. Hyperinflation caused by emphysema causes decreased sound transmission as a result of the destruction of the acinar units and causes increased air as a result of the loss of normal lung structure. The loss of lung compliance resulting from pulmonary fibrosis also may produce decreased or absent breath sounds. Extrapulmonary causes include tumors, neuromuscular weakness (i.e., muscular dystrophy), and musculoskeletal deformities (i.e., kyphoscoliosis). Pain is a common cause for decreased or absent breath sounds. When the patient attempts to take a deep breath, the volume is limited because of the onset of pain. The causes of the pain can be varied—from incisional (e.g., midsternotomy) to traumatic (e.g., fractured ribs). If no underlying pathologies are present, decreased breath sounds may be a reflection of the depth of respiration or the thickness of the chest wall (e.g., in obesity or with the presence of bandages). The skill of auscultation lies in the differentiation between normal and abnormal breath sounds.

ADVENTITIOUS BREATH SOUNDS

Adventitious breath sounds are the extraneous noises produced over the bronchopulmonary tree and are an indication of an abnormal process or condition. These sounds may be more easily identifiable than abnormal sounds. Adventitious sounds are classified as crackles (rales), rhonchi, and wheezes. Crackles (rales) are described as discontinuous, low-pitched sounds. They occur predominantly during inspiration. The sound of rubbing hair between the fingers or of Velcro popping simulates crackles. Crackles usually indicate a peripheral airway process. Rhonchi are low-pitched but continuous sounds. These occur in both inspiration and expiration. *Snoring* is a term used to describe its quality. Rhonchi are attributed to an obstructive process in the larger, more central airways. Wheezes are continuous but high-pitched. A hissing or whistling quality is present. Wheezes that occur predominantly during inspiration are an indication of bronchospasm; wheezes during exhalation are an indication of airway secretions. The airways get larger on inspiration and smaller on exhalation. Consequently, when the patient has bronchospasm, a high-pitched wheeze is heard on inspiration. During exhalation, the airways become more narrow, consequently when air goes past secretions in a narrowed airway, an expiratory wheeze is heard on auscultation. Being able to identify the difference between inspiratory and expiratory wheezing is very important because this will help to determine what treatment is indicated. Inspiratory wheezing indicates that a bronchodilator is needed, whereas expiratory wheezing suggests the need for airway clearance techniques.

EXTRAPULMONARY SOUNDS

An adventitious sound that is nonpulmonary is the friction rub. It can be described as a rubbing or leathery sound, and it occurs during both inspiration and expiration. The sound is produced when the visceral (inner) pleural lining rubs against the parietal (outer) pleura and is a sign of a primary pleural process, such as inflammation or neoplasm. Pain is usually associated with a friction rub.

VOICE SOUNDS

Voice sounds are vibrations heard through a stethoscope and produced by the speaking voice as it travels down the tracheobronchial tree and through the lung parenchyma. These sounds, over the normal lung, are low-pitched and have a muffled or mumbled quality. The transmission of these vocal vibrations can be increased or decreased in the presence of an underlying pulmonary pathologic process. Bronchophony describes the phenomenon of increased vocal transmission. Words or letters are louder and clearer. It is caused by conditions in which there is increased lung density, as in consolidation due to pneumonia. To assess for bronchophony, the patient is usually asked to repeat "blue moon" or "one, two, three." Egophony may also be present when there is increased transmission of the vocal vibrations. In this case, the patient is asked to say "eeee." The underlying process distorts the e sound so that an "aaa" sound is heard over the peripheral area by the examiner. Egophony coexists with bronchophony.

Whispered voice sounds also produce low-pitched vibrations over the chest that are muffled by normal lung parenchyma. In whispered pectoriloquy, these whispered voice sounds become distinct and clear; "one, two, three" or "ninety-nine" are used to evaluate this sound. Whispered pectoriloquy can be present when bronchophony and egophony are absent. This sign is helpful in identifying smaller or patchy areas of lung consolidation.

Voice sounds are a method of confirming abnormal breath sounds. If a patient with significant atelectasis secondary to compression of lung tissue presents with bronchial breath sounds, then egophony and bronchophony are also audible.

Websites are available that allow the beginner in auscultation to hear actual lung sounds. The two websites included in this chapter's references have links to these auditory sites. Other sites may be found by doing an online search (using Google or another search engine) with key words such as "auscultation of breath sounds."

Heart Sounds

As with lung sounds, superficial topographic landmarks assist the therapist in auscultation of heart sounds and murmurs. The left ventricular apex is normally located at the midclavicular line (MCL) in the fifth intercostal space (ICS). The cardiac apex is also known as the point of maximum impulse (PMI), where the pulse is most strongly heard. There are four reference areas for cardiac auscultation; they do not correspond directly to the underlying cardiac anatomy. On the other hand, these areas do relate to the events arising at the individual cardiac valves. These four areas are defined as the following.

- Aortic: second ICS, at right sternal border (RSB)
- Pulmonic: second ICS, at left sternal border (LSB)
- Tricuspid: fourth and fifth ICS, LSB
- Mitral: cardiac apex, fifth ICS, MCL

Technique

An environment that is as quiet as possible is recommended. Positions used for cardiac auscultation include the following: supine—used for all areas; left lateral decubitus (side-lying)—listening to cardiac apex or mitral area, bell usually used; and sitting—used for all areas. Clinically, there are times when positions may be limited. In those cases, the therapist must listen with the patient in the best position available. However, if possible, the left side-lying position is most valuable because the pathological S_3 and S_4 sounds are heard most clearly. If the patient is in a sitting position, a leaning-forward position may also be used for better auscultation.

Normal Heart Sounds

The first heart sound (S_1) signifies the closing of the atrioventricular valves. Its duration is 0.10 seconds; it is heard the loudest at the cardiac apex. The two components of S_1 are tricuspid and mitral. Both the diaphragm and the bell of the stethoscope can be used to hear S_1. Its loudness is enhanced by any condition in which the heart is closer to the chest wall (i.e., thin chest wall) or in which there is an increased force to the ventricular contraction (e.g., tachycardia resulting from exercise; Figure 15-9).

The second heart sound (S_2) represents the closing of the semilunar valves and the end of ventricular systole. Its components are aortic and pulmonic. During expiration, these two components are not distinct because the time difference in the closure of the valves is less than 30 milliseconds. However, during inspiration, a splitting of S_2 is audible. This physiologic split results from the increased venous return to the right heart secondary to the decreased intrathoracic pressure that occurs during inspiration. The pulmonic valve closure is delayed as the right ventricular systolic time is lengthened. A split S_2 is heard commonly in children and young adults. The diaphragm of the stethoscope should be used to hear the split. The pulmonic component is the softer sound and is best heard at the LSB, in the second to fourth ICS. The two components may be heard best in the aortic and pulmonic areas, respectively. When the split is heard in both phases of respiration, an underlying cardiac abnormality is suspected. Causes may include right bundle branch block and pulmonary hypertension.[2,7]

Gallops

The third heart sound (S_3) is a faint, low-frequency sound and reflects the early (diastolic) ventricular filling that occurs after the atrioventricular valves open. S_3 is normal in children and young adults; however, it is usually abnormal in individuals

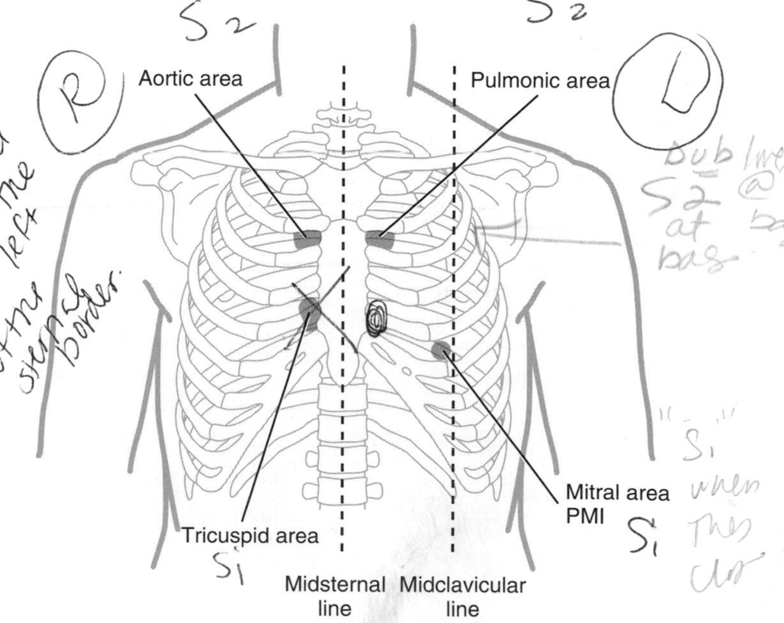

Fig. 15-9 Cardiac auscultation. *(From http://www.kumc.edu/kumcpeds/cardiology/tofmsllecture/auscultaitonareas.gif.)*

over age 40. An extra effort must be made to auscultate S_3; the bell of the stethoscope should be used. The ideal position to hear S_3 is left side-lying; the bell should be placed over the cardiac apex. Causes of a pathological S_3 may include ventricular failure, tachycardia, or mitral regurgitation. "Ken-TUCK-y" is one sound that has been used to approximate the sound sequencing of S_3 in the cardiac cycle (S_1, S_2, S_3).

The fourth heart sound (S_4) signifies the rapid ventricular filling that occurs after atrial contraction. When present, it is heard before S_1. S_4 may be heard in the "normal" individual with left ventricular hypertrophy. The location of S_4 is similar to that of S_3. Its sound can be described as dull because of the sudden motion of stiff ventricles in response to increased atrial contraction. Pathologies eliciting an S_4 may include systemic hypertension, cardiomyopathies, and coarctation of the aorta. "TENN-es-see" is a sound that approximates the sound sequencing when S_4 is present (S_4, S_1, S_2).

Murmurs

Cardiac murmurs are the vibrations resulting from turbulent blood flow. They may be described based on position in cardiac cycle (systole, diastole), duration, and loudness. Systolic murmurs occur between S_1 and S_2; diastolic murmurs occur between S_2 and S_1. A continuous murmur starts in S_1 and lasts through S_2 for a portion or all of diastole. The loudness of a murmur is a factor of the velocity of blood flow and the turbulence created as it flows through a specific opening such as a valve. Grades I to VI are described in Table 15-1.

Murmurs that are grade III or higher are usually associated with cardiovascular pathology.

Mediate Percussion

Mediate, or indirect, percussion allows the therapist to assess the density of the underlying organs. Striking the chest wall produces vibrations in the underlying structures that, in turn, give rise to sound waves or percussion tones. The quality of tone depends on the density of the tissue or organ (i.e., it becomes louder over air-filled structures). These tones are described by the following terms:

- Resonant: loud or high amplitude, low pitch, longer duration; heard over air-filled organs such as the lungs
- Dull: low amplitude, medium to high pitch, short duration; heard over solid organs such as the liver
- Flat: high pitch, short duration; heard over muscle mass such as the thigh
- Tympanic: high pitch, medium duration; heard over hollow structures such as the stomach
- Hyperresonant: very low pitch, prolonged duration; heard over tissue with decreased density (increased air-to-tissue ratio); abnormal in adults; heard over lungs with emphysema

Table 15-1 Grading of Heart Murmurs

Grade	Loudness	Comments
I	Faint	Requires concentrated effort to hear
II	Faint	Audible immediately
III	Louder than II	Intermediate intensity
IV	Loud	Intermediate intensity; associated with palpable vibration (thrill)
V	Very loud	Thrill present
VI	Audible without stethoscope	

Technique

The middle finger of the nondominant hand is placed firmly on the chest wall in an intercostal space and parallel to the ribs. The top of the middle finger of the dominant hand strikes the distal phalanx of the stationary hand with a quick, sharp motion. The impetus of the blow comes from the wrist rather than the elbow and has been likened to that of a paddle ball player (Figure 15-10).[2] As with auscultation, the therapist must follow the sequence of apices to bases and side to side so that comparisons can be made. This technique is not usually used in infants because percussion is too easily transmitted by a small chest.

Diaphragmatic Excursion

Assessment of diaphragmatic movement can be made with mediate percussion. The patient is asked to breathe deeply and hold that breath. The lowest level of the diaphragm on maximal inspiration coincides with the lowest point where a resonant tone is heard. The patient is then asked to exhale, and mediate percussion is repeated. The lowest area of resonance now moves higher, as the diaphragm ascends with relaxation. The distance between these two points is described as the diaphragmatic excursion; the normal range is 3 to 5 cm (Figure 15-11). Diaphragmatic movement is decreased in patients with COPD.

Palpation

Physical therapists use palpation in all areas of practice. Touch is an integral part of physical therapy. As part of the chest examination, palpation is used to assess areas of tenderness, abnormalities, chest wall excursion, edema, tactile fremitus,

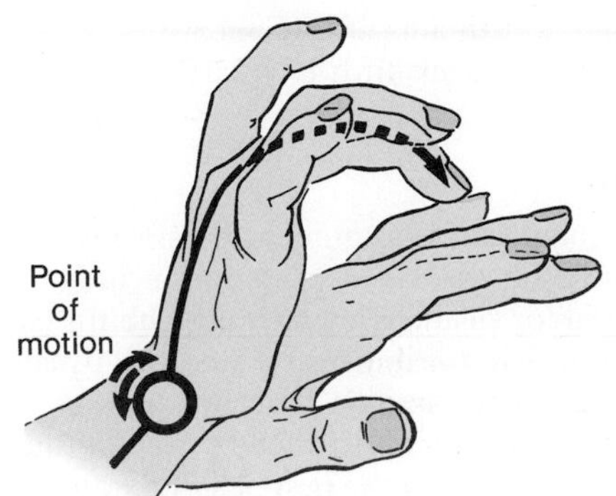

Fig. 15-10 Mediate percussion technique. *(Adapted from Buckingham EB: A primer of clinical diagnosis, ed 2, New York, 1979, Harper & Row. In Cameron MH, Monroe LG: Physical rehabilitation: Evidence-based examination, evaluation, and intervention, St Louis, 2007, Saunders.)*

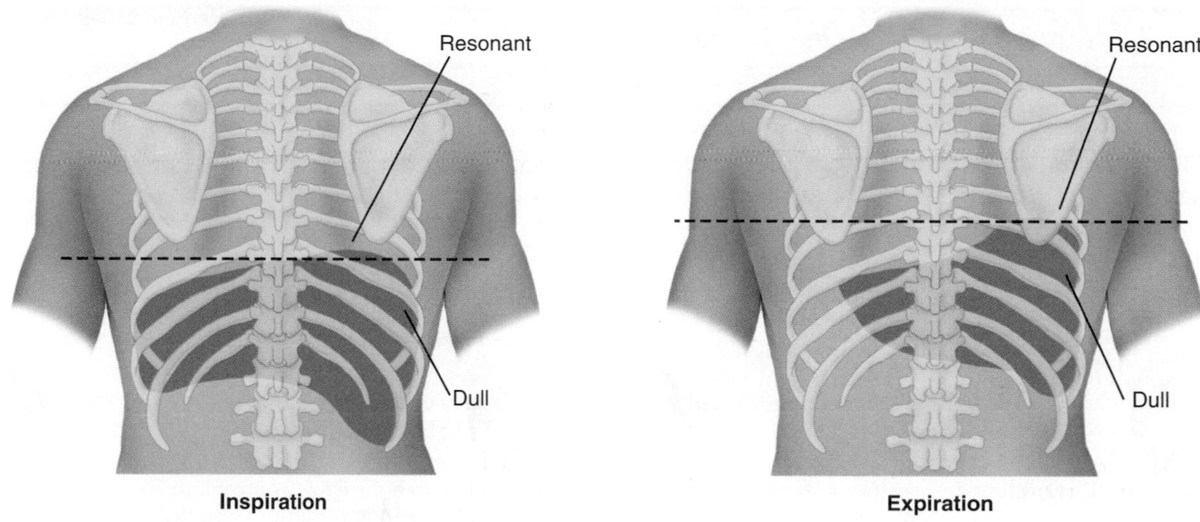

Fig. 15-11 Diaphragmatic excursion. *(From Schwartz MH:* Textbook of physical diagnosis: History and examination, *ed 6, St Louis, 2010, Saunders.)*

and tracheal deviation. It can help to differentiate between musculoskeletal impairments and pulmonary impairments.

Tenderness

Specific superficial or deep landmarks are identified by means of palpation. Determination of gross spinal alignment can be performed by tracing the spinous processes in a cephalocaudal direction. Certain structures can be identified, such as the T4 vertebra or the sternal angle; this augments the physical therapist's evaluation. Areas of tenderness can be assessed for degree of discomfort and reproducibility. Differentiation of chest wall discomfort of an organic nature, such as in angina, from that of a musculoskeletal condition may be made through palpation. In a patient complaining of chest pain, angina may be ruled out if the physical therapist can reproduce or increase the discomfort by increasing tactile pressure. However, one must also determine that corroborating symptoms (e.g., diaphoresis, tachycardia) are not present. Angina or chest pain secondary to myocardial ischemia usually results from exertion and may be relieved by rest. Crepitus is a crunchy sound often associated with articular structures. However, when bubbles of air occur within subcutaneous tissue, a crackling sensation can be palpated. An air leak from a chest-tube site is one circumstance in which crepitus is palpated over the chest wall. Crepitus can also be secondary to a pleural or friction rub.

Edema

Palpation allows the physical therapist to assess peripheral edema. Dependency of body parts such as lower extremities or sacrum can cause swelling related to cardiac and noncardiac conditions. Assessment of edema is performed by pressing two fingers into the particular areas for 2 to 3 seconds. If an impression is left once the fingers are removed, then pitting or dependent edema is present. The degree of edema is based on the length of time that the indentation lasts. 1+ is the least degree; 4+ is the worst.

Chest Wall Excursion

Evaluation of thoracic expansion allows the therapist to observe a baseline level by which to measure progress or decline in a patient's condition. Chest wall movement can be restricted unilaterally as a result of lobar pneumonia, scoliosis, muscle weakness, paralysis or a surgical incision. A symmetrical decrease in chest wall motion occurs in the patient with COPD.

The hyperinflation associated with COPD produces an increase in the anteroposterior diameter with a progressive loss of diaphragmatic excursion. Normal chest wall excursion is about 3.25 inches (8.5 cm) in a young adult between 20 and 30 years of age. One method is to use a tape measure at the level of the axilla and xiphoid. In a study of 120 normal subjects, ages ranging from 20 years to 70+ years, Kinney LaPier[8] performed tape measure readings of subjects in a sitting or standing position at rest and at maximal inspiration (vital capacity) breaths. They found that subjects 20 to 29 years of age had 5.1 ± 6.2 CM excursion. In subjects 70 years and older, the excursion was only 2.5 ± 2.9 cm. The study found a definite decrease in chest wall excursion with age and recommends not utilizing chest wall excursion by tape measure in patients over 65.[8]

The most common method involves direct hand contact. This technique is performed in all planes and from top to bottom. Symmetry and extent of movement are noted. The procedures for this method are found in Table 15-2.

Tactile Fremitus

Spoken words produce vibration over the chest wall. Voice sounds have been previously discussed under auscultation. When the physical therapist's hands are placed on the chest wall, the vibrations of spoken words can be felt; these are described as tactile fremitus. The presence or absence of tactile fremitus provides information about the density of the underlying lungs and thoracic cavity.[2]

Table 15-2 **Methods for Evaluating Thoracic Expansion**

Method	Steps
Apical or upper lobe motion (Figure 15-12, *A*)	1. The physical therapist faces the patient. The area to be examined is exposed and draped as needed. 2. The physical therapist's hands are placed over the anterior chest. The heel of the hand is at about the level of the fourth rib and the fingertips reach toward the upper trapezii. 3. The thumbs lie horizontal at about the level of the sternal angle and meet at the midline, slightly stretching the skin. 4. The patient is asked to inhale. 5. The hands should be relaxed to allow for movement beneath. 6. The symmetry and extent of movement are assessed.
Anterolateral or middle lobe/lingula motion (Figure 15-12, *B*)	1. See step 1 of Apical, above. 2. The physical therapist's hands are placed with the palms distal to the nipple line and the thumbs meeting in the midline. The fingers lie in the posterior axillary fold. 3. See steps 4 to 6 of Apical, above.
Posterior excursion/lower lobe motion (Figure 15-12, *C*)	1. The physical therapist stands behind the patient. 2. The area to be examined is exposed with draping used as appropriate. 3. The physical therapist's hands are placed flat on the posterior chest wall at the level of the tenth rib. The thumbs meet at the midline; fingers reaching toward the anterior axillary fold. 4. See steps 4 to 6 of Apical, above.

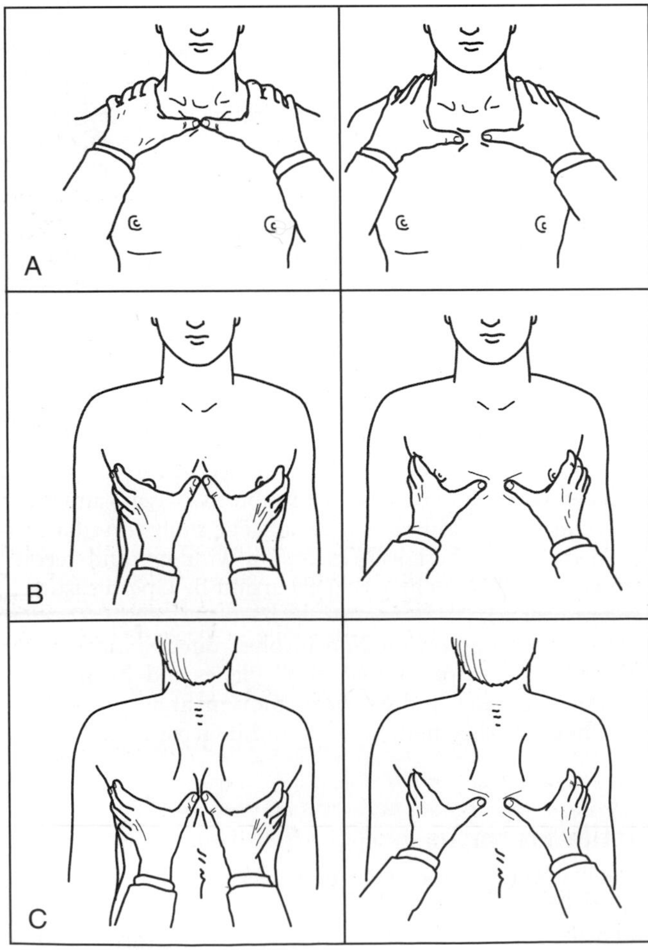

Fig. 15-12 Palpation of upper lobe motion (**A**), right middle and left lingula lobe motion (**B**), and lower lobe motion (**C**). *(Redrawn from Cherniack RM, Cherniack L:* Respiration in health and disease, *ed 2, Philadelphia, WB Saunders, 1972.)*

Technique

Two methods can be used to evaluate for tactile fremitus (Figure 15-13). In the first technique, the therapist uses the palmar surface of one or both hands. The second method involves the use of the ulnar border of one hand. With both techniques, the sequence is, again, cephalocaudal and side to side. In either method, the next step is to ask that the patient speak a predetermined phrase. The two most commonly used phrases are "ninety-nine" and "one, two, three." A light but firm touch is recommended.

Tracheal Deviation

The trachea's midline position can be examined anteriorly (Figure 15-14). The physical therapist places an index finger in the medial aspect of the suprasternal notch. This is repeated on the opposite side. An equal distance between the clavicle and the trachea should exist bilaterally. Tracheal deviation may be caused by a pneumothorax, atelectasis, or a tumor. Whether the deviation is ipsilateral or contralateral depends on the underlying cause. A right pneumothorax or pleural effusion deviates the trachea away from the affected side (i.e., the left); a left lower lobe atelectasis, however, deviates the trachea toward the affected side (i.e., the left).

Case Studies

Case Study 15-1

A 30-year-old man with cystic fibrosis presents with a 1-week history of increased sputum production, loss of appetite, fatigue, and a 3-pound (6.6-kg) weight loss. With a system review of the chest (visual inspection) and the tests and measures of auscultation, mediate percussion, and palpation, the following findings are shown:

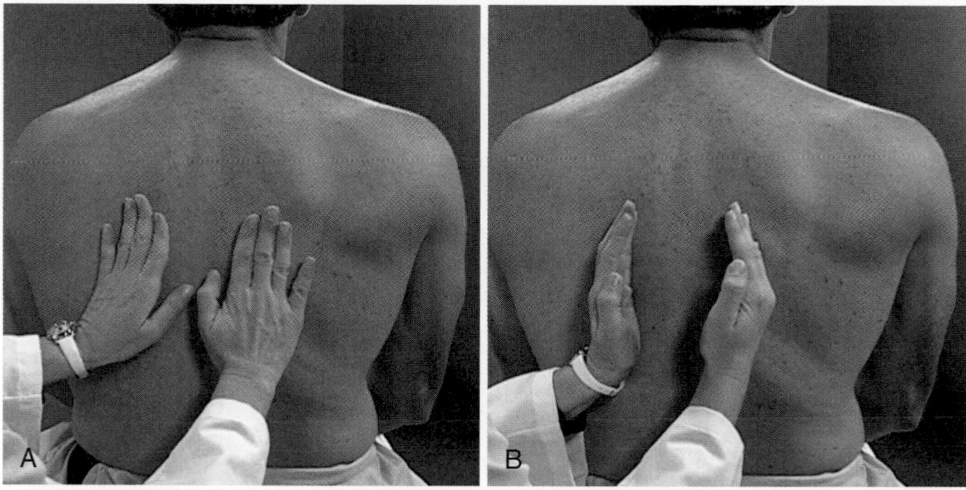

Fig. 15-13 Technique for evaluating fremitus. **A,** Method one. **B,** Method two. *(**B** from Schwartz MH. Textbook of Physical Diagnosis: History and Examination, ed 6. St. Louis, 2010, Saunders.)*

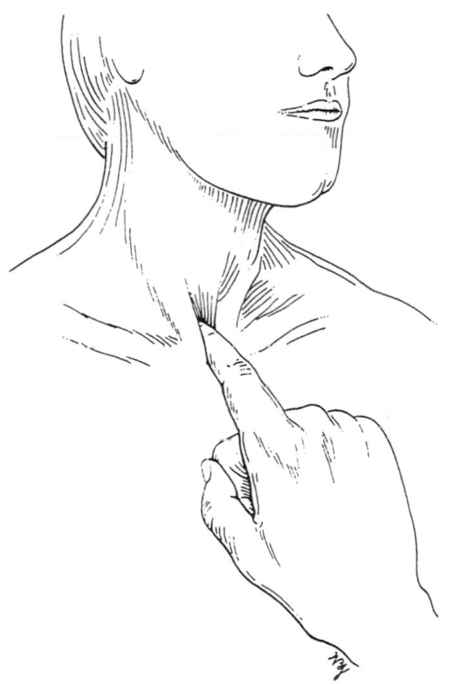

Fig. 15-14 Technique for determining the position of the trachea. *(From Schwartz MH.* Textbook of physical diagnosis: History and examination, *ed 6, St Louis, 2010, Saunders.)*

- Visual inspection: Forward head and neck, protracted shoulders, kyphotic posture, and increased anteroposterior diameter are present; the patient appears thin and fatigued; respiratory rate 24, use of accessory muscles observed; the patient has an effective and wet cough producing green thick mucus
- Auscultation: Decreased breath sounds with scattered crackles throughout all lung fields, especially over right posterior upper lobe and right middle lobe
- Palpation: Limited chest wall excursion (CWE), especially laterally on right
- Mediate percussion: Dull over right middle and lower chest, especially laterally

The evaluation component utilizes the above findings to identify the appropriate outcomes and treatment interventions. Based on the acuity of the examination, acute exacerbation of cystic fibrosis may be the diagnosis. The focus may be on secretion clearance and identification of the most appropriate airway clearance techniques. Would the high-frequency chest oscillations (ThAIRapy Vest) or manual techniques of chest percussion, vibration/shaking, and specific postural drainage positions be the choice for this patient? Scheduling airway clearance techniques and coordination treatments with respiratory therapy and inhaled medications is indicated as well. Ongoing daily reexamination will determine whether the treatment interventions need to be modified or continued as is. The patient's home exercise and airway clearance program should be reevaluated to prevent recurrence. The use of a daytime device such as Acapella or Flutter or other easy-to-use equipment may be helpful to enhance the patient's airway clearance program (see Chapter 21).

For more information about musculoskeletal issues in people with cystic fibrosis, see the article by Massery (2005).[9]

Case Study 15-2

An 8-year-old female admitted to the pediatric inpatient unit presents on chart review (history) with a 4-day history of recurrent fevers, shortness of breath, and lethargy. A chest radiogram shows a right middle lobe infiltrate, based on the following findings:

- Visual inspection: Tachypnea; RR 44; I:E ratio 1:1; weak, shallow cough
- Auscultation: Bronchial over right midanterior chest; egophony also present
- Mediate percussion: Dull over affected area
- Palpation: Trachea midline, markedly decreased CWE on right side

Anticipated outcomes may include the following.

1. The patient will demonstrate an effective cough.
2. The patient will demonstrate decreased work of breathing.

Treatment interventions may include manual chest percussion, vibration/shaking, postural drainage to right middle lobe

Table 15-3 Differentiation of Common Pulmonary Conditions

Condition	Inspection	Palpation	Percussion	Auscultation
Emphysema	Increased anteroposterior diameter; use of accessory muscles; thin individual	Decreased tactile fremitus	Increased resonance; decreased excursion of diaphragm	Decreased lung sounds; decreased vocal fremitus
Chronic bronchitis	Possible cyanosis; short, stocky individual	Often normal	Often normal	Early crackles
Pneumonia	Possible cyanosis	Increased tactile fremitus; splinting on affected side	Dull	Late crackles; bronchial breath sounds
Pulmonary embolism	Sudden onset of dyspnea; chest pain	Usually normal	Usually normal	Usually normal
Pneumothorax	Rapid onset	Absent fremitus; trachea may be shifted to other side; may have decreased chest wall excursion on affected side	Hyperresonant	Absent breath sounds
Pleural effusion	May be no outward clinical sign	Decreased fremitus; trachea shifted to other side; decreased chest wall excursion on affected side	Dullness	Absent breath sounds
Atelectasis	Often no outward clinical sign	Decreased fremitus; trachea shifted to same side; decreased chest wall excursion on affected side	Dullness	Absent breath sounds

Modified with permission from Swartz MH: *Textbook of physical diagnoses—History and examination,* ed 2, Philadelphia, 1994, WB Saunders.

area and instruction in huff coughing. Games that may be incorporated to facilitate the huffing and also increase the I:E ratio include blowing bubbles, windmills, kazoos. Handheld airway clearance devices, such as the Flutter, TheraPEP, or Acapella, may also be used.

Case Study 3

A 72-year-old woman presents with symptoms of persistent fevers, left chest wall discomfort, and history of a fall 1 week ago. A CT scan shows a loculated pleural effusion on the left. A left chest tube has been inserted for drainage. The working medical diagnosis is empyema. The patient is a nonsmoker. The following information is learned during the examination component of the patient management model:

- Visual inspection: RR 30; I:E ratio 1:2; epidural catheter for pain control; effective dry cough
- Auscultation: Absent breath sounds halfway up left lower lateral chest wall
- Mediate percussion: Flat over left lower lateral chest wall
- Palpation: Trachea deviated to right; decreased CWE on left; range of motion of left shoulder joint limited in flexion and abduction at about 90 degrees maximum; no preadmission shoulder limitations

Outcomes and treatment interventions must expand beyond the pulmonary diagnosis of empyema because the surgical insertion of a chest tube and the fall itself have impacted the musculoskeletal system as well.

An anticipated outcome would be for the patient to demonstrate no abnormal lung sounds as a result of increased lung volumes. Interventions would include breathing strategies (i.e., left lateral costal and diaphragmatic breathing). Ventilatory strategies could be incorporated into range-of-motion exercises for the shoulder. Incentive spirometry may also facilitate increased lung volumes. Finally, as the patient's condition becomes less acute, further evaluation may determine whether a balance impairment was the cause of the initial fall.

Table 15-3 presents differentiation of diagnoses by the elements of a chest physical examination.

Summary

As demonstrated in the case studies, each of the examination skills discussed contributes to the physical therapist's evaluation of the individual patient. This initial examination component of the patient management model makes it possible to perform the remaining components of evaluation, diagnosis, and prognosis.

Review Questions

1. Describe the sequence used to auscultate lung sounds.
2. Name two causes for decreased breath sounds.
3. What do bronchial breath sounds indicate if found where normal vesicular breath sound should be heard?
4. Name two causes for a pathologic S_3.
5. Why is it more appropriate to have the patient in a left side-lying position to evaluate heart sounds?
6. Formulate a plan for the evaluation of a patient with an acute right lower lobe pneumonia.
7. Which components of the chest physical examination might a physical therapist include in the initial assessment of an older adult patient with a recent left total hip replacement and a history of COPD and CHF?

References

1. American Physical Therapy Association: *The guide to physical therapist practice*, ed 2, Arlington, West Virginia, 2001, APTA.
2. Swartz, MH: *Textbook of physical diagnoses—history and examination*, ed 4, Philadelphia, 2002, WB Saunders.
3. George, RB, Light, RW, Matthay, MA, et al: *Chest medicine*, ed 2, Baltimore, 1990, Williams and Wilkins.
4. Seidel, HM, Ball, JW, Dains, JE, et al: *Mosby's guide to physical examination*, ed 5, Philadelphia, 2003, Mosby.
5. Bickley, LS, Szilagyi, PG: *Bates' guide to physical examination and history taking*, ed 8, Philadelphia, 2003, Lippincott Williams & Wilkins.
6. Gurunga, A, Scrafford CG, Tielsch JM, et al: Computerized lung sound analysis as diagnostic aid for the detection of abnormal lung sounds: a systematic review and meta analysis. *Respir Med* 105(9):1396-1403, 2011 Sept, E Pub 2011 June 14.
7. Tilkian, AG, Conover, MD: *Understanding heart sounds and murmurs*, ed 3, Philadelphia, 1993, WB Saunders.
8. Kinney LaPier, TL: Chest wall expansion values in subjects without impairment across the adult lifespan. *Phys Occupational Ther Geriatrics* 21(1):65-81, 2002.
9. Massery M: Musculoskeletal and neuromuscular interventions: a physical approach to cystic fibrosis. *J R Soc Med* 98(Suppl 45):55-66, 2005.

II

Chapter **16**

Monitoring Systems, Catheters, and Devices in the Intensive Care Unit

Elizabeth Dean and Christiane Perme

KEY TERMS

Acid-base balance
Arousal
Critical illness polyneuropathy
ECG monitoring
Fluid and electrolyte status
Hemodynamic status
ICU-acquired weakness
Intracardiac pressures
Intracranial pressure monitoring
Neuropsychological status
Ventricular assist devices

CHAPTER OUTLINE

The primary goal of the intensive care unit (ICU) team is to achieve hemodynamic stability and optimal oxygen transport for each patient who is critically ill, keeping a view toward the patient's eventual return to maximal functional participation in life and activity. This chapter introduces monitoring systems used in the evaluation of cardiovascular and pulmonary status in patients in the ICU and describes some related elements of cardiovascular and pulmonary regulation and control that are relevant to the assessment of risk and oxygen transport status, and to physical therapy intervention.

ICUs are highly specialized. Medical advances now preserve lives that would have been lost in the past. Patients admitted to the ICU require intense and often invasive yet life-preserving medical management. ICUs can be categorized as either general or specific. In major hospital centers, units are often designed and staffed for the exclusive management of specific types of conditions such as medical, surgical, trauma, burns, coronary care, and neonatal care. Although monitoring priorities may differ among specialized ICUs, the principles are similar and relate either directly or indirectly to the foremost goal of preserving life by maximizing oxygen transport and minimizing threat to it and by preventing the risks associated with recumbency and restricted mobility. In recent years, attention has focused on long-term outcomes of people who have had ICU stays—that is, the emphasis is on patients thriving after, rather than simply surviving, a course of ICU care.

The cardiovascular and pulmonary status of the patient in the ICU is often jeopardized by fluid and electrolyte disturbances and acid-base imbalance. This chapter describes the regulation of these systems and the clinical implications of imbalance relevant to the physical therapist. The principal monitoring systems used in assessing cardiovascular and pulmonary sufficiency in the ICU are highlighted. These include the electrocardiogram (ECG), arterial and venous lines, intracardiac monitoring, and the intracranial pressure (ICP) monitor. Although not monitoring systems per se, ventricular-assist devices (e.g., the intraaortic counterpulsation technique) are used to augment myocardial efficiency. These

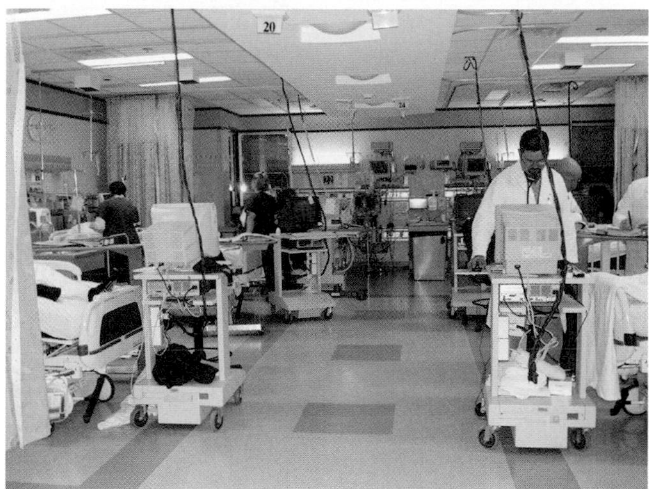

Fig. 16-1 General view of an intensive care unit.

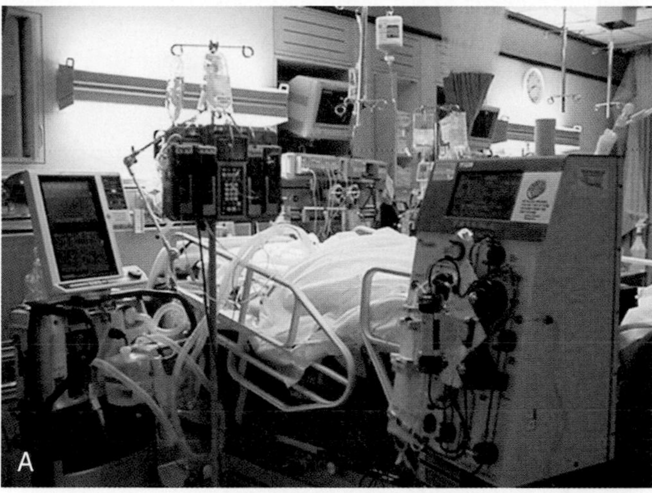

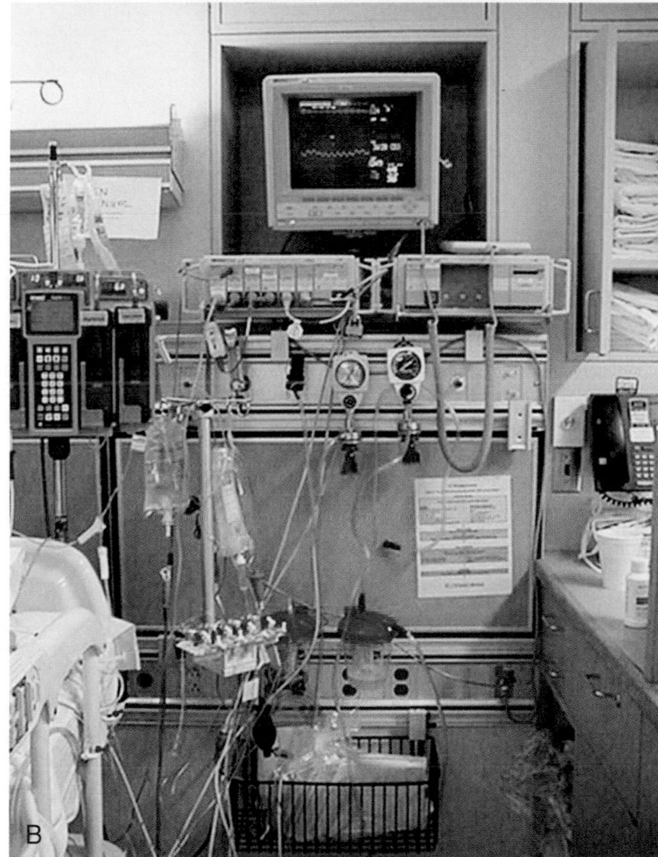

Fig. 16-2 **A,** Closer bedside view of a patient in the intensive care unit. Note that with all the equipment, the patient is almost lost. **B,** Bedside monitoring equipment.

warrant special attention by the physical therapist with respect to determining the patient's readiness for treatment, establishing treatment parameters, and assessing safety.

Familiarity with the extensive monitoring facilities in the ICU relieves some of the apprehensions the physical therapist may have about practicing in this setting. Such monitoring is central to the standard of physical therapy care in the ICU to guide progressive mobilization and management overall.[1] On introduction to the unit, the physical therapist is immediately struck by the high-tech environment. Quality care in this setting depends on harnessing the potential of high-tech monitoring equipment to optimize assessment, evaluate treatment parameters, and establish anticipated and actual effectiveness of intervention, as well as to reduce untoward risk for the patient.

Figure 16-1 illustrates a general view of a typical ICU. A view of a patient's bedside area in the ICU shows life-support equipment and the various lines and catheters that are in place (Figure 16-2). A closer view of the patient demonstrates precisely where the various lines and catheters are positioned and identifies where caution must be observed. Treatments are modified according to the types and positions of the lines and catheters for each patient (Figure 16-3).

Intravenous Lines

Intravenous (IV) lines are routinely established in the superficial veins, such as those on the back of the hand, often before admission to the ICU if the patient is admitted through the emergency department or transferred from the ward. These lines provide an immediate route for fluids, electrolytes, nutrition, and medications. The choice of specific lines to use depends on the patient's needs based on the history, laboratory tests, clinical and physical examinations, and ongoing evaluation.

Fluid and Electrolyte Balance

When the normal regulation of fluid intake, utilization, and excretion are disrupted, fluid, electrolytes, and acid-base imbalances result. Essentially, all medical and surgical conditions threaten these life-dependent mechanisms to some degree. Minor imbalances may be corrected with modification of the patient's nutrition and fluid intake. Major imbalances can be life-threatening, necessitating immediate, highly invasive medical intervention.

Imbalances are reflected as excesses, deficits, or as an abnormal distribution of fluids within the body.[2] Excesses result from increased intake and decreased loss of fluid and electrolytes. Deficits result from abnormal shifts of fluid and electrolytes among the intravascular and extravascular fluid

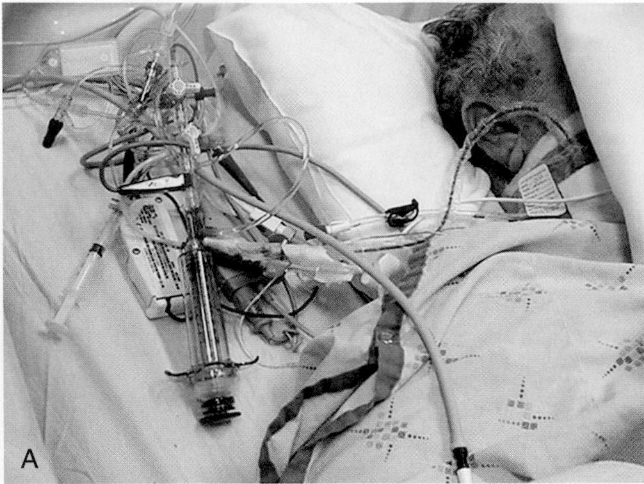

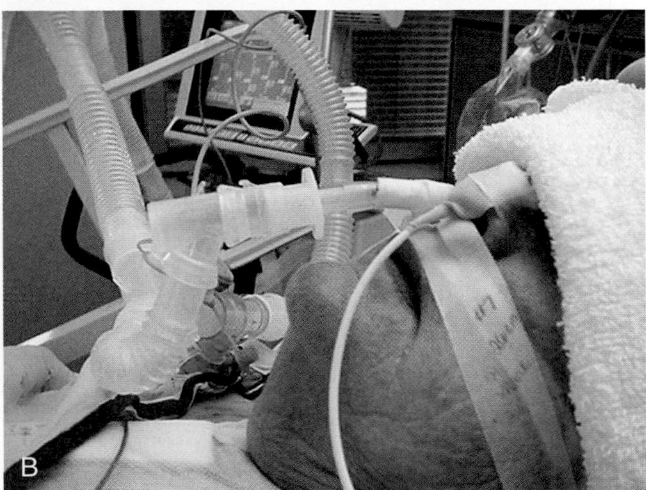

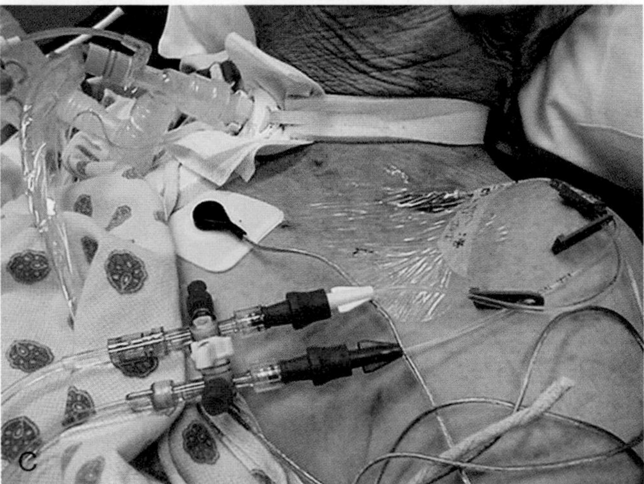

Fig. 16-3 A, Note the Swan-Ganz catheter on the right jugular vein. **B,** The patient is on a ventilator with a nasoendotracheal tube in place. **C,** Tracheostomy and left subclavian central venous catheter.

compartments of the body. Excesses can occur with kidney dysfunction, promoting fluid retention, and with respiratory dysfunction, which promotes carbon dioxide retention. Deficits are commonly associated with reduced intake of fluids and nutrition. Diaphoresis and wounds can also contribute to major fluid loss. Diarrhea and vomiting drain the gastrointestinal tract of fluid. Hemorrhage always results in fluid and electrolyte loss. Deficits may be secondary to fluid entrapment and localized edema within the body (third-spacing), making this source of fluid unavailable for regulation of homeostasis.

Moderate to severe fluid imbalance can be reflected in the systemic blood pressure and central (jugular) venous pressure (CVP). Elevated blood pressure can be indicative of fluid overload, but an intravascular fluid deficit of 15% to 25% must develop before blood pressure drops significantly. The jugular vein becomes distended with fluid overload. Normally, the jugular pulse is not visible 2 cm above the sternal angle when the individual rests at a 45-degree angle. If the jugular pulse is noted, this can be a sign of fluid overload.

Fluid replacement is based on a detailed assessment of the patient's needs. Whole blood is preferred for replacing blood loss. Plasma, albumin, and plasma volume expanders such as Dextran can be used to substitute for blood loss and to help reestablish blood volume. Albumin and substances such as dextran increase plasma volume by increasing the osmotic pressure of the blood, hence the reabsorption of fluid from the interstitial space. Low-molecular-weight dextran has the added advantage of augmenting capillary blood flow by decreasing blood viscosity and is therefore particularly useful in treating shock.

Excesses and deficits of fluids and electrolytes can be determined on the basis of laboratory determinations of serum levels of the specific electrolytes. Electrolyte levels and hematocrit are decreased with fluid excess (hemodilution) and are increased with fluid loss (hemoconcentration).

Excess fluid can be managed by controlled fluid intake, normal diuresis, and diuretic medications. Replacement of fluid and electrolyte losses can be achieved by oral intake, tube feeding, IV infusion, and parenteral hyperalimentation.

Assessment of fluid and electrolyte balance is based on both subjective and objective findings (Table 16-1). At the bedside, the physical therapist must be alert to complaints of headache, thirst, and nausea, as well as changes in dyspnea, skin turgor, and muscle strength. More objective assessment is based on fluid intake, output, and body weight. Fluid balance is so critical to physical well-being and cardiovascular and pulmonary sufficiency that fluid input and output records are routinely maintained at bedside. These records also include fluid volume lost in urine and feces, wound drainage, and fluids aspirated from any body cavity (e.g., abdomen and pleural space).

A patient's weight may increase by several kilograms before edema is apparent. The dependent areas of the body manifest the first signs of fluid excess. Patients on bed rest show sacral swelling; patients who can sit on the edge of the bed or in a chair for prolonged periods tend to show swelling of the feet and hands.

Decreased skin turgor can indicate fluid deficit. Tenting of the skin over the anterior chest in response to pinching may suggest fluid depletion. Wrinkled, toneless skin is more common in younger patients.

In contemporary ICU care, supplemental nutrition is a priority to maintain fluid and electrolyte balance, minimize weight loss, preserve strength and stamina, and support healing and recovery. Prescribing nutritional supplements for the patient in the ICU is a specialty in the field of nutrition and can take various forms depending on the patient's needs.

Table 16-1 **Assessment of Fluid and Electrolyte Imbalance**

Area	Fluid Excess/ Electrolyte Imbalance	Fluid Loss/ Electrolyte Imbalance
Head and neck	Distended neck veins, facial edema	Thirst, dry mucous membranes
Extremities	Dependent edema "pitting," discomfort from weight of bed covers	Muscle weakness, tingling, tetany
Skin	Warm, moist, taut, cool feeling when edematous	Dry, decreased turgor
Respiration	Dyspnea, orthopnea, productive cough, moist breath sounds	Changes in rate and depth of breathing
Circulation	Hypertension, jugular pulse visible at 45-degree sitting angle, atrial dysrhythmias	Pulse rate irregularities, dysrhythmia, postural hypotension, sinus tachycardia
Abdomen	Increased girth, fluid wave	Abdominal cramps

Modified from Phipps WJ, Long BC, Woods NF, editors: *Medical-surgical nursing: Concepts and clinical practice,* ed 6, Philadelphia, 1999, Elsevier.

The cardiovascular and pulmonary assessments can reveal changes in fluid balance. Lung sounds are valuable in identifying fluid overload. Vesicular sounds may become more bronchovesicular. Crackles may increase in coarseness. In the presence of fluid retention involving the pleurae, breath sounds diminish to the bases. Dyspnea and orthopnea may also be symptomatic of fluid excess.

An early sign of congestive heart failure (CHF) with underlying fluid overload is an S_3 gallop (Ken-TUCK-y) caused by rapid ventricular filling.

Vigilance by the physical therapist with respect to fluid and electrolyte balance is essential in all areas of practice, not only in the ICU. Fluid imbalance is common in older people and in young children, so it needs to be watched for on the ward, in the home, and in the community.

Chest Tube Drainage and Fluid Collection Systems

Chest tubes are large catheters placed in the pleural cavity to evacuate fluid and air and to drain into a graduated collection reservoir at bedside.[2] A typical chest tube drainage and collection system is shown in Figure 16-4, *A*. The removal of thick fluids such as blood and organized exudates by chest tubes is often indicated to prevent entrapment and loculation. Chest tubes are commonly inserted in the sixth intercostal space in the mid- or posterior axillary line. Chest tubes inserted into the pleural space are used to evacuate air or exudate. Chest tubes can also be inserted into the mediastinum to evacuate blood such as after open heart surgery (Figure 16-4, *B*).

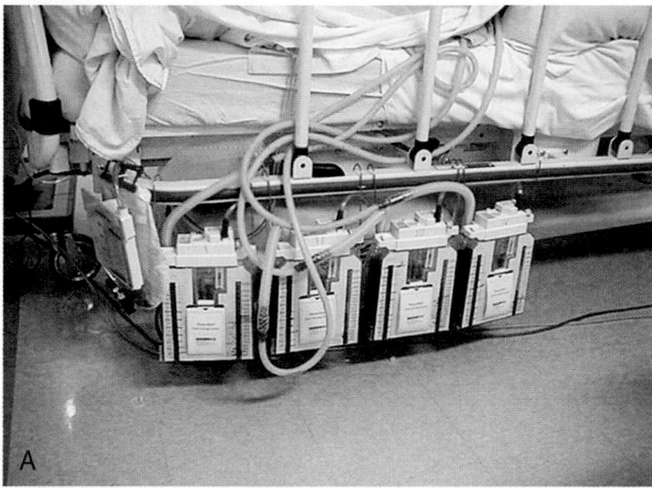

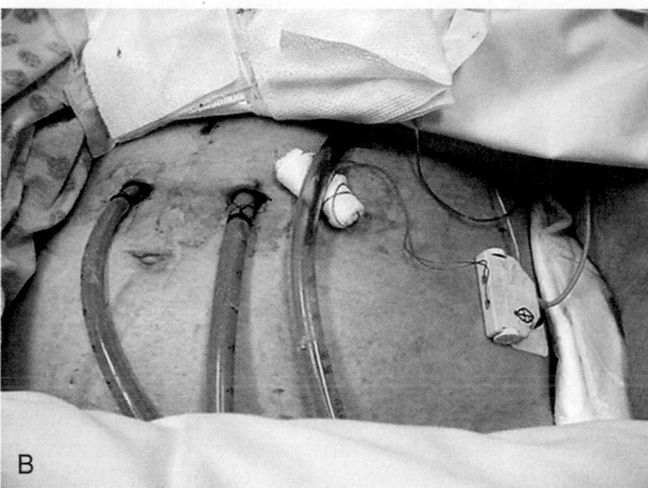

Fig. 16-4 A, Chest tube drainage. **B,** Anterior view; mediastinal drains.

Any collection system is designed to seal the drainage site from the atmosphere and offer minimal resistance to the drainage of fluid and gas. This is accomplished by immersing the end of the collection tube in water. This is referred to as an underwater seal system. Additional reservoirs are included to decrease the resistance to fluid leaving the chest. This resistance is greater in a single-reservoir system in which the reservoir serves as both the collection receptacle and the underwater seal. A third reservoir can be added to the system; it is attached to the suction and serves as a pressure regulator. The more elaborate drainage systems are used for precise measurement of fluid loss in patients after thoracic and cardiovascular surgery.

The amount of exudate collected in the reservoir is measured every several hours or more often if the patient is losing considerable amounts of fluid or less than the amount predicted. This information is incorporated into the overall fluid-balance assessment. In addition, changes in the quantity and quality of exudates should be noted by the physical therapist before, during, and after changes in position and therapeutic interventions. Chest drainage systems should always be upright and below level of tube insertion. Keeping the container lower than chest level facilitates fluid drainage. It also prevents fluids from flowing back into the chest cavity. Continuous bubbling in water-seal bottle/chamber indicates an air leak. Physical therapists mobilizing patients with chest tubes should be alert to sudden severe respiratory distress and/or pain, which can indicate a tension pneumothorax. If a chest tube is accidently dislodged during physical therapy, the site needs to be immediately compressed, and the nurse must be called.

Acid-Base Balance

Control of acid-base balance in the body is achieved by regulation of the hydrogen ion concentration in the body fluids.[3,4] The pH of the body is normally maintained within a narrow range of 7.35 to 7.45 or slightly alkaline. When pH of the blood drops below 7.35, a state of acidosis exists; above 7.45, a state of alkalosis exists. Regulation of pH is vital because even slight deviations from the normal range cause marked changes in the rate of cellular chemical reactions. A pH below 6.8 or above 8 is incompatible with life.

Acid-base balance is controlled by several regulatory buffer systems, primarily the carbonic acid-bicarbonate, phosphate, and protein buffer systems. These systems act very quickly to prevent moment-to-moment changes in pH. In compensation, pH is returned to normal by altering the component not primarily affected. If the primary cause is respiratory, the compensating mechanism is metabolic. If the primary cause is metabolic, the compensating mechanism is respiratory. The lungs compensate for metabolic problems over hours, whereas the kidneys compensate for respiratory problems over days (see Chapter 10).

A guide to the clinical presentation of acid-base imbalances is shown in Table 16-2. Along with the major distinguishing characteristics of acid-base imbalance described in this chapter and elsewhere in this volume, potassium excess (hyperkalemia) is associated with both respiratory and metabolic acidosis, and neuromuscular hyperexcitability is associated with both respiratory and metabolic alkalosis.

Table 16-2 Signs and Symptoms of Common Acid-Base Disturbances

	Respiratory Disturbances	Metabolic Disturbances
Acidosis	Hypercapnia Hypoventilation Headache Visual disturbances Confusion Drowsiness Coma Hyperkalemia Ventricular fibrillation (secondary to hyperkalemia) Depressed tendon reflexes	Bicarbonate deficit Hyperventilation Headache Mental dullness Deep respirations Stupor Coma Hyperkalemia Cardiac dysrhythmias (secondary to hyperkalemia)
Alkalosis	Hypocapnia Lightheadedness Numbness/tingling of digits Tetany Convulsions Hypokalemia Cardiac dysrhythmias (secondary to hypokalemia)	Bicarbonate excess Depressed respirations Mental confusion Dizziness Numbness/tingling of digits Muscle twitching Tetany Convulsions Hypokalemia Cardiac dysrhythmias (secondary to hypokalemia)

Blood Gases

Analysis of the composition of arterial and mixed venous blood provides vital information about respiratory, cardiac, and metabolic function (see Chapter 10).[5,6] For this reason, blood gases are usually analyzed in the ICU. In cases in which the patient's condition is changing for better or worse over a short period of time or when a specific treatment response is of interest, blood gases may be analyzed several times daily. With an arterial line in place, frequent blood gas analysis is feasible and not traumatic for the patient. Should the patient be anemic, however, blood loss associated with repeated arterial blood sampling may mean that it is contraindicated. Thus requests for arterial blood gas analysis need to be particularly stringent in patients who are anemic.

Arterial saturation ($Sa{O_2}$), the proportion of hemoglobin combined with oxygen, can be readily monitored noninvasively by a pulse oximeter ($Sp{O_2}$). The earlobe or a finger is warmed by rubbing before the oximeter sensor is attached. Within seconds, the $Sp{O_2}$ can be read directly from the monitor. Pulse oximetry is a useful adjunct for routine evaluation of the effectiveness of mechanical ventilation, the effect of anesthesia, and the treatment response. Continuous estimation of $Sa{O_2}$ is particularly useful before, during, and after mobilization and exercise, position changes, and other therapeutic interventions. The $Sa{O_2}$ may appear to be reduced in patients who are anemic or jaundiced or those who have reduced cardiac output. The $Sp{O_2}$ reading may be inaccurate in patients with poor peripheral perfusion, who have cold extremities, or who have pigmented skin. The oxygenation of patients in the ICU varies considerably over time and even moment-to-moment, irrespective of sedation, high post end-expiratory pressure, or inverse ventilation.[7]

Mixed venous oxygen saturation ($S\bar{v}{O_2}$) provides a useful index of oxygen delivery and utilization at the tissue level.[8] $S\bar{v}{O_2}$ is highly correlated to tissue oxygen extraction, and thus is a good index of the adequacy of oxygen delivery. The $S\bar{v}{O_2}$ is particularly useful as a significant warning sign, a guide to myocardial function, and a tool to titrate positive end-expiratory pressure support. The normal value of $S\bar{v}{O_2}$ is 75%. Concern is raised by $S\bar{v}{O_2}$ values of less than 60% or a drop of 10% for several minutes. Excessive $S\bar{v}{O_2}$ values above 80% are also cause for concern. High $S\bar{v}{O_2}$ values may occur in patients with left-to-right shunts in the heart, hyperoxia, hypothermia, cyanide toxicity, sepsis, anesthesia, and drug-induced paralysis. Despite its general clinical usefulness, $S\bar{v}{O_2}$ is a nonspecific indicator of the adequacy of oxygen transport (i.e., of the balance between oxygen supply and demand). Abnormal $S\bar{v}{O_2}$ values do not indicate precisely where the problem lies; so other hemodynamic variables need to be considered. Further, $S\bar{v}{O_2}$ has been reported to fluctuate as much as ±6% in patients in the ICU in response to routine activity and treatment.[9] Maintaining normal $S\bar{v}{O_2}$ in patients with multiple trauma improves survival rates over those in whom oxygen transport values are maintained at above normal levels.[10] Enhancing cardiac output and hemoglobin as well as $S\bar{v}O_2$ is essential to increase oxygen delivery (DO_2) above its critical level and avoid tissue oxygen debt.[11] Impaired extraction at the tissue level has been attributed to heterogeneity of oxygen delivery.[12]

Hypoxemia

In health, age and body position are factors that reduce arterial oxygen tension.[13] Arterial oxygen levels diminish with age as a result of reduced alveolar surface area, pulmonary capillary blood volume, and diffusing capacity. Normal PaO_2 levels expressed in mm Hg in older people should exceed the value of 110-0.5 (age). In a young adult, PaO_2 ranges from 90 to 100 mm Hg in the upright seated position. In the supine position, this range is reduced to 85 to 95 mm Hg; in sleeping, to 70 to 85 mm Hg. These values are clinically significant because in older people, smokers, and people with pathology, these positional effects are accentuated. Despite sedation in patients who are critically ill, spontaneous variability of PaO_2 is considerable, and factors unduly influencing it must be controlled when using PaO_2 as an outcome.[7]

Hypoxemia refers to reduced oxygen tension in the blood. Some common signs and symptoms of various degrees of hypoxemia in adults appear in Table 16-3. Although the brain is protected by autoregulatory mechanisms, an arterial oxygen tension of 60 mm Hg produces signs of marked depression of the central nervous system, reflecting the extreme sensitivity of cerebral tissue to hypoxia.

Hypoxemia is compensated primarily by increased cardiac output, improved perfusion of vital organs, and in the long term, polycythemia. Secondary mechanisms of compensation include improved unloading of oxygen at the tissue level as a result of tissue acidosis and anaerobic metabolism, which is achieved through a rightward shift of the oxyhemoglobin dissociation curve.

The progressive physiological deterioration observed at decreasing arterial oxygen levels will occur at higher oxygen levels if any one of the major compensating mechanisms for hypoxemia is defective. Even a mild drop in PaO_2, for example, is poorly tolerated by a patient with reduced hemoglobin and impaired cardiac output. Alternatively, the signs and symptoms of hypoxemia may appear at lower arterial oxygen levels (e.g., in patients with chronic airflow limitation who have adapted to reduced PaO_2 levels).

Monitoring oxygen kinetics is essential to understanding oxygen transport status in patients who are critically ill and thus ensuring early intervention.[12,14] DO_2 and $\dot{V}O_2$ and their constituents can be measured directly or indirectly with calorimetry. Patients who survive heart failure have distinct oxygen kinetic profiles.[15] In response to improved cardiac index and DO_2 in survivors, $\dot{V}O_2$ did not change, whereas the oxygen extraction ratio (OER) decreased. In nonsurvivors, $\dot{V}O_2$ increased and the OER did not change. Such profiles can assist in establishing baseline information, detecting changes early, and modifying physical therapy interventions.

Table 16-3 Signs and Symptoms of Hypoxemia

PaO_2	Signs and Symptoms
80-100 mm Hg	Normal
60-80 mm Hg	Moderate tachycardia, possible onset of respiratory distress
50-60 mm Hg	Malaise Lightheadedness Nausea Vertigo Impaired judgment Incoordination Restless Increased minute ventilation
35-50 mm Hg	Marked confusion Cardiac dysrhythmias Labored respiration
25-35 mm Hg	Cardiac arrest Decreased renal blood flow Decreased urine output Lactic acidosis Poor oxygenation Lethargy Maximal minute ventilation Loss of consciousness
<25 mm Hg	Decreased minute ventilation (secondary to depression of respiratory center)

Hyperoxia

Mean tissue oxygen tensions rise less than 10 mm Hg when pure oxygen is administered to a healthy person under normal conditions. Therefore the function of nonpulmonary tissues is little altered. In the lung, high concentrations of oxygen replace nitrogen in poorly ventilated regions. This results in collapse of areas with reduced ventilation-perfusion matching (de-nitrogen atelectasis). Lung compliance is diminished.

High concentrations of oxygen (inspired oxygen fractions greater than 50%) can directly injure bronchial and parenchymal lung tissue. The toxic effect of oxygen is both time- and concentration-dependent. Very high concentrations of oxygen may be tolerated for up to 48 hours. However, high concentrations of oxygen in combination with positive pressure breathing can predispose the patient to oxygen toxicity and lung parenchymal injury. At concentrations of inspired oxygen less than 50%, clinically detectable oxygen toxicity is unusual regardless of the duration of oxygen therapy.

Hypocapnia

Acute reductions in arterial carbon dioxide levels (hypocapnia) result in alkalosis and diminished cerebral blood flow secondary to cerebral vasoconstriction. The major consequences of abrupt lowering of $PaCO_2$ are altered peripheral and central nerve function. Mechanical ventilation may initially cause an abrupt decrease in arterial PCO_2 and lead to a life-threatening situation. In addition to blood gas analysis, end tidal CO_2 measurement is useful in that it provides an index of $PaCO_2$.

Hypercapnia

CO_2, the principal end product of metabolism, is a relatively benign gas. CO_2 has a key role in ventilation and in regulating changes in cerebral blood flow, pH, and sympathetic tone.

Acute increases in CO_2 (hypercapnia) depress the level of consciousness secondary to the effect of acidosis on the nervous system. Similar but slowly developing increases in CO_2, however, are relatively well tolerated. A high $Pa{CO_2}$ is suggestive of alveolar hypoventilation, which causes a reduction in alveolar and arterial Po_2. Some patients with severe chronic airflow obstruction have been reported to be able to lead relatively normal lives with $Pa{CO_2}$ in excess of 90 mm Hg if hypoxemia is countered with supplemental oxygen. Acute administration of oxygen to patients with chronic obstructive lung disease, however, may be hazardous, because it interferes with their hypoxic drive to breathe, on which they are reliant.

Acute hypercapnia enhances sympathetic stimulation, causing an increase in cardiac output and in peripheral vascular resistance. These effects offset the effect of excess hydrogen ions on the cardiovascular system, allowing better tolerance of low pH than with metabolic acidosis of a similar degree. At extreme levels of hypercapnia, muscle twitching and seizures may be observed. Trends in $Pa{CO_2}$ can be monitored indirectly using end tidal CO_2 measures.

ECG Monitoring

A single-channel ECG monitor with an oscilloscope, strip recorder, and digital heart rate display is typically located above the patient at bedside in the ICU (Figure 16-5). Often, the ECG can be observed at bedside and at a central monitoring console, where the ECGs of all patients in the ICU can be observed simultaneously.

The ECG monitor allows for continuous surveillance of heart rate and rhythm regardless of activity. Low and high heart rates are determined; rates below and above those rates will trigger an alarm. For routine monitoring in the coronary care unit, a modified chest lead is often used. Depending on the lead configuration desired, as few as three electrodes can be positioned on the chest to provide optimal information regarding changes in heart rate and rhythm, and thereby ensure close patient monitoring. The positive electrode is positioned at the fourth intercostal space at the right sternal border. The negative electrode is positioned at the first intercostal space in the left midclavicular line. The ground electrode, used to dissipate electrical interference, is often positioned at the first intercostal space in the right midclavicular line, although the ground electrode may be positioned wherever convenient. Other electrode placements may be required, for example, in patients with pacemakers or chest burns.

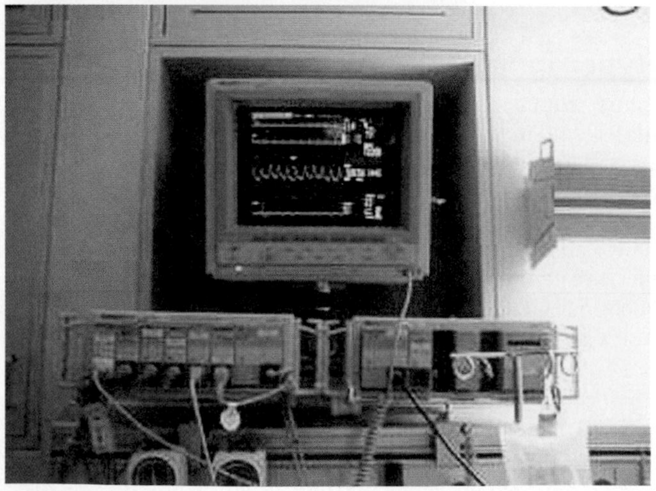

Fig. 16-5 ECG monitor.

Problems with the ECG monitor usually result from faulty technique, electrical interference, or movement artifact. A thickened baseline can be caused by 60-cycle electrical interference. An erratic signal often results from coughing and movement. The cause of any irregularity must be explained and abnormal electrical activity of the myocardium ruled out. It is a dangerous practice for the physical therapist to turn off the ECG alarm system during treatment.

Cardiac dysrhythmias can be broadly categorized into tachydysrhythmias and bradydysrhythmias. Tachydysrhythmias are subdivided into supraventricular and subjunctional tachycardias. Bradydysrhythmias are subdivided into sinus bradycardia and those related to heart block and conduction abnormalities. The subjunctional tachycardias and ventricular dysrhythmias are particularly life-threatening. Ventricular tachycardia and ventricular fibrillation are medical emergencies requiring immediate recognition and treatment.

The characteristic features of common dysrhythmias are illustrated in Chapter 12. Physical therapists specializing in ICU management should be thoroughly familiar with ECG interpretation and the implications of the various dysrhythmias on patient management. For further elaboration of ECG application and interpretation, refer to Kinney and Packa[16] and Dubin.[17]

The clinical picture associated with cardiac dysrhythmias depends on the nature of the dysrhythmia, the age and condition of the patient, the medications, and specifically, the absence or presence of underlying heart disease. The distinguishing clinical features of common atrial and ventricular dysrhythmias are outlined in Table 16-4.

The subjunctional or ventricular dysrhythmias are typically associated with severe illness. Cyanosis and duskiness of the mucosal linings and periphery may be apparent. The patient is unresponsive, the pulse is ineffective, and spontaneous respirations are likely to be absent. In this case, defibrillation is initiated by the nursing and medical staff to restore an effective, more normal rhythm. The high incidence of myocardial conduction irregularities warrants a defibrillator being present in the ICU for rapid implementation of this common cardioversion procedure by the medical and nursing staff. Ventricular dysrhythmias may be better tolerated if ventricular rate is low, thereby improving cardiac output. Even in this circumstance, however, these dysrhythmias present an emergency.

The ECG of a patient with a pacemaker reflects either an imposed fixed or intermittent rhythm and rate, depending on whether a fixed rate or a demand pacemaker has been inserted. The electrical impulse from the pacemaker has a unique ECG wave form.

Hemodynamic Monitoring

Hemodynamic status reflects the adequacy of blood volume and electromechanical coupling of the myocardium to effect adequate cardiac output and peripheral perfusion

Table 16-4 **Clinical Picture of Common Dysrhythmias**

Dysrhythmia	No Underlying Cardiovascular Disease	Underlying Cardiovascular Disease
TACHYCARDIAS		
A. Supraventricular tachycardia	No symptoms Abrupt-onset palpitations, lightheadedness, nausea, fatigue	May precipitate congestive heart failure, acute coronary insufficiency, myocardial infarction, pulmonary edema
1. Sinus tachycardia	Awareness of the heart on exertion or with anxiety	Secondary to some precipitating factor, such as fever, electrolyte imbalance, anemia, blood and fluid loss, infection, persistent hypoxemia in COPD, acute MI, congestive heart failure, thyrotoxicosis
2. Paroxysmal atrial tachycardia (PAT)	Prevalent, sudden onset, precipitated by coffee, smoking, and exhaustion	Common supraventricular tachycardia Spontaneous onset of regular palpitations that can last for several hours May be obscured by myocardial insufficiency and CHF in older patients Increased anxiety and report of fatigue
3. Atrial flutter	Rare May be difficult to distinguish from PAT May be precipitated by alcohol, smoking, physical and emotional strain	Rapid regular-irregular rate Suggests block at AV node Atrial flutter waves in jugular venous pulse
4. Atrial fibrillation	Rare, occasionally with alcohol excess in the young	Usually secondary to a variety of cardiac disorders
5. Paroxysmal atrial tachycardia with block	Rare	Common arrhythmia seen with digitalis toxicity
B. Subjunctional	Rare	Usually related to MI, pulmonary embolus, severe CHF Often unconscious, cyanotic; ineffective pulse, blood pressure, and respiration
1. Ventricular tachycardia	Rare	Predisposed to ventricular fibrillation
2. Ventricular fibrillation	Rare	Ineffective cardiac output, unconscious, dusky; cardiac arrest threat
BRADYCARDIAS		
A. Sinus bradycardia	Physiological in very fit young adults	In older patients, may suggest sinus node and conduction system pathology; can produce syncope or CHF
B. Heart block	Rare	Hypotension, dizziness, lightheadedness, syncope In chronic block with sustained bradycardia, CHF may be more frequent Most common dysrhythmia iatrogenically produced with digitalis excess Associated with numerous cardiac conditions; commonly in age-related degenerative disease in conducting system, inferior and occasionally anterior MIs

commensurate with changing metabolic demand. In individuals who are not critically ill, monitoring fluid input and output, heart rate, and blood pressure may suffice in providing a profile. To monitor a patient's hemodynamics more closely in the ICU, however, the insertion of various invasive lines may be indicated in addition to the lines and leads needed to monitor basic fluid and electrolyte balance and ECG. These require invasive arterial and venous lines.

Intraarterial Lines

An arterial line is established by direct arterial puncture. It is usually in the radial artery; however, it can be seen in the femoral, axillary, or brachial artery (Figure 16-6, *A, B*). Blood pressure can be measured directly from this line. A digital monitor displays systolic and diastolic blood pressures above the patient at bedside. High and low blood pressure levels are set, above and below which the alarm will sound. Blood gas analysis can be performed routinely with an intraarterial line in place without repeating the puncture of a blood vessel.

Pulmonary Artery Balloon Flotation Catheter

The pulmonary artery balloon flotation (Swan-Ganz) catheter is designed to provide an accurate and convenient means of hemodynamic assessment in the ICU by monitoring intracardiac pressures and, in combination with other measures, assessing cardiac reserve, an important determinant of outcome following critical illness.[18] The catheter is usually inserted into the internal jugular vein, the subclavian vein, or

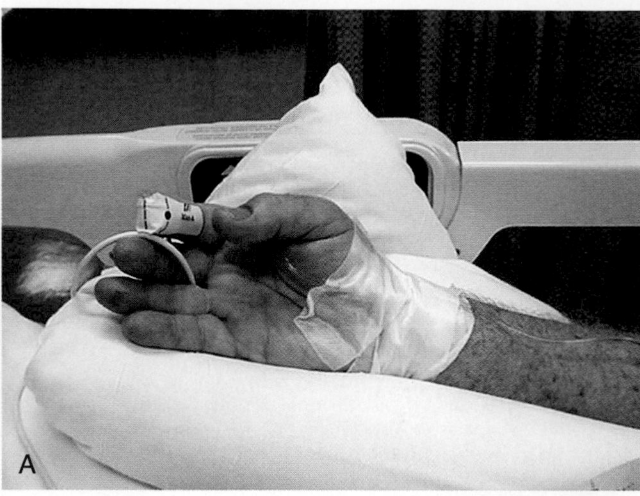

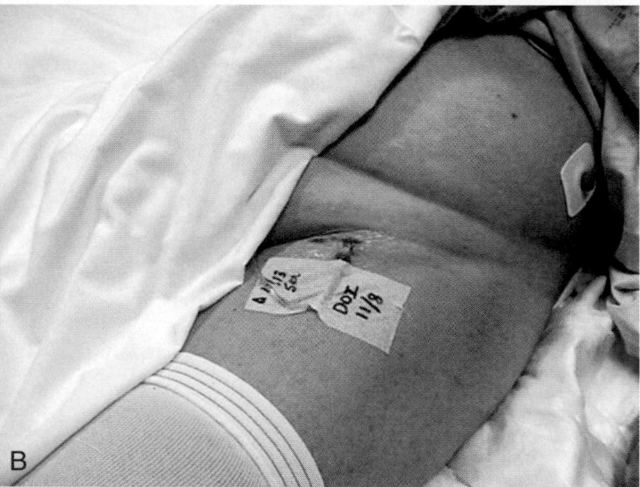

Fig. 16-6 **A,** Radial arterial line. Also note the pulse oximeter sensor on the finger. **B,** Femoral arterial line.

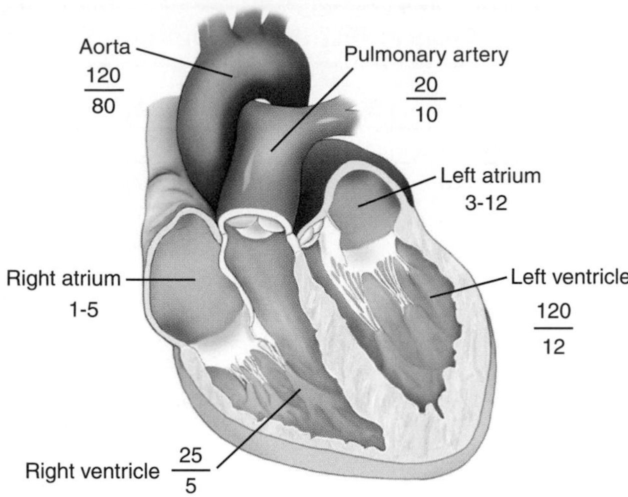

Fig. 16-7 Normal cardiac pressures in each heart chamber.

a large peripheral arm vein and is directed by the flow of blood into the right ventricle and pulmonary artery (see Figure 16-3, *A*). The catheter is carefully secured to prevent dislodging. Some of the complications that have been associated with pulmonary artery catheterization, however, include infection, venous thrombosis, myocardial irritation, air embolism, and pulmonary ischemia or infarct to segmental lung tissue.[19]

Complex catheters are available for monitoring a variety of parameters. In a two-lumen catheter, the first lumen is used to measure pulmonary artery pressure (PAP) and obtain mixed venous blood samples. The second lumen terminates in a balloon with a volume of less than 1 mL, which is inflated and deflated to obtain pulmonary artery occlusion or wedge pressure (PAOP or PAWP, respectively). The normal range of the systolic PAP is 20 to 30 mm Hg, and it normally reflects right ventricular pressure (RVP). The diastolic PAP ranges from 7 to 12 mm Hg and reflects left ventricular pressure in the absence of pulmonary disease. The average range of PAWP is 8 to 12 mm Hg and gives an estimation of mean left atrial pressure (LAP) and the pressure in the left ventricle (LVP). Figure 16-7 shows the normal cardiac pressures in each heart chamber. More elaborate catheters have pacing wires, thermistors for cardiac output determination, and sensors for arterial saturation.

The PAP increases as a result of elevated pulmonary blood flow, increased pulmonary arteriolar resistance secondary to primary pulmonary hypertension or mitral stenosis, and left ventricular failure. Measurement of PAP and PAWP, in particular, allows for more prudent management of heart failure and cardiogenic shock.

The PAP, PAWP, and end-diastolic LVP are directly related. Impaired left ventricular contractility that compromises normal emptying (e.g., left ventricular failure, mitral stenosis, or mitral insufficiency) results in an elevated end-diastolic LVP, which in turn, elevates PAWP and PAP. An end-diastolic PAP greater than 20 mm Hg or a PAWP greater than 12 mm Hg is considered abnormal.

The PAP and PAWP are low during hypotension secondary to hypovolemia. Infusion of normal saline, whole blood, or low-molecular-weight dextran elevates the blood volume and blood pressure. Restoration of blood volume returns end-diastolic PAP and PAWP to normal.

Elevation of the end-diastolic PAP secondary to heart failure with pulmonary edema can typically be reduced with appropriate medication. The effectiveness of a drug and its prescription parameters can be assessed by the observed changes in the end-diastolic PAP.

Deterioration of cardiovascular status and worsening of the clinical signs and symptoms of heart failure elevate end-diastolic PAP and PAWP, decrease cardiac output, decrease arterial and right atrial oxygen tension, and increase the oxygen difference between arterial and venous blood. As the heart pump continues to fail, arterial oxygen tension decreases, suggesting abnormal lung function and probably elevated LAP. Pulmonary dysfunction at this stage includes diffusion abnormalities, redistribution of pulmonary blood flow into the less well-ventilated upper lobes, and right-to-left shunting, which causes deoxygenated blood to bypass well-ventilated regions of the lungs. All patients with acute infarction or shock have reduced arterial oxygen tension. When the failing heart is unable to effectively eject blood through the aorta to the systemic circulation, fluid may back up into the lungs. Pulmonary congestion must be cleared before the patient can appropriately respond to oxygen administration.

Despite the enormous benefits of direct invasive hemodynamic monitoring to patient assessment and management, the benefits of basic hemodynamic assessment are a fundamental part of the cardiovascular and pulmonary assessment, regardless of whether the patient has an invasive line inserted.[20] Basic hemodynamic monitoring includes heart rate, ECG, blood pressure, and peripheral tissue perfusion. These are fundamental to the physical therapy assessment of all patients across settings. Even though ECG may not necessarily be monitored by the physical therapist directly in non-ICU settings, knowledge of its status is imperative in order to establish whether an individual is safe to treat and, if so, how treatment should be modified and what precautions should be taken.

Central Venous Pressure Monitoring

CVP is monitored by means of a venous line or catheter inserted into the subclavian, basilic, jugular, or femoral vein (see Figure 16-3, *C*). The catheter is advanced to the right atrium by way of the inferior or superior vena cava, depending on the site of insertion. Minimal risk for phlebitis or infection is associated with this procedure.

CVP is the blood pressure measured in the vena cavae or right atrium. Normal CVP ranges from 0 to 5 cm H_2O or from 5 to 10 cm H_2O if measured at the sternal notch or midaxillary line, respectively. Essentially, the CVP provides information about the adequacy of right heart function, including effective circulating blood volume, effectiveness of the heart as a pump, vascular tone, and venous return. Measurement of CVP is particularly useful in assessing fluid volume and fluid replacement. If the patient has chronic airflow limitation, ventricular ischemia, or infarction, the CVP will reflect changes in pathology rather than fluid volume.

Specifically, CVP provides an index of right atrial pressure (RAP). The relationship between RAP and end-diastolic LVP is unreliable; therefore end-diastolic PAP and PAWP are used as the principal indicators of cardiovascular and pulmonary sufficiency in patients in failure and shock.

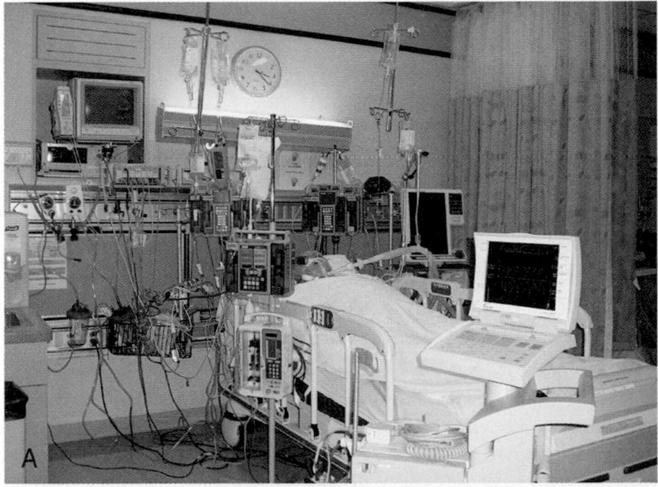

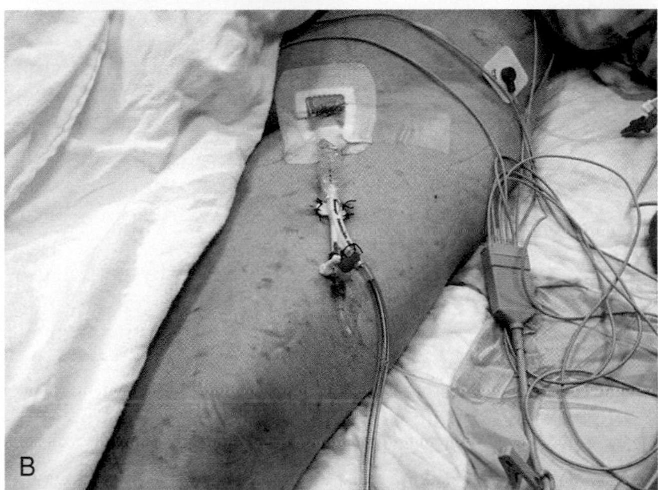

Fig. 16-8 A, Patient on an intraaortic balloon pump (IABP) support. **B,** Close-up of the IABP insertion on the femoral artery.

Intraaortic Balloon Counterpulsation Device

Intraaortic balloon counterpulsation (Figure 16-8, *A*) provides mechanical circulatory assistance by using an intraaortic balloon. The balloon is inserted into the femoral artery (see Figure 16-8, *B*). To maintain proper placement and good circulation, the patient's leg must be extended. The presence of an intraaortic balloon must be taken into consideration whenever the patient is being treated and positioned. Inflation and deflation of the balloon with helium is correlated with the ECG. The intraaortic balloon is deflated during ventricular systole and assists the emptying of the aorta. Stroke volume is potentiated, afterload is reduced (hence reducing ventricular pressure), and myocardial oxygen delivery enhanced. The balloon is inflated during diastole, thereby restoring arterial pressure and coronary perfusion. Counterpulsation improves cardiac output, reduces evidence of myocardial ischemia, and reduces ST-segment elevation. Intraaortic balloon counterpulsation is commonly used after open-heart surgery and for CHF, medically refractory myocardial ischemia, ventricular septal defects, and left main coronary stenosis in patients who are in shock. The intraaortic balloon pump provides protection for the myocardium in many instances until surgery can be performed. Limb ischemia, the most common complication, occurs in 10% to 15% of patients.

Left ventricular assist devices are used when patients develop cardiogenic shock and are unresponsive to conventional management. These devices take over the pumping action of the left ventricle and decrease myocardial workload and oxygen consumption. These types of assistive devices may have considerable potential in the management of refractory heart failure.

Intracranial Pressure Monitoring

Increased ICP results from neurological insults such as head injury, hypoxic brain damage, aneurysm, hemorrhage, and cerebral tumor. If severe and unrelenting, the pressure may need to be decompressed with surgery; otherwise, brain tissue may be irreversibly damaged, leading to permanent neurological deficits. In the adult, the cranial vault is rigid and noncompliant. Increases in the volume of the cranial contents from tissue edema result in an elevated ICP and decreased cerebral perfusion pressure.

Changes in consciousness are the earliest and most sensitive indicators of increased ICP.[21] Altered consciousness reflects herniation of the brainstem and compression of the midbrain. Compression of the oculomotor nerve and the pupilloconstrictor fibers results in abnormal pupillary reactions that are associated with brain damage.

The effects of ICP on blood pressure and pulse are variable. Blood pressure may be elevated secondary to elevated ICP and hypoxia of the vasomotor center. A reflex decrease in pulse occurs as blood pressure rises.

Compression of upper motor neuron pathways interrupts the transmission of impulses to lower motor neurons; progressive muscle weakness results. A contralateral weakened hand grasp, for example, may progress to hemiparesis or hemiplegia. The Babinski sign, hyperreflexia, and rigidity are additional motor signs that provide evidence of decreasing motor function as a result of upper motor neuron involvement.

Herniation can produce incoordinate respirations that are correlated with the level of brainstem compression. Cerebrate rigidity results from tentorial herniation of the upper brainstem. This results in the blocking of the motor inhibitory fibers and the familiar extended body posture. Seizures may be present. These neuromuscular changes may further compound existing cardiovascular and pulmonary complications in the patient in the ICU.

Clinically, increased ICP is best detected by altered consciousness, blood pressure, pulse, pupillary responses, movement, temperature, and respiration. The ICP monitor provides direct measurement of ICP. A hollow screw is positioned through the skull into the subarachnoid space. The screw is attached to a Luer-Lok, which is connected to a transducer and oscilloscope for continuous monitoring.

The prevention of further increase in ICP and a corresponding reduction in cerebral perfusion pressure is a treatment priority. High ICP and low cerebral perfusion pressure are highly correlated with brain injury. Measures to reduce venous volume are maintained until ICP has stabilized within normal range. Prudent body positioning is used to enhance venous drainage by elevating the bed 15 to 30 degrees and maintaining the head above heart level. Neck flexion is avoided by the placement of a neck support or sand bags. Fluid intake and output are carefully regulated and monitored; the patient may need to be fluid restricted. Stimulation of the Valsalva maneuver is avoided because intrathoracic pressure and ICP may increase correspondingly.

The normal range of the ICP is 0 to 10 mm Hg for adults and 0 to 5 mm Hg for patients under 6 years of age. The ICP may reach 50 mm Hg in the normal brain; typically, however, this pressure returns to baseline levels instantaneously. In patients with high levels of ICP and low cerebral compliance, extra care must be exercised during routine management and therapy. An ICP up to 30 mm Hg that is elicited by turning or suctioning may be acceptable, provided the pressure drops immediately following removal of the pressure-potentiating stimulus. Patients may be mechanically hyperventilated to keep arterial P_{CO_2} at low levels, because hypercapnia dilates cerebral vessels and hypocapnia constricts them.

To establish whether a patient will tolerate a treatment that requires movement or body positioning, an indication of cerebral compliance is needed. This can be obtained by observing changes in ICP during routine nursing procedures or by titrating small degrees of movement or position change and observing the rate at which the ICP returns to baseline following the challenge. Rapid return to baseline minimizes the risk for reduced cerebral perfusion pressure secondary to the increased ICP. A slow return to baseline or sustained elevation of ICP is consistent with poor cerebral compliance and indicates that treatment should be modified or possibly not performed at all, depending on the absolute level of the ICP. Physical therapy assessment only may be indicated until compliance improves.

Assessment of Arousal and Brain Activity

Patients in the ICU tend to have low arousal directly or indirectly related to underlying pathology, as well as from induced sedation and antianxiety medications.[22] Although medication is often indicated to reduce arousal, a balance must be maintained by the medical staff to avoid under- or oversedating the patient. To benefit maximally from physical therapy and actively participate in treatment, patients need to be as consciously aware as possible. Tools such as the Richmond Agitation-Sedation Scale[23] have been developed to quantify arousal state, which can be helpful in directing the course of treatment.

The Glasgow Coma Scale is a common tool for the clinical assessment and evaluation of the adequacy of basic brain function; it includes review of motor, sensory, pain, arousal, and cognitive status. An electroencephalogram (EEG), provides useful information about gross cerebral functioning and changes in level of consciousness. A single-channel EEG monitor can be readily used in the ICU to reveal evidence of posttraumatic epilepsy when the clinical signs may be inhibited by muscle relaxants. An EEG assessment may be of benefit in assessing arousal, prognosis, the response to treatment of cerebral function, and the planning and prescribing of treatment.

Neuromuscular Assessment

The neuromuscular assessment is a fundamental component of the assessment of the patient in the ICU. The patient may have been admitted for a primary neuromuscular condition with risk for respiratory failure. In addition, all patients in the ICU are at risk for ICU-acquired weakness. ICU-acquired weakness is defined as weakness developing in a patient who is critically ill with no identifiable cause other than nonspecific inflammation.[24] It has been associated with the administration of steroids, neuromuscular blockade, hyperglycemia, sepsis, multiple organ failure, bedrest (recumbency), and restricted mobility. The terms critical illness polyneuropathy (CIP) and critical illness myopathy (CIM) are commonly used in the ICU. The neuromuscular manifestations of CIP and CIM are difficult to assess in a valid manner. Despite this, their early identification is essential in order to avoid significant weakness, irreversible deterioration, delayed recovery, and prolonged dependence on mechanical ventilation.[25] Other causes need to be ruled out. Prognosis is good if ICU-acquired weakness is detected early and rehabilitation is instituted.

Because many patients in the ICU are administered sedatives and muscle relaxants, placing them at increased risk for ICU-acquired weakness, the physical therapist needs to monitor level of arousal and sedation. The use of agitation and sedation scales can be useful in monitoring arousal and the patient's capacity to cooperate with treatment.[23,26] The physical therapist has an important role in minimizing the need for pharmacological sedation by optimizing pain control, relaxation, comfort, and the individual's perception of control.

Peripheral-nerve electrical stimulation (e.g., of the median nerve) is used to monitor potential neuropathies in a patient in a coma or under neuromuscular blockade. Such stimulation is sufficient to activate the pathways of the ascending reticular activating system associated with consciousness and to hasten awaking from coma.[27] In addition, patients score better on repeated assessment with the Glasgow Coma Scale initially and at 1 month after injury, and they have shorter ICU stays.

There is no specific treatment for ICU-acquired weakness. It is prudent to consider reducing patients' exposure to the risk factors. Recent studies have demonstrated that the most promising management of ICU-acquired weakness is physical therapy, even while the patient is receiving life-and-organ support interventions.[28,29]

Cognitive Assessment

The ICU experience can contribute to cognitive impairment or worsen it in patients who are already impaired.[30,31] These effects can extend for several months beyond the ICU stay.[32] Risk factors include functional dependence and low body mass, as well as previous cognitive impairment.[33] Preexisting cognitive impairment must be identified and changes in cognition should be monitored so they can be detected early. Strategies can be implemented to avoid cognitive impairment, including frequent orientation of the patient to time and place, surrounding the individual with familiar objects and family and friends, using familiar tape recordings (voices or music), taking time to talk to the patient, and being reassuring. Further, strategies to reduce anxiety, stress, restlessness, and negative mood states can reduce the duration of hospitalization in patients in the ICU.[34]

Acute distress disorder comparable to traumatic stress syndrome has been described recently in individuals after accidental injuries. In addition to the nature of the accident itself and the associated threat to life, factors contributing to an individual's overall stress include hospitalization, length of the ICU stay, the ICU experience, and pain management.[35,36] Thus optimizing the patient's perception of care is important in preventing and offsetting symptoms of acute distress.

With improvement in the management of acute respiratory distress syndrome (ARDS), long-term studies have examined the relationship between cognitive performance, employability, and return to work in survivors. These patients may exhibit long-term cognitive deficits and impaired health status, which contribute to disability and marked reduction in health-related quality of life.[37] An understanding of these potential consequences will help their prevention and the comprehensive management of ARDS.

Pain Assessment

Pain has been described as one of the vital signs. Assessing pain in the ICU is particularly challenging, given that patients cannot readily communicate their discomfort and pain. Physical therapists need to monitor discomfort and pain as part of the ongoing assessment to ensure not only that the patient is comfortable but also that therapeutic interventions do not contribute to compromised oxygen transport by increasing distress and that they do not interfere with sleep and recovery. Further, noninvasive interventions should be used as much as possible to reduce the necessity of pharmacological agents that can compromise the patient's capacity to cooperate with treatment. Optimal management can be achieved only with accurate assessment and ongoing evaluation as the basis for progressing treatment. Pain assessment tools include the McGill Pain Questionnaire, a pain analog scale, the Wong-Baker FACES pain scale, and others.[38] The therapist should choose the format to which the patient can most readily respond.

Long-Term Outcomes Related to ICU Care

The study of outcomes of patients who have experienced ICU stays has become a focus of research. In previous decades, if a patient survived the ICU stay, this was viewed as the primary outcome. These days, most patients survive the ICU; however, outcomes related to their return to a full and active life may be less favorable.[39] Focusing on long-term outcomes can be integrated into the physical therapy care in the ICU. This includes assessment and evaluation of some aspects of functional status, as well as a premorbid evaluation based on the patient's self-report, if possible, or that of family members. In addition, the practice of physical therapy needs to extend from the ICU to the ward and then to the home, with judicious follow up after the patient has returned to the community. Depending on the age of the patient, the reason for ICU admission, and comorbidity, return to a maximal level of functioning could take a year or more.

Summary

The capacity of patients in the ICU to participate in life and perform the requisite activities is severely compromised because of life-threatening illness or injury (i.e., involving the oxygen transport system). The immediate goal of the ICU is to provide intense life-preserving, specialized care with the view of ultimately returning the individual to a healthy and productive life. Monitoring cardiovascular and pulmonary functions and oxygen transport is an essential component of management. Regulation of homeostasis is disrupted in disease or following highly invasive medical and surgical interventions. Physical therapists practicing in the ICU need to have a thorough understanding of homeostatic regulation and the monitoring of fluid and electrolyte balance, acid-base balance, and blood gases. Physical therapy has an essential role in restoring homeostasis in patients requiring intensive care by using conservative, noninvasive approaches, in addition to averting the musculoskeletal, neuromuscular, and multisystem complications associated with recumbency and restricted mobility. The selection of treatment and the assessment of treatment response are based on quantitative evaluation of the parameters affecting oxygen transport and cardiovascular and pulmonary functions, as well as the patient's subjective sense of well-being. Detailed monitoring is necessary to provide well reasoned and informed management of the patient in the ICU, as well as to prevent deterioration and detect complications early. In the ICU, where a patient's status may change from moment to moment, the information gathered from monitoring is essential to maximize physical therapy effectiveness and minimize deleterious effects. This information is critical in establishing the indications for physical therapy, prescribing treatment parameters, and determining when to progress, withhold, or discontinue treatment. The windows of opportunity for intervention are often narrow, so the physical therapist must be able to identify these expeditiously on the basis of frequent serial assessment and to intervene appropriately.

Further, psychosocial assessment is fundamental to eliciting the most favorable outcomes. Other anticipated outcomes include reduced requirement for invasive care (i.e., drugs and surgery) and shorter length of stay in the ICU and in hospital afterwards. Physical therapists have a major role in employing noninvasive, ethical interventions in the ICU and in helping to minimize the costs of this expensive, high-tech, labor-intense area of care. Databases and longitudinal studies of the profiles and long-term outcomes of patients following various critical illnesses after return to the community are needed. Such prognostic information would help to refine the assessment of patients by physical therapists, as well as the short- and long-term management of patients in the ICU. Finally, the physical therapist has a primary role in ensuring that the patient has returned as fully as possible to life in the community in the following months after discharge. ICU outcomes have now extended from merely surviving an ICU stay to thriving afterwards—even if this outcome takes a year or more to achieve.

Review Questions

1. Explain how the International Classification of Functioning, Disability and Health (see Chapters 1, 7 and 17) relates to physical therapy goals for patients in the ICU and how this classification can be applied in this setting with special reference to the role of monitoring.
2. Explain the determinants of fluid and electrolyte balance and factors that contribute to fluid excesses and deficits.
3. Describe the basis of acid-base balance.
4. Describe the physiological effects of hypoxia and hypercapnia.
5. Explain the physiological basis of ECG monitoring and common supraventricular and ventricular dysrhythmias.
6. Explain (a) the physiological basis of the pulmonary artery balloon flotation catheter, and (b) what is represented by altered CVP, RAP (systolic and diastolic), PAP (systolic and diastolic), and PAWP.
7. Describe the basis of the intraaortic balloon counterpulsation device with respect to improving myocardial function.
8. Describe intracranial pressure monitoring, its physiological basis, and the clinical implications of such monitoring.
9. What is ICU-acquired weakness? What is its clinical significance in the ICU? What are the implications for the physical therapist?
10. Provide the rationale for cognitive assessment in the ICU.
11. What is the physical therapist's role in pain assessment in the ICU environment?
12. As primarily a noninvasive practitioner, the physical therapist plays what role in patient management in the high-tech ICU environment?

References

1. Perme C, Chandrashekar R: Early mobility and walking program for patients in intensive care units: creating a standard of care. *American Journal of Critical Care* 18:212–221, 2009.
2. Phipps WJ, Long BC, Woods NF, editors: *Medical-surgical nursing: concepts and clinical practice*, ed 6, Philadelphia, 1999, Elsevier.
3. Hall JE: *Guyton and Hall textbook of medical physiology*, ed 12, Philadelphia, 2010, Elsevier.
4. Shapiro BA, Peruzzi WT, Kozelowski-Templin R: *Clinical application of blood gases*, ed 5, St. Louis, 1994, Mosby.
5. Barrett KE, Brooks H, Boitano S, et al: *Ganong's review of medical physiology*, ed 23, New York, 2009, McGraw-Hill Professional Publishing.
6. West JB: *Respiratory physiology: The essentials*, ed 8, Baltimore, 2008, Williams & Wilkins.
7. Tsai YH, Lin MC, Hsieh MJ, et al: Spontaneous variability of arterial oxygenation in critically ill mechanically ventilated patients. *Intensive Care Medicine* 25:37–43, 1999.
8. Copel LC, Stolarik A: Continuous Svo2 monitoring: a research review. *Dimensions of Critical Care Nursing* 10:202–209, 1991.
9. Noll ML, Fountain RL, Duncan CA, et al: Fluctuation in mixed venous oxygen saturation in critically ill medical patients: a pilot study. *American Journal of Critical Care* 1:102–106, 1992.
10. Kremzar B, Spec-Marn A, Kompan L, et al: Normal values of Svo2 as a therapeutic goal in patients with multiple injuries. *Intensive Care Medicine* 23:65–70, 1997.
11. Vallett B, Tavernier B, Lund N: Assessment of tissue oxygenation in the critically-ill. *European Journal of Anaesthesiology* 17:221–229, 2000.
12. Walley KR: Heterogeneity of oxygen delivery impairs oxygen extraction by peripheral tissues: theory. *Journal of Applied Physiology* 81:885–894, 1996.
13. Oakes DF: *Clinical practitioners pocket guide to respiratory care*, ed 6, Orono, 2004, Health Education Publications.
14. Wiedemann HP, Matthay MA, Matthay RA: Cardiovascular-pulmonary monitoring in the intensive care unit (Part 1). *Chest* 85:537–549, 1984.
15. Inoue T, Morooka S, Sakai Y, et al: Oxygen demand-supply relationship in peripheral tissues as a therapeutic indicator in acute myocardial infarction with advanced heart failure. *Cardiology* 82:30–35, 1993.
16. Kinney MR, Packa DR: *Andreoli's comprehensive cardiac care*, ed 8, Philadelphia, 1996, Elsevier.
17. Dubin D: *Rapid interpretation of EKGs: a programmed course*, ed 6, Tampa, Fla, 2000, Cover Publishing.
18. Timmins AC, Hayes M, Yau E, et al: The relationship between cardiac reserve and survival in critically ill patients receiving treatment aimed at achieving supranormal oxygen delivery and consumption. *Postgraduate Medical Journal* 68(Suppl 2):S34–S40, 1992.
19. Puri VK, Carlson RW, Bander JJ, et al: Complications of vascular catheterization in the critically ill: a prospective study. *Critical Care Medicine* 8:495–499, 1980.
20. Civetta JM, Taylor RW, Kirby RR: *Critical care*, ed 3, Philadelphia, 1997, Lippincott Williams & Wilkins.
21. Borozny ML: Intracranial hypertension: implications for the physiotherapist. *Physiotherapy Canada* 39:360–366, 1987.
22. Weinert CR, Calvin AD: Epidemiology of sedation and sedation adequacy for mechanically ventilated patients in a medical and surgical intensive care unit. *Critical Care Medicine* 35:393–401, 2007.

23. Ely EW, Truman B, Shintani A, et al: Monitoring sedation status over time in ICU patients: reliability and validity of the Richmond Agitation-Sedation Scale (RASS). *Journal of the American Medical Association* 289:2983–2991, 2003.
24. Winkelman C: The role of inflammation in ICU-acquired weakness. *Critical Care* 14:186, 2010.
25. Hund EF, Fogel W, Krieger D, et al: Critical illness polyneuropathy: clinical findings and outcomes of a frequent cause of neuromuscular weaning failure. *Critical Care Medicine* 24:1328–1333, 1996.
26. Detriche O, Berre J, Massaut J, et al: The Brussels sedation scale: use of a simple clinical sedation scale can avoid excessive sedation in patients undergoing mechanical ventilation in the intensive care unit. *British Journal of Anaesthesia* 83:698–701, 1999.
27. Cooper JB, Jane JA, Alves WM, et al: Right median nerve electrical stimulation to hasten awakening from coma. *Brain Injury* 13:261–267, 1999.
28. Griffiths R, Hall J: Intensive care unit acquired weakness. *Critical Care Medicine* 38:779–787, 2010.
29. Vincent JL, Norenberg M: Intensive care unit acquired weakness: Framing the topic. *Critical Care Medicine* 37(Suppl):S296–S298, 2009.
30. Di Carlo A, Perna AM, Pantoni L, et al: Clinically relevant cognitive impairment after cardiac surgery: 6-month follow-up study. *Journal of Neurological Science* 188:85–93, 2001.
31. Pisani MA, Inouye SK, McNicoll L, et al: Screening for preexisting cognitive impairment in older intensity care unit patients: use of proxy assessment. *Journal of the American Geriatric Society* 51:689–693, 2003.
32. Jackson JC, Hart RP, Gordon SM, et al: Six-month neuropsychological outcome of medical intensive care unit patients. *Critical Care Medicine* 31:1226–1234, 2003.
33. Bo M, Massaia M, Raspo S, et al: Predictive factors of in-hospital mortality in older patients admitted to a medical intensive care unit. *Journal of the American Geriatric Society* 51:529–533, 2003.
34. Shi SF, Munjas BA, Wan TT, et al: The effects of preparatory sensory information on ICU patients. *Journal of Medical Systems* 27:191–204, 2003.
35. Fuglsang AK, Moergeli H, Hepp-Beg S, et al: Who develops acute stress disorder after accidental injuries? *Psychotherapy and Psychosomatics* 71:214–222, 2002.
36. Rundshagen I, Schnabel K, Wegner C, et al: Incidence of recall, nightmares, and hallucinations during analgosedation in intensive care. *Intensive Care Medicine* 28:38–43, 2002.
37. Rothenhausler HB, Ehrentraut S, Stoll C, et al: The relationship between cognitive performance and employment and health status in long-term survivors of the acute respiratory distress syndrome: results of an exploratory study. *General Hospital Psychiatry* 23:90–96, 2001.
38. Blenkharn A, Faughnan S, Morgan A: Developing a pain assessment tool for use by nurses in an adult intensive care unit. *Intensive Critical Care Nursing* 18:332–341, 2002.
39. Herridge MS, Cheung AM, Tansey CM, et al: One-year outcomes in survivors of the acute respiratory distress syndrome. *New England Journal of Medicine* 348:683–693, 2003.

Part III

Cardiovascular and Pulmonary Physical Therapy: Interventions

PART III OUTLINE

Chapter 17 III

Maximizing Outcomes: Relating Interventions to an Individual's Needs

Elizabeth Dean and Donna Frownfelter

KEY TERMS

- Activity
- Clinical decision making
- Clinical judgment
- Clinical reasoning
- Diagnosis
- Extrinsic factors
- International Classification of Functioning, Disability and Health
- Intrinsic factors
- Oxygen transport limitations
- Oxygen transport threats
- Participation
- Pathophysiological factors
- Problem definition
- Restricted mobility and recumbency factors
- Structures and functions
- Intervention prescription

CHAPTER OUTLINE

As direct access to patients becomes globally accepted, the capacity of the physical therapist to diagnose problems that are amenable to, as well as not amenable to, physical therapy is crucial for effective, safe, and responsible care. After formulating the diagnoses in partnership, as much as possible, with the patient and consistent with the health care team overall, the physical therapist prioritizes the diagnoses to address those most critical to the patient. These diagnoses may not necessarily be the reason the individual initially sought care from, or was referred to, a physical therapist. This is the essence of evidence-informed practice in the context of epidemiological indicators as distinct from evidence-based practice that supports the effectiveness of specific interventions (see Chapter 1).

This chapter provides a basis for clinical decision making and intervention prescription in physical therapy for patients ranging from the individual who is medically unstable and critically ill to the individual who is medically stable with cardiovascular and pulmonary dysfunction or at risk and living in the community. In addition, physical therapists have an active role in wellness and its promotion in the form of structured programs as well as one-on-one care. Thus the individuals they counsel include those with cardiovascular and pulmonary pathologies secondary to impairments or threats of other organ systems as well as those with primary impairments or threats of the cardiovascular and pulmonary systems (see Chapter 6).

Clinical reasoning is the process of critically analyzing the patient's status (participation in life and activities, as well as anatomic structures or physiological function) with respect to the individual's psychosocial, cultural, and environmental contexts (see Chapters 1 and 17). What is the individual able to do (and not able to do)? What is the status of the organ systems? How do these two interrelate? The answers to these questions serve as the basis of the detailed diagnostic work-up by the physical therapist. This process results in the diagnoses or problems that are then prioritized to ensure that the patient's needs are addressed appropriately—that is, "the right interventions targeted at the right problems at the right time." Initial priorities include life-preserving interventions (including addressing threats) and the minimizing of physical and psychological distress. Facilitators and barriers to the patient's adhering to the intervention recommendations, including health literacy and lifestyle education, are clearly identified, and education and interventions are adapted to meet the needs of the individual. With this database, the physical therapist prescribes interventions so that their outcomes are maximized in the short term and the long term.

International Classification of Functioning, Disability and Health

Participation

For most individuals, the highest priority is the capacity to live a life consistent with their needs and wants according to their sociocultural norms. The World Health Organization (WHO) acknowledges this in its International Classification of Functioning, Disability and Health, which emphasizes the interrelationship among structure and function, activity, and participation in life. Health has been defined by WHO as emotional, spiritual, intellectual, and physical well-being—not merely the absence of pathology.[1] Participation refers to the capacity of individuals to fulfill these needs in a social context and thereby fulfill the multiple roles in their lives—as parent, child, sibling, employee, employer, student, or homemaker, as well as in avocational pursuits (Figure 17-1). Participation in life is assessed by open-ended questions asked during the history and interview. In addition, an increasing number of questionnaire tools and scales are available for clinical use. Table 17-1 outlines some common generic and condition-specific tools that can be used to assess quality of life, life satisfaction, sickness impact, and subjective sense of well-being. These can be useful outcome measures (technically, these scales provide scores that are indexes rather than actual measures of the constructs) for the physical therapist and the patient. Many of these scales have been shown to be reliable as well as valid. Validating these scales is conceptually and methodologically challenging; hence their limitations must be recognized.

Activity

Participation in life and fulfilling one's roles and obligations require the ability to perform a range of certain activities to some level of proficiency (see Figure 17-1). The role of a parent, for example, requires being able to identify the needs of children, as well as to plan and coordinate activities involved with their care (e.g., picking them up, bathing and dressing them, performing physical activities and playing with them, and taking them to school). With respect to occupational roles, for example, to fulfill the needs of being a truck driver, the individual needs to be able to get to work, climb into the truck, check the engine, crawl under the truck, load and unload the truck, read a map, and operate a standard

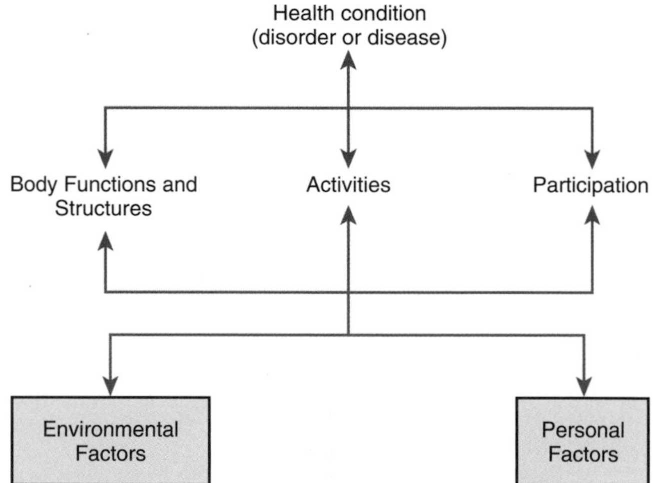

Fig. 17-1 Model of ability. *(Modified from the Model of Disablement, World Health Organization, 2002).*

Table 17-1 Tools for Evaluating Domains of Quality of Life (Activity and Participation)

Type of Tool	Name of Specific Tools	Developers
General well-being scales, questionnaires, profiles, inventories	Medical Outcomes Study, Short Form (SF-36) Sickness Impact Profile (SIP) Quality of Well-Being Scale Quality of Life Systemic Inventory Nottingham Health Profile Dartmouth Primary Care Cooperative Information Multidimensional Health Locus of Control Inventory Symptom Questionnaire	Stewart et al, 1988[2] Gibson et al, 1975[3] Kaplan et al, 1984[4] McGavin et al, 1977[5] Hunt et al, 1980[6] Wasson et al, 1992[7] Wallston and Wallston, 1981[8] Kellner, 1987[9]
Cardiac-specific scales and questionnaires	Minnesota Living with Heart Failure Questionnaire Outcomes Institute Angina Type Specification Quality of Life after Myocardial Infarction	Rector et al, 1987[10] Rogers et al, 1994[11] Oldridge et al, 1991[12]
Pulmonary-specific scales and questionnaires	Chronic Respiratory Disease Questionnaire St. George's Respiratory Questionnaire Pulmonary Functional Status Scale Pulmonary Functional Status and Dyspnea Questionnaire Living with Asthma Questionnaire	Guyatt et al, 1987[13] Jones et al, 1992[14] Weaver and Narsavage, 1992[15] Lareau et al, 1994[16] Hyland, 1991[17]
Cardiac rehabilitation questionnaire	EuroQol Questionnaire	Schweikert et al, 2006[18]
Heart disease questionnaire	MacNew Heart Disease Quality of Life Questionnaire (MacNew)	Höfer et al, 2004[19]

transmission. To be an elementary school teacher requires being able to move around the classroom, help children with physical tasks, and anticipate their needs, stay alert to danger, and respond quickly. The physical therapist's assessment must identify the composite activities that are limited and that affect an individual's capacity to participate in fulfilling his or her roles.

Structure and Function

Limitations of anatomic structure and physiological function often interfere with the performance of specific activities that are involved in fulfilling roles and obligations in life (i.e., participating in life) (see Figure 17-1). Some limitations may be specific to a particular role, and some may interfere across roles. The physical therapy assessment identifies the limitations of structure and function and the degree to which they interfere with given activities and roles in life. Some limitations of structure and function related to oxygen transport do not necessarily limit activity or participation; yet they can be the most clinically important, life-threatening problems (e.g., high blood pressure, cardiac dysrhythmias, abnormal clotting factors, high blood glucose, and aerobic deconditioning). Given the prevalence of lifestyle-related conditions and their risk factors, each individual needs to be assessed for risk for heart disease, smoking-related conditions, hypertension and stroke, diabetes, and cancers (see Chapter 1). Assessment of a patient's bone health and risk for osteoporosis and arthritis is also prudent, especially now that individuals are generally living longer and often have lifestyles that predispose them to osteopenia and osteoporosis. Physical therapists have a primary role in assessing these risks for several reasons:

First, these problems can be the most important clinically in terms of health and threat to life (chronic morbidity and premature death) for the patient, either directly or indirectly.

Second, identifying these problems enables the physical therapist to work collaboratively with the health care team in addressing and following the patient in a coordinated, integrated manner. If a patient was not referred and new problems are detected, the physician needs to be alerted. With direct-access practice, this is a primary responsibility of the contemporary physical therapist. If risk factors have been identified or have manifested clinically, the patient may be taking medication or may be a candidate for surgery. The physical therapist has a primary role in avoiding or minimizing the need for invasive care (specifically, drugs and surgery)—this is a particularly important and often underestimated goal of the physical therapist, who is committed to using and promoting noninvasive care. The physical therapist must closely monitor a patient's responses to invasive care (i.e., drugs and surgery) in relation to problems of direct relevance to them, with the intention of reducing such intervention.

Third, the physical therapist needs to institute relevant and targeted health education for lifelong behavior change (i.e., assess the patient's needs, including health literacy, knowledge deficits about health and health status, learning readiness, and learning style; tailor the education materials to the learner; and assess the outcome of the educational intervention comparable to other physical therapy interventions) (see Chapters 1 and 27).

Fourth, the presence of risk factors may require a higher level of patient monitoring, including the results of invasive testing (e.g., blood work for cholesterol, triglycerides, and blood glucose) and other tests such as imaging results and ECGs.

Fifth, physical therapy interventions and their prescriptive parameters may need to be modified based on an individual's risk factors for lifestyle-related conditions.

Sixth, special attention to medications may be indicated, and these may need to be coordinated with physical therapy management.

Seventh, the presence of risk factors for lifestyle-related conditions requires long-term management and follow-up.

Psychosocial and cultural factors are assessed to identify beliefs, attitudes, lifestyle behaviors, and expectations of care (see Chapter 1). A learning assessment (see Chapter 28) is conducted to identify health literacy and knowledge deficits, the learning style of the patient, and readiness to participate in intervention. Identifying facilitators and barriers that will impact the outcome of the therapeutic relationship is central to ensuring maximal therapeutic outcomes, including an individual's subjective sense of well-being and empowerment.

Clinical decision making and intervention prescription are based on the answers to several questions related to oxygen transport status, which underpins an individual's capacity for activity and participation, as well as threats to health. With respect to a given patient, the following must be considered:

- What are the problems with respect to participation, activity, and structure and function (impairments)? What are the interrelationships among these problems? (Remember: The interrelationships will be specific to the individual).
- What is the prognosis—with and without intervention?
- What is the relationship between the prognosis for each problem and the objectives of intervention and prescription?
- What are the intervention priorities, and why?
- What are the interventions of choice, and why?
- What are the prescriptive parameters for each, and why? How should they be sequenced, and why?
- What is the course of intervention, and why? What are the requirements for follow-up in the short and long term, and why?
- What are the boundaries of knowledge that would guide a physical therapist to refer a patient to another health care professional (e.g., counselor, nutritionist, personal trainer, physician, psychologist)?

Considering that a patient can have oxygen transport limitations in the absence of participation and activity limitations—and the fact that, based on epidemiological evidence, this is true for many people—oxygen transport limitations and risks need to be evaluated in every patient. Underlying risk, without overt manifestation clinically or in daily life, can constitute significant risk to the patient and the potential for significant impact on participation and activity. Furthermore, physical therapy, by definition, emphasizes the physiological aspects of the patient, so awareness of the possibility of such underlying threats is essential to ensure that the appropriate monitoring is instituted to maximize safety and that interventions are modified to maximize therapeutic outcome in the short and long term.

The principles involved in relating cardiovascular and pulmonary physical therapy interventions to the patient's needs depend on an analysis of those needs with respect to the patient's level of participation in life and ability to perform the identified composite activities. The degree to which limitations of anatomic structure and physiological function (with a focus on impairments of the steps in the oxygen transport pathway; Chapter 2) affect activity and participation is assessed. The relationship of impairment to an individual's ability and participation cannot be assumed. Verification can be extracted from the history and overall assessment, including measures and indexes of the individual's capacity to perform activities and participate in life. These aspects of the assessment can be obtained through the use of standardized questionnaire tools that reveal the impact of health-related quality of life and sickness; these tools can be used as outcome measures in conjunction with measures of anatomic structure and physiological function (see Table 17-1). Changes in structure and function with intervention may or may not have a corresponding effect on health-related quality of life or sickness. For example, high blood pressure is most often asymptomatic, but the patient may be prescribed a stringent exercise program and education program. Such knowledge may help to identify those individuals whose quality of life is most likely to improve, as well as where intervention should be targeted.[20]

The physical therapist formulates a physiologically based intervention hierarchy based on the premise that physiological function, including oxygen transport, is optimal when humans are upright and moving (see Chapters 18, 19, and 20). Applying a systematic physiological approach to diagnosis and the analysis of the patient's problems, with respect to limitations in the oxygen transport pathway, leads directly to identifying effective interventions. Such an approach provides a rational basis for modifying or discontinuing intervention based on the use of appropriate outcome measures.

What Is the Problem?

Consistent with the International Classification of Functioning, Disability and Health, there are three primary levels of analysis:[21]

Structure and function (impairment)
Ability (disability)
Participation in life (handicap)

These components are affected by facilitating factors and barriers (see Figure 17-1).[21] Structure and function refer to the underlying anatomic and physiological limitations that may or may not contribute to the patient's symptoms but are clinically important and warrant remediation or being addressed in management. Limitation of activities contributes to a compromised capacity to fulfill one's roles in life, such as those of occupation, profession, parent, and member of various groups that make up an individual's identity. Usually, a patient presents clinically with complaints of being unable to complete tasks or fulfill roles because of pathophysiological, psychological, or environmental and physical barriers and limitations.

Measures and tools are standardized (concerning validity and reliability, see Chapter 7) for the assessment of each of these levels. With an increased focus on the quality of participation in life, numerous scales have emerged to quantify the subjective sense of well-being and health-related quality of life (see Table 17-1 for some examples).

Oxygen transport is determined by a multitude of factors that affect the steps in the oxygen transport pathway, thereby affecting participation in life and related activities (see Figure 17-1; see Chapter 2).[22-24] For intervention to be directed specifically to the underlying problems, the physical therapist needs to consider several levels of analysis of the deficits contributing to impaired or threatened oxygen transport. To be proficient in such analysis, the physical therapist must have a thorough knowledge of the multiple factors that contribute to normal gas exchange and those that contribute to abnormal gas exchange. This knowledge base includes a thorough understanding of the relevant anatomy and physiology; the multisystem and integrative pathophysiology; the impact of medical, surgical, and nursing procedures; the effects of various laboratory tests and procedures; and the impact of pharmacological agents on cardiovascular and pulmonary function (Box 17-1). Assessment of oxygen transport reserve and reserve capacity is fundamental to the management of all patients[25] and their risk factors,[26] regardless of disease acuity. Routine procedures contribute to fluctuations in oxygen demands.[27] Maximizing the ratio of oxygen delivery to consumption improves clinical outcomes in patients who range from being medically stable to being unstable.[28,29,30]

For a given patient, the cardiovascular and pulmonary physical therapist prescribes intervention by extracting the relevant information from the history, the laboratory tests and investigative procedures, and the assessment (Box 17-2; see Part II). Although physical therapists are primarily noninvasive practitioners, they use and request the results of invasive

Box 17-1 Fundamental Knowledge and Expertise to Diagnose Limitations in Oxygen Transport and Risk Factors

- Oxygen transport deficits and how they affect or threaten participation and activity
- Normal cardiopulmonary and cardiovascular anatomy and physiology
- Knowledge about how the above are affected by normal conditions such as aging and lifestyle habits (e.g., smoking, stress, and the physical environment)
- Physiological adaptation to hypoxia and cardiopulmonary impairment
- Cardiopulmonary and cardiovascular pathophysiology and disease processes; how they affect normal cardiopulmonary and cardiovascular function
- Multisystem and integrative pathophysiology that can have a secondary effect on cardiopulmonary function and oxygen transport
- Effects of medical, surgical, and nursing procedures on oxygen transport and gas exchange
- Investigative laboratory procedures and tests and their effects on cardiopulmonary function
- Pharmacological effects on cardiopulmonary function of any medication

Box 17-2 Steps in Diagnosing Limitations in Oxygen Transport

1. Determine what factors are specifically contributing to impaired oxygen transport and which steps in the pathway are affected.
2. Determine those factors that threaten oxygen transport and the steps in the pathway that are involved.
3. Determine the relative magnitude of the effect of each factor that is either impairing or threatening oxygen transport; prioritize the importance of each.
4. Distinguish those factors that are amenable to, and those that are not amenable to, physical therapy. In the case of the latter, intervention may have to be modified and the type and level of monitoring may have to be reevaluated.
5. Based on the answers to 1 through 4, select, prioritize, and apply specific interventions prescriptively, addressing each factor that contributes to cardiopulmonary dysfunction and is amenable to physical therapy.

From World Health Organization: Definition of health. 2011. http://www.who.int/suggestions/faq/en/.

tests and investigations in their assessments and evaluations. Problems are prioritized on the basis of the relative magnitude of each problem's threat or effect on oxygen transport limitation, along with the evidence supporting the effectiveness of various noninvasive interventions in addressing each diagnosis or problem. Once the mechanisms of the cardiovascular and pulmonary dysfunction have been identified, specific interventions are selected and prioritized and the prescriptive parameters of each intervention are then defined. With respect to education, a learning assessment is an essential component of the overall assessment; it identifies health status knowledge deficits and prescribes learning interventions consistent with the patient's needs (see Chapter 28).

The Diagnoses or Problems

The diagnostic work-up is designed to relate oxygen transport limitations and threats to an individual's participation in life and its composite activities. The components of the analysis of oxygen transport limitations (impairment diagnoses) follow. Physical therapists have a particular interest and focus of care related to the interrelationships among limitations (impairments) of structure and function and an individual's activity and his or her participation in life (i.e., limitation or improvement at one level and its association with limitation or improvement in the other levels).

Impaired Oxygen Transport

Two levels of problems must be identified: functional and physiological limitations. Functional limitations are those that affect the patient's ability to perform activities of daily living (ADLs), such as reduced activity or exercise tolerance as a result of reduced peripheral oxygenation; reduced mobility related to deconditioning resulting from resting in bed; extremity or internal injury; anticoagulant therapy; drug-induced paralysis; impaired physical mobility related to muscle weakness and partial paralysis; paralysis; depressed consciousness; or anemia.

Anatomic and physiological limitations are the individual's overall deficits in oxygen transport and those that specifically arise at the individual steps in the pathway. Examples of the limitations at each step in the pathway appear in Tables 17-2 and 17-3.

Threatened Oxygen Transport

Although the complications of restricted mobility and static body positions are well understood, the precise prescription parameters for mobilization and body positioning to avoid these complications have not been defined in detail (see Chapters 18, 19, and 20). With respect to cardiovascular and pulmonary complications, a 1- or 2-hourly turning regimen is commonly accepted. For the patient who is flaccid or comatose, range-of-motion (ROM) exercises every several hours facilitates blood flow through dependent areas and enhances alveolar ventilation, as well as mobilizing joints and muscles. Antiembolic stockings and pneumatic compression devices are routinely used to minimize circulatory stasis in the legs and thereby the potential for thrombi formation.

The physical therapist has a major role in preventing infection of all types but particularly cardiovascular and pulmonary infections. Cardiovascular and pulmonary assessment and intervention involve handling and close contact with patients. Thus the risk for nosocomial infection is high in patients who are hospitalized. Some standard means of preventing infection include meticulous handwashing before and after visiting each patient, avoiding contact with open wounds and body fluids, and using clean technique in proximity to invasive lines and catheters. The physical therapist moves and repositions patients often, so it is essential that the positions of lines, leads, and catheters be continuously monitored to avoid displacement. The physical therapist must consider when it is appropriate to gown, mask, and use gloves so as to protect and be protected from the patient adequately.

Factors That Contribute to or Threaten Oxygen Transport

The factors that can impair oxygen transport directly or can threaten it fall into four primary categories (Table 17-4): the underlying cardiovascular and pulmonary pathophysiology, restricted mobility (loss of physical exercise stress), recumbency (loss of vertical gravitational stress), extrinsic factors (i.e., factors related to the patient's care), and intrinsic factors (i.e., factors related to the patient).

Restricted Mobility and Recumbency

Although bed rest can be considered an extrinsic factor (i.e., a therapeutic intervention that contributes to cardiovascular and pulmonary dysfunction), the negative consequences of this intervention are often not appreciated fully because of the widespread use of rest in bed. To emphasize the importance of considering the effects of this intervention with each patient, the effects of restricted mobility and recumbency are analyzed separately (see Chapters 18, 19, and 20).

Table 17-2 Examples of Limitations and Threats to the Steps in the Oxygen Transport Pathway

Area of Limitation	Specific Threats
Central control of breathing	Altered central nervous system (CNS) afferent input and control of breathing Impaired efferent pathways Pharmacological depression Substance-abuse depression
Airways	Aspiration related to lack of gastrointestinal (GI) motility Aspiration secondary to esophageal reflux Obstruction secondary to airway edema, bronchospasm, or mucus Inhaled foreign bodies
Lungs	Altered breathing pattern secondary to decreased lung compliance Ineffective breathing pattern related to decreased diaphragmatic function and increased lung volumes, respiratory muscle weakness, respiratory muscle fatigue, CNS dysfunction, guarding, reflex, fatigue, and respiratory inflammatory process Ineffective airway clearance related to restricted mobility, immobility, sedation, and pulmonary dysfunction secondary to long smoking history, impaired mucociliary transport, absent cilia, or dyskinesia of cilia, retained secretions, ineffective cough and mucociliary mechanisms, infection, inability to cough efficiently, artificial airway/intubation and endotracheal tube, drug-induced paralysis, and sedation Large airway obstruction secondary to compliant oropharyngeal structures Chest wall rigidity and decreased compliance Loss of normal chest wall excursion movements (pump- and bucket-handle motions) and capacity to move appropriately in all three planes of motion Chest wall and spinal deformity Impaired lung fluid balance and acute lung injury
Blood	Bleeding abnormalities, altered body temperature (hypothermia, hyperthermia), fever, inflammation, hypermetabolism secondary to mediator systems Altered body temperature related to integumentary disruption Low hematocrit secondary to GI bleed (more prone to hypoxia) Anemia Thrombocytopenia Disseminated intravascular coagulation Abnormal clotting factors (i.e., balance between clotting and not clotting, sludging of blood) Thromboemboli Bleeding disorders with liver disease; abnormal clotting factors
Gas exchange	Alveolar collapse, atelectasis, intrapulmonary shunting or pulmonary edema, shallow breathing and tenacious mucus, body position, consolidation and alveolar collapse, ventilation/perfusion mismatch, airway constriction, fluid volume excess, pleural effusions, breathing at low lung volumes, abdominal distension and guarding, ineffective airway clearance, pulmonary microvascular thrombi and altered capillary permeability secondary to circulating mediators, closure of small airways secondary to dynamic airway compression, decreased functional residual capacity, and intrapulmonary shunting, increased lung surface tension Diffusion defects
Respiratory muscles	Upper abdominal surgery, weakness, fatigue, neuromuscular disease, ileus related to gastric distension, mechanical dysfunction
Myocardial perfusion	Coronary artery occlusion Tachycardia Potential for cardiac dysrhythmia related to reperfusion Cardiac dysrhythmia related to myocardial hypoxia Compression by edema or space-occupying lesions
Heart	Decreased venous return and cardiac output secondary to volume deficit, ascites, myocardial ischemia, hemorrhage, and coagulopathies Conduction defects Mechanical defects Defects in electromechanical coupling Abnormal distension characteristics and myocardial wall compliance Abnormal afterload

Table 17-2 Examples of Limitations and Threats to the Steps in the Oxygen Transport Pathway—cont'd

Area of Limitation	Specific Threats
Systemic hemodynamic	Blood pressure Volume deficit (related to volume losses during surgery and inadequate oral intake, blood loss, internal injuries (e.g., hematoma and third-spacing phenomenon); hormonal imbalance; increased intestinal motility; vomiting; diarrhea; fluid sequestration in tissues; nasogastric [NG] suction and diarrhea; hypovolemia; sepsis and shock; surface capillary leak and fluid loss as in burns and excoriated wounds; fluid shifts, and secondary to recumbency and restricted mobility; or some combination) Alteration in peripheral tissue perfusion related to acute myocardial infarction, myocardial depression, maldistribution of blood volume, and altered cellular metabolism Volume excess (related to excessive intravenous administration, impaired excretion, renal failure, water intoxication, therapeutic volume expansion, acute myocardial infarction (MI) and acute renal failure related to renal retention of sodium and water and increased levels of aldosterone, renin, angiotensin II, and catecholamines; or some combination)
Tissue perfusion	Impaired cardiac output Impaired due to disseminated microvascular thrombi Atherosclerosis and thromboembolic events, decreased circulating blood volume, decreased vascular integrity, and inflammatory process Decreased cardiac output related to reduced venous return, impaired right ventricular function, dysrhythmias, increased afterload, and bradycardia Low oxygen content in the blood Thromboembolism, vasoconstriction secondary to toxins, sepsis, etc., blood flow alterations and hypermetabolism secondary to mediator systems
Tissue oxygenation	Multisystem organ failure with altered peripheral tissue perfusion and gas exchange at the cellular level

Table 17-3 Factors That Can Contribute Indirectly to Oxygen Transport Limitations or Impairments

Type of Factors	Specific Limitations or Impairments
Factors related to infection	Pulmonary and nonpulmonary infections increase the demands on the oxygen transport system
Cognitive factors	Impaired neurological status and central cardiopulmonary control Alteration in mental status secondary to inadequate cerebral perfusion with hypotension and cardiogenic shock Sleep pattern disturbance; altered blood gases, and fatigue Anxiety and agitation related to powerlessness and lack of knowledge, breathlessness, pharmacological paralysis, impaired verbal community secondary to intubation, paralysis
Psychosocial factors	Anxiety related to the condition, shortness of breath, hospitalization Social isolation secondary to impaired communication Fear and hopelessness Pain response
Nutritional factors	Altered nutritional needs secondary to greater need than resting state (i.e., increased caloric need and nutrients associated with illness, inability to ingest food, inability to absorb food) Restricted ingestion of food and water High caloric needs secondary to infectious process and protein catabolism

Table 17-4 Factors That Can Limit or Impair Oxygen Transport

Factors	Type of Limitation or Impairment
Cardiopulmonary pathophysiology (see Chapter 5)	Primary (acute, chronic, acute on chronic) Secondary (chronic, acute on chronic)
Noncardiopulmonary pathophysiology (abnormalities in other systems that can impair oxygen transport [see Chapter 6])	Central nervous system Musculoskeletal Gastrointestinal Endocrine (diabetes) Renal Liver abnormalities Nutritional deficits and obesity
Restricted mobility	Loss of physical-exercise stress (see Chapter 18) Recumbency Loss of vertical-gravitational stress (see Chapter 19)
Extrinsic factors	Those related to the patient's care (see Chapter 2)
Intrinsic factors	Those related to the patient (see Chapter 2)

Intervention Goals

Once the deficits and threats to oxygen transport have been determined by the physical therapist, the goals of intervention fall into three categories: short-term, long-term, and preventive (Table 17-5). In addition to improving the outcomes of primary physical therapy interventions, physical therapists seek to eliminate, reduce, or delay the need for invasive care (i.e., drugs and surgery) as much as possible. These are core contemporary physical therapy goals.

Practice Patterns

The American Physical Therapy Association's (APTA's) Guide to Physical Therapist Practice (2003)[31] has evolved over the past couple of decades, and it currently reflects a broad scope of practice. The Guide describes examination (history, systems review, and tests and measures), evaluation, diagnosis, prognosis (including plan of care), and intervention (with anticipated goals and expected outcomes). Each physical therapy area of practice has multiple associated practice patterns. Each practice pattern addresses reexamination, global outcomes, and criteria for termination of physical therapy services. Given the APTA's adoption of the International Classification of Functioning, Disability and Health,[21] the evaluation consists of a review of health rather than strictly a primary focus on illness. The iterative cycle of clinical decision making based on outcomes and the modification of interventions is designed to achieve the expected outcomes within a prescribed time frame (Figure 17-2). Based on the consensus of several hundred clinicians in the United States, several primary practice patterns have been defined for each specialty. Once patients are evaluated, their profiles may be described by one or more practice patterns, within one or more specialty areas of practice. There are eight practice patterns in the cardiovascular and pulmonary area (Box 17-3). These patterns and the Guide (2003)[31] provide an overall frame of reference for practice rather than serving as a basis for practice. Patients are increasingly complex, given increasing life expectancy and concomitant comorbidities, coupled with lifestyle-related factors and their impact on the patient's presenting complaint or underlying risk factors. Therefore categorizing a patient in one or more practice patterns may be insufficient to address the patient's complaints. These patterns serve as guides only.

Box 17-3 Cardiovascular and Pulmonary Preferred Practice Patterns Based on Oxygen Transport Limitations and Risks

Pattern A: Primary Prevention/Risk Reduction for Cardiovascular/Pulmonary Disorders

Pattern B: Impaired Aerobic Capacity/Endurance Associated with Deconditioning

Pattern C: Impaired Ventilation, Respiration/Gas Exchange, and Aerobic Capacity/Endurance Associated with Airway Clearance Dysfunction

Pattern D: Impaired Aerobic Capacity/Endurance Associated with Cardiovascular Pump Dysfunction or Failure

Pattern E: Impaired Ventilation and Respiration/Gas Exchange Associated with Ventilatory Pump Dysfunction or Failure

Pattern F: Impaired Ventilation and Respiration/Gas Exchange Associated with Respiratory Failure

Pattern G: Impaired Ventilation, Respiration/Gas Exchange, and Aerobic Capacity/Endurance Associated with Respiratory Failure in the Neonate

Pattern H: Impaired Circulation and Anthropometric Dimensions Associated with Lymphatic Systems Disorders

Data from American Physical Therapy Association: Guide to physical therapist practice, ed 2, Washington, DC, 2003, APTA.

Table 17-5 Short-Term, Long-Term, and Preventive Intervention Goals for Patients With Oxygen Transport Deficit or Its Risk

Short-Term Goals	Long-Term Goals	Preventive Goals
Empower the patient to manage symptoms and learn strategies to reduce health risk through effective education for life-long health. Correct or reverse cardiovascular and pulmonary dysfunction that underlies the threat to or limitations on participation in life and its composite activities. Reduce the rate of deterioration. Avoid worsening the patient's condition. Avoid, reduce, or postpone the need for drugs (including supplemental oxygen) and surgery.	Empower the patient through health education that promotes life-long health and well-being and minimizes the likelihood of the recurrence of problems. Enhance the efficiency of the steps in the oxygen transport pathway overall. Enhance the efficiency of those specific steps in the oxygen transport pathway that compensate for impaired steps that may or may not be reversibly affected. Maximize oxygen transport capacity to sustain and optimize healing and allow for maximal functional activity. Avoid, reduce, or postpone the need for drugs (including supplemental oxygen) and surgery. Minimize the need for doctor- and hospital-based care. Reduce the cost of invasive doctor- and hospital-based care and related health care costs.	Promote life-long health (full participation in life and its activities) and subjective well-being through patient empowerment and self-responsibility—health and participation for all; in so doing, increase the threshold for chronic conditions and their rates of progression, thereby increasing the threshold for morbidity and premature mortality. Maximize oxygen transport and aerobic conditioning to prevent cardiovascular and pulmonary dysfunction. Prevent multisystem organ complications and all-cause infection that will lead to restricted movement, recumbency, and potential deterioration. Provide supportive palliative care for patients at the end of life. Reduce the impact and burden of lifestyle-related conditions on individuals, their families, their communities, society as a whole, and the health of the population as a whole.

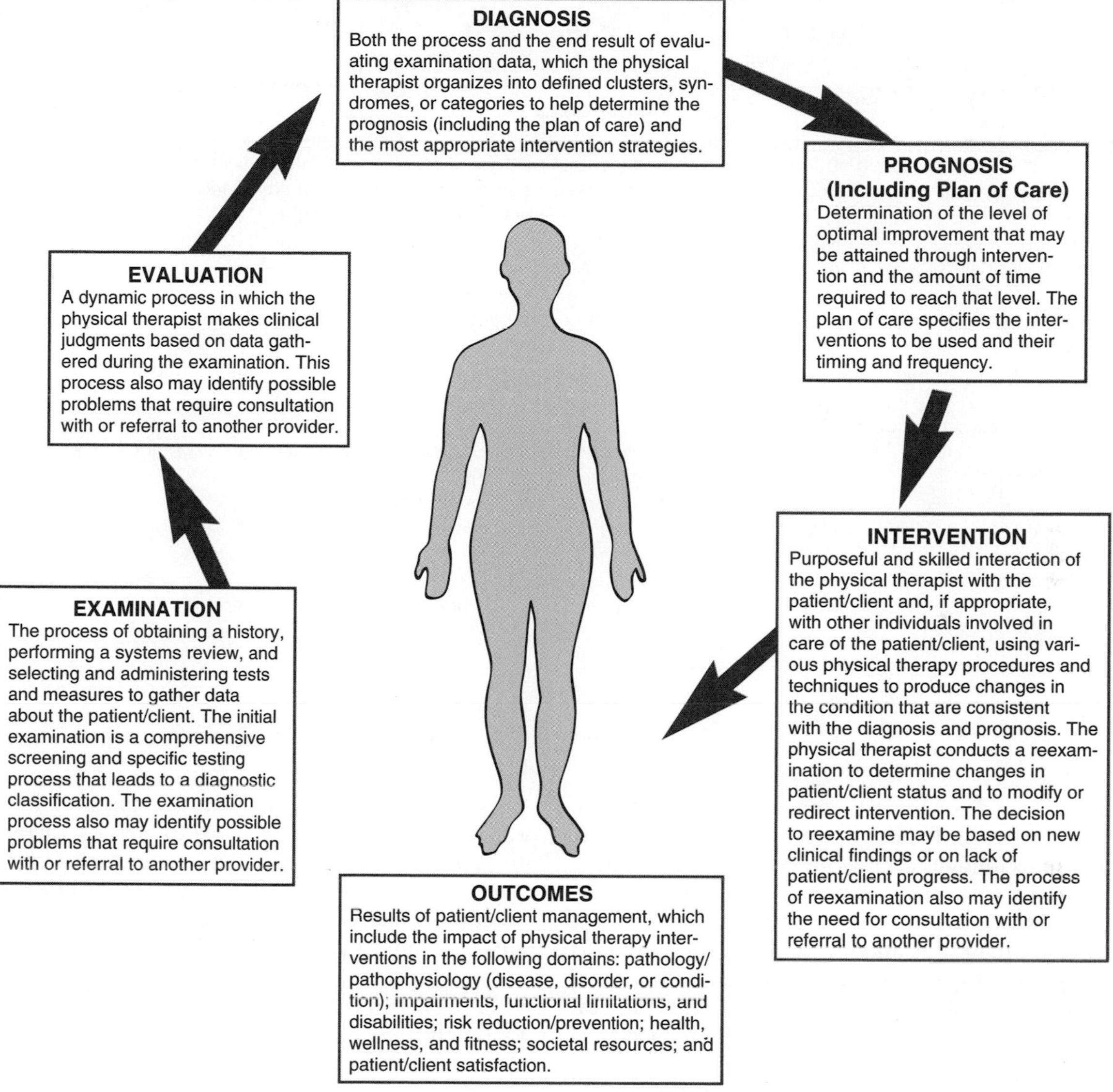

Fig. 17-2 Iterative process of clinical reasoning and decision making. *(From American Physical Therapy Association:* Guide to physical therapist practice, *ed 2, Alexandria, VA, 2003, APTA.)*

They are not diagnoses, nor do they replace sound clinical reasoning and judgment.

What is the Intervention, and Why?

Clinical Decision Making

The basis for clinical decision making in the management of the patient with cardiovascular and pulmonary dysfunction or its risk is to pair the most effective interventions with impaired or threatened steps in the oxygen transport pathway. Considerable time may pass between interventions, so a maximal therapeutic effect is dependent on the effectiveness of between-intervention interventions (i.e., teaching the patient to carry out prescriptive intervention whenever possible, motivating the patient to adhere to and follow the intervention plan, and eliciting the assistance of the patient's family or nursing staff in supporting the patient in doing so).

When confined to hospital, patients may spend excessive time recumbent and in restricted body positions; they tend to turn and move less frequently and are not upright or moving much of time. Depending on the particular oxygen transport deficits of a patient, the body positions the patient assumes can have a positive, negative, or neutral effect on oxygen transport. Thus the patient's position and his or her reduced activity level must be monitored and adverse effects anticipated, countered or, preferably, prevented.

Examples of some common intervention goals in managing the patient with cardiovascular and pulmonary dysfunction are shown in Box 17-4. Specific interventions are identified to address these goals and for each deficit or threat to oxygen transport. Intervention goals and specific interventions are prioritized according to the relative significance of the impact of each on oxygen transport.

A physiologically based intervention hierarchy is shown in Table 17-6. The intervention hierarchy is based on the premise that physiological function, including oxygen transport, is optimal when a person is upright and moving. Thus the purpose of the hierarchy is to implement the interventions that are most physical first: active movement and exercise in

Box 17-4 Common Intervention Goals in the Management of a Patient with Cardiovascular and Pulmonary Dysfunction or Its Risk

Overall Goals

Direct intervention at maximizing or preserving participation and activity by addressing structural and functional deficits in oxygen transport and gas exchange

- Direct intervention at specific steps involved
- Increase efficiency of all steps in the pathway
- Augment medical management
- Use medical management to augment physical therapy outcomes
- Use physical therapy to augment medical management
- Coordinate with nursing management (e.g., in critical care)

Specific Goals

Direct intervention at specific steps in the oxygen transport pathway

- Increase air entry and alveolar ventilation (minimize airflow resistance)
- Increase air distribution (optimize lung compliance and chest wall compliance and reduce airway resistance)
- Increase ventilation and perfusion matching
- Increase diffusion
- Increase oxyhemoglobin saturation
- Decrease work of breathing (from increased resistance, reduced or excessive compliance)
- Decrease work of the heart (from increased preload, contraction, increased afterload)
- Increase efficiency of heart mechanics
- Minimize ECG irregularities (identify factors that contribute to irregularities; anticipate problems)
- Optimize blood flow distribution
- Optimize oxygen extraction ratio
- Decrease excessive or unnecessary energy expenditure
- Optimize CO_2 removal
- Optimize blood volume and distribution to maintain hemodynamic status
- Support nutrition and hydration initiatives where possible

the upright position. The hierarchy ranges from these to the interventions that are the least physical: conventional chest physical therapy techniques such as ROM, postural drainage and percussion, and suctioning. The latter may simulate some of the physiological effects of being upright and moving, but their effects are more limited and less scientifically substantiated, and they facilitate fewer steps in the oxygen transport pathway. They do not substitute for the more active physical interventions that are higher in the intervention hierarchy. Each of the interventions in the hierarchy has a role in the management of cardiovascular and pulmonary dysfunction or its risks, but they are implemented in descending order to ensure that the most effective interventions are used first.

Intervention Plan

The intervention plan consists of interventions that will most expediently and efficiently remediate the problems that have been identified. These interventions are prioritized according to the greatest effect they are predicted to have on remediating the oxygen transport deficit or minimizing any threat to oxygen transport and on maximizing their benefit-to-risk ratio given the specific patient's presentation. Depending on the specific intervention goals and the adequacy of balance between oxygen supply and demand, the coordination of physical therapy interventions with other care (e.g., nursing care and certain tests and procedures) is commonly indicated.

Intervention Prescription

Once the specific pathophysiological problems underlying deficits or threats to oxygen transport have been identified, they are differentiated into (1) those that can be addressed by physical therapy (i.e., noninvasive physical interventions); (2) those that are not amenable to physical therapy but need to be considered during intervention to determine whether intervention is contraindicated or needs to be modified and whether specific outcome and intervention-response measures are indicated; and (3) those that are best managed invasively, which may necessitate referral to a physician.

Problems amenable to physical therapy are prioritized. Optimal interventions are identified for each problem, and their parameters are prescribed. The intervention goals are identified: to reverse pathophysiological mechanisms contributing to impaired oxygen transport: to compensate for irreversible pathophysiological deficits (improve the efficiency of other steps in the oxygen transport pathway); to decelerate deterioration; to avoid making the patient worse; to provide palliative care, support, and comfort; and to prevent the occurrence of problems in the future (see Intervention Goals, earlier in this chapter). Based on the goals of intervention, the parameters of the intervention are defined. Intervention parameters in the management of a patient with cardiovascular and pulmonary problems are shown in Box 17-5. To achieve these goals, a range of modalities and aids may be needed in the short term and in the long term (Box 17-6).

What Is the Course of Intervention?

Once an intervention has been prescribed, the prescription must be reviewed at each intervention session and modified accordingly (i.e., the prescription parameters change as the patient's condition changes). In addition, the parameters may be modified within an intervention on the basis of the patient's response. The physical therapist also decides when to discontinue a given intervention, as well as which cardiovascular and

Table 17-6 **Physiological Intervention Hierarchy for Management of Limited Oxygen Transport to Optimize Participation and Activity**

Order of Interventions	Goal	Specific Type of Interventions or Effects
I. Mobilization and exercise	Elicit an exercise stimulus that addresses one of the three effects on the various steps in the oxygen transport pathway, or some combination thereof	Acute effects Long-term effect Preventive effects
II. Body positioning	Elicit a gravitational stimulus that simulates being upright and moving as much as possible: active, active-assisted, or passive	Hemodynamic effects related to fluid shifts Cardiopulmonary effects on ventilation and its distribution, perfusion, ventilation, and perfusion matching and gas exchange
III. Breathing control maneuvers	Augment alveolar ventilation, facilitate mucociliary transport, and stimulate coughing	Coordinated breathing with activity and exercise Spontaneous eucapnic hyperventilation Maximal tidal breaths and movement in three dimensions Sustained maximal inspiration Pursed-lip breathing to end-tidal expiration Incentive spirometry
IV. Coughing maneuvers	Facilitate mucociliary clearance with the least effect on dynamic airway compression and the fewest adverse cardiovascular effects	Active and spontaneous cough with closed glottis Active-assisted (self-supported or supported by other) Modified coughing interventions with open glottis (e.g., forced expiratory technique, huff)
V. Relaxation and energy-conservation interventions	Minimize the work of breathing and of the heart and minimize undue oxygen demand	Relaxation procedures at rest and during activity Energy conservation, (i.e., balance of activity and rest, performing activities in an energy-efficient manner, improved movement economy during activity) Pain-control interventions
VI. ROM exercises (cardiopulmonary indications)	Stimulate alveolar ventilation and alter its distribution	Active Assisted-active Passive
VII. Postural drainage positioning	Facilitate airway clearance using gravitational effects	Bronchopulmonary segmental drainage positions
VIII. Manual techniques	Facilitate airway clearance in conjunction with specific body positioning	Autogenic drainage Manual percussion Shaking and vibration Deep breathing and coughing
IX. Suctioning	Facilitate the removal of airway secretions collected centrally	Open suction system Closed suction system Tracheal tickle Instillation with saline Use of manual hyperinflation bag (bagging)

pulmonary physical therapy interventions to employ; again, these decisions are based on the patient's responses to the intervention and on the outcome. Some change in intervention should be effected with one or two intervention sessions, confirming that improvement is being maximized. If no improvement is noted, an explanation is found and the intervention is changed to elicit improvement. When no improvement is demonstrated, particularly in patients who are seriously ill, physical therapy may still have a role in preventing deterioration, so it should not necessarily be withdrawn. However, a rationale should always be proposed for continued intervention in the event of no demonstrable change. Continued intervention may be indicated, for example, in a patient in an induced coma. Hemodynamic and oxygen transport status must be maintained in anticipation of the induced coma being reversed. In most other situations, however, some improvement toward the eventual goal of maximizing activity and participation status should be expected from every intervention.

Measures to assess response and outcome to interventions are selected so that they reflect (1) activity and participation status, (2) the status of oxygen transport overall, and (3) the integrity of the step or steps in the oxygen transport pathway that were identified as being the primary problems contributing to cardiovascular and/or pulmonary dysfunction in the original assessment (Table 17-7; see Part II). Cardiovascular and pulmonary dysfunction is determined on the basis of the history, assessment, and laboratory investigations such as pulmonary function testing, breathing pattern, cardiac function testing, fluid balance and renal function, arterial blood gases, arterial saturation, vital signs, and hemodynamic variables, including heart rate and ECG, blood pressure, and rate pressure product. Subjective reports are also clinically relevant, such as subjective ratings of perceived exertion, breathlessness,

Box 17-5 Parameters of the Intervention Prescription in the Management of a Patient with Cardiovascular and Pulmonary Dysfunction or Its Risk

Determine whether to intervene or not to intervene at this time
Define measures and outcomes on which intervention progression and determination of whether goals have been met are based
Define parameters of intervention based on history, laboratory investigations, tests, and assessment
Intervention types
Intensity of each intervention (if applicable)
Duration of each intervention
Frequency of each intervention
Instruct patient in the between-intervention intervention and, if applicable, also instruct the nurse, a family member, or both
Reassess every intervention
Modify as necessary within each intervention
Modify and progress interventions as indicated
Determine when intervention is to be discontinued
Request additional supportive information, tests, and investigations as indicated throughout the course of intervention
Predict time course for optimal effects and course of intervention to determine intervention efficacy; modify as necessary
Schedule and coordinate interventions in conjunction with other interventions: medical, surgical, nursing; respiratory therapy (weaning); oxygen supplementation; sympathomimetic drugs; ADLs; balance with sleep and rest periods; food intake and feeds; peak energy times; peak of drug potency and effects (e.g., pain, reduced sedation, reduced neuromuscular blockade)

Box 17-6 Use of Modalities and Aids

Goal: To incorporate the use of the modalities and aids that enhance the prescribed interventions over the short and the long term

Modalities	**Pharmacological Agents**
Treadmill, ergometer, rowing machine	Oxygen
Weights	Bronchodilators
Pulleys	Vasodilators
Nebulizers and aerosols	Antihypertensives
Flutter valve	Antiinflammatories
BIPAP* and CPAP†	Mucolytics
Incentive spirometer	Surfactant
Orthoses, braces, and supports	Analgesics

**Bilevel positive airway pressure.*
†Continuous positive airway pressure.

musculoskeletal or wound pain, angina, and fatigue. These same measures are used as outcome measures to detect improved oxygen transport and gas exchange.

Considering that clinical decision making is based largely on the results of tests and measures, it is essential that these measures have certain characteristics. Measurements must be objective and their procedures standardized to maximize test validity and reliability. Although physical therapists specialize in noninvasive assessment procedures as well as interventions, noninvasive measures are prone to imprecision, thereby leading to measurement error and unreliability. It is therefore essential that assessment measurements be performed in a systematic manner and according to measurement guidelines in order to maximize their quality and usefulness in guiding and directing intervention (Chapter 7). Invasive interventions, including blood work, scans, and radiographs, are also fundamental to the physical therapist's assessment and ongoing evaluation. Assessment measurements always precede intervention to ensure that the intervention and its prescriptive parameters are appropriate. Measurements during intervention provide information about the patient's responses, both beneficial and detrimental. This feedback determines the parameters of intervention and whether the intervention should be modified in some way or possibly discontinued. The overall intervention response is established by further monitoring and assessment at the termination of intervention and often at periodic intervals post-intervention so that delayed effects can be monitored. Frequent and periodic measurements over time are referred to as serial measurements and provide useful trend data. The pre- and post-intervention responses and any noteworthy responses during intervention are charted, along with sufficient information about the procedures that were used (i.e., assessment, as well as intervention procedures).

Physical therapists often require the results of invasive tests such as blood work or invasive hemodynamic monitoring to establish intervention response and outcome; thus these may need to be requested.

Assessment and reevaluation data provide feedback to the physical therapist about her or his clinical decision making and the therapeutic outcomes, as well as about the effectiveness of the prescribed interventions in the management of a given patient. Patient satisfaction with the physical therapist and with management, elicited by means of a formal evaluation by the patient, is also critical for evaluating service and the overall outcome of physical therapy for each individual.

Summary

This chapter provides a framework for clinical reasoning and decision making based on oxygen transport characteristics that underlie a limitation in activity and participation in life as defined by the model of ability advocated by the World Health Organization.[21] Carried out in partnership with the patient, as much as possible, the process includes diagnoses and intervention prescriptions in the management of patients with cardiovascular and pulmonary dysfunction, who range from the individual who is medically unstable and critically ill to the individual who is medically stable with cardiovascular and pulmonary dysfunction, or its risk, and living in the community. The purpose of a systematic approach to clinical decision making is to maximize intervention outcome and cost effectiveness. This is done by focusing on physiological and evidence-based practice within the context of evidence-informed practice (i.e., informed by epidemiology) and monitoring to gauge improvement after every intervention so as to

Table 17-7 **Measures and Outcomes to Assess Limitations in the Steps in the Oxygen Transport Pathway**

Status or Function	Measures or Outcomes
Central control of breathing	Central drive to breathe test Arterial blood gases Cerebral perfusion and pressure
Ambient air	Partial pressures of O_2, N_2 and CO_2 Air pollution and quality Humidity
Airways	Clinical assessment including auscultation Pulmonary function tests Arterial blood gases Chest radiograph Histamine challenge exercise tests
Lungs	Clinical assessment, including inspection, percussion, palpation, and auscultation Pulmonary function tests Ventilation and perfusion scans Diffusion capacity test Arterial blood gases Chest radiograph Immunological status Respiratory muscle assessment Assessment of the structure and integrity of chest wall Lung water studies
Blood	Circulating blood volume and cardiac output Arterial oxygen content Venous oxygen content Plasma volume Red and white blood cell counts Protein constituents Platelets Hemoglobin Coagulability Viscosity Stasis Hydration Immunological status
Pulmonary circulation	Perfusion scan Pulmonary artery balloon floatation catheter to assess central venous pressure, pulmonary artery pressures, wedge pressure
Heart	Clinical assessment, including percussion, palpation, and auscultation Inspection and clinical observation tests, including jugular venous distension test Heart rate, systolic and diastolic blood pressures, and rate pressure product ECG Hemodynamic studies to assess cardiac output, stroke volume, cardiac distensibility, and ejection fraction Ultrasound procedures to examine mechanical integrity Scans Coordination of electromechanical behavior of heart Coronary artery perfusion studies Stress test Hemodynamic monitoring including central venous pressure, pulmonary artery pressures, and wedge pressure Angiography Chest radiograph
Peripheral circulation	Clinical assessment findings Segmental blood pressures of the extremities Ultrasound studies Arterial and venous lab studies and investigations Adequacy and efficiency of lymphatic drainage system of the heart and lungs, and peripheral circulation Stress test
Tissue	Enzyme studies Tissue biopsies Vascularization of tissue Adequacy and efficiency of arterial and venous tissue Blood flow Tissue fluid balance; hydrostatic pressure, oncotic pressure, and lymphatic pressure Blood work including serum lactates and $S\dot{V}O_2$ Tissue oxygenation and pH Nutritional and hydration status

ensure that the patient is progressing and time is not wasted. The clinical decision-making process involves diagnosis (i.e., specific analysis of the patient's problems—limitations in activity and participation) in relation to the physiology and underling pathophysiology, the contribution of restricted mobility and recumbency, and extrinsic (related to the patient's care) and intrinsic (related to the patient's characteristics) factors. Based on this analysis, interventions and their parameters are prescribed so that they have the greatest physiological and scientific justification for being likely to return an individual to health and participation in life. Interventions and their prescription parameters should have clear and justifiable rationales. Specific monitoring of the impaired steps in the oxygen transport pathway is essential to establishing and confirming the diagnoses, determining the potentially most effective interventions, evaluating the intervention response, refining and progressing the intervention, and determining when to discontinue intervention and physical therapy overall or to discharge the patient from care. The specific components of the intervention prescription include the intervention, its intensity (if applicable), duration, and frequency, as well as its course and progression. A problem-solving approach to patient care has become essential across health care professions, given the prohibitive cost of such care and the need for health care to be physiological, evidence-based, cost-effective, and ethically justifiable. As noninvasive practitioners, physical therapists need to evaluate their effectiveness in avoiding, reducing, or postponing the need for invasive care (i.e., drugs and surgery). Although these outcomes are exceptionally important, they all too often are underestimated in practice.

Review Questions

1. Describe the three levels of assessment, based on the World Health Organization's model of ability and participation.[21]
2. Describe the use of the oxygen transport pathway as a conceptual model of cardiovascular and pulmonary practice and as the basis for defining problems related to cardiovascular and pulmonary dysfunction and risk (structure and function level).
3. Distinguish among the short-term goals, long-term goals, and preventive goals of cardiovascular and pulmonary physical therapy management. Relate to participation, activity, and structure and function.
4. Discuss the significance of the reduction of invasive care (avoidance, reduction, and postponement of drugs and surgery) as a primary outcome for patients under the care of physical therapists who specialize largely in noninvasive management.
5. Distinguish the four categories of factors that contribute to cardiovascular and pulmonary dysfunction or threat (i.e., pathophysiology, restricted mobility and recumbency, extrinsic factors, and intrinsic factors).
6. Describe the factors that need to be considered in intervention prescription.
7. Describe the factors that need to be considered in determining the course of intervention.
8. Describe the process of modifying, progressing, or discontinuing intervention with respect to the iterative process of evaluation and modifying intervention prescription.
9. What is the role of prognosis in intervention planning in the short term and long term?
10. Describe why physical therapists prescribe interventions rather than administer interventions with standard protocols for given limitations of oxygen transport and address restrictions in activity and participation.

References

1. World Health Organization: Definition of health. 2011. http://www.who.int/suggestions/faq/en/.
2. Stewart A, Hays R, Ware JJ: The MOS short-form general health survey: Reliability and validity in a patient population. *Medical Care* 26:724–735, 1988.
3. Gibson B, Gibson J, Bergner M: The sickness impact profile: Development of an outcome measure of health care. *Annals of Internal Medicine* 65:1304–1310, 1975.
4. Kaplan R, Atkins C, Timms R: Validity of a quality-of-well-being scale as an outcome measure in chronic obstructive pulmonary disease. *Journal of Chronic Diseases* 37:85–95, 1984.
5. McGavin C, Gupta S, Lloyd E, et al: Physical rehabilitation for the chronic bronchitic: Results of a controlled trial of exercises in the home. *Thorax* 32:307–311, 1977.
6. Hunt S, McEwen J, McKenna S: A quantitative approach to perceived health. *Journal of Epidemiology and Community Health* 34:281–295, 1980.
7. Wasson J, Keller A, Rubenstein L, et al: Benefits and obstacles of health status assessment in ambulatory settings: the clinician's points of view. The Dartmouth Primary Care COOP Project. *Medical Care* 30:42–49, 1992.
8. Wallston KA, Wallston BS: Health locus of control scales. In Lefcourt HM, editor: *Research with the locus of control construct*, New York, 1981, Academic Press.
9. Kellner R: *Manual of the symptom questionnaire.* Albuquerque, NM: Department of Psychiatry, School of Medicine, 1987, University of New Mexico, unpublished.
10. Rector T, Kubo S, Cohn J: Patients' self-assessment of their congestive heart failure. *Heart Failure* October/November: 198–209, 1987.
11. Rogers WJ, Johnstone DE, Yusuf S, et al: Quality of life among 5025 patients with left ventricular dysfunction randomized between placebo and enalapril: The Studies of Left Ventricular Dysfunction. The SOLVD Investigators. *J Am Coll Cardiol* 23(2):393–400, 1994 Feb.
12. Oldridge N, Guyatt G, Jones N, et al: Effects on quality of life with comprehensive rehabilitation after acute myocardial infarction. *American Journal of Cardiology* 67:1084–1089, 1991.
13. Guyatt G, Berman L, Townsend M, et al: A measure of quality of life for clinical trials in chronic lung disease. *Thorax* 42:773–778, 1987.
14. Jones P, Quirk F, Baveystock C, et al: A self-complete measure of health status for chronic airflow limitation. *American Review of Respiratory Disease* 145:1321–1327, 1992.
15. Weaver T, Narsavage G: Physiological and psychological variables related to functional status in chronic obstructive pulmonary disease. *Nursing Research* 41:286–291, 1992.
16. Lareau S, Carrieri-Kohlman V, Janson-Bjerklie S, et al: Development and testing of the Pulmonary Functional Status and Dyspnea Questionnaire. *Heart Lung* 23:242–250, 1994.
17. Hyland M: The living with asthma questionnaire. *Respiratory Medicine* 85:13–16, 1991.
18. Schweikert B, Hahmann H, Leidl R: Validation of the EuroQol questionnaire in cardiac rehabilitation. *Heart* 92:62–67, 2006.
19. Höfer S, Lim L, Guyatt G, et al: The MacNew Heart Disease Health-Related Quality of Life Instrument: A summary. *Health and Quality of Life Outcomes* 2:3, 2004.
20. Ferrucci L, Baldasseroni S, Bandinelli S, et al: Disease severity and health-related quality of life across different chronic conditions. *Journal of the American Geriatric Society* 48:1490–1495, 2000.
21. World Health Organization: International Classification of Functioning, Disability and Health. 2002. http://www.who.int/classifications/icf/en/index.htmlarch/ICIDH-2PFDec-2000.pdf.
22. Dean E: Oxygen transport: A physiologically based conceptual framework for the practice of cardiopulmonary physiotherapy. *Physiotherapy* 80:347–355, 1994.

23. Dean E: Preferred practice patterns in cardiopulmonary physical therapy: A guide to physiologic measures. *Cardiopulmonary Physical Therapy Journal* 10:124–134, 1999.
24. Epstein CD, Henning RJ: Oxygen transport variables in the identification and treatment of tissue hypoxia. *Heart & Lung* 22:328–348, 1993.
25. Weissman C, Kemper M, Harding J: Response of critically ill patients to increased oxygen demand: hemodynamic subsets. *Critical Care Medicine* 22:1809–1816, 1994.
26. Goldhill DR, Worthington L, Mulcahy A, et al: The patient-at-risk team: Identifying and managing seriously ill ward patients. *Anaesthesia* 54:853–860, 1999.
27. Jerusum J: Tissue oxygenation and routine nursing procedures in critically ill patients. *Journal of Cardiovascular Nursing* 11:12–30, 1997.
28. Corriveau ML, Rosen BJ, Dolan GF: Oxygen transport and oxygen consumption during supplemental oxygen administration in patients with chronic obstructive pulmonary disease. *American Journal of Medicine* 87:633–637, 1989.
29. Kelly KM: Does increasing oxygen delivery improve outcome? Yes. *Critical Care Clinics* 12:635–644, 1996.
30. Lugo G, Arizpe D, Dominguez G, et al: Relationship between oxygen consumption and oxygen delivery during anesthesia in high-risk surgical patients. *Critical Care Medicine* 21:64–69, 1993.
31. American Physical Therapy Association: Guide to physical therapist practice, ed 2, Washington, DC, 2003, American Physical Therapy Association.

III

Chapter 18

Mobilization and Exercise: Physiological Basis for Assessment, Evaluation, and Training

Elizabeth Dean and Scotty Butcher

KEY TERMS

Exercise
Metabolic demand
Mobilization
Oxygen transport
Physical activity
Prescription
Recumbency
Restricted mobility
Sedentary activity

CHAPTER OUTLINE

Physical therapists use mobilization and exercise as the basis for patient assessment, evaluation, and intervention; the two concepts in conjunction are a therapist's primary tools. These tools are used to prevent, remediate, or delay limitations in participation and activity. They can also be used to assess and evaluate limitations in structure and function or in exercise capacity. This chapter will begin with an overview of the terminology, then move into the basic physiology of mobilization and exercise. The bulk of the chapter will use those introductory concepts to look at the physiology as a basis for assessment, evaluation, and training.

The routine application of mobilization and exercise should be distinguished from the prescriptive application of mobilization and exercise; the three objectives of prescribing mobilization and exercise for the purpose of maximizing oxygen transport are differentiated in this chapter. The detrimental multisystem effects of prolonged sedentary activity and restricted activity (bed rest) in the general population are outlined, and techniques to counter those effects are described. The acute and chronic responses to exercise described in this chapter are typical for individuals without pathology. Chapter 19 outlines testing and training prescription principles and practical details for exercise testing and prescription. Special considerations in common patient populations with respect to exercise testing and training prescription are described in Chapters 24 and 25.

Terminology in Mobilization and Exercise

Before moving into the physiology of mobilization and exercise, a few definitions are necessary to clarify the discussion. Strict definitions are important when discussing the following concepts:

Mobilization
Exercise versus physical activity
Training
Oxygen consumption

Mobilization

Mobilization is the therapeutic and prescriptive application of low work load activity in the management of cardiovascular and pulmonary dysfunction. Primarily, the goal of mobilization is to exploit the acute effects of exercise in order to optimize oxygen transport. Although this activity is considered low work load, it can elicit high patient-specific relative metabolic demand. Even a relatively low dose of a mobilization stimulus can impose considerable metabolic demand on a patient with cardiovascular or pulmonary compromise, which is why it is prescribed for patients who are acutely ill. Mobilization is also used because of its beneficial effects on other organ systems such as the musculoskeletal, neurological, integumentary, gastrointestinal, and renal systems. Whenever possible, mobilization is performed in the upright position, which is the physiological position (Chapter 20), to optimize gravitational stress on fluid shifts and central and peripheral hemodynamics. Mobilization is thus prescribed as both a gravitational stimulus and an exercise stimulus.

Exercise Versus Physical Activity

Physical activity is defined as bodily movement produced by muscle contraction that increases metabolic demand substantially over the resting state. Exercise, then, is defined as a form of physical activity that is structured and repetitive. Exercise typically requires at least moderate physical exertion, such that respiratory rate and heart rate are noticeably accelerated, especially when performed to develop or maintain fitness. Exercise is prescribed by physical therapists in the management of subacute and chronic cardiovascular or pulmonary dysfunction. The ultimate goal of exercise is the maximization of function in all steps of the oxygen transport pathway down to supporting structures (i.e., muscles and other tissues). A short-term goal of exercise is the exploitation of its cumulative physiological effects to adapt to long-term exercise.

Training

Although specific principles of training have been designed for athletes involved in performance-based activities, these principles also apply to any patient that physical therapists encounter. Training in both cases, is defined as the systematic application of progressive exercise stimuli to elicit a specific physiological, functional, or skill-based goal (or goals). Typically, to achieve specific patient-based goals, the application of multiple exercise modes and training guidelines is required. This type of training often involves both aerobic and anaerobic exercise using cyclic and resistance-based exercises. Application of training principles to exercise testing and prescription is discussed further in Chapter 19.

Oxygen Consumption

The amount of oxygen taken in during a given activity is measured as oxygen consumption ($\dot{V}O_2$). Oxygen consumption is dictated by fluctuating metabolic requirements: demand is at its lowest point when the body is rest but increases to intermediate levels during submaximal activity and reaches a peak at the maximal level of exercise an individual can volitionally tolerate. Metabolic cost increases with illness or injury as a result of healing and repair. Two abbreviations frequently appear in the exercise physiology literature to denote oxygen consumption: $\dot{V}O_{2max}$ and $\dot{V}O_{2peak}$. Although often used interchangeably, these terms are technically distinct.

$\dot{V}O_{2max}$ Versus $\dot{V}O_{2peak}$

A true "maximal" value would reflect the oxygen consumption of *all* muscles working maximally: the value would be the product of cardiac output (CO) × arteriovenous oxygen content difference (a–v O_2 content difference) (see Figure 2-2). This is documented as $\dot{V}O_{2max}$.

The problem with using $\dot{V}O_{2max}$, however, is that most exercise activities, including exercise tests, are selective in their focus and tend to work just the legs or the arms, or work the legs in different ways (i.e., cycling a lower-extremity ergometer versus walking on a treadmill). $\dot{V}O_{2peak}$, then, measures oxygen consumption in the context of the exercise: where $\dot{V}O_{2max}$ is then a theoretical value, $\dot{V}O_{2peak}$ is a practical one.

Maximal effort resulting from leg work generates a greater $\dot{V}O_{2peak}$ than maximal effort resulting from arm work; further, maximal effort resulting from treadmill walking or running generates a greater $\dot{V}O_{2peak}$ than maximal leg work on a cycle ergometer (about 10% more). This greater $\dot{V}O_{2peak}$ may be explained by the larger muscle mass of the legs than the arms in the first situation, and the arm work and requirement for increased postural stabilization in the second situation. The more a patient's muscle groups work simultaneously, the closer $\dot{V}O_{2peak}$ approximates true $\dot{V}O_{2max}$.

Whether $\dot{V}O_{2max}$ can be achieved is an academic question. Maximal effort exerted during Nordic (cross-country) skiing approximates theoretical $\dot{V}O_{2max}$ most closely in that the activity requires strenuous arm and leg work coupled with marked postural stabilization. In the laboratory, $\dot{V}O_{2max}$ is obtained based on a maximal exercise test in which metabolic evaluation is performed. Such evaluation indicates when the individual's maximal level of physiological capacity is reached, including the attainment of age-predicted maximal heart rate. The evaluation may also include a plateau of or decrement in $\dot{V}O_2$ with increasing work rate.

In the update of the literature in this and other chapters, the term used is the same term used by the cited investigators in describing their work. Literature published in recent years tends to adopt the more precise terminology, $\dot{V}O_{2peak}$, when describing the $\dot{V}O_2$ achieved by an individual when performing a maximal effort during a specified exercise testing condition.

Aerobic Capacity

An additional problematic term typically used in exercise physiology literature is *aerobic capacity.* $\dot{V}O_{2max}$ represents the maximal rate of aerobic glycolysis (or maximal aerobic power). Though aerobic capacity is often used to describe $\dot{V}O_{2max}$, aerobic capacity actually refers to the total amount of energy produced aerobically and better reflects aerobic endurance than $\dot{V}O_{2max}$. The term *maximal aerobic power* is more appropriate to describe $\dot{V}O_{2max}$.

Basic Principles of Mobilization and Exercise

Exercise as an Assessment and Evaluation Tool

Exercise has been the basis for physical therapy for more than 100 years, but exercise science has only emerged as a discipline within the past 60 years. Over this time, typical responses of various organ systems to both short- and long-term exercise stress have been detailed by researchers. The main question being addressed pertains to what physiological changes can be expected when an individual initiates exercise (particularly in a test with a standardized protocol). Changes in breathing, heart rate, blood pressure arterial saturation, $\dot{V}O_2$, and $\dot{V}O_{2max}$, as well as subjective responses of exertion and fatigue, are all aspects of this study. An understanding of these responses has enabled physical therapists to use exercise as a tool in the assessment, evaluation, and training of patients.

Physiological response can vary in deconditioned people where a given work rate is perceived as highly strenuous, yet the absolute work rate is relatively low. These responses can be markedly altered in people with a range of pathologies (depending on their types and severities) and these differences need to be anticipated and considered (see Chapters 24 and 25) in the assessment of a patient.

For evaluation, exercise tests can serve as standardized outcome measures. As evaluation tools, tests are repeated periodically (e.g., every few weeks) in order to progress the exercise or training prescription until the target conditioning goal is achieved. Special attention is paid in these cases to pre-exercise conditions and the standardization of both exercise procedures and measurement procedures (Chapter 19).

Clinically, physical therapists select which test outcomes are relevant based on the patient's needs and goals. In some patients, objective responses such as HR or SpO_2 may be primarily of interest, whereas subjective responses such as breathlessness, fatigue, or pain may be of particular interest. Some pathologies can limit the level of conditioning that is achievable with training; thus a comprehensive multisystem assessment is needed to establish realistic goals for the training, along with parameters to maximize its benefits and limit potential adverse effects.

Often for people with chronic conditions, many of whom may be older, submaximal tests can be used to compare responses from one time to another for given work rates. In other cases, the physical therapist may wish to estimate $\dot{V}O_{2max}$ by conducting a $\dot{V}O_{2peak}$ test, which can be done directly or indirectly. Direct measurement of $\dot{V}O_2$ requires metabolic measurement with a cart and capacity for expired gas analysis for O_2 and CO_2 (Figure 18-1). Such carts require pretest gas calibration in addition to calibration of the exercise modality (treadmill or ergometer). The patient needs to be familiarized and habituated to the tester(s) and testing situation, and practice beforehand, to ensure the results are valid. Indirect assessment of $\dot{V}O_{2max}$ is imprecise but can provide an index of general conditioning if methods are tightly standardized; this is particularly important when test results are used as outcome measures. Practices related to exercise testing and training prescription are detailed in Chapter 19.

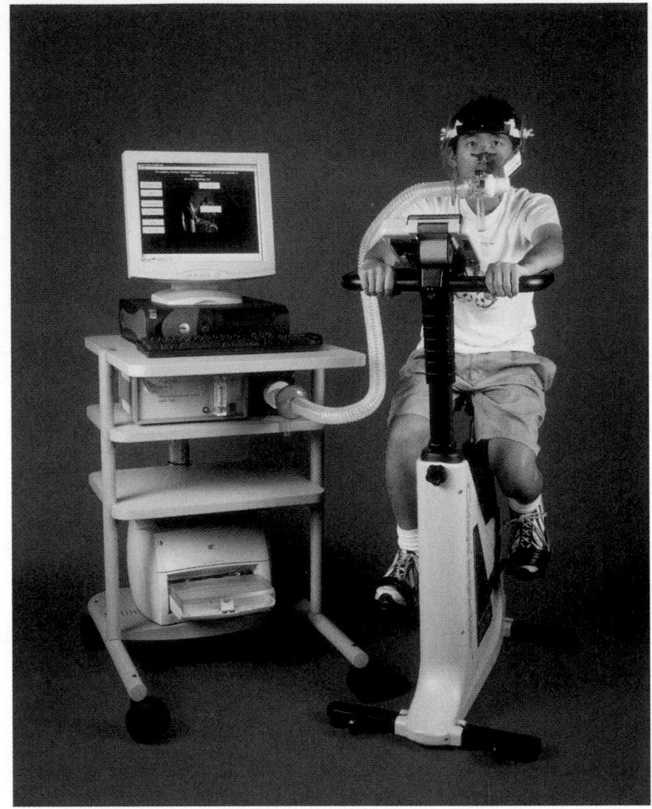

Fig. 18-1 Patient being exercise tested and assessed with a metabolic measurement cart. Note the apparatus interfacing with patient for expiratory gas analysis during the phases of the exercise test.

Oxygen Transport and Metabolic Demand of Patients

In health, when individuals have a typical reserve capacity, the acute and long-term responses to an exercise stimulus can be largely predicted. Specifically, minute ventilation (VE), cardiac output (CO), and each of their components (hence, DO_2) increase commensurate with work rate and oxygen demand.

In patients whose oxygen transport capacity is reduced or threatened, mobilization and exercise constitute a metabolic load that is superimposed on other factors that increase metabolic cost (Table 18-1). Hospitalized patients may be hypermetabolic. In addition to their basal metabolic demands, their energy demands are increased secondarily to factors such as pain, anxiety, increased body temperature, healing and repair processes, increased work of breathing, and increased work of the heart, as well as in response to interventions and

Table 18-1 **Factors That Contribute to Increased Metabolic Demand and Oxygen Consumption in Patient Populations**

Type of Factors	Specific Factors
Pathophysiological Factors	Fever (secondary to an infectious agent or inflammation, surgery, multiple trauma, severe illness) Thermoregulatory challenges (too hot or too cold, altered ambient temperature and humidity) Healing and repairing (secondary to illness, trauma, surgery) Combating infection
Intervention-Related Factors	Alerting, noxious, and painful responses to routine nursing, medical, and physical therapy interventions, including injections, insertion of lines, procedures, and neurological checks Feeding, enterally or parenterally Being handled physically (by health care workers) Body position Changing body position (passive, active assist, or active changes) Range of motion exercises (passive, active assist, or active) Mobilization and exercise Pharmacological agents
Psychosocial Factors	Social contact (with health care workers, family) Anxiety Discomfort Pain
Miscellaneous	Noise Disrupted circadian rhythms when ill, hospitalized, or away from daylight

procedures such as physical therapy. The goal, therefore, in prescribing mobilization and exercise is to ensure a safety margin wherein the patient's demand for oxygen does not exceed the available normal supply or delivery. This can be indicated clinically if the patient's oxygen transport levels worsen by either objective or subjective measurement.

Several interventions can increase $\dot{V}O_2$ and overall metabolic demand;[1,2] therefore the capacity of the oxygen transport system to meet the patient's metabolic demands needs to be established in the assessment. These interventions include:

- Mobilization
- Exercise
- Body positioning
- Arousal
- Breathing control maneuvers
- Coughing
- Postural drainage
- Manual techniques
- Bagging
- Suctioning
- Range-of-motion (ROM) exercises

Questions to ask include the following: Can the oxygen transport system support the patient's metabolic demands? If so, what reserve capacity is available to support a mobilization or exercise stimulus? The exercise stimulus is designed to exploit the potential of the reserve capacity. Estimating reserve capacity is essential so that the effectiveness of the therapeutic exercise stimulus (i.e., neither subthreshold or suprathreshold) can be maximized.

Metabolic demand and $\dot{V}O_2$ are determined by many factors. In patients, the effect of arousal, anxiety, pain, and noxious stimulation, in addition to the hypermetabolic demands of recovery, contribute to energy cost and demand on the oxygen transport system. Thus relaxing and calming patients are central components of physical therapy because these interventions reduce oxygen demand, as do physical therapy interventions for pain management. Although relaxation, often coupled with sedation or analgesia, is central to physical therapy management in other settings, relaxation procedures should be applied in the management of patients with cardiovascular and pulmonary dysfunction in situations in which agitation, anxiety, and pain contribute to increased oxygen demand. This is especially true in intensive care, where oxygen transport is compromised or threatened in most patients (see Chapters 34 and 35).

The typical method for prescribing exercise to achieve desired acute and long-term adaptations is longer duration, whole-body aerobic exercise at a moderate-vigorous intensity. This type of stimulus appropriately optimizes both central (cardiac, blood volume, oxygen delivery) and peripheral (oxygen extraction, glycolytic/mitochondrial enzyme function, capillarization) components for increasing $\dot{V}O_{2max}$. This type of training, however, also requires an adequate central response of the cardiovascular and/or respiratory systems to produce a high level of cardiac output during exercise. In patients with compromised cardiovascular or respiratory function, this type of exercise is extremely difficult and can often lead to undue fatigue. The stimulus for increasing metabolic demand with exercise can be achieved in ways that can help minimize $\dot{V}O_2$, thus reducing the impact of reduced cardiovascular and/or respiratory function.[3] For example, in patients with chronic obstructive lung disease, breathing a low-density helium gas mixture relieves some of the respiratory loading, resulting in increases in exercise tolerance[4] and peripheral muscle trainability.[5] Use of such breathing gases is not usually practical in clinical settings, however. Other methods such as single limb training and high-intensity interval training, have been shown to reduce central demand and optimize peripheral load (see Chapter 19).

Cellular Energetics in Response to Acute Mobilization and Exercise

The integrity of the cardiopulmonary unit is fundamental to maximize oxygen transport and cellular respiration. Oxygen is continuously being used by every cell in the body for oxidative phosphorylation and the synthesis of adenosine triphosphate (ATP). The splitting of a phosphate bond from ATP to form adenosine diphosphate yields a considerable amount of energy for metabolism. The energy for this process comes from the reduction of hydrogen in the formation of water and carbon dioxide, which are the end products of the Krebs cycle and the electron transfer chain (i.e., cellular respiration). These metabolic processes, which make up oxidative phosphorylation, take place in the mitochondria of the cells (see Chapter 2).

The balance between oxygen consumption and oxygen delivery is precisely regulated to ensure not only that there is an adequate supply of oxygen but also that, under typical resting conditions, approximately four times as much oxygen is delivered to the tissues as is used. This safety margin permits the immediate availability of oxygen when the system is perturbed by physical, gravitational, or psychological challenges (see Chapter 2).

Anaerobic metabolism is prevalent at the initiation of all movement/activity/exercise and also during intense, short, sprint-type activities (i.e., sports such as hockey, soccer, and volleyball or functional activities such as stair climbing, heavy lifting/carrying, and vigorous walking/running). Physical therapists tend to focus on aerobic rather than anaerobic exercise; however, in situations where tasks to be improved involve high levels of intensity, training programs may be designed to elicit anaerobic adaptations. In conditions for which Do_2 is compromised, patients may rely on anaerobic metabolism to sustain ATP production and breakdown to provide energy. Anaerobic capacity and, specifically, the anaerobic threshold can increase with training; however, anaerobic training effects are less than aerobic training effects achieved with aerobic training.

Although the term *anaerobic* implies that the exercise is performed in the absence of oxygen, anaerobic metabolism provides a short-term means of supporting phosphorylation, using substrates other than oxygen to generate and split ATP. If insufficient oxygen is available, the amount of ATP that can be generated anaerobically is limited; thus this process can be sustained for only a short period.

Lactic acid accumulates in the blood during anaerobic metabolism. In healthy, untrained individuals lactic acid increases exponentially at an exercise intensity of about 55% of maximal aerobic power.[6]

Anaerobic metabolism is thought to be triggered by tissue hypoxia, though the term *anaerobic* is somewhat a misnomer: oxygen is still needed to pay the oxygen debt. In healthy patients the need for oxygen is delayed rather than eliminated; in patients with disease, anaerobic metabolism occurs when a patient's oxygen transport system cannot meet the metabolic demand required (i.e., patients with sepsis and multisystem organ dysfunction). Serum lactate levels are elevated in these patients, resulting in metabolic acidosis, which is unfavorable to the maintenance of homeostasis.

During exercise, the cellular Po_2 is lower than the surrounding interstitial fluid Po_2 and oxygen diffuses rapidly through cell membranes. At the onset of physical exercise, the increased metabolic demand of the muscle and supporting tissues increases the oxygen diffusion gradient. Feedback mechanisms are triggered to increase Do_2, which depends primarily on arterial oxygen content and CO.

The first line of defense is the response to an increase in pericellular pH. The concentration of carbon dioxide is increased, and this, as a result of the decrease in pH, facilitates the dissociation of oxygen from hemoglobin (i.e., it shifts the oxyhemoglobin dissociation curve to the right). CO, the product of stroke volume and heart rate (SV × HR), increases commensurate with metabolic demand. The immediate response to oxygen utilization and lowered tissue oxygen is an increase in CO to increase Do_2. This averts arterial desaturation that is not typically observed in health, even with extreme exertion. With progressive exercise intensity, SV increases disproportionately at lower intensities to increase CO, with HR contributing to a greater extent at moderate and high exercise intensities. However, older individuals exercising at high intensity in upright positions rely more on the Frank-Starling effect than on HR.[7] In health, exercise-induced cardiac fatigue has been proposed as a limiter to prolonged exercise.[8] The mechanisms of the associated reduced left ventricular systolic and diastolic function are unclear.

The increase in systemic CO results in increased venous return and pulmonary CO. The SV plateaus at 40% of $\dot{V}o_{2max}$, and thereafter CO is augmented by increases in HR (Figure 18-2). One exception in health is in elite athletes, whose SV may continue to increase commensurate with exercise intensity.[9] To oxygenate a greater volume of blood in the lungs, an increased volume of air must be inspired. To increase $\dot{V}_E$, tidal volume (V_T) and respiratory rate (RR) increase. At low intensities of exercise, V_T increases disproportionately to RR, whereas at moderate to high intensities, V_T plateaus and further increases in $\dot{V}_E$ are effected by an increase in RR (Figure 18-3).[10] Exercise is associated with a small increase in airway diameter and length of pulmonary structures, hence, a reduction in airway resistance. Zone 2, the zone of greatest alveolar ventilation to perfusion ($\dot{V}_A/Q$) matching in the lungs, is increased as a result of pulmonary capillary dilation and recruitment. Diaphragmatic excursion is enhanced, and the distributions of ventilation and perfusion become more uniform throughout the lungs, which minimizes airway closure and atelectasis. Exercise increases diaphragmatic excursion, which leads to inflation of the lungs in three planes (anteroposterior, transverse, and cephalocaudal, particularly in the upright position).

Rhythmic inflation and deflation of the lungs associated with physical activity has several clinically important effects:

- First, this action increases alveolar ventilation ($\dot{V}_A$) by a primary increase in V_T.
- Second, exercise-induced lung motion facilitates lymphatic flow and drainage. Optimal lymphatic drainage is essential for lung water balance with the increased volume of blood being processed through the pulmonary circulation and lung parenchyma. This action may explain, in part, the beneficial effect of mobilization on the distribution and function of pulmonary immune factors.[11] The increased movement of the lungs during exercise has a primary effect on mucociliary transport and mucus clearance.[12] Physical activity may also minimize bacterial colonization in the airways, hence reducing the risk for pulmonary infection.[13]
- Finally, lung movement stimulates surfactant production and its distribution over parenchymal tissue. Surfactant is essential for reducing surface tension in the alveoli, maintaining alveolar stability, and maintaining lung compliance, thereby minimizing airway closure and areas of lung collapse.

Circulation to the heart and periphery is primed and responds to the increased demands of acute exercise. Hemodynamic adjustments occur immediately with the onset of exercise stress and in fact may precede it due to a typical anticipatory response. To maximize the availability of CO to working muscle (e.g., the legs), blood shifts from the venous capacitance reservoirs, such as the venous compartments of the gut and extremities. At rest, most of the circulation (70%) is contained within the highly compliant venous circulation. The

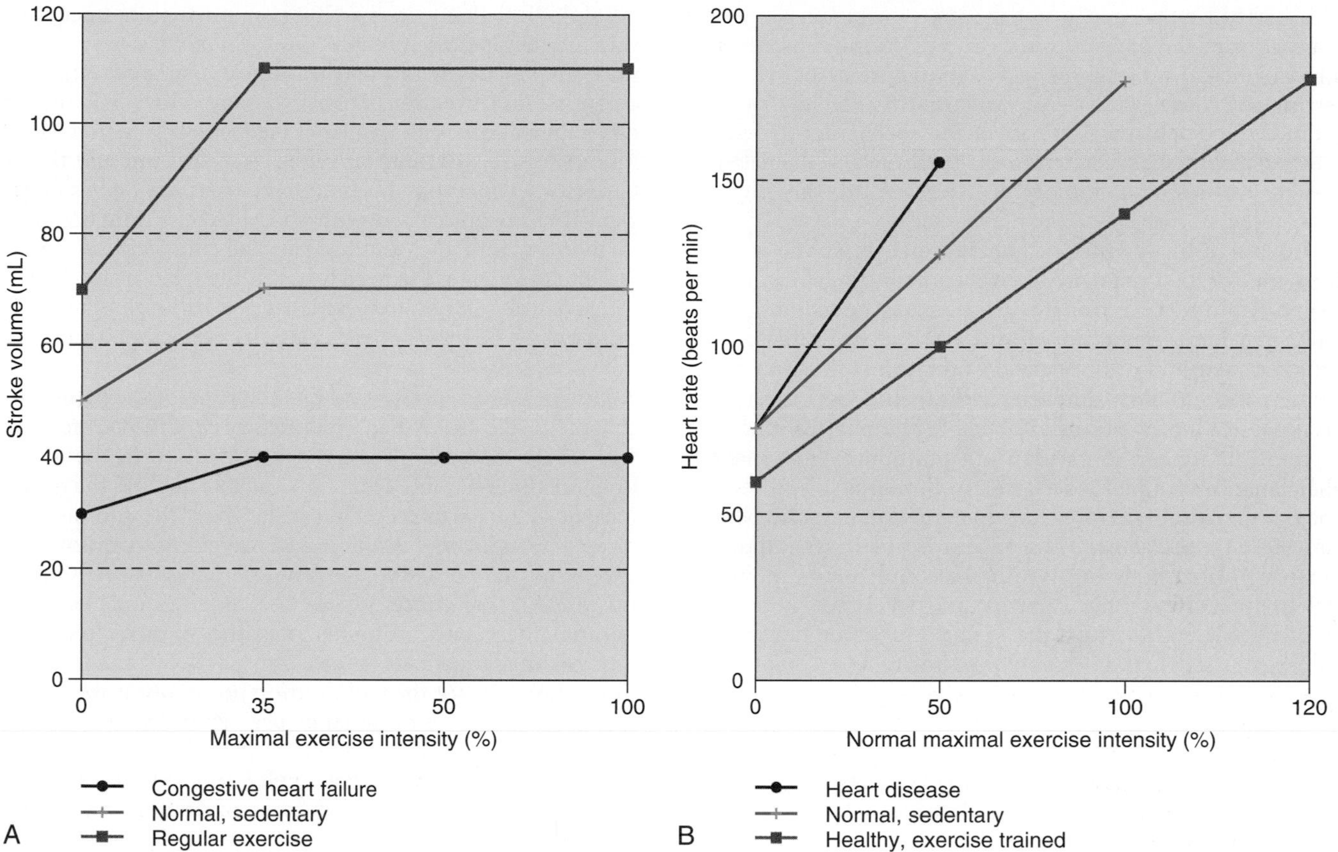

Fig. 18-2 Relationship between stroke volume (SV) and heart rate (HR) with increasing cardiac output (CO) or exercise intensity. Horizontal axis represents O_2 consumption ($\dot{V}O_2$) corresponding to exercise intensity; left vertical axis is stroke volume (*dashed lines*); right vertical axis represents heart rate (*solid lines*). *Light lines,* Before aerobic training; *dark lines,* after aerobic training.

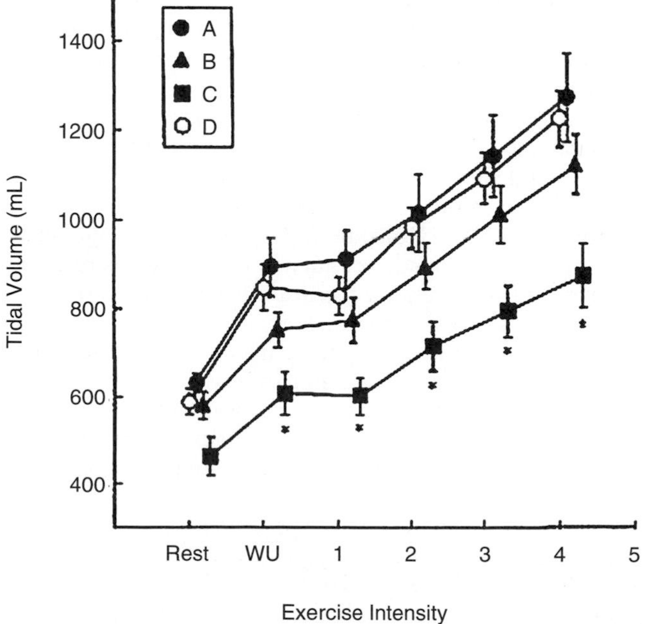

Fig. 18-3 Relationship between tidal volume (V_T) and respiratory rate (RR) with increasing minute ventilation (V_E) or exercise intensity. Horizontal axis represents minute ventilation corresponding to exercise intensity; left vertical axis represents V_T (*solid line*); right vertical axis represents RR (*dashed line*).

Starling law of the heart regulates the forward movement of blood commensurate with the volume of blood that is received. The heart chambers are normally distensible; they adjust to changing volumes of blood returning to the heart and pump more forcefully when stretched than at rest, in order to eject blood through the pulmonary and peripheral circulations. Muscle enzymes that extract oxygen at the cellular level are also primed and are synthesized commensurate with chronic metabolic demand.

Effects of Mobilization and Exercise on Oxygen Transport

In health, optimal oxygen transport depends on the integrity of each step in the oxygen transport pathway and the interdependency of these steps. Cardiovascular and pulmonary dysfunction can lead to dysfunction in one or more steps in the oxygen transport pathway. Because of the interdependence of these steps and the ability of functional steps to compensate for dysfunctional steps, gross measures of gas exchange and oxygenation can be normal. The number of steps in the pathway that are affected by pathology and its severity determine the impairment of oxygen transport overall and the degree to which this impairment is reflected in gross measures of oxygen transport.

To maximize the capacity of the steps in the oxygen transport pathway, the oxygen transport system must be exposed to two principal stressors: (1) gravitational stress and (2) exercise stress. These stressors are essential to life in that they enhance the biochemical, physical, and mechanical efficiency of the steps in the oxygen transport pathway and the patient's capacity to respond rapidly to changes in the physical environment.

Conversely, the absence of gravitational stress and exercise stress are the two primary factors contributing to impaired oxygen transport secondary to bed rest deconditioning. Exploiting both gravitational and exercise stress to prevent cardiovascular and pulmonary dysfunction is thus indicated. Further, mobilization and exercise are the two most vital physiological interventions available to the physical therapist for remediating cardiovascular and pulmonary dysfunction. Body position has marked effects on pulmonary and cardiovascular function (Chapter 20) and thus on exercise performance. The more acutely ill a patient is, the more important it is that upright body positioning be coupled with mobilization to increase aerobic capacity and tolerance to exercise stress. The degree to which this is done, however, depends on the patient's status and ongoing monitoring (see Chapters 16, 34, and 35).

The Prescription of Mobilization and Exercise

The prescription of exercise is fundamental to the management of primary and secondary cardiovascular and pulmonary dysfunction. Guidelines have been well developed for prescribing exercise to maximize functional work capacity or aerobic power for healthy people and individuals with chronic heart and lung conditions.[14-21]

As clinical exercise specialists, physical therapists strive to take advantage of the effects of exercise in most patients and adapt the prescription based on the patient's clinical presentation and needs. Exercise training is typically based on a person's responses to a maximum graded exercise test. Although somewhat less precise, exercise training intensity can be prescribed based on a proportion of the individual's age-predicted maximum heart rate provided there is no significant medical history. Submaximal exercise testing is often indicated for patients with severely impaired functional work capacity because of the inherent risks associated with maximal testing and the potential for invalid test results.[22] Submaximal exercise testing has had a greater role in patient assessment and evaluation than as a basis for exercise prescription. Because of the greater utility of submaximal exercise testing in patient populations, guidelines for the latter warrant being better elucidated.

The prescription of mobilization for the patient with acute cardiovascular and pulmonary dysfunction has been a relatively neglected research priority when compared with the number of studies concerning the prescription of exercise. This is surprising, given that early mobilization is generally a key component of cardiovascular and pulmonary physical therapy for patients who are acutely ill. Orlava (1959)[23] was among the first to report the beneficial use of mobilization to manage acute cardiovascular and pulmonary compromise; specifically, bronchopulmonary pneumonia. In addition, the physiological literature has long supported an unequivocal role for therapeutic mobilization to maximize oxygen transport in patients with acute cardiovascular and pulmonary dysfunction.[24] Even for patients who are critically ill, the goal of mobilization is to evaluate the patient's responses with respect to oxygen transport reserve capacity and use this as a basis for estimating the limits of a patient's physiological capacity to be mobilized, with a view to returning the patient to living within the community. The more critically ill the patient, the greater the need to assess the relationship between the patient's $\dot{V}O_2$ and oxygen delivery (DO_2) (see Chapter 2);[25] this ensures that the patient's capacity for oxygen transport is not exceeded.

Unlike exercise testing and prescription for the patient with chronic cardiovascular and pulmonary conditions, the patient with acute dysfunction is not exercise-tested in the conventional manner because of understandable risk and the patient's incapacity to perform such a test. Given the profound and direct effects of mobilization and exercise on cardiovascular and pulmonary function, the physical therapist needs to identify the specific effects of exercise required and define the optimal therapeutic stimulus (i.e., the stimulus that yields the maximal benefit to oxygen transport with the least risk). The parameters for the mobilization prescription are based on factors other than a maximal or peak effort (see Chapters 16, 34, and 35).

Acute and chronic cardiovascular and pulmonary pathology have the additional challenges of compromising functional capacity in two ways. First, in acute illness, the patient tends to be recumbent in bed a great proportion of the time; second, in both acute and chronic illnesses, the patient's physical activity is reduced. Recumbency and restricted mobility have physiologically distinct effects on oxygen transport that contribute jointly to bed rest deconditioning; recumbency, however, has been considered to be the primary determinant of bed rest deconditioning.[26-28] The impact of these factors is exaggerated in smokers, young people, older adults, obese individuals, and patients who are mechanically ventilated.

The goals of mobilization and exercise are directed at correcting impairments and enhancing the patient's capacity for activity and participation (see overview of the WHO International Classification of Function, Disability and Health in Chapters 1 and 17). Outcomes related to improving abilities and participation include self-care, home management, return to work, and resumption of avocational activities. Return to work warrants special mention. Return to work is often related to oxygen transport capacity in terms of aerobic and muscle power. However, there are economic, psychosocial, and environmental factors that need to be considered. These factors, too, should be part of the overall assessment and incorporated when setting overall goals and establishing the appropriate outcomes for a given patient.

Preventive Effects of Exercise

The preventive effects of exercise are evident in prehabilitation. The term *prehabilitation* can be used to refer to patient conditioning before a surgical intervention or hospital admission.[29] Individuals can be prescribed exercise programs commensurate with their age, functional status, and anticipated procedure or surgery. The purpose is to reduce complications, speed recovery, minimize the time until discharge, and promote a complete return to daily living as soon as possible.

Although it is widely accepted that exercise provides profound preventive benefits for most patients, these benefits have not been adequately researched for the critically ill. Some general practices, however, have become accepted clinically for patients who are acutely ill, including the practice of turning patients. The turning frequency that is widely accepted is every 2 hours, though there is no literature to support evidence of greater preventive effects when a patient is turned every 2 hours rather than hourly or every 4 hours. Sitting up and ambulating are two other practices that are used. The timing of these interventions, however, is often based on convenience, on the patient's other needs, or on a once- or twice-a-day regimen, rather than on a prescriptive basis with consideration of rest or recovery periods between treatments. Patients who sit or walk for preventive reasons may assume suboptimal and even deleterious slumped or asymmetric positions. Patients and their caregivers need to be reminded about the importance of proper body position at all times, and patients should be provided with appropriately supported chairs, firm bolsters, and adjustable beds that maintain optimal body positions. The benefits can be augmented by scheduling such interventions when the patient is rested, or coordinating them with medications, e.g., analgesics or delay of sedating medication.

When prescribing exercise to elicit its optimal preventive effects, the physical therapist needs to consider the same variables as when prescribing exercise for its beneficial acute and long-term effects—that is, the patient's age, capabilities, premorbid functional work capacity, and the type, distribution, and severity of the patient's underlying condition(s). Such preventive mobilization or exercise must be prescribed in such a way as to avoid having any deleterious effects on the patient's overall condition. Even after highly invasive investigative procedures such as heart catheterization, patients can benefit from safe early ambulation.[30]

Prescription of Prehabilitation Exercise

Although much is known about the protective benefits of cardiovascular and pulmonary fitness and conditioning and about the negative effects of bed rest and restricted mobility (discussed later in this section), little has been documented about prescribing exercise to counter orthostatic intolerance in a given patient.[31] The characteristics of deconditioning or detraining in a given individual are determined by age, sex, conditioning status before bed rest, underlying pathophysiology, fluid and electrolyte balance, medications, and the duration of bed rest.[32]

The preventive effects of an exercise stimulus can be defined as that exercise dose that will maintain the patient's conditioning level and prevent deterioration. At present, the prescription of preventive mobilization and exercise is nonspecific. Aerobic exercise and resistance muscle training have differential effects in countering the effects of restricted mobility.[33,34] Although the upright position is the primary means of countering orthostatic changes associated with recumbency, exercise may have a limited role.[35] Even though high-intensity, short-duration, isotonic cycle ergometry training (ITE) and intermittent resistive isokinetic training (IKE) have no effect on orthostatic intolerance associated with recumbency in healthy people, ITE maintains plasma volume, red blood cells, and positive fluid balance, and IKE has no effect on plasma loss but mitigates red blood cell loss.

These differential training effects are of considerable clinical interest; however, they are the result of high-intensity training, and further recumbent exercise should not be considered a substitute for the gravitational stress associated with the upright position. Although patients who are severely ill are not usually capable of performing intense exercise, it is important to note that the responses to upright exercise by healthy people after 5 days of bed rest can be maintained with a daily 30-minute session of intense interval upright exercise training.[36] Further, moderately intense exercise performed against lower body negative pressure to simulate an upright 1-g environment fails to counter orthostatic intolerance after 15 days of bed rest.[37] Also, aerobic pedaling exercise in the supine position during bed rest may be inadequate to maintain hemodynamic function and $\dot{V}O_{2max}$.[38] With respect to the parameters for prescription of mobilization, the intensity of training appears to be singularly important in attenuating the deconditioning effects associated with bed rest. In terms of importance, intensity is followed by frequency.[39]

Resistance training fails to counter the cardiovascular deconditioning associated with bed rest.[40] Some evidence suggests that isometric exercise during bed rest can attenuate the decrement in $\dot{V}O_{2peak}$ and maintain muscle integrity better than isotonic exercise.[41] Markers of lactic dehydrogenase, hence anaerobic threshold, increase with both types of exercise. Over time, however, reduced hydrostatic stress contributes to reduced lactic dehydrogenase in both types of training.

Research is needed to refine exercise prescription for the preventive effects of exercise in recumbent patients whose mobility is restricted. For example, the following questions need to be answered:

- What preventive mobilization/exercise is best for which individuals and under what conditions (i.e., what are the principles of prescription)?
- How do different types of exercise compare with respect to their preventive effects when all else is constant (i.e., patient's age and demographic profile, smoking history, general health, presenting illness and severity, body weight, nutritional status, aerobic condition, stress levels, cognitive status, and medication schedule)?
- Does exercising in some body positions elicit better preventive effects than exercise in other body positions?
- What principles establish the mobilization/exercise intensity, duration, and frequency that are optimal for a given individual whose mobility is restricted?
- What types of exercise are best suited for cross-transfer of their effects between the ipsilateral and contralateral limbs, to limit deconditioning when one limb is immobilized?
- What are the parameters that should guide physical activity during the day to limit prolonged periods of sitting (i.e., maximal duration of periods of inactivity, degree of physical activity needed to offset the deleterious effects of sedentary periods)?
- What constitutes an adequate stimulus to maximize the preventive effects of exercise for a given patient, particularly a patient who is critically ill?

Hazards of Sedentary Activity

Cardiorespiratory conditioning or fitness is related to the volume of regular physical activity; however, its relationship to health measures is less strong.[42] Physical inactivity has been causally implicated in lifestyle-related conditions (Chapter 1), but in general, it is not known whether a precise dose of activity or exercise exists that can provide protection against these conditions. One exception to this occurs with ischemic heart disease, in which a threshold intensity of 6 metabolic equivalents (METs) in conjunction with a minimal volume of regular physical activity is recommended for optimal cardiovascular health.[43] The precise dose for prevention of hypertension and stroke is less clear.[44] Moderate as opposed to heavy exercise has been recommended.[43] The choice of relative or absolute intensity of effort depends on the desired preventive outcomes, as well as the patient's specific characteristics and history.

More and more, life in the developed world tends to be characterized not only by inactivity but by prolonged periods of sedentary behavior. Although an individual may adhere, for example, to a routine exercise program that includes aerobic exercise 3 to 5 days a week at moderate intensity for 20 to 40 minutes, this does not entirely offset the deleterious effects of prolonged periods of inactivity that are characteristic of many people's activity patterns throughout the day, week, year, or their overall lives. The negative effects of inactivity may be particularly injurious for older adults and those with disabilities, who may be less able to perform even the basic activities of daily living. This further contributes to the downward spiral of inactivity, often combined with weight gain, which makes it even more challenging for someone to move and be physically active.

Although a person may exercise an hour a day, the question arises about the remaining 23 hours. Over the past decade, investigators have focused on the health consequences not only of physical inactivity but of prolonged periods of sedentary behavior as well. Research has shown that in addition to regular physical exercise, breaks during periods of sedentary activity (including screen-based activities) are essential to offset the effects of chronic inactivity.[45,46] With the advent of screen-based entertainment, children today are at serious risk for the consequences of hours of sedentary activity; furthermore, sedentary children are more likely to become sedentary adults. Conversely, children who are active and move frequently are more likely to do so as adolescents and adults.[47]

Chronic inactivity increases the risk for chronic lifestyle-related conditions and promotes premature aging. Alternatively, a physically active lifestyle promotes health and well-being, even offsetting lifestyle-related chronic conditions, as people age.[48]

Physiological Effects of Bed Rest

Humans are designed to be upright and moving; indeed "upright and moving" can be described as the normal physiological position. The deconditioning associated with restricted activity in patients is comparable to detraining in athletes,[32,39] yet is distinct from bed rest deconditioning, which is associated with recumbency as well as restricted mobility.

When people are recumbent *and* inactive, gravitational stress (the vertical gravitational gradient) and exercise stress are removed. Bed rest, which requires patients to remain in this recumbent and inactive state, is one of the most commonly used yet seldom questioned therapeutic practices. Despite its widespread acceptance, the body positions it promotes are nonphysiological (Chapter 20). The harmful sequelae of this posture have been well documented;[24,39,49-56] yet the more severely ill the patient is, the more confined that individual is to the bed—thereby the greater the risk for multisystem complications (Table 18-2).

The classic study by Saltin and colleagues (1968)[57] demonstrated marked multisystem deterioration within 3 weeks of bed rest in five healthy young men and the restoration of aerobic capacity with strenuous training afterwards. In a follow-up of the same subjects 30 years later,[58] all were found to have an age-related decrement in aerobic power. When their exercise responses were compared over that time frame, it was revealed that bed rest had had a more profound impact on physical work capacity than 30 years of aging.

Table 18-2 Physiological Consequences of Bed Rest

Bed Rest Consequence	Potential Mechanisms
I. Fluid volume redistribution	Decreased plasma and blood volume Decreased total heart and left ventricular volumes Increased hematocrit Diuresis and natriuresis Venous stasis
II. Muscular inactivity	Increased insulin resistance Decreased muscle mass Decreased muscle strength Decreased muscle endurance
III. Altered distribution of body weight and pressure	Urine stasis, retention, tendency toward calculus formation Hypercalciuria Bone demineralization Local skin changes
IV. Aerobic deconditioning	Increased HR at rest and at all levels of activity Decreased resting and maximum stroke volume Decreased maximum cardiac output Increased risk for venous thrombosis and thromboembolism Decreased orthostatic tolerance Decreased aerobic conditioning Decreased $\dot{V}O_{2max}$ Increased venous compliance
V. Other	Catabolism Anorexia Paralytic ileus Constipation Increased sensitivity to thermal stimuli; increased sweating and hyperemia Increased anxiety, hostility, depression, psychosis Increased auditory threshold Increased focal point, decreased near point of visual acuity Alteration in clearance of some drugs

Adapted from Woods SL: Cardiac nursing, ed 5, Philadelphia, 2010, JB Lippincott, Williams & Wilkins.

Of clinical importance is the fact that deterioration of cardiovascular and pulmonary function occurs at a faster rate than musculoskeletal deterioration and that the rate of recovery from the negative effects of bed rest is generally slower than the rate of impairment.[59,60] These effects of bed rest are accentuated in older adults[61] and are likely to further compound the oxygen transport and other deficits of patients with pathology.

Oxidative stress has been implicated in age-related physiological changes.[62] Disuse deconditioning has been implicated as an oxidative stressor contributing to aging, especially when combined with the effects of smoking and a Western-type diet (see Chapter 1). In fact, half of the physical decline associated with aging has been attributed to lack of physical activity.[63] With regular physical activity and prescribed aerobic and strengthening programs, these changes can be substantially offset. As a result, functional capacity is maximized and, in the event of illness, the individual has better physiological reserve to deal with the pathophysiological insult. Regardless of age, however, exercise-induced physiological and health advantages are lost following cessation of exercise.[64] Restricted mobility in older adults has been also associated with clinical depression.[65] Thus the evidence supports the need for sustained physical activity and exercise throughout life to derive their functional and health benefits.

The recumbent, immobile positions associated with bed rest adversely affect most organ systems by means of an apparent down-regulation of the oxygen transport system.[66] This is clinically important because in conventional patient management, there is a direct relationship between how sick the patient is and the amount of time she or he is confined to bed. In addition, the musculoskeletal, neurological, gastrointestinal, and genitourinary systems are adversely affected.

Cardiovascular and Pulmonary Effects

A primary effect of mobilization and exercise on the cardiovascular and pulmonary systems is enhanced mucociliary transport and airway clearance.[12] Frequent changes in body position augment airway clearance and minimize the pooling and stagnation of bronchial secretions, hence reducing airway obstruction and airflow resistance (Chapter 20). The benefits of frequent body position changes to prevent the accumulation of secretions or resolve them can be augmented when combined with mobilization.

The cardiovascular deconditioning resulting from bed rest includes the loss of fluid-volume and pressure regulating mechanisms, the loss of plasma volume, and diuresis.[67-70] In turn, the hematocrit is increased, and the risk for developing deep vein thromboses and thromboemboli is increased. This is exacerbated by increases in blood viscosity, platelet count, platelet stickiness, plasma fibrinogen,[71] and stasis of venous blood flow.

Venous thromboembolic disease is preventable with conservative management, including prophylactic anticoagulation in some instances.[72] In addition to restricted mobility, other risk factors include being older, undergoing venous catheterization, and hormone replacement therapy. Conditions that are associated with risk include previous thromboembolus, myocardial infarction, heart failure, severe lung disease, cancer, obesity, and paralytic conditions such as stroke. After acute stroke, patients are particularly at risk due to paresis, recumbency, restricted mobility, and circulatory stasis.[73] The work of the heart is increased in a patient who is immobile and recumbent, as is the work of breathing. The work of the heart is greater as a result of the increased filling pressures and heart rate associated with chronic recumbency and the increased blood viscosity. The work of breathing is increased because of reduced lung volumes secondary to visceral encroachment on the underside of the diaphragm, increased intrathoracic blood volume, and restricted chest wall motion.

Pulmonary sequelae of recumbency include reduced lung volumes and capacities, particularly functional residual capacity (FRC), residual volumes (RV), and forced expiratory volumes.[74-78] A reduction in FRC in the supine position compared with the sitting position has been attributed to both a decrease in thoracic volume and an increase in thoracic blood volume, thereby increasing pulmonary venous engorgement.[79] Thus alveolar-arterial oxygen difference and arterial oxygen tension are reduced during bed rest.[80-82] Closing volumes are increased, precipitating arterial desaturation in recumbent positions and subsequent complications.

With bed rest, the blood vessels of the muscles and splanchnic circulation dilate. With prolonged bed rest, they may lose their ability to constrict. The ability of these vessels to constrict is essential for preventing the pooling of blood and maintaining circulating blood volume when the patient assumes the upright position. Following bed rest, a patient may feel lightheaded or dizzy and may faint. Individual differences in terms of orthostatic intolerance have been reported and need to be assessed.[67,68,83,84] Individuals with greater venous compliance in the legs recruit mechanisms to compensate, such as activation of the renin-angiotensin-aldosterone system, activation of the sympathetic nervous system, and inhibition of the parasympathetic nervous system, so they tolerate orthostatic challenges better.

Musculoskeletal Effects

With only a few days of bed rest, muscle atrophy is initiated, leading to weakness, discoordination, and balance difficulty.[57,85] With severe weakness, excessive strain may be placed on ligaments and joints. Muscles and their inert structures are differentially affected. In the knee extensors, for example, tendon stiffness is reduced and their hysteresis characteristics become exaggerated, whereas this does not occur in the plantar flexors.[86] Muscle mass and strength may be lost, and muscle and ligament shortening may occur along with joint contractures, skin lesions, and decubitus ulcers.[87,88]

At the cellular level, disuse atrophy begins within 4 hours of bed rest. Compared with type IIa muscle fibers in vastus lateralis, type I fibers have been reported to be more seriously affected by bed rest, and they respond less favorably to muscle-resistance training.[89] Differences in fiber type may explain why muscles in the lower limbs are differentially affected; for example, the plantar flexors are particularly affected.[90] Also, sex differences in muscle strength loss with bed rest have been reported.[91] Muscle imbalance may result from poor postural alignment.

Skeletal muscle protein synthesis is compromised by bed rest, aging, nutritional deficit, uncontrolled diabetes mellitus, and sepsis.[92] Disuse osteoporosis results from reduction of the mechanical stress caused by gravity and from lack of active muscle contraction across joints. Prevention is a primary goal because recovery of mineral loss in bone is prolonged and its loss is largely irreversible.[93] Bone mass is restored later than muscle mass and function after a period of restricted mobility, which contributes to fracture risk.[94]

The limited positioning alternatives in bed may contribute to poor postural alignment, stiffness, and soreness. Bed rest allocates weight bearing to various body parts not adapted for weight bearing. Skin breakdown most commonly occurs over bony prominences, such as the sacrum, trochanters, elbows, scapulae, and heels. Risk factors for pressure ulcers include age, prolonged hospitalization, restricted mobility and general debility, low body weight, low diastolic BP, and surgical intervention.[95]

Immobile patients are at risk for bone demineralization. An issue of particular importance in older populations, patients with disabilities, postmenopausal women, and patients on steroids is calcium loss. Prevention of disuse osteoporosis is the primary aim because remineralization of bone, even with aggressive exercise, body positioning, electrical stimulation, and possible pharmaceutical agents, is unlikely.[93] In patients who are critically ill, cytokines have been implicated in inactivity-related inflammation and muscle injury and atrophy. Activity has been proposed as a countermeasure.[96]

Renal Effects

Bed rest–induced diuresis increases renal load. Patients with renal insufficiency are particularly seriously affected by this effect, as well as by other sequelae of bed rest.[97] As a result, they may exhibit dysrhythmias, muscle wasting, weakness, neuropathy, glucose intolerance, and reduced bone density.

Central Nervous System Effects

With bed rest and recumbency, orthostatic intolerance in combination with resting tachycardia and reduced exercise capacity occur, reflecting diminished reflex activity of the sympathetic nervous system. Baroreceptor-mediated activity is blunted and appears to involve abnormal processing in the central nervous system at the level of the ventrolateral medulla.[98] CNS changes include slowed electrical activity of the brain, emotional and behavioral changes, slowed reaction times, sleep disturbances, and impaired psychomotor performance.[88,99] Diminished sympathetic activity is the primary factor responsible for orthostatic intolerance along with hypovolemia; the net result is bed rest deconditioning.[100]

Metabolic Effects

Metabolic changes that occur during periods of bed rest and the relative absence of muscle contraction include glucose intolerance and reduced insulin sensitivity;[101] increased calcium excretion due to bone loss; and increased nitrogen excretion secondary to protein loss from atrophying muscle.[102,103] In sedentary people, plasma lipids are elevated and skeletal muscle becomes insulin resistant.[104] Insulin sensitivity and triglyceride levels are highly responsive to changes in diet, activity level, and thermogenic state. Fit people are highly insulin sensitive, whereas unfit sedentary people tend to be insulin insensitive. Reversal and the normalizing of insulin sensitivity are dependent on increasing muscle contraction.

Immunological Effects

Bed rest has been associated with reduced cytokine function and antibody counts, hence, reduced immunity and an increased risk for infection.[105,106] Lymph flow is reduced with bed rest, which may predispose patients to further risk for infection.[107]

Psychological Effects

Bed rest also affects psychological status. Patients may become depressed or sensorily deprived or may develop a psychoneurosis.[108]

Alternatives to the Nonspecific Use of Bed Rest

The evidence supports the following:

1. Bed rest as an effective intervention is lacking.
2. The use of bed rest remains nonspecific and excessive.
3. Bed rest has multisystemic negative effects and thus must be prescribed as specifically and judiciously as medication.
4. Methods other than bed rest to manage very ill patients such as those in the intensive care unit (ICU) must be developed.

Given this evidence, alternatives need to be exploited within and outside physical therapy treatment. Physical therapists, for example, need to become active in designing furniture and devices that are better suited to patients' normal physiological functioning and to the needs of patients' courses of recovery. Such appliances would include the presence in ICUs of a greater number of stretcher chairs that enable easy transfer of patients from bed to chair and upright positioning and a greater availability of patient-lifting devices. Greater attention needs to be given to chair design in settings where patients may be immobile; effective chair design could augment the mobilization process in addition to promoting body position changes.

Kinetic and rotating beds are electromechanical beds that turn the patient through an arc of about 30 degrees to both sides from the supine position over several minutes.[109,110] These beds are used for heavy-care patients who are critically ill and are unable or difficult to turn. Even though studies have shown these beds can enhance oxygenation in severely compromised patients such as those with acute respiratory distress syndrome,[111,112] they need to be used selectively judiciously.[113] Reliance on passive positioning by the bed should not substitute for more active and active-assisted patient positioning. Such interventions constitute the initial stages of mobilization and ambulation.

The use of tilt tables to promote mobilization may be hazardous because the muscle pumping action when the legs are dependent is minimal. Passive standing on a tilt table constitutes a greater hemodynamic stress than does active standing. Upright sitting postures with the legs dependent may elicit greater physiological benefit than passive standing and with less risk because of the resulting increased hemodynamic stress. Leg movement elicited by stepping in place, however, can counter the marked fluid shifts associated with the upright position.

Even in patients who are seriously acutely ill (e.g., those in the ICU), body positioning and mobilization are essential to offset the deleterious effects of loss of gravitational stimulation from being upright and loss of exercise stimulation from restricted mobility (Chapters 33, 34, 35, and 36).[114]

Indications for Bed Rest

Despite the universal acceptance of bed rest as a medically therapeutic intervention, indications for its therapeutic use have not been well documented, and its effectiveness continues to be questioned.[39] Further, much more is known about the adverse and potentially life-threatening hazards of bed rest than about its benefits. Bed rest should clearly be used as selectively and prescriptively as other medical interventions to ensure that specific benefits are being derived and that the multisystemic negative sequelae are minimized.

Many procedures such as surgery are associated with considerable pain, so being relatively immobile and recumbent in bed is believed to minimize postsurgical discomfort. Minimizing the effects of gravity and the need to bear weight is commonly indicated in patients after orthopedic surgery. Likewise, the bed enables a patient with multiple wounds and fractures to be immobilized and supported in a fixed position that is believed to promote healing.

Conditions that are associated with edema require minimizing the effect of gravity on the affected limbs. Whether edema can be controlled by localized elevation rather than bed rest must be established. Certain conditions may require some activity restriction, particularly in their acute stages in order to reduce the work of the heart, as in cases of myocardial infarction. However, 50 years ago, restriction to a chair was reported to be more beneficial than restriction to bed in patients with heart disease.[115] Despite this finding, many patients continue to recline in beds rather than sit upright in chairs and initiate ambulation. Mobilizing patients and permitting bathroom privileges has also been reported to be less stressful than having to use a bedpan.[116]

Acute Effects of Mobilization and Exercise

Physiology of Acute Exercise

A comprehensive list of the physiological benefits of acute exercise is presented in Table 18-3. The principal benefits include:

- Increased $\dot{V}_E$ secondary to increased V_T, RR, or both
- Improved airflow rates
- Improved mucus transport
- Improved CO secondary to increased SV, HR, or both
- Increased tissue oxygen extraction

The particular benefits of acute mobilization and exercise can be directed at each patient's specific pathophysiological deficits.

After decades of research in exercise science, based in particular on college-aged male students, an increasing number of studies have identified sex differences in exercise responses. Higher $\dot{V}O_2$ peak and muscle strength are found in men compared with women even when adjusted for body weight. These are explained primarily by hormonal differences, specifically estrogen and progesterone in women and testosterone and androgen in men. Differences in autonomic function contribute to the reduced risk by women for heart disease and to their increased longevity.[117] Women have greater

Table 18-3 Acute Physiological Effects of Mobilization and Exercise

Body System	Effects
Pulmonary	Increased regional ventilation Increased regional perfusion Increased regional diffusion Increased zone 2 (i.e., area of ventilation-perfusion matching) Increased tidal volume Altered breathing frequency Increased minute ventilation Increased efficiency of respiratory mechanics Decreased airflow resistance Increased flow rates Increased strength and quality of a cough Increased mucociliary transport and airway clearance Increased distribution and function of pulmonary immune factors
Cardiovascular	Hemodynamic effects Increased venous return Increased stroke volume Increased heart rate Increased myocardial contractility Increased stroke volume, heart rate, and cardiac output Increased coronary perfusion Increased circulating blood volume Increased chest tube drainage Peripheral circulatory effects Decreased peripheral vascular resistance Increased peripheral blood flow Increased peripheral tissue oxygen extraction
Lymphatic	Increased pulmonary lymphatic flow Increased pulmonary lymphatic drainage
Hematological	Increased circulatory transit times Decreased circulatory stasis
Neurological	Increased arousal Increased cerebral electrical activity Increased stimulus to breathe Increased sympathetic stimulation Increased postural reflexes
Neuromuscular	Increased regional blood flow Increased oxygen extraction
Endocrine	Increased release, distribution, and degradation of catecholamines
Genitourinary	Increased glomerular filtration Increased urinary output Decreased renal stasis
Gastrointestinal	Increased gut motility Decreased constipation
Integumentary	Increased cutaneous circulation for thermoregulation
Multisystemic Effects	Decreased effects of anesthesia and sedation Decreased deleterious cardiopulmonary effects of surgery Decreased risk for loss of gravitational stimulus in conjunction with the upright position

parasympathetic control of the heart and less sympathetic activity.

CARDIOVASCULAR AND PULMONARY EFFECTS

Respiratory muscle fitness may affect exercise performance in healthy individuals. Isolated respiratory muscle training increases respiratory muscle endurance and endurance time in response to whole-body exercise.[118-120] Although $\dot{V}O_{2max}$ is unaffected, $\dot{V}_E$ and blood lactate decrease after training. In addition, respiratory muscle training can attenuate breathlessness in healthy people during exercise. However, improved respiratory muscle strength and endurance with specific training have been reported not to transfer to $\dot{V}O_{2max}$ in athletes.[121] Although optimizing respiratory muscle fitness through whole-body functional exercise is the goal in patient care, these findings have some clinical implications.

The increased metabolic demand of acute exercise results in a slight increase in airway diameter and increases in:

- Minute alveolar ventilation
- Alveolar ventilation
- Tidal volume
- Respiratory rate
- Air flow rates
- Cardiac output
- Stroke volume
- Heart rate
- Blood pressure
- Rate pressure product (RPP; the product of heart rate and systolic BP)

In healthy people and those with heart disease, RPP is highly correlated with myocardial $\dot{V}O_2$ and thus with myocardial work[122]), $\dot{V}O_2$, and carbon dioxide production ($\dot{V}CO_2$). Generally, SV increases disproportionately more than HR at low intensities of exercise to effect CO. With increasing intensity, SV contributes proportionately less to HR, which continues to increase until the maximum HR is achieved with incremental exercise. In moderately active young women, however, SV plateaus through moderate to heavy exercise intensity and then undergoes a secondary increase at very heavy work loads.[123] With endurance training, SV is increased, largely reflecting increased diastolic filling and emptying rates and an increase in blood volume. Older people may not increase their maximal CO and SV in response to training, in favor of peripheral adaptation.[124] The area of greatest ventilation-to-perfusion matching in the midzones of the lungs, zone 2, is increased secondary to increased dilation and recruitment of pulmonary capillaries.[125]

The hemodynamic benefits of exercise are maximized in the upright position (as opposed to recumbent positions) because exercise alone fails to counter the loss of volume-regulating mechanisms associated with recumbency.[126] Most important is the role of gravitational stress on maintaining BP control and reducing orthostatic intolerance (see Chapter 19 for the effects of position changes on hemodynamics). During exercise, end-diastolic volume and SV have been reported to be greater in the upright position than the supine position in endurance athletes, which supports greater reliance on the Frank-Starling law.[127] Thus body position determines the relative contributions of HR, myocardial contractility, and the Frank-Starling mechanism to CO during exercise. Patients with impaired venous return and myocardial contractility may benefit from moderate-intensity recumbent cycling in which central circulation and local vasodilation are favored.[128] Plasma volume increases with acute intense exercise, and this has been shown to be position-dependent.[129] Plasma albumen content increases in upright compared with supine positions, and this is thought to be responsible for the increase in plasma volume. By coupling upright positioning with exercise, the physical therapist may directly help to normalize fluid balance and hemodynamics in patients whose fluid homeostasis is threatened.

The effect of acute exercise on blood coagulation and platelet aggregability is of particular interest in individuals with existing risk factors for clotting. The risk for stroke, for example, is of clinical importance in people with atrial fibrillation. Moderate levels of activity are associated with minimal procoagulatory effects compared with high-intensity exercise, which increases platelet activity.[130] Whether this increased platelet activity constitutes a risk factor clinically has yet to be determined.

The role of exercise in preventing deep vein thrombosis is well established. Although controversy has existed regarding its role in managing deep vein thrombosis, aggressive approaches, including walking based on judicious assessment, have been proposed.[131] Recent evidence has shown that leg compression coupled with walking is superior to bed rest in the management of acute deep vein thrombosis in outpatients.[132] Further, a systematic review and metaanalysis have corroborated that mobilization does not increase the rate of pulmonary embolism or complications above that found with bed rest.[133]

ENDOCRINE EFFECTS

Mobilization and exercise stimulate the endocrine system. Catecholamines, released to support the cardiovascular system, sustain a given exercise work rate. Increased sympathetic activity secondary to mobilization can help reduce the patient's need for sympathomimetic pharmacological agents,[134] an important physical therapy outcome. Sympathetic nerve stimulation is increased, resulting in sympathetic neurotransmitters being processed more efficiently (i.e., synthesized and biodegraded). This is a significant effect that can be used as a goal when prescribing mobilization. When exogenous catecholamines are used to augment DO_2 (optimally to 600 mL/min/m^2) in patients in surgical ICUs, the survival rate is improved and there are no increases in cardiac events over those in control patients.[135] Whether this effect, which is probably mediated by improved cardiac reserve, could be achieved by exercise-induced sympathetic stimulation warrants study. An additional benefit of sympathetic arousal in patients who are critically ill may include antiinflammatory effects associated with increased catecholamines.[136]

MUSCULOSKELETAL EFFECTS

Resistance muscle training in patients who are critically ill has been shown to have general and local benefits in terms of acute and long-term effects, as well as its preventive effects. Peripheral and respiratory muscles are important targets of exercise prescription in this patient population, and such training may have implications for avoiding mechanical ventilation or, if mechanical ventilation is indicated, facilitating weaning.[137] Resistance exercise is an effective countermeasure to muscle atrophy when a patient is recumbent.[33,138]

Resistance muscle training has been a mainstay of physical therapy for motor recovery and conditioning effects in patient populations. There has been an increasing interest in the hemodynamic effects of resistance training and their interactions. Notably, after a resistance training program, healthy older adults show improved aerobic exercise responses. Cardiovascular responses to exertion are reduced, peak responses are delayed, and recovery from maximum exertion is faster.[139] Training effect is determined by a dose-dependent relationship between intensity of resistance training and aerobic exercise responses, in addition to the individual's pretraining status.[140] These effects are of benefit to patients with primary cardiovascular and pulmonary dysfunction; thus modified resistance training has become an integral component of traditional cardiac and pulmonary rehabilitation programs (see Chapter 24). Resistance muscle training, however, is associated with increased arterial wall stiffness, hence reduced compliance and increased pulse pressure.[141] Increased pulse pressure is a risk factor for ischemic heart disease, which suggests the need for caution in prescribing exercise that has a selective effect on pulse pressure.

Caution should be taken with high-resistance exercise, which is defined relative to the individual's strength and endurance status. Sit-ups, for example, require relatively strong abdominal contraction and can elicit a heavy resistance contraction or strong isometric effort in weak individuals. In turn, intrathoracic pressure increases, SV decreases, and vascular injury may be precipitated. There have been reports of catastrophic neurological consequences (stroke and spinal epidural hematoma) in two healthy young men.[142] Thus before abdominal exercise is prescribed, patients should be screened for risk factors. Breathing control should be incorporated to reduce intrathoracic and intraabdominal pressure. The physical therapist needs to be vigilant about detecting neurological signs and symptoms early.

Upper-body and lower-body work have distinct physiological characteristics.[143] These responses may have to be avoided (as in the hemodynamic stress of upper-body work in an individual with myocardial dysfunction) or exploited (as in an individual with lower-body paralysis). Oxygen kinetics differ for the two types of work, as do their hemodynamic responses. $\dot{V}O_2$ kinetics are prolonged in arm cranking compared with leg cycling. This change is consistent with increased type II fiber recruitment. Type II fibers are metabolically inefficient compared with fast, glycolytic, type I fibers.

CENTRAL NERVOUS SYSTEM EFFECTS

CNS responses to mobilization include arousal via activation of the reticular activating system and priming of the various organ systems involved.[144] With respect to autonomic function, parasympathetic inhibition occurs at the start of exercise, followed by sympathetic activation to augment the force and rate of myocardial contraction. Substrate utilization and transfer to working tissue, as well as the capacity for oxygen to be supplied to muscle, are precisely regulated through coordinated control of body temperature, breathing, cardiac function, and vasoactivity, both systemically and locally; at the tissue level, they are regulated by the control of local metabolism and the production of vasoactive and chemoactive substances.

METABOLIC EFFECTS

The metabolic effects of acute exercise, in particular, on glucose metabolism and growth hormone synthesis are of considerable clinical relevance because these functions are fundamental to health and recovery. Restricted physical activity causes hyperinsulinemia and hyperglycemia and reduces growth hormone synthesis.[145] Thus the acute effects of exercise are instrumental in offsetting these changes.

IMMUNOLOGICAL EFFECTS

Acute exercise has profound effects on the immune system. Even a single bout of moderate exercise has a positive effect on immunity.[146] Whether there is a dose-dependent effect is not known. Also unknown is whether there is a cumulative effect of short periods of less intense exercise, such as for the patient who is acutely ill or who has a low functional capacity.

Exercise induces white blood cell production, so it may optimize natural immunity.[147] Generally, moderate levels of regular aerobic exercise are associated with improved immune function.[148] Within the first 10 minutes of intense exercise, leukocytosis increases, as do the thrombocytes responsible for increasing platelet production. These changes are not associated with exercise-related hypovolemia or hyperthermia. Whether leukocytosis and exercise are dependent on dose or whether there is a critical exercise intensity that has to be achieved to stimulate leukocytosis has yet to be established. Prolonged exhaustive exercise has been associated with compromised immunity, which may be avoided with optimal rest and recovery, along with good nutrition and possibly vitamin C supplements.[149] After prolonged heavy exercise in athletes, an "open window" of susceptibility to infection lasting 3 to 72 hours after exercise has been described.[150] The risk for infection may be exacerbated by lack of rest and sleep, inappropriate diet, weight loss, and mental strain, and it may be prevented or reversed by better rest and diet and exercise.[151] Training strategies recommended for athletes to optimize their immunocompetence have relevance for clinical populations. Exercise sessions are monitored for individuals' susceptibility to infection, their general health, and the intensity and duration of the exercise session, as well as recovery, rest, optimal diet, and stress management.[152,153]

PSYCHOLOGICAL EFFECTS

Acute exercise has also been reported to improve psychological well-being and mood.[154] Despite the well-established benefits of exercise on mental health (e.g., reducing anxiety and tension and relieving depression),[155] it is not utilized often enough. To take full advantage of these nonpharmaceutical cost-effective benefits, exercise needs to be a more frequent recommendation.

Prescribing Exercise and Mobilization

The clinical decision-making process involved in defining the optimal mobilization and exercise stimulus for a given patient is multifactorial. The integrity of each step in the oxygen transport pathway and the overall integrity of the system in preserving arterial oxygenation and pH, are determined based on the:

Patient's history
History of the current illness
Assessment
Lab test results
Diagnostic procedure results

Once the necessary specific effects of acute mobilization or exercise are identified and matched to the patient's underlying pathophysiology (Box 18-1), the mobilization or exercise stimulus can be prescribed. Rather than a rigidly structured regimen, the prescription must evolve as the patient progresses in order to maximize its benefits (Table 18-4).

There are two primary components in assessing acute exercise responses:

1. Establishing a stable baseline founded on standardizing the preexercise conditions; and
2. Determining the appropriateness of the quantitative and qualitative changes in the objective and subjective responses during the onset of activity, the steady-state phase of activity, cool-down, and recovery.

Recovery is an important part of the exercise response assessment; postexercise hypotension in a healthy person, for example, is greater and longer after intense exercise.[156] After

Box 18-1 Common Conditions Associated with Acute Cardiovascular and Pulmonary Dysfunction That May Be Helped by the Acute Effects of Mobilization and Exercise

Atelectasis
Pulmonary consolidation
Pulmonary infiltrates
Bronchopulmonary and lobar pneumonias
Bronchiolitis
Alveolitis
Pleural effusions
Acute lung injury and pulmonary edema
Hemothorax
Pneumothorax
Cardiopulmonary insufficiency
Cardiopulmonary sequelae of surgery
Cardiopulmonary sequelae of restricted mobility

Table 18-4 Acute Mobilization and Exercise: The Clinical Decision-Making Process Underlying Mobilization Prescription

Step 1	A. Identify all factors contributing to deficits in oxygen transport (Chapter 2): 1. The underlying pathophysiology of the disease or condition 2. Restricted mobility and recumbency 3. Extrinsic factors related to the patient's care 4. Intrinsic factors related to the individual patient B. Identify the parameters that need monitoring before, during, and after each session
Step 2	Determine whether mobilization and exercise are indicated and, if so, which form of either will specifically address the oxygen transport deficits identified in step 1.
Step 3	Match the appropriate mobilization or exercise stimulus to patient's oxygen transport capacity. Examples: activities of daily living, walking unassisted, standing erect with assist and taking a few steps, transferring from bed to chair,* seated dangling position over bed side, moving in bed†
Step 4	Set the intensity within therapeutic and safe limits of the patient's oxygen transport capacity.
Step 5	Combine the various body positions, especially the erect position, with the following maneuvers: 1. Thoracic mobility exercises (flexion, extension, side flexion, and rotation) 2. Active, active assist, or passive range of motion exercises 3. Breathing control exercises, especially when coordinated with body movements 4. Coughing, spontaneous and voluntary, supported by self or others
Step 6	Set the duration of the mobilization sessions according to the patient's responses, such as changes in the measures and indexes of oxygen transport, rather than according to time.
Step 7	Repeat the mobilization sessions as often as possible according to their beneficial effects and their being safely tolerated by the patient.
Step 8	A. Increase the intensity of the mobilization stimulus, the duration of the session, or both, commensurate with the patient's capacity to maintain optimal oxygen transport when confronted with an increased mobilization stressor, and in the absence of distress; monitored variables should remain within the predetermined threshold range. B. Adjust the frequency based on patient response—in general, shorter treatments and increased frequencies (see Table 18-7).
Step 9	Continue progression until: A. The patient's functional status provides a base for resuming activities and full participation in life, with or without further physical therapy, and B. The threat to the oxygen transport system is minimized.

*All sitting positions require upright erect sitting. Propped up, semirecumbent, slouched, or slumped positions, although approximating the upright position, are not physiologically comparable.

†No amount of movement or activity is too small to derive acute or long-term benefits.

the cessation of intense exercise, CO is initially maintained by increased SV; after low-intensity exercise, it is maintained by HR.

Understanding the patient's capacity to respond to maximal or submaximal exercise is fundamental to the physical therapy assessment of most patients:

- $\dot{V}O_{2max}$ reflects the sum of the conductances of an integrated system of oxygen transport from the inspired air to the mitochondria.
- CO is in part passively regulated by the elastic characteristics of the peripheral circulation,[157] so its anatomic and physiological integrity is essential to DO_2.

The diffusive conductance of muscle is a particularly important component of oxygen transport and has become a focus of research related to impaired exercise capacity in patients with chronic heart, lung, and renal disease.[158] This may explain why the correction of central cardiovascular defects in oxygen transport can fail to restore exercise capacity in these patients.

To evaluate an apparently healthy individual who is beginning an exercise program, the Physical Activity Readiness Questionnaire (PAR-Q) is an established screening device (Figure 18-4). The answers help establish whether a progressive exercise program is indicated or whether there are contraindications to the individual's undertaking a progressive exercise program. The person may require a medical workup if cardiovascular and pulmonary risk factors or musculoskeletal limitations exist. Underlying conditions may have to be addressed beforehand or concurrently.

The prescription of mobilization and exercise to stimulate their acute benefits parallels that of the prescription of exercise for its long-term, central, and peripheral aerobic effects. The exercise parameters for achieving long-term adaptations in healthy people have been defined[14] (Table 18-5) and are generally well accepted: the individual engages in aerobic exercise at a heart rate intensity of 40%-85% of heart rate reserve (HRR) for 20 to 40 minutes, 3 to 5 days a week (HRR based on the Karvonen formula: HR_{rest} + 40%-85% [HR_{peak}/HR_{max} – HR_{rest}]). The traditional formula of training exercise (HR 70%-85% of age-predicted maximum or tested maximum, for 20 to 40 minutes, 3 to 5 days a week) may have greater utility in people with mild chronic conditions. Aerobic training effects are usually observed within 2 months.

In severely deconditioned individuals and in some other patient populations, however, such a prescription would not be realistic, ethical, or indicated. Thus exercise is prescribed that is sufficient to elicit progressive oxygen transport adaptation within defined limits of certain objective responses and subjective responses such as perceived exertion, shortness of breath, angina, discomfort/pain, and general fatigue. Considerable research however is needed to refine the prescription of mobilization and exercise for their acute effects in patients with acute cardiovascular and pulmonary dysfunction. Furthermore, specifications for the low-level exercise needed to effect long-term aerobic adaptation have not been elucidated in detail. Nonetheless, based on physiological understanding of acute exercise responses and of cardiovascular and pulmonary pathophysiology, principles for prescribing mobilization to exploit its acute effects related to oxygen transport can be formulated.

Early mobilization has been reported not only to reduce the risk for restricted mobility, but also to initiate the rehabilitation process along its continuum toward return to daily function. After an acute stroke, for example, patients undergo threat to oxygen transport in addition to the risks for restricted mobility during the acute period. A recent review of patients during this period reported low activity levels.[159]

Differences in acute aerobic exercise responses exist between men and women; one example is in those with hypertension.[160] The lower $\dot{V}O_{2max}$ in women has been attributed to both central and peripheral factors. The higher $S\bar{v}O_2$ observed in women contributes to their reduced arteriovenous oxygen difference. These findings can be explained by women's smaller muscle mass, capillary density, and oxidative capacity. Older women show depressed cardiac function compared with

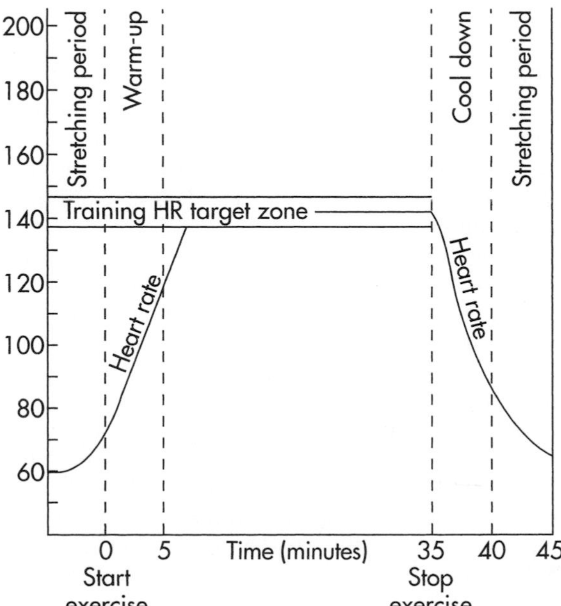

Fig. 18-4 Components of the exercise training session: stretching, warm-up, training zone, cool-down, and stretching. *(From American College of Sports Medicine:* Guidelines for exercise testing and prescription, *ed 6, Philadelphia, 2010, Lippincott, Williams & Wilkins.)*

Table 18-5 Exercise Prescription Parameters to Elicit Long-Term Aerobic Benefits in Generally Healthy People

Parameter	Specification
Exercise type	Rhythmic activity involving the large muscle groups—legs, arms, or both
Intensity	40% to 85% of HRR using predicted HR_{max} or observed HR_{max} (based on Karvonen formula)
Duration	20 to 40 minutes
Frequency	3 to 5 days/week
Course	6 to 8 weeks

HRR, Heart rate reserve, which equals (HR_{max} – HR_{rest}) × desired exercise intensity + HR_{rest}.

Modified from the American College of Sports Medicine: Guidelines for exercise testing and prescription, *ed 8, Philadelphia, 2010, Lippincott, Williams & Wilkins.*

young women; however, this difference is not observed between older and younger men.[161] Specifically, the percentage of increase in ejection fraction and the decrease in vascular resistance are depressed. This may be explained by endothelial dysfunction in postmenopausal women, which impairs peripheral vascular function during exercise.

Acute aerobic exercise responses to resistance muscle training have become more interesting clinically because the aerobic responses may have to be used as a guide to the muscle training prescription, particularly in individuals with cardiovascular risk factors and in those who are severely ill. One study examined the metabolic and cardiorespiratory responses of healthy people to maximal intermittent knee isokinetic exercise at 60 degrees/sec and 180 degrees/sec.[162] In the last 2 minutes of exercise, $\dot{V}O_2$, $\dot{V}_E$, HR, and BP were comparable, consistent with a steady rate. The slope for the increase in $\dot{V}O_2$ was steeper in the 60 degrees/sec protocol than in the 180 degrees/sec, whereas HR was unaffected by angular velocity. Neither systolic nor diastolic BP was related to exercise intensity or angular velocity of exercise. Although the metabolic and cardiorespiratory responses to intermittent isokinetic exercise of the knee mimic dynamic exercise, qualitative differences likely reflect an isometric component associated with postural stabilization. Thus the cardiorespiratory capacity of patients must be screened to ensure that they can safely meet this demand or, conversely, so that the resistance training program can secondarily augment cardiovascular conditioning.

The acute hemodynamic responses to isolated muscle testing and training are seldom considered when such training is prescribed for clinical populations such as people with low back pain. These patients tend to have weak muscle strength and poor physical conditioning.[163] Repetitive McKenzie exercises are commonly used in management; these include forward flexion of the trunk in standing and lying and back extension in standing and lying. The hemodynamic responses to these exercises have been reported to be distinct.[164] The hemodynamic stress (i.e., the effect on HR and BP) is greater in horizontal lying positions (trunk flexion greater than extension) than in the standing position (trunk flexion greater than extension). These differences may reflect the degree of postural stabilization associated with each exercise, thereby explaining the isometric muscle contraction and disproportionate changes in hemodynamic responses compared with aerobic exercise. Thus both the aerobic and isometric hemodynamic consequences of such isolated muscle exercises must be considered, regardless of whether the training is intended for managing back pain or heart disease.

Mobilization Testing for Progression

Evaluating a patient's response to a mobilization stimulus can be assessed in two ways: through challenges or through observation.

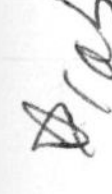

If stable, the patient can be exposed to a mobilization challenge test. The patient is monitored before, during, and after mobilization activities comparable to monitoring for a graded exercise test. Box 18-2 outlines levels of mobilization and devices that can be used (by the physical therapist or the patient) to augment the patient's performance; these are factors included in the overall prescription and are likely to be revised frequently from one treatment session to the next, or even within a session. Relatively low-intensity activities, such as bed exercises, moving in bed, changing body position, sitting up, dangling over the bed's side, transferring to a chair, doing chair exercises, and taking short walks with assistance, constitute a sufficient stimulus to elicit the acute effects of exercise, as well as gravitational stimulus. The degree of assistance required to perform the activity should be noted because it demonstrates the patient's individual effort.

Box 18-2 Examples of Activities Used to Exploit the Acute Effects of Mobilization

Mobilization Stimuli

Ambulation (independently, with one or more assisting)
Cycle ergometry (lower and upper extremities)
Activities of daily living (independently, with one or more assisting)
Standing (independently, with one or more assisting)
Transferring (independently, with one or more assisting)
Dangling (independently, with one or more assisting)
Cycle ergometry in bed (lower extremity)
Turning in bed
Bed exercises

Mobilization Aids

For the patient:
- Walking aids (crutches, cane, IV pole for support, orthoses)
- Weights
- Pulleys
- Monkey bar
- Grab bars
- Grab rope
- Portable oxygen
- Portable ventilator

For the physical therapist:
- Transfer belts
- Mechanical lifts for patients

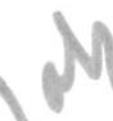

If a patient's status is unstable and oxygen transport is jeopardized, monitoring that patient during usual care, such as when turning the patient, performing daily activities, and implementing nursing and medical procedures, can provide an indication of the patient's physiological responses to mobilization and the capacity of the oxygen transport system to meet metabolic demand. Any movement that is sufficient to perturb the oxygen transport system, no matter how minimal, is sufficient to elicit short- and long-term gains. Similarly, responses should be observed during and after the imposed body position change or movement and observed for recovery time to baseline.

Patients who are acutely ill may benefit from recumbent exercise for mobilization testing and training if upright positioning is not tolerated. Body position affects exercise parameters, as well as resting parameters. End-diastolic and end-systolic left ventricular volumes and SVs are larger in the supine position than in a 70-degree upright tilt, at rest, or during exercise.[165] CO was comparable, given an increase in HR in the semirecumbent position. When subjects were tested maximally, the left ventricular ejection fraction was greater in the semirecumbent position than in the supine position. Overall, exercise capacity was greater in the supine and full upright positions than in the semirecumbent position. Thus body position affects exercise responses directly by its effect on hemodynamics and cardiac function. Careful patient monitoring is essential, given that recumbent exercise can be more physiologically stressful than exercise conducted upright.

It is important to note for the purposes of progressing a patient's mobilization and exercise prescription that differences between sexes exist in response to bed rest. The types of muscle-function changes that occur, for example, differ between men and women. Mechanical efficiency when cycling decreases in both healthy men and women after 20 days of horizontal bed rest,[166] but delta efficiency (i.e., change in work output/change in energy expended) in upright exercise compared with supine exercise is greater for men and goes unchanged in women. This is thought to reflect a selective decrement in slow-twitch muscle fibers associated with a decrease in leg muscle mass in men during bed rest.

MONITORING FOR PROGRESSION

Patients for whom mobilization is prescribed require monitoring. Because of the stress to the oxygen transport system that mobilization elicits, the following variables, in addition to oxygen transport variables, are useful:

- HR
- Systolic and diastolic BP
- RPP
- RR
- SaO_2
- Arterial blood gases
- ECG

The RPP is an index of myocardial $\dot{V}O_2$ during exercise and an indicator of the work of the heart.[167] In individuals with ischemic heart disease, the anginal threshold often can be defined by the RPP. After bed rest, healthy individuals have blunted sympathetic responses to isometric exercise in the antigravity muscles;[168] thus patients who have had periods of recumbency and restricted activity may show similar abnormal responses to exercise. Subjective responses, including discomfort and pain, fatigue, exertion, and breathlessness, can be recorded as needed. Visual analog scales are commonly used, as are modified Borg scales: 0 (nothing at all) to 10 (maximal exertion).[169] Subjective responses are more inherently variable and unreliable, therefore potentially less valid.[170] Nonetheless, intrasubject reliability may be acceptable if measures are conducted in a standardized manner and thus can serve as supplementary outcome measures.

Prescription of a Mobilization Stimulus

Prescribing a mobilization stimulus for its acute effects parallels the prescription of exercise for its long-term effects but with some important differences. In patients with acute disease, a mobilization stimulus often results in a greater response gain than is found with such a stimulus in patients with subacute or chronic illness. In addition to the rapid favorable response an acutely ill patient may have to acute exercise, the patient may exhibit a negative response just as quickly. Thus judicious monitoring of treatment responses in these patients is essential; the prescription is driven by patient response.

Patients for whom mobilization is indicated have had variable periods of recumbency that can alter their hemodynamics and autonomic function, as well as their capacity to respond normally to mobilization.[171] Hemodynamic responses even to static exercise can be blunted, and this may vary from day to day. Further, such responses can vary from hour to hour in acutely ill patients, and day to day in patients with chronic dysfunction. In patients who are severely and acutely ill, passive rather than active exercise may be the only feasible option. Little research has been done to examine the acute and chronic effects of such exercise, although when passive cycling is compared with active cycling (10% of $\dot{V}O_{2max}$) in healthy people, $\dot{V}O_2$, HR, exertion, and electromyographic (EMG) activity are predictably lower.[172] The shortening of the duration of the preejection period and the length of this period in relation to ejection time, however, is similar. Plasma catecholamines remain at resting levels for both types of exercise, but blood lactates increase in both, with higher levels occurring in active cycling. Thus the inotropic response to exercise probably depends on both skeletal muscle mechanoreceptors and the Frank-Starling effect (preload and shortening in the preejection period).

The optimal therapeutic dose of the acute mobilization stimulus, particularly the initial dose, is based on the patient's presentation and history; the specific parameters are determined by the goals of the treatment and the acute effects of exercise that are indicated. The intensity of mobilization necessary for many patients will be the intensity that elicits the reactions outlined in Box 18-3.

Over time, exposure to an acute exercise stimulus of an appropriate intensity, for an appropriate duration and at an appropriate frequency, will stimulate long-term aerobic adaptation to that stimulus. Underprescribing the exercise stimulus results in less potent effects; overprescribing results in excessive, deleterious effects. Although the latter may be tolerated in the short run, the patient's well-being may be jeopardized by suboptimal treatment responses, overtraining signs and symptoms, and risk.

The duration of each mobilization session and the frequency of sessions are response-dependent rather than time-dependent. The optimal mobilization threshold, in which physiological variables increase but not in excess of predetermined acceptable and safe limits, should be maintained for as long as possible within the patient's fatigue and comfort levels and in the absence of adverse responses (determined by ongoing monitoring). The mobilization sessions should be repeated as often as the patient can tolerate them (i.e., as often as the patient exhibits beneficial responses or no deterioration and adequately recovers between treatments). Treatment sessions for acute cardiovascular and pulmonary dysfunction are usually shorter and more frequent than for patients with chronic cardiovascular and pulmonary dysfunction. The patient's condition changes rapidly with respect to both

Box 18-3 Physiological Reactions to Appropriate Mobilization Intensity

- Optimal V_Ts
- Optimal $\dot{V}_A$
- Increased RR
- Increased air flow rates
- Enhanced mucociliary transport
- Cough stimulation

Note: All of the reactions above should occur without arterial desaturation, hemodynamic instability, or respiratory distress.

improvement and deterioration. Progression of mobilization for its immediate acute effects is usually rapid. Progression of exercise for its long-term effects may occur every several weeks, whereas progression of mobilization for its acute effects may occur as frequently as every treatment to every few days. Over time, exposure to a progressive mobilization stimulus leads to long-term physiological adaptations throughout the oxygen transport pathway. The goal is to achieve the oxygen transport status that is consistent with being able to discharge the patient from care to home or from one level of care to the next lowest level of care (e.g., from critical care to the ward).

The Mobilization Session

The scheduling of and preparation for a mobilization session is crucial to the response that can be expected. The conditions outlined in Table 18-6 should be adhered to as closely as possible, and their details should be recorded so that any factor that influences the response to treatment can be identified.

Circadian rhythms refer to physiological changes that occur in response to the fluctuating synthesis and secretion of hormones and other endocrine regulators over time (usually over 24 hours). These have a profound effect on physiological function. Circadian rhythms can be exploited in optimizing functional performance. Younger people may want to exercise later in the day, whereas older people might optimize their activity and exercise in the morning.[174] These differences are important to the physical therapist concerned with optimizing performance in patient populations whose response to activity and functional capacities may be dependent on time of day. Growth hormone production is determined by circadian fluctuations, sleep, and exercise.[175] Growth hormone is implicated in metabolism and physical performance throughout life. Thus exercise-induced growth hormone is an important effect of exercise that can optimize levels of growth hormone for general health, well-being, and successful aging. Circadian rhythms can be desynchronized during illness and, in particular, during hospitalization. That is why normal day and night cycles should be maintained, even in critical care units, so as to augment patients' recovery.

The basic components of a mobilization session should approximate the components of an exercise session described by the American College of Sports Medicine for long-term training effects[14] (Figure 18-5). Wherever possible, the session should include warm-up, steady-rate, cool-down, and recovery. These components are less distinct when a patient has minimal functional capacity or is being mobilized to remediate acute cardiovascular and pulmonary dysfunction. The rhythmic movement of large muscle groups is still ideal. Prolonged static maneuvers are usually avoided, particularly if the patient is severely ill, because of their disproportionate hemodynamic response. The movements that are usually

Table 18-6 Preparation for Mobilization

Preparation Recommendation	Specific Considerations
The patient should be physically prepared.	The patient should be rested, should not have eaten heavily in the previous couple of hours, should be as attentive and aroused as possible, and should be experiencing minimal pain, discomfort, or other distress. The patient's clothing should not be restrictive.
The patient's medication schedule should be reviewed.	A review of a patient's medication schedule will ensure that treatments are well timed with respect to analgesia and medications that interfere with an optimal treatment response, such as narcotics.
Any equipment should be noted and positioned appropriately.	Equipment, monitors, or arterial and intravenous lines (including arterial lines, intravenous lines, and catheters) should be positioned to avoid disconnections or mishaps. Mobilizing a patient in intensive care requires the positioning of the mechanical ventilator and other supports before moving the patient. Portable ventilators facilitate mobilizing and ambulating patients.[173]
Move procedures and techniques should be discussed with the team before implementation.	The physical therapist must prepare assistants before moving a patient, particularly if assistance is required. Despite the number of people assisting, the goal is usually to have the patient perform as much of the mobilization activity as possible (within the margins of safety and maximal therapeutic response). To be beneficial, even small degrees of physical movement can provide sufficient stress to the cardiovascular and pulmonary systems.

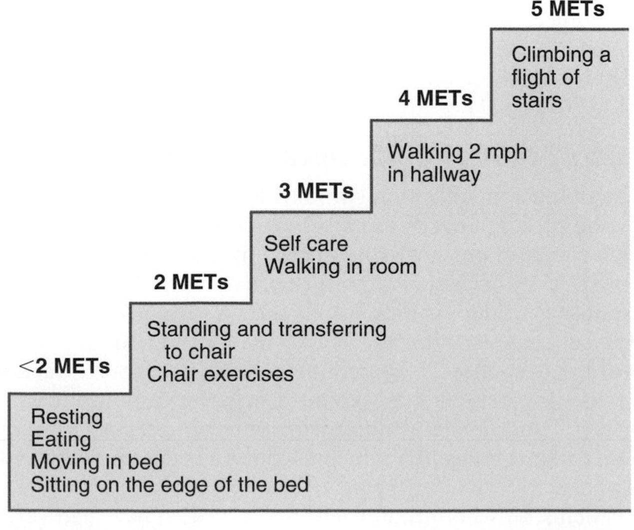

Fig. 18-5 Progression of mobilization in patients with acute medical and surgical conditions, based on a consideration of METs. *(Modified from Woods SL:* Cardiac nursing, *ed 5, Philadelphia, 2005, Lippincott, Williams & Wilkins.)*

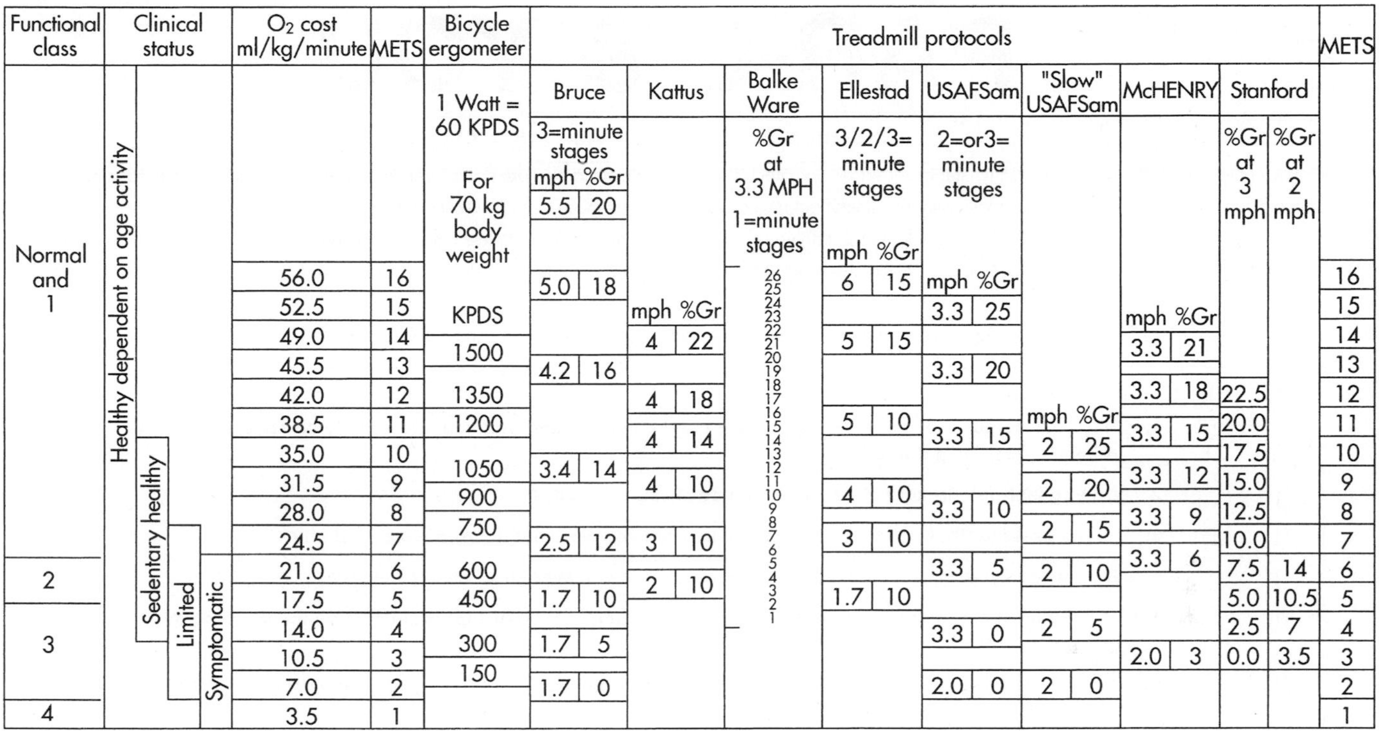

Functional class	Clinical status	O_2 cost ml/kg/minute	METS	Bicycle ergometer	Treadmill protocols: Bruce	Kattus	Balke Ware	Ellestad	USAFSam	"Slow" USAFSam	McHENRY	Stanford		METS
				1 Watt = 60 KPDS For 70 kg body weight KPDS	3=minute stages mph %Gr 5.5 20	mph %Gr	%Gr at 3.3 MPH 1=minute stages	3/2/3= minute stages mph %Gr	2=or3= minute stages mph %Gr	mph %Gr	mph %Gr	%Gr at 3 mph	%Gr at 2 mph	
Normal and 1	Healthy dependent on age activity	56.0	16		5.0 18		26 25 24 23 22 21 20 19 18 17 16 15 14 13 12 11 10 9 8 7 6 5 4 3 2 1	6 15						16
		52.5	15						3.3 25					15
		49.0	14	1500		4 22		5 15			3.3 21			14
		45.5	13		4.2 16				3.3 20					13
		42.0	12	1350		4 18					3.3 18	22.5		12
		38.5	11	1200		4 14		5 10	3.3 15		3.3 15	20.0		11
	Sedentary healthy	35.0	10	1050	3.4 14					2 25		17.5		10
		31.5	9	900		4 10				2 20	3.3 12	15.0		9
		28.0	8	750				4 10	3.3 10		3.3 9	12.5		8
	Limited	24.5	7		2.5 12	3 10		3 10		2 15		10.0		7
2	Symptomatic	21.0	6	600		2 10			3.3 5	2 10	3.3 6	7.5	14	6
		17.5	5	450	1.7 10			1.7 10				5.0	10.5	5
3		14.0	4	300					3.3 0	2 5		2.5	7	4
		10.5	3		1.7 5						2.0 3	0.0	3.5	3
		7.0	2	150	1.7 0				2.0 0	2 0				2
4		3.5	1											1

Fig. 18-6 Oxygen cost of work stages of some commonly used exercise test protocols. *(From Froehlicher VF, Myers JN:* Exercise and the heart, *ed 4, Philadelphia, 2000 Elsevier.)*

considered when mobilizing a patient include turning, sitting up, shifting, transferring, standing, and taking some steps. The progression of the levels of mobilization and exercise for medical and surgical patients, based on a consideration of metabolic cost (up to light to moderate activity), is illustrated in Figure 18-6. This schema represents the low end of the incremental staircase of activities based on the MET level shown in Figure 18-7 for a broader range of physical activities (up to very heavy activity).

Patients progress from one level to the next on the basis of their objective and subjective responses. Mobilization can be metabolically demanding for patients with acute cardiovascular and pulmonary dysfunction. Thus pacing the mobilization session allows the patient to rest between stages. The patient is reassured and encouraged to relax and coordinate deep breathing and coughing with the activity. Throughout the session, attention is given to the patient's biomechanical alignment, postural erectness, and stability. Back extension or body positioning minimizes the slumping of the chest wall and compromised ventilation. In this way, chest wall expansion is maximized in three dimensions. The erect position is efficient and requires the least amount of energy to maintain. Less demand is placed on the accessory muscles of respiration in erect sitting, and this effect is enhanced further by leaning forward and supporting the arms.

This chapter emphasizes the principles of mobilization and progression for the patient who is acutely ill but medically stable. Patients who are medically unstable, including those in the ICU, warrant special consideration, which is addressed in Chapters 33, 34, 35, and 36. Regardless of the clinical setting, however, the rate at which progression occurs typically depends on a patient's response rather than a structured protocol.

MONITORING IN THE MOBILIZATION SESSION

The more acute the patient's condition, the more important it is that physiological variables be recorded as outlined previously. The capacity to measure multiple objective measures is available in special care and intensive care units, and often these are continuously monitored. Subjective responses are also vital to refine the adequacy of the mobilization stimulus (not too much and not too little); however, severely ill patients are often unable to respond effectively or may respond unpredictably. Compared with the condition of chronic patients, the condition of acute patients tends to vary more within and between sessions and afterwards, which necessitates greater monitoring.

Monitoring should be performed continuously or at least frequently in patients for whom acute mobilization has been prescribed. First, a baseline of the patient's resting metabolic state must be established. Second, the metabolic responses to stimuli that perturb oxygen transport and the lability of these responses must be established. Obtaining such a profile provides some indication of the upper limit for the target intensity range of mobilization. The target intensity range can be defined in terms of an upper and a lower level of various physiological variables. The variables to be measured depend on the patient (see Chapters 2 and 17). Most commonly, the values described in Box 18-4 are considered basic measures and indexes of exercise response that require no invasive procedures.

Physical Activity Readiness Questionnaire - PAR-Q (revised 2002)

PAR-Q & YOU

(A Questionnaire for People Aged 15 to 69)

Regular physical activity is fun and healthy, and increasingly more people are starting to become more active every day. Being more active is very safe for most people. However, some people should check with their doctor before they start becoming much more physically active.

If you are planning to become much more physically active than you are now, start by answering the seven questions in the box below. If you are between the ages of 15 and 69, the PAR-Q will tell you if you should check with your doctor before you start. If you are over 69 year of age, and you are not used to being very active, check with your doctor.

Common sense is your best guide when you answer these questions. Please read the questions carefully and answer each one honestly: check YES or NO.

YES	NO		
☐	☐	1.	**Has your doctor ever said that you have a heart condition and that you should only do physical activity recommended by a doctor?**
☐	☐	2.	**Do you feel pain in your chest when you do physical activity?**
☐	☐	3.	**In the past month, have you had chest pain when you were not doing physical activity?**
☐	☐	4.	**Do you lose your balance because of dizziness or do you ever lose consciousness?**
☐	☐	5.	**Do you have a bone or joint problem (for example, back, knee or hip) that could be made worse by a change in your physical activity?**
☐	☐	6.	**Is your doctor currently prescribing drugs (for example, water pills) for your blood pressure or heart condition?**
☐	☐	7.	**Do you know of any other reason why you should not do physical activity?**

If you answered

YES to one or more questions

Talk with your doctor by phone or in person BEFORE you start becoming much more physically active or BEFORE you have a fitness appraisal. Tell your doctor about the PAR-Q and which questions you answered YES.

- You may be able to do any activity you want — as long as you start slowly and build up gradually. Or, you may need to restrict your activities to those which are safe for you. Talk with your doctor about the kinds of activities you wish to participate in and follow his/her advice.
- Find out which community programs are safe and helpful for you.

NO to all questions

If you answered NO honestly to all PAR-Q questions, you can be reasonably sure that you can:

- start becoming much more physically active – begin slowly and build up gradually. This is the safest and easiest way to go.
- take part in a fitness appraisal – this is an excellent way to determine your basic fitness so that you can plan the best way for you to live actively. It is also highly recommended that you have your blood pressure evaluated. If your reading is over 144/94, talk with your doctor before you start becoming much more physically active.

DELAY BECOMING MUCH MORE ACTIVE:

- if you are not feeling well because of a temporary illness such as a cold or a fever – wait until you feel better; or
- if you are or may be pregnant – talk to your doctor before you start becoming more active.

PLEASE NOTE: if your health changes so that you then answer YES to any of the above questions, tell your fitness or health professional. Ask whether you should change your physical activity plan.

Informed Use of the PAR-Q: The Canadian Society for Exercise Physiology, Health Canada, and their agents assume no liability for persons who undertake physical activity, and if in doubt after completing this questionnaire, consult your doctor prior to physical activity.

No changes permitted. You are encouraged to photocopy the PAR-Q but only if you use the entire form.

NOTE: if the PAR-Q is being given to a person before he or she participates in a physical activity program or a fitness appraisal, this section may be used for legal or administrative purposes.

"I have read, understood and completed this questionnaire. Any questions I had were answerd to my full satisfaction."

NAME ____

SIGNATURE ____ DATE ____________________

SIGNATURE OF PARENT ____ WITNESS ____________________
or GUARDIAN (for participants under the age of majority)

Note: This physical activity clearance is valid for a maximum of 12 months from the date it is completed and becomes invalid if your condition changes so that you would answer YES to any of the seven questions.

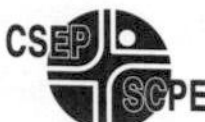

Supported by:  Health Canada Santé Canada

Fig. 18-7 The Physical Activity Readiness Questionnaire (PAR-Q). *(From Health Canada: Canadian Society for Exercise Physiology, 2005, www.csep.ca.)*

Box 18-4 Commonly Used Monitoring Variables

HR
ECG
BP
RPP
RR
Perceived exertion
Breathlessness
Discomfort/pain
Fatigue

Box 18-5 Qualitative Assessment in Monitoring

The patient's response compared with resting baseline measures
The quality as well as the immediacy of the response
The characteristics of the quality of response
- Is the response commensurate with the intensity of the exercise stimulus?
- With cessation of exercise, do the responses revert to baseline? If so, how fast?
- Do the variables return to baseline or remain above baseline?

Table 18-7 Relationships Among Mobilization and Exercise Prescription Parameters: Examples of Inverse Relationship Between Session Duration and Frequency

Incremental Activity	Session Duration	Session Frequency
Mobilization activities (e.g., self-care, moving in bed, bed exercises, sitting up in bed, sitting on the edge of the bed, standing, transferring to chair, walking)	Short (5 min) Long (20 min)	Once/1 to 2 hours 4 to 6 times/day
Interval continuous aerobic exercise	Short (5 min) Long (20 min)	Once/1 to 2 hours 4 to 6 times/day
Continuous aerobic exercise (light)	Short (5 min) Long (20 min)	Once/1 to 2 hours 4 to 6 times/day
Continuous aerobic exercise (moderate)	Short (10 min) Long (30 min)	2 to 3 times/day Once/1 to 2 days
Continuous aerobic exercise (heavy)	Short (20 min) Long (30 to 45 min)	Daily 3 to 5 days/week

Note: Intensity is set to the needs of the individual (i.e., oxygen transport and aerobic capacity are being stressed sufficiently to meet the treatment goals, with risk being minimized). The duration and frequency of treatments are based on the individual's responses and tolerance, with these being maintained within an optimal margin of safety and of recovery profiles.

At the other end of the spectrum is the critically ill patient who has various invasive lines and monitoring equipment, including hemodynamic monitoring and intracranial pressure monitoring. This patient requires more specific and frequent measurement of oxygen transport status. Several measures in high-dependency care areas can be monitored continuously, such as cardiac rhythm, HR, and BP, and arterial saturation. The use of transcutaneous oxygen and carbon dioxide tensions as indexes of gas exchange has been considered limited in exercise testing; yet their use would overcome the need for arterial cannulation.[176] The use of these measures as estimates of gas exchange has been shown to be reliable, provided the electrodes are heated and the workload changes are gradually increased to allow for latency in response time.

Monitoring during nursing procedures and other types of routine care provides an indication of the patient's functional capacity without having to conduct a modified exercise test. Detailed monitoring is conducted during a mobilization or exercise challenge. Qualitative assessments can be made based on the physical therapist's subjective impressions (Box 18-5). The patient's self-reports are also important.

Adaptation to an Acute Mobilization Stimulus

When an individual is exposed to repeated exercise stress of a specific threshold intensity and for a response-dependent duration and frequency, there is a cumulative adaptive response to that repeated stimulation, or a long-term training response. The goal is to adapt the patient to multiple short mobilization sessions per day, as frequently as once per hour as indicated and as tolerated, and progressively increase the intensity of these sessions, reduce the duration, and correspondingly reduce the frequency of sessions. Table 18-7 illustrates the inverse relationship between exercise duration and frequency of the sessions.

Mobilization activities prescribed to enhance oxygen transport can be coupled with resistive muscle work to increase muscle strength and endurance (e.g., weights, use of a monkey bar for moving in bed and sitting up, manual resistive exercise, the use of wrist or ankle weights, ergometry, and walking). Coordinating postural changes, thoracic mobility, and upper-extremity exercises with inspiratory and expiratory efforts can be effective in stimulating increased V_T and improving ventilation-perfusion matching. Chapters 22 and 23 illustrate how such movement and breathing patterns can be combined in order to maximize oxygen transport in patients with neurological conditions. Such coordinated exercise, however, can also be used in patients with acute cardiovascular and pulmonary conditions. Isometric exercises, postures that require increased muscle work for stabilization, and activities that elicit the Valsalva maneuver produce disproportionate hemodynamic responses, which could be detrimental. The capacity of the patient to respond appropriately to these loads must be assessed beforehand to minimize risk.

In deconditioned individuals and in those whose oxygen transport system has been pathologically compromised, the exercise intensity associated with relatively low-intensity mobilizing activities (such as bed exercises, moving in bed, sitting up, dangling over bedside, transferring to chair, chair exercises, and short walks with assistance) constitute sufficient progressive gravitational and exercise stimuli to initiate adaptation to being upright and moving. However, it is important to stress that optimal adaptation occurs only if these activities are prescribed at the requisite intensity, duration, and frequency, and the exercise prescription progresses commensurate with the individual's adaptation. Mechanical ventilation is not a contraindication to mobilization; new generations of mechanical ventilators are portable and perform comparably to conventional ventilation. They are associated with minimal adverse effects on hemodynamic variables and oxygen transport[173] and can facilitate mobilization and ambulation.

In the management of acute cardiovascular and pulmonary dysfunction, the parameters of mobilization stimuli include a relatively low intensity (although it is often perceived as intense by the patient), short duration, and high frequency of sessions. If the patient is severely compromised, as in end-stage heart or lung disease, interrupted or interval training is indicated. This type of training is characterized by either on-off exercise, which allows for rest in between bouts of exercise, or high-low intensities of activity. The volume of work that can be achieved in an interrupted protocol by a severely compromised patient is greater than that achievable during continuous activity. With physiological adaptation over time, the exercise period can be increased and the rest period decreased and possibly eliminated. When high- and low-intensity exercises are alternated, the workload can be progressed by increasing the respective loads in each phase or by increasing the duration of the higher load period. If the patient has a low functional work capacity but sufficient physiological reserve, adaptation can be rapid, necessitating small, frequent progressions. As the patient's aerobic capacity increases, the response gains are correspondingly smaller. If the patient has both poor functional capacity and poor physiological reserve capacity, progress would be correspondingly slower.

When mobilization is prescribed to remediate acute cardiovascular and pulmonary dysfunction, particularly in patients in the ICU, extensive and often invasive monitoring is required. This permits detailed assessment and ongoing metabolic assessment of the patient's treatment responses and recovery. With these supports, mobilization and exercise can be prescribed effectively for these patients. Judicious monitoring minimizes inherent risks for either under- or overprescribing the intensity of the exercise stimulus (see Part II). Monitoring leads, lines, and catheters may restrict body positions and activities. Such encumbrances, however, do not preclude most activities, including ambulation. Moving relatively immobile patients who are confined to their beds with lines and leads is crucial, because it is these patients who benefit significantly from exercise stress and succumb most severely to its removal.

Long-Term Effects of Mobilization and Exercise

In health, the long-term effects of exercise occur in response to a specific and sufficient exercise stimulus to which the individual is exposed for a finite period. With respect to aerobic training or adaptation, the essential training parameters for generally healthy people are shown in Table 18-5. As central and peripheral adaptation to the exercise stimulus occurs, each step in the oxygen transport system becomes more efficient in facilitating DO_2, $\dot{V}O_{2max}$, and extraction at the cellular level.[6,15,19] The long-term effects of aerobic exercise are summarized in Table 18-8.

CARDIOVASCULAR AND PULMONARY EFFECTS

In addition to an increase in $\dot{V}O_{2max}$, training results in exercise-induced bradycardia and increased SV at rest and in reduction in the physiological demands of submaximal work

Table 18-8 Long-Term Physiological Effects of Mobilization and Exercise

Body System Affected	Specific Effects
Pulmonary	Decreased submaximal minute ventilation Increased respiratory muscle strength and endurance Increased collateral ventilation Increased pulmonary vascularization
Cardiovascular	Increased myocardial muscle mass Increased myocardial efficiency Exercise-induced bradycardia Decreased stroke volume at rest and submaximal work rates Decreased resting heart rate and blood pressure Decreased submaximal heart rate, blood pressure, and rate pressure product Decreased submaximal perceived exertion and breathlessness Increased efficiency of thermoregulation Decreased orthostatic intolerance when performed in the upright position
Hematological	Increased circulating blood volume Increased number of red blood cells Optimize hematocrit Optimize cholesterol Decreased blood lipids
Central Nervous	Increased sense of well-being Increased concentration
Neuromuscular	Enhance neuromotor control Increased efficiency of postural reflexes associated with type of exercise Increased efficiency of reflex control Increased movement efficiency and economy
Musculoskeletal	Increased muscle vascularization Increased myoglobin Increased muscle metabolic enzymes Increased glycogen storage capacity Increased biomechanical efficiency Increased movement economy Muscle hypertrophy Increased muscle strength and endurance Increased ligament tensile strength Maintain bone density
Endocrine	Increased efficiency of hormone production and degradation to support exercise
Immunological	Increased resistance to infection
Integumentary	Increased efficiency of skin as a heat exchanger Increased sweating efficiency Decreased skin abrasions and breakdown Increased healing

rates. Specifically, ventilation and hemodynamic responses to submaximal exercise are decreased. Endurance training increases parasympathetic activity and decreases sympathetic activity at rest.[177] Arterial stiffness is decreased,[178] and microcirculatory function and tissue perfusion are improved.[179] The subjective experience of exercise stress is also reduced. These training effects are commensurate with increases in the efficiency of oxygen transport at each step in the pathway. Unlike the effects in patients with low functional work capacity, however, exercise does not improve ventilatory performance, as is evidenced by the relationship between ventilation and the production of carbon dioxide:[180]

$$\dot{V}_E - \dot{V}CO_2 \text{ slope}$$

and

$$\dot{V}_E/\dot{V}CO_2$$

Because of the marked ventilatory reserve in health, it is normally CO, rather than ventilation, that limits exercise. However, there is some evidence that the respiratory system can limit endurance in healthy sedentary people, in athletes (especially women) with a higher fitness level, and in patients with chronic respiratory disease.[181-183]

Although change in $\dot{V}O_{2peak}$ is the gold standard for aerobic conditioning, theoretically, submaximal $\dot{V}O_2$ values for given work rates do not change with training[184] unless improvement in movement efficiency and economy has occurred. With training, an individual reduces the physiological responses to each exercise load on an incremental exercise test and so is able to achieve a higher work load, thus a higher $\dot{V}O_{2peak}$ with training.

The theory that maximum HR (HR_{max}) is genetically determined and does not change with training has been challenged.[185] Factors that down-regulate HR have been implicated in resetting maximum heart rate. Such factors include the baroreceptors, autonomic function, electrophysiology of the sinoatrial node, and a reduction in the number and density of beta-adrenergic receptors.

The rheology of blood plays an important role in cardiovascular disease. Platelet adhesiveness and aggregation are reduced with regular aerobic exercise.[71] Optimal platelet adhesiveness along with blood volume maintain optimal blood viscosity, which is important for blood flow through the heart and blood vessels and for perfusion of peripheral tissue. Increased plasma viscosity and hematocrit have been attributed to exercise-induced hemoconcentration as a result of the shift of fluid from the blood to the interstitium.[186] With long-term endurance training, the plasma volume expands, which may reduce the resistance of blood flow to working muscle.

Exercise is a powerful controller of normal BP and an effective intervention to control high BP in patients with hypertension. The antihypertensive effects of long-term aerobic exercise are mediated through a reduction in total peripheral resistance and altered blood rheology. In addition, exercise may lead to weight loss, which contributes to lower BP. Individuals who are normotensive experience no changes in BP with an aerobic exercise program, even though peripheral resistance is reduced.[187]

Aerobic exercise improves the hemodynamic responses and lipid profiles of individuals with cardiac disease (see Chapter 24). Walking, cycling, and running are common types of aerobic exercise. However, patients from other cultures and those who do not enjoy these types of exercise may prefer tai chi, which also has been shown to have beneficial effects on BP, lipid profiles, and relaxation.[188,189]

Hemoglobin concentration and the number of circulating red blood cells are essential to effecting optimal oxygen transport (see Chapters 2 and 13). A single bout of exercise, as well as long-term exercise, can influence the erythropoietin processes in bone marrow.[190] In the extreme, exercise can interfere with these processes and result in "sports anemia." This condition can reflect postexercise plasma expansion, increased hemolysis with intense exercise, iron deficiency, bleeding into the digestive and urinary systems, and abnormal erythropoiesis.

Changes in cardiac structure and function after prolonged exercise by healthy people have been of interest to researchers in their attempt to understand changes during ill health. Questions such as "Does the heart muscle show signs of fatigue and impaired function with such exercise?" have been posed. One study of highly trained male athletes showed some cardiac damage, along with reduced diastolic filling and contractility of the left ventricle, after completion of a half-ironman triathlon.[191]

CENTRAL NERVOUS SYSTEM EFFECTS

The responses of the CNS to training include autonomic nervous system conditioning that is associated with BP control and thermoregulation.[192] Training is associated with a more sensitive vascular response to stress, which may reflect greater alpha-adrenergic sensitivity.[193] The capacity to sweat is primed in response to exercise, which ensures that the muscle and internal organs remain at a temperature that is metabolically and energetically optimal for a given workload.

As the body adapts to the exercise training stimulus (overload principle), the intensity is increased to elicit further training benefit. This is the basis for the physiological adaptation to a training stimulus. Depending on the goals of the exercise prescription, a decision is made after several weeks about whether the exercise intensity should be raised to further increase aerobic capacity or whether a maintenance program is indicated. The training program is progressed by establishing a new exercise intensity, which usually is based on 40% to 85% of the HRR achieved in a repeat of the initial exercise test.

METABOLIC EFFECTS

The effect of exercise on glucose kinetics is clinically important for several reasons. First, illness creates metabolic stress on glucose metabolism; second, bed rest reduces insulin sensitivity; third, sedentary lifestyle and high-glycemic diets contribute to hyperglycemia and insulin insensitivity; and fourth, physical therapy's primary drug, exercise, places stress on energy substrates, including glucose metabolism, commensurate with the type, intensity, and duration of exercise. The time course of changes in glucose metabolism is important to the physical therapist because the patient must be protected from hypoglycemia and the effects of training on the muscles' sensitivity to insulin must be optimized. Even though these changes are well known to occur with multiple weeks of aerobic training, serial measures over the training period show that after 10 days there are benefits to glucose kinetics.[194]

EFFECTS IN SPECIAL POPULATIONS

Aggressive mobilization/exercise has been reported to have significant functional impact in the management of patients in the ICU. Prolonged intensive physical training, for example, has been reported to result in the regeneration of skeletal muscle after prolonged catabolism and weight loss.[195] Despite studies supporting aggressive mobilization, the physical therapist needs to establish the optimal dose at any given time and to monitor to ensure the best response and the least risk.

Aerobic power declines with age. The capacity to train, however, is not age-limited; training effects have been reported in octogenarians.[196] Often older people show greater gains in response to training because of their reduced levels of baseline conditioning. Oxygen kinetics may be slowed with aging. Training responses reflect an increasing contribution to aerobic training by peripheral as opposed to central adaptations.[197] Furthermore, based on a 30-year follow-up study, age-related decline in aerobic power over the course of 30 years was reversible with aerobic training.[197] Tasks and exercises that involve various physiological systems are differentially affected by aging as well as by training. Training profiles of young and middle-aged adults show an age-related performance decline in cardiorespiratory endurance but not in muscle endurance.[198] This finding has implications for norms of fitness and prognosis for recovery. Finally, lack of exercise has been implicated in the incidence of cognitive impairment in older adults.[199] Physiological changes associated with aging, particularly those related to exercise capacity, are often confounded by deconditioning and related physical deterioration in older adults rather than being an immutable consequence of aging.[200]

Summary

Physical therapists are clinical exercise physiologists whose primary interventions include mobilization and exercise to address limitations in participation and activity irrespective of whether these limitations result from primary or secondary cardiovascular/pulmonary dysfunction. This chapter first distinguishes mobilization, physical activity, and exercise. The role of mobilization and exercise in assessment and evaluation is addressed. Next, the chapter describes three distinct goals associated with the prescription of mobilization and exercise in the management of impaired oxygen transport: to exploit the preventive effects, acute effects, and long-term effects of mobilization and exercise so as to maximize an individual's oxygen transport capacity and his or her capacity for activity and participation in life when that person is limited by impairment of oxygen transport at the structural and functional levels. Special attention is given to prolonged sedentary behavior and to bed rest, focusing on how their injurious effects can be prevented.

The physical therapist needs a comprehensive and detailed understanding of the potent and direct effects of mobilization and exercise on oxygen transport preventively, acutely, and in the long term, as well as their multisystem effects. The specific mobilization or exercise prescription is based on a comprehensive multisystem assessment, an analysis of oxygen transport dysfunction or failure, and the treatment goals for a given patient. Ongoing monitoring is essential for defining the starting point of a mobilization or exercise program, progressing it over time, and evaluating time for discontinuation. Progression is response-dependent rather than protocol-dependent; thus patients will progress at varying rates.

Review Questions

1. Describe how the physical therapy exploitation of the effects of mobilization and exercise is congruent with the levels of the WHO International Classification of Functioning, Disability and Health (i.e., structure and function, activity, and participation).
2. Distinguish among mobilization, physical activity, and exercise.
3. Describe (a) the effect of sedentary activity on health and (b) the implications of prolonged periods of inactivity for people who may exercise regularly according to established guidelines—for example, 40% to 85% of heart rate reserve (based on the Karvonen formula) for 20 to 40 minutes, 3 to 5 days a week.
4. Describe the negative sequelae of restricted mobility and bed rest.
5. Describe the physiological changes that take place as an individual undertakes acute exercise and that must occur to effect a conditioning response.
6. Describe the distinction between "prescriptive" mobilization or exercise and its "routine" clinical use to prevent the sequelae of recumbency and restricted activity.
7. Describe the clinical relevance of physical therapists' prescribing response-dependent versus protocol-dependent mobilization.

References

1. Dean E, Murphy S, Parrent L, et al: Metabolic consequences of physical therapy in critically ill patients. Proceedings of the World Confederation of Physical Therapy Congress, Washington, DC, 1995.
2. Weissman C, Kemper M, Damask MC, et al: Effect of routine intensive care interactions on metabolic rate. *Chest* 86:815–818, 1984.
3. Butcher SJ, Jones RL: The impact of exercise training intensity on change in physiological function in patients with chronic obstructive pulmonary disease. *Sports Medicine* 36:307–325, 2006.
4. Marciniuk DD, Butcher SJ, Reid JK, et al: The effects of helium-hyperoxia on 6-min walking distance in COPD: a randomized controlled trial. *Chest* 131:1659–1665, 2007.
5. Butcher SJ, Lagerquist O, Marciniuk DD, et al: Relationship between ventilatory constraint and muscle fatigue during exercise in COPD. *European Respiratory Journal* 33:763–770, 2009.
6. McArdle WD, Katch FI, Katch VL: *Essentials of exercise physiology*, ed 3, Philadelphia, 2005, Lippincott Williams & Wilkins.
7. Rodeheffer RJ, Gerstenblith G, Beard E, et al: Postural changes in cardiac volumes in men in relation to adult age. *Experimental Gerontology* 21:367–378, 1986.
8. Dawson E, George K, Shave R, et al: Does the human heart fatigue subsequent to prolonged exercise? *Sports Medicine* 33:365–380, 2003.
9. Zhou B, Conlee RK, Jensen R, et al: Stroke volume does not plateau during graded exercise in elite male distance runners. *Medicine and Science in Sport and Exercise* 33:1849–1854, 2001.
10. Jones NL, Fletcher I: *Clinical exercise testing*, ed 4, Philadelphia, 1997, Elsevier.
11. Pyne DB: Regulation of neutrophil function during exercise. *Sports Medicine* 17:245–258, 1994.
12. Wolff RK, Dolovich MB, Obminski G, et al: Effects of exercise and eucapnic hyperventilation on bronchial clearance in man. *Journal of Applied Physiology* 43:46–50, 1977.

13. Skerrett SJ, Niederman MS, Fein AM: Respiratory infections and acute lung injury in systemic illness. *Clinics in Chest Medicine* 10:469–502, 1989.
14. American College of Sports Medicine: *ACSM's guidelines for exercise testing and prescription*, ed 8, Philadelphia, 2010, Lippincott Williams & Wilkins.
15. Astrand PO, Rodahl K, Dahl H, et al: *Textbook of work physiology: Physiological basis of exercise*, ed 4, Philadelphia, 2003, Human Kinetics.
16. Belman MJ, Wasserman K: Exercise training and testing in patients with chronic obstructive lung disease. *Basics of Respiratory Disease* 10:1–6, 1981.
17. Ehrman JK, De Jong A, editors: American College of Sports Medicine. *Resource manual for guidelines for exercise testing and training*, ed 6, Philadelphia, 2010, Wolters Kluwer Health/Lippincott Williams & Wilkins.
18. Ehrman JK, Gordon PM, Visich PS, et al, editors: *Clinical exercise physiology*, ed 2, Champaign, Ill, 2009, Human Kinetics.
19. Froelicher VF, Myers JN: *Exercise and the heart*, ed 5, Philadelphia, 2006, Elsevier.
20. Irwin S, Tecklin JS, editors: *Cardiopulmonary physical therapy*, ed 4, Philadelphia, 2004, Elsevier.
21. Woods SL: *Cardiac nursing*, ed 5, Philadelphia, 2010, Lippincott, Wolters Kluwer Health/Lippincott Williams & Wilkins.
22. Noonan V, Dean E: Submaximal exercise testing: Clinical application and interpretation. *Physical Therapy* 80:782–807, 2000.
23. Orlava OE: Therapeutic physical culture in the complex treatment of pneumonia. *Physical Therapy Review* 39:153–160, 1959.
24. Dean E, Ross J: Discordance between cardiopulmonary physiology and physical therapy. Toward a rational basis for practice. *Chest* 101:1694–1698, 1992.
25. Weissman C, Kemper M: The oxygen uptake-oxygen delivery relationship during ICU interventions. *Chest* 99:430–435, 1991.
26. Chase GA, Grave C, Rowell LB: Independence of changes in functional and performance capacities attending prolonged bed rest. *Aerospace Medicine* 17:1232–1237, 1966.
27. Convertino VA, Hung J, Goldwater D, et al: Cardiovascular responses to exercise in middle-aged men after 10 days of bed rest. *Circulation* 65:134–140, 1982.
28. Winslow EH: Cardiovascular consequences of bed rest. *Heart Lung* 14:236–246, 1985.
29. Topp R, Ditmyer M, King K, et al: The effect of bed rest and potential of prehabilitation on patient in the intensive care unit. *AACN Clinical Issues* 13:263–276, 2002.
30. Rosenstein G, Cafri C, Weinstein JM, et al: Simple clinical risk stratification and the safety of ambulation two hours after 6 French diagnostic heart catheterization. *Journal of Invasive Cardiology* 16:126–128, 2004.
31. Convertino VA: Cardiovascular consequences of bed rest: effect on maximal oxygen uptake. *Medicine and Science in Sport and Exercise* 2:191–196, 1997.
32. Mujika I, Padilla S: Detraining: loss of training-induced physiological and performance adaptations. I: Short-term insufficient training stimulus. *Sports Medicine* 30:79–87, 2000a.
33. Alkner BA, Tesch PA: Efficacy of a gravity-independent resistance exercise device as a countermeasure to muscle atrophy during 29-day bed rest. *Acta Physiologica Scandinavica* 181:345–357, 2004.
34. Shackelford LC, LeBlanc AD, Driscoll TB, et al: Resistance exercise as a countermeasure to disuse-induced bone loss. *Journal of Applied Physiology* 97:119–129, 2004.
35. Greenleaf JE: Intensive exercise training during bed rest attenuates deconditioning. *Medicine and Science in Sports and Exercise* 29:207–215, 1997.
36. Lee SM, Bennett BS, Hargens AR, et al: Upright exercise or supine lower body negative pressure exercise maintains exercise responses after bed rest. *Medicine and Science in Sport and Exercise* 29:892–900, 1997.
37. Schneider SM, Watenpaugh DE, Lee SM, et al: Lower-body negative pressure exercise and bed-rest-mediated orthostatic intolerance. *Medicine and Science in Sport and Exercise* 34:1446–1453, 2002b.
38. Suzuki Y, Kashihara H, Takenaka K, et al: Effects of daily mild supine exercise on physical performance after 20 days of bed rest in young persons. *Acta Astraunaut* 33:101–111, 1994.
39. Mujika I, Padilla S: Detraining: loss of training-induced physiological and performance adaptations. II: Long-term insufficient training stimulus. *Sports Medicine* 30:145–154, 2000b.
40. Belin De Chantemele E, Blanc S, Pellet N, et al: Does resistance exercise prevent body fluid changes after a 90-day bed rest? *European Journal of Applied Physiology* 29:555–564, 2004.
41. Greenleaf JE, Juhos LT, Young HL: Plasma lactic dehydrogenase activities in men during bed rest with exercise training. *Aviation and Space Environmental Medicine* 56:193–198, 1985.
42. Oja P: Dose response between total volume of physical activity and health and fitness. *Medicine and Science in Sports and Exercise* 33(6 Suppl):S428–S437, 2001.
43. Shepherd RJ: Absolute versus relative intensity of physical activity in a dose response context. *Medicine and Science in Sports and Exercise* 33(6 Suppl):S400–S418, 2001.
44. Kohl HW III: Physical activity and cardiovascular disease: Evidence for a dose response. *Medicine & Science in Sports & Exercise* 33(6 Suppl):S472–S483, 2001.
45. Healy GN, Dunstan DW, Salmon J, et al: Breaks in sedentary time. Beneficial associations with metabolic risk. *Diabetes Care* 31:661–666, 2008.
46. Thorp AA, Healy GN, Owen N, et al: Deleterious associations of sitting time and television viewing time with cardiometabolic risk biomarkers. *Diabetes Care* 33:327–334, 2010.
47. Biddle SJH, Pearson N, Ross GM, et al: Tracking of sedentary behaviors of young people: A systematic review. *Preventive Medicine* 51:345–351, 2010.
48. Ryan AS: Exercise in aging: its important role in mortality, obesity and insulin resistance. *Aging Health* 6:551–563, 2010.
49. Allen C, Glasziou P, Del Mar C: Bed rest: a potentially harmful treatment needing more careful evaluation. *Lancet* 354:1229–1233, 1999.
50. Bassey EJ, Fentem PH: Extent of deterioration in physical condition during postoperative bed rest and its reversal by rehabilitation. *British Medical Journal* 4:194–196, 1974.
51. Chobanian AV, Lille RD, Tercyak A, et al: The metabolic and hemodynamic effects of prolonged bed rest in normal subjects. *Circulation* 49:551–559, 1974.
52. Dock W: The evil sequelae of complete bed rest. *Journal of the American Medical Association* 125:1083–1085, 1944.
53. Harrison TR: The abuse of rest as a therapeutic measure for patients with cardiovascular disease. *Journal of the American Medical Association* 125;1075–1077, 1944.
54. Knight J, Nigam Y, Jones A: Effects of bedrest 1: Cardiovascular, respiratory and haematological systems. 2009. wwwNursingtimesNet/nursing-practice/clinical-specialisms/cardiology/effects-of-bedrest-1-cardiovascular-respiratory-and-haematological-systems/5002005Article, retrieved February 2011.
55. Levine BD, Zuckerman JH, Pawelczyk JA: Cardiac atrophy after bed-rest deconditioning. A nonneural mechanism for orthostatic intolerance. *Circulation* 96:517–525, 1997.
56. Ross J, Dean E: Integrating physiological principles into the comprehensive management of cardiopulmonary dysfunction. *Physical Therapy* 69:255–259, 1989.
57. Saltin B, Blomqvist G, Mitchell JH, et al: Response to exercise after bed rest and after training. *Circulation* 38(VII):S1–S78, 1968.
58. McGuire DK, Levine BD, Williamson JW, et al: A 30-year follow-up of the Dallas Bedrest and Training Study: I. Effect of age on the cardiovascular response to exercise. *Circulation* 104:1350–1357, 2001a.
59. Kottke FJ: The effects of limitation of activity upon the human body. *Journal of the American Medical Association* 196:825–830, 1966.
60. Sandler H, Popp RL, Harrison DC: The hemodynamic effects of repeated bed rest exposure. *Aerospace Medicine* 59:1047–1053, 1988.
61. Harper CM, Lyles YM: Physiology and complications of bed rest. *Journal of the American Geriatrics Society* 36:1047–1054, 1988.
62. Bejma J, Ramires P, Ji LL: Free radical generation and oxidative stress with ageing and exercise: Differential effects in the myocardium and liver. *Acta Physiologica Scandinavica* 169:434–351, 2000.
63. Landin RJ, Linnemeier TJ, Rothbaum DA, et al: Exercise testing and training of the elderly patient. *Cardiovascular Clinics* 15:201–218, 1985.
64. Lennon S, Quindry JC, Hamilton KL, et al: Loss of exercise-induced cardioprotection following cessation of exercise. *Journal of Applied Physiology* 96:1299–1305, 2004.
65. Lampinen P, Heikkinen E: Reduced mobility and physical activity as predictors of depressive symptoms among community-dwelling older adults: An eight-year follow-up study. *Aging Clinical and Experimental Research* 15:205–211, 2003.
66. Ferretti G, Girardis M, Moia C, et al: Effects of prolonged bed rest on cardiovascular oxygen transport during submaximal exercise in humans. *European Journal of Applied Physiology and Occupational Physiology* 78:398–402, 1998.
67. Grenon SM, Hurwitz S, Sheynberg N, et al: Role of individual predisposition in orthostatic intolerance before and after simulated microgravity. *Journal of Applied Physiology* 96:1714–1722, 2004a.
68. Grenon SM, Sheynberg N, Hurwitz S, et al: Renal, endocrine, and cardiovascular responses to bed rest in male subjects on a constant diet. *Journal of Investigative Medicine* 52:117–128, 2004b.

69. Hirayanagi K, Iwase S, Kamiya A, et al: Functional changes in autonomic nervous system and baroreceptor reflex induced by 14 days of 6 degrees head-down bed rest. *European Journal of Applied Physiology* 92:160–167, 2004.
70. Hirayanagi K, Kamiya A, Iwase S, et al: Autonomic cardiovascular changes during and after 14 days of head-down bed rest. *Autonomic Neuroscience* 27:110:121–128, 2004.
71. Wang JS, Jen CJ, Chen HI: Effects of exercise training and deconditioning on platelet function in men. *Arteriosclerosis and Thrombosis* 15:1668–1674, 1995.
72. Jacobs LG: Prophylactic anticoagulation for venous thromboembolic disease in geriatric patients. *Journal of the American Gerontological Society* 51:1472–1478, 2003.
73. Harvey RL: Prevention of venous thromboembolism after stroke. *Topics in Stroke Rehabilitation* 10:61–69, 2003.
74. Blair E, Hickman JB: The effect of change in body position on lung volumes and intrapulmonary gas mixing in normal subjects. *Journal of Clinical Investigation* 34:383–389, 1995.
75. Craig DB, Wahba WM, Don H, et al: "Closing volume" and its relationship to gas exchange in the seated and supine positions. *Journal of Applied Physiology* 31:717–721, 1971.
76. Hsu HO, Hickey RF: Effect of posture on functional residual capacity postoperatively. *Anesthesiology* 44:520–521, 1976.
77. Powers, JH: The abuse of rest as a therapeutic measure in surgery. *Journal of the American Medical Association* 125:1079–1083, 1944.
78. Svanberg L: Influence of position on the lung volumes, ventilation and circulation in normals. *Scandinavian Journal of Clinical and Laboratory Investigations* 25:1–195, 1957.
79. Sjostrand T: Determination of changes in the intrathoracic blood volume in man. *Acta Physiologica Scandinavica* 22:116–128, 1951.
80. Cardus D: O_2 alveolar-arterial tension differences after 10 days' recumbency in man. *Journal of Applied Physiology* 23:934–937, 1967.
81. Clauss RH, Scalabrini BY, Ray JF, et al: Effects of changing body positions upon improved ventilation-perfusion relationships. *Circulation* 37(Suppl 4):214–217, 1968.
82. Ray JF, Yost L, Moallem S, et al: Immobility, hypoxemia, and pulmonary arteriovenous shunting. *Archives of Surgery* 109:537–541, 1974.
83. Bleeker MWP, De Groot PCE, Pawelczyk JA, et al: Effects of 18 days of bed rest on leg and arm venous properties. *Journal of Applied Physiology* 96:840–847, 2004.
84. Zhang R, Zuckerman JH, Pawelczyk JA, et al: Effects of head-down-tilt bed rest on cerebral hemodynamics during orthostatic stress. *Journal of Applied Physiology* 83:2139–2145, 1997.
85. Lentz, M: Selected aspects of deconditioning secondary to immobilization. *Nursing Clinics of North America* 16:729–737, 1981.
86. Kubo K, Akima H, Ushiyama J, et al: Effects of 20 days of bed rest on the viscoelastic properties of tendon structures in lower limb muscles. *British Journal of Sports Medicine* 38:324–330, 2004.
87. Kasper CE, Talbot LA, Gaines JM: Skeletal muscle damage and recovery. *AACN Clinical Issues* 13:237–247, 2002.
88. Rubin M: The physiology of bed rest. *American Journal of Nursing* 88:50–56, 1988.
89. Trappe S, Trappe T, Gallagher P, et al: Human single muscle fibre function with 84 day bed-rest and resistance exercise. *Journal of Physiology* 557: 501–513, 2004.
90. Akima H, Kuno S, Suzuki Y, et al: Effects of 20 days of bed rest on physiological cross-sectional area of human thigh and leg muscles evaluated by magnetic resonance imaging. *Journal of Gravitational Physiology* 4:S15–S21, 1997.
91. Yamamoto T, Sekiya N, Miyashita S, et al: Gender differences in effects of 20 days horizontal bed rest on muscle strength in young subjects. *Journal of Gravitational Physiology* 4:S31–S36, 1997.
92. Farrell PA: Protein metabolism and age: Influence of insulin and resistance exercise. *International Journal of Sport, Nutrition and Exercise Metabolism* 11(Suppl):S150–S163, 2001.
93. Takata S, Yasui N: Disuse osteoporosis. *Journal of Medical Investigation* 48:147–156, 2001.
94. Bloomfield SA: Changes in musculoskeletal structure and function with prolonged bed rest. *Medicine and Science in Sports and Exercise* 29:197–206, 1997.
95. Lindgren M, Unosson M, Fredrikson M, et al: Immobility—a major risk factor for development of pressure ulcers among adult hospitalized patients: A prospective study. *Scandinavian Journal of Caring Science* 18:57–64, 2004.
96. Winkelman C: Inactivity and inflammation: Selected cytokines as biologic mediators in muscle dysfunction during critical illness. *AACN Clinical Issues* 15:74–82, 2004.
97. Krasnoff J, Painter P: The physiologic consequences of bed rest and inactivity. *Advances in Renal Replacement Therapy* 6:124–132, 1999.
98. Hasser EM, Moffitt JA: Regulation of sympathetic nervous system function after cardiovascular deconditioning. *Annals of the New York Academy of Science* 940:454–468, 2001.
99. Ryback RS, Lewis OF, Lessard CS: Psychobiologic effects of prolonged bed rest (weightless) in young healthy volunteers. Study II. *Aerospace Medicine* 42:529–535, 1971.
100. Kamiya A, Michikami D, Fu Q, et al: Pathophysiology or orthostatic hypotension after bed rest: paradoxical sympathetic withdrawal. *American Journal of Physiology. Heart and Circulatory Physiology* 285:H1158–H1167, 2003.
101. Mikines KJ, Richter EA, Dela F, et al: Seven days of bed rest decrease insulin action on glucose uptake in leg and whole body. *Journal of Applied Physiology* 70:1245–1254, 1991.
102. Deitrick JE, Whedon GD, Shorr E: Effects of immobilization upon various metabolic and physiologic functions of normal man. *American Journal of Medicine* 4:3–36, 1948.
103. Hulley SB, Vogel JM, Donaldson CL, et al: The effect of supplemental oral phosphate on the bone mineral changes during prolonged bed rest. *Journal of Clinical Investigation* 50:2506–2518, 1971.
104. Stannard SR, Johnson NA: Insulin resistance and elevated triglyceride in muscle: more important for survival than 'thrifty' genes? *Journal of Physiology* 554:595–607, 2004.
105. Ahlinder S, Birke G, Norberg R, et al: Metabolism and distribution of IgG in patients confined to prolonged strict bed rest. *Acta Medica Scandinavica* 187:267–270, 1970.
106. Sonnfeld G: Space flight, microgravity, stress, and immune responses. *Advances in Space Research* 23:1945–1953, 1999.
107. Havas E, Komulainen J, Vihko V: Exercise-induced increase in serum creatine kinase is modified by subsequent bed rest. *International Journal of Sports Medicine* 18:578–582, 1997.
108. Ishizaki Y, Fukuoka H, Ishizaki T, et al: Evaluation of psychological effects due to bed rest. *Journal of Gravitational Physiology* 7:183–184, 2000.
109. Powers J, Daniels D: Turning points: implementing kinetic therapy in the ICU. *Nursing Management* 35(Suppl):1–7, 2004.
110. Schimmel L, Civetta JM, Kirby RR: A new mechanical method to influence pulmonary perfusion in critically ill patients. *Critical Care Medicine* 5:277–279, 1977.
111. Nelson LD, Anderson HB: Physiologic effects of steep positioning in the surgical intensive care unit. *Archives of Surgery* 124:352–355, 1989.
112. Summer WR, Curry P, Haponik EF, et al: Continuous mechanical turning of intensive care unit patients shortens length of stay in some diagnostic-related groups. *Journal of Critical Care* 4:45–53, 1989.
113. Delaney A, Gray H, Laupland KB, et al: Kinetic bed therapy to prevent nosocomial pneumonia in mechanically ventilated patients: a systematic review and meta-analysis. *Critical Care* 10:R70:1–12, 2006.
114. Needham DM: Mobilizing patients in the intensive care unit. Improving neuromuscular weakness and physical function. *Journal of the American Medical Association* 305:437–522, 2011.
115. Levin SA, Lown B: Armchair treatment of acute coronary thrombosis. *Journal of the American Medical Association* 148:1365–1369, 1952.
116. Kinney MR, Packa DR: *Andreoli's comprehensive cardiac care*, ed 7, Philadelphia, 1996, Elsevier.
117. Carter JB: Effect of endurance exercise on autonomic control of heart rate. *Sports Medicine* 33:33–46, 2003.
118. Boutellier U: Respiratory muscle fitness and exercise endurance in healthy humans. *Medicine and Science in Sport and Exercise* 30:1169–1172, 1998.
119. Inbar O, Weinter P, Azgad Y, et al: Specific inspiratory muscle training in well-trained endurance athletes. *Medicine and Science in Sport and Exercise* 32:1233–1237, 2000.
120. Markov G, Spengler CM, Knopfli-Lenzin C, et al: Respiratory muscle training increases cycling endurance without affecting cardiovascular responses to exercise. *European Journal of Applied Physiology* 85:233–239, 2001.
121. Williams JS, Wongsathikun J, Boon SM, et al: Inspiratory muscle training fails to improve endurance capacity in athletes. *Medicine and Science in Sport and Exercise* 34:1194–1198, 2002.
122. Gobel FL, Norstrom LA, Nelson RR, et al: The rate-pressure product as an index of myocardial oxygen consumption during exercise in patients with angina pectoris. *Circulation* 57:549–556, 1978.

123. Ferguson S, Gledhill N, Jamnik VK, et al: Cardiac performance in endurance-trained and moderately active young women. *Medicine and Science in Sports and Exercise* 33:1114–1119, 2001.
124. Spina RJ, Rashid S, Davila-Roman VG, et al: Adaptations in beta-adrenergic cardiovascular responses to training in older women. *Journal of Applied Physiology* 89:2300–2305, 2000.
125. West JB: *Respiratory physiology: The essentials*, ed 8, Philadelphia, 2008, Wolters Kluwer Health/Williams & Wilkins.
126. Sandler H: Cardiovascular effects of inactivity. In Sandler H, Vernikos J, editors: *Inactivity physiological effects*, New York, 1986, Academic Press.
127. Warburton DE, Haykowsky MJ, Quinney HA, et al: Myocardial responses to incremental exercise in endurance-trained athletes: influence of heart rate, contractility and the Frank-Starling effect. *Experimental Physiology* 87:613–622, 2002.
128. Leyk D, Essfeld D, Hoffmann U, et al: Postural effect on cardiac output, oxygen uptake and lactate during cycle exercise of varying intensity. *European Journal of Applied Physiology and Occupational Physiology* 68:30–35, 1994.
129. Nagashima K, Mack GW, Haskell A, et al: Mechanism for the posture-specific plasma volume increase after a single intense exercise protocol. *Journal of Applied Physiology* 86:867–873, 1999.
130. Goette A, Weber M, Lendeckel U, et al: Effect of physical exercise on platelet activity and the von-Willebrand factor in patients with persistent lone atrial fibrillation. *Journal of Interventionistic Cardiology and Electrophysiology* 10:39–46, 2004.
131. Aldrich D, Hunt DP: When can the patient with deep vein thrombosis begin to ambulate? *Physical Therapy* 84:268–273, 2004.
132. Blattner W, Partsch H: Leg compression and ambulation is better than bed rest for the treatment of acute deep vein thrombosis. *International Angiology* 22:393–400.
133. Trujilio-Santos AJ, Martos-Perez F, Perea-Milla E: Bed rest or early mobilization as treatment of deep vein thrombosis: A systematic review and meta-analysis. *Medical Clinics (Barcelona)* 122:641–647, English abstract.
134. Bydgeman S, Wahren J: Influence of body position on the anginal threshold during leg exercise. *European Journal of Clinical Investigation* 4:201–206, 1974.
135. Yu M, Takanishi D, Myers SA, et al: Frequency of mortality and myocardial infarction during maximizing oxygen delivery: A prospective, randomized trial. *Critical Care Medicine* 23:1025–1032, 1995.
136. Uusaro A, Russell JA: Could anti-inflammatory actions of catecholamines explain the possible beneficial effects of supranormal oxygen delivery in critically ill surgical patients? *Intensive Care Medicine* 26:299–304, 2000.
137. Cirio S, Piaggi GC, De Mattia E, et al: Muscle retraining in ICU patients. *Monaldi Archives of Chest Diseases* 59:300–303, 2003.
138. Reeves NJ, Maganaris CN, Rerretti G, et al: Influence of simulated microgravity on human skeletal muscle architecture and function. *Journal of Gravitational Physiology* 9:P153–P154, 2002.
139. Vincent KR, Vincent HK, Braith RW, et al: Strength training and hemodynamic responses to exercise. *American Journal of Geriatric Cardiology* 12:97–106, 2003.
140. Izquierdo M, Hakkinen K, Ibanez J, et al: Effects of strength training on submaximal and maximal endurance performance capacity in middle-aged and older men. *Journal of Strength Conditioning Research* 17:129–139, 2003.
141. Dart AM, Kingwell BA: Pulse pressure: A review of mechanisms and clinical relevance. *Journal of the American College of Cardiology* 37:975–984, 2001.
142. Uber-zak LD, Venkatesh YS: Neurologic complications of sit-ups associated with the Valsalva maneuver: 2 case reports. *Archives of Physical Medicine and Rehabilitation* 83:278–282, 2002.
143. Schneider DA, Wing AN, Morris NR: Oxygen uptake and heart rate kinetics during heavy exercise comparison between arm cranking and leg cycling. *European Journal of Applied Physiology* 88:100–106. 2002a.
144. Browse NL: *The physiology and pathology of bed rest*, Springfield, Ill, 1965, Charles C. Thomas.
145. Smorawinski J, Kaciuba-Uscilko H, Nazar K, et al: Comparison of changes in glucose tolerance and insulin secretion induced by three-day bed rest in sedentary subjects and endurance or strength trained athletes. *Journal of Gravitational Physiology* 5:P103–P104, 1998.
146. Nieman DC: Current perspective on exercise immunology. *Current Sports Medicine Review* 2:239–242, 2003.
147. McKenzie MA, Greenleaf JE, Looft-Wilson R, et al: Leucocytosis, thrombocytosis, and plasma osmolality during rest and exercise: An hypothesis. *Journal of Physiology and Pharmacology* 50:259–273, 1999.
148. MacKinnon LT: Special features for the Olympics: effects of exercise on the immune system: overtraining effects on immunity and performance in athletes. *Immunology and Cell Biology* 78:502–509, 2000a.
149. MacKinnon LT: Chronic exercise training: effects on immune function. *Medicine and Science in Sport and Exercise* 32:S369–S376, 2000b.
150. Nieman DC: Special feature for the Olympics: Effects of exercise on the immune system: exercise effects on systemic immunity. *Immunology and Cell Biology* 78:496–501, 2000.
151. Mascitelli L, Pezzetta F: Anti-inflammatory effects of physical exercise. *Archives of Internal Medicine* 163:1682–1688, 2003.
152. Gleeson M: The scientific basis of practical strategies to maintain immunocompetence in elite athletes. *Exercise Immunology Review* 6:75–101, 2000.
153. Pyne DB, Gleeson M, McDonald WA, et al: Training strategies to maintain immunocompetence in athletes. *International Journal of Sports Medicine* 21(Suppl 1):S51–S60, 2000.
154. Yeung RR: The acute effects of exercise on mood state. *Journal of Psychosomatic Research* 40:123–141, 1996.
155. Byrne A, Byrne DG: The effect of exercise on depression, anxiety and other mood states: A review. *Journal of Psychosomatic Research* 37:565–574, 1993.
156. Forjaz CL, Cardosa CG Jr, Rezk CC, et al: Postexercise hypotension and hemodynamics: The role of exercise intensity. *Journal of Sports Medicine and Physical Fitness* 44:54–62, 2004.
157. Sheriff DD, Mendoza JR: Passive regulation of cardiac output during exercise by the elastic characteristics of the peripheral circulation. *Exercise and Sports Science Review* 32:31–35, 2004.
158. Wagner PD: Determinants of maximal oxygen transport and utilization. *Annual Review of Physiology* 58:21–50, 1996.
159. Bernhardt J, Dewey H, Thrift A, et al: Inactive and alone: Physical activity within the first 14 days of acute stroke unit care. *Stroke* 35:1005–1009, 2004.
160. Reybrouck T, Fagard R: Gender differences in the oxygen transport system during maximal exercise in hypertensive subjects. *Chest* 115:788–792, 1999.
161. Yoshioka J, Node K, Hasegawa S, et al: Impaired cardiac response to exercise in post-menopausal women: relationship with peripheral vascular function. *Nuclear Medicine Communication* 24:383–389, 2003.
162. Marzorati M, Perini R, Milesi S, et al: Metabolic and cardiorespiratory responses to maximal intermittent knee and isokinetic exercise in young health humans. *European Journal of Applied Physiology* 81:275–280, 2000.
163. Smeets RJEM, Wittink H, Hidding A, et al: Do patients With chronic low back pain have a lower level of aerobic fitness than healthy controls? Are pain, disability, fear of injury, working status, or level of leisure time activity associated with the difference in aerobic fitness level? *Spine* 31:90–97, 2006.
164. Al-Obaidi S, Anthony J, Dean E, et al: Cardiovascular responses to repetitive McKenzie lumbar spine exercise. *Physical Therapy* 81:1524–1533, 2001.
165. Cotsamire DL, Sullivan MJ, Bashore TM, et al: Position as a variable for cardiovascular responses during exercise. *Clinics in Cardiology* 10:137–142, 1987.
166. Suzuki Y, Iwamoto S, Haruna Y, et al: Effects of 20 days horizontal bed rest on mechanical efficiency during steady-state exercise at mild-moderate work intensities in young subjects. *Journal of Gravitational Physiology* 4:S46–S52, 1997.
167. Steele PP, Maddoux G, Kirch DL, et al: Effects of propranolol and nitroglycerin on left ventricular performance in patients with coronary arterial disease. *Chest* 73:19–23, 1978.
168. Kamiya A, Michikami D, Shiozawa T, et al: Bed rest attenuates sympathetic and pressor responses to isometric exercise in antigravity leg muscles in humans. *American Journal of Physiology, Regulation, Integration and Comparative Physiology* 286:R844–R850, 2004.
169. Borg G: Psychophysical basis of perceived exertion. *Medical Science in Sports and Exercise* 14:377–381, 1982.
170. Whaley MH, Brubaker PH, Kaminsky LA, et al: Validity of rating of perceived exertion during graded exercise testing in apparently healthy adults and cardiac patients. *Journal of Cardiopulmonary Rehabilitation* 17:261–267, 1997.
171. Kacin A, Mekjavic IB, Rodman S, et al: Influence of active recovery followed prolonged bed rest on static exercise pressure response. *Journal of Gravitational Physiology* 9:91–92, 2002.
172. Krzeminski K, Kruk B, Nazar K, et al: Cardiovascular, metabolic and plasma catecholamine responses to passive and active exercise. *Journal of Physiology and Pharmacology* 51:267–278, 2000.
173. McCluskey A, Gwinnutt CL, Hardy L, et al: Evaluation of the Pneupac Ventipac portable ventilator in critically ill patients. *Anaesthesia* 56:1073–1081, 2001.
174. Atkinson G, Reilly T: Circadian variation in sports performance. *Sports Medicine* 21:292–312, 1996.
175. Godfrey RJ, Madgwick Z, Whyte GP: The exercise-induced growth hormone response in athletes. *Sports Medicine* 33:599–613, 2003.

176. Carter R, Banham SW: Use of transcutaneous oxygen and carbon dioxide tensions for assessing indices of gas exchange during exercise testing. *Respiratory Medicine* 94:350–355, 2000.
177. Carter R, Holiday DB, Nwasuruba C, et al: Six-minute walk work for assessment of functional capacity in patients with COPD. *Chest* 123:1408–1415, 2003.
178. Gates PE, Tanaka H, Graves J, et al: Left ventricular structure and diastolic function with human aging: relation to habitual exercise and arterial stiffness. *European Heart Journal* 24:2213–2220, 2003.
179. Franzoni F, Galetta F, Morizzo C, et al: Effects of age and physical fitness on microcirculatory function. *Clinical Science (London)* 106:329–335, 2004.
180. Clark AL, Skypala I, Coats AJ: Ventilatory efficiency is unchanged after physical training in healthy persons despite an increase exercise tolerance. *Journal of Cardiovascular Risk* 1:347–351, 1994.
181. Boutellier U, Piwko P: The respiratory system as an exercise limiting factor in normal sedentary subjects. *European Journal of Applied Physiology and Occupational Physiology* 64:145–152, 1992.
182. Guenette JA, Witt JD, McKenzie DC, et al: Respiratory mechanics during exercise in endurance-trained men and women. *Journal of Physiology* 581.3:1309–1322, 2007.
183. O'Donnell DE: Hyperinflation, dyspnea, and exercise intolerance in chronic obstructive pulmonary disease. *Proceeds of the American Thoracic Society* 3:180–184, 2006.
184. Williams DH, Williams C: Cardiovascular and metabolic responses of trained and untrained middle-aged men to a graded treadmill walking test. *British Journal of Sports Medicine* 17:110–116, 1983.
185. Zavorsky GS: Evidence and possible mechanisms of altered maximum heart rate with endurance training and tapering. *Sports Medicine* 29:13–26, 2000.
186. El-Sayed MS: Effects of exercise and training on blood rheology. *Sports Medicine* 26:281–292, 1998.
187. Jones AYM, Dean E, Scudds R: Effectiveness of a community-based t'ai chi program and implications for public health initiatives. *Archives of Physical Medicine and Rehabilitation* 86:619–625, 2005.
188. Wijnen JA, Kool MJ, van Baak MA, et al: Effect of exercise training on ambulatory blood pressure. *International Journal of Sports Medicine* 15:10–15, 1994.
189. Tsai JC, Wang WH, Chan P, et al: The beneficial effects of Tai Chi Chuan on blood pressure and lipid profile and anxiety states in a randomized controlled clinical trial. *Journal of Alternative and Complementary Medicine* 9:747–754, 2003.
190. Szygula Z: Erythrocytic system under the influence of physical exercise and training. *Sports Medicine* 10:181–197, 1990.
191. Shave R, Dawson E, Whyte G, et al: Altered cardiac function and minimal cardiac damage during prolonged exercise. *Medicine and Science in Sports and Exercise* 36:1098–1103, 2004.
192. Kreider RB: Physiologic consideration of ultraendurance performance. *International Journal of Sports and Nutrition* 1:3–27, 1991.
193. Boutcher SH, Nurhayati Y, McLaren PF: Cardiovascular response of trained and untrained old men to mental challenge. *Medicine and Science in Sports and Exercise* 33:659–664, 2001.
194. Mendenhall LA, Swanson SC, Habash DL, et al: Ten days of exercise training reduces glucose production and utilization during moderate-intensity exercise. *American Journal of Physiology* 266:E136–E143, 1994.
195. Bulow HH, Kanstrup L, Henriksen O, et al: CT and magnetic resonance imaging and spectroscopy for noninvasive study of regeneration of skeletal musculature after intensive therapy. *Ugeskrift for Laeger* 19:2273–2276, 1993. English abstract.
196. Ehsani AA, Spina RJ, Peterson LR, et al: Attenuation of cardiovascular adaptations to exercise in frail octogenarians. *Journal of Applied Physiology* 95:1781–1788, 2003.
197. McGuire DK, Levine BD, Williamson JW, et al: A 30-year follow-up of the Dallas Bedrest and Training Study: II. Effect of age on cardiovascular adaptation to exercise training. *Circulation* 104:1358–1366, 2001b.
198. Knapik JJ, Banderet LE, Vogel JA, et al: Influence of age and physical training on measures of cardiorespiratory and muscle endurance. *European Journal of Applied Physiology and Occupational Physiology* 72:490–495, 1996.
199. Ho SC, Woo J, Sham A, et al: A 3-year follow-up study of social, lifestyle and health predictors of cognitive impairment in a Chinese older cohort. *International Journal of Epidemiology* 30:1389–1396, 2001.
200. Zeleznik J: Normative aging of the respiratory system. *Clinics in Geriatric Medicine* 19:1–18, 2003.

Mobilization and Exercise: Testing and Training

Elizabeth Dean and Scotty Butcher

KEY TERMS

Conditioning
Exercise testing
Exercise prescription
Metabolic demand
Mobilization
Training

CHAPTER OUTLINE

This chapter describes the principles and practices for exploiting the preventive, acute, and long-term effects of mobilization, exercise, and training. Mobilization and exercise are prescribed to elicit whichever of these distinct effects is indicated. They are prescribed on the basis of their indications, contraindications, and potential side effects for a given individual. Exercise to exploit each of these effects can be prescribed to address limitations in specific organ systems, as well as augment activity ability and participation. Chapters 24 and 25 expand on these topics, describing special considerations for patient populations with an emphasis on targeting exercise testing and prescription for training based on *people with conditions* rather than for the condition(s) a patient has.

Pre-exercise Test Evaluation

In addition to exercise test indications and contraindications (see next section), a detailed history and examination need to be conducted to determine the appropriateness of test selection, to quantify the relative risk associated with exercise testing, and to determine the level of supervision required. This includes the usual medical and surgical histories to define the types of pathology a patient may have and that may limit his or her exercise capacity. In addition, all medications need to be considered. Which medications impact exercise performance either positively or adversely? Which medications may need to be taken prophylactically? What medications was the patient taking on previous exercise tests? Are these being taken this time? How will this affect the current exercise test results in terms of their comparison? Can medications be withheld? (And should they be?) When is the patient exercising in relation to the timing of medication administration? How might this affect exercise performance? Is this different from a previous test? What about time of day? Does this differ from the time of day when a previous test was performed? Cumulative fatigue and/or discomfort or pain over the course of a day are often reported by patients with certain chronic conditions, thus warranting the establishment of a standard time of day for testing. Other issues must be considered. For instance, how well did the patient sleep last night? How well hydrated is the patient? What and when was the most recent meal? Is the patient a smoker? If so, when was the last cigarette smoked? Additional external factors such as the ambient temperature of the test location and the presence of noise, distraction, and disruption need to be controlled.

Pre-exercise Screening for Minimizing Cardiovascular Risk During Testing

Exercise testing can pose a risk to the patient, so exercise testing must have clear indications, and any contraindications must be ruled out. On the other hand, earlier guidelines for exercise testing in patients, particularly those with cardiac conditions, were too conservative.[1] Patients can be exercised aggressively provided that the indications are based on a comprehensive assessment and a judiciously selected exercise test and protocol and provided that the patient is appropriately monitored throughout testing. The American College of Sports Medicine (ACSM)[2] has developed an algorithm (Figure 19-1, *A*) to determine the risk for cardiovascular events during exercise testing (Table 19-1) as well as guidelines for test selection and level of supervision required based on the risk assessment (Figure 19-1, *B*). As shown in Figure 19-1, *A*, patients with known cardiovascular, metabolic, or pulmonary disease are classified as having a high risk for sustaining a cardiovascular event during exercise. For these individuals, a comprehensive medical examination and physician-supervised exercise testing is recommended before starting a moderate or vigorous intensity exercise program (see Figure 19-1, *B*). For individuals who do not have the conditions listed above, the remainder of the algorithm describes how patient signs and symptoms and coronary artery disease risk factors determine the risk classification and exercise testing and supervision requirements. Physical therapists need to screen patients systematically before exercise testing or prescription.

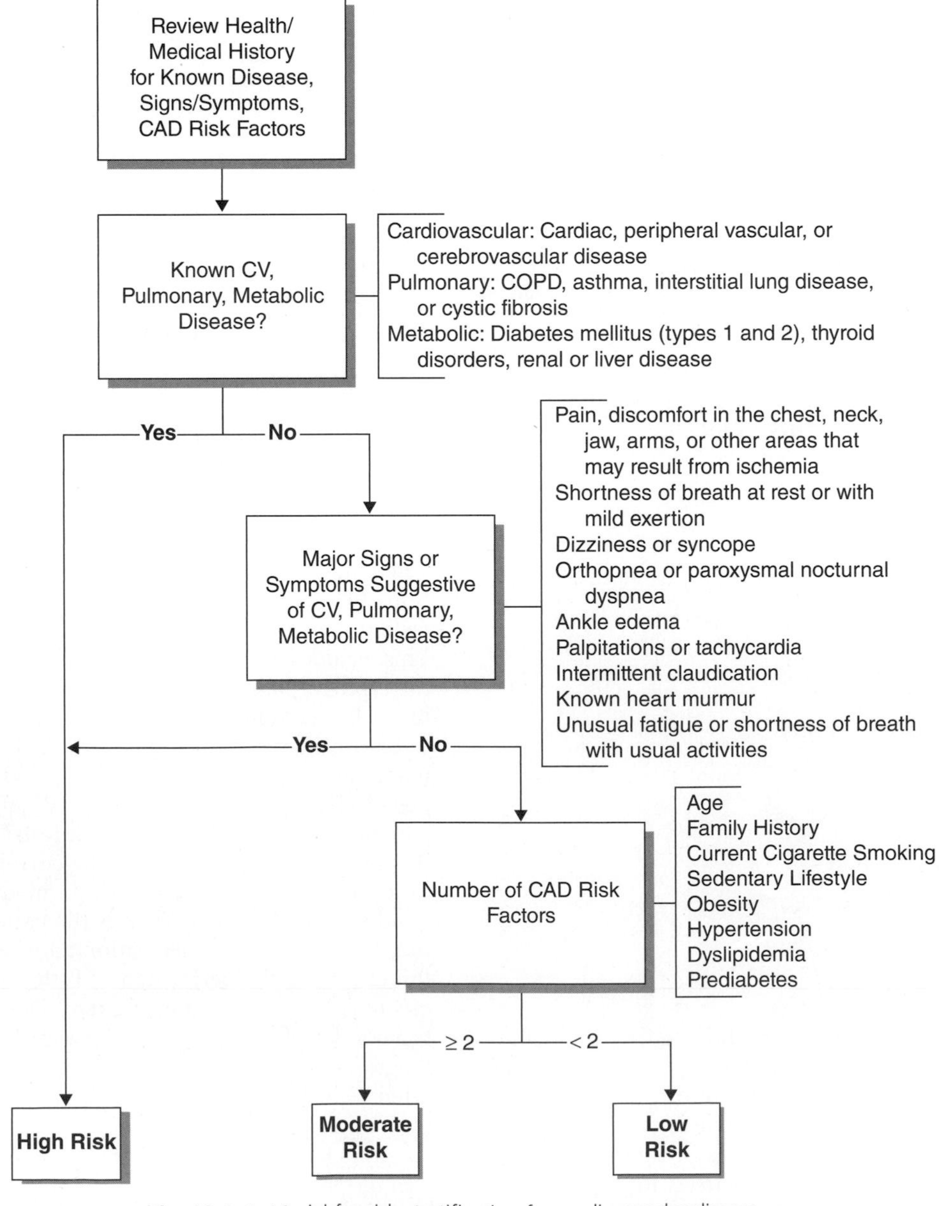

Fig. 19-1 A, Model for risk stratification for cardiovascular disease.

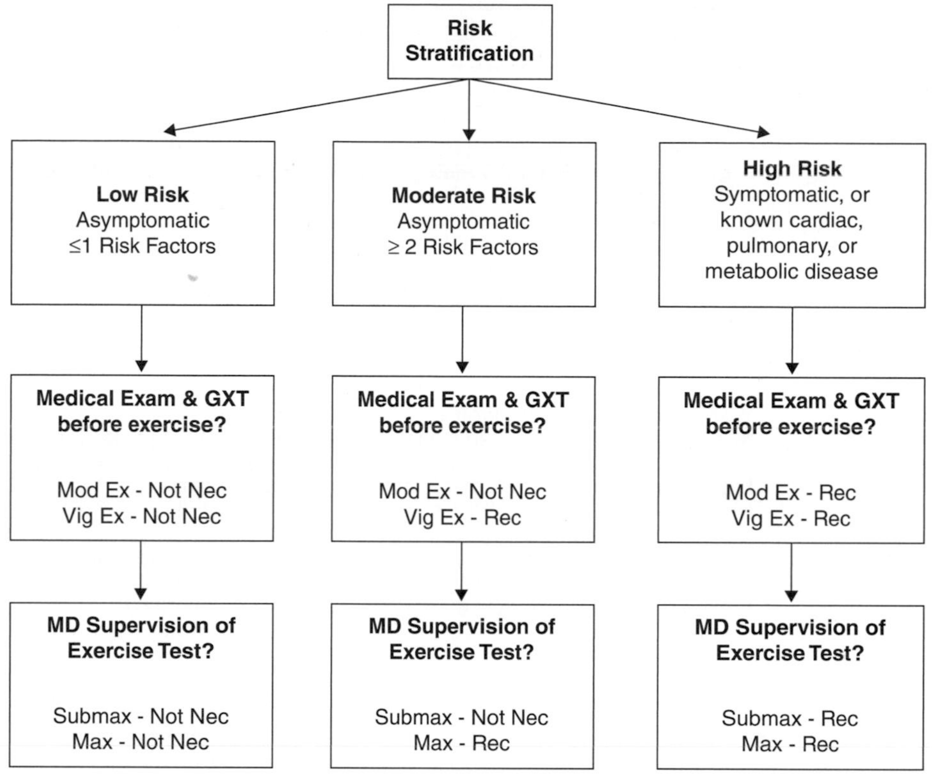

Mod Ex: Moderate intensity exercise; 40-60% of $\dot{V}O_{2max}$; 3-6 METs; "an intensity well within the individual's capacity, one which can be comfortably sustained for a prolonged period of time (~45 minutes)"

Vig Ex: Vigorous intensity exercise; > 60% of $\dot{V}O_{2max}$; 6 METs; "exercise intense enough to represent a substantial cardiorespiratory challenge"

Not Nec: Not necessary; reflects the notion that a medical examination, exercise test, and physician supervision of exercise testing would not be essential in the preparticipation screening, however, they should not be viewed as inappropriate

Rec: Recommended; when MD supervision of exercise testing is "Recommended," the MD should be in close proximity and readily available should there be an emergent need

B

Fig. 19-1, cont'd B, Guidelines for test selection and level of supervision required based on the risk assessment. *(From American College of Sports Medicine, 2010.)*

Exercise Testing

Numerous conditions, including nonprimary cardiovascular and pulmonary conditions, have been shown to benefit from the long-term effects of aerobic exercise (Table 19-2) (see Chapters 24 and 25). Thus for each patient with these conditions, the exercise prescription differs. Comparable with prescribing mobilization in acute conditions, prescribing exercise for long-term adaptations is based on the patient's presentation, history, premorbid status and conditioning level, lab and investigative reports related to physiological reserve capacity, the exercise test, and the goals of the exercise prescription. To promote health, as few as 30 minutes of moderately intense exercise a day on most days of the week is required.[3] However, based on ACSM (2010)[2] guidelines, optimal aerobic exercise adaptation requires an exercise stimulus of 70% to 85% of HR_{max} for 20 to 40 minutes, 3 to 5 times a week for at least 6 to 8 weeks. However, the effect of exercise intensity on $\dot{V}O_{2max}$ and on CO continues to be studied.[4] Improvement in $\dot{V}O_{2max}$ does not appear to be achieved by the same central and peripheral adaptations across a range of exercise intensities. Some individuals have high $\dot{V}O_{2max}$, CO, and SV without a history of training.[5] This may reflect a genetically determined greater blood volume.

The indications for exercise testing are numerous (Box 19-1). They range from quantifying maximum functional, aerobic, or oxygen transport capacities to assessing endurance during low-level activities of daily living (ADLs). The capacity of the oxygen transport system is the most important determinant of maximum oxygen uptake in healthy people. Metabolic studies including $\dot{V}O_2$ provide a link between impairment and functional capacity[6] and can distinguish cardiac versus

Table 19-1 Cardiovascular Risk Factor Threshold for Risk Stratification

	Risk Factors	Defining Criteria
Positive	Age	Men ≥45 years; Women ≥55 years
	Family history	Myocardial infarction, coronary revascularization, or sudden death before 55 years of age in father or other male first-degree relative, or before 65 years of age in mother or other female first-degree relative
	Cigarette smoking	Current cigarette smoker or those who quit within the previous 6 months or exposure to environmental tobacco smoke
	Sedentary lifestyle	Not participating in at least 30 minutes of moderate intensity (40% to 60% $\dot{V}O_2R$) physical activity on at least 3 days of the week for at least 3 months
	Obesity[a]	Body mass index: ≥30 kg × m^2 – or – Waist girth: >102 cm (40 inches) for men >88 cm (35 inches) for women
	Hypertension	Systolic blood pressure ≥140 mm Hg and/or diastolic ≥90 mm Hg, confirmed by measurements on at least two separate occasions, or on antihypertensive medication
	Dyslipidemia	Low-density lipoprotein (LDL-C) cholesterol ≥130 mg × dL-1 (3.37 mmol × L-1) – or – High-density lipoprotein (HDL-C) cholesterol <40 mg × dL-1 (1.04 mmol × L-1) – or – On lipid-lowering medication If total serum cholesterol is all that is available, use ≥200 mg × dL-1 (5.18 mmol × L-1)
	Prediabetes	Impaired fasting glucose (IFG) = fasting plasma glucose ≥100 mg × dL-1 (5.50 mmol × L-1) – or – Impaired glucose tolerance (IGT) = 2-hour values in oral glucose tolerance test (OGTT) ≥140 mg × dL-1 (7.70 mmol × L-1) but <200 mg × dL-1 (11.00 mmol × L-1) confirmed by measurements on at least two separate occasions
Negative	High-serum HDL cholesterol	≥60 mg × dL-1 (1.55 mmol × L-1)

Note: It is common to sum risk factors in making clinical judgments. If HDL is high, subtract one risk factor from the sum of positive risk factors, because high HDL decreases CVD risk.

[a]Professional opinions vary regarding the most appropriate markers and thresholds for obesity; therefore allied health professionals should use clinical judgment when evaluating the risk factor.

Modified from the American College of Sports Medicine. (2010). Guidelines for exercise testing and prescription, ed 8. Philadelphia: Williams and Wilkins.

Box 19-1 Common Indications for Exercise Testing in Patient Populations

Diagnosis of Limitations of Structure and Function

- Primary cardiovascular and pulmonary dysfunction
- Secondary cardiovascular and pulmonary dysfunction

Diagnosis of Factors Contributing to Limitations of Activity and Participation

- Assessment
  - Maximal functional work capacity
  - Submaximal functional work capacity
  - Endurance
  - Dyspnea
  - Chest pain
  - Ability to work
  - Employment options
  - Cardiopulmonary and cardiovascular conditioning
  - Limitations due to noncardiovascular and pulmonary factors
  - Movement economy
  - Effect of medication (supplemental oxygen, blood pressure medication, antianginal medication, oral hypoglycemic agents and insulin, analgesics, bronchodilators)
  - Adequacy of diabetes management
  - Adequacy of orthotics, walking aids, and prostheses
- Prescription
  - Exercise program
  - Medications (effects and regulation)

pulmonary contribution to exercise intolerance.[7] $\dot{V}O_2$ studies require the use of a nose clip or face mask, which may contribute to perceived exertion in addition to the increased dead space that is created by the inspiratory circuit. In a study comparing the two devices in patients with congestive heart failure, no difference in gas-exchange measurements was observed.[8] Perceived exertion, however, was not reported. This is an important finding given that $\dot{V}O_{2peak}$ is a strong predictor of survival (see Chapter 24).

Contraindications to Exercise Testing

Contraindications to exercise testing and, in particular, maximal testing are classified as relative or absolute (Box 19-2). Absolute contraindications prohibit the safe conduction of an exercise test, whereas the presence of relative contraindications requires that the test, protocol, physiological variables monitored, or end point of the test be modified. Both the indications for the test and any contraindications must be clearly established before performing an exercise test.

The guidelines used to test and train healthy people with no disease are not directly generalizable to patients with chronic illness who are medically stable. Because of functional impairments in these patients (secondary to cardiopulmonary, cardiovascular, neuromuscular, or musculoskeletal dysfunction), exercise testing and training must be modified. Moreover, patients who are physically challenged experience more subjective symptoms in response to exercise than do healthy people, so monitoring the subjective responses to exercise is essential. The Borg scale of rating perceived exertion

Table 19-2 **Chronic Conditions That Benefit from the Long-Term Effects of Mobilization and Exercise**

Cardiovascular conditions	Congenital heart disease Acquired heart disease Postsurgical heart conditions Angina Hypertension Hyperlipidemia Hypercholesterolemia Chronic heart failure Heart transplantation Peripheral vascular disease
Cardiopulmonary conditions	Chronic obstructive pulmonary disease Chronic ventilatory insufficiency and failure Interstitial lung disease Asthma Cystic fibrosis Postthoracotomy conditions Lung transplantation
Neurological conditions	Stroke Parkinson syndrome Quadriplegia Paraplegia Cerebral palsy Down syndrome Multiple sclerosis Poliomyelitis and post polio syndrome
Endocrine conditions	Thyroid dysfunction Diabetes mellitus
Neoplastic conditions	General conditioning Prevention in some cases
Musculoskeletal conditions	Osteoarthritis Rheumatoid arthritis Ankylosing spondylitis Osteopenia and osteoporosis
Connective tissue conditions	Systemic lupus erythematosus Scleroderma
Nutritional disorders	Insulin resistance associated with physical inactivity Obesity Anorexia
Conditions requiring organ transplantation	Pre- and postsurgical stages
Other systemic conditions	Chronic fatigue syndrome Chronic depression Renal disease Liver disease Alcoholism Nonalcoholic and alcoholic cirrhosis of the liver
Other	Pregnancy

can be modified for clinical use to score breathlessness, discomfort, pain, and fatigue (Table 19-3).[9,10] If the end points of the scale have been well described and are understood by the patient, the ratings can be used to compare the patient's subjective exercise responses over repeated tests. The patient's subjective reports can be correlated with the exercise response and so can provide a basis for exercise prescription as well as avoiding adverse responses.

Box 19-2 **Relative and Absolute Contraindications to Exercise Testing**

Absolute Contraindications	Relative Contraindications
Congestive heart failure Acute electrocardiogram changes in myocardial ischemia Unstable angina Ventricular or dissecting aneurysm Ventricular tachycardia Multifocal ectopic beats Repetitive ventricular ectopic activity Untreated or refractory tachycardia Supraventricular dysrhythmia Recent thromboembolic event (pulmonary or other) Uncontrolled asthma Uncontrolled heart failure Pulmonary edema Uncontrolled hypertension (>250 mm Hg systolic, >120 mm Hg diastolic) Acute infections	Recent myocardial infarction (less than 4 weeks earlier) Aortic valve disease Severe cardiomegaly Pulmonary hypertension Resting tachycardia Resting electrocardiogram abnormalities Poorly controlled diabetes Severe electrolyte disturbance Severe systemic hypertension Significant conduction disturbance Complete atrioventricular block Fixed-rate pacemakers Acute cerebrovascular disease Respiratory failure Left ventricular failure Epilepsy

Adapted from Jones NL, Fletcher J: *Clinical exercise testing,* ed 4, Philadelphia, 1997, WB Saunders.

The functional impairments and capacities of the patient determine the nature of the exercise test; it can be one of various types, depending on the objective of testing and potential training. If exercise training is an objective of the exercise test, the activity used in the test should be comparable to that to be used in training. Physiological responses and adaptation to exercise are specific to the training stimulus (the specificity-of-exercise principle). Thus if walking is to be the training activity, the test should be a walking test, not a cycling test.

Standardization of Exercise Tests and General Procedures

There are numerous variants of standard exercise tests (Table 19-4). They are categorized as continuous tests or interrupted tests. Continuous tests include maximal and submaximal incremental tests and steady-rate tests; interrupted tests include maximal interval and submaximal interval tests. Interrupted tests are designed for patients with low functional work capacity who cannot sustain prolonged periods of aerobic exercise. These patients can perform more work over time when the workload is intermittent. Specifically, the test allows for alternating fixed periods of work and rest or of high and low intensities of exercise. The proportion of work to rest or high to low exercise intensity is set according to the patient's level of impairment. One patient, for example, may be able to tolerate 3 to 5 minutes of relatively high-intensity work alternated with bouts of 1 to 2 minutes of low-intensity work, whereas another patient may be able to tolerate only 1 minute of low-intensity work alternated with 10 to 20 seconds of rest.

For maximal standardization and the capacity to perform comprehensive monitoring, stationary exercise modalities such as the treadmill, ergometer, or step are recommended.

Table 19-3 Subjective Scales of Exercise Responses

	Perceived Exertion	Breathlessness	Discomfort/Pain	Fatigue
0	Nothing at all	Nothing at all	Nothing at all	Nothing at all
0.5	Very very weak	Very very light	Very very light	Very very light
1	Very weak	Very light	Very weak	Very light
2	Weak	Light	Weak	Light
3	Moderate	Moderate	Moderate	Moderate
4	Somewhat strong	Somewhat hard	Somewhat strong	Somewhat hard
5	Strong	Hard	Strong	Hard
6				
7	Very strong	Very heavy	Very strong	Very heavy
8				
9				
10	Very very strong	Very very hard	Very very strong	Very very hard
	Maximal	Maximal	Maximal	Maximal

Based on the Borg rating of perceived exertion scale.

Table 19-4 Exercise Tests Applicable to Patient Populations

Test Type	Indications
CONTINUOUS TESTS	
Maximal	Generally medically stable patient No significant musculoskeletal abnormalities Test maximal functional capacity Basis for aerobic exercise program
Incremental	Incremental work rates, usually 2 to 5 minutes in duration
Steady rate	Endurance test at a given work rate, usually a comfortable walking or cycling speed
Submaximal	For patients in whom maximal testing is contraindicated
Incremental	Approximate maximal exercise testing Test of near-maximal functional capacity or some significant proportion of maximum
Steady rate	Establish baseline of response to steady-rate exercise, usually at 61% to 75% of predicted HR_{max} Establishes an index of endurance, cardiopulmonary conditioning and may give an index of movement economy
INTERRUPTED TESTS	
Maximal or submaximal	Establish level of functional capacity in patients with extremely low functional work capacity On-off protocol or high-low intensity protocol, such as 5 min on to 1 min off, alternate high- and low-intensity exercise in cycles, such as 1 minute high to 15 seconds low

However, there may be indications to perform an exercise test without a modality, such as the 12-minute walk test or some variant like 6 or 3 minutes.[11-13] Standardization of such tests, however, is more challenging. Practice has a significant effect on the results of the 12-minute walk test, so this test must be repeated to achieve a valid test. Also, the instructions for this test are less well standardized clinically than are those for the treadmill or ergometer; this jeopardizes stringent test control and thus must be tightly standardized.[14]

Like other diagnostic and testing procedures, the validity and reliability of the exercise test depend on standardization of the procedures. Test validity and reliability can easily be compromised in the absence of repeated testing and controls.[15,16] Early ergometer training responses at rest along with submaximal heart rates and reduction in EMG activity in the arms and legs can reflect familiarization.[17] Repeated exercise tests reflect the marked effects of practice. Practice reduces energy output, improves practice-related coordination, and reduces muscle activation.[18] However, with good quality control, a test's validity and reliability can be maximized, even in patients with severe disease such as chronic heart failure.[19] The pre-exercise test conditions and the preparation and testing procedures must be standardized (Box 19-3).

The test is terminated as soon as the sign or symptom criteria for terminating the test are reached or when the criteria for prematurely terminating the test are reached (Table 19-5). Recording the test conditions and procedures in detail is essential. An example of an exercise test data sheet that can be modified to any testing protocol that includes an exercise modality is shown in Figure 19-2, *A*. Many patients are unable to be exercise-tested using a modality; these patients can walk on a marked circuit, and the results are recorded on an exercise test data sheet similar to the one shown in Figure 19-2, *B*. Systematic and detailed record keeping will maximize the test's validity and its interpretation and will ensure that the same procedures are used in follow-up tests, thereby maximizing the comparability of the results of repeated tests. It is imperative that retests be comparable in every respect to the

Box 19-3 Pre-exercise Test Conditions

- Establish the indications for an exercise test.
- Determine absolute and relative contraindications to conducting an exercise test.
- Ensure that patient is free of any acute illnesses, including influenza and colds for 48 hours.
- Ensure that patient understands the purpose of the test and provides signed consent.
- Ensure that patient has not eaten heavily, has avoided caffeinated beverages, and has refrained from smoking for at least 3 hours before testing.
- Ensure that patient is rested and has not exercised or been excessively exerted for at least 24 hours before testing.
- Standardize time of day and the influence of circadian rhythm.
- Ensure that patient is appropriately dressed: shorts, nonbinding clothes, short-sleeve shirt, socks, running or walking shoes that have proper support, and secured laces or fastenings.
- Orthoses should be worn unless the test is evaluating changes in functional capacity with and without an orthosis.
- Ensure that patient understands the subjective rating scales and is able to read them when they are held at an appropriate distance.
- Select the type of exercise test, the protocol, and the exercise test termination criteria beforehand.
- Ensure that the patient is familiar with and has practiced performing the test or test activity, preferably before the test day, so as to reduce arousal, improve movement efficiency, and maximize test validity.
- Based on purpose of the test, determine beforehand the premedication status of the patient. If medicated (e.g., bronchodilators or analgesics), ensure that they are at peak effect during test.
- Room temperature (standardized and recorded).

Preparation for an Exercise Test

- Patient changes into exercise clothes and shoes (not new); ensure that laces are secure.
- If the ergometer is used, the seat-to-pedal distance must be established before the test, and the seat should be adjusted to allow for 15 degrees of knee extension when the foot is lowermost in the pedal in the revolution cycle; the knee must not extend fully.
- Patient sits quietly in a supported chair to establish a resting baseline.
- Monitors are attached (e.g., heart rate, electrocardiogram, blood pressure cuff, pulse oximeter), and the subjective rating scales are explained.
- Testing procedures are explained and demonstrated; the patient has an opportunity to ask questions.

General Procedures for an Exercise Test

- Unnecessary conversation and interaction with the patient are kept to a minimum throughout all stages of the test, including postexercise recovery, so as to optimize the validity of the measurements and the test results overall.
- Resting baseline measures are taken over 5 minutes or until they have reached a plateau.
- Patient stands on treadmill or sits erect on cycle ergometer with feet securely strapped into place on the pedals; the metatarsal heads should be positioned comfortably over the pedals.
- Patient uses two fingers for balance on one side, if possible, when walking on the treadmill, rather than a hand grip; if on the ergometer, does not excessively grasp the handlebar.
- Additional baseline measures are recorded in this position for 2 to 3 minutes or until the baseline is stable.
- The test timer is started.
- The warm-up portion of the protocol begins.
- The selected protocol is carried out.
- Patient is monitored objectively and subjectively at least every couple of minutes throughout all stages of the test, including postexercise recovery.
- The test is terminated when the preset exercise test termination criteria or any of the criteria for prematurely terminating an exercise test are reached.
- The cool-down begins.
- When the cool-down portion of the protocol is complete, the patient moves to the supported chair for the postexercise recovery phase, with legs slightly elevated and uncrossed.
- Postexercise recovery continues until resting baseline measures have been reached or are within 5% to 10%.
- Obtain a report from patient about how patient feels.
- Disconnect the monitoring equipment.
- Continue to observe patient for any untoward postexercise signs or symptoms.

original test in terms of the preparation of the patient and the procedures.

Nutrition and preexercise meals as they relate to exercise testing and training of individuals with pathology have been given little attention in the literature compared with the attention given to the nutrition of healthy people and athletes. Nutritional preparation in respect to macro- and micronutrients and the timing of meals with respect to activity and exercise could have a major impact on the functional capacity of an individual with oxygen transport impairments and low functional capacity. The performance by healthy people in a session of moderate- to high-intensity exercise for 35 to 40 minutes is improved if they consume a meal moderately high in carbohydrates and low in fat and protein 3 hours before exercise, rather than 6 hours before.[20] Missing or delaying meals could alter performance on a test or the outcome of training. Because it has been relatively overlooked in patient populations, nutrition as well as hydration should be a focus of the physical therapy assessment and standardized for the pretest and posttest and training sessions.

Exercise testing is considered resource-intense because of the need for highly qualified individuals to perform tests that are safe, valid, and reliable. In addition, pretest conditions must be met, and the patient has to devote a significant amount of time to taking one or more repeated tests. As a means of streamlining such testing, one study, using two different protocols, compared arterial blood gases and respiratory and metabolic measures in patients who reported

Table 19-5 Criteria for Prematurely Terminating an Exercise Test

Miscellaneous	Wish of individual for any reason Failure of monitoring equipment
General signs and symptoms	Fatigue Lightheadedness, confusion, ataxia, pallor, cyanosis, dyspnea, nausea, or peripheral vascular insufficiency Onset of angina
Electrocardiogram signs	Symptomatic supraventricular tachycardia Sinus tachycardia displacement (3 mm) horizontal or downsloping from rest Ventricular tachycardia Exercise-induced left bundle branch block Onset of second- or third-degree atrioventricular block R wave on T wave premature ventricular contractions (one) Frequent multifocal premature ventricular contractions (frequent runs of three or more) Atrial fibrillation when absent at rest Appearance of a Q wave
Other cardiovascular signs	Any fall in blood pressure below the resting level Exercise hypotension (>20 mm Hg drop in systolic blood pressure) Excessive blood pressure increase (systolic ≥220 or diastolic ≥110 mm Hg) Inappropriate bradycardia (drop in heart rate greater than 10 beats/min with increase or no change in work load)

Modified from the American College of Sports Medicine. (2010). Guidelines for exercise testing and prescription, ed 8. Philadelphia: Williams and Wilkins; and Jones, N.L., & Fletcher, J. (1997). Clinical exercise testing, ed 4. Philadelphia: WB Saunders.

shortness of breath.[21] One protocol was an incremental exercise test and the other a constant-work protocol. The data generated by both protocols were comparable; however, $PaCO_2$ was somewhat higher during the incremental test, as were exercise stress indexes when compared above the anaerobic threshold. No differences were observed below this threshold.

Exercise Tests and Protocols

Common exercise tests and protocols, along with their psychometric properties, are shown in Appendixes C and D for both maximal and submaximal exercise testing. These serve as an easy reference for the clinician regarding the patients for whom they are suited, their protocols and means of standardizing these tests, and how the results can be interpreted.[16] The type of exercise test or tests depends on the patient's needs and the suitability of various tests to achieve the outcomes of interest. Exercise tests can be used for diagnosis, assessment and evaluation, prognosis, and exercise prescription. The purpose is one major consideration in selecting the specific test and its protocol. The exercise test can be a continuous maximal, a submaximal incremental or steady-rate, or an interrupted maximal or submaximal test. Submaximal tests can be used either evaluatively on their own, or they can be used to predict a maximal exercise response. The protocol for the test and the end points to be used in terminating the test are determined beforehand on the basis of the indications for the test and the objectives. Some commonly used protocols are shown in Figure 18-6, along with a comparison of the energy expenditure required by the various work stages in their protocols.

Evaluative Submaximal Exercise Tests

Step tests, an example of a fixed-rate exercise test in that the load and rate remain constant, emerged as practical field tests several decades ago. With the emergence of a range of field tests since then, step tests are being used less commonly. Nonetheless, when well standardized and selected appropriately for a given person, step tests can provide valuable information about aerobic fitness because they can elicit vigorous exercise intensities. People who are obese and/or physically deconditioned may require supervision when performing a step test.[22]

The 12-minute walk test and its variants, 6-minute and 3-minute walk tests, were designed to test patients with lung disease.[12] These tests have been favored clinically, because they are functional and do not require exercise equipment. However, these tests are often used for patients who have extremely impaired exercise capacity and are unable to tolerate being tested on an exercise modality. A major disadvantage, therefore, is that the patient cannot be as comprehensively monitored. Thus patients who are to undergo a 12-minute walk test or one of its variants must be selected with care.

When the 6-minute walk test is applied to healthy older adults, it has been shown to be reliable; two familiarization tests are needed to minimize arousal and the learning effect.[23] In the same trial, the subjects walked, on average, at 80% of $\dot{V}O_{2max}$. Based on a comparison with the performance of patients with chronic obstructive pulmonary disease (COPD) to an "encouraged" 6-minute walk test and a standard incremental cycling test, the prognostic value of the walk test was reported to be high.[24] Patients achieved a high steady-rate $\dot{V}O_2$ in the walk test. No differences were reported in $\dot{V}O_2$, HR, and arterial blood gases between the two tests at peak. However, $\dot{V}_E$ and $\dot{V}CO_2$ were lower in the walk test. When performance was "encouraged," the 6-minute walk test was reported to have good prognostic value.

The 6-minute walk test has been favored as an expedient and inexpensive means of evaluating the functional capacity of older adults with multiple comorbidities. A short distance walked by this cohort is associated with having a low level of education; being non-Caucasian; having a reduced capacity to perform activities of daily living; self-reporting poor health; having a history of heart disease, stroke, or diabetes; and showing abnormal levels of C-reactive protein, fibrinogen, and white blood cell count.[25]

The 6-minute walk test can provide a useful measure of the distance an individual can walk. Because it fails to account for body weight, which is a determinant of exercise capacity, the validity of the 6-minute walk test has been questioned.[26] To enhance its usefulness, Carter and colleagues (2003)[27]

A

Patient name:		
Patient number:		
Date:		
Weight (kg):	Height (cm):	Body mass index:
Waist (cm):	Hip (cm):	Waist-to-hip ratio:
Reason for test:		
Type of test:		
Resting HR:	Resting BP:	
FEV1:	FVC:	FEV1/FVC:
Spo_2:		
Medications and timing in relation to test:		
Review of pre-exercise checklist:		
Level of handrail support:	N/A	YES
Level		
Use of orthotics and types:	N/A	YES
Type		
What was the reason for test?		
How often does the patient experience the level of exertion reached on the test in daily life (e.g., 1x/wk, 1x/month, 3x/day, never, other)?		

Minute or stage	Speed or tension	Grade or RPM	Heart rate and/or ECG changes	Blood pressure	Rate pressure product	Spo_2	Rating of perceived exertion or breathlessness	Discomfort/pain (not anginal)	Comments

B

Patient name:		
Patient number:		
Date:		
Weight (kg):	Height (cm):	Body mass index:
Waist (cm):	Hip (cm):	Waist-to-hip ratio:
Reason for test:		
Type of test:		
Resting HR:	Resting BP:	
FEV1:	FVC:	FEV1/FVC:
Spo_2:		
Medications and timing in relation to test:		
Review of pre-exercise checklist:		
Use of orthotics and types:	N/A	YES
Type		
Use of walking aids during the test:	N/A	YES
Type		
What was the reason for test?		
How often does the patient experience the level of exertion reached on the test in daily life (e.g., 1x/wk, 1x/month, 3x/day, never, other)?		
What was the reason for test termination?		

Minute	Runway or circuit distance	Heart rate and/or ECG changes	Blood pressure	Rate pressure product	Spo_2	Rating of perceived exertion or breathlessness	Discomfort/pain (not anginal)	Comments

Fig. 19-2 Exercise test data sheets for **(A)** treadmill or ergometer, and **(B)** for walk or circuit test.

proposed the use of the product of the distance of the 6-minute walk and the body weight, to yield the work involved in the 6-minute walk. This measure provides a more valid measure of exercise performance and, in addition, can be converted to provide an index of calorie expenditure, hence serving as a standardized basis of comparison across exercise modalities.

Recently, the 6-minute walk test has been conducted on a treadmill. Although there are advantages of treadmill tests over field tests, the results of the two types of test may differ, at least in people after cardiac surgery.[28]

The shuttle test has been another commonly used exercise test for patients with disabilities. When performance on this test is compared with the 6-minute walk distance in patients with COPD, the two tests appear to assess different pathophysiological processes.[29] The shuttle test is considered a more accurate predictor of maximal exercise capacity than is the 6-minute walk test.

Predictive Submaximal Exercise Testing

One application of exercise testing in patient populations that has been of interest is to predict $\dot{V}O_{2peak}$.[16] Prediction of $\dot{V}O_{2peak}$ involves a large margin of error in healthy populations, and that margin could be expected to be greater in patients who are likely to be more deconditioned, have comorbidities, and are prone to greater variations in their exercise responses. The Astrand-Ryhming Cycle Ergometer Test continues to be one of the most frequently used submaximal tests for exercise prescription as well as for prediction of $\dot{V}O_{2peak}$.[30] Prediction of $\dot{V}O_{2peak}$ is obtained from a nomogram in which the $\dot{V}O_{2peak}$ is estimated from the submaximal HR. To improve its accuracy, an age-correction factor is used to adjust for the age-dependent decrement in HR_{peak}.[31] This ergometer test has the clinical advantage of being applicable to less ambulatory people.

Three equations have been compared to predict $\dot{V}O_{2peak}$ in patients with hypertension and fibromyalgia:[32] one equation is from the ACSM; one equation is from the Fitness and Arthritis in Seniors Trial (FAST); and the third equation was developed by Foster and colleagues (FOSTER). Predicted $\dot{V}O_{2peak}$ for all equations was different from the actual measured values. However, the FAST and FOSTER equations predicted values within 1 MET for both patient groups; the ACSM equation predicted values that were different by more than 2 METs.

The distance walked in the 6-minute walk test can provide valid information regarding the functional capacity of elderly patients with chronic heart failure.[33] The results are highly correlated with $\dot{V}O_{2max}$ and can differentiate between classes III and IV of the New York Hospital Association classification of functional capacity.

The heart rate index has recently been described as a means of predicting energy expenditure with the equation $METs = 6 \times HR_{index} - 5$.[34] This equation was based on secondary analysis of 220 data sets (n = 11,257 of multiple ages, pathophysiology and presence/absence of beta blocker therapy) from 60 published exercise studies. These studies reported resting HR (HR_{rest}), a measured-activity HR ($HR_{absolute}$), and measured oxygen consumption (mL O_2/kg/min) associated with the $HR_{absolute}$. HR_{index} ($HR_{absolute}/HR_{rest}$) was calculated. Regression analysis of oxygen consumption (expressed as METs) was performed against HR_{index} to derive the equation to predict METs. Simple tools are compelling for clinical use and warrant further study.

The oxygen uptake efficiency slope (OUES), which is based on a submaximal test, has been proposed as a valid and reliable index of exercise performance in patients with congestive heart failure.[35] This method was tested on older healthy individuals and on patients on the basis of the rationale that maximal testing is not always valid, feasible, or safe. The OUES involves plotting $\dot{V}O_2$ against the logarithm of total ventilation at submaximal work rates. On repeated tests, the OUES is less variable than endurance or $\dot{V}O_{2peak}$. Thus the OUES is an objective and reproducible measure of cardiorespiratory reserve based on submaximal effort. The measure reflects ventilatory-circulatory-metabolic coupling and is influenced primarily by pulmonary dead-space ventilation and exercise-induced lactic acidosis.

Maximal Exercise Testing

With respect to exercise capacity in patient populations, maximal aerobic performance has been of primary interest for diagnosis, assessment, evaluation, and prognosis. Maximal incremental exercise tests (graded exercise tests, or GXTs) can be highly useful in patient populations as long as consideration for the higher level of motivation required to achieve a maximal response is taken. In addition, because maximal exercise testing inherently involves a higher risk for cardiovascular complications than does submaximal testing, it should be used judiciously.

$\dot{V}O_2$ studies (also called cardiopulmonary exercise tests, or CPETs) have become a primary component of the workup of patients with abnormal exercise tolerance for diagnostic and assessment purposes and for exercise prescription. Metabolic measurement carts are used to conduct these studies. To ensure valid and reliable data, the gases used by the cart must be calibrated and testing procedures tightly standardized before the test as well as during it. A practice session is recommended to reduce learning effects and sympathetic arousal.[36] Before the commencement of the test, a couple of minutes of baseline measures are taken, against which the acute exercise responses and the recovery responses can be compared. The metabolic measurement cart can be programmed to display a variety of exercise variables and graphs of interest. The exercise test results are interpreted according to an evaluation of the resting baseline values, the responses of the exercise variables to changes in the exercise test protocol (qualitatively and quantitatively appropriate), the interrelationship of these changes, and whether they achieve some peak value, such as HR or perceived exertion. Beforehand, a decision is made with respect to whether the test is sign- or symptom-limited. Any unusual responses or events during the test are documented. The full impact of the test may not be manifested for several hours or even the next day; thus the patient is followed so that these changes or effects can be evaluated as well. In some patients, lactate measures that require invasive blood work or, minimally, a finger prick, may be indicated.

From the results of CPETs, there are several important variables that can be used clinically. First, determination of the exercise limitation(s) can be made. As described in Chapter 18, the normal limitation to aerobic exercise performance is usually considered to be cardiac output, more specifically, stroke volume. In this case, subjects will exhibit a near maximal heart rate (>90% of age predicted maximum), evidence of a high metabolic demand involving anaerobic energy (respiratory exchange ratio – $\dot{V}CO_2/\dot{V}O_2$ – >1.1; or blood lactate levels >8 mmol/L), and near maximal perceptions of effort (rate of perceived exertion >8/10 or >17/20). If these factors are present, a cardiovascular limitation is presumed. In this case, if $\dot{V}O_{2max}$ values are well below the predicted maximal values, the patient may have some degree of underlying cardiovascular pathology or may simply be deconditioned. Examination of the pre-exercise history, the exercise ECG findings, and the levels of O_2 saturation can determine whether the cardiovascular limitation is due to disease or deconditioning. Another common limitation to aerobic exercise observed in clinical exercise testing is due to an inadequate ability to achieve an appropriate level of ventilation. Ventilatory limitations can be detected by the use of pre-exercise spirometry and exercise tidal flow volume loops; or may be detected by comparing the $\dot{V}_E$ achieved at maximal exercise to the predicted or measured maximal voluntary ventilation (MVV). $\dot{V}_E$/MVV >90% is considered to indicate a ventilatory limitation. The interested reader is referred to the ATS/ACCP Statement on Cardiopulmonary exercise testing[37] for more information on these topics.

Second, CPETs provide a range of exercise performance data, including anaerobic threshold, which is often ignored. Recently, however, the anaerobic threshold has been considered an important marker of cardiovascular insufficiency and exercise performance that has importance in evaluating the performance of individuals with low functional work capacity, such as older adults and patients with left ventricular dysfunction, and in prescribing exercise for them.[38,39] In addition, examining the anaerobic threshold may have particular relevance to individuals in these groups, who may be ill-advised to undergo maximal stress tests. From CPET, anaerobic threshold can be determined by the following criteria:

1. $\dot{V}_E/\dot{V}CO_2$ plateau
2. $\dot{V}_E/\dot{V}O_2$ reaching a nadir and increasing incrementally after this point
3. RER approximately 1.0[39]

Third, CPETs can provide valuable information related to the cardiovascular health and fitness of an individual. $\dot{V}O_{2max}$ is considered by many to be the gold standard for determination of fitness. Although this point is debatable, $\dot{V}O_{2max}$ reference values that are specific to age and gender are widely used to determine an individual's level of fitness. In terms of prescribing exercise training, values at peak exercise such as HR_{max} and work rate maximum can be used to help set appropriate levels of intensity.

In the case of a practitioner who wishes to perform maximal testing, but who does not have access to the required equipment and/or expertise to measure respiratory gases (and $\dot{V}O_2$), a maximal GXT may be conducted. A maximal GXT without respiratory monitoring holds the same level of risk associated with CPETs, but it will still provide valid information on maximal work rate attained and also on a subject and modality specific maximal heart rate. In this case, an achieved maximal heart rate or maximal work rate can be used to prescribe exercise training intensity more accurately than using an age-predicted maximal heart rate or a predicted maximal work rate based on submaximal testing. In addition, if all of the monitoring requirements other than $\dot{V}O_2$ are maintained (ECG, SpO_2, dyspnea, etc.), the safety of using vigorous to high-intensity exercise as a training technique can be ascertained.

General Testing Considerations

Reproducibility of exercise test results is a particular concern in patient populations whose status may change from day to day. When tested weekly for 4 weeks, patients with stable COPD have been reported to have reproducible submaximal physiological exercise responses and ratings of perceived exertion in response to a constant work rate.[40] Exercise performance at a constant work rate is a functional indicator of endurance. On serial exercise testing of patients with chronic heart failure, the mechanical efficiency of walking markedly improves, giving rise to an apparent placebo effect, which has been reported to be independent of motivation and changes in conditioning.[41] This factor can invalidate the findings of a single test. Highly trained individuals show a more marked neuroendocrine (sympathoadrenal and hypothalamopituitary adrenal) response in a second bout than in the first bout of exercise performed on the same day.[42] Study is needed on the implications of neuroendocrine changes with repeated exercise tests in patient populations.

Knowledge of the patient's functional ability based on verbal report is useful and serves as a guideline for selecting the type of exercise test, its parameters, and the test termination criteria. Although these verbal reports do not replace an exercise test, they can be used as an adjunct. The diagram of oxygen cost is shown in Figure 19-3. This visual analog scale is constructed of a 100-mm line with physical activities hierarchically sequenced based on oxygen cost; the high end of the scale represents strenuous activity (walking briskly uphill) and the low end of the scale represents no activity, or sleep. The patient crosses the line at the point where breathlessness does not allow continuation at the patient's best (see Figure 19-3). Figure 19-4 shows incremental workloads associated with step increments in metabolic cost—that is, multiples of resting or near resting metabolic rate (resting metabolic rate = 1 MET, or 3.5 mL O_2/min/kg of body weight). Metabolic costs of activities range from very light to very heavy activities. One limitation of such charts in indicating the metabolic costs of various activities and exercises is that they can be used only as a general guide in patients with cardiopulmonary compromise, as they do not take into consideration the increased work of breathing and the work of the heart that is observed in patients with cardiopulmonary dysfunction, or the increased energy cost associated with abnormal biomechanics as observed in patients with neuromuscular and musculoskeletal conditions.

Exercise testing and training can be challenging in individuals with physical disabilities, such as those with stroke. Because of this limitation, many patients are denied the potential benefits of diagnostic exercise testing and exercise training. The use of external body supports is one means of providing support during standardized exercise testing on a treadmill. One study examined the metabolic effects of a 15% body-weight support in individuals without impairments.[43] End-expiratory gas variables were not affected, except for maximal V_T, which was lower with body support; however, time to achieve peak values was increased. The responses of patient populations who would require variable levels of body support have yet to be determined. Another dimension of exercise

Brisk walking uphill	100	
Medium walking uphill		
		Brisk walking on the level
Slow walking uphill		
		Heavy shopping
		Medium shopping
Bedmaking		
		Light shopping
Washing yourself		
		Slow walking on the level
Sitting		
		Standing
	0	Sleeping

Fig 19-3 Oxygen cost diagram used to assess breathlessness on exertion *(From McGavin CR, Artivini M, Naoe H, et al: Dyspnea, disability, and distance walked: Comparison of estimates of exercise performance in respiratory disease, British Medical Journal, 22:241-243, 1978.)*

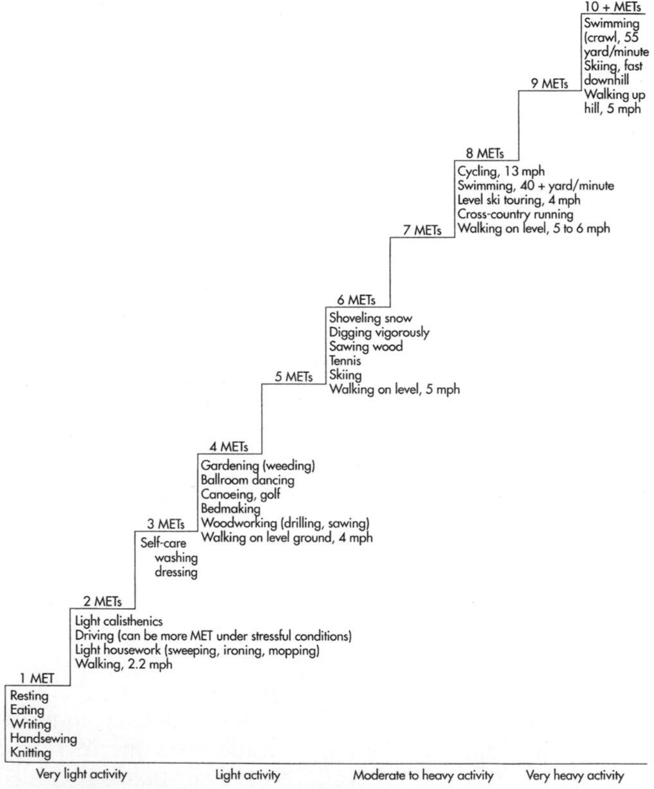

Fig. 19-4 Energy cost in METs of activity and exercise. *(From Woods SL:* Cardiac nursing, *ed 5, Philadelphia, 2010, JB Lippincott, Williams & Wilkins.)*

testing in people with disabilities is the assessment of gait speed, which is associated with physical independence and in activities such as crossing an intersection safely. In addition, gait speed has been proposed as a means of predicting discharge for people with acute stroke. Within the first 5 weeks following stroke, the 5-meter walk test at a comfortable pace (as opposed to the 10-meter walk test, the timed up-and-go test, and other common functional assessment indexes) is the measure of choice for detecting change in walking ability.[44] Finally, movement economy can be compromised in people with physical disabilities, given that their movements are biomechanically inefficient (e.g., people with the residua of poliomyelitis).[45] Abnormal postural alignment and movement asymmetry need to be considered in patient populations because these impairments can increase the energy cost of a given work rate based on norms.

Exercise testing has a role in preoperative assessment. In combination with other tests and examination, exercise testing in patients as a component of the workup for abdominal aortic aneurysm repair with measurement of $P\bar{v}O_2$ can identify patients at risk for perioperative complications.[46] Exercise testing has been used to define a gas-exchange threshold for patients with COPD who are being considered for thoracic surgery.[47] A $\dot{V}O_{2peak}$ of less than 20 mL O_2/kg/min has been recommended as the threshold for predicting perioperative complications. Routine preoperative exercise testing has been advocated. Exercise testing has also been recommended to assist in determining the operability of a patient with lung cancer.[48,49] Patients may be excluded from lung resection surgery based on conventional medical criteria, yet included based on their $\dot{V}O_{2peak}$. These patients have shown survival benefit.

Monitoring

Common variables measured during an exercise test include HR, ECG, systolic and diastolic BP, rate pressure product (RPP), RR, SpO_2, and subjective responses such as perceived exertion, breathlessness, discomfort, pain, and fatigue (see Chapter 18). Assessment of dyspnea is central to monitoring individuals with breathing and exertional impairments. The Borg scale and the visual analog scale are applicable to individuals with dyspnea, and if assessed in a systematic manner, they can provide valid and reliable measures when used in the patient groups for which they were designed, so they should be used routinely.[50] Measures are taken every few minutes after the patient has been exercising at a given intensity for a few minutes when a response to steady-rate exercise is being assessed. This allows for relative stabilization of oxygen kinetics during dynamic exercise. Subjective responses to exercise and daily activities are often the most important to the patient because these typically interfere with their social participation and its composite activities.

Pulse pressure (SBP − DBP) is known to be influenced by aging and arterial wall elasticity.[51] Pulse pressure is also influenced by lifestyle interventions, including exercise and diet.

Therefore it may serve as an index of changes in arterial wall stiffness with exercise training.

More detailed analysis can be done, depending on the testing or training goals. Noninvasive measures, including transcutaneous oxygen and carbon dioxide tensions, can be readily used to assess gas exchange during testing.[52] Invasive monitoring can be done in conjunction with metabolic testing. Such monitoring requires blood sampling through an intra-arterial line to examine serial changes in oxygen and carbon dioxide tensions, acid base balance, and arterial saturation, as well as to provide a means for conducting the thermodilution method that yields an index of CO.

The short- and long-term recovery responses, both quantitative and qualitative, in patient populations are important components of the exercise testing profile. The physical therapist must have a thorough understanding of normal physiological recovery responses in order to benchmark abnormal and atypical responses. Sustained elevated BP after cessation of exercise, for example, has been reported to be more sensitive than ECG for detecting myocardial insufficiency. Further, systolic BP after exercise is a strong predictor of hypertension, coronary artery disease, and cardiovascular mortality. An increase in systolic BP and the percent maximum systolic BP 2 minutes after exercise is directly and independently related to risk for stroke.[53]

Exercise Training Prescription

Physical therapists have a long history of prescribing exercise for health and rehabilitation. As mentioned previously, physical therapists are clinical exercise physiologists who are in a prime position to lead the charge against sedentarism, to utilize well-developed and monitored exercise programs for disease prevention, and to promote rehabilitation in any care setting. It must be stressed that exercise testing and prescription/training are essential components of the physical therapy assessment and treatment plan in every setting—from the ICU to the acute care hospital, to the community program, and finally to the private practice clinics. All patients, regardless of their illness and injury (with the exception of those for whom exercise is contraindicated, unsafe, or impractical), should first be encouraged to be as active as possible, and physical therapists play an essential role in providing comprehensive individualized prescription for each patient.

Exercise Prescription for Health and General Fitness

The components of exercise training for patients for general physical conditioning are the same as those for healthy people: selection of the type of exercise; its intensity, duration, and frequency; and the course of training and its progression. An individualized, rather than standardized, exercise prescription is essential to maximize outcomes in the same way that a physician individualizes a drug prescription.[54] The word *prescription* implies individualization to a person's needs and goals, including his or her social participation and its composite activities. The selection of the type of exercise used for training and the type used in the exercise test is based on the specific objectives of training.

Several expert organizations provide general guidelines for exercise prescription for health and general fitness. Arguably, the foremost of these organizations is the American College of Sports Medicine. The ACSM guidelines are well established and updated frequently; they provide enough guidance to give a comprehensive prescription, but allow enough flexibility to suit the demands of each individual patient. Table 19-6 provides a wide array of examples of how to approach exercise prescription for patients based on their individual level of habitual activity and physical fitness. The FITT approach (frequency, intensity, time, type/mode) to providing exercise prescription ensures that each prescription is detailed enough to be performed by each patient. Although guidelines are just examples, they provide a good starting point from which to design an exercise prescription. These principles are purposefully vague in terms of the exact numbers to use. This range of potential values, particularly for intensity, reflects the fact that improvements in cardiovascular health and fitness can occur with almost any type of exercise prescription within the designated ranges.

Intensity

The intensity of exercise is arguably the most important aspect of exercise prescription and is usually set at some proportion of the HR response or some other response, to a maximum or near-maximum work rate that was safely tolerated during an exercise test. The training intensity for a relatively fit individual who is able to tolerate several incremental work stages on a graded exercise test may be optimal between 65% and 85% of the heart rate reserve (HRR) achieved in the test. The HRR is calculated by taking the percentage intensity within the physiological range from rest to maximum. Thus HRR is equal to $(HR_{max} - HR_{rest}) \times$ intensity fraction + resting heart rate. HR_{max} can be estimated based on a predicted HR_{max} such as 220 − age. This predicted maximum is associated with significant error ± 10 beats (i.e., deviation from the actual HR_{max} achieved in a maximal test), thus the HR at which training is eventually conducted is refined on the basis of other indexes, such as the talk test and general responses. The ratio of HR_{max} (actual or predicted) and resting HR (the heart rate ratio method) provides a good estimate of $\dot{V}O_{2max}$ in healthy men and may have some application in some patient populations.[55]

A patient who is unable to tolerate a couple of increases in work stage is more likely to benefit from an exercise intensity range of 30% to 50% of HRR. In some patients, HR is an invalid indicator of exercise intensity because of the pathology or medications.[45,56] Thus other responses, such as BP, arterial saturation, or subjective parameters such as rating of perceived exertion or breathlessness, can be used. Use of subjective symptoms to supplement the training parameters is useful in patients whose objective exercise responses may be spurious and less valid (e.g., patients on medications that alter autonomic activity).

Time and Frequency

The duration (time) and frequency of the exercise program are established based on the patient's functional capacity, physiological reserve capacity, and exercise responses (see Table 19-6 for general guidelines). Patients with low

Table 19-6 **Recommended FITT Framework for the Frequency, Intensity, and Time of Aerobic Exercise for Apparently Healthy Adults**[a]

		Frequency		Intensity[b]			Time		
Habitual Physical Activity/ Exercise Level	**Physical Fitness Classification**[c]	*kcal/week 1*	*days/week1*	*HRR/$\dot{V}O_2R$ where R is reserve capacity*	*% HR_{max}*	*Perception of Effort*	*Total Duration Per Day (min)*	*Total Daily Steps During Exercise*[d]	*Weekly Duration (min)*
Sedentary/no habitual activity or exercise/extremely deconditioned	Poor	500-1000	3-5	30%-45%	57%-67%	Light-moderate	20-30	3000-3500	60-150
Minimal physical activity/no exercise/moderately highly deconditioned	Poor-fair	1000-1500	3-5	40%-55%	64%-74%	Light-moderate	30-60	3000-4000	150-200
Sporadic physical activity/no or suboptimal exercise/moderately to mildly deconditioned	Fair-average	1500-2000	3-5	55%-70%	74%-84%	Moderate-hard	30-90	≥3000-4000	200-300
Habitual physical activity/regular moderate to vigorous intensity exercise	Average-good	>2000	3-5	65%-80%	80%-91%	Moderate-hard	30-90	≥3000-4000	200-300
High amounts of habitual activity/regular vigorous intensity exercise	>Good-excellent	>2000	3-5	70%-85%	84%-94%	Somewhat hard-hard	30-90	≥3000-4000	200-300

kcal, Kilocalories; *$\dot{V}O_2R$*, oxygen uptake reserve; *HRR,* heart rate reserve; *$\%HR_{max}$*, percentage of age-predicted maximal heart rate.

[a]The various methods to quantify exercise intensity in this table may not necessarily be equivalent to each other.

[b]Fitness classification based on normative fitness data categorized by $\dot{V}O_{2max}$

[c]Perception of effort using the ratings of perceived exertion (RPE), OMNI, talk test, or feeling scale.

[d]Total steps based on counts from a pedometer.

Note: These recommendations are consistent with the U.S. Department of Health and Human Services Physical Activity Guidelines.

functional capacities but with adequate physiological reserve capacity respond quickly to a training stimulus (short training course), so they should be progressed accordingly. However, patients with low functional capacities and with limited physiological reserve capacity adapt more slowly (long training course). The shorter the training course, the sooner a retest is indicated to progress and reset the training parameters. To ensure that the patient continues to be trained safely and optimally, the training parameters should be progressed based on an exercise retest.

Type

The type or mode of exercise should be specific to the individual goals of the client, but should involve a large amount of muscle mass and should be relatively functional. For these reasons, walking, cycling, running, and swimming are often prescribed. Hemodynamic exercise responses depend on the type of exercise and the degree of static exercise and postural stabilization involved and on the muscle mass recruited. Depending on the patient's status and diagnoses, hemodynamic responses have to be considered. The HR response to ergometer rowing using the arms and legs, for example, is lower than running for the same relative workload.[57] Correspondingly, venous return, $\dot{V}O_{2max}$ and O_2 pulse are also greater in rowing.

Water exercise, including chair exercise in the water and running, are undergoing a revival in physical therapy for the management of chronic conditions. Water provides buoyancy, prevents injury, reduces spinal loading and lower extremity loading, minimizes muscle soreness, and optimizes temperature control to facilitate exercise performance. Long-term effects of water exercise such as deep-water running include increased blood volume, increased stroke volume, and increased cardiac output.[58] Water exercise for strength or cardiovascular endurance has benefits for training and for recovery from injury. Aquatic exercise programs have the advantage of being offered to groups as a way of improving fitness in healthy individuals and in people with pathologies such as stroke.[59]

Cross-training principles analogous to those used in athletes apply to patients.[60,61] Based on the assessment of oxygen transport deficits and threats and goals for the individual (e.g., function, health, fitness, prevention, or a combination), a decision is made regarding the prescription of a single mode or a dissimilar mode of training. Because of the specificity of exercise principles, the generalization of a single-mode exercise cannot be assumed; thus, other types of exercise, including task-specific exercise, may have to be included. Also, consideration should be given to the cross-transfer effects of exercising one side of the body. Cross-transfer between ipsilateral and contralateral limbs should be considered when focusing attention on one side of the body or to limit detraining during periods of unilateral immobilization.

Developing exercise programs for the masses of sedentary people in the community constitutes one of the greatest challenges to the physical therapist. Motivating people to be physically active in their daily lives and undertake a formal program of exercise is a skill in itself (see physical activity pyramid in Chapter 1). Intermittent bouts of exercise accumulated throughout the day are showing acceptance by the public and are producing favorable results. The 10,000-steps-per-day program encourages individuals to wear a pedometer and become conscious of how closely they approximate this guideline, which has been associated with an "active" lifestyle.[62] With this objective information, people may be more inclined to increase the number of their daily steps so as to improve their health by elevating the range of their daily steps from the inactive to the active lifestyle. Another creative public health initiative is a stair-climbing program in the community. Such a program has been directed toward sedentary young women.[63] The 7-week program of stair climbing involves progressing from one flight to several flights daily using a public-access stairway of 199 steps. This short-term exercise program resulted in aerobic conditioning as evidence by reduced $\dot{V}O_2$, HR, and lactate during stair climbing and by improved cholesterol levels. Such innovative approaches have enormous potential for improving public health.

Exercise Training to Improve Tasks or Performance

Contrary to the wide range of variables listed above related to exercise prescription for general health and fitness, performing exercise training for improvements in tasks or performance requires the use of a much more specific prescription. This specific prescription needs to be tailored to each individual patient and usually requires the use of specific exercise or functional tests. The use of the physical therapy history or interview, then, represents a crucial aspect of determining the tests and training program design. If there is a specific functional task or performance goal that is identified by the patient or the physical therapist, the exercise test(s) should attempt to, as closely as possible, reflect the requirements of the task or performance. Exercise training program design should then reflect the task/performance, as well as the results of the exercise test. For example, in a private practice setting, a worker who is recovering from a low back injury due to fatigue which caused abnormal lifting mechanics might have the goal of reducing fatigue so that he may maintain proper lifting mechanics throughout his day. Exercise testing, then, should mimic the movement pattern used (lifting) and attempt to determine his endurance in performing lifting related tasks. The training program should be suited to his current level of performance and progressed appropriately to allow optimal adaptation.

Another example of how training programs are designed might be a patient with obesity who needs to increase her sustained walking speed. An appropriate test might be to perform a graded exercise test with $\dot{V}O_2$ measurement to allow the estimation of this individual's anaerobic threshold (as a marker of maximal sustainable pace). The exercise training program would be designed to have the patient increase her anaerobic threshold (using an intensity of exercise at or around anaerobic threshold).

A significant difference between exercise prescription for health and training program design is that training programs often require long-term periodization in order to address multiple needs. Usually, this type of training design involves structuring periods of training that progress from more general to more task- or performance-specific. In the example of the patient wanting to increase anaerobic threshold, the physical therapist would usually begin the program with some lower intensity aerobic exercise for 3 to 8 weeks designed to increase overall endurance and tolerance to walking. After this initial period of "aerobic base" training, the physical therapist would progress the program by prescribing training to increase anaerobic threshold. This type of training program design is complex, and a full description is beyond the scope of this chapter; however, physical therapists working with patients requiring improvements in specific tasks/performance should be competent in comprehensive program design.[64]

Emerging Alternate Types of Exercise Prescription

For many patients, continuous aerobic training as described above is either ineffective, inefficient, or intolerable (see Chapters 18, 34, and 35). There are a few promising methods of altering aerobic exercise prescription techniques that help to minimize these limitations. One example is the use of single-limb training (as opposed to double-limb). As mentioned in Chapter 18, patients who exhibit inability to exercise at high enough intensities to elicit significant physiological benefit due to impairments of central cardiovascular or respiratory responses can increase their muscle specific peripheral load by restraining exercise in one limb. Dolmage and Goldstein (2008)[65] found that single-limb cycling in patients with COPD allowed patients to rapidly progress single-limb workload, resulting in a significantly greater increase in $\dot{V}O_{2max}$ than the group who trained using two-legged cycling (22% versus 1%, respectively). This increase in $\dot{V}O_{2max}$ was achieved during a double-legged cycling GXT. What is most striking about this study is the fact that the overall training time between the two groups was the same. The double-legged training group cycled for 30 minutes continuously, whereas the single-limb group exercised one leg for 15 minutes, then switched legs for the remaining 15 minutes. There are two main conclusions that can be made in regard to the physiological adaptations achieved with single-limb training. First, it appears that progression of overall intensity beyond what is capable through double-legged training in this population is much more important than overall training time. Second, because $\dot{V}O_{2max}$ increased in the single-limb group on a double-limbed test, the mechanisms for increases in $\dot{V}O_{2max}$ are likely due to peripheral adaptations. It has been proposed that adaptations at the level of muscle mitochondria are most apparent with maximizing the amount of tissue oxygenation to minimize the circulating PO_2.[66,65]

Another example of a promising method of exercise training is the use of high-intensity interval training. Although typically thought of as an "athletic" type of training, high-intensity interval training has been used successfully in patients with cardiovascular and respiratory disease. In patients with COPD, for example, ventilatory limitations prevent continuous exercise performance at high intensities.[67] As such, interval exercise models can be used to attempt to increase overall workload during exercise and to enhance muscular adaptation.[68,69] Interval exercise involves alternating periods of higher intensity work bouts (termed work phase) with those of lower intensity (termed recovery phase). The results of training studies reported to date in COPD indicate that high-intensity interval training (at a work phase of 90% to 100% of peak aerobic power) increases muscle performance and exercise tolerance to a similar degree as continuous training, with less ventilatory limitation and dyspnea.[68,69] In addition, the adaptations achieved in skeletal muscle are comparable to those achieved by continuous training. Meyer and colleagues (1996)[70] used high-intensity interval training at a work phase of approximately 120% of peak aerobic power compared with a continuous exercise protocol at 75% of peak power in patients with chronic heart failure. The interval exercise protocol resulted in greater exercise times, with reduced levels of ventilatory and cardiac stress and reduced symptoms of fatigue and dyspnea. After only 3 weeks of training at this high intensity, these patients achieved remarkable increases in maximal aerobic power and leg muscle performance, with reduced symptoms and stress during training.[70]

Recovery and Overtraining

The prescription of the parameters for optimal physiological recovery has not been described in detail. However, the practice of progressive, decremental exercise intensity in the form of a warm-up is supported. Such activity facilitates venous return and the return of HR and other exercise parameters to baseline values.[71] In addition, light activity after exercise promotes the degradation of circulating catecholamines. Priming exercise in athletes improves performance,[72] and this result can be expected in nonathletes as well. However, the parameters (i.e., exercise type, intensity, and duration) of an optimal warm-up have yet to be defined, and they may depend on the individual, general health and fitness, weight, age, and morbidity.

New advances in athletic training may have application to clinical populations, including titrating, or periodizing, training day by day, week by week, or month by month. Periodization has two primary goals: to structure a training program to achieve optimal, multiple physiological adaptations and to prevent overtraining. An overtraining phenomenon has been described in healthy people. Athletes whose performance has dropped off may improve performance outcomes with several weeks of rest.[73] Prevention of overtraining is achieved through a detailed analysis of the responses to and recovery from the previous exercise session. This method is based on modeling the effects of training, detraining, and overtraining.[74,75] This method does not assume that the interval between exercise sessions is the same across individuals or the same for a given individual from one day to the next. The proponents of the model believe that training is optimized by the avoidance of under- or overtraining and that training effects are better if they are accumulated over time, rather than according to the conventional methods that subscribe to a rigid exercise intensity, duration, and frequency over some interval (e.g., 6 to 8 weeks).

The role of overtraining in people with underlying pathology, whether induced by the pathology or resulting from an excessive therapeutic exercise prescription, is not well understood. The extent to which some severely compromised patients are, in fact, overtrained as a mere consequence of their activities of daily living is not known. It is possible that the syndrome of inability to maintain work performance, persistent fatigue, frequent illness (in particular upper respiratory tract infections), disturbed sleep, and altered mood states may reflect overwork in patients that is analogous to overtraining in athletes.[76,77] With respect to immunity, reduced neutrophil function may be implicated in both situations. In athletes, this overtraining syndrome due to excessive physical exertion and inadequate recovery has been related to autonomic dysfunction and increased cytokine production. Because regular intense exercise can suppress mucosal immunity and because saliva is the most commonly used secretion for assessing mucosal immunity, monitoring the saliva of athletes during critical training periods provides an index of risk status. The usefulness of mucosal assessment in clinical populations warrants investigation. Relaxation has been shown to offset the exercise-induced suppression of secretory immunoglobulin associated with upper respiratory tract infection in healthy people.[78] The role of relaxation and its immune protection warrants exploitation in clinical populations. Immunity may be optimized with an appropriate balance of exercise, rest, and recovery. Achieving an optimal balance of exercise and rest or recovery warrants study in patient populations as a means of maximizing a patient's social participation.

Prescriptive rest periods between bouts of exercise and optimal sleep in patient populations, comparable to the training of athletes, should be considered as carefully as the prescriptive parameters of exercise itself to maximize functional performance.

Exercise Prescription

General Procedures

Before an exercise session, the patient needs to review a checklist to ensure that exercise is not contraindicated on that day. This is particularly important for patients whose conditions change rapidly or whose disease course tends to fluctuate, as in multiple sclerosis, cystic fibrosis, chronic fatigue syndrome, and congestive heart failure. Box 19-4 provides a checklist to be used in preparation for exercise testing and training sessions. Such a checklist, however, must be tailored to each patient. Aids and devices for older patients must provide assistance that is optimal and safe and promotes the most independence. Inappropriate aids are associated with poor patient outcomes in this population, and their use requires more surveillance by carers.[79]

Active exercise is always selected to elicit optimal oxygen transport stress for improving aerobic and muscle power. Passive exercise, however, may have a limited role in some patients. Compared with active exercise, little is known about the physiological responses to passive exercise. When low-intensity active and passive cycling are compared in healthy people, inotropic changes are elicited primarily with active exercise, thus are dependent on mechanoreflexes stimulated by the metabolic products of skeletal muscle.[80] Cardiac output is increased by an increase in HR during active cycling and by an increase in stroke volume during passive cycling. It is interesting to note that blood lactate increases in both active and passive cycling but is higher during active cycling. These findings are of some physiological interest and may have potential therapeutic application; however, active exercise is the therapeutic priority, no matter how minimal the absolute intensity, duration, and frequency may be initially. The degree to which passive exercise could be exploited in individuals unable to cooperate with an exercise program, or whether passive exercise could augment active exercise, warrants further study.

Box 19-4 Patient's Checklist Before an Exercise Testing or Training Session

- Feeling well over the past 48 hours
- No infections (e.g., upper respiratory tract infection) or influenza
- No fever
- No unaccustomed muscle or joint discomfort or pain
- No chest tightness or pain
- No unaccustomed breathing difficulty or fatigue
- Adequate night's sleep
- Has not eaten heavily within past 3 hours
- Best time of day
- Wearing or using orthoses, walking aids, and devices
- Clothing appropriate for exercise conditions (indoors or outdoors)
- Appropriate socks and footwear that is comfortable, well-fitting, and has secured laces (double-knotted)
- Has water within reach
- Taken preexercise medications at specified time
- Has nitroglycerine within reach (patients with cardiac dysfunction)
- Has inhaler within reach (patients with pulmonary dysfunction)
- Has sugar supply within reach (patients with diabetes)
- Standardize and record the use of orthotics and walking aids

Specific Procedures

In a supervised setting, the general procedures used in exercise training are comparable to those used for testing. Specifically, the patient prepares for the training session in a standardized manner and is monitored according to his or her condition. The components of the session are the same with respect to warm-up, cool-down, and recovery. The main part of the exercise program, however, will usually be steady-rate or interrupted exercise. Varying work rates may be indicated for some patients.

In the majority of situations, the goal is to transfer the responsibility of surveillance and monitoring from the physical therapist to the patient. Depending on the patient's pathology and ability to learn how to monitor exercise responses accurately, this process takes varying amounts of time. Planning of transition to home and the community is considered from the beginning. The patient's daily needs at home serve as the basis for the exercise program; his or her skills need to be transferred from the physical therapist and clinic to the home environment.

Monitoring

For safety reasons and to ensure that the patient is within the target training range of the variables selected to set exercise intensity, the patient must be closely monitored. This is particularly true if the patient has any risk for untoward or adverse reactions to exercise. If a patient is considered to be at any risk, exercise training should take place only in a supervised setting. A stable patient may begin an exercise program in a supervised setting, but with training and education can usually be transferred to an unsupervised setting. Education includes self-monitoring of exercise responses, maintaining exercise intensity within the appropriate limits, and keeping a record of the details of their exercise sessions. When the patient is safely carrying out the exercise program independently in the community, some mechanism is needed to follow up on the patient's progress. If the objective is continued conditioning, the patient should be rescheduled for a retest. If the patient is on a maintenance program, the physical therapist is responsible for reminders about exercise and injury precautions and about notifying the physical therapist or physician if significant adverse effects are observed.

The HR, BP, RR, and other measure are taken according to standardized procedures. Electronic equipment and mechanical devices must be calibrated. A break point in the double product (HR × systolic BP) and work-rate relationship can provide a good estimate of the anaerobic threshold in patients with exercise intolerance as well as in healthy persons.[81]

Patients on sympathomimetic drugs or with various pathologies will have abnormal exercise responses. Thus knowledge of these factors is essential to determine whether a measure is valid.

The World Health Organization recommends repeated BP measurements be performed in the sitting or supine position followed by standing[82] and that the cuff be positioned at the level of the right atrium, irrespective of body position. One concern about this recommendation is that systolic and diastolic BP is lower in a sitting than in a supine position, so the two readings are not equivalent.[83] Blood pressure may be under- or overestimated if the level of the cuff is not at the level of the right atrium, regardless of body position. Further, this effect may be amplified in patients with autonomic dysfunction such as that found in patients with diabetes.

Nutritional status and rest/sleep status must be assessed in patient populations by physical therapists to maximize exercise capacity and function comparable to competitive athletes. Mobilization and exercise must be prescribed to maximize these effects during acute and chronic long-term exercise.

Most evidence related to exercise and health has focused on cardiovascular conditioning. The relationship between other dimensions of health is being increasingly studied—for example, immunological status[84] and mental health.[85] With respect to mental health, little is known about the parameters of exercise that are optimally antidepressive, other than benefits may be associated with regular physical activity, preferably engaged in with other people. Although there is an association between depressive symptoms and reduced activity in community-living older adults, research is needed to establish the role of exercise training in preventing or attenuating these symptoms.[85]

Summary

Although the principles of prescribing mobilization and exercise for their optimal preventive effects have not been scientifically elucidated in comparison with their general health benefits, physical activity and exercise in some form are indicated to offset the deleterious effects of deconditioning associated with lack of activity.

When the long-term effects of exercise are indicated, the exercise stimulus is defined in an appropriate prescription, generally involving higher intensity, longer duration, and less frequency when compared with the exercise prescription for acute effects. A long-term prescription is designed to be followed for several weeks or more before demonstrable physiological adaptation can be observed and the exercise parameters redefined based on an a subsequent exercise test for progression of conditioning. The precise parameters are based on considerations such as the patient's age, smoking history, body mass index, waist-to-hip ratio, cognitive status, the goals of physical activity and exercise for the patient, and his or her needs and wants,

The three levels of prescription of exercise are physiologically distinct and need to be prescribed specifically by the physical therapist for a given patient, taking into consideration the indications, contraindications, and side effects for that individual.

Finally, the physical therapist needs to be proficient in the assessment of nutritional status and sleep/rest status in every patient. These are important variables in facilitating and inhibiting response to exercise comparable to that in athletic training.

Review Questions

1. Describe the differences in exercise prescription parameters (i.e., type of exercise stimulus, intensity, duration, frequency, and course) when prescribing exercise for its (a) preventive effects, (b) acute effects, and (c) chronic effects.
2. Distinguish between submaximal and maximal exercise tests. Name two of each, their psychometric characteristics, their protocols, and their outcomes.
3. Describe the factors that can invalidate exercise test results and jeopardize test reliability and thus must be tightly controlled by the physical therapist.
4. Describe how the physical therapy assessment of nutrition and sleep/rest can be used to augment clinical outcomes.

References

1. Fletcher BJ, Dunbar S, Coleman J, et al: Cardiac precautions for non-acute inpatient settings. *American Journal of Physical Medicine and Rehabilitation* 72:140–143, 1993.
2. American College of Sports Medicine: *Guidelines for exercise testing and prescription*, ed 8, Philadelphia, 2010, Lippincott Williams & Wilkins.
3. Varo Cenarruzabeitia JJ, Martinez Hernandez JA, Martinez-Gonzalez MA: Benefits of physical activity and harms of inactivity. *Medical Clinics (Barcelona)* 121:665–672, 2003.
4. Lepretre PM, Koralsztein JP, Billat VL: Effect of exercise intensity on relationship between $\dot{V}O_{2max}$ and cardiac output. *Medicine and Science in Sports and Exercise* 36:1357–1363, 2004.
5. Martino M, Gledhill N, Jamnik V: High VO2max with no history of training is primarily due to high blood volume. *Medicine and Science in Sports and Exercise* 4:966–971, 2002.
6. Singh VN: The role of gas exchange analysis with exercise testing. *Primary Care* 28:159–179, 2001.
7. Myers J, Madhavan R: Exercise testing with gas exchange analysis. *Cardiology Clinics* 19:433–445, 2001.
8. Baran DA, Rosenwinkel E, Spierer DK, et al: Validating facemask use for gas exchange analysis in patients with congestive heart failure. *Journal of Cardiopulmonary Rehabilitation* 21:94–100, 2001.
9. Borg GAV: Psychophysiological bases of perceived exertion. *Scandinavian Journal of Rehabilitation Medicine* 2:92–98, 1970.
10. Borg G: Psychophysical basis of perceived exertion. *Medical Science in Sports and Exercise* 14:377–381, 1982.
11. Butland RJA, Pang J, Gross ER, et al: Two-, six-, and 12-minute walking tests in respiratory disease. *British Medical Journal* 284:818–822, 1982.

12. McGavin CR, Gupta SP, McHardy GJR: Twelve-minute walking test for assessing disability in chronic bronchitis. *British Medical Journal* 1:822–823, 1976.
13. McGavin CR, Artvinli M, Naoe H, et al: Dyspnoea, disability, and distance walked: Comparison of estimates of exercise performance in respiratory disease. *British Medical Journal* 2:241–243, 1978.
14. Dean E, Ross J: Mobilization and exercise conditioning. In Zadai C, editor: (1992). *Clinics in physical therapy. Pulmonary management in physical therapy*, New York, 1992a, Churchill Livingstone.
15. Kraemer MD, Sullivan M, Atwood JE, et al: Reproducibility of treadmill exercise data in patients with atrial fibrillation. *Cardiology* 76:234–242, 1989.
16. Noonan V, Dean E: Submaximal exercise testing: clinical application and interpretation. *Physical Therapy* 80:782–807, 2000.
17. Ziemba AW, Chwalbińska-Moneta J, Kaciuba-Uścilko H, et al: Early effects of short-term aerobic training. Physiological responses to graded exercise. *Journal of Sports Medicine and Physical Fitness* 43:57–63, 2003.
18. Lay BS, Sparrow WA, Hughes KM, et al: Practice effects on coordination and control, metabolic energy expenditure, and muscle activation. *Human Movement Science* 21:807–830, 2002.
19. Meyer K, Westbrook S, Schwaibold M, et al: Short-term reproducibility of cardiopulmonary measurements during exercise testing in patients with severe chronic heart failure. *American Heart Journal* 134:20–26, 1997.
20. Maffucci DM, McMurray RG: Towards optimizing the timing of the pre-exercise meal. *International Journal of Sport Nutrition and Exercise Metabolism* 10:103–113, 2000.
21. Zeballos RJ, Weisman IM, Connery SM: Comparison of pulmonary gas exchange measurements between incremental and constant work exercise above the anaerobic threshold. *Chest* 113:602–611, 1998.
22. Hansen D, Jacobs N, Bex S, et al: Are fixed-rate step tests medically safe for assessing physical fitness? *European Journal of Applied Physiology*. Mar 4 [Epub ahead of print], 2011.
23. Kervio G, Carre F, Ville NS: Reliability and intensity of the six-minute walk test in healthy elderly subjects. *Medicine & Science in Sports and Exercise* 35:169–174, 2003.
24. Troosters T, Vilaro J, Rabinovich R, et al: Physiological responses to the 6-min walk test in patients with chronic obstructive lung disease. *European Respiratory Journal* 20:564–569, 2002.
25. Enright PL, McBurnie MA, Bittner V, et al: The 6-min walk test: A quick measure of functional status in elderly adults. *Chest* 123:387–398, 2003.
26. Gylfadottir S: *The six-minute walk test: A methodologic perspective and with special reference to individuals with poliomyelitis*, 2003, University of British Columbia, Canada, thesis.
27. Carter R, Holiday DB, Nwasuruba C, et al: Six-minute walk work for assessment of functional capacity in patients with COPD. *Chest* 123:1408–1415, 2003.
28. Olper L, Cervi P, De Santi F, et al: Validation of the treadmill six-minute walk test in people following cardiac surgery. *Physical Therapy* Feb 10 [Epub ahead of print], 2011.
29. Onorati P, Antonucci R, Valli G, et al: Non-invasive evaluation of gas exchange during a shuttle walk test vs. a 6-min walking test to assess exercise tolerance in COPD patients. *European Journal of Applied Physiology* 89:331–336, 2003.
30. Astrand PO, Ryhming I: A nomogram for calculation of aerobic capacity from pulse rate during submaximal work. *Journal of Applied Physiology* 7:218–221, 1954.
31. Astrand I: Aerobic capacity in men and women with special reference to age. *Acta Physiologica Scandinavica* 49(Suppl) 169:2–92, 1960.
32. Dominick KL, Gullette EC, Babyak MA, et al: Predicting peak oxygen uptake among older patients with chronic illness. *Journal of Cardiopulmonary Rehabilitation* 19:81–89, 1999.
33. Peeters P, Mets T: The 6-minute walk as an appropriate exercise test in elderly patients with chronic heart failure. *Journal of Gerontology. A. Biological Sciences and Medical Sciences* 51:147–151, 1996.
34. Wicks JR, Oldridge NB, Nielsen LK, et al: Heart rate index: A simple method for prediction of oxygen uptake. *Medicine and Science and Sports and Exercise* Feb 28 [Epub ahead of print], 2011.
35. Hollenberg M, Tager IB: Oxygen update efficiency slope: An index of exercise performance and cardiopulmonary reserve requiring only submaximal exercise. *Journal of the American College of Cardiology* 36:194–201, 2000.
36. Dean E, Ross J, Bartz J, Purves S: Improving the validity of clinical exercise testing: The relationship between practice and performance. *Archives of Physical Medicine and Rehabilitation* 70:599–604, 1989.
37. American Thoracic Society / American College of Chest Physicians: ATS/ACCP statement on cardiopulmonary exercise testing. *American Journal of Respiratory and Critical Care Medicine* 167:211–277, 2003.
38. Nappi A, Cuocolo A, Imbriaco M, et al: Ambulatory monitoring of left ventricular function: Walk and bicycle exercise in congestive heart failure. *Journal of Nuclear Medicine* 38:948–953, 1997.
39. Wasserman K: Anaerobic threshold and cardiovascular function. *Monaldi Archives of Chest Diseases* 58:1–5, 2002.
40. Covey MK, Larson JL, Wirtz S: Reliability of submaximal exercise tests in patients with COPD. Chronic obstructive lung disease. *Medicine and Science in Sports and Exercise* 31:1257–1264, 1999.
41. Russell SD, McNeer FR, Beere PA, et al: Improvement in the mechanical efficiency of walking: An explanation for the "placebo effect" seen during repeated exercise testing of patients with heart failure. Duke University Clinical Cardiology Studies (DUCCS) Exercise Group. *American Heart Journal* 135:107–114, 1998.
42. Ronsen O, Haug E, Pedersen BK, et al: Increased neuroendocrine response to a repeated bout of endurance exercise. *Medicine and Science in Sport and Exercise* 33:568–575, 2001.
43. MacKay-Lyons M, Makrides L, Speth S: Effect of a 15% body weight support on exercise capacity of adults without impairments. *Physical Therapy* 81:1790–1800, 2001.
44. Salbach NM, Mayo NE, Higgins J, et al: Responsiveness and predictability of gait speed and other disability measures in acute stroke. *Archives of Physical Medicine and Rehabilitation* 82:1204–1212, 2001.
45. Dean E, Ross J: Movement energetics of individuals with a history of poliomyelitis. *Archives of Physical Medicine and Rehabilitation* 74:478–483, 1993.
46. Nugent AM, Riley M, Megarry J, et al: Cardiopulmonary exercise testing in the pre-operative assessment of patients for repair of abdominal aortic aneurysm. *Irish Journal of Medical Science* 167:238–241, 1998.
47. Torchio R, Gulotta C, Parvis M, et al: Gas exchange threshold as a predictor of severe postoperative complications after lung resection in mild-to-moderate chronic obstructive lung disease. *Monaldi Archives of Chest Diseases* 53:127–133, 1998.
48. Gilbreth EM, Weisman IM: Role of exercise stress testing in preoperative evaluation of patients for lung resection. *Clinics in Chest Medicine* 15:389–403, 1994.
49. Walsh GL, Morice RC, Putman JB, et al: Resection of lung cancer is justified in high-risk patients selected by exercise oxygen consumption. *Annals of Thoracic Surgery* 58:704–710, 1994.
50. Cullen DL, Rodak B: Clinical utility of measures of breathlessness. *Respiratory Care* 47: 986–993, 2002.
51. Dart AM, Kingwell BA: Pulse pressure: a review of mechanisms and clinical relevance. *Journal of the American College of Cardiology* 37:975–984, 2001.
52. Carter R, Banham SW: Use of transcutaneous oxygen and carbon dioxide tensions for assessing indices of gas exchange during exercise testing. *Respiratory Medicine* 94:350–355, 2000.
53. Kurl S, Laukkanen JA, Rauramaa R, et al: Systolic blood pressure response to exercise stress test and risk of stroke. *Stroke* 32:2036–2041, 2001.
54. Vallet G, Ahmaidi S, Serres I, et al: Comparison of two training programmes in chronic airway limitation patients: Standardized versus individualized protocols. *European Respiratory Journal* 10:114–122, 1997.
55. Uth N, Sorensen H, Overgaard K, et al: Estimation of $\dot{V}O_{2max}$ from the ratio between HR_{max} and HR_{rest}: The Heart Rate Ratio Method. *European Journal of Applied Physiology* 91:111–115, 2004.
56. Dean E, Ross J: Discordance between cardiopulmonary physiology and physical therapy. Toward a rational basis for practice. *Chest* 101:1694–1698, 1992b.
57. Yoshiga CC, Higuchi M: Heart rate is lower during ergometer rowing than during treadmill running. *European Journal of Applied Physiology* 87:97–100, 2002.
58. Reilly T, Dowzer CN, Cable NT: The physiology of deep-water running. *Journal of Sports Science* 21:959–972, 2003.
59. Chu KS, Eng JJ, Dawson AS, et al: Water-based exercise for cardiovascular fitness in people with chronic stroke: A randomized controlled trial. *Archives of Physical Medicine and Rehabilitation* 85:870–874, 2004.
60. Mujika I, Padilla S: Detraining: loss of training-induced physiological and performance adaptations. I: Short-term insufficient training stimulus. *Sports Medicine* 30:79–87, 2000a.
61. Mujika I, Padilla S: Detraining: Loss of training-induced physiological and performance adaptations. II: Long-term insufficient training stimulus. *Sports Medicine* 30:145–154, 2000b.
62. Tudor-Locke C, Bassett DR, Jr: How many steps/day are enough? Preliminary pedometer indices for public health. *Sports Medicine* 34:1–8, 2004.
63. Boreham CA, Wallace WF, Nevill A: Training effects of accumulated daily stair-climbing exercise in previously sedentary young women. *Preventive Medicine* 30:277–281, 2000.

64. Bompa TO, Haff GG: *Periodization: Theory and methodology of training*, ed 5, Champaign, IL, Human Kinetics.
65. Dolmage TE, Goldstein RS: Effects of one-legged exercise training of patients with COPD. *Chest* 133:370–376, 2008.
66. Butcher SJ, Jones RL: The impact of exercise training intensity on change in physiological function in patients with chronic obstructive pulmonary disease. *Sports Medicine* 36:307–325, 2006.
67. Neder AJ, Jones PW, Nery LE, et al: Determinants of the exercise endurance capacity in patients with chronic obstructive pulmonary disease: The power-duration relationship. *American Journal of Respiratory and Critical Care Medicine* 162:497–504, 2000.
68. Puhan MA, Busching G, Schunemann HJ, et al: Interval versus continuous high-intensity exercise in chronic obstructive pulmonary disease: A randomized trial. *Annuls of Internal Medicine* 145:816–825, 2006.
69. Vogiatzis I, Terzis G, Nanas S, et al: Skeletal muscle adaptations to interval training in patients with advanced COPD. *Chest* 128:3838–3845, 2005.
70. Meyer K, Samek L, Schwaibold M, et al: Physical responses to different modes of interval exercise in patients with chronic heart failure: Application to exercise training. *European Heart Journal* 17:1040–1047, 1996.
71. Takahashi T, Miyamoto Y: Influence of light physical activity on cardiac responses during recovery from exercise in humans. *European Journal of Physiology and Occupational Physiology* 77:305–311, 1998.
72. Jones AM, Koppo K, Burnley M: Effects of prior exercise on metabolic and gas exchange responses to exercise. *Sports Medicine* 33:949–971, 2003.
73. Koutedakis Y, Budgett R, Faulmann L: Rest in underperforming elite competitors. *British Journal of Sports Medicine* 24:248–252, 1990.
74. Banister EW: Dose/response effects of exercise modeled from training: Physical and biochemical measures. *Annals of Physiology and Anthropology* 11:345–356, 1992.
75. Morton RH: Modeling training and overtraining. *J Sports Science* 15:335–340, 1997.
76. MacKinnon LT: Special features for the Olympics: Effects of exercise on the immune system: Overtraining effects on immunity and performance in athletes. *Immunology and Cell Biology* 78:502–509, 2000a.
77. MacKinnon LT: Chronic exercise training: effects on immune function. *Medicine and Science in Sport and Exercise* 32:S369–S376, 2000b.
78. Reid MR, Drummond PD, MacKinnon LT: The effect of moderate aerobic exercise and relaxation on secretory immunoglobulin A. *International Journal of Sports Medicine* 22:132–137, 2001.
79. Taylor DH, Hoenig H: The effect of equipment usage and residual task difficulty on use of personal assistance, days in bed, and nursing home placement. *Journal of the American Gerontological Society* 52:72–79, 2004.
80. Krzeminski K, Kruk B, Nazar K, et al: Cardiovascular, metabolic and plasma catecholamine responses to passive and active exercise. *Journal of Physiology and Pharmacology* 51:267–278, 2000.
81. Riley M, Maehara K, Porszasz J, et al: Association between the anaerobic threshold and the break-point in the double product-work rate relationship. *European Journal of Applied Physiology and Occupational Physiology* 75:14–21, 1997.
82. World Health Organization: Bulletin of the World Health Organization, 77; and International Society of Hypertension (1999). Guidelines for the management of hypertension. *Hypertension* 17:183–293, 1999.
83. Netea RT, Elving LD, Lutterman JA, et al: Body position and blood pressure measurement in patients with diabetes mellitus. *Journal of Internal Medicine* 25:393–399, 2002.
84. Nieman DC: Current perspective on exercise immunology. *Current Sports Medicine Review* 2:239–242, 2003.
85. Lampinen P, Heikkinen E: Reduced mobility and physical activity as predictors of depressive symptoms among community-dwelling older adults: An eight-year follow-up study. *Aging Clinical and Experimental Research* 15:205–211, 2003.

Chapter 20 III

Body Positioning

Elizabeth Dean

KEY TERMS

Body position changes
Cardiovascular and pulmonary function
Gravitational gradients
Oxygen transport
Prescriptive body positioning
Routine body positioning
Static body positioning

CHAPTER OUTLINE

The purpose of this chapter is threefold. First, therapeutic body positioning prescribed by physical therapists to optimize cardiovascular and pulmonary function and oxygen transport is differentiated from routine body positioning. Second, the physiological effects of static body positions as opposed to dynamic body position changes on cardiovascular and pulmonary function and oxygen transport are described. Third, the principles for prescribing therapeutic versus routine body positioning are presented.

Body positions that simulate the normal physiological effects of gravity and position change on oxygen transport are the clinical priority; being "upright and moving" is the physiological body position. When, because of disease or injury, patients are unable to be upright and moving consistent with the demands of normal living, the physical therapist simulates the patient's being upright and moving by means of specific body positions. Whether body positions are assumed actively by the patient or the patient is positioned passively by the physical therapist depends on the patient's status and needs.

Specific indications for body positioning and the decision-making process are highlighted. The chapter does not provide treatment prescriptions for given conditions because no specific patient is being considered. Understanding the physiological effects of body position on oxygen transport and how pathophysiology disrupts these normal processes is fundamental to prescribing body positioning for a given patient. An optimal body position can be prescribed only on the basis of consideration of all factors that impact on oxygen transport: the effects of the patient's pathophysiology and its specific presentation in that individual, the effect of restricted mobility and recumbency, the effect of extrinsic factors related to the patient's care, and the effect of intrinsic factors related to the patient (Chapter 17). It is only with an integrated analysis of these factors overall that (1) the most beneficial body positions can be predicted; (2) the least beneficial body positions can be identified and used minimally; and (3) the appropriate outcome measures can be selected.

Gravity and Normal Physiological Function: Physical Therapy Implications

The human is an orthograde organism. From moment to moment, gravity exerts its influence on the human body and particularly affects oxygen transport. The combined effects of gravity on the lungs, heart, and peripheral circulation are central to their interdependent function and to establishing normal oxygen transport. Knowledge of the effects of gravity on cardiovascular and pulmonary function in health and the deleterious effects of pathophysiological states on cardiovascular and pulmonary function (both primary pathology of the cardiovascular and pulmonary system and pathology of this system secondary to pathology in one or more other systems, as described in Chapter 6) provides a foundation for therapeutic body positioning as a primary intervention to optimize oxygen transport. Because of its potent and direct effect on oxygen transport, therapeutic body positioning can maintain or augment arterial oxygenation so that invasive, mechanical, and pharmacological forms of respiratory support can be postponed, reduced, or avoided—a primary objective of cardiovascular and pulmonary physical therapy.

In health, normal oxygen transport is maintained by being upright and moving—the physiological body position. A patient who may have prolonged periods of recumbency is also exposed to gravity continuously, but not to the same extent as in the upright position. Each body position the patient assumes differentially affects the steps of the oxygen transport pathway as a result of alterations in gravitational stress. Oxygen transport can be improved, maintained, or worsened with changes in body position. Despite being essential to normal cardiovascular and pulmonary function, gravity is the principal contributor to inhomogeneity of physiological function down the lungs.[1] Figure 20-1 illustrates the effect of this gradient with respect to alveolar ventilation ($\dot{V}_A$), perfusion (Q), ventilation and perfusion ratio ($\dot{V}_A/Q$), PaO_2, PCO_2, PN_2, oxygen content, carbon dioxide (CO_2) content, pH, and the flow of oxygen and CO_2 in and out of the lungs. Thus the lungs should not be likened to balloons, either physiologically or anatomically.

Based on a detailed analysis of all factors contributing to impaired oxygen transport and gas exchange (Chapter 17), the body positions that will have an optimal effect on oxygenation and those that may be deleterious must be distinguished from one another. In this way, a greater proportion of time can be spent by the patient in beneficial positions and less time in deleterious positions. Body positions themselves are associated with energetic stress, particularly in positions with greater gravitational stress, so the upright position can be more energetically demanding than supine positions, which are more demanding than lateral positions.[2] Compression forces also affect the heart and cardiac output. Lying on the left side, for example, can compromise cardiac output, particularly within 12 hours after surgery in patients whose cardiac index is less than 2.3 L/min/m^2.[3]

In health, gravitational effects and movement continually perturb the distributions of ventilation ($\dot{V}_A$) and perfusion (Q), and optimize $\dot{V}_A/Q$ matching commensurate with physiological demand. When body positions that are initially beneficial to the patient are assumed for too long, hydrostatic, gravitational, and compression forces acting on the heart, blood volume, lymphatic system, lungs, and chest wall, including the diaphragm, eventually compromise oxygen transport, offsetting any benefit. Therefore close monitoring is essential to ensure that the patient is turned to another position before the effects become detrimental. Frequent changes in body position and avoidance of prolonged periods in any single position minimize this risk.

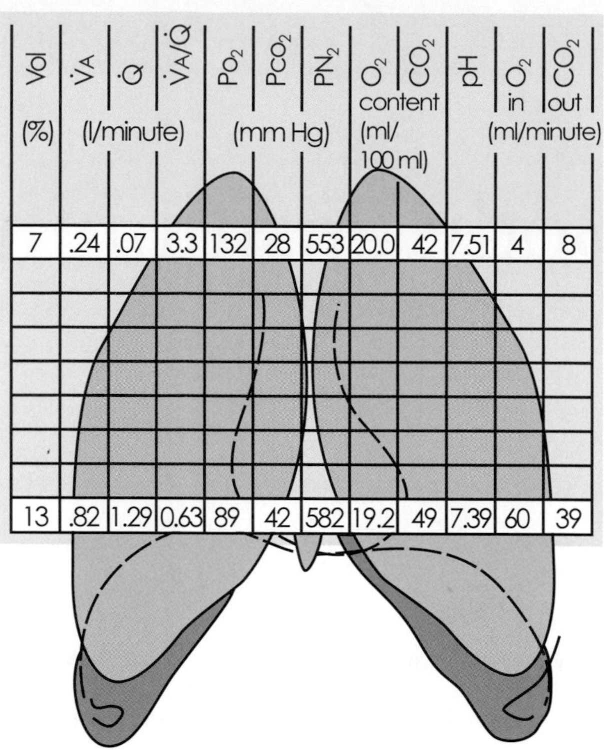

Fig. 20-1 Regional physiological differences down the upright lung. *VA*, Alveolar ventilation; *Q*, perfusion; $\dot{V}_A/Q$, ventilation-perfusion ratio. *(From West JB:* Respiratory physiology: The essentials, *ed 7, Baltimore, 2008, Williams & Wilkins.)*

The length of time a body position is maintained is response-dependent rather than time-dependent,[4] and it reflects individual differences, including pathology, severity, age, and body mass. Knowledge of the deleterious effects of prolonged periods in a single position supports the prescription of both frequent body position changes and extreme sequential body positions. These perturbations simulate the normal perturbations that the cardiovascular and pulmonary systems experience in health during normal mobility and body position changes in daily life. The ability to weigh the relative beneficial and deleterious effects of each possible body position (through 360 degrees in the horizontal plane and 180 degrees in the vertical plane, ranging from approximately 20 degrees head down to 20 degrees leaning forward) on a given patient's gas exchange is critical in prescribing body positioning.

Prescriptive Versus Routine Body Positioning

The literature supports the benefits of frequent body position changes, particularly for a patient who is relatively immobile, not alert, severely debilitated, obtunded, breathing at low lung volumes, obese, aged or very young, or has lost the sigh mechanism. Even though the effectiveness of routinely turning patients every 2 hours has not been firmly established, it continues to be an accepted standard of care (although intensive care units fall short of this minimal guideline).[5] The practice is based on the belief that the deleterious consequences associated with assuming a static position for a prolonged period will be prevented. More frequent turning, however, may have greater physiological benefits in patients who are critically ill, and this suggests that patients who are less severely ill may also benefit from being gravitationally challenged systematically. The preventive effects of a routine turning regimen are distinct from the acute effects of body positioning on oxygen transport, which is the primary focus of this chapter.

Physiological Effects of Various Body Positions

Body positioning has potent and direct effects on most steps of the oxygen transport pathway, so it can be prescribed to elicit these effects preferentially. Because humans function optimally when upright and moving, therapeutic interventions that elicit or simulate being upright and moving (i.e., elicit both gravitational and exercise stress) are most justified physiologically (see Chapter 17). The recumbent supine position, a common position assumed by patients who are hospitalized, is nonphysiological and is deleterious to oxygen transport. The side-lying positions have an effect that is intermediate between that of upright and supine. The prone position, which is underutilized clinically, can have such a significant powerful effect on oxygen transport that a good rationale must be made for not incorporating this position into the treatment prescription.

The indications for therapeutic body positioning and for frequent body position changes to optimize oxygen transport are shown in Tables 20-1 and 20-2. For each of the indications listed, an optimal therapeutic body position can be selected for a given patient. A description of the physiological effects of several primary body positions follow, namely, the upright/supine, side-lying, head-down, and prone positions. However, this information cannot be applied out of context. The specific positions prescribed for a given patient are based on consideration of the multiple factors that impair oxygen transport (Chapter 17) in conjunction with a physiological analysis of the most justifiable positions.

Because of the potent and direct effects of body positioning on the steps in the oxygen transport pathway in health and in disease, it is unknown whether the beneficial effects reported with the use of postural drainage are attributable to enhanced mucociliary transport; or to the direct effect of positioning the good lung down on improving the gas exchange of that lung by increasing alveolar volume of the affected, nondependent lung; or to both of these mechanisms. Typically, studies evaluating conventional chest physical therapy, including postural drainage, have failed to control for the direct effect of body positioning on oxygen transport or for the direct effects of increased arousal and mobilization that occur when a patient's body position is changed.[6,7] This is a serious methodological problem that pervades the literature evaluating conventional practices, so-called chest physical therapy, and one that has to be considered when interpreting the results of studies of these

Table 20-1 Indications for Body Positioning to Optimize Oxygen Transport

Cardiopulmonary Indications	Decreased regional alveolar volume Decreased regional ventilation Decreased regional perfusion Decreased regional diffusion Compromised ventilation to perfusion matching Pulmonary shunting Decreased lung volumes and capacities, particularly functional residual capacity, vital capacity, and tidal volume Closure of dependent airways Abnormal breathing frequency Abnormal minute ventilation Monotonous pattern of tidal ventilation Suboptimal position of the hemidiaphragms Decreased respiratory muscle efficiency Airway resistance Suboptimal lung compliance Suboptimal flow rates Weak ineffective cough Poor biomechanical efficiency of cough's strength and productivity Increased work of breathing Abnormal arterial blood gases, gas exchange, and oxygenation Impaired mucociliary transport and mucus clearance Untoward gravitational, mechanical, and compression forces on the lungs, chest wall, diaphragm, and the gut Impaired viscerodiaphragmatic breathing Suboptimal pattern of breathing
Cardiovascular and Lymphatic Indications	Suboptimal preload and afterload Increased work of the heart Impaired systolic ejection fraction to pulmonary and systemic circulations Suboptimal venous return Untoward gravitational, mechanical, and compression forces on the myocardium, great vessels, mediastinal structures, and lymphatic system Suboptimal fluid shift from central to dependent areas (extremities) and vice versa to maintain fluid volume regulating mechanisms
Other Systemic Indications	Decreased patient arousal Undue energy expenditure Discomfort Pain Posturally increased muscle tone Increased intrathoracic pressure Increased intraabdominal pressure Increased intracranial pressure Biomechanically suboptimal body positions Decreased chest tube drainage Decreased urinary drainage Impaired peripheral perfusion

Table 20-2 Indications for Frequent Changing of Body Position

Cardiopulmonary Indications	Alter chest wall configuration Shift distribution of alveolar volume Shift distribution of ventilation Shift distribution of perfusion Shift distribution of diffusion Shift distribution of ventilation to perfusion matching Shift mechanical physical compression of the heart on adjacent alveoli Shift position of the heart, thereby altering chamber end diastolic filling pressures, preload, afterload, and work of the heart Shift distribution of mucus transport and accumulation Stimulate effective and productive cough Facilitate pumping action needed for optimal lymphatic drainage Perturb pattern of monotonous tidal ventilation Perturb breathing pattern Shift gravitational, mechanical, and compression forces on the lungs, chest wall, diaphragm, and gut Simulate normal inflation-deflation sigh cycles Shift intraabdominal pressure
Cardiovascular Indications	Shift gravitational, mechanical, and compression forces on the myocardium, great vessels, mediastinal structures, and lymphatic system Stimulate fluid volume shifts particularly to the dependent limbs
Other Systemic Indications	Alter arousal state Promote relaxation Promote comfort Control pain Prevent skin breakdown, risk for infection, and resulting positioning limitations Shift abnormal postural tone patterns Optimize chest tube drainage Promote urinary drainage

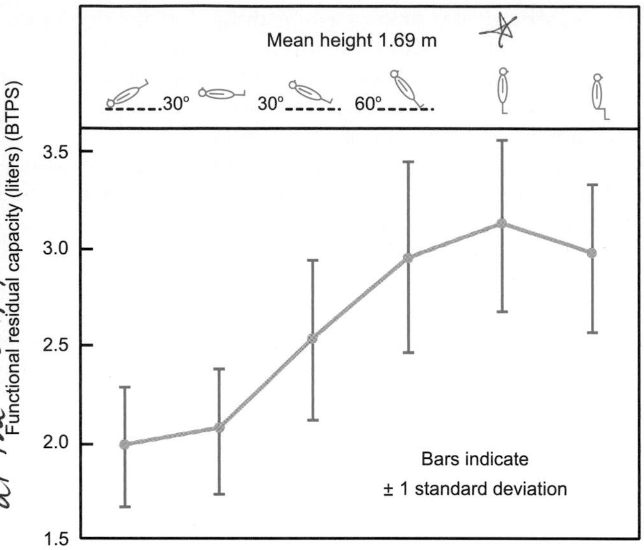

Fig. 20-2 Changes in functional residual capacity in various body positions. *(From Lumb AB, Pearl RG: Nunn's applied respiratory physiology, ed 6, Philadelphia, 2005, Butterworth Heinemann).*

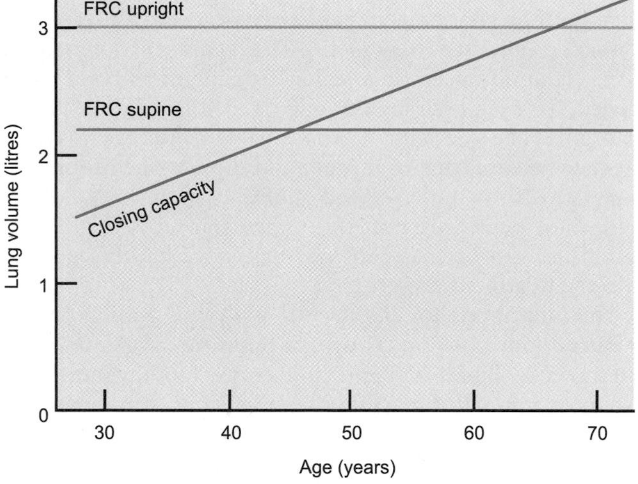

Fig. 20-3 Functional residual capacity (FRC) and closing capacity as a function of age. *(From Lumb AB, Pearl RG: Nunn's applied respiratory physiology, ed 6, Philadelphia, 2005, Butterworth Heinemann).*

procedures. Unless these potent confounding variables are controlled, the degree to which conventional chest physical therapy has a beneficial effect over and above the effects of positioning, as well as of mobilization and increased arousal, cannot be established.[8]

Upright Positions

Although the upright position is common to the physiological and anatomical positions, movement in the upright constitutes the true physiological position in that the upright position coupled with movement (e.g., walking, cycling, or movement in sitting) is consistent with the requirements of daily activities. To meet the energetic demands of these activities, oxygen transport is optimized to the greatest degree, in that ventilation and perfusion are more uniform than they would be without the additional exercise stimulus. The upright standing position maximizes lung volumes and capacities, with the exception of closing volume, which is decreased.[9] Functional residual capacity (FRC), the volume of air remaining in the lungs at the end of end-tidal expiration, is greater in standing than in sitting and exceeds that in the supine position by as much as 50% (Figure 20-2). Maximizing FRC is associated with reduced airway closure and maximal arterial oxygenation.[10,11] Figure 20-3 illustrates the relationship of FRC and closing capacity as a function of age. Because of age-related pulmonary changes, the closing capacity of the dependent airways increases with age; this effect is further accentuated with recumbency. Airway closure is evident in the supine position in the healthy 45-year-old person and in the upright seated position in the healthy 65-year-old person.[12] Compression atelectasis results from cardiac weight, abdominal pressure, and pleural effusions, the effects of which are determined by the specific position of the patient.[13] These positional

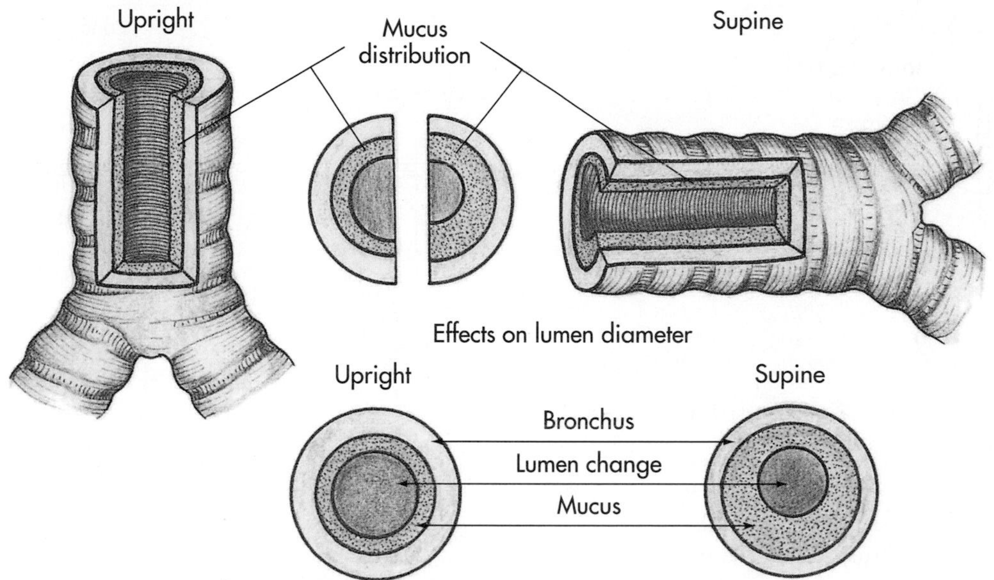

Fig. 20-4 Effect of recumbency and gravity on distribution of respiratory tract and diameter of bronchiolar lumen. *(From Gröer MW, Shekleton ME:* Basic pathophysiology: A holistic approach, *ed 3, St Louis, 1989, Mosby.)*

effects are further accentuated in patient populations with cardiovascular and pulmonary, thoracic, and abdominal pathologies, so the upright position is favored, and the supine position should be minimized so as to prevent airway closure and impaired gas exchange.

With respect to pulmonary function testing, the upright sitting position with legs dependent is the standard reference position.[14,15] When upright, the diameter of the main airways increases slightly. If the airways are obstructed, even small degrees of airway narrowing induced by recumbency can increase airway resistance (Figure 20-4). When a person is upright, the vertical gravitational gradient is maximal, the anteroposterior dimension of the chest wall is the greatest, and compression of the heart and lungs is minimized.[16] The shortened position of the diaphragmatic fibers is countered by an increase in the neural drive to breathe when a person is in the upright position.[17] Maximal expiratory pressure is augmented with progressively upright positions in patients with chronic obstructive lung disease, as well as in those in health; standing results in the highest values and head-down positions the lowest.[18] Thus coughing and other forced expiratory maneuvers should be encouraged when the individual is in the optimal erect, upright position.

The distribution of ventilation is determined primarily by the effect of gravity, which changes down the lung because of the anatomical position and the suspension of the lungs within the chest. At FRC in the upright position, the intrapleural pressure at the apex is −10 cm H_2O and at the base −2.5 cm H_2O (Figure 20-5). The intrapleural pressure is less negative in the base because of the suspended mass of the lungs. As a result of the greater negative intrapleural pressure in the apices, thus low compliance, these lung units have a larger initial volume; hence smaller volume changes occur during respiration. Because the lung units at the base have a smaller initial volume, thus high compliance, larger volume changes occur during respiration. Therefore, depending on their relative position with respect to gravity, different regions of the lung are at different points on the pressure volume curve.

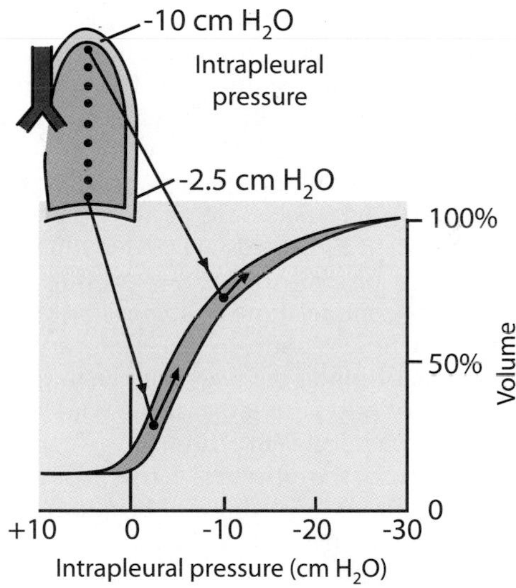

Fig. 20-5 Schematic of the regional differences in ventilation down the upright lung. *(From West JB:* Ventilation/bloodflow and gas exchange, *ed 4, Oxford, 1985, Blackwell Scientific.)*

A common clinical concern is patients breathing at low lung volumes—for example, patients in pain, patients who have undergone thoracic or abdominal incisions, older and younger patients, obese patients, pregnant patients, patients with gastrointestinal dysfunction (such as paralytic ileus and ascites, organomegaly, or intrathoracic or intraabdominal masses) patients who are malnourished, and patients who are mechanically ventilated or have spinal cord injuries). Breathing at low lung volumes reverses the normal intrapleural pressure gradient such that in the upright lung the apices have a negative intrapleural pressure compared with the bases, which have a positive intrapleural pressure (i.e., exceeding airway pressure) (Figure 20-6). This results in the apices being more compliant, thus better ventilated, than the bases. The bases are prone to airway closure in individuals breathing at low lung volumes.

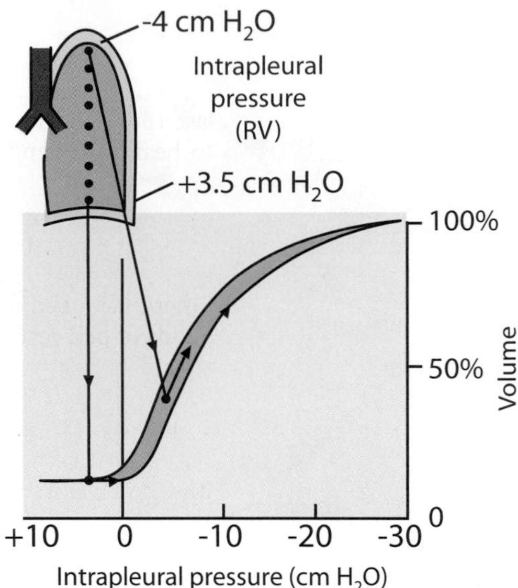

Fig. 20-6 Schematic of the regional differences in ventilation at low lung volumes. *(From West JB:* Ventilation/bloodflow and gas exchange, *ed 4, Oxford, 1985, Blackwell Scientific.)*

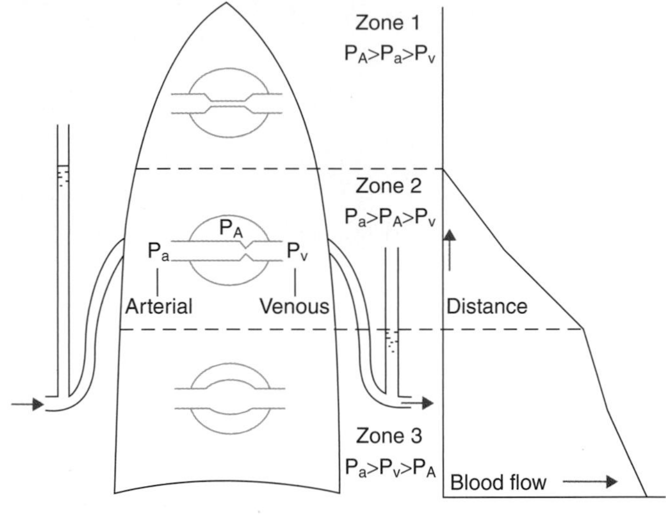

Fig. 20-7 Schematic of pressures affecting the pulmonary capillaries and blood flow. *(From West JB:* Ventilation/bloodflow and gas exchange, *ed 4, Oxford, 1985, Blackwell Scientific.)*

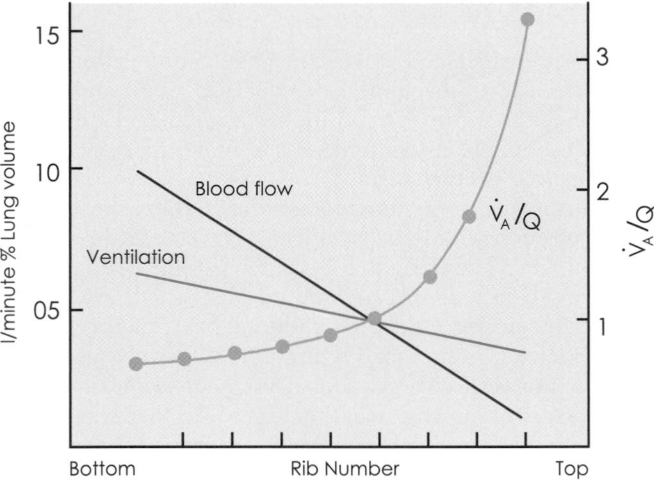

Fig. 20-8 Distributions of ventilation and blood flow down the upright lung and the distribution of ventilation perfusion matching down the upright lung. *(From West JB:* Ventilation/bloodflow and gas exchange, *ed 4, Oxford, 1985, Blackwell Scientific.)*

Another factor that reverses the normal intrapleural pressure gradient is mechanical ventilation. Despite its necessity in the management of patients in respiratory failure, mechanical ventilation can contribute to hypoxemia in several ways. First, it reverses the normal intrapleural pressure gradient so that the uppermost lung fields are preferentially ventilated. Because the dependent lung fields are preferentially perfused, $\dot{V}_A/Q$ mismatch is promoted. Positive pressure ventilation has the additional complication of increasing intrathoracic pressure and reducing venous return and cardiac output. These factors, in addition to the negative pressure required to open the inspiratory valve, can increase the work of breathing associated with mechanical ventilation.[19-21]

Although gravity is the primary determinant of interregional differences in the distribution of ventilation in the healthy lung, intraregional differences, secondary to differences in compliance and resistance of contiguous lung units, also contribute.[22] These effects are exaggerated in patient populations.[23]

The distribution of perfusion down the upright lung is also primarily dependent on gravity (Figure 20-7). The pressures affecting blood flow through the pulmonary capillaries and resulting in the typical uneven distribution (inhomogeneity) of blood flow are alveolar pressure and the arterial and venous pressures. In zone 1, at the apex, alveolar pressure predominates over arterial and venous pressures, so there is little or no blood flow. Zone 2, in the middle zone, reflects the blood flow from the recruitment of pulmonary vessels. Arterial pressure exceeds alveolar pressure and blood flow. Zone 3, in the lower area of the lung, reflects the blood flow from the distension of pulmonary vessels; arterial and venous pressures exceed alveolar pressure. And zone 4 (not illustrated), in the most dependent portion of the lung, has little or no pulmonary blood flow because of the interstitial pressure acting on the pulmonary blood vessels and creating a compression force.[1]

The matching of $\dot{V}_A$ and Q reflects the interfacing of the distributions of $\dot{V}_A$ and Q down the upright lung. Both $\dot{V}_A$ and Q increase down the upright lung; however, $\dot{V}_A$ increases disproportionately more than Q (Figure 20-8). As a result, the optimal area for $\dot{V}_A/Q$ matching is in the midzone, where the ratio is about 1.0.[24]

The upright position is associated with marked hemodynamic effects. These effects reflect primarily the central blood volume, which is shifted from the thoracic compartment to the dependent venous compartments when a person assumes the upright position from the supine.[25-27] End-diastolic volume and stroke volume are decreased, which results in a compensatory increase in heart rate.[28] Cardiac output is correspondingly decreased. The net effect of these physiological changes is a reduction in myocardial work.[29] This finding is corroborated by the observation that the anginal threshold is increased in patients with cardiac conditions when they are upright.[30] Further, intermittent gravitational stress following myocardial infarction or bypass surgery maintains orthostatic tolerance and thereby prevents bed rest deconditioning.[31]

Peripheral vascular resistance increases and blood flow decreases with the assumption of an upright position greater than 45 degrees to offset dependent fluid shifts and potential blood pressure drop (Figure 20-9). An upright angle of at least 60 degrees is needed to optimize cardiac output and sympathetic tone.[32] Another important effect of body position on fluid volume is the promotion of urinary drainage from the renal pelvi to the bladder when in the upright position, as a result of the reduced area for urinary stasis when in this position as opposed to the supine position (Figure 20-10). Optimal renal function is essential to preserving normal hemodynamic status.

Older individuals who are relatively immobile tend to sit for prolonged periods. Without frequent exposure to standing upright, however, the phenomenon of seated postural hypotension may result.[33] In addition, dependent circulatory stasis and other consequences of restricted mobility such as deconditioning are promoted in this position.

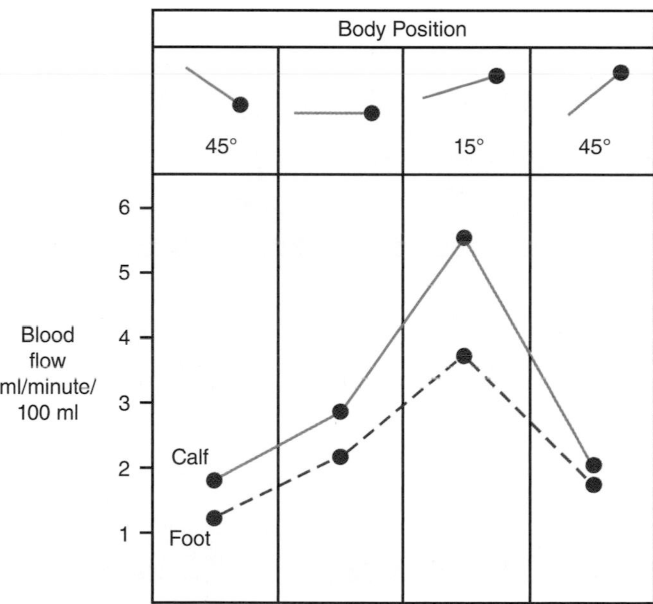

Fig. 20-9 *Effect of body position on peripheral blood flow.*

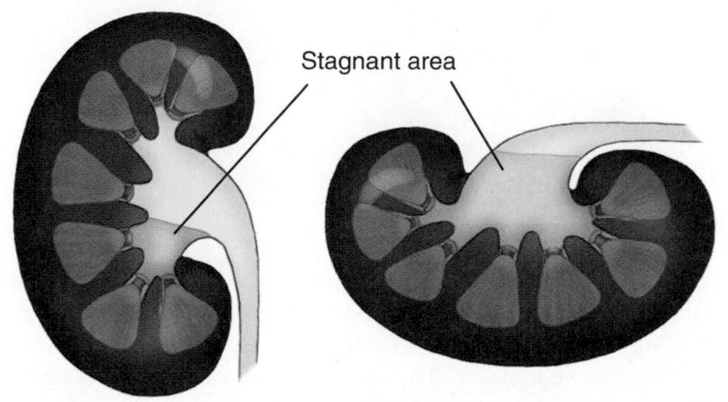

Fig. 20-10 Effect of body position on drainage from the pelvis of the kidney. *(From Browse NL:* The physiology and pathology of bed rest, *Springfield, Ill, 1965, Charles C. Thomas.)*

Supine Position

The indiscriminate use and overwhelming acceptance of bed rest evolved historically over the past 150 years. In the mid-1800s, the use of immobilization to heal bones and injuries was extended to the management of other conditions in the belief that internal organs could be rested as a therapeutic intervention as well. The injudicious application and overuse of bed rest to address medical problems has been challenged over several decades.[34-38] Although there has been a marked decrease in the use of prolonged periods of bed rest based on innumerable studies over the past several decades of its negative sequelae,[39] its use is still quite common despite the fact that its merits as a therapeutic modality and the parameters for its prescription (i.e., indications and specifications to achieving healing and recovery without deterioration) have not been scientifically established.

The supine position inherent in bed rest alters the configuration of the chest wall, the anteroposterior position of the hemidiaphragms, the intrathoracic pressure, the intraabdominal pressure secondary to the shifting of the abdominal viscera in this position, and the mechanics of cardiac function.[40-45] The normal anteroposterior configuration becomes more transverse. The hemidiaphragms are displaced cephalad, which reduces FRC in this position.[10] Prefaut and Engel[46] observed that hypoxic vasoconstriction secondary to closure of the dependent airways in the supine position contributed to preferential perfusion of the nondependent lung zones. Finally, in the supine position, excess pulmonary secretions tend to pool on the dependent sides of the airways. The upper side may dry out, exposing the patient to infection and obstruction (see Figure 20-4).

An increase in intrathoracic blood volume in the supine position also contributes to a reduction in FRC and lung compliance and to increased airway resistance.[47,48] Collectively, these effects predispose the patient to airway closure and an increase in the work of breathing. Although a healthy person can accommodate to these physiological changes, a healthy person does not assume this position for prolonged periods without unconsciously shifting. A hospitalized patient, however, is less likely to adapt to these immediate changes and their long-term effects. They may be less responsive to the need to shift position or unable to respond to afferent stimuli prompting a need to change position. These effects are accentuated in older people whose arterial oxygen tensions progressively diminish with age.[47,49] Compared with younger people, the arterial oxygen tensions of older people are particularly lower in the supine position compared with the reference sitting position.[50]

Several cardiovascular changes occur when the supine position is assumed (e.g., hemodynamic or intolerance to position change). A central shift of blood volume from the extremities to the central circulation initiates orthostatism.[27,51] This fluid shift increases both the preload and the afterload of the right side of the heart. This increased volume tends to distort the interventricular septum and reduce left ventricular volume and preload. The relatively increased central blood volume inhibits the release of antidiuretic hormone and atrial natriuretic peptide from the right side of the heart[52] and diuresis is stimulated.[53] Between 10% and 15% of fluid is lost within 24 hours,[27] which can manifest clinically as cardiac underfilling, orthostatic intolerance, and negative fluid balance.[54]

Altered autonomic nervous system function also has been implicated in the etiology of bed rest deconditioning.[55,56] Individuals with impaired autonomic control (those with high spinal cord lesions) exhibit greater reductions in mean arterial pressure and stroke volume compared with able-bodied individuals.[57] Because of local vascular regulation, cerebral circulation can be maintained. Finally, when individuals are confined to bed rest abruptly, they show more dehydration than do individuals confined to bed rest for a longer term, and it occurs faster, possibly because of less opportunity to compensate.[58] Although the prescriptive parameters regarding the optimal gravitational stress required to offset the hemodynamic changes that occur with the supine position have yet to be elucidated (degree of upright angle, duration, and frequency),[59] there are other effects of the upright position that support its frequent use in patients whose mobility is restricted. Anatomical regions adapt to the relative microgravity effects of the supine position differently according to the redistribution of transmural pressures and flows within the various vascular beds.[60] Knowledge of these physiological adaptations is essential for refining therapeutic countermeasures.

Although lower body negative pressure (LBNP) may have a role in space exploration for maintaining orthostatic stability and has been shown to offset change with bed rest such that exercise capacity is maintained,[61] LBNP will not likely be a feasible or practical modality in acute management. Despite its reported benefit in countering the adverse fluid shifts associated with recumbency, LBNP does not address other negative effects of bed rest.

Because of a reduction in the vertical gravitational gradient, and therefore in the intrapleural pressure gradient of the lung, in the supine position, the distribution of $\dot{V}_A/Q$ matching appears more uniform and evenly matched in horizontal positions.[62,63] These changes, however, must be considered in conjunction with other changes associated with the supine position: namely, reduced FRC, reduced vital capacity, reduced flow rates, increased area of dependent lung, and increased closure of the dependent airways, as well as its associated hemodynamic consequences. These deleterious factors offset any theoretical benefit of the supine position on V/Q matching.[64] However, in a patient who is unresponsive, hemodynamically unstable, and clinging to life, a recumbent position may be the only alternative (see end-of-life issues in Chapter 33).

The position of the diaphragm and its function are dependent on body position. Figure 20-11 illustrates the effect of body position on the level and movement of the diaphragm consistent with compromised lung function recorded in recumbent positions. In the supine position, the resting level of the diaphragm is influenced differentially by anesthesia and neuromuscular blockade.[65] Figure 20-12 illustrates these effects. In the spontaneously breathing subject, the excursion of the diaphragm is greater posteriorly because of the dependent viscera beneath the posterior portion of the diaphragm. During anesthesia with or without paralysis, the diaphragm ascends 2 cm into the chest. When paralysis is induced, the loss of diaphragmatic tone results in greater excursion of the nondependent rather than the dependent part of the diaphragm.

A study of hemodynamic postural effects in healthy subjects supports that the horizontal position maximizes central blood

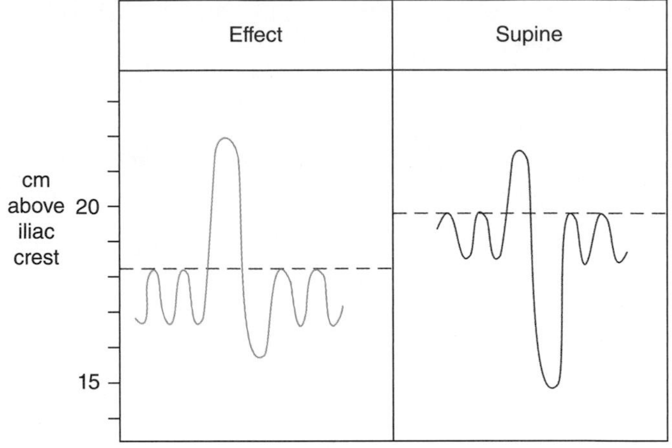

Fig. 20-11 Effect of body position on the level and movements of the diaphragm during respiration. *(From Browse NL:* The physiology and pathology of bed rest, *Springfield, Ill, 1965, Charles C. Thomas.)*

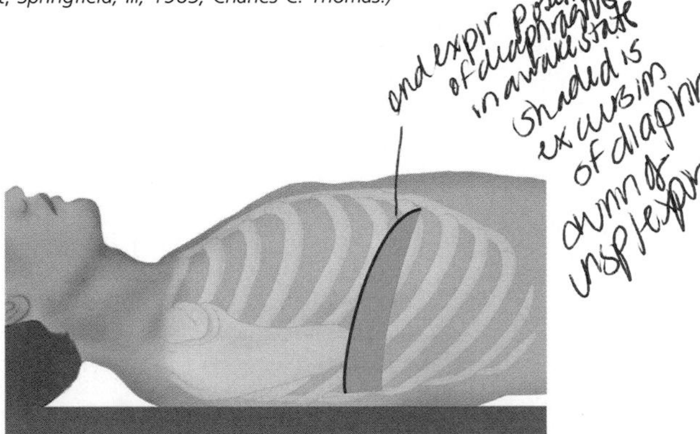

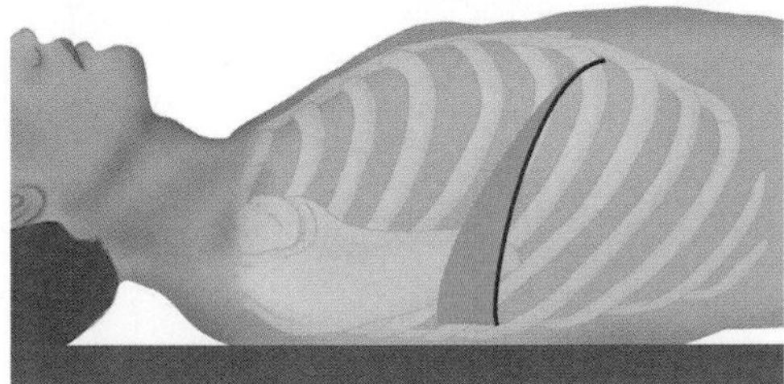

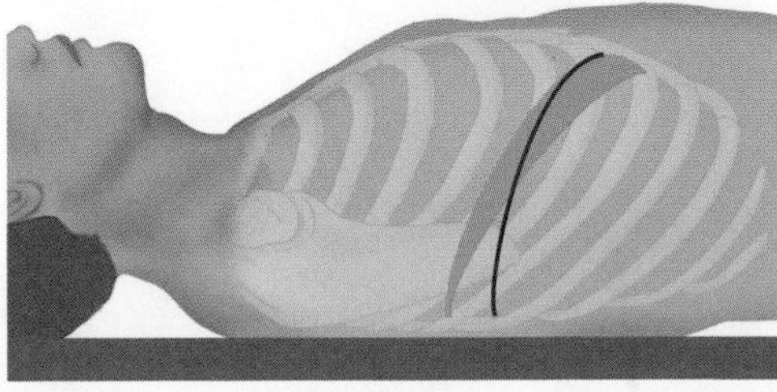

Fig. 20-12 Position of the diaphragm in an awake, spontaneously breathing subject and in anesthetized subjects with and without paralysis. The line is the end-expiratory position of the diaphragm in the awake state in the supine position. The shaded area shows the excursion of the diaphragm during inspiration and expiration. *(From Froese AB, Bryan AC: Effects of anesthesia and paralysis on diaphragmatic mechanics in man,* Anesthesiology *41:242-255, 1974.)*

volume.[66] This position, however, cannot be considered clinically optimal because of such effects as intrathoracic and intraabdominal compression.

Side-Lying Positions

Side-lying may be theoretically less deleterious compared with the supine position.[22,45,67] The side-lying position accentuates anteroposterior expansion at the expense of transverse excursion of the dependent chest wall. In this position, the dependent hemidiaphragm is displaced cephalad because of the compression of the viscera beneath it. This results in a greater excursion during respiration and to greater contribution to the ventilation of that lung and to gas exchange as a whole. The FRC in side-lying falls between that in the upright and supine positions. Compared with supine, in side-lying compliance is increased, resistance is reduced, and the work of breathing is reduced, whereas these measures are reversed when side-lying is compared with the upright position. Figure 20-13 illustrates the difference in lung volumes between maximal inspiration and FRC in a spontaneously breathing subject in right side-lying. Although ventilation is enhanced to the dependent lung, inspiratory lung volume and FRC are reduced. Compared with the reference sitting position, FEV_1 and FVC are reduced similarly in left and right side-lying, with no differential effects of side-lying on diffusing capacity and closing volume.[68] These lung-function effects in side-lying may reflect altered lung geometry with position change and a reduction in the vertical diameter of each lung in side-lying compared with that which occurs in the supine position.[69]

Side-lying increases end-diastolic ventricular pressure on the dependent side secondary to compression of the viscera beneath the diaphragm and to reduced lung compliance on that side.[70] Although such changes can be readily accommodated in health, they may further impair gas exchange in individuals with oxygen transport deficits.

Optimal $\dot{V}_A/Q$ matching occurs in the upper one-third of each lung in the side-lying position.[71] The total area for optimal $\dot{V}_A/Q$ matching, therefore, is likely greater than that in the upright position, which contributes theoretically to

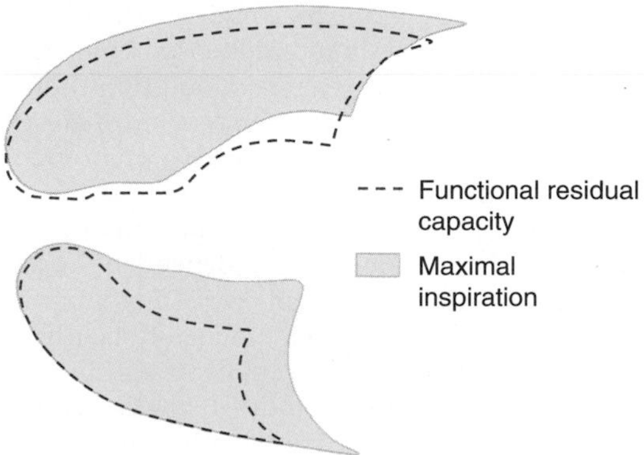

Fig. 20-13 Outlines of the lungs at two lung volumes in a conscious, spontaneously breathing subject in the right side-lying position. *(From Lumb AB, Pearl RG:* Nunn's applied respiratory physiology, *ed 6, Philadelphia, 2005, Butterworth Heinemann).*

an improved $\dot{V}_A/Q$ matching. These apparent improvements, however, are offset by reduced lung volumes and airflow rates in this position.

In healthy people and in patients, arterial oxygen tension is greater in side-lying than in supine position.[72] This is true for patients receiving supplemental oxygen, as well as for those who are not. Thus side-lying can be used to enhance the efficiency of gas exchange and thereby minimize or avoid the use of supplemental oxygen. Arterial blood gases have been reported to be improved in patients with unilateral lung disease[73,74] when they are positioned with the good lung down and worsened when the affected lung is down. When lung pathology is bilateral, arterial blood gas values are better when patients lie on the right side than when they lie on the left. This can be explained by the greater size of the right lung and the reduced compression of the heart on the lung in this position compared with left side-lying.[75,76] The practice of "down with the good lung," however, has been questioned in patients with unilateral lung collapse secondary to central airway lesions.[77] Not all patients respond favorably when the good lung is down. Research is necessary to distinguish the characteristics of responders and nonresponders to refine the prescription of body positions.

The side-lying rather than the supine position is often a preferred position for patients who are hospitalized; yet its physiological consequences are not well understood. The pulmonary effects of side-lying have been reported for healthy older people.[68] FEV_1 and FVC are reduced comparably for right and left side-lying compared with a reference sitting position. Although diffusing capacity and homogeneity of ventilation appear to be unchanged, they may be adversely affected in patient populations with single and combined pathologies that affect oxygen transport.

Patients who are hemodynamically unstable require special consideration with respect to body positioning. These patients may be less able to benefit from active mobilization and are more reliant on positional perturbation than on movement to promote optimal gas exchange. In one study of patients with severe respiratory failure and receiving inotropic support, the extreme left lateral position contributed to a hyperdynamic state, and the right lateral position predisposed the patients to hypotension, likely as a result of impaired right ventricular preload.[78] Spirometric evidence from patients who were intubated supports decreased dynamic lung compliance in the lateral and prone positions compared with supine.[79] Body positioning warrants judicious prescription, with particular attention to the angle of the lateral position and the duration and to monitoring to observe the effect.

Prolonged side-lying has been shown to mobilize lung water in patients with pulmonary edema, and to a lesser extent in patients with pulmonary inflammation.[80] Physical therapy interventions that entail gravitational challenges, therefore, can have a direct effect on lung water distribution and possibly compartmentalization, which in turn, may affect pulmonary compliance and gas exchange. Similarly, pleural effusions respond to the effect of gravity. In patients with unilateral effusions, when the effusion is positioned lowermost in side-lying, oxygenation is lower than when the effusion is positioned uppermost.[81] This may be explained by the effusion impairing $\dot{V}_A/Q$ matching and gas exchange in the lowermost lung.

Head-Down Position

The head-down position augments oxygen transport in some patients by improving pulmonary mechanics. Patients with chronic airflow limitation, for example, tend to have hyperinflated chests and flattened diaphragms in which the contraction of the diaphragm is inefficient because of the position of its muscle fibers on the length tension curve. The head-down position causes the viscera to be displaced cephalad beneath the diaphragm. The diaphragm is positioned more normally and rests at a higher and more mechanically efficient position in the chest.[82,83] In this position, patients may experience relief from dyspnea, reduced accessory muscle use, reduced upper chest breathing patterns, and reduced minute ventilation. Patients with pathology in the lung bases may also benefit from the head-down position in that this position favors gas exchange in the more functional upper lung fields and promotes alveolar distension of bases, which are uppermost in the head-down position. Other patients, however, such as those with respiratory muscle fatigue, may have increased respiratory distress in this position due to the added resistive loading of the diaphragm because of the weight of the viscera beneath. These observations support the need to prescribe body positioning on an individual basis with consideration of the multiple factors that may impair oxygenation as well as enhance it.

Prone Position

There is mounting physiological and scientific justification for use of the prone position to enhance arterial oxygenation and reduce the work of breathing in patients with cardiovascular and pulmonary dysfunction who may or may not be mechanically ventilated. The prone position shifts the mobile structures of the thoracic and abdominal cavities.[84,85] The heart and great vessels are displaced anteriorly. The liver, spleen, and kidney shift anteriorly and caudally.

The prone position increases arterial oxygen tension, tidal volume, and dynamic lung compliance.[86-88] The pleural pressure gradient is homogenized; hence the distribution of $\dot{V}_A$ and alveolar inflation are augmented. Ventilation to perfusion matching has been shown to be more uniform in horizontal positions,[62] reflecting more uniform pleural pressure gradient and less lung compression by the heart.[89] In addition, the prone position reduces stroke volume, increases sympathetic activity, and augments urine output.[90] There has been increasing interest in exploiting these benefits in patients who are critically ill where mobilizing options are more limited (see Chapters 34 and 35). The prone position has some role in avoiding mechanical ventilation in patients who are conscious and alert, thereby reducing the risk for ventilator-associated complications.[88] Over the years, studies of prone positioning have been conducted largely in patients with acute respiratory distress syndrome (see Chapter 36).[91-93] Prone is associated with improving oxygenation in 70% to 80% of cases.[94] The effect of prolonged duration in the prone position has been studied, and the benefits appear to be dose-dependent.[95] The physiological outcomes of prone positioning in the management of acute lung injury are thought to reflect the particular pathoetiology.

Complications associated with prolonged periods in the prone position, particularly skin breakdown, are common; thus close monitoring of skin over bony prominences is essential. To prevent or manage these complications, intermittent prone positioning has been advocated. Intermittent prone positioning of patients with acute respiratory distress syndrome and best positive end-expiratory pressure (PEEP) therapy can reduce FIO_2 levels to less than 0.50, the critical level for oxygen toxicity.[96]

In a study using a canine model of acute lung injury, the prone position was observed to augment oxygenation in conjunction with low PEEP and to offset the negative hemodynamic effects of high PEEP.[97] This finding is consistent with clinical outcome studies. The two common variants of the prone position are prone abdomen-restricted and prone abdomen-free. Prone abdomen-restricted refers to lying prone with the abdomen in contact with the bed, whereas in the prone abdomen-free position, the patient's hips and chest are elevated so that the abdomen is free. Both prone positions augment gas exchange, but the prone abdomen-free position, comparable to the hands-and-knees position,[98] enhances lung compliance, tidal volume, FRC, and diaphragmatic excursion to a greater degree and minimizes compression of the heart and abdominal viscera on the lungs.[13] In one study, use of supplemental oxygen was reduced in four of five patients who were mechanically ventilated and whose positioning regimen included the prone abdomen-free position.[99]

Although patients in respiratory failure have been shown to benefit from the prone position, certain precautions must be observed. The patient must be positioned so that all pressure point stress (particularly on the head and face), as well as stress on the tubing and circuitry of the mechanical ventilator tubing, is minimized. The patient should be monitored continuously. A semiprone position can provide many of the physiological benefits of a full prone position and can minimize the risks, particularly in patients who are mechanically ventilated and those with cervical spine pathology. In addition, the semiprone position simulates the prone abdomen-free position. The semiprone position may be more conservative, more comfortable, and safer for the patient who is severely ill, potentially hemodynamically unstable, older, or has a protruding abdomen.

For patients unable to be mobilized, use of some variant of the prone position is even more important. Excessive recumbency, particularly in patients who are being positioned through a restricted arc (e.g., supine and one-quarter turns to either side), should be offset by some variant of the prone position, and this position should be incorporated often. Inevitably, patients exposed to a restricted arc of positioning may readily develop atelectasis in the dependent lung fields. Patients who are mechanically ventilated and have monotonous patterns of tidal ventilation are at particular risk. The only means of preventing and countering compression and hydrostatically induced atelectasis is by positioning dependent areas uppermost and repositioning the patient frequently.

The time course for the development of such hydrostatic complications is dependent on the patient's status, which may change from hour to hour in an individual who is critically ill. Although it is essential to monitor objective measures of oxygen transport and the adequacy of the steps in the oxygen transport pathway, subclinical changes will precede clinically measurable changes. By the time changes manifest in clinical measures, significant pathology may be present. Prevention, anticipation, and early detection are key.

Physiological Effects of Frequent Changes in Body Position

Table 20-2 lists some of the physiological effects of frequent changes in body position that are mediated primarily through their effects on respiratory mechanics, cardiac mechanics, airway closure, mucociliary transport, lymphatic drainage, and altered neural activation of the diaphragm. These effects, resulting from a change in position, are distinct from the benefits derived from a particular static body position. The benefits of changing position can be enhanced by moving to an extreme position (i.e., moving from supine to prone, rather than moving from supine to side-lying). Extreme body position changes simulate, but do not replace, the physiological "stir-up" and perturbations that occur with normal mobility and being upright. When the stir-up regimen was originally proposed, Dripps and Waters[100] did not appreciate fully the physiological implications of regular upright standing.[101] The net effect of changing body position is a stirring-up of the constituent distributions of $\dot{V}_A$, Q, and $\dot{V}_A/Q$ matching and shifting of internal organs and their compression on the structures of the cardiovascular and pulmonary unit. Areas of dependent atelectasis, physiological dead space and shunting, and mucus distribution are dramatically shifted.[102] The stir-up stimulates lymphatic drainage, surfactant production and distribution through stretching of the lung parenchyma, and the distribution and function of pulmonary immune factors.[103] Frequent physical perturbations also may inhibit bacterial colonization.[104] In addition, frequent body position changes shift and redistribute compression forces acting on the diaphragm, myocardium, and mediastinal structures and the compression of the lungs by the myocardium and mediastinal structures.

Frequent body position changes are used by physical therapists to stimulate the patient and increase arousal to a more alert and wakeful state (Figure 20-14). The more upright the patient, the greater the neurological arousal and the greater the stimulus to breathe; this effect is augmented by encouraging the patient to be self-supporting. Commensurate with an increase in arousal, the patient is stimulated to take deeper breaths and, hence, to increase $\dot{V}_A$. When body positioning is coupled with mobilization, vasodilation and recruitment of the pulmonary capillaries are stimulated, and this, in turn, improves the homogeneity of the distributions of $\dot{V}_A$ and Q, hence augmenting $\dot{V}_A/Q$ matching.

Prescription of Therapeutic Body Positions and Body Position Changes

Prescription of body positioning is based on an analysis of the factors that contribute to impaired oxygen transport for each patient.[105] Specific positions are selected to simulate as closely as possible the physiological function of the normal, healthy, upright cardiovascular and pulmonary unit and oxygen transport, and the perturbations and stirring-up that occurs hemodynamically during normal mobility and being upright.[101] A hierarchy of body positioning alternatives based on the physiological justification of the various positions appears in Table 20-3. These positions range from the most to the least physiological. The hierarchy is based on the premise that oxygen transport is optimal when upright and moving. Mobilization in the upright position increases tidal volume and respiratory rate, hence increasing minute ventilation, flow rates, and mucociliary transport and clearance and enhances the efficiency and effectiveness of airway clearance and coughing. Thus incorporating active movement into the body position change is optimal.

Despite the well-documented benefits of the judicious application of therapeutic body positioning to enhance oxygen transport, it does not replace the more physiological intervention of mobilization and exercise to maximize oxygen transport. Rather, once the effects of mobilization/exercise have been maximally exploited, body positioning is the next best physiological approximation to a mobilized upright state. However, even the mobilized patient benefits from therapeutic body positioning between mobilization sessions and during the night and rest periods. The progressive sequence of body positioning with movement is considered from the outset in planning for fully functional recovery and return to daily life.

Body position should first be exploited when coupled with movement followed by the erect sitting positions with legs dependent. Figure 20-15 illustrates several variants of the sitting position. Each of these positions has distinct effects on oxygen transport, so the specific upright position has to be prescribed specifically, because the supported and propped-up positions in bed do not substitute for upright, erect sitting. These variants have a role only when the patient deteriorates while being positioned upright or when in that position. Sitting with the feet down and supported is preferable to the propped up long sit because of the gravitationally induced

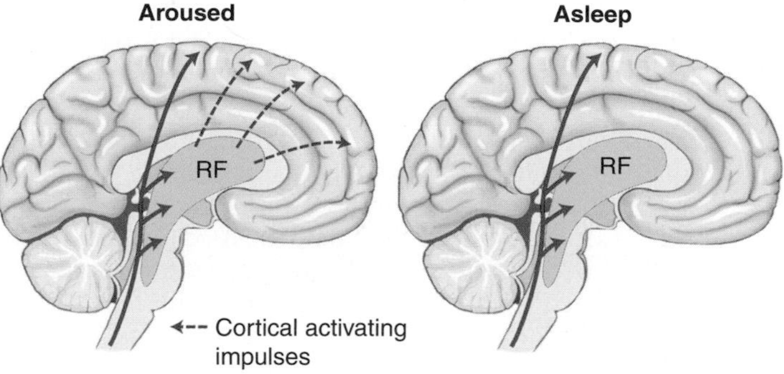

Fig. 20-14 Effect of arousal on cerebral activity. *(From Browse NL: The physiology and pathology of bed rest, Springfield, Ill, 1965, Charles C. Thomas.)*

Table 20-3 Physiological Hierarchy of Body Positions

Most Physiological Body Position	Least Physiological Body Position (Provisos)
Upright and moving in a 1-g gravitational field and exposed to a range of body positions and body-position changes over time	The upright erect sitting position implies that the back, head, and neck are vertical and aligned, with flexion only at the hips; the patient is not slumped or recumbent.
Relaxed erect standing (not too prolonged)	The less able the patient is to assist in positioning, the greater the need for more extreme positions and greater turning frequency.
Erect sitting (self-supported or with assist) with feet moving (e.g., active, active assisted, or passive cycling motion)	If the patient is totally unable to move (i.e., in a coma or paralyzed), extreme body positions are indicated if they are not contraindicated because of hemodynamic instability or increased intracerebral pressure.
Erect sitting (self-supported or with assist) with feet dependent	The upright position is used as much as possible, provided the patient is physically supported for safety and monitored in terms of treatment response.
Lean-forward sitting, with arms supported and feet dependent	Passive standing on a tilt table is hemodynamically questionable; it is preferable that patients be placed in a high Fowler position, with legs positioned dependently, using the knee breaks in the bed.
≥45-degree sitting with legs dependent	Regimens of 360-degree horizontal turning and 180-degree vertical turning (ranging from 20 degrees head-down to 20 degrees lean-forward) are used unless contraindicated. Positioning through a maximal arc simulates as closely as possible the three-dimensional movement of the chest wall during normal respiration.
Erect long sitting (legs nondependent)	
<45-degree sitting (legs nondependent)	
Prone and semiprone/side-lying	
Supine	

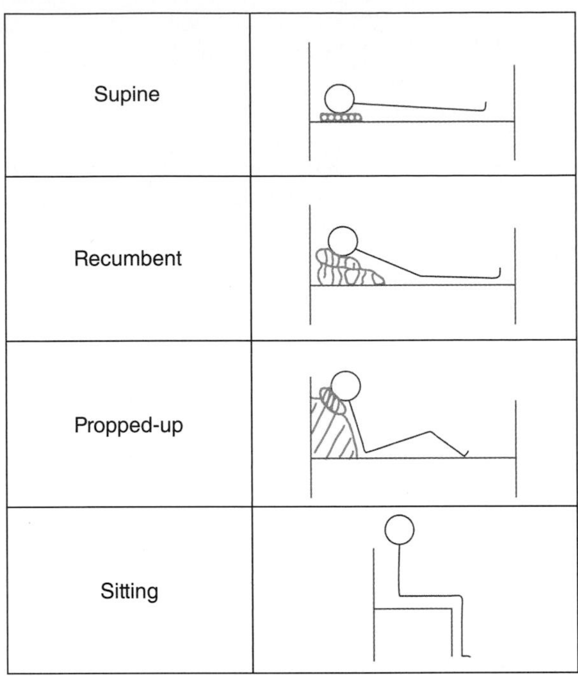

Fig. 20-15 Approximations of the upright position from supine. The recumbent and propped-up positions are not comparable physiologically to the upright sitting position. *(From Browse NL:* The physiology and pathology of bed rest, *Springfield, Ill, 1965, Charles C. Thomas.)*

hemodynamic benefits associated with this position. Sitting up in bed fails to position the patient in a perfectly vertical upright position. The head-up position in bed can be maximized, and the use of knee breaks in the bed provides a gravitational stimulus to the circulating blood volume.

One challenge when positioning patients in bed is the tendency to lose the position, usually from the compliance of the mattress and supporting pillows. Patients lose optimal positions in bed very quickly, so they should be monitored to ensure that the specific positions are maintained. An uncorrected slumped position can compromise pulmonary function and gas exchange. Pillows should not be used to maintain a body position because they are easily compressed and shifted. Blankets and sheets tightly rolled and secured with tape and rigid bolsters are more effective in maintaining a patient's body position.

Although there is a role for modified positions such as half side-lying, these positions are often overused at the expense of full turns to each side or prone or semiprone positions. Patients can be positioned safely (with appropriate supervision and monitoring) and comfortably in these full positions by observing the normal precautions of passive positioning.

A common practice is to progressively turn patients in one-quarter turns, such as from supine to side-lying and back to supine and so forth. However, the use of extreme positions and extreme position changes may yield greater physiological benefit with respect to the degree of perturbation and stir-up elicited.[106] Extreme position changes result in significant alterations in the distributions of $\dot{V}_A$, Q, and $\dot{V}_A/Q$ matching. Mucociliary transport is stimulated, and secretion accumulation and stagnation is minimized. In addition, the more extreme the body position, the greater the degree of arousal stimulated, particularly in the upright positions, and arousal is essential in patients who are critically ill.

Another important consideration is the time course of changes in oxygen transport with positions and position changes. There are three plausible outcomes: a favorable response, no response, or an unfavorable response. With the passage of time, all three outcomes will deteriorate. The specific time depends on the multitude of factors contributing to impaired oxygen transport. With judicious monitoring, the duration of a position can be maintained as long as the patient responds favorably, and it is modified before or at the first sign of deteriorating gas exchange.

Because of the marked changes that can be expected with body positioning and body positioning changes, the physical therapist has a narrow window of opportunity to assess and treat the patient before, during, and after position changes (immediate and delayed effects).

Mechanical Body Positioning

Kinetic or mechanically turning beds have long been known to benefit oxygen transport in patients who are severely ill.[107-111] These beds are indicated for those patients who are moderately hemodynamically unstable and on neuromuscular blockers and thus tolerate manual turns poorly. Such turning frames are contraindicated, however, for patients who are less ill. Even for patients who require multiple assistants and extra caution and time to turn and position effectively, these issues should never deny a patient a much-needed treatment with proven effectiveness.

The benefit of these beds on oxygen transport in patients who are critically ill has implications for the management of patients who are less severely ill. Continuous mechanical rotation can be simulated by increasing the frequency and arc of positions when manually positioning patients.

Practical Considerations in Positioning Patients

Prescriptive body positioning can require a significant amount of the physical therapist's time, as well as that of other team members. Such prescriptive positioning is based on clear indications and well-defined parameters; it is not to be confused with "routine" positioning. For any hospitalized patient who is recumbent and inactive, body positioning is a 24-hour concern, both during and between treatments. Such patients are at risk for impaired oxygen transport. The team as a whole has a responsibility to ensure that complications related to static positioning and restricted mobility are prevented.[112]

Despite the time and labor involved in turning a patient to the prone position, particularly if the patient is mechanically ventilated, the benefits of this position (even for short periods) outweigh the time and effort required. Given the benefits that can be derived from the prone position, justification has to be made for not doing so. Frequently, therapeutic body positioning can be effectively coordinated with nursing interventions and other procedures. With all body positions, but especially with the prone position in patients who are severely ill, potential inclusion and exclusion criteria should be reviewed, along with preturn considerations, the turning technique, assistants, monitoring the effectiveness of the prone position, passive movements, and limb positioning.[91] Finally, any problems or adverse responses to the prone, as to other positions, are documented.

Extreme body positions and body position changes are the interventions of choice after mobilization has been fully exploited or in the event that the role of mobilization is limited for a given patient. When extreme positions are less feasible, modified positions may be used. Even though the greatest benefits will be derived from extreme changes because they simulate the normal range of changes the human body is exposed to in health, small changes can be effective in altering intrapleural gradients slightly so that previously closed alveoli will be opened, even though previously opened ones may close. Although modified positions and small degrees of position change should not be relied on, their potential benefits should not be minimized in patients for whom extreme positions are contraindicated. Before and after each position change are prime opportunities to assess the patient and to encourage deep breathing and coughing or to suction the patient, as indicated.

Monitoring Responses to a Body Position or Position Changes

The prescriptive parameters of body positioning and body position changes include the positions selected, the duration in each position, the sequence of position changes, the cycle of all positions, and position changes overall. Because a patient necessarily assumes a body position at all times (is never free of gravitational forces), positioning patients between treatments can contribute as much to the overall treatment response as the treatment itself because the patient spends more time in the between-treatment positions than in the within-treatment positions.

The duration and frequency of the positions and the frequency of body position changes are response-dependent rather than time-dependent. Monitoring is the basis for defining and modifying the body positioning prescription. The physiological variables to be monitored depend on the patient's specific presentation and on cardiovascular and pulmonary dysfunction and its severity and distribution. Monitoring the patient who is not critically ill includes subjective and objective evaluation of indexes of the adequacy of oxygen transport (Part II). Among the most important are oxygen delivery, oxygen consumption, oxygen extraction, and gas exchange indicators such as the A/aO_2 difference and the PAO_2/PaO_2. Subjectively, the patient's facial expression, respiratory distress, dyspnea, anxiety, peripheral edema, discomfort, and pain are assessed. Objectively, heart rate, blood pressure, respiratory rate, SaO_2, flow rates, and bedside spirometry can be readily assessed. The appropriate standardization and procedures need to be used to ensure that the measures are both valid and reliable (see Chapter 7). Because physiological variables change from moment to moment, serial measures over a period of time should be taken to establish an average value, rather than using peak or discrete measures, which may misrepresent a treatment effect.

To interpret and compare various measures, the FIO_2 and any change in FIO_2 must be recorded. The use of the ratio PaO_2:FIO_2 enables comparison of gas exchange within and between patients when FIO_2 levels differ or change.[113] Similarly, for patients who are mechanically ventilated, any changes in the ventilatory parameters must be noted, in addition to other interventions that have a direct effect on oxygen transport. Only in this way will the clinician be able to reasonably conclude that the position or position change was instrumental in enhancing oxygen transport.

Measures and outcomes are recorded before (pretreatment baseline), during, and at periodic intervals following the treatment. A valid stable pretreatment baseline is essential to determine the therapeutic effect of a given position on oxygen transport. Variables monitored during the treatment are focused on ensuring that the treatment is having a beneficial effect, in addition to its not having any deleterious effect on the patient subjectively or with respect to any parameter of oxygen transport. As long as beneficial effects are being recorded, a position can usually be safely maintained in the absence of other contraindications; however, diminishing returns can be expected as the period becomes prolonged.

Patients maintained in static positions for more than 1 to 2 hours need to be monitored closely. A position change is physiologically defensible after this duration, rather than risking diminishing returns and potentially worsening the patient's condition.

The patient who is critically ill has the "advantage" of having more monitoring devices and lines in place. These provide access to several measures and indexes of oxygen transport, and certain hemodynamic and pulmonary variables are available continuously to ensure that the outcome is therapeutic and the patient is safe.

Summary

The premise underlying body positioning is that the physiological body position consistent with social participation and activity is "upright and moving." The specific purpose of this chapter is to differentiate therapeutic body positioning, which is prescribed by the physical therapist to optimize oxygen transport, from "routine" body positioning, which has the primary objective of maintaining gas exchange and preventing complications. The physiological effects on cardiovascular and pulmonary function and oxygen transport of different body positions and of changing body positions are described. The primary goal is to strive toward the physiological position for optimizing oxygen transport (i.e., upright and preferably moving). Issues related to optimizing the prescription of therapeutic body positioning and monitoring treatment outcome are presented.

This chapter focuses on the physiological effects of body positioning, an intervention that has well-documented, direct, and potent effects on oxygen transport. Establishing a clear rationale for prescribing a specific body position or body position changes is essential. The rationale, however, is based on multiple factors in addition to the physiological considerations presented. This chapter highlights the principles that must be considered in the decision-making process for prescribing therapeutic body positioning.

Review Questions

1. Relate the physiological body position of being upright and moving to the categories of participation and activity in the WHO International Classification of Functioning, Disability and Health.
2. Describe the effects of gravity on cardiovascular and pulmonary function and oxygen transport.
3. Distinguish prescriptive from routine body positioning.
4. In reference to the seated upright position, describe the effects of each of the following body positions on cardiovascular and pulmonary function and oxygen transport in health: supine, side-lying, head-down, and prone.
5. In reference to the seated upright position, describe the effects of each of the following body positions on cardiovascular and pulmonary function and oxygen transport in disease: supine, side-lying, head-down, and prone.
6. Explain how a physiologically ideal body position with respect to oxygen transport can be deleterious over time.
7. Distinguish between the prescription of therapeutic body positions and the frequency of body position changes.
8. Describe the principles of monitoring oxygen transport variables before, during, and after positioning a patient.
9. Explain why body positioning protocols cannot be defined for the management of specific pathological conditions, although this is often the way in which it is studied scientifically.

References

1. West JB: *Respiratory physiology: The essentials*, ed 8, Philadelphia, 2008, Lippincott Williams, Wilkins.
2. Jones AYM, Dean E: Body position change and its effect on hemodynamic and metabolic stress. *Heart and Lung* 33:281–290, 2004.
3. Doering L, Dracup K: Comparisons of cardiac output in supine and lateral positions. *Nursing Research* 37:114–118, 1988.
4. Bliss MR: The rationale for sitting elderly patients in hospital out of bed for long periods is medically unsubstantiated and detrimental to their recovery. *Medical Hypotheses* 62:471–478, 2004.
5. Krishnagopalan S, Johnson EW, Low LL, et al: Body positioning of intensive care patients: Clinical practice versus standards. *Critical Care Medicine* 30:2588–2592, 2002.
6. Dean E: Invited commentary to "Are incentive spirometry, intermittent positive pressure breathing, and deep breathing exercises effective in the prevention of postoperative pulmonary complications after upper abdominal surgery? A systematic overview and meta-analysis." *Physical Therapy* 74:10–15, 1994.
7. Ross J, Dean E: Integrating physiologic principles into the comprehensive management of cardiopulmonary dysfunction. *Physical Therapy* 69:255–259, 1989.
8. Dean E: Tightening up physical therapy practice: the confounding variable: Friend or foe? *Physiotherapy Canada* 46:77–78, editorial, 1994.
9. Svanberg L: Influence of posture on lung volumes, ventilation and circulation of normals. *Scandinavian Journal of Clinical Laboratory Investigations* 25:1–195, 1957.
10. Hsu HO, Hickey RF: Effect of posture on functional residual capacity postoperatively. *Anesthesiology* 44:520–521, 1976.
11. Ray JF, 3rd, Yost L, Moallem S, et al: Immobility, hypoxemia, and pulmonary arteriovenous shunting. *Archives of Surgery* 109:537–541, 1974.
12. Leblanc P, Ruff F, Milic-Emili J: Effects of age and body position on airway closure in man. *Journal of Applied Physiology* 28:448–451, 1970.
13. Rouby JJ, Puybasset L, Nieszkowska A, et al: Acute respiratory distress syndrome: lessons from computed tomography of the whole lung. *Critical Care Medicine* 31(Suppl):S285–S295, 2003.
14. American Thoracic Society: Standardization of spirometry. *American Journal of Respiratory and Critical Care Medicine* 152:1107–1136, 1995. 1994 Update.
15. Hankinson JL, Odencrantz JR, Fedan KB: Spirometric reference values from a sample of the general U.S. population. *American Journal of Respiratory and Critical Care Medicine* 159:179–187, 1999.
16. Weber KT, Janicki JS, Shroff SG, et al: The cardiopulmonary unit: The body's gas exchange system. *Clinics in Chest Medicine* 4:101–110, 1983.
17. Druz WS, Sharp JT: Electrical and mechanical activity of the diaphragm accompanying body position in severe chronic obstructive pulmonary disease. *American Review of Respiratory Diseases* 125:275–280, 1982.
18. Badr C, Elkins MR, et al: The effect of body position on maximal expiratory pressure and flow. *Australia Journal of Physiotherapy* 48:95–102, 2002.
19. Brochard L, Rua F, Lorino H, et al: Inspiratory pressure support compensates for the additional work of breathing caused by the endotracheal tube. *Anesthesiology* 75:739–745, 1991.
20. García Vicente E, Sandoval Almengor JC, Díaz Caballero LA, et al: Invasive mechanical ventilation in COPD and asthma. *Medicina Intensiva* Jan 7. [Epub ahead of print], 2011.
21. Tobin MJ: Mechanical ventilation. *New England Journal of Medicine* 330:1056–1061, 1994.

22. Ross J, Dean E: Body positioning. In Zadai CC, editor: *Clinics in physical therapy, pulmonary management in physical therapy*, New York, 1992, Churchill Livingstone.
23. Mason RJ, Broaddus VC, Martin T, et al: *Murray and Nadel's textbook of respiratory medicine*, ed 5, Philadelphia, 2010, Elsevier.
24. West JB: *Pulmonary pathophysiology: The essentials*, ed 7, Philadelphia, 2007, Lippincott Williams and Wilkins.
25. Blomqvist CG, Stone HL: Cardiovascular adjustments to gravitational stress. In Shepherd JT, Abboud FM, editors: Handbook of physiology, section 2: Circulation, vol 2, Bethesda, Md., 1963, American Physiological Society.
26. Gauer OH, Thron HL: Postural changes in the circulation. In Hamilton WF, editor: *Handbook of Physiology*, Washington, 1965, American Physiological Society.
27. Sandler H: Cardiovascular effects of inactivity. In Sandler H, Vernikos J, editors: *Inactivity: Physiological effects*, Orlando, 1986, Academic Press.
28. Thandani U, Parker JO: Hemodynamics at rest and during supine and sitting bicycle exercise in normal subjects. *American Journal of Cardiology* 41:52–58, 1978.
29. Langou RA, Wolfson S, Olson EG, et al: Effect of orthostatic postural changes on myocardial oxygen demands. *American Journal of Cardiology* 39:418–421, 1977.
30. Prakash R, Parmely WW, Dikshit K, et al: Hemodynamic effects of postural changes in patients with acute myocardial infarction. *Chest* 64:7–9, 1973.
31. Convertino VA: Value of orthostatic stress in maintaining function status soon after myocardial infarction or cardiac artery bypass grafting. Journal of Cardiovascular *Nursing* 18:124–130, 2003.
32. Zaidi A, Benitez D, Gaydecki PA, et al: Haemodynamic effects of increasing angle of head up tilt. *Heart* 83:181–184, 2000.
33. Cohen N, Gorelik O, Fishlev G, et al: Seated postural hypotension is common among older inpatients. *Clinical Autonomic Research* 13:447–449, 2003.
34. Dock W: The evil sequelae of complete bed rest. *Journal of the American Medical Association* 125:1083–1085, 1944.
35. Harrison TR: The abuse of rest as a therapeutic measure for patients with cardiovascular disease. *Journal of the American Medical Association* 125:1075–1077, 1944.
36. Moreno F, Lyons HA: Effect of body posture on lung volumes. *Journal of Applied Physiology* 16:27–29, 1961.
37. Powers JH: The abuse of rest as the therapeutic measure in surgery. *Journal of the American Medical Association* 125:1079–1083, 1944.
38. Winslow EH: Cardiovascular consequences of bed rest. *Heart Lung* 14:236–246, 1985.
39. Dean E, Ross J: Discordance between cardiopulmonary physiology and physical therapy: Toward a rational basis for practice. *Chest* 101:1694–1698, 1992b.
40. Behrakis PK, Baydur A, Jaeger MJ, et al: Lung mechanics in sitting and horizontal body positions. *Chest* 83:643–646, 1983.
41. Craig DB, Wahba WM, Don HF, et al: Closing volume and its relationship to gas exchange in seated and supine positions. *Journal of Applied Physiology* 31:717–721, 1971.
42. Don HF, Craig DB, Wahba WM, et al: The measurement of gas trapped in the lungs at functional residual capacity and the effect of posture. *Anesthesiology* 35:582–590, 1971.
43. Druz WS, Sharp JT: Activity of respiratory muscles in upright and recumbent humans. *Journal of Applied Physiology* 51:1552–1561, 1981.
44. Klingstedt C, Hedenstierna G, Baehrendtz S, et al: Ventilation-perfusion relationships and atelectasis formation in the supine and lateral positions during conventional mechanical and differential ventilation. *Acta Anaesthesiologica Scandinavica* 34:421–429, 1990.
45. Roussos CH, Fukuchi Y, Macklem PT, et al: Influence on diaphragmatic contraction on ventilation distribution in horizontal man. *Journal of Applied Physiology* 40:417–424, 1976.
46. Prefaut CH, Engel LA: Vertical distribution of perfusion and inspired gas in supine man. *Respiratory Physiology* 43:209–219, 1981.
47. Lumb AB, Pearl RG: *Nunn's applied respiratory physiology*, ed 6, Philadelphia, 2005, Elsevier/Butterworth Heinemann.
48. Sjostrand T: Determination of changes in the intrathoracic blood volume in man. *Acta Physiologica Scandinavica* 22:116–128, 1951.
49. Creditor MC: Hazards of hospitalization of the elderly. *Annals of Internal Medicine* 118:219–223, 1993.
50. Hardie JA, Morkve O, Ellingsen I: Effect of body position on arterial oxygen tension in the elderly. *Respiration* 69:123–128, 2002.
51. Matzen S, Perko G, Groth S, et al: Blood volume distribution during head-up tilt induced central hypovolaemia in man. *Clinical Physiology* 11:411–422, 1991.
52. Perko G, Payne G, Linkis P, et al: Thoracic impedance and pulmonary atrial natriuretic peptide during head-up tilt induced hypovolemic shock in humans. *Acta Physiologica Scandinavica* 150:449–454, 1994.
53. Norsk P: Renal adjustment to microgravity. *Pflugers Archives* 441(Suppl):R62–R65, 2000.
54. Dean E, Ross J: Mobilization and exercise conditioning. In Zadai CC, editor: *Clinics in physical therapy. Pulmonary management in physical therapy*, New York, 1992, Churchill Livingstone.
55. Hasser EM, Moffitt JA: Regulation of sympathetic nervous system function after cardiovascular deconditioning. *Annals of the New York Academy of Science* 940:454–468, 2001.
56. Hughson RL, Yamamoto Y, Maillet A, et al: Altered autonomic regulation of cardiac function during head-up tilt after 28-day head-down bed-rest with counter-measures. *Clinical Physiology* 14:291–304, 1994.
57. Houtman S, Colier WN, Oeseburg B, et al: Systemic circulation and cerebral oxygenation during head-up tilt in spinal cord injured individuals. *Spinal Cord* 38:158–163, 2000.
58. Zorbas YG, Yarullin VL, Denogratov SD, et al: Fluid volume measurements in normal subjects to disclose body hydration during acute bed rest. *International Urology and Nephrology* 35:457–465, 2003.
59. Zhang LN, Gao F, Ma J, et al: Daily head-up tilt, standing or centrifugation can prevent vasoreactivity changes in arteries of simulated weightless rats. *Journal of Gravitational Physiology* 7:P143–P144, 2000.
60. Zhang LF: Vascular adaptation to microgravity: What have we learned? *Journal of Applied Physiology* 91:2415–2430, 2001.
61. Watenpaugh DE, Ballard RE, Schneider SM, et al: Supine lower body negative pressure exercise during bed rest maintains upright exercise capacity. *Journal of Applied Physiology* 89:218–227, 2000.
62. Mure M, Domino KB, Lindahl SGE, et al: Regional ventilation-perfusion distribution is more uniform in the prone position. *Journal of Applied Physiology* 88: 1076–1083, 2000.
63. Nyrén S, Mure M, Jacobsson H, et al: Pulmonary perfusion is more uniform in the prone than in the supine position: scintigraphy in healthy humans. *Journal of Applied Physiology* 86:1135–1141, 1999.
64. Ross J, Dean E, Abboud RT: The effect of postural drainage positioning on ventilation homogeneity in healthy subjects. *Physical Therapy* 72:794–799, 1992.
65. Froese AB, Bryan AC: Effects of anesthesia and paralysis on diaphragmatic mechanics in man. *Anesthesiology* 41:242–255, 1974.
66. Harms MP, vanLieshout JJ, Jenstrup M, et al: Postural effects on cardiac output and mixed venous oxygen saturation in humans. *Experimental Physiology* 88:611–616, 2003.
67. Hurewitz AN, Susskind H, Harold WH: Obesity alters regional variation in lateral decubitus position. *Journal of Applied Physiology* 59:774–783, 1985.
68. Manning F, Dean E, Ross J, et al: Effects of side lying on lung function in older individuals. *Physical Therapy* 79:456–466, 1999.
69. Klingstedt C, Hedenstierna G, Lundqvist H, et al: The influence of body position and differential ventilation on lung dimensions and atelectasis formation in anaesthetized man. *Acta Anaethesiologica Scandinavica* 34:315–322, 1990b.
70. Lange RA, Katz J, McBride W, et al: Effects of supine and lateral positions on cardiac output and intracardiac pressures. *American Journal of Cardiology* 62:330–333, 1988.
71. Kaneko K, Milic-Emili J, Dolovich MB, et al: Regional distribution of ventilation and perfusion as a function of body position. *Journal of Applied Physiology* 21:767–777, 1966.
72. Clauss RH, Scalabrini BY, Ray JF, et al: Effects of changing body position upon improved ventilation-perfusion relationships. *Circulation* 37(Suppl 2):214–217, 1968.
73. Remolina C, Khan AU, Santiago TV, et al: Positional hypoxemia in unilateral lung disease. *New England Journal of Medicine* 304:523–526, 1981.
74. Sonneblick M, Meltzer E, Rosin AJ: Body positional effect on gas exchange in unilaeral pleural effusion. *Chest* 83:784–786, 1983.
75. Dean E: Effect of body position on pulmonary function. *Physical Therapy* 65:613–618, 1985.
76. Zach MB, Pontoppidan H, Kazemi H: The effect of lateral positions on gas exchange in pulmonary disease. *American Review of Respiratory Diseases* 110:49–53, 1974.
77. Chang SC, Chang HI, Shiao GM, et al: Effect of body position on gas exchange in patients with unilateral central airway lesions: Down with the good lung? *Chest* 103:787–791, 1993.

78. Bein T, Metz C, Keyl C, et al: Effects of extreme lateral posture on hemodynamics and plasma atrial natriuretic peptide levels in critically ill patients. *Intensive Care Medicine* 22:651–655, 1996.
79. Tanskanen P, Kytta J, Randell T: The effect of patient positioning on dynamic lung compliance. *Acta Anaesthesiologica Scandinavica* 41:602–606, 1997.
80. Zimmerman JE, Goodman LR, St Andre AC, et al: Radiographic detection of mobilizable lung water: the gravitational shift test. *American Journal of Roentgenology* 138:59–64, 1982.
81. Duan LF, Lu SY, Ling AZ: Effect of position change on the PaO_2 in patients with unilateral tuberculous pleural effusion. *Zhonghua Hu Li Za Zhi* 32:190–191, English abstract, 1997.
82. Barach AL, Beck GJ: Ventilatory effects of head-down position in pulmonary emphysema. *American Journal of Medicine* 16:55–60, 1954.
83. De Troyer A: Mechanical role of the abdominal muscles in relation to posture. *Respiratory Physiology* 53:341–353, 1983.
84. Ball WS, Wicks JD, Mettler FA, Jr: Prone-supine change in organ position: CT demonstration. *American Journal of Roentgenology* 135:815–820, 1980.
85. Albert RK, Hubmayr RD: The prone position eliminates compression of the lungs by the heart. *American Journal of Respiratory Critical Care Medicine* 16:1660–1665, 2000.
86. Gattinoni L, Caironi P: Prone positioning: beyond physiology. *Anesthesiology* 113:1262–1264, 2010.
87. Jolliet P, Bulpa P, Chevrolet JC: Effects of the prone position on gas exchange and hemodynamics in severe acute respiratory distress syndrome. *Critical Care Medicine* 26:1934–1935, 1998.
88. Valter C, Christensen AM, Tollund C, et al: Response to the prone position in spontaneously breathing patients with hypoxemic respiratory failure. *Acta Anaesthesiologica Scandinavica* 47:416–418, 2003.
89. Fessler HE, Talmor DS: Should prone positioning be routinely used for lung protection during mechanical ventilation? *Respiratory Care* 55:88–99, 2010.
90. Pump B, Talleruphuus U, Christensen NJ, et al: Effects of supine, prone, and lateral positions on cardiovascular and renal variables in humans. *American Journal of Physiology. Regulatory, Integrative and Comparative Physiology* 283:R174–R180, 2002.
91. Ball C, Adams J, Boyce S, et al: Clinical guidelines for the use of the prone position in acute respiratory distress syndrome. *Intensive Critical Care Nursing* 17:94–104, 2001.
92. Flaatten H, Aardal S, Hevroy O: Improved oxygenation using the prone position in patients with ARDS. *Acta Anaesthesiologica Scandinavica* 42: 329–334, 1998.
93. Langer M, Mascheroni D, Marcolin R, et al: The prone position in ARDS patients. *Chest* 94:103–107, 1988.
94. Pelosi P, Brazzi L, Gattinoni L: Prone position in acute respiratory distress syndrome. *European Respiratory Journal* 20:1017–1028, 2002.
95. McAuley DF, Giles S, Fichter H, et al: What is the optimal duration of ventilation in the prone position in acute lung injury and acute respiratory distress syndrome? *Intensive Care Medicine* 28:414–418, 2002.
96. Michaels AJ, Wanek SM, Dreifuss BA, et al: A protocolized approach to pulmonary failure and the role of intermittent prone positioning. *Journal of Trauma* 52:1037–1047, 2002.
97. Lim CM, Koh Y, Chin JY, et al: Respiratory and haemodynamic effects of the prone position at two different levels of PEEP in a canine lung injury model. *European Respiratory Journal* 13:163–168, 1999.
98. Mellins RB: Pulmonary physiotherapy in the pediatric age group. *American Review of Respiratory Diseases* 110(Suppl 1):37–142, 1974.
99. Douglas WW, Rehder K, Beynen FM, et al: Improved oxygenation in patients with acute respiratory failure: The prone position. *American Review of Respiratory Diseases* 115:559–566, 1977.
100. Dripps RD, Waters RM: Nursing care of surgical patients. I. The "stir-up." *American Journal of Nursing* 41:530–534, 1941.
101. Convertino VA: Effects of exercise and inactivity on intravascular volume and cardiovascular control mechanisms. *Acta Astronaut* 27:123–129, 1992.
102. Gattinoni L, Pelosi P, Vitale G, et al: Body position changes redistribute lung computed-tomographic density in patients with acute respiratory failure. *Anesthesiology* 74:15–23, 1991.
103. Pyne DB: Regulation of neutrophil function during exercise. *Sports Medicine* 17:245–258, 1994.
104. Skerrett SJ, Niederman MS, Fein AM: Respiratory infections and acute lung injury in systemic illness. *Clinics in Chest Medicine* 10:469–502, 1989.
105. Doering LV: The effect of positioning on hemodynamics and gas exchange in the critically ill: A review. *American Journal of Critical Care* 2:208–216, 1993.
106. Piehl MA, Brown RS: Use of extreme position changes in acute respiratory failure. *Critical Care Medicine* 4:13–14, 1977.
107. Fink MP, Helsmoortel CM, Stein KL, et al: The efficacy of an oscillating bed in the prevention of lower respiratory tract infection in critically ill victims of blunt trauma: A prospective study. *Chest* 97:132–137, 1990.
108. Gentillelo L, Thompson DA, Tonnesen AS: Effect of a rotating bed on the incidence of pulmonary complications in critically ill patients. *Critical Care Medicine* 16:783–786, 1988.
109. Summer WR, Curry P, Haponik EF, et al: Continuous mechanical turning of intensive care patients shortens length of stay in some diagnostic-related groups. *Journal of Critical Care* 4:45–53, 1989.
110. Ahrens T, Kollef M, Stewart J, et al: Effect of kinetic therapy on pulmonary complications. *American Journal of Critical Care* 13:376–383, 2004.
111. Delaney A, Gray H, Laupland KB, et al: Kinetic bed therapy to prevent nosocomial pneumonia in mechanically ventilated patients: A systematic review and meta-analysis. *Critical Care* 10:R70, 2006.
112. Markey DW, Brown RJ: An interdisciplinary approach to addressing patient activity and mobility in the medical-surgical patient. *Journal of Nursing Care Quality* 16:1–12, 2002.
113. Dean E, Ross J: Oxygen transport: The basis for contemporary cardiopulmonary physical therapy and its optimization with body positioning and mobilization. *Physical Therapy Practice* 1:34–44, 1992.

Chapter 21 III

Airway Clearance Techniques

Anne Mejia-Downs

KEY TERMS

Active cycle of breathing technique
Acoustic airway clearance
Airway clearance techniques
Autogenic drainage
Forced expiratory technique
High-frequency chest wall oscillation
Intrapulmonary percussive ventilation
Manual hyperventilation
Percussion
Positive expiratory pressure
Postural drainage
Shaking
Vibration

CHAPTER OUTLINE

Oxygen transport from the lungs to body tissues can be limited in patients with an ineffective cough or an impairment of normal mechanisms of mucociliary clearance. An array of techniques for assisting the mobilization of airway secretions is available for patients and caregivers to augment a patient's own mechanisms. When prescribing an optimal method of airway clearance, the caregiver must consider the pathophysiology and the clinical manifestations of the disease, the physiological basis of the method, availability of the technique to the patient, and the patient's acceptance of the technique.

This chapter reviews the physiological basis of each airway clearance technique (ACT), the history of its use, and research on its effectiveness. An introduction to the application of these techniques to patients is presented. Also addressed are the benefits and burdens of each technique, contraindications and precautions, and practical concerns regarding patient care.

Evidence for the use of airway clearance techniques is often difficult to evaluate, in part due to agreement that top-level evidence on this topic is lacking.[1a-b] The components of a given treatment have not been standardized and the literature refers to ACTs using a variety of terms, including chest physiotherapy, chest physical therapy (CPT), bronchial drainage, postural drainage (PD) therapy, and bronchial hygiene. In addition, the availability of equipment and cultural differences in its application confound research results. Differences in the outcome measures for a given technique also occur—some studies use wet or dry (dehydrated) sputum volume or radioaerosol clearance, whereas other studies use pulmonary function tests, radiographic evidence, or arterial blood gases to asses the effectiveness of a specific technique. The majority of secretion clearance research has been focused on patients with cystic fibrosis, as the need for ongoing secretion removal is apparent in this population. However, results showing a treatment to be effective in one cross section of patients must not be generalized to apply to the treatment across all patients with pulmonary disease.

Historically, the gold standard of airway clearance has been a combination of postural drainage, percussion, and vibration with cough. This has been challenged[1b-c] as more techniques have been demonstrated to be effective. Postural drainage and percussion have been shown to be ineffective in some cases and, in fact, to be detrimental to pulmonary status in others. Caregivers have also been shown to suffer from the performance of percussion; repetitive-motion injuries of the wrists have been documented as a result of regular performance of percussion.[2,3]

Alternative techniques have arisen out of the need to find effective methods for those patients not responsive to traditional methods. A desire to increase adherence with airway clearance, especially in patients approaching adolescence and adulthood, has led to an investigation of more independent techniques.[4] Many of these techniques have been practiced longer in other countries, but are now commonly used by practitioners in the United States.

It is important to remember, however, that secretion clearance is just one step toward realizing effective gas exchange in the complex oxygen transport pathway.[5] Airway clearance, when indicated, should be integrated into a comprehensive plan of care, including positioning and mobilization, to optimize oxygen transport.

Conditions That May Indicate Airway Clearance

Oxygen transport is the primary purpose of the cardiopulmonary system (see Chapter 2). Ventilation of the alveoli is an important step in the oxygen transport chain; it allows optimal delivery of oxygen to the tissues. Several medical and surgical conditions may interfere with this process. Retained secretions or mucus plugs in the airways may interfere with the exchange of oxygen. The secretions must be mobilized from the peripheral, or smaller, airways to the larger, more central airways, where coughing or suction may remove them.

The following conditions may be associated with difficulty in mobilizing airway secretions. Difficulty in effectively mobilizing secretions can result from a combination of factors including impaired ciliary motion, reduced lung inflation, impaired lung elasticity, impaired chest wall mobility and biomechanics, and weak or fatigued respiratory muscles. These factors can be coupled with increased viscosity of airway secretions.

- Cystic fibrosis
- Bronchiectasis
- Atelectasis
- Respiratory muscle weakness
- Mechanical ventilation
- Neonatal respiratory distress syndrome
- Asthma

Cystic Fibrosis

In this multisystem genetic disease of exocrine gland dysfunction, copious (often purulent), thick secretions and mucus plugs block the peripheral and central airways. Even infants diagnosed with cystic fibrosis, whether symptomatic or not, show evidence of small airway obstruction in the form of bronchial mucus casts.[6] Recurrent bacterial infections combined with this mucus hypersecretion in the lungs leads to destruction of the bronchial walls, or bronchiectasis. Airway clearance is recommended for all patients with CF and continues to be an important therapy in the treatment of cystic fibrosis.[1b,6a] This practice is supported by evidence of deteriorating lung function when regular treatments of postural drainage and percussion have been stopped.[7,8]

Bronchiectasis

This condition results in a breakdown of the elastic tissue in the bronchial walls, causing severe dilation. Inflamed mucosa and copious purulent secretions are present in this condition. Airway clearance has been shown to benefit patients with bronchiectasis in the mobilization of sputum.[9,10]

Atelectasis

This condition is caused by the collapse of alveolar segments, often by retained pulmonary secretions. It has been documented in patients who have undergone surgery under general anesthesia, especially in cases of thoracic or abdominal surgery. ACTs are indicated in cases of atelectasis due to mucus plugging.[11,12]

Respiratory Muscle Weakness

Many patients with neurological or metastatic diseases or general debilitation tend to hypoventilate or have increased work of breathing. They are unable to maintain adequate control of respiratory secretions and often have weak, ineffective coughing mechanisms.[13] This is especially true in patients with diminished diaphragm innervation resulting from spinal cord injuries.[14]

Mechanical Ventilation

Patients requiring ventilatory support for any reason, including patients who are obtunded or comatose, are at risk for atelectasis and are unable to manage their secretions independently.[15] Airway clearance is considered standard practice in the management of patients on mechanical ventilation.[15a]

Neonatal Respiratory Distress Syndrome

These infants are born lacking surfactant in the lungs, which results in atelectasis. ACTs may be useful in clearing secretions and preventing atelectasis, but there should be a clear indication for this procedure and it must be monitored carefully in this population.[16,17]

Asthma

This condition is characterized by the presence of hyperreactive airways and mucus plugging. ACTs may be beneficial to assist in the mobilization of mucus plugs but are not helpful in treating uncomplicated acute exacerbations.[18]

There are several conditions that do not appear to benefit from ACTs. Patients with pneumonia or chronic bronchitis without large amounts of secretion production do not appear to benefit from airway clearance. No differences in outcome were found when these populations were treated with postural drainage and percussion.[19-22] Viral bronchiolitis is an asthma-like lung disease occurring in infants less than 2 years of age. These patients do not appear to benefit from ACTs.[23] Also of little benefit, and possibly harmful, is the inclusion of airway clearance in the routine care of postoperative patients without extensive secretions.[18] Even in patients with a history of lung disease, the use of ACTs has failed to affect the incidence of atelectasis as a postoperative complication.[24]

Airway Clearance Techniques

Airway clearance techniques differ with respect to equipment needs, the skill level required to perform them, and their usefulness with various clinical problems. Matching a patient with an appropriate method or combination of methods may increase effectiveness, reduce complications, and promote long-term adherence to the treatment. This will, in turn, assist with achieving the goals of airway clearance: reducing airway obstruction, improving ventilation, and optimizing gas exchange.

Preparation for any secretion removal technique should include evaluation of the patient's pulmonary status so that measures may be compared before and after a treatment is provided. A physical examination, including inspection, palpation, measurement of vital signs, and chest auscultation, provides assessment of a treatment's effectiveness. Other outcome measures include chest radiographs, arterial blood gas measurements, and pulmonary function studies. An adequate intake of fluids (as allowed) decreases the viscosity of the secretions, allowing easier mobilization.

Several factors must be taken into account when scheduling an optimal time for airway clearance. At least 30 minutes to 1 hour should be allowed for the completion of tube feedings or meals. The inhalation of bronchodilator medications should take place before airway clearance maneuvers to improve secretion removal by opening the airways. Inhaled antibiotics are best scheduled after airway clearance has taken place for optimal deposition of medication. If necessary, adequate pain control should be provided to receive a patient's best effort and cooperation with a treatment.

Exercise for Airway Clearance

In addition to improving many outcomes in patients with lung disease, exercise has been shown to assist in secretion clearance.[25-28] Exercise increases mucociliary transport in patients with chronic bronchitis.[28] Higher transpulmonary pressure with aerobic exercise may open closed bronchi, as well as increase collateral ventilation to allow mucus to be moved.[26] It has also been shown that exercise-induced hyperventilation is more effective than eucapnic hyperventilation in mobilizing bronchial secretions.[29] The contribution of increased expiratory airflow and exercise-induced coughing are other factors in improving secretion removal. Exercise for secretion clearance has focused on aerobic or endurance exercise; however, any form of exercise must be adapted to the individual patient's status and abilities.

Based on a lack of decrease in lung function following the cessation of PD and percussion but the continuation of an exercise program, or based on the improvement in pulmonary function, exercise has been recommended as a replacement for a conventional chest physiotherapy routine in some patients or at some stages of lung disease.[26,27,30,31] In hospitalized patients with cystic fibrosis, no significant change in pulmonary function was reported when exercise was substituted for two of three daily treatments of PD, percussion, and vibration, and the weight of the sputum produced was equivalent.[30] In terms of mucus cleared, no significant differences were found among exercise on a cycle ergometer, postural drainage, and PEP mask breathing.[32] Increases in sputum expectoration on exercise days as opposed to nonexercise days have also been reported.[27,33]

However, other studies conclude that exercise alone is not sufficient and recommend its use as a complement to other forms of airway clearance. Airway clearance using PD and FET was shown to be more effective than exercise with a cycle ergometer in inducing sputum expectoration.[34] Results from Bilton and colleagues[35] demonstrated that any modality that included the active cycle of breathing technique (ACBT) in PD positions alone or in combination with exercise is better than exercise alone at clearing sputum.

It is difficult to compare these studies, however, because the mode and length of exercise differ, as do the outcome measures of effectiveness of airway clearance. Exercise as an airway clearance technique is not suitable for the very young (younger than 4 to 5 years of age), for patients with neuromuscular limitations, or for patients with limited exercise tolerance. Moreover, the potential need for supplemental oxygen during exercise should be monitored. Nonetheless, evidence suggests that an exercise program, in addition to clearing secretions, may decrease morbidity and mortality by improving exercise capacity.[36,37]

Treatment with Exercise

- A walking program requires only a suitable pair of shoes and a safe location. Higher-impact exercise, because of increased stress on the knees, requires shoes specifically for that purpose. Clothing should be appropriate for the weather if exercising outdoors.
- Exercise equipment suitable for a patient who is beginning an exercise program includes the treadmill, bicycle ergometer, elliptical trainer, mini-trampoline, or arm ergometer. For more accomplished exercisers or patients with a higher exercise tolerance, equipment may include a stair climber, cross-country ski machine, or rowing machine. Numerous other exercise equipment options are available; the patient's interests should be the primary factor for choosing.
- Tools to monitor a patient's response to exercise include a sphygmomanometer, stethoscope, heart rate monitor, pulse oximeter, and a scale to measure patient's level of perceived exertion (Figure 21-1). In a home setting, patients should be knowledgeable in self-monitoring exercise intensity. For those patients who require closer monitoring, a pulse oximeter may be rented from an oxygen supply company. Monitoring of vital signs before and during exercise, and during recovery, will allow titration of the workload for optimal performance.
- Supplemental oxygen and oxygen delivery supplies will be necessary for those patients who exhibit oxygen desaturation during exercise.
- Patients with hyperreactive airways should be premedicated with a prescribed bronchodilator before an exercise session.
- The principles of an exercise prescription addressing mode, intensity, duration, and frequency, as well as principles of "warm up" and "cool down," should be followed

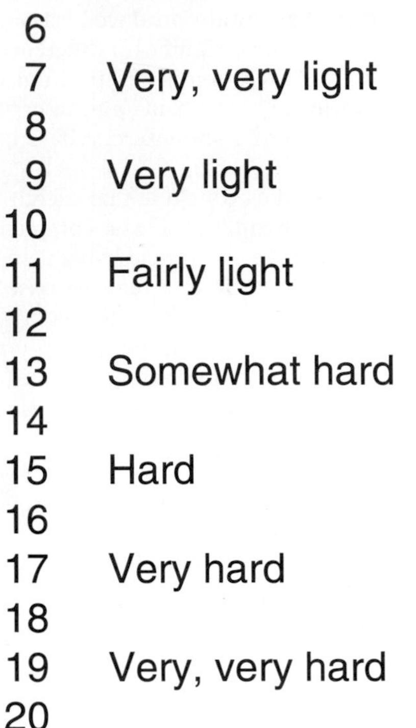

Fig. 21-1 Original perceived exertion scale. *(From Borg G: Psychophysical basis of perceived exertion,* Medicine and Science in Sports and Exercise *14:377, 1982.)*

when using exercise as a form of airway clearance. Individualizing an exercise program for each patient is of the utmost importance.

- Patients hospitalized for an acute exacerbation may not be able to initially perform endurance exercise. These patients should be started slowly and progressed as tolerated; consider using interval training.
- The patient should be instructed in huffing or controlled coughing to expectorate secretions as they are loosened.
- A regular, consistent program of exercise should be scheduled around the patient's daily activities to achieve adherence (e.g., walking the dog, sports at school, stopping by the health club after work).

Advantages and Disadvantages of Exercise

Exercise has the advantage of being the only airway clearance technique that is performed regularly by people without lung disease. This factor can make it appealing to those patients who do not want to call attention to their differences from their peers. Exercise may improve self-esteem, a sense of well-being, and quality of life. Higher levels of exercise tolerance in patients with cystic fibrosis have been demonstrated to improve survival.[37]

Some patients may not tolerate the amount or frequency of exercise necessary for this to be the sole method of airway clearance. Thus various airway clearance techniques can be used as adjuncts to exercise. This is particularly true during an acute exacerbation when activity tolerance is limited, or in infants or patients with neurological or musculoskeletal limitations. Andreasson[26] observed that regular contact with a caregiver seems to be necessary for successful exercise training, as does family support, especially in young children. This points out the difficulty with adherence to a home program. Adherence will also be affected by a patient's preference for a particular activity, scheduling conflicts, and commitment by friends and family members.

Precautions for Using Exercise

Several precautions must be observed when using exercise as a form of airway clearance. Care must be taken in prescribing exercise to patients with hyperreactive airways or a tendency toward oxygen desaturation. Desaturation has been shown to occur with exercise in individuals with pulmonary disease,[38,39] and therefore it becomes prudent to monitor oxygen saturation, providing supplemental oxygen for the exercise period when indicated. Exercise-induced bronchospasm must also be considered when pulmonary compromise is seen with exercise, especially with higher-intensity exercise.[40] When medication is indicated, it is recommended to provide an inhaled bronchodilator 20 to 30 minutes before exercise to alleviate this symptom.[41] Use of bronchodilator medication and supplemental oxygen may be necessary to improve exercise tolerance, but these patients require closer monitoring as well. Andreasson[26] reports a risk for pneumothorax associated with exercise in patients with extensive bullae.

Contraindications and Precautions for Manual and Mechanical Airway Clearance Techniques

In patients who are very young, who have limited ability to cooperate, or who are not adherent to other ACTs, percussion, shaking, and vibration offer methods for dislodging retained secretions. However, because of the force transmitted to the thoracic cage with these techniques, there are many precautions and contraindications to consider. The therapist should not make this decision alone but should seek direction from the medical team. These treatments are not completely benign and should not be performed in the absence of good indications.[42]

Percussion has been shown to contribute to a fall in PaO_2 in acutely ill patients,[43] especially in patients with cardiovascular instability[44] and in neonates.[45] The factor that seems most closely associated with or predictive of this effect is the patient's baseline PaO_2.[42] Cardiac dysrhythmias have been associated with chest percussion for bronchial drainage[11] and Huseby[46] hypothesizes that hypoxemia may be the underlying mechanism of CPT-caused cardiac arrhythmias.

Patients with hyperreactive airways (e.g., asthma) show intolerance for percussion as part of airway clearance. Campbell and colleagues[47] demonstrated a fall in FEV_1 associated with percussion; it was not evident when percussion was omitted. Administration of a bronchodilator before treatment with percussion precluded the fall in FEV_1. Wheezing has also been associated with percussion and vibration in patients with cystic fibrosis and COPD.[48,49]

Box 21-1 summarizes the precautions and contraindications for external manipulation of the thorax associated with percussion, shaking, and high-frequency chest compression.

Box 21-1 Contraindications to External Manipulation of the Thorax in Addition to Contraindications for Postural Drainage

- Subcutaneous emphysema
- Recent epidural spinal infusion or spinal anesthesia
- Recent skin grafts or flaps on the thorax
- Burns, open wounds, and skin infections of the thorax
- Recently placed pacemaker
- Suspected pulmonary tuberculosis
- Lung contusion
- Bronchospasm
- Osteomyelitis of the ribs
- Osteoporosis
- Coagulopathy
- Complaint of chest-wall pain
- Additional contraindications for percussion of a neonate
  - Intolerance to treatment as indicated by low oxygen saturation values
  - Rib fracture
  - Hemoptysis

From AARC Clinical Practice Guideline: Postural drainage therapy, Respiratory Care *36:1418-1426, 1991; and Crane L: Physical therapy for the neonate with respiratory disease. In Irwin S, Tecklin JS, editors:* Cardiopulmonary physical therapy, *St. Louis, 1985, Mosby.*

Vibration involves less force to the thorax and may be better tolerated than the aforementioned techniques. A nebulized bronchodilator may be administered during a treatment of high-frequency chest compression to avoid the consequences of hyperreactive airways.

Postural Drainage

Postural drainage, also known as bronchial drainage, is a passive technique in which the patient is placed in positions that allow gravity to assist with the drainage of secretions from the bronchopulmonary tree. PD is accomplished by positioning the patient so that the angle of the lung segment to be drained allows gravity to have its greatest effect (Figure 21-2). Positioning the patient to assist the flow of bronchial secretions from the airways has been a standard treatment for some time in patients with retained secretions.[50]

Knowledge of the anatomy of the tracheobronchial tree is vital to effective treatment. Each lobe to be drained must be aligned so that gravity can mobilize the secretions from the periphery to the larger, more central airways. The mechanism of postural drainage is considered to be a direct effect of gravity on bronchial secretions, although observations made by Lannefors (1992)[32] that gravity also influences regional lung ventilation and volume suggest that these mechanisms are also involved.

PD has been shown to be effective in mobilizing secretions in patients with cystic fibrosis,[51,52] bronchiectasis,[10] and other pulmonary diseases.[53,54] Other treatments, such as percussion, vibration, and the active cycle of breathing technique (ACBT), may be used while the patient is in postural drainage positions.

There are, however, many contraindications to gravity-enhancing positioning for PD. Recent studies have reported adverse effects of head-down or Trendelenburg positions required for the lower lobes. Modified positions should be used for head-down positions unless it has been shown to be effective in a particular patient. The head of the bed should remain flat instead of being tipped into the Trendelenburg (head down) position.

Preparation for Postural Drainage

- For the hospitalized patient, electric beds allow patients to be positioned more easily. Air therapy beds, most often used in the intensive care unit (ICU), are valuable aids for positioning, especially in patients who are large or unresponsive.
- In the ICU, it is imperative to be familiar with the multiple lines, tubes, and other devices attached to the patient (see Chapter 16). Allow enough slack from each device to position a patient for postural drainage.
- Ensure there are enough staff members to position the patient with as little stress to both patient and staff as possible.[55]
- For treatment in the clinic, have foam wedges or pillows available for positioning.
- For home treatment, aids in positioning might include pillows, sofa cushions, or a bean-bag chair.
- Nebulized bronchodilators or mucolytics before PD may facilitate the mobilization of sputum.
- For the patient with an adequate cough to expectorate secretions, have tissues or a specimen cup available. Have suctioning equipment ready to remove secretions from an artificial airway or the patient's oral or nasal cavity after the treatment. Refer to Chapter 43 for a discussion of suctioning.

Treatment with Postural Drainage

- After determining the lobe of the lung to be treated by auscultation and chest x-ray, position the patient in the appropriate position, supporting the patient comfortably in the position indicated (see Figure 21-2).
- If postural drainage is used exclusively, each position should be maintained for 5 to 10 minutes, if tolerated, or longer when focusing on a specific lobe. Coordinating the positioning with nursing care for skin pressure relief may allow the time spent in a position to be extended. If postural drainage is used in conjunction with another technique, the time in each position may be decreased. For example, if percussion and vibration are performed while the patient is in each PD position, 3 to 5 minutes is sufficient.
- A patient who requires close monitoring should not be left unattended, but this may be appropriate if a patient is alert and able to reposition himself or herself.
- It is not always necessary to treat each affected lung segment during every treatment; this may prove to be too fatiguing for the patient. The most affected lobes should be addressed with the first treatment of the day, with the other affected areas addressed during subsequent treatment(s).
- The patient should be encouraged to take deep breaths and cough after each position, if possible, and again after the

treatment is completed. Having the patient sit upright or lean forward optimizes this effort by allowing the use of the abdominals for a stronger cough.[55]

- Mobilization of secretions may not be apparent immediately after the treatment, but this may occur up to 1 hour later. The patient should be thus informed and reminded to clear secretions at a later time. A health care practitioner or family member should be included in this aspect of treatment, especially with patients who need encouragement.[55]

Advantages and Disadvantages of Postural Drainage

Postural drainage is relatively easy to learn; the patient and/or caregiver must be familiar with the appropriate positioning for the affected lung fields. Treatment in the hospital may be coordinated with other patient activities, such as positioning for skin pressure relief, bathing, or positioning for a test or procedure. Home treatment can be coordinated with activities such as reading or watching television.

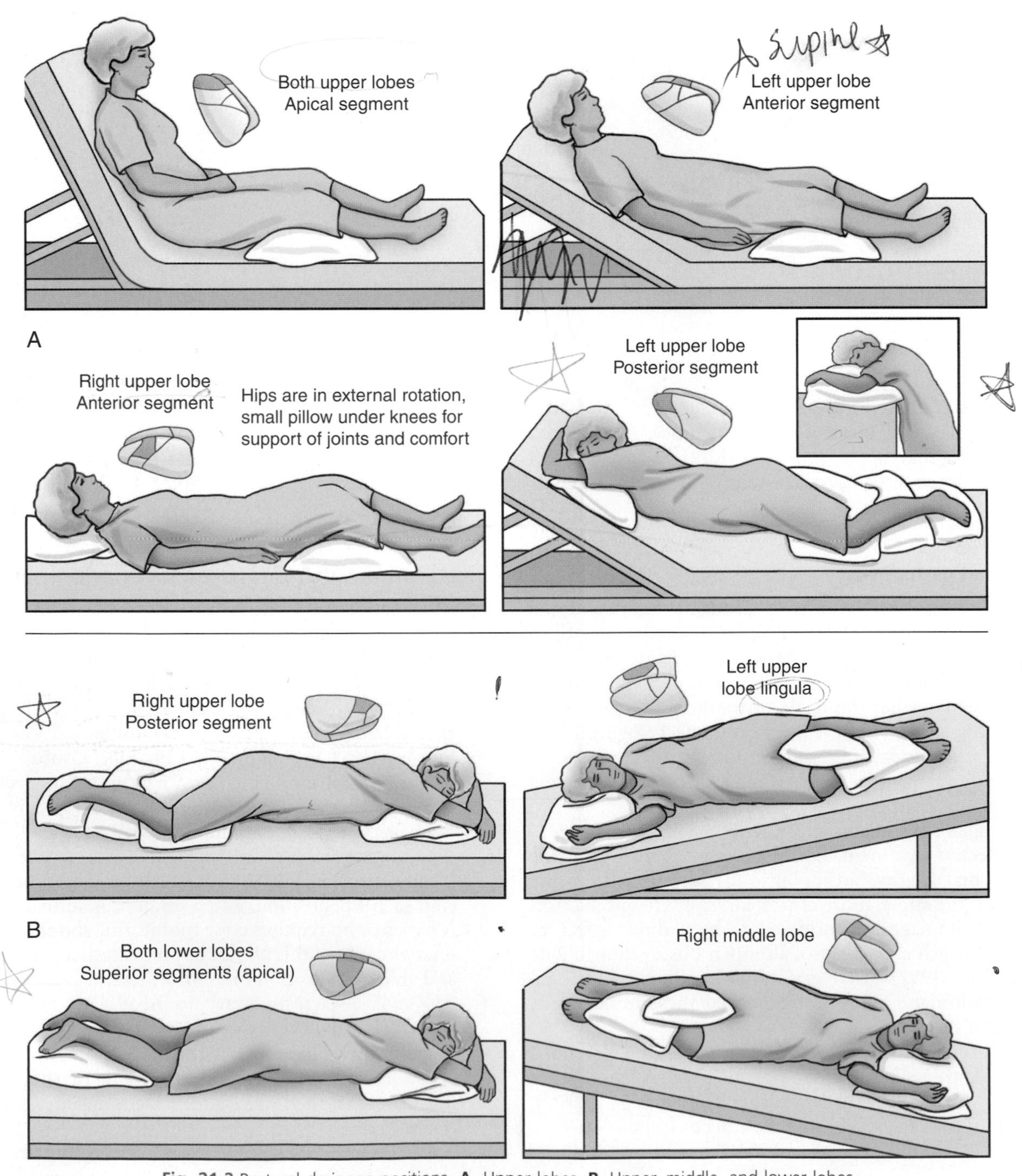

Fig. 21-2 Postural drainage positions. **A,** Upper lobes. **B,** Upper, middle, and lower lobes.

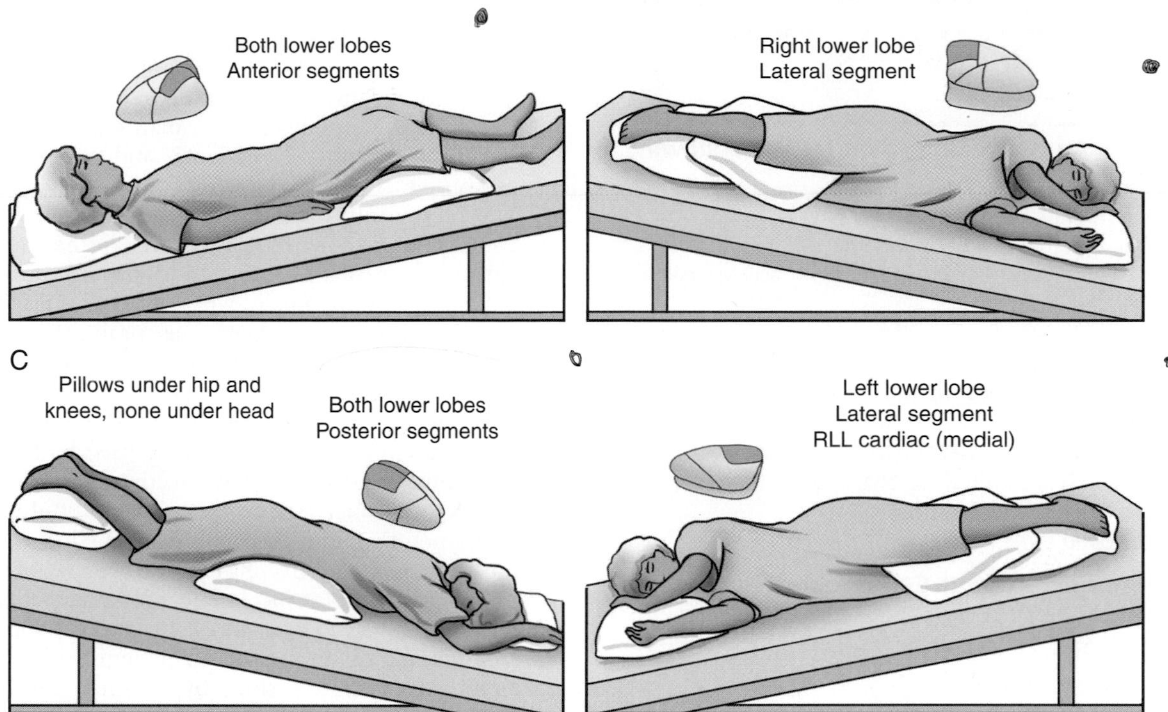

Fig. 21-2, cont'd C, Lower lobes.

For many patients, optimal PD positions will be contraindicated for a variety of reasons and modified positions should be used. Adherence to PD may be a challenge because of the length of the treatment; this is especially challenging in the pediatric population, who will require considerable distraction to maintain a desired position for the appropriate length of time. Children who are able to role-play the treatment—for instance, with a doll or stuffed toy—may better understand what is expected and be more cooperative with therapy.

The cost of the equipment required for PD is minimal. The cost of a caregiver's time to provide the treatment, however, especially in the case of a chronic disease, may be substantial. A family member should be taught the procedure, if possible, to decrease the cost and provide flexibility in scheduling.

General Precautions and Contraindications to Postural Drainage Positioning

It is essential that the therapist and the health care team discuss treatment priorities when deciding to use PD positions. A decision to use postural drainage might be made despite a contraindication if the benefits are thought to outweigh the risks in a particular case. For example, it is known that use of the Trendelenburg (head-down) position increases intracranial pressure in patients after neurosurgery.[56] However, if the patient develops atelectasis, the stress of respiratory embarrassment may also increase intracranial pressure. In this instance, the decision may be made to position the patient to clear the atelectasis and subsequently return to a modified conservative regimen.[55]

A fall in arterial O_2 saturation has been reported with the use of postural drainage for airway clearance, although the effects of PD were not separated from additional techniques.[46,57] Therefore O_2 saturation levels should be monitored during treatment, especially in patients with known low PaO_2 values.

Caution must also be used in treating a patient with end-stage lung disease in postural drainage positions because of the risk for hemoptysis.[58,59] Decreased cardiac output[60,61] has been associated with chest physiotherapy treatment; however, the effects of postural drainage were not separated from those of percussion and vibration.

Many physical therapists working with the pediatric population almost never use the head-down position in treating infants but rather a modified routine that excludes the Trendelenburg position. The head-down position has been shown to increase the incidence of gastroesophageal reflux in neonates.[16] Button and colleagues[62] found that the head-down position is associated with gastroesophageal reflux, distressed behavior, and lower oxygen saturation in infants with cystic fibrosis. It should be noted that a finding of gastroesophageal reflux can occur even 1 hour after treatment. A modified routine that eliminates head-down positioning is associated with fewer respiratory complications.[63] Box 21-2 summarizes the precautions and contraindications concerning postural drainage.

Percussion

Percussion, sometimes referred to as chest clapping, is a traditional approach to secretion mobilization. A rhythmical force is applied with a caregiver's cupped hands against the thorax, over the involved lung segments, trapping air between the patient's thorax and the caregiver's hands (Figure 21-3), with the aim of dislodging or loosening bronchial secretions from the airways so they may be removed by suctioning or expectoration. This technique is performed during both the inspiratory and expiratory phases of breathing. Percussion is

Box 21-2 Contraindications for Postural Drainage

All Positions Are Contraindicated for the Following:

- Intracranial pressure (ICP) >20 mm Hg
- Head and neck injury until stabilized
- Active hemorrhage with hemodynamic instability
- Recent spinal surgery (e.g., laminectomy) or acute spinal injury
- Active hemoptysis
- Empyema
- Bronchopleural fistula
- Pulmonary edema associated with heart failure (HF)
- Large pleural effusions
- Pulmonary embolism
- Older, confused, or anxious patients
- Rib fracture, with or without flail chest
- Surgical wound or healing tissue

Trendelenburg Position Is Contraindicated for the Following:

- Patients in whom increased ICP is to be avoided
- Uncontrolled hypertension
- Distended abdomen
- Esophageal surgery
- Recent gross hemoptysis related to recent lung carcinoma
- Uncontrolled airway at risk for aspiration

Trendelenburg Position Is Contraindicated for the Following Cases in Neonates:

- Untreated tension pneumothorax
- Recent tracheoesophageal fistula repair
- Recent eye or intracranial surgery
- Intraventricular hemorrhage (grades III and IV)
- Acute heart failure or cor pulmonale

From AARC Clinical Practice Guideline: Postural drainage therapy, Respiratory Care *36:1418-1426, 1991; and Crane L: Physical therapy for the neonate with respiratory disease. In Irwin S, Tecklin JS, editors:* Cardiopulmonary physical therapy, *St. Louis, 1985, Mosby.*

used in postural drainage positions for increased effectiveness[64,65] and may also be used during ACBT. For individuals with pulmonary disease, percussion in conjunction with postural drainage continues to be a mainstay of the treatment, especially for pediatric patients and patients who are unresponsive.

The proposed mechanism of action of percussion is the transmission of a wave of energy through the chest wall into the lung. This wave loosens secretions from the bronchial wall and moves them proximally, where ciliary motion and cough (or suction) can remove them. The combination of postural drainage and percussion has been shown to be effective in secretion removal.[66-68]

A handheld mechanical percussor can be used by a caregiver to minimize fatigue or may be used by the patient to self-administer percussion. The effectiveness of mechanical as opposed to manual percussion has been studied. Maxwell and Redmond[69] found mechanical percussion equivalent to manual percussion in effecting removal of secretions. Although there was a significant increase in pulmonary function with manual techniques, Pryor and colleagues[70,71] supported the use of mechanical percussion in patients, using the forced expiration technique. A study by Rossman and colleagues[72] was in disagreement, finding that mechanical percussion did not enhance postural drainage in secretion removal.

There are contraindications to percussion. If a patient's pulmonary status is of greater concern than the relative contraindications, a decision may be made to administer the treatment, with appropriate modifications.

Preparation for Percussion

- The only equipment required for manual percussion is the caregiver's cupped hands to deliver the force to mobilize secretions.
- For the adult and older pediatric population, electric or pneumatic percussors that mechanically simulate percussion are available. This enables a patient to apply

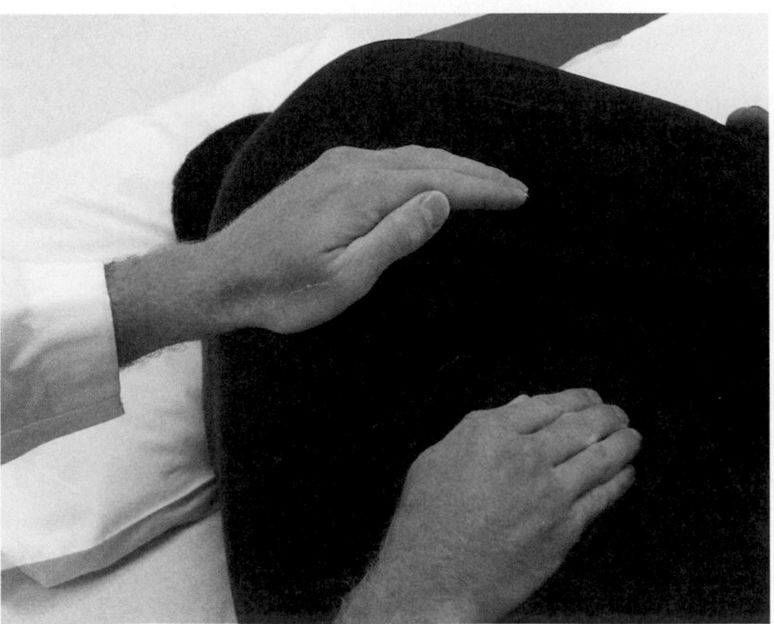

Fig. 21-3 Chest percussion.

self-percussion more effectively. Several models have variable frequencies of percussion, as well as different levels of intensity.

- Several devices, including padded rubber nipples, pediatric anesthesia masks, padded medicine cups, or the bell end of a stethoscope may be used to provide percussion to infants whose chest walls are too small to accommodate the size of an adult's hand.
- Placing the patient in appropriate PD positions (as the patient's condition allows) enhances the effect of percussion.
- A thin towel or hospital gown should cover the patient's skin where the percussion is to be applied. The force of percussion over bare skin may be uncomfortable; however, padding that is too thick absorbs the force of the percussion without benefit to the patient.
- Adjust the level of the bed so that the caregiver may use proper body mechanics during the treatment. The caregiver may become excessively fatigued or injured as a result of lengthy or numerous treatments if proper body mechanics are ignored.

Treatment with Percussion

- Position the hand in the shape of a cup with the fingers and thumb adducted. It is important to maintain this cupped position with the hands throughout the treatment, while letting the wrists, arms, and shoulders stay relaxed.
- The sound of percussion should be hollow as opposed to a slapping sound. If erythema occurs with percussion, it is usually a result of slapping or not trapping enough air between the hand and the chest wall.[73]
- The patient will better tolerate an even, steady rhythm. The rate of manual percussion delivered by caregivers can vary between 100 and 480 times per minute.[73]
- The force applied to the chest wall from each hand should be equal. If the nondominant hand is not able to keep up with the dominant hand, the rate should be slowed to match that of the slower hand. It might be helpful to start with the nondominant hand and let the dominant hand match the nondominant hand.[55] The force does not have to be excessive to be effective; the amount of force should be adapted to the patient's comfort.
- If the size of an infant does not allow use of a full hand, percussion may be done manually with four fingers cupped, three fingers with the middle finger "tented," or the thenar and hypothenar surfaces of the hand.[74]
- Hand position should be such that percussion does not occur over bony prominences of the patient. The spinous processes of the vertebrae, the spine of the scapula, and the clavicle should all be avoided. Percussion over the floating ribs should also be avoided because these ribs have only a single attachment.
- Percussion should not be performed over breast tissue. This will produce discomfort and diminish the effectiveness of the treatment. In the case of very large breasts, it may be necessary to move the breast out of the way with one hand (or ask the patient to do this) and percuss with the other hand.
- A patient may be taught to perform one-handed self-percussion to those areas that can be reached comfortably, either manually or with a mechanical percussor. This does, however, virtually preclude the treatment of the posterior lung segments.

Advantages and Disadvantages of Percussion

The addition of percussion to a PD treatment may enhance secretion clearance and shorten the treatment. Patients, especially young children and infants, often find the rhythm soothing and are relaxed and sedated by percussion.

Patients with chronic lung disease who have used PD and percussion for many years and have found it effective may be reluctant to try an alternative method of airway clearance. Acceptance of this method is dependent on the consistent availability of a family member or other caregiver to provide the treatment. Mechanical percussors allow a patient more independence or decrease fatigue of a caregiver, and they are especially useful in patients requiring ongoing treatment at home.

Percussion is not well tolerated by many patients postoperatively without adequate pain control. The force of percussion may also be contraindicated in patients with osteoporosis or coagulopathy. Percussion has been associated with a fall in oxygen saturation, which can be eliminated with concurrent thoracic expansion exercises and pauses for breathing control.[75]

Delivering percussion for extended periods on an ongoing basis can result in injury to the caregiver, whether a family member or a health care provider; repetitive motion injuries of the upper extremities may occur in long-term delivery of percussion for airway clearance.

The expense of a mechanical device for percussion is minimal compared with the ongoing cost of a caregiver to provide percussion and PD, either in the hospital setting or at home. In the case of young children or unresponsive patients, there are few choices for airway clearance. For other populations, however, a more independent method can prove to be more cost-effective if adequate adherence is achieved.

Vibration and Shaking

The techniques of vibration and shaking are on opposite ends of a spectrum. Vibration involves a gentle, high-frequency force, whereas shaking is more vigorous in nature. Vibration is delivered through a sustained co-contraction of the caregiver's upper extremities to produce a vibratory force while applying pressure to the chest wall over the involved lung segment. Shaking is similar in application to vibration, and is described as a bouncing maneuver, sometimes referred to as "rib springing," supplying a concurrent, compressive force to the chest wall. Like percussion, vibration and shaking are used in conjunction with PD positioning. Unlike percussion, they are performed only during the expiratory phase of breathing, starting with peak inspiration and continuing until the end of expiration. The compressive forces follow the movement of the chest wall. Both techniques require the assistance of a caregiver, but a mechanical vibrator may be used in place of manual vibration.

It is proposed that vibration and shaking enhance mucociliary transport from the periphery of the lung fields to the larger, central airways. Because the compressive force to the thorax is greater with shaking than vibration, it produces increased chest wall displacement, and the stretch of the respiratory muscles may produce an increased inspiratory effort and lung volume.[76] The same relative contraindications for percussion should be observed for shaking, because it involves the application of force to the thorax.

Pavia[77] demonstrated a higher, though not statistically significant, rate of secretion clearance and sputum production with vibration. However, this study was conducted while subjects were in the upright position only, which does not replicate the use of vibration clinically. Many studies do not separate the effects of vibration from the components of PD and percussion because they are often used in conjunction. In fact, many studies describe the techniques of PD, percussion, and vibration or shaking as a single entity and refer to the treatment as chest physical therapy or postural drainage therapy. Mackenzie and colleagues[78] demonstrated significant improvement in total lung/thorax compliance after treatment with postural drainage, percussion, and vibration in mechanically ventilated patients. Feldman and colleagues[48] demonstrated improved ventilatory function by improved expiratory flow rates in patients receiving postural drainage, percussion, vibration, and directed coughing.

Preparation for Vibration and Shaking

- For manual techniques, the caregiver's hands are the only "equipment" required.
- Mechanical vibrators are available to administer the treatment and are useful for self-treatment by a patient or to reduce fatigue in the caregiver.
- For infants, a padded electric toothbrush may be used.[74]
- Place the patient in the appropriate PD position or modified position, as the patient's status allows.
- Place a thin towel or hospital gown over the patient's skin. The material should not be thick enough to absorb the effect of the vibration or shaking.
- Proper body position of the caregiver is important to deliver an effective treatment and to decrease caregiver fatigue.

Treatment with Vibration and Shaking

- For vibration, the hands may be placed side by side or on top of each other, as shown in Figure 21-4. As with shaking, the patient is instructed to take in a deep breath while in a proper PD position. A gentle but steady co-contraction of the upper extremities is performed to vibrate the chest wall, beginning at the peak of inspiration and following the movement of chest deflation. The frequency of manual vibration is between 12 and 20 Hz.[44,53]
- For shaking, with the patient in the appropriate PD position, place your hands over the lobe of the lung to be treated and instruct the patient to take in a deep breath. At the peak of inspiration, apply a slow (approximately 2 times per second), rhythmic bouncing pressure to the chest wall until the end of expiration. The hands follow the movement of the chest as the air is exhaled. The frequency of shaking is 2 Hz.[44,53]
- If the patient is mechanically ventilated, the previously described techniques needs to be coordinated with ventilator-controlled exhalation.
- If the patient has a rapid respiratory rate, either voluntary or ventilator-controlled, it may be necessary to apply vibration or shaking only during every other exhalation.
- A mobile chest wall is necessary to apply a compressive force without causing discomfort. If a patient has limited chest wall compliance, vibration will probably be better tolerated than shaking.
- Mechanical vibrators may be used by the unattended patient, although only limited attention can be paid to the posterior portions of the lungs.

Advantages and Disadvantages of Vibration and Shaking

The use of vibration and/or shaking in addition to PD may enhance the mobilization of secretions. Shaking or vibration may be better tolerated than percussion, especially in the postsurgical patient. Manual vibration and shaking allows the caregiver to assess the pattern and depth of respiration. The stretch on the muscles of respiration during expiration may encourage a deeper subsequent inspiration. A mechanical vibrator, more commonly used with pediatric patients, may be preferable for delivery of airway clearance in the long-term.

The patient cannot apply these techniques without assistance, except in a limited manner with a mechanical vibrator, so adherence and regular administration of vibration depends on caregiver availability.

The same contraindications for percussion apply because shaking and vibration involve compression to the thorax. The technique of vibration is less constrained by these contraindications than is shaking.

Manual Hyperinflation

The technique of manual hyperinflation was used more commonly in the past for patients requiring mechanical ventilation. However there is not enough evidence to promote the regular use of this technique that has many contraindications and that is not well known in the United States.[80] A brief description of the technique and its precautions follows. Two caregivers are needed to perform the technique with the patient placed in PD positions.[79] One caregiver uses a manual inflation bag to hyperinflate the lungs with a slow, deep inspiration and, after a short pause, provides a quick release to allow rapid exhalation. A second caregiver applies shaking or vibration at the beginning of exhalation to mobilize secretions. The technique is promoted to mobilize secretions and reinflate collapsed areas of the lung and is likened to simulating a cough—deep inspiration, pause, and forceful exhalation.

Clement[80] reported that this method of airway clearance enabled patients to be maintained on ventilators for long periods while retaining normal lung function. It was also demonstrated that the addition of positioning and vibrations enhanced the treatment of atelectasis by hyperinflation and suctioning.[81]

The risks to using manual hyperinflation are numerous. There are several adverse hemodynamic effects of this technique and hyperinflation has the potential to cause barotraumas.[61,80,83]

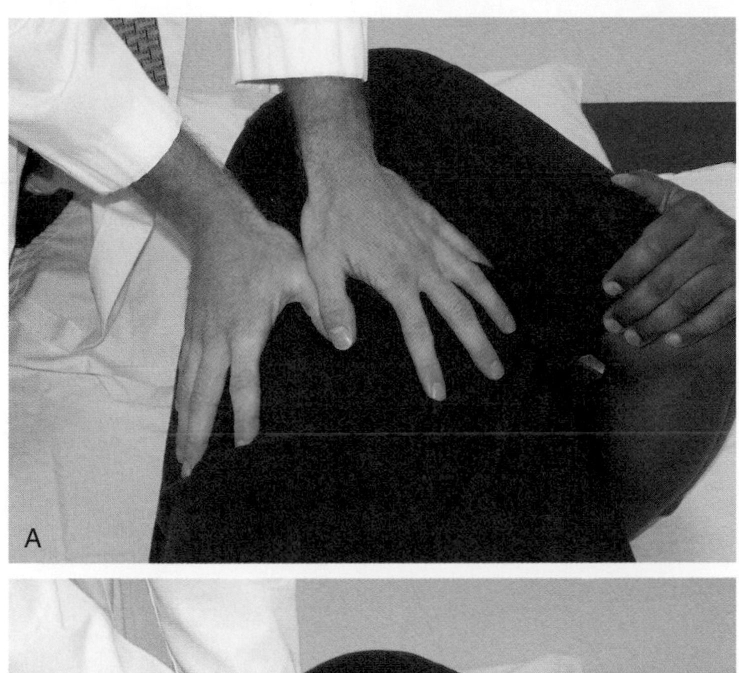

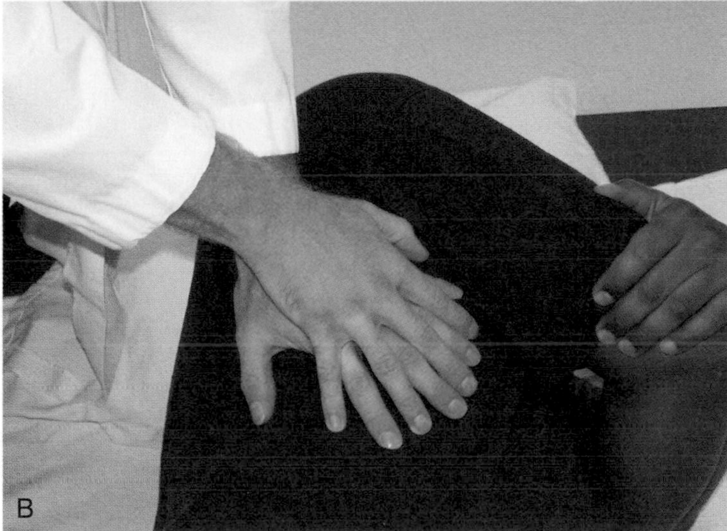

Fig. 21-4 Vibration techniques. **A,** With hands positioned on both sides of the chest. **B,** With hands placed one on top of the other.

Active Cycle of Breathing Technique

In New Zealand, Thompson[85] described clearing bronchial secretions in patients with asthma by using a technique of forced expirations and diaphragmatic breathing. British physiotherapists modified the technique and further described it in the literature, first as the forced expiration technique (FET)[70] and later as the active cycle of breathing technique.[86]

As described by Webber and Pryor,[86] ACBT consists of repeated cycles of three ventilatory phases: breathing control, thoracic expansion exercises, and FET. Breathing control is described as gentle tidal volume breathing with relaxation of the upper chest and shoulders. The thoracic expansion phase consists of deep inspiration and may be accompanied by percussion or vibration performed by a caregiver or the patient. This phase helps to loosen secretions. The forced expiration technique involves one or two huffs, as when fogging a window or cleaning glasses with one's breath. Slow huffing from a middle lung volume (a medium-sized inspiration) down to a low lung volume moves secretions from the peripheral to the upper airways, whereas upper airway secretions may be cleared by a quicker huff from a high lung volume or deeper inspiration.[86]

The period of breathing control between the other phases is essential in order to prevent bronchospasm.[87] The period of thoracic expansion, which increases lung volume and promotes collateral ventilation, allows air to get behind secretions and assist in their mobilization.[88] Mead and colleagues[89] described the physiological theory of the equal pressure point (EPP), which is the basis for FET. EPP is the point in the airways where the pressure is equal to the pleural pressure. The forced expiratory maneuver produces compression of the airway peripherally to EPP. A huff from high lung volume causes compression within the trachea and bronchi, which moves secretions from these larger airways. A huff continued to low lung volume shifts the EPP more peripherally, which mobilizes more peripheral secretions.[84]

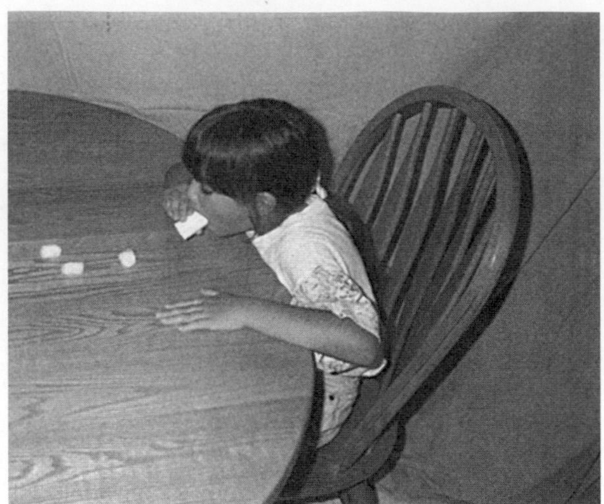

Fig. 21-5 Using a peak flow meter mouthpiece for huffing.

Because huffing has been shown to stabilize collapsible bronchial walls, it increases the expiratory flow in patients with obstruction without causing airway collapse.[90] Another benefit of this technique is its ability to maintain oxygen saturation. The decrease in oxygen saturation that has been demonstrated with postural drainage and percussion has been prevented by the use of ACBT.[75] Hassani and colleagues (1994)[91] showed that unproductive cough and FET resulted in the movement of secretions proximally from all regions of the lung in patients with mild hyposecretion. Therefore, FET may help to avoid prolonged retention of secretions, even in patients who produce little sputum.

ACBT may be performed in the sitting position but has been shown to be more effective in gravity-assisted positions; although horizontal side lying may have fewer adverse effects than the head-down position.[50,92] This method encourages active participation of the patient and has been shown to be as effective when performed by the patient alone or with the aid of a caregiver.[70] FET performed by patients independently has been shown to clear more sputum in a shorter amount of time than PD with self-percussion combined with percussion and shaking by a physical therapist.[70] Improvements in pulmonary function[93] and sputum clearance[94] have been demonstrated in patients with cystic fibrosis who incorporated FET into their postural drainage treatments. ACBT has been shown to be equally effective as positive expiratory pressure (PEP) in a year-long study.[50] Additionally, this method of airway clearance may be used with some children as young as 3 or 4 years of age. The sequence of ACBT is shown in Box 21-3.

Box 21-3 Active Cycle of Breathing Technique

- Breathing control
- Diaphragmatic breathing at normal tidal volume
- 3-4 thoracic expansion exercises
- Deep inhalation with relaxed exhalation at vital capacity, with or without chest percussion
- Breathing control
- 3-4 thoracic expansion exercises
- Breathing control
- Forced expiratory technique
- 1-2 huffs at middle to low lung volume
- Abdominal muscle contraction to produce forced exhalation
- Breathing control

Modified from Webber B, Pryor J: Physiotherapy skills: Techniques and adjuncts. In Webber B, Pryor J, editors: Physiotherapy for respiratory and cardiac problems, *Edinburgh, 1993, Churchill Livingstone.*

Preparation for Active Cycle of Breathing Technique

- The only equipment required for this manual technique is the patient's or caregiver's hands to percuss or shake/vibrate the chest wall during the thoracic expansion phase.
- Mechanical percussors or vibrators may be used during the thoracic expansion phase, either for self-percussion by the patient or for use by the caregiver.
- To teach the huffing maneuver (part of FET), it may be helpful to use a peak flow meter mouthpiece to maintain the mouth and glottis open (Figure 21-5). Young children may be taught games of huffing at cotton balls or tissue to improve the effect of the technique.[86] To help them focus on the expiratory maneuver, small children may also be taught to flap their arms to their lateral chest as they perform the huff, a technique referred to as the "chicken breath."[95]
- The patient should be in a PD position to stimulate drainage of a productive area of the lungs, although the entire treatment may also be performed in the upright sitting position. If PD positions are used, equipment for positioning will be required.
- Most patients tolerate treatment of two or three productive areas during one session.
- A minimum of 10 minutes in any productive position may be necessary to clear a patient with a moderate amount of secretions. Patients after surgery or with minimal secretions may not require as much time, and very ill patients may fatigue before optimal treatment is given.[86]

Treatment with Active Cycle of Breathing Technique

- During the breathing control phase, the patient is instructed to breathe in a relaxed manner using normal tidal volume. The upper chest and shoulders should remain relaxed, and the lower chest and abdomen should be active. The breathing control phase should last as long as is required for the patient to relax and prepare for the next phases, usually 5 to 10 seconds.
- The emphasis during the thoracic expansion phase is on inspiration. The patient is instructed to take in a deep breath to the inspiratory reserve volume; expiration is passive and relaxed. The caregiver or the patient may place a hand over the area of the thorax being treated to facilitate increased chest wall movement.
- Chest percussion, shaking, or vibration may be performed in combination with thoracic expansion as the patient exhales. For surgical patients or those with lung collapse, a breath hold or a sniff at the end of inspiration encourages collateral ventilation to redistribute air into collapsed segments and assist with reexpansion of the lung.
- The FET phase consists of huffing interspersed with breathing control. A huff is a rapid, forced exhalation without maximal effort. This maneuver is comparable to fogging a pair of eyeglasses with warm breath so they may be cleaned. Unlike a cough, in which the glottis is closed, a huff requires the glottis to remain open. In an effective huff, the muscles of the abdomen should contract to provide greater expiratory force. Other characteristics of effective versus ineffective huffing are shown in Box 21-4.
- Two different levels of huffing are characterized in FET. To mobilize secretions from peripheral airways, a huff after a medium-sized inspiration will be effective. This huff will be longer and quieter. To clear secretions that have reached the larger, proximal airways, a huff after a deep inspiration will be effective. This huff will be shorter and louder.
- The patient must pause for breathing control after one or two huffs. This will prevent any increase in airflow obstruction.
- ACBT should be adapted to the individual patient's needs. If secretions are tenacious, two cycles of the thoracic expansion phase may be necessary to loosen secretions before FET can follow. In a patient with bronchospasm or unstable airways, the breathing control phase may be as long as 10 to 20 seconds.[86] After surgery, the patient may be shown how to support the incision with her hands during FET to achieve sufficient expiratory force.
- When a huff from a medium-sized inspiration through complete expiration is nonproductive and dry sounding for two cycles in a row, the treatment may be concluded.[96]

Box 21-4 Effective Versus Ineffective Huffing

Effective Huffing	Ineffective Huffing
Mouth open, O-shaped to keep glottis open	Mouth half or almost closed
Forced expiration	Expiration always starting from high lung volume
From middle to low lung volume moves peripheral secretions	Abdominal muscles not used
From high to middle lung volume moves proximal secretions	Sound more like hissing or blowing
Muscles of the chest wall and abdomen contract	Mouth shaped as for "E" sound
Sound is like a sigh, but forced	Incorrect quality of expiration
Rate of expiratory flow varies with the following	Too vigorous or long, producing paroxysmal coughing
The individual	Too gentle
The disease	Too short
The degree of airflow obstruction	"Catching" or "grunting" at the back of the throat
Crackles heard if excess secretions are present	

From Partridge C, Pryor J, Webber B: Characteristics of the forced expiration technique, Physiotherapy *75:193-194, 1989.*

Advantages and Disadvantages of Active Cycle of Breathing

Incorporation of ACBT into a treatment of PD and percussion allows the patient to participate actively in secretion mobilization and offers the prospect of independently managing airway clearance. ACBT may be introduced at 3 or 4 years of age, with a child becoming independent in the technique at 8 to 10 years of age.

The technique may be adapted for patients with gastroesophageal reflux, bronchospasm, and an acute exacerbation of their pulmonary disease. A decrease in oxygen saturation caused by chest percussion may be avoided by using ACBT.[75] When the technique is performed independently, the cost of using ACBT for the long term is minimal.

In young children or extremely ill adults, it may be necessary for a caregiver to assist the patient with this technique. An assistant will also be required for the patient in whom percussion or shaking during the thoracic expansion phase increases the effectiveness of the treatment.

Autogenic Drainage

In Belgium in 1976, Chevaillier introduced autogenic drainage (AD), or self-drainage, for the treatment of asthmatic patients. He observed that during sleep, as well as while playing and laughing during the day, mucus was mobilized better than it was during PD and clapping. AD is an "antidyspnea" technique based on quiet expirations in a relaxed state and without use of postural drainage positions.[97]

Schoni[98] eloquently explained the physiology of AD's three phases, which use diaphragmatic breathing to mobilize secretions by varying expiratory airflow (Figure 21-6). The first phase starts with a normal inspiration and is followed by a breath hold to ensure equal filling of lung segments by collateral filling; then a deep exhalation is made into the expiratory reserve volume range. By lowering the middle tidal volume below the functional residual capacity level, secretions from peripheral lung regions are mobilized by the compression of peripheral alveolar ducts. Mid-expiratory tidal volume is lowered in the range of normal expiratory reserve volume. Chevaillier[97] named this phase the "unsticking" phase. The second phase of AD consists of tidal volume breathing

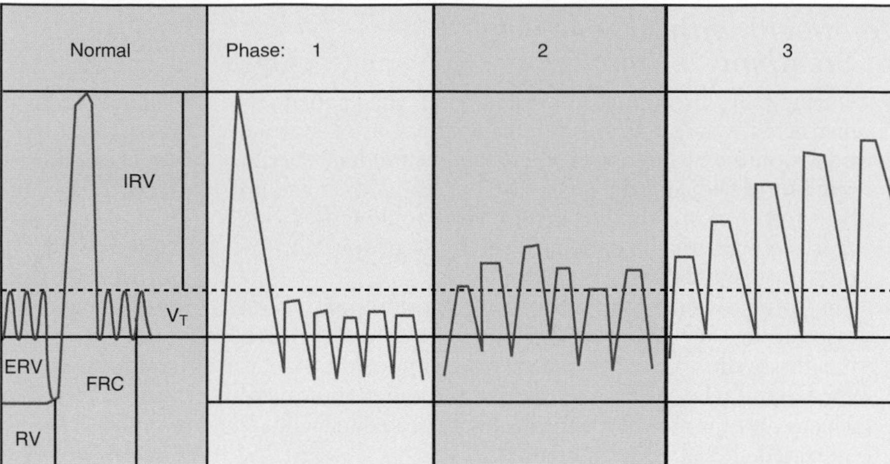

Fig. 21-6 Phases of autogenic drainage shown on a spirogram of a normal person. Phase 1: unstick; phase 2: collect; phase 3: evacuate. *VT,* Tidal volume; *ERV,* expiratory reserve volume; *RV,* reserve volume; *FRC,* functional residual capacity; IRV, inspiratory reserve volume; *IRV + VT + ERV,* vital capacity. *(From Schoni MH: Autogenic drainage: A modern approach to physiotherapy in cystic fibrosis,* Journal of the Royal Society of Medicine *82(Suppl 16):32-37, 1989.)*

gradually changing from the expiratory reserve volume into the inspiratory reserve volume range, which mobilizes secretions from the apical parts of the lungs. The velocity of the airflow must be adjusted at each level of inspiration so that the maximal expiratory airflow is reached without being high enough to cause collapse of the airways. Flow volume curves show that higher flows of longer duration can be achieved with AD,[99] demonstrating that mucus can be moved farther and at a faster rate. This is the "collecting" phase[97] The third phase consists of deeper inspiration into the inspiratory reserve volume, with huffing often used to help in evacuating the mobilized secretions. Control of airflow during this final phase is essential to the avoidance of uncontrolled, unproductive coughing. Chevaillier[97] named this phase the "evacuating" phase.

The Belgian method of AD has been modified by German practitioners using a combination of diaphragmatic and costosternal breathing in a treatment that is not separated into phases.[100] This modification resulted from the observation that many patients had difficulty breathing in the expiratory reserve volume range. The patient varies his or her mid-tidal volume in a passive exhalation followed by an active exhalation through pursed lips or through the nose. The German method of airway clearance includes other maneuvers in conjunction with AD, including inhalation therapy, FET, chest wall exercises, and physical activity.

Assisted AD has been described for use in treating infants and patients who are unable to participate.[50] Gentle manual pressure is applied to the chest during inspiration in an effort to vary the volume of breath inhaled; no pressure is applied during exhalation. This technique is often applied while gently bouncing the infant on a therapy ball.

AD has been compared with positive expiratory pressure and PD with percussion and/or vibration. It was reported that more sputum was produced with AD in patients with hyperreactive airways.[101] In a 2-year crossover trial, AD was found to be as effective as conventional CPT among patients with cystic fibrosis for improving pulmonary function.[102] However, patients exhibited a strong preference for AD over CPT, increasing the likelihood of adherence. Miller[103] showed greater clearance of inhaled radioisotopes with AD than with ACBT, with no significant differences in sputum weight, spirometry, or transcutaneous oxygen saturation. Giles[104] also studied oxygen saturation in AD and found greater levels with AD than with PD with percussion; there was also greater sputum evacuated with AD.

Preparation for Autogenic Drainage

- No equipment is needed for a patient to perform the technique of AD. The patient must possess good proprioceptive, tactile, and auditory perception of the mucus moving—this feedback makes it possible to adjust the technique of AD.
- To teach this method to a patient, a caregiver needs keen tactile and auditory senses to coach a patient to move between the phases by listening to and palpating the chest to identify the location and the quality of the secretions.
- The patient should be seated upright in a chair with a back for support. The surroundings should be devoid of distractions, allowing the patient to concentrate on the breathing technique.
- The upper airways (nose and throat) should be cleared of secretions by huffing or blowing the nose.
- The caregiver should be seated to the side and slightly behind the patient, close enough to hear the patient's breathing. One hand should be placed to feel the work of the abdominal muscles and the other hand placed on the upper chest (Figure 21-7).

Treatment with Autogenic Drainage

- In all phases, inhalation should be done slowly, through the nose if possible, using the diaphragm or lower chest. A 2- to 3-second breath hold should follow, allowing collateral ventilation to get air behind the secretions.
- Exhalation should occur actively with the mouth and glottis open, listening for the movement of mucus while avoiding a wheeze. The vibrations of the mucus may also be felt with the hand placed on the upper chest. The frequency of these vibrations reveals their location. High frequencies mean that the secretions are located in the small airways; low frequencies mean that the secretions have moved to the large airways.[97]
- In practice, inspiration is followed by a deep expiration into the expiratory reserve volume. The patient attempts to exhale as far into the expiratory reserve volume as possible, contracting the abdominal muscles to achieve this.

This low lung volume breathing continues until the mucus is loosened and starts to move into the larger airways.

- The second phase collects the mucus in the middle airways by increasing the lung volume to a greater level than in the initial phase. Tidal volume breathing is then changed gradually from expiratory reserve volume toward the inspiratory reserve volume range[98] so that the lungs are expanded more with each inspiration. The patient increases both inspiration and expiration to move a greater volume of air. This low to middle lung volume breathing continues until the sound of the mucus decreases, signaling its movement into the central airways to be evacuated.
- In the evacuation phase, the patient increases inspiration into the inspiratory reserve volume range. This middle-to-high lung volume breathing continues until the secretions are in the trachea and are ready to be expectorated. The collected mucus can be evacuated by a stronger expiration or a high-volume huff. Nonproductive coughing should be avoided, since it may result in collapse of airways. See Figure 21-6 for a diagram of the three phases of AD.
- Compression of the airways should be avoided. If wheezing is heard, the expiratory flow rate must be decreased. Beginners may have to use pursed lips to avoid airway compression.[97] Instructing the patient to roll the tongue (if possible) may assist in controlling the expiratory flow rate.
- In the simplified German procedure, the patient begins by varying the mid-tidal volume without excessive effort. After a passive but rapid expiration, an actively performed expiration follows, achieving exhalation to a low expiratory reserve volume (Figure 21-8).
- The duration of each phase of AD depends on the location of the secretions. The duration of a session depends on the amount and viscosity of the secretions. An average treatment will be 30 to 45 minutes in length. However, a patient who is experienced in performing AD will clear secretions in a shorter amount of time than a beginner.

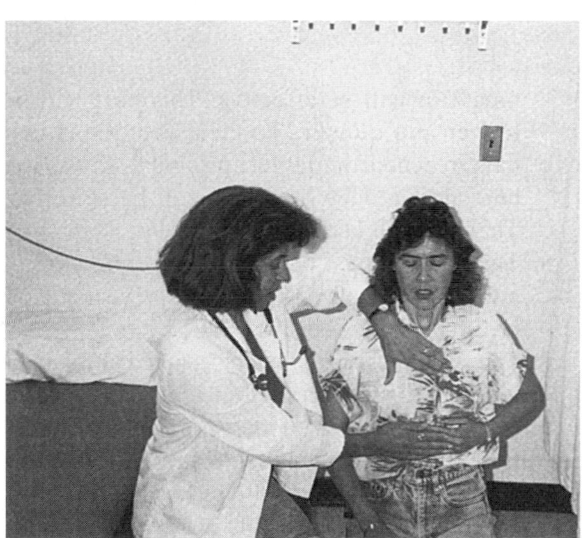

Fig. 21-7 Autogenic drainage.

Advantages and Disadvantages of Autogenic Drainage

When learned effectively, AD may be performed independently by patients over 12 years of age and requires no additional equipment. It is ideal for the adolescent or adult who prefers an independent method. Because it does not require the use of PD positions, it is appropriate for patients with gastroesophageal reflux. It is also recommended for use in patients with airway hyperreactivity.[105] The technique of AD requires attention to airflow and volume and to cough suppression until secretions are mobilized; this is a key factor to success.[106] Learning AD requires tactile and auditory feedback and continued modifications of the patient's technique, at least initially, to achieve a good result.

Although widely used in Europe, the use of AD in the United States is limited by the lack of trained caregivers but is growing in popularity. To learn this technique, patients must demonstrate good self-discipline and concentration. This method takes more practice than others. AD is not the treatment of choice for a patient who is unmotivated or uncooperative, and a study of flow volume curves suggests that AD would not be appropriate for small children even if they were cooperative.[99] A patient must also be available for periodic reevaluation and refinement of the technique. During early hospitalization for patients admitted with an acute exacerbation is a challenging time in terms of learning AD. Patients who are skilled in the technique may choose a more passive

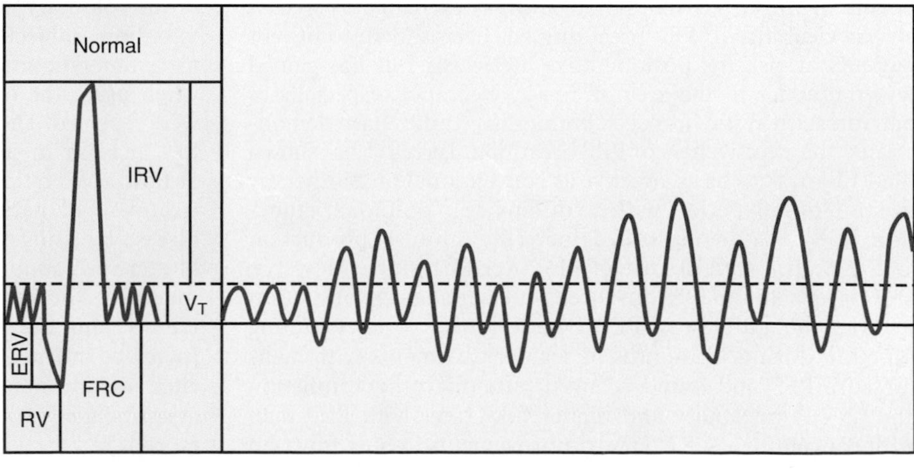

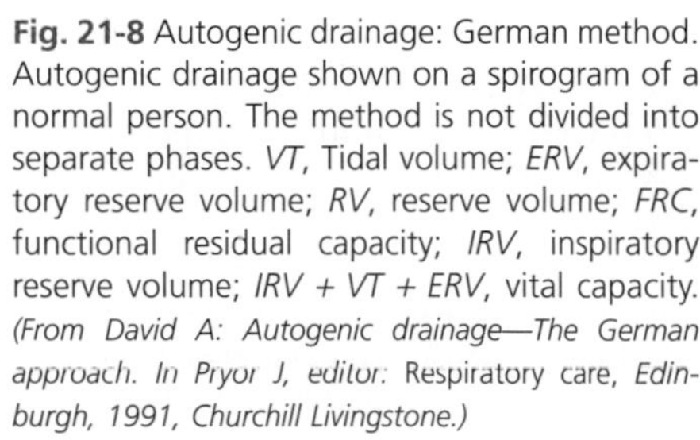

Fig. 21-8 Autogenic drainage: German method. Autogenic drainage shown on a spirogram of a normal person. The method is not divided into separate phases. *VT*, Tidal volume; *ERV*, expiratory reserve volume; *RV*, reserve volume; *FRC*, functional residual capacity; *IRV*, inspiratory reserve volume; *IRV + VT + ERV*, vital capacity. *(From David A: Autogenic drainage—The German approach. In Pryor J, editor:* Respiratory care, *Edinburgh, 1991, Churchill Livingstone.)*

form (one consuming less energy) of airway clearance at such times until they return to their baseline pulmonary status.

Positive Expiratory Pressure

The development and use of positive expiratory pressure (PEP) breathing came about in the 1980s in Denmark and is now widely used in the United States. Although high- or low-pressure PEP is prescribed worldwide, only low-pressure PEP is approved in the United States. Several devices deliver PEP in either oscillatory or smooth flow methods. Oscillatory PEP provides (1) positive expiratory pressure, (2) oscillation of the airways and (3) accelerated expiratory flow rates to loosen secretions and move them centrally.

Positive expiratory pressure includes a one-way breathing valve and an adjustable level of expiratory resistance that creates a back pressure to stent the airways open during exhalation. It is theorized that PEP breathing reinflates collapsed alveoli by allowing air to be redistributed through collateral channels—the pores of Kohn and the Lambert canals—allowing pressure to build up distal to the obstruction and promoting the movement of secretions toward the larger airways.[107,108] In addition, supplemental oxygen and nebulized medication can be effectively delivered during treatment with PEP.[109] A manometer in the circuit determines and monitors the pressure generated by the patient. In low-pressure PEP breathing, the resistance is regulated to achieve 10 to 20 cm of H_2O during slightly active expiration. The appropriate resistor is one that produces a flow volume curve demonstrating a maximal forced vital capacity, good plateau, and no curvilinearity.[88] Low-pressure PEP breathing is used more often than high-pressure PEP, as it offers equal effectiveness at a lower presumed risk for pneumothorax.

High-pressure PEP uses the same principles but at much higher levels of pressure (50 to 120 cm H_2O). Inspiration is performed to total lung capacity; this is followed by a forced expiratory maneuver against the PEP mask, which is connected to a spirometer. For high-pressure PEP therapy, the Pep/Rmt (Astra Tech Healthcare, Molndal, Sweden) mask is used. The equipment consists of a ventilation mask, a one-way valve, and various resistors. Spirometry is used to determine the appropriate resistance for each individual patient, but generally, a 1½-mm resistor is used for infants, a resistor of up to 2½ to 3 mm for older children and adults, and 3½ mm for adults with COPD.

Airway stability is maintained with PEP breathing, which results in improved ventilation and gas exchange as well as airway clearance.[110] PEP breathing has been shown to benefit patients at risk for postoperative atelectasis but has gained wider practice in the area of airway clearance, especially in patients with cystic fibrosis.[95] Numerous studies have demonstrated the effectiveness of PEP breathing. Tyrrell[111] has shown the PEP mask to be as effective as conventional physiotherapy over a 1-month period, with no difference in pulmonary function. Falk[112,113] demonstrated increased sputum production and clearance with the use of PEP over FET alone. However, Hofmeyer[114] found FET produced a greater quantity of sputum without the addition of PEP. Oberwaldner[115] evaluated lung function during 10 months of regular treatments with high-pressure PEP and found reduced pulmonary hyperinflation and airway instability and higher flow rates with PEP than with conventional CPT. These improvements in lung function deteriorated only 2 months after a return to conventional CPT. A study by Pfleger and colleagues[105] compared PEP with AD and found that PEP cleared higher amounts of sputum and demonstrated increased lung function. Finally, decreased duration of hospitalization has been cited as a benefit of using PEP breathing for airway clearance.[116]

Two of the most commonly used devices in the United States are the Acapella (Figure 21-9, *A* and *B*) and TheraPEP (DHD Healthcare, Wampsville, New York) (Figure 21-9, *C*). The TheraPEP device consists of a mouthpiece and an expiratory resistor that can accommodate many levels of expiratory flow. It comes with a detachable pressure monitoring port and indicator to show 10 to 20 cm of H_2O. The TheraPEP can accommodate a mask of different sizes. The Acapella has performance characteristics similar to those of the Flutter.[117] It comes in several models: green for patients who can maintain an expiratory flow of 15 L/min or more, blue for patients whose expiratory flow rate is less than 15 L/min, and the Acapella Choice. The Acapella Choice disassembles more easily than the original models for ease of cleaning (Figure 21-9, *D*). The Acapella consists of a mouthpiece attached to the body of the unit that uses a counterweighted plug and magnet to create airflow oscillation and a dial for expiratory resistance at the other end.

A device developed in Switzerland to deliver high-frequency oscillation PEP breathing and decrease the collapsibility of the airways is the Flutter VRP1 (VarioRaw, Aubonne, Switzerland). Axcan Pharma (Birmingham, Alabama) markets the Flutter VRP1 valve in the United States, the first oscillatory PEP device available in this country. This pipelike device consists of a steel ball, a plastic cone, a perforated cover, and a mouthpiece. Exhaled air causes the steel ball to roll up and down the cone causing airflow vibration. The PEP maintained by the Flutter (5 to 35 cm of H_2O) prevents dynamic airway compression and improves airflow acceleration.[118] The full effects of the vibration induced by the Flutter (6 to 20 Hz) may be received by changing the angle of the device. Movement of the Flutter upward increases the pressure and frequency while movement of the device downward results in lower pressure and frequency.[118] The vibration of the chest can be palpated to provide feedback as to the optimal angle of the device. The recommended procedure for use of the Flutter is shown in Box 21-5.

This early form of oscillatory PEP has been well studied. Konstan and colleagues[119] compared the amount of sputum expectorated with the Flutter with that expectorated with vigorous voluntary cough, with PD, with percussion, and with vibration. Subjects with cystic fibrosis produced more than three times the amount of sputum when using the Flutter than when using the other two methods, and no adverse effects were reported. The improvement in expectoration is based on the increase in airway diameter and the improvement in airflow acceleration.[120] Ambrosino[121] reported success in the treatment of patients with chronic obstructive pulmonary disease by using the device. When compared with AD, the Flutter was found to produce equal amounts of expectorated mucus.[122] The advantages of the Flutter device lie in its portability and the ease with which its use can be learned. Increased independence and better compliance have also been cited as advantages of this technique. However, frequent assessment of patient technique and appropriate level of resistance is recommended.[87]

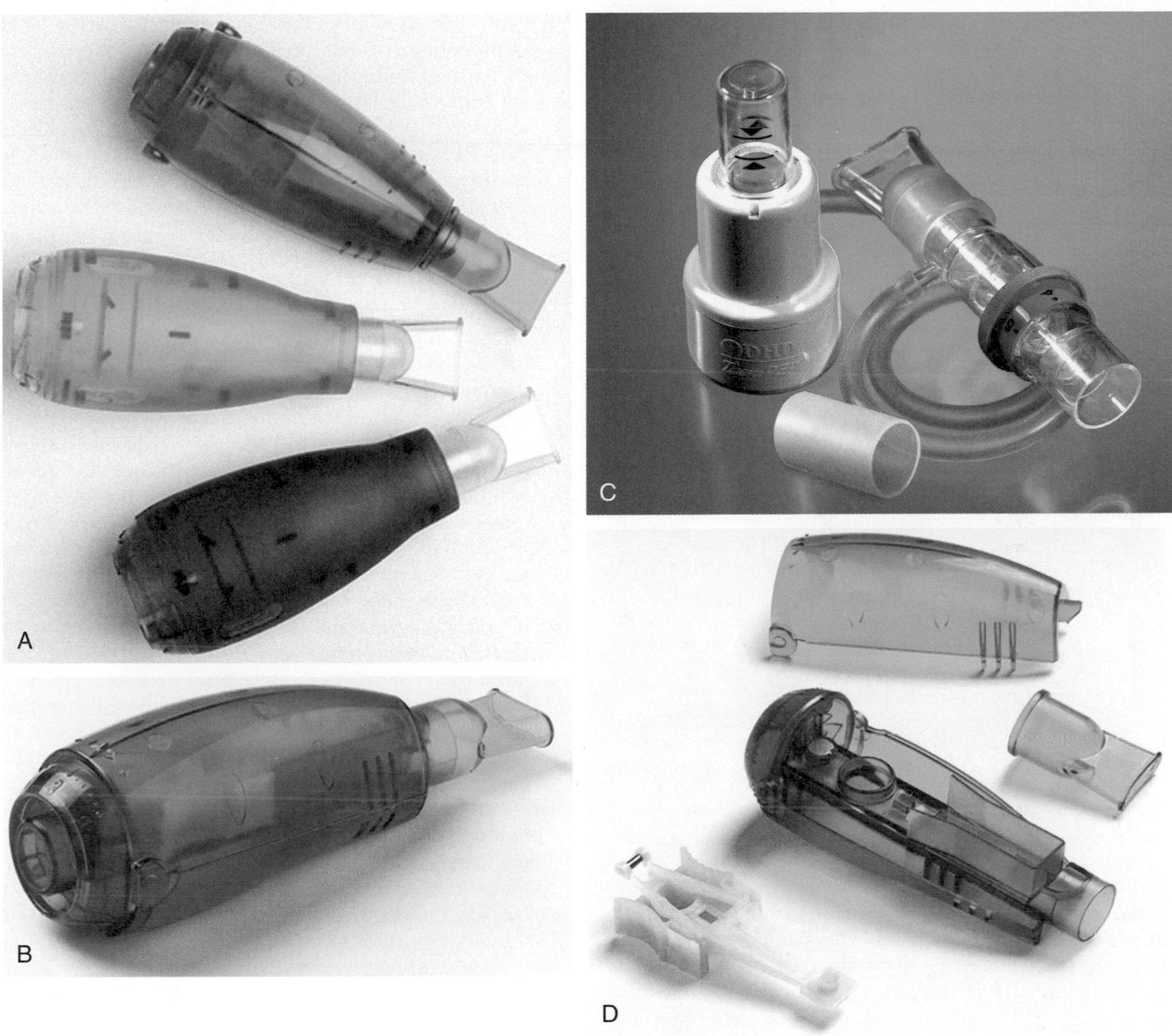

Fig. 21-9 A-D, Positive expiratory pressure devices: TheraPEP and Acapella.

Another device that provides PEP with oscillations is the Quake (Thayer Medical, Tucson, Arizona), which consists of a mouthpiece integrated into the outer housing and a crank that interrupts airflow and allows the user to manually adjust the frequency of the vibration. This allows a wider range of oscillation frequencies than other devices, such as the Flutter. When using the Quake, it is recommended to rotate the handle at a steady and comfortable rate of about 1 to 2 rotations per second during exhalation. At the end of exhalation, the user may either remove the Quake from the mouth to inhale or continue to rotate the handle and slowly begin to breathe in deeply, then repeat the exhalation cycle. Both the inhalation and exhalation rate and the speed of the handle rotation may be varied to produce the ideal level of vibration in the lungs. This device can be used with a mouthpiece or a facemask, whereas the Flutter can only be used with a mouthpiece. The disadvantage of the Quake is that it requires both hands—one to hold the device and one to turn the crank. The other devices can be used with only one hand.

Preparation for Positive Expiratory Pressure

- Several different devices are available to deliver positive expiratory pressure with a steady level of resistance or oscillatory flow. The practitioner should be familiar with the specific device being used to provide adequate instructions to the patient and family.
- A mask can be used in place of the mouthpiece on most PEP devices (for adults and children) and is preferred by some practitioners. The rationale for using a mask is that the lung volumes should be increased during the entire phase of exhalation through the PEP device, which is more difficult to achieve when using a mouthpiece because the patient may open the mouth around the mouthpiece at the

Box 21-5 **Proper Patient Technique for Using Flutter***

- Gather supplies, relax, and assume proper posture and position. Begin stage 1, mucus loosening and mucus mobilization.
- Slowly inhale beyond a normal breath, but do not fill lungs completely.
- Hold breath for 2 to 3 seconds.
- Place Flutter in mouth, adjust tilt, and keep cheeks stiff.
- Exhale through Flutter at a reasonably fast but not too forceful speed.
- Exhale beyond a normal breath, but do not empty lungs completely.
- Attempt to suppress cough.
- Repeat steps 2 through 7 for 5 to 10 breaths. Begin stage 2, mucus elimination.
- Slowly inhale, filling lungs completely.
- Hold breath for 2 to 3 seconds.
- Place Flutter in mouth, adjust tilt, and keep cheeks stiff.
- Exhale forcefully through Flutter as completely as possible.
- Repeat steps 9 through 12 for 1 to 2 breaths.
- Initiate cough (or "huff" maneuver). Return to step 2 and repeat full sequence until lungs are clear or therapy is over.
- Additional sessions may be added if necessary.
- Clean Flutter and store in clean, dry location.

*For more information about Flutter, contact Axcan Pharma, 22 Inverness Center Parkway, Birmingham, AL 35242; phone 205-991-8085

end of expiration causing a fall in lung volumes.[123] The use of nose clips is recommended when using a mouthpiece.

- A manometer can be placed proximal to the resistor in the initial stages of instruction in the use of PEP in most devices. First, the manometer helps to determine and monitor the appropriate level of resistance needed for the patient to achieve 10 to 20 cm of H_2O throughout exhalation. Second, the visual display of the manometer serves as feedback to assist the patient in mastering the technique.[95]
- Aerosol medication delivered by nebulizer may be placed inline in many devices to be delivered simultaneously with PEP for airway clearance, improving the deposition of medication.[109,124] If aerosolized medication is to be used simultaneously, the patient should be instructed in how to stop the flow of the aerosol when the mask or mouthpiece is removed during the PEP treatment session for coughing. Supplemental oxygen may also be placed inline in many devices for patients who require this.
- Bubble PEP is a variation of positive expiratory pressure that is particularly useful when treating children. Equipment needed includes a length of tubing 15 to 18 inches long and a plastic container filled with a column of water 13 cm high (this will generate a positive expiratory pressure of around 20 cm of H_2O). A few drops of food coloring and/or 3 to 6 squirts of liquid detergent or bubble liquid may be added to make the treatment more entertaining. Place the tubing at the very bottom of the container—it is important that the tube remain at the base of the column of water to generate the required expiratory pressure. If detergent or bubbles are included, place the container in a large bowl or on a towel to contain the overflow.[123]
- All PEP devices should be cleaned regularly with hot, soapy water; many can be cleaned in a dishwasher. In the hospital, the equipment should be sterilized according to infection control recommendations.

Treatment with Positive Expiratory Pressure

- To determine the correct level of resistance for PEP, the patient inhales using tidal volume and exhales actively into the mask or mouthpiece. The resistor valve is adjusted while the level of PEP is monitored on the manometer. The resistance is gradually decreased until the PEP level supplying 10 to 20 cm of water pressure has been identified.[113] Mahlmeister[95] reports most patients achieve this pressure range with flow resistors of 2.5 to 4.0 mm in diameter. Selection of the proper resistor produces the desired inspiratory to expiratory ratio of 1:3 or 1:4.[95] The use of too great a resistance will create an increased respiratory rate or too low a pressure, whereas too small a resistor will create a slow respiratory rate or too high a pressure.[125]
- For high-pressure PEP, appropriate resistance is determined by connecting the outlet of the PEP mask to a spirometer. The resistor producing the highest forced vital capacity through the PEP mask is selected for continued use.[115] The patient breathes in and out through the mask at tidal volume for 6 to 10 breaths; then inspiration is done to total lung capacity and a forced expiratory maneuver is performed against the PEP mask. This is repeated until all the mucus is mobilized.[125]
- For a PEP therapy treatment, the patient should be seated upright with elbows resting on a table. Use of a mask may require securing the device with both hands for a tight seal. If needed, the patient may be in a reclining position for all PEP devices except the Flutter, which is position dependent. To use the Flutter valve, the patient should be seated upright (Figure 21-10).
- The patient should be instructed to breathe into the mask or mouthpiece to tidal volume, using the lower chest and abdomen, and pause for an inspiratory hold for 2 to 3 seconds to equalize ventilation before exhaling.[123] Exhalation into the mask or mouthpiece should be slightly active but not forced. The patient continues breathing into the mask or mouthpiece for 10 to 15 breaths, using a normal respiratory rate. After a series of 10 to 15 breaths, the mask or mouthpiece is removed from the face and the patient performs a series of huffs and/or coughing to expectorate any mucus that has been mobilized.[126] It may be necessary to pause every 5 to 10 exhalations before resuming the session.[118]
- The series of PEP breaths followed by huffs should be repeated about four to six times. The total treatment lasts about 15 to 20 minutes and should be performed twice during the day or as needed. The frequency and duration of the treatment must be individualized for each patient. During periods of pulmonary exacerbation, patients are encouraged to increase the frequency of PEP treatments rather than extend the length of individual sessions.[95]

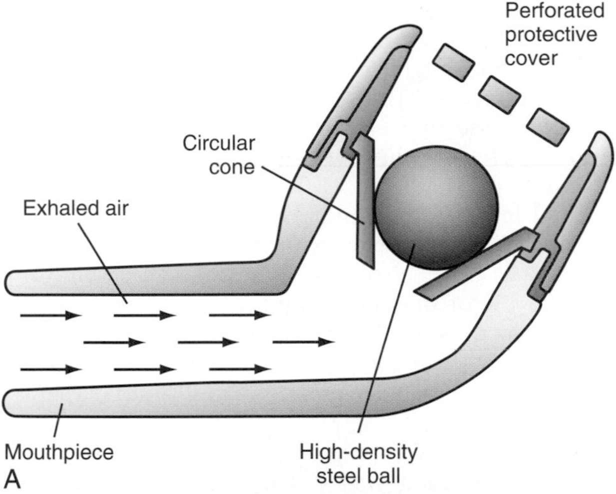

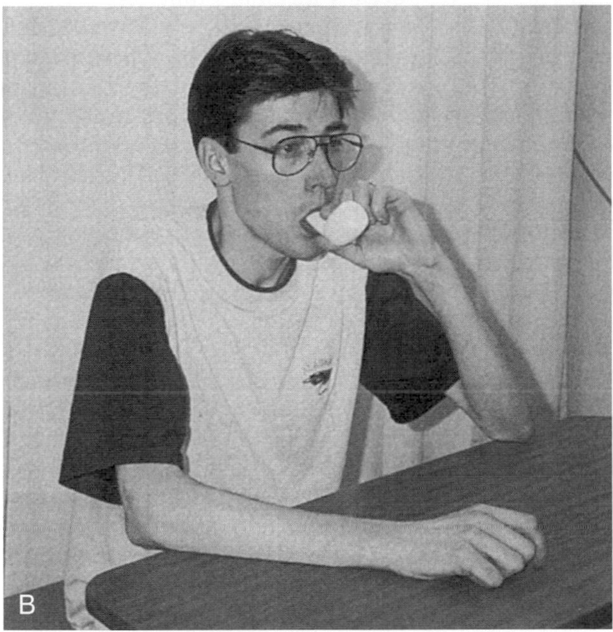

Fig. 21-10 Use of Flutter valve.

Some patients have a tendency to hyperventilate and become dizzy; an inspiratory pause will prevent this.[123]

- Initially, the patient and caregiver monitor the effort by means of the manometer, ensuring that a pressure of 10 to 20 cm of H_2O is achieved throughout exhalation (this is not possible with the Flutter). After the technique is mastered with the appropriate resistor, the manometer may be removed from the system. The appropriate resistance should be rechecked periodically during clinical visits or periods of hospitalization.
- For Bubble PEP, the patient is instructed to blow through the tube with enough force to cause the bubbles to rise up to the top of the container. After a number of breaths, the patient is asked to do huffing or coughing before resuming the treatment. The therapist may prescribe the height of the column of water to alter the pressure, the number of breaths taken, and the huffs or coughs needed to tailor the treatment to each patient.[123]

Advantages and Disadvantages of Positive Expiratory Pressure

PEP therapy does not possess some of the limitations of conventional PD and percussion for secretion clearance and is therefore applicable to a wider patient population. It is relatively easy to learn in one or two sessions and may be applied equally to the pediatric (children over 4 years of age) and adult populations. PEP is appropriate for use during acute episodes in hospitalized patients, as well as for long-term use for chronic pulmonary conditions. The expense of the equipment is minimal, and once the patient is competent in the technique, it provides independence (except for small children). All PEP devices are quite portable, making airway clearance easier to perform during travel or when away from home during the day. PEP devices can be used in any position except the Flutter, which is position dependent. Some musical instruments can provide a form of PEP therapy because of the manner in which they are played, with an inspiratory pause and resisted exhalation.[123] These instruments include the clarinet, oboe, bassoon, French horn, trumpet, flute, and voice. Low-pressure PEP is more commonly used in North America because it is believed to be not only as effective as high-pressure PEP, but also easier and safer to use and monitor. In those patients in whom PEP is an appropriate airway clearance technique, a high degree of acceptance has been shown.[112,117,127] This may translate into better adherence in the long term.

A decision to use PEP should be carefully evaluated in cases of acute sinusitis, ear infection, epistaxis, and recent oral or facial surgery or injury.[95] For PEP therapy to be effective, a patient should be able to cooperate and actively participate with the treatment. Although rare, pneumothorax has been reported with high-pressure PEP.[115]

Precautions for Positive Expiratory Pressure

The use of PEP for airway clearance carries an increased risk for pneumothorax.[115] Bronchodilator premedication should be considered when applying PEP in patients who show clinical or physiological signs of airway hyperreactivity.[105]

The increased airflow produced by the huff cough, as in the ACBT, may aggravate bronchospasm.[90] Additionally, Hietpas[90] cautions that the movement of secretions into the larger airways by the huff cough may precipitate spontaneous explosive coughing.

High-Frequency Chest Wall Oscillation

Efforts aimed at mucus clearance by creating a differential airflow rate led to the development of a high-frequency chest wall oscillation (HFCWO) system. Hansen and Warwick[128] designed a large-volume, variable-frequency air-pulse delivery system that can be used by patients with obstructive lung disease to promote mucus clearance.

High-frequency chest wall oscillation, also referred to as high-frequency chest compression, consists of an inflatable vest linked to an air-pulse generator. Although the sensation of the device is somewhat akin to mechanical percussion, it differs significantly in its mechanism of action. HFCWO works by differential airflow (i.e., the expiratory flow rate is higher than the inspiratory flow rate), allowing the mucus to be transported from the periphery to the central airways for

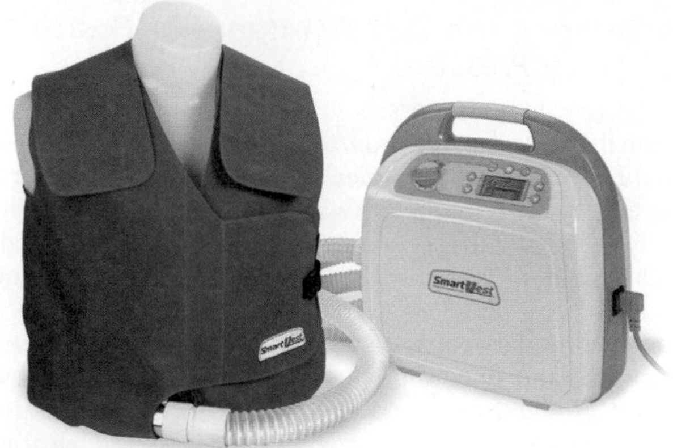

Fig. 21-11 SmartVest® high-frequency chest wall oscillation (HFCWO) system for airway clearance. *(Courtesy Electromed, Inc. New Prague, Minn.)*

expectoration (Figure 21-11). HFCWO has also been shown to decrease the viscosity of mucus, making it easier to mobilize.

The first HFCWO system developed was the Vest (Hill ROM, St. Paul, Minnesota), consisting of an inflatable fitted vest connected to an air-pulse generator by flexible tubing. This device provides oscillation of the entire thoracic cavity at varying frequencies (5 to 25 Hz). The lung volume expired tends to increase with lower frequencies (less than 10 to 12 Hz), whereas the flow rates tend to increase with higher frequencies (12 to 20 Hz). Continuous aerosolized medication or saline administered concurrently may assist with secretion mobilization.[129] The original, larger unit of the Vest is best used in a clinical setting; it can be placed on a wheeled stand for easy mobility. Newer models weigh as little as 17 pounds, providing more mobility than earlier models; these units fit under an airplane seat and are easier to manage during travel.

Two probable mechanisms of action have been offered to explain the significant increase in sputum mobilization that occurs with HFCWO.[130] One mechanism proposes that oscillatory airflow leads to changes in the consistency of mucus, which results in increased mobilization of secretions. Considerable decreases in mucus viscoelasticity were observed during administration of oscillatory airflow.[131] Another mechanism proposes that the difference between the expiratory and inspiratory velocities produces shear forces strong enough to move mucus. Chang and colleagues[132] demonstrated that nonsymmetrical airflow (peak expiratory flow rates greater than inspiratory flow rates) could be an important factor leading to increases in mucus clearance during the administration of HFCWO. The chest compressions produce a transient flow pulse similar to that observed during coughing, and by using the flows with the greatest rates and volumes, sufficient force is obtained to move mucus in the airway.[133]

HFCWO has been shown to increase mucus clearance rates in animal models, with the most pronounced effect in the 11 to 15 Hz frequency range.[134] Radford and colleagues[68] used bronchoscopy to demonstrate a marked increase in the speed and flow of mucus produced by oscillations at even higher frequencies than those attainable by manual percussion. Results of short-term use of the Vest have been mixed, but they show HFCWO to be at least as effective as conventional CPT. Robinson[135] showed no significant improvement or deterioration of lung function with its use. In additional studies, Kluft and Faverio[136,137] demonstrated increased wet and dry sputum weights using HFCWO as opposed to manual CPT, and Arens (1993)[138] showed similar dry sputum weight but an increase in wet sputum weight and a significant improvement in pulmonary function with HFCWO as opposed to conventional CPT. One 2-year study showed improved lung function and greater sputum production in subjects with cystic fibrosis with the use of HFCWO rather than manual CPT.[133] No adverse effects were observed with long-term use of the Vest. Hospitalized patients with acute exacerbation of lung disease have been shown to tolerate HFCWO well,[139] and the safety and tolerance of this method have been demonstrated in long-term mechanically ventilated patients.[140]

The fit of the vest requires attention because nausea, abdominal and chest wall discomfort, and complaints of urinary urgency may occur with an ill-fitting vest.[106] HFCWO systems are much more costly than other mechanical aids for airway clearance; thus expense may be a deterrent for some potential users. However, in a study of HFCWO users insured by Blue Cross and Blue Shield, a 49% reduction in health care costs was shown in the year following initial use of the vest as compared with the year before HFCWO use.[141] The impact of the use of the HFCWO device in a hospital department demonstrated a substantial savings resulting from therapy self-administration by patients.[142]

Preparation for High-Frequency Chest Wall Oscillation

- In order to provide adequate instructions to the patient and family, the practitioner should be familiar with the specific HFCWO device being used. The various models of inflatable vests are constructed to fit the thorax differently and are available in different sizes (from toddler to large adult). A full vest model should extend to the top of the thigh when the patient is sitting upright. A shorter vest (chest vest) is also available, resulting in less pressure to the abdominal area and less gastric discomfort. The vest should fit properly, but breathing should not feel restricted while the vest is deflated. A single layer of clothing or patient gown should be worn under the vest. For the hospital setting, adjustable vests are available for use with multiple patients (following appropriate infection control guidelines for cleaning). For home use, each patient should be fitted for his or her own vest.
- Simultaneous use of aerosolized medication is recommended for use throughout the treatment. This humidifies the air to counteract the drying effect of the increased airflow.

Treatment with High-Frequency Chest Wall Oscillation

- The patient should be seated upright in a chair, and the tubing should be securely connected to the air pulse generator. Start the aerosol therapy before turning on the HFCWO system.
- The pressure control setting should be adjusted according to patient comfort, opting for the highest pressure that is well tolerated.

- The treatment should progress through different frequencies, from low (7 to 10 Hz) to medium (10 to 14 Hz) and then to high (14 to 20 Hz), to achieve both higher flow rates and increased lung volume. Warwick[133] reported that the frequencies associated with the highest flow rates were usually greater than 13 Hz, whereas those associated with the largest volume were usually less than 10 Hz. The average length of time spent at each frequency is 10 minutes, but this will vary according to patient tolerance, amount and consistency of secretions, and the acuity of the patient's illness. After treatment at each frequency for the prescribed length of time, the patient should be instructed to huff or cough to clear loosened secretions.
- HFCWO has also been used with patients requiring long-term mechanical ventilation. Whitman and colleagues[140] found use of HFCWO to be safe and effective and concluded that it resulted in time savings over conventional PD and percussion.
- Patients with long-term central intravenous access such as a Porta-Cath or Hickman are able to use HFCWO with sufficient padding (such as a foam doughnut pillow) to relieve pressure around the access site.

Advantages and Disadvantages of High-Frequency Chest Wall Oscillation

This method of airway clearance allows independence and is easily learned in a short period. HFCWO can accommodate children as young as 2 years of age, and a vest may be custom-made for very large or obese adults. HFCWO is appropriate for those patients in whom PD positions are contraindicated, and it has also been used successfully in reclining patients who are unable to tolerate the upright sitting position. Use of HFCWO may result in time savings at home, as well as in a hospital or long-term care facility, because nebulized medications may be administered concurrently with the airway clearance treatment and all lobes of the lungs are treated simultaneously. The amount of time for patient contact required for a hospital caregiver is much less with this method than with conventional PD and percussion. This efficiency would also benefit families in which there is more than one member requiring airway clearance (such as siblings with cystic fibrosis). In those patients for whom it is appropriate (and reimbursable), HFCWO is an effective method of airway clearance. It provides independence for long-term use at home, as well as for acute exacerbations in the hospital.

A disadvantage of HFCWO as a method of airway clearance is the cost of the equipment. A study by Ohnsorg,[141] however, demonstrated a decline in total health care costs for the year after HFCWO was put into use by 11 patients. A study of the impact of the device in a hospital setting[142] reported a substantial savings as a result of therapy self-administration. Replacement of the equipment should not be a factor, because a lifetime warranty is available for the devices.

Intrapulmonary Percussive Ventilation

Intrapulmonary percussive ventilation (IPV) is an airway clearance method that simultaneously delivers intrathoracic percussion and aerosolized solution for bronchodilation.[143] An apparatus known as the Phasitron is the functional component in the intrapulmonary percussive ventilator. The Phasitron provides high-frequency impulses during inspiration, while positive expiratory pressure is maintained throughout passive exhalation. The pressure generated is between 10 and 30 cm of H_2O.

The intrapulmonary percussive ventilation device made by Percussionaire (Sandpoint, Idaho) works in a manner similar to that of the HFCWO except that a pneumatic device delivers the oscillation internally instead of externally. A mouthpiece delivers high flow rate mini-bursts of gases into the lungs at rates of 100 to 240 cycles per minute. Continuous pressure in the airways is maintained while pulsatile, percussive intraairway pressure rises and dilates the airways, enhancing intrabronchial secretion mobilization. This device provides percussion at 6 to 14 Hz, with a positive expiratory pressure of 10 to 20 cm of water pressure and simultaneous delivery of an aerosol. The aerosol mist within the lungs reduces adhesive forces of retained secretions.

It is theorized that changes in the frequency and pressure of the airflow delivered through the IPV device assist in stabilizing the airways and decrease the viscosity of the secretions; this results in increased sputum mobilization.[106] IPV has been found to be as effective as postural drainage and percussion in improving pulmonary function and sputum expectoration.[144] Marks[145] found no difference between IPV and Flutter in number of hospital or antibiotic days required to treat an exacerbation and reported good acceptance of this method of airway clearance by patients. IPV may be beneficial for patients with asthma and neuromuscular disease, as well as those with cystic fibrosis.[146,147]

Treatment with Intrapulmonary Percussive Ventilation

- One IPV model meant for institutional use is the Percussionaire Model IPV-1, which is powered by 50 psi of gas. Percussive rates or frequencies range from less than 100 to greater than 225 cycles per minute. This model has the capability to be used with an endotracheal tube and can be installed on a wheeled stand for greater mobility. Use of the hospital unit must be supervised by a respiratory care practitioner.
- The Percussionaire Impulsator is self-contained for home use and powered by a compressor, but it may also be used in a clinical situation. It generates 40-psi source pressure, which provides for efficient delivery of impulses and aerosolized medication. Condensation is minimal compared with institutional models, so maintenance on the unit is low. The patient and caregivers must receive training to use the home unit.
- A new model by Percussionaire, the HC Impulsator, is a portable IPV device that weighs less than 15 pounds, allowing patients to use it when traveling.
- Aerosolized medication in saline solution is delivered via the nebulizer component of the IPV unit.
- Treatment with IPV is titrated for patient comfort and visible thoracic movement. A thumb button is held for 5- to 10-second intervals to initiate the percussive impulses and released after an interval to allow exhalation. After each deep exhalation, the percussive interval starts again. When the patient needs to cough or expectorate, the thumb button is released until coughing is completed or secretions are cleared.

- The clinician or the patient at home programs each percussive interval. An average treatment lasts about 20 minutes.

Advantages and Disadvantages of Intrapulmonary Percussive Ventilation

IPV is available for home use and can be continued during hospitalization. IPV allows for greater independence for adolescents and adults with long-term need for airway clearance. Homnick[143] reported that three-fourths of the patients using IPV in one study estimated increased sputum production, and satisfaction was high for comfort and independence. IPV provides a safe and effective form of airway clearance.[148]

IPV is neither appropriate for nor tolerated by young children. In other patients, a feeling of claustrophobia or chest fullness may be a factor in deciding whether to use IPV.[106] The IPV device is more expensive than a PEP device but less costly than a unit for HFCWO. The availability of IPV in the clinical setting is not as common as other airway clearance devices; therefore, respiratory care practitioners may not be as familiar or comfortable with its application. The use of IPV may increase as more patients request alternative methods of airway clearance and as more research is done to demonstrate its benefits.

Acoustic Airway Clearance

A recent form of airway clearance uses acoustic vibrations to clear secretions from the lungs. The Frequencer (Dymedso Inc., Boisbriand, Quebec) is a device that provides mechanical vibration in addition to acoustic oscillation to mobilize secretions through a variety of tissue depths. The sound level (56-78 dB) generated at maximal power is below the level that would cause hearing damage.[149] Normal human hearing is limited to frequencies of 20 to 20,000 Hz, and the Frequencer operates between 20 and 65 Hz. The device adjusts to the resonant frequency of the airways of the lungs and is able to target small portions of the lungs as opposed to affecting the entire lung fields at once. It is similar to HFCWO in that the vibrations thin the viscosity of the pulmonary secretions. However, unlike HFCWO, which has an upper frequency of 25 Hz, the frequency of oscillation provided by the Frequencer is substantially higher at 20 to 65 Hz.

In a pilot study comparing the Frequencer with traditional postural drainage and percussion, the amount of sputum produced by the Frequencer was the same as or more than PD and patients reported less discomfort.[149] Another small study by Vallejos[150] described the use of the Frequencer in a clinical environment; treatment with the device produced sputum 75% of the time, and patients showed a preference for ACT by this method.

Treatment with Acoustic Airway Clearance

- The Frequencer consists of a control unit that generates acoustic waves in a range of frequencies and a transducer head to deliver the oscillation to a specific area of the lung. The treatment settings are changed by using a touch screen, and the settings can be locked to prevent accidental alterations. Intensity and frequency levels can be adjusted by sliding buttons up and down.
- Four sizes of adapters for the transducer are available to accommodate patients of varying body sizes. The control unit displays suggested levels of treatment for babies, children, and adults.
- There are six suggested chest treatment areas with a recommended 3-minute duration for each area.

Advantages and Disadvantages of Acoustic Airway Clearance

Use of the Frequencer does not require the patient to alter breathing patterns, and allows the treatment to be focused on the specific lung areas. It has the same effect of thinning the mucus as does HFCWO; furthermore, nebulized medication or supplemental oxygen can be administered concurrently. It appears to be appropriate for all ages and body sizes and can be applied in the upright position.

The Frequencer device is far more expensive than the PEP devices; the cost is similar to that of the HFCWO. In addition, it is less well known than other techniques. A relatively small number of patients with pulmonary disease has been exposed to acoustic airway clearance, and a few studies have been conducted on its efficacy across conditions.

Factors Affecting Selection of Airway Clearance Techniques

The process of prescribing an appropriate technique for secretion mobilization should be ongoing, with periodic reevaluation of the method and its effects on the patient. Mobilization and exercise are exploited to the maximal degree to mobilize secretions as indicated, and its effects may need to be augmented with manual or mechanical airway clearance techniques. Clinical judgment is needed to establish whether mobilization or exercise is sufficient or whether additional airway clearance support is needed. If it is determined that additional airway clearance techniques are warranted, clinical judgment must also be used to decide which specific techniques are indicated.

Among patients with pulmonary disorders, poor adherence to the performance of airway clearance on a regular basis has been well documented.[4,151-153] Litt[151] has shown that the complexity and increased duration of a prescribed treatment has a negative influence on patient adherence. It has been suggested that better adherence may be achieved if the treatment is specifically tailored to the individual patient's needs with regard to clinical status, family functioning, and family concerns (Box 21-6). Negotiation between the patient and the caregiver is also effective; patients are more likely to adhere to a prescribed treatment regimen to which they have agreed in collaboration with their caregiver.[154] The regular use of a particular ACT by a patient is governed by personal belief in the effectiveness of the method for his or her own disease process, the manner in which the method affects the family's life habits, and the patient's willingness to use the technique on a daily basis. Adherence is ultimately the best index of an ACT's effectiveness. For this reason, it is incumbent upon caregivers to consider the many factors that may alter a patient's adherence to a particular method when recommending a specific technique, especially in a patient with a chronic disease. These factors include the availability of the caregiver to teach the technique and the willingness of the patient to learn it; the patient's concurrent medical problems; the effectiveness of the technique (subjective and objective); support for the technique from family, friends, and health care personnel; age and lifestyle of the patient; and the cost of the treatment.[106] Table 21-1 summarizes factors that can influence the choice of an airway clearance technique.

Box 21-6 Factors to Be Considered When Selecting an Airway Clearance Technique

- Motivation
- Patient's goals
- Physician/caregiver's goals
- Effectiveness (of considered technique)
- Patient's age
- Patient's ability to learn
- Skill of therapists/teachers
- Fatigue or work required
- Need for assistants or equipment
- Limitations of technique based on disease type and severity
- Costs (direct and indirect)
- Desirability of combining methods

From Hardy KA: A review of airway clearance: new techniques, indications, and recommendations, Respiratory Care *39:440-452, 1994.*

Availability

Accessibility of equipment or trained personnel limits the use of some ACTs. Some techniques of airway clearance that have been used in other countries for some time are new to health care providers and patients in the United States. Use of a method may be limited by the lack of caregivers trained to instruct patients in a particular technique. In the case of AD, the number of instructors available to teach the technique to patients and the time the health care team member must spend to learn it limits the method. AD takes longer for a caregiver to learn how to teach than does PEP or HFCWO. For IPV or acoustic airway clearance, the equipment and trained personnel must be available in the hospital; if a home unit is to be used, proper training of the patient and caregiver must be included. The ACBT is easily incorporated into conventional chest physical therapy by learning the FET and modifying the use of percussion or shaking. Exercise for airway clearance may be out of the realm of a respiratory therapist who is trained in respiratory care but not familiar with principles of exercise testing and prescription.

The patient's availability must also be taken into consideration. Proper instruction and review of a patient's technique are imperative to achieving optimal results. Instruction in PEP, ACBT, and HFCWO can be initiated during a single outpatient clinic visit, and further training can be provided during return visits. On the other hand, instruction in AD takes several training sessions. The patient needs to allow time to

Table 21-1 Considerations When Selecting an Airway Clearance Technique

Technique	Age of Patient	Assistant Needed	Equipment Needed	During Acute Exacerbation	Concurrent Nebulizer	Precautions	Cost
PD, percussion, vibration/shaking	Any age	Yes	Positioning aids; percussor/vibrator; devices for infants	Yes	Only in upright or side-lying	May need to modify positions; repetitive motion injuries	Expensive if performed by caregiver over long term
ACBT	Begin to teach at 3-4 years of age	Until 8-10 years of age	Positioning aids; percussor/vibrator	Yes	Only in upright or side-lying	Precautions for head-down positions	Inexpensive if done independently
AD	Age ≥12 years	No	None	Best to use an alternative	No	Takes time to learn	No cost
HFCWO	Age ≥2-3 years	For young children	Air pulse generator; appropriately sized vest	Yes	Yes	Chest tube, indwelling catheter, or other device in chest area	Very expensive
IPV	Adolescents and adults	While in hospital	Home unit or hospital unit	May not be well tolerated	Yes	Titrate for comfort and visible chest movement	Moderately expensive
Acoustic Airway Clearance	All ages	For children	Acoustic generator and appropriate size transducer	Possibly; further studies are needed	Yes	Further studies are needed	Very expensive
Exercise	Children, adolescents, and adults	For young children	Variable	No	Premedicate before exercise	Exercise-induced bronchospasm; oxygen desaturation; adjunct to ACT	Depends on type of exercise

learn the method and be available and willing to fine-tune the technique with the therapist periodically. Unlike a clinic visit, hospital admission for an exacerbation of a pulmonary disease makes the patient a captive audience for instruction in a variety of techniques, including AD or a home exercise program after the acute stage has passed.

The key to success of airway clearance is the reevaluation of any technique used. The patient and caregiver must be available to demonstrate and review of the technique periodically so that modifications can be made. For example, in the case of PEP, reassessment of its resistance is recommended. A change in a patient's level of independence or motivation, a decline or marked improvement in pulmonary status, or a decrease in the effectiveness of a technique all necessitate reevaluation of the current method.

Effectiveness

The age of the patient can influence the effectiveness of a particular technique. Infants and very young children are limited to conventional postural drainage, percussion, and vibration performed by a caretaker, because they are not able to cooperate with other methods of airway clearance. A vest for HFCWO can be fitted for children as young as 2 or 3 years of age. After the age of 3 or 4, a youngster may be taught huffing and breathing control and can be assisted with the ACBT. PEP and exercise are also suitable for this age group, depending on the child's attention span and cooperation. As the child grows older and the variety of appropriate techniques increases, close supervision remains necessary. In the adolescent, even when physical assistance is no longer required, emotional support from family and friends is paramount to continued success with a technique. Children 12 years of age and older are capable of using any of the ACTs, including AD, which requires more concentration than a younger child is typically able to exhibit consistently. The company manufacturing the Frequencer claims that its device is suitable for all ages.

Another consideration in selecting a technique is the effectiveness of the technique measured both subjectively and objectively. A patient's subjective response to the treatment has implications for adherence to it. The ease of sputum mobilization and the quantity of sputum expectorated are important to a patient; this measure provides immediate feedback without a visit to the hospital or clinic. Although it is difficult to quantify, many patients rely on the amount of sputum production to guide their choices of secretion clearance methods. The effort that a treatment requires, or even more important, the amount of energy remaining after completion of the treatment, will affect the patient's willingness to continue with a technique.

Objective clinical measures to assess the effectiveness of an ACT can be followed during clinic appointments or periods of hospitalization. Radiographic changes, breath sounds, and pulmonary function tests may demonstrate adequate airway clearance or the need to reassess the appropriateness of the technique and its application. In addition to the quantity of sputum measured, other changes to monitor in sputum quality are color and viscosity. Hemodynamic values and measures of oxygenation—for instance, heart rate, blood pressure, O_2 saturation, changes in mechanical ventilator settings and arterial blood gas values—can be monitored to assess a patient's response to a particular intervention. The ultimate indicator of a favorable response is patient adherence, as this will determine to a degree to which benefit is sustained.

Clinical Status

The clinical status of a patient is key to determining the appropriateness of a particular ACT and the need to modify a technique. In addition, complications that occur as a result of a technique or precautions associated with a particular method must guide a patient and caregiver to find an alternate technique. For example, PD and percussion could worsen airway hyperreactivity, and although exercise should be preceded by an inhaled bronchodilator, in this case, HFCWO, PEP, acoustic airway clearance, and IPV can be performed concurrently with bronchodilator administration. AD lends itself well to use by patients with airway hyperreactivity. Gastroesophageal reflux prohibits patients from performing airway clearance in conventional PD positions. In this instance, AD, PEP, HFCWO, IPV, acoustic airway clearance and exercise, or ACBT in upright positions, are the preferred treatments. In infants or neurologically impaired patients in whom PD and percussion are the treatments of choice, modified PD positions are used, with exclusion of the Trendelenberg position, and sufficient time is allowed between a feeding and a treatment with PD. Sinus surgery may make use of a PEP mask intolerable, and the placement of a chest tube may necessitate a temporary replacement for HFCWO.

The severity of a patient's lung disease affects the choice of ACT. A patient hospitalized with an acute pulmonary exacerbation may need to be assisted with a passive method of secretion clearance until the patient's condition allows a return to a more independent technique. Similarly, a patient with end-stage lung disease might not have the energy to perform an ACT such as AD or ACBT, in which case a more passive technique would be appropriate. Also, a marked decrease in pulmonary function may limit the airflow control necessary for AD and PEP.

Lifestyle

A patient's living situation and the support of family and friends may influence a preference for a method of airway clearance. Many patients adopt a multifaceted approach to secretion clearance, becoming adept at several methods and using them as their conditions dictate. Patients who primarily use AD or exercise may use an alternate form of airway clearance during an acute exacerbation. Patients who use HFCWO at home may use a more portable technique when away from home. Patients who rely on assistance to perform percussion may need to learn a more independent method when assistance is not available. The lack of an assistant to provide airway clearance is a factor that prompts many patients to seek methods other than postural drainage and percussion. HFCWO, PEP, ACBT, acoustic airway clearance, exercise, and AD are techniques that provide independence from a caregiver. Adolescents eager for self-reliance, students away at school, and adults living alone frequently choose these independent methods. For optimal results, a health care team member who is skilled in airway clearance must regularly reevaluate each technique's effectiveness after it has been agreed that a patient exhibits independence in a given technique. The support received from health care providers is vital to the patient's motivation to continue with a technique or to learn a new one.

When airway clearance is indicated daily, it becomes necessary to accommodate a patient's schedule. A patient may have a preference for the most effective treatment performed in the least time. A patient may also be interested in performing another activity during the airway clearance treatment—for example, AD or PEP may be performed while riding in a car (as a passenger); HFCWO can be conducted while studying for an examination or surfing the Internet; and a patient can be watching the news on TV while running on a treadmill or during percussion by an assistant.

Expense

In this era of skyrocketing health care costs, especially for long-term care and chronic disease, the expense of an airway clearance technique must be considered. The initial cost of equipment, replacement costs, and the expense of any required assistance all figure into the total cost of treatment. Often the choice of a technique is limited by the reimbursement available by a third-party payer. Nonetheless, the caregiver must strike a balance between economic and clinical considerations in choosing a mode of therapy. If several methods prove to be equally effective, it would be prudent to select the least expensive method. Although a common form of airway clearance in the United States continues to be postural drainage and percussion by a caregiver, this often proves to be quite expensive if a family member is not available for ongoing home treatments. Payment of a trained assistant for home use of PD and percussion is a great expense. Depending on the duration and frequency of treatment, this cost may outweigh that for other ACTs long-term. The equipment costs for ACTs vary. The generator required for HFCWO is more expensive to purchase or rent on a monthly basis than an IPV unit, but replacement should not be necessary. The Frequencer device used to deliver acoustic airway clearance is also expensive. Mechanical percussors or vibrators are moderately priced, and PEP devices are the least expensive of the techniques requiring equipment, with replacement of a unit expected to be necessary occasionally during a lifetime of use. A patient independently using ACBT or AD consumes the fewest financial resources.

Summary

Numerous ACTs have been shown to reduce obstruction, enhance mucociliary clearance, and improve ventilation, accomplishing the goal of improved oxygen transport. The effectiveness of various techniques has been demonstrated in multiple studies and evaluated with numerous outcome measures. In some cases, routine application of ACTs has not been shown to be effective in achieving improved oxygen transport. Acute asthma, bronchitis, pneumonia without copious secretions, bronchiolitis, and routine postoperative conditions were not shown to benefit from PD, percussion, and vibration.[18,21] ACTs are not without side effects or complications; routine use of these methods is not recommended without clear indications. Indications for ACTs have been established for acute illness and for chronic conditions. In acute illness, traditional methods (i.e., PD, percussion, and vibration) have been shown to be beneficial in patients with copious secretions and in the treatment of atelectasis.[155] For patients with cystic fibrosis, treatment with PEP and exercise in conjunction with PD, percussion, and vibration were also shown to be effective in an acute exacerbation.[156] In chronic disease states, patients with cystic fibrosis and bronchiectasis have been found to benefit from PD, percussion, and vibration, as well as PEP, autogenic drainage, ACBT, acoustic airway clearance, IPV, and exercise.[106,149,155,156]

The health care provider needs to consider many factors in recommending a technique of airway clearance for a patient. In addition to the availability of the technique and its effectiveness, these factors include consideration of several variables—physiological, psychological, and practical—that affect a patient's response to treatment. Treatments aimed at secretion clearance require monitoring the response of a patient to treatment and periodic reevaluation of this response. Caregivers need to incorporate this information into the real life situations presented by patients and choose a technique or combination of techniques that best suits each patient's needs. Acceptance of a specific treatment technique by the patient and family is paramount; adherence is the key to achieving effective treatment, especially in chronic lung conditions.

Health care providers are challenged to keep abreast of techniques and their modifications to best meet the patient's needs. The role of the caregiver involves more than technical expertise. The caregiver is uniquely positioned to simplify medical language for patients and families and encourage adherence to airway clearance. Support of a treatment by a health care provider can increase the benefit derived from the treatment.

Further research in the area of airway clearance is needed to compare and standardize techniques, follow long-term outcomes, and establish optimal treatment guidelines. This information will assist caregivers in evaluating and recommending a given technique of airway clearance for a particular patient or clinical population.

Review Questions

1. Which ACTs can be performed without purchasing specialized equipment?
2. Which ACTs would be appropriate to use during a hospitalization for a pulmonary exacerbation?
3. Which ACTs are most suited for instruction during a single outpatient clinic visit?
4. What outcome measures do you have at your disposal for evaluating the effectiveness of airway clearance?
5. Which ACT(s) would be appropriate for:
   - A 3-year-old newly diagnosed with cystic fibrosis?
   - An adolescent with bronchiectasis desiring independence from parental assistance?
   - A young adult with a spinal cord injury living alone?
   - An older adult with chronic bronchitis living in an extended care facility?
6. What are contraindications to chest percussion and/or postural drainage?
7. What factors should be considered in introducing a new method of airway clearance to a patient?

References

1a. Hess DR: Airway clearance: Physiology, pharmacology, techniques, and practice. *Respir Care* 52(10):1392–1396, 2007.

1b. Flume PA, Robison KA, O'Sullivan BP, et al: Cystic fibrosis pulmonary guidelines: Airway clearance therapies. *Resir Care* 54(4):522–537, 2009.

1c. Main E, Prasad A, Schans C: Conventional chest physiotherapy compared to other airway clearance techniques for cystic fibrosis. *Cochrane Database Syst Rev* (1):CD00201, 2005.

2. Ford RM, Godreau KM, Burns DM: Carpal tunnel syndrome as a manifestation of cumulative trauma disorder in respiratory care practitioners [abstract]. *Respiratory Care* 36:137, 1991.
3. MMWR Publication from the Centers for Disease Control: Occupational disease surveillance: carpal tunnel syndrome. *Journal of the American Medical Association* 282:886–889, 1989.
4. Currie DC: Practice, problems and compliance with postural drainage: a survey of chronic sputum producers. *British Journal of Diseases of the Chest* 80:249–253, 1986.
5. Dean E, Ross J: Discordance between cardiopulmonary physiology and physical therapy. *Chest* 101:1694–1698, 1992.
6. Wood RE: Treatment of cystic fibrosis lung disease in the first two years. *Pediatric Pulmonology* 4:685–690, 1989.

6a. Yankaskas JR, Marshall BC, Sufian B, et al: Cystic Fibrosis Adult Care. *Chest* 125:1S–39S, 2004.

7. Desmond K, Schwenk WF, Thomas E, et al: Immediate and long-term effects of chest physical therapy in patients with cystic fibrosis. *Journal of Pediatrics* 103:538–542, 1983.
8. Reisman J, Rivington-Law B, Corey M, et al: Role of conventional therapy in cystic fibrosis. *Journal of Pediatrics* 113:632–636, 1988.
9. Gallon A: Evaluation of chest percussion in the treatment of patients with copious sputum production. *Respiratory Medicine* 85:45–51, 1991.
10. Mazzocco MC, Owens GR, Kirilloff LH, et al: Chest percussion and postural drainage in patients with bronchiectasis. *Chest* 88:360–363, 1985.
11. Hammon WE, Martin RJ: Chest physical therapy for acute atelectasis. *Physical Therapy* 61:217–220, 1981.
12. Marini JJ, Pierson DJ, Hudson LD: Acute lobar atelectasis: a prospective comparison of fiberoptic bronchoscopy and respiratory therapy. *American Review of Respiratory Diseases* 119:971–978, 1979.
13. Massery M: Respiratory rehabilitation secondary to neurological deficits: understanding the deficits. In Frownfelter D, editor: *Chest physical therapy and pulmonary rehabilitation*, ed 2, Chicago, 1987, Year Book Medical.
14. Wetzel JL, Lunsford BR, Peterson MJ, et al: Respiratory rehabilitation of the patient with a spinal cord injury. In Irwin S, Tecklin JS, editors: *Cardiopulmonary physical therapy*, ed 3, St. Louis, 1995, Mosby.
15. Dickman C, Wilchynski JA: Respiratory failure. In Frownfelter D, editor: *Chest physical therapy and pulmonary rehabilitation*, ed 2, Chicago, 1987, Year Book Medical.

15a. Branson RD: Secretion management in the mechanically ventilated patient. *Respir Care* 52(10):1328–1347, 2007.

16. Crane L: Physical therapy for the neonate with respiratory disease. In Irwin S, Tecklin JS, editors: *Cardiopulmonary physical therapy*, ed 3, St. Louis, 1995, Mosby.
17. Finer N, Boyd J: Chest physiotherapy in the neonate: a controlled study. *Pediatrics* 61:282–285, 1978.
18. Eid N, Buchheit MD, Neuling M, et al: Chest physiotherapy in review. *Respiratory Care* 36:270–282, 1991.
19. Britton S, Bejstedt M, Vedin L: Chest physiotherapy in primary pneumonia. *British Medical Journal* 290:1703–1704, 1985.
20. Rochester DF, Goldberg SK: Techniques of respiratory physical therapy. *American Review of Respiratory Diseases* 122:133–146, 1980.
21. Sutton PP, Pavia D, Bateman JR, Clarke SW: Chest physiotherapy: a review. *European Journal of Respiratory Diseases* 63:188–201, 1982.
22. Wollmer P, Ursing K, Midgren B, et al: Inefficiency of chest percussion in the physical therapy of chronic bronchitis. *European Journal of Respiratory Disease* 66:233–239, 1985.
23. Webb MSC, Martin JA, Cartlidge PH, et al: Chest physiotherapy in acute bronchiolitis. *Archives of Diseases of Childhood* 60:1078–1079, 1985.
24. Torrington K, Sorenson D, Sherwood L: Postoperative chest percussion with postural drainage in obese patients following gastric stapling. *Chest* 86: 891–895, 1984.
25. Orenstein DM, Franklin BA, Doershuk CF, et al: Exercise conditioning and cardiopulmonary fitness in cystic fibrosis. *Chest* 80:392–398, 1981.
26. Andreasson B, Jonson B, Kornfalt R, et al: Long-term effects of physical exercise on working capacity and pulmonary function in cystic fibrosis. *Acta Paediatr Scand* 76:70–75, 1987.
27. Zach MS, Purrer B, Oberwaldner B: Effect of swimming on forced expiration and sputum clearance in cystic fibrosis. *Lancet* 11:1201–1203, 1981.
28. Oldenberg FA Jr, Dolovich MB, Montgomery JM, et al: Effects of postural drainage, exercise, and cough on mucus clearance in chronic bronchitis. *American Review of Respiratory Diseases* 120:739–745, 1979.
29. Wolff RK, Dolovich MB, Obminski G, et al: Effects of exercise and eucapnic hyperventilation on bronchial clearance in man. *Journal of Applied Physiology: Respiratory Environment Exercise Physiology* 43:46–50, 1977.
30. Cerny FJ: Relative effects of bronchial drainage and exercise for in-hospital care of patients with cystic fibrosis. *Physical Therapy* 69:633–639, 1989.
31. Zach M, Oberwaldner B, Hausler F: Cystic fibrosis: physical exercise versus chest physiotherapy. *Archives of Diseases of Childhood* 57:587–589, 1982.
32. Lannefors L, Wollmer P: Mucus clearance with three chest physiotherapy regimes in cystic fibrosis: a comparison between postural drainage, PEP, and physical exercise. *European Respiratory Journal* 5:748–753, 1992.
33. Baldwin DR: Effect of addition of exercise to chest physiotherapy on sputum expectoration and lung function in adults with cystic fibrosis. *Respiratory Medicine* 88:49–53, 1994.
34. Salh W, Bilton D, Dodd M, et al: Effect of exercise and physiotherapy in aiding sputum expectoration in adults with cystic fibrosis. *Thorax* 44:1006–1008, 1989.
35. Bilton D, Dodd ME, Abbot JV, et al: The benefits of exercise combined with physiotherapy in the treatment of adults with cystic fibrosis. *Respiratory Medicine* 86:507–511, 1992.
36. Lapin CD: *Is exercise a substitute for airway clearance techniques?* Dallas, 1993, Seventh Annual North American Cystic Fibrosis Conference (symposium).
37. Nixon PA: The prognostic value of exercise testing in patients with cystic fibrosis. *New England Journal of Medicine* 327:1785–1788, 1992.
38. Henke KG, Orenstein DM: Oxygen saturation during exercise in cystic fibrosis. *American Review of Respirator Diseases* 129:708–711, 1984.
39. Lane R, Cockroft A, Adams L, et al: Arterial oxygen saturation and breath issues in patients with cardiovascular disease. *Clinical Science* 72:693–698, 1987.
40. Godfrey S, Silverman M, Anderson S: The use of the treadmill for assessing exercise-induced asthma and the effect of varying the severity and duration of exercise. *Pediatrics* 56(Suppl):893–898, 1975.
41. Orenstein DM, Reed ME, Grogan FT Jr., et al: Exercise conditioning in children with asthma. *Journal of Pediatrics* 106:556–560, 1985.
42. McDonnell T, McNicholas WT, Fitzgerald MX: Hypoxaemia during chest physiotherapy in patients with cystic fibrosis. *Irish Journal of Medical Sciences* 155:345–348, 1986.
43. Connors AF Jr., Hammon WE, Martin RJ, et al: Chest physical therapy: the immediate effect on oxygenation in acutely ill patients. *Chest* 78:559–564, 1980.
44. Gormenzano J, Branthwaite MA: Pulmonary physiotherapy with assisted ventilation. *Anaesthesia* 27:249–257, 1972.
45. Fox WW, Schwartz JG, Shaffer TH: Pulmonary physiotherapy in neonates: physiologic changes and respiratory management. *Journal of Pediatrics* 92:977–981, 1978.
46. Huseby J, Hudson L, Stark K, et al: Oxygenation during chest physiotherapy [abstract]. *Chest* 70:430, 1976.
47. Campbell AH, O'Connell JM, Wilson F: The effect of chest physiotherapy upon the FEV1 in chronic bronchitis. *Medical Journal of Australia* 1:33–35, 1975.
48. Feldman J, Traver GA, Taussig LM: Maximal expiratory flows after postural drainage. *American Review of Respiratory Disease* 119:239–245, 1979.
49. Tecklin JS, Holsclaw DS: Evaluation of bronchial drainage in patients with cystic fibrosis. *Physical Therapy* 55:1081–1084, 1975.
50. Holland A, editor: Physotherapy for Cystic Fibrosis in Australia: A Consensus Statement. March 2008. Accessed 4/1/2011. Available at: http://www.thoracic.org.au/professional-information/position-papers-guidelines/cystic-fibrosis/
51. Lorin MI, Denning CR: Evaluation of postural drainage by measurement of sputum volume and consistency. *American Journal of Physical Medicine* 50:215–219, 1971.
52. Wong JW, Keens TG, Wannamaker EM, et al: Effects of gravity in tracheal transport rates in normal subjects and in patients with cystic fibrosis. *Pediatrics* 60:146–152, 1977.
53. Bateman JR, Newman SP, Daunt KM, et al: Is cough as effective as chest physiotherapy in the removal of excessive tracheobronchial secretions? *Thorax* 36:683–687, 1981.
54. Zausmer E: Bronchial drainage: evidence supporting the procedures. *Physical Therapy* 48:586–591, 1968.

55. Frownfelter D: Postural drainage. In Frownfelter D, editor: *Chest physical therapy and pulmonary rehabilitation*, ed 2, Chicago, 1987, Year Book Medical Publishers, pp 265–290.
56. Humberstone N: Respiratory assessment and treatment. In Irwin S, Tecklin JS, editors: *Cardiopulmonary physical therapy*, ed 2, St. Louis, 1990, Mosby.
57. Selsby D, Jones JG: Some physiological and clinical aspects of chest physiotherapy. *British Journal of Anaesthesia* 64:621–631, 1990.
58. Hammon WE, Martin RJ: Fatal pulmonary hemorrhage associated with chest physical therapy. *Physical Therapy* 59:1247–1248, 1979.
59. Stern RC, Wood RE, Boat TF, et al: Treatment and prognosis of massive hemoptysis in cystic fibrosis. *American Review of Respiratory Diseases* 117:825–828, 1978.
60. Barrell SE, Abbas HM: Monitoring during physiotherapy after open heart surgery. *Physiotherapy* 64:272–273, 1978.
61. Laws AK, McIntyre RW: Chest physiotherapy: a physiological assessment during intermittent positive pressure ventilation in respiratory failure. *Canadian Anaesthetists' Society Journal* 16:487–493, 1969.
62. Button BM, Heine RG, Catto-Smith AG, et al: Chest physiotherapy, gastro-oesophageal reflux, and arousal in infants with cystic fibrosis. *Archives of Disease in Childhood* 89:435–439, 2004.
63. Button BM, Heine RG, Catto-Smith AG, et al: Chest physiotherapy in infants with cystic fibrosis: to tip or not? A five-year study. *Pediatric Pulmonology* 35:208–213, 2003.
64. Sutton PP, Lopez-Vidriero MT, Panà D, et al: Assessment of percussion, vibratory-shaking and breathing exercise in chest physical therapy. *European Journal of Respiratory Diseases* 66:147–152, 1985.
65. Bateman J, Newman SP, Daunt KM, et al: Regional lung clearance of excessive bronchial secretions during chest physical therapy in patients with stable chronic airways obstruction. *Lancet* 1:294–297, 1979.
66. Denton R: Bronchial secretions in cystic fibrosis. *American Review of Respiratory Disease* 86:41–46, 1962.
67. May DB, Munt PW: Physiologic effects of chest percussion and postural drainage in patients with stable chronic bronchitis. *Chest* 75:29–32, 1979.
68. Radford R, Barutt J, Billingsley JG, et al: A rational basis for percussion-augmented mucociliary clearance. *Respiratory Care* 27:556–563, 1982.
69. Maxwell M, Redmond A: Comparative trial of manual and mechanical percussion technique with gravity-assisted bronchial drainage in patients with cystic fibrosis. *Archives of Diseases of the Childhood* 54:542–544, 1979.
70. Pryor JA, Webber BA, Hodson ME, et al: Evaluation of the forced expiration technique as an adjunct to postural drainage in treatment of cystic fibrosis. *British Medical Journal* 18:417–418, 1979.
71. Pryor JA, Parker RA, Webber BA: A comparison of mechanical and manual percussion as adjuncts to postural drainage in the treatment of cystic fibrosis in adolescents and adults. *Physiotherapy* 67:140–141, 1981.
72. Rossman CM, Waldes R, Sampson D, et al: Effect of chest physiotherapy on the removal of mucus in patients with cystic fibrosis. *American Review of Respiratory Diseases* 126:131–135, 1982.
73. Imle PC: Percussion and vibration. In Mackenzie, editor: *Chest physical therapy in the intensive care unit*, ed 2, Baltimore, 1989, Williams & Wilkins, pp 134–152.
74. Crane LD: Physical therapy for the neonate with respiratory disease. In Irwin S, Tecklin JS, editors: *Cardiopulmonary physical therapy*. St. Louis, 1990, Mosby, pp 409–410.
75. Pryor JA, Webber BA, Hodson ME: Effect of chest physiotherapy on oxygen saturation in patients with cystic fibrosis. 45:77, 1990.
76. Levenson CR: Breathing exercises. In Zadai CC, editors: *Pulmonary management in physical therapy*, New York, 1992, Churchill Livingstone.
77. Pavia D, Thomson ML, Phillipakos D: A preliminary study of the effect of a vibrating pad on bronchial clearance. *American Review of Respiratory Diseases* 113:92–96, 1976.
78. MacKenzie CF, Shin B, Hadi F, et al: Changes in total lung/thorax compliance following chest physiotherapy. *Anesthesia and Analgesia*, 59:207–210, 1980.
79. Webber BA: Physiotherapy for patients receiving mechanical ventilation. In Webber BA, editor: *The Brompton Hospital Guide to Chest Physiotherapy*, ed 5, Oxford, 1988, Blackwell.
80. Clement AJ, Hubsch SK: Chest physiotherapy by the "bag squeezing" method: A guide to technique. *Physiotherapy* 54:355–359, 1968.
81. Stiller K, Geake T, Taylor J, Grant R, Hall B: Acute lobar atelectasis: A comparison of two chest physiotherapy regimens. *Chest* 98:1336–1340, 1990.
82. Reference deleted in proofs.
83. Garradd J, Bullock M: The effect of respiratory therapy on intracranial pressure in ventilated neurosurgical patients. *Australian Journal of Physiology* 32:107–111, 1986.
84. Reference deleted in proofs.
85. Thompson BJ: The physiotherapist's role in the rehabilitation of the asthmatic. *New Zealand Journal of Physiotherapy* 4:11–16, 1973.
86. Webber B, Pryor J, editors: Active cycle of breathing techniques. In *Bronchial hypersecretion: current chest physiotherapy in cystic fibrosis (CF)*, 1993, International Physiotherapy Committee for Cystic Fibrosis (IPC/CF), pp 113–116.
87. Lapin A: Physical therapy in cystic fibrosis: a review. *Cardiopulmonary Physical Therapy* 1:11–12, 1990.
88. Prasad SA: Current concepts in physiotherapy. *Journal of the Royal Society of Medicine* 86(Suppl 20):23–29, 1993.
89. Mead J, Turner JM, Macklem PT, et al: Significance of the relationship between lung recoil and maximum expiratory flow. *Journal of Applied Physiology* 22:95–108, 1967.
90. Hietpas BG, Roth RD, Jensen WM: Huff coughing and airway patency. *European Journal of Respiratory of Disease* 24:710–713, 1979.
91. Hasani A, Pavia D, Agnew J, et al: Regional mucus transport following unproductive cough and FET in patients with airways obstruction. *Chest* 105:1420–1425, 1994.
92. Steven MH, Pryor JA, Webber BA: Physiotherapy versus cough alone in the treatment of cystic fibrosis. *New Zealand Journal of Physiotherapy* 20:31–37, 1992.
93. Webber BA, Hofmeyer JL, Morgan MDL, et al: Effect of postural drainage, incorporating the forced expiration technique, on pulmonary function in cystic fibrosis. *British Journal of Diseases of the Chest* 80:353–359, 1986.
94. Sutton PP, Parker RA, Webber BA, et al: Assessment of the forced expiration technique, postural drainage and directed coughing in chest physiotherapy. *European Journal of Respiratory Diseases* 64:62–68, 1983.
95. Mahlmeister MJ, Fink JB, Hoffman GL, et al: Positive-expiratory-pressure mask therapy: theoretical and practical considerations and a review of the literature. *Respiratory Care* 36:1218–1229, 1991.
96. Pryor JA: The forced expiration technique. In Pryor JA, editor: *Respiratory care*, Edinburgh, 1991, Churchill Livingstone, pp 79–100.
97. Chevaillier J: *Airway clearance techniques*, Dallas, 1992, Presented at Sixth Annual North American Cystic Fibrosis Conference.
98. Schoni MH: Autogenic drainage: a modern approach to physiotherapy in cystic fibrosis. *Journal of the Royal Society of Medicine* 82(Suppl 16):32–37, 1989.
99. Dab I, Alexander F: The mechanism of autogenic drainage studied with flow volume curves. *Mon Paed* 10:50–53, 1979.
100. David A: Autogenic drainage: The German approach. In Pryor J, editor: *Respiratory care*, Edinburgh, 1991, Churchill Livingstone.
101. Davidson NGT: Physiotherapy in cystic fibrosis: a comparative trial of PEP, AD, and conventional percussion and drainage techniques [abstract]. *Pediatric Pulmonology* 2(Suppl):132, 1988.
102. Davidson AGF, Wong LTK, Piric GE, et al: Long-term comparative trial of conventional percussion and drainage physiotherapy versus AD in cystic fibrosis [abstract]. *Pediatric Pulmonology* 8(Suppl):235, 1992.
103. Miller S, Hall D, Clayton CB, et al: Chest physiotherapy in cystic fibrosis (CF): a comparative study of autogenic drainage (AD) and active cycle of breathing technique (ACBT) (formerly FET). *Pediatric Pulmonology* 9(Suppl):240, 1993.
104. Giles DR, Acurso FJ, Wagener JS: Acute effects of PD and clapping versus AD on oxygen saturation and sputum recovery in cystic fibrosis. *Pediatric Pulmonology* 9(Suppl):252, 1993.
105. Pfleger A, Theissl B, Oberwaldner B, et al: Self-administered chest physiotherapy in cystic fibrosis: a comparative study of high-pressure PEP and autogenic drainage. *Lung* 170:323–330, 1992.
106. Downs AM, Lindsay KLB: Physical therapy associated with airway clearance dysfunction. In DeTurk, WE, Cahalin LP, editors: *Cardiovascular and pulmonary physical therapy: An evidence-based approach*, New York, 2004, McGraw Hill, pp 463–490.
107. Andersen JB, Qvist J, Kann T: Recruiting collapsed lung through collateral channels with positive end-expiratory pressure. *Scandinavian Journal of Respiratory Diseases* 4: 260–266, 1979.
108. Groth S, Stafanger G, Dirksen H, et al: PEP (PEP-mask) physiotherapy improves ventilation and reduces volume of trapped gas in cystic fibrosis. *Bulletin of European Physiopathology and Respiratory* 21:339–343, 1985.
109. Andersen JB, Klausen NO: A new mode of administration of nebulized bronchodilator in severe bronchospasm. *European Journal of Respiratory Diseases* 119(Suppl 63):97–100, 1982.
110. Hardy KA: A review of airway clearance: new techniques, indications, and recommendations. *Respiratory Care* 39:440–452, 1994.
111. Tyrrell JC, Hill EJ, Martin J: Face mask physiotherapy in cystic fibrosis. *Archives of Diseases of Childhood* 61:598–611, 1986.

112. Falk M, Kelstrup M, Andersen JB, et al: Improving the ketchup bottle method with PEP, PEP in cystic fibrosis. *European Journal of Respiratory Diseases* 65:423–432, 1984.
113. Falk M, Mortensen J, Kelstrup M, et al: Short-term effects of PEP and the FET on mucus clearance and lung function in cystic fibrosis [abstract]. *Pediatric Pulmonology* 9(Suppl):241, 1993.
114. Hofmeyer JL, Webber BA, Hodson ME: Evaluation of PEP as an adjunct to chest physiotherapy in the treatment of cystic fibrosis. *Thorax* 41:951–954, 1986.
115. Oberwaldner B, Evans JC, Zach MS: Forced expirations against a variable resistance: a new chest physiotherapy method in cystic fibrosis. *Pediatric Pulmonology* 2:358–367, 1986.
116. Simonova O, Kapranov N, Smirnova E, et al: PEP-mask therapy in complex treatment of cystic fibrosis patients. *Pediatric Pulmonology* 8(Suppl):245, 1992.
117. Volsko TA, DiFiore J, Chatburn RL: Performance comparison of two oscillating positive expiratory pressure devices: Acapella versus Flutter. *Resp Care* 48:124–130, 2003.
118. Althaus P: Oscillating PEP. In *Bronchial hypersecretion: current chest physiotherapy in cystic fibrosis (CF)*, International Committee for CF (IPC/CF), 1993.
119. Konstan MW, Stern RC, Doershuk CF: Efficacy of the Flutter device for airway mucus clearance in patients with cystic fibrosis. *Journal of Pediatrics* 124:689–693, 1994.
120. Schibler A, Casaulta C, Kraemer R: Rationale of oscillatory breathing as chest physiotherapy performed by the Flutter in patients with cystic fibrosis (CF) [abstract]. *Pediatric Pulmonology* 8(Suppl):244, 1992.
121. Ambrosino N: Clinical evaluation of a new device for home chest physiotherapy in nonhypersecretive COPD patients. *American Review of Respiratory Diseases* 4:260, 1991.
122. Lindemann H: Evaluation of VRP1 physiotherapy. *Pneumology* 46:626–630, 1992.
123. Button B, McIlwaine M: *Airway clearance techniques training class*, New Orleans, 2002, Presented at the Sixteenth Annual North American Cystic Fibrosis Conference.
124. Frischknecht-Christensen E, Norregaard O, Dahl R: Treatment of bronchial asthma with terbutaline inhaled by conespacer combined with positive expiratory pressure mask. *Chest* 100:317–321, 1991.
125. McIlwaine M: *Airway clearance techniques (ACT) refresher class*, Dallas, 1993, Presented at Seventh Annual North American Cystic Fibrosis Conference.
126. Falk M, Kelstrup M: PEP. In *Physiotherapy in the treatment of cystic fibrosis (CF)*, International Physiotherapy Group for Cystic Fibrosis (IPC/CF), 1995.
127. Steen HF, Redmond AO, O'Neill D, et al: Evaluation of the PEP mask in cystic fibrosis. *Acta Paediatr Scand* 80:51–56, 1991.
128. Hansen LG, Warwick WJ: High-frequency chest compression system to aid in clearance of mucus from the lung. *Biomedical Instrumentation and Technology* 24:289–294, 1990.
129. Warwick WJ: *Airway clearance by high-frequency chest compression*, Washington, D.C., 1992, Sixth Annual North American Cystic Fibrosis Conference (symposium).
130. Klous DR: *High-frequency chest wall oscillation: Principles and applications*, St. Paul, 1994, Published by American Biosystems, Inc., pp 626–630.
131. Tomkiewicz R, Bivij A, King M: *Rheologic studies regarding high-frequency chest compression (HFCC) and improvements of mucus clearance in cystic fibrosis*, Boston, 1994, ATS International Conference (abstract).
132. Chang HK, Weber ME, King M: Mucus transport by high-frequency nonsymmetrical oscillatory airflow. *Journal of Applied Physiology* 65:1203–1209, 1988.
133. Warwick WJ, Hansen LG: The long-term effect of high-frequency chest compression therapy on pulmonary complications of cystic fibrosis. *Pediatric Pulmonology* 11:265–271, 1991.
134. King M, Phillips DM, Gross D, et al: Enhanced tracheal mucus clearance with high-frequency chest wall compression. *American Review of Respiratory Disease* 128:511–515, 1983.
135. Robinson C, Hernried L: Evaluation of a high-frequency chest compression device in cystic fibrosis. *Pediatric Pulmonology* 8(Suppl):255, 1992.
136. Kluft J, Becker L, Castagnino M, et al: Comparison of bronchial drainage treatments in cystic fibrosis. *Pediatric Pulmonology* 22:271–274, 1996.
137. Faverio L, Kluft J, Fink R, et al: A comparison of bronchial drainage treatments in patients with cystic fibrosis [abstract]. *American Journal of Respiratory and Critical Care Medicine* 149:A669, 1994.
138. Arens R, Gozal D, Omlin KJ, et al: Comparative efficacy of high-frequency chest compression and conventional chest physiotherapy in hospitalized patients with cystic fibrosis. *Pediatric Pulmonology* (suppl. 9):239, 1993.
139. Burnett M: Comparative efficacy of manual chest physiotherapy and a high-frequency chest compression vest in treatment of cystic fibrosis [abstract]. *American Review of Respiratory Disease* 147(Suppl):A30, 1993.
140. Whitman J, Van Beusekom R, Olson S, et al: Preliminary evaluation of high-frequency chest compression for secretion clearance in mechanically ventilated patients. *Respiratory Care* 38:1081–1087, 1993.
141. Ohnsorg F: *A cost analysis of high-frequency chest wall oscillation in cystic fibrosis*, Boston, 1994, Abstract presented at the ALA/ATS International Conference.
142. Klous D, Boyle M, Hazelwood A, et al: Chest vest and cystic fibrosis: Better care for patients. *Advanced Respiratory Care Management* 3:44–50, 1993.
143. Homnick D, Spillers C, White F: The intrapulmonary percussive ventilator compared to standard aerosol therapy and chest physiotherapy in the treatment of patients with cystic fibrosis. *Abstracted in Pediatric Pulmonology* 10(Suppl):266, 1994.
144. Natale JE, Pfeifle J, Homnick DN: Comparison of intrapulmonary percussive ventilation and chest physiotherapy: A pilot study in patients with cystic fibrosis. *Chest* 105:1789–1895, 1994.
145. Marks JH, Homnick DN, Hare K, et al: The PercussiveTech HF compared to the Flutter device in cystic fibrosis patients: A six-month pilot study. *Pediatric Pulmonology* 22(Suppl):309, 2001.
146. Hardy KA, Anderson BD: Noninvasive clearance of airway secretions. *Respiratory Care Clinics of North America* 2:323–345, 1996.
147. Homnick DN, White F, de Castro C: Comparison of effects of an IPV to standard aerosol and chest physiotherapy treatment in cystic fibrosis. *Pediatric Pulmonology* 20:50–55, 1995.
148. Marks JH, Homnick DN: Safety and effectiveness of IPV compared to standard chest physiotherapy. *Pediatric Pulmonology* 19(Suppl):290, 1999.
149. Cantin AM, Bacon M, Berthiaume B: Mechanical airway clearance using the Frequencer electro-acoustical transducer in cystic fibrosis. *Clin Invest Med* 29(3):159–165, 2006.
150. TS, Kindel S, Phillips-Clar J: Evaluation of Sputum Production with the use of the Frequencer with the Adult Cystic Fibrosis Patients. *Respir Care* 2010:149 [Abstract], 2010.
151. Litt IF, Cushey WR: Compliance with medical regimens during adolescence. *Pediatric Clinics of North America* 27:3–15, 1980.
152. Muszynski-Kwan AT, Perlman R, Rivington-Law BA: Compliance with and effectiveness of chest physiotherapy in cystic fibrosis: a review. *Physiotherapy of Canada* 40:28–32, 1988.
153. Passero MA, Remor B, Salomon J: Patient-reported compliance with cystic fibrosis therapy. *Clinical Pediatrics* 20:265–268, 1981.
154. Shultz K: Compliance with therapeutic regimens in pediatrics: a review of implications for social work practice. *Social Work Health Care* 5:267–278, 1980.
155. Kirifoff LH, Owens GR, Rogers RM, et al: Does chest physical therapy work? *Chest* 88:436–444, 1985.
156. Boyd S, Brooks D, Agnew-Coughlin J, et al: Evaluation of the literature on the effectiveness of physical therapy modalities in the management of children with cystic fibrosis. *Pediatric Physical Therapy* 70–74, 1994.

Chapter 22

III

Facilitating Airway Clearance with Coughing Techniques

Donna Frownfelter and Mary Massery

KEY TERMS

Mucociliary blanket
Cough
Cough pump
Cough stages
Reflex cough
Smoker's cough
Complications of coughing
Airway clearance deficits
Assisted cough
Cough assist machine
Suctioning
Swallowing dysfunction
Throat clearing

CHAPTER OUTLINE

Cough truly serves many purposes: a therapeutic technique, a diagnostic signpost, and a social necessity. If it didn't already exist, we would have to invent it.

—Glen A. Lillington, MD

Cough is one of the most frequently reported symptoms in patients with pulmonary impairments. It is important to get a good history and physical examination to determine the cause and course of the patient's cough.[1] History should include sudden onset versus chronic; duration and type of cough—productive, nonproductive, or wheezy; whether the cough disturbs sleep and function; and what relieves or aggravates it. Diagnostic testing may include chest imaging, pulmonary function tests, bronchoscopy, and evaluation for gastroesophageal reflux (GER).[2] GER is said to be the causative factor in up to 41% of adults with chronic cough.[3]

The cough is an interesting phenomenon. It can either be a reflex or a voluntary action. Generally, in healthy individuals, a cough is rarely heard unless a person has a cold, or an irritant is inhaled and a sneeze or a cough ensues to evacuate the foreign body. The mucociliary escalator functions as the primary means to clear secretions and inhaled particulate matter. Except in certain circumstances—for instance, the mucus is very thick, as in individuals with dehydration or abnormal secretions; or a foreign body is inhaled; or a bolus of food "goes down the wrong hole," that is, into the trachea rather than the esophagus—a cough is not the usual mechanism to clear mucus. The mucus blanket and the support of the cough mechanism are the two means promoting normal airway clearance.

Frequent coughing or throat clearing may signal that the airways are irritated, that mucus is not clearing normally, or that the person is in an uncomfortable situation. This is something to be aware of, especially when treating patients with cystic fibrosis or asthma and patients with psychogenic issues. Depending on the reason for a cough, a variety of different approaches might be utilized. In most patients with primary pulmonary disease, the cough is related to the need for improved hydration and airway clearance. With patients who have psychogenic coughs, psychotherapy, biofeedback, and relaxation techniques have proven to be effective.[4] Medications to suppress a cough are used rarely, primarily in the case of nonproductive, inflamed airways. Future directions are moving toward better medical management of cough reflex hypersensitivity through better diagnosis and medication.[5] If the cough is productive, hydration and coughing are necessary to expel secretions to prevent pneumonia from occurring.

Many people who have habitual coughs are unaware of their coughing. For example, when asked whether they cough, smokers with typical morning and ongoing smoker's coughs may deny coughing. Often, a spouse will chime in, saying, "He coughs and hacks all the time." An individual might constantly clear his or her throat and swallow mucus but will claim to be unproductive of mucus and free of a cough. It is important for therapists to be aware of both the reflex and the voluntary nature of their patients' coughs and observe for throat clearing and swallowing of mucus.

Frequent coughing or throat clearing may indicate other problems besides airway clearance deficits. For example, a patient may have postnasal drip from a sinus infection or allergy. When the mucus drips down into the back of the throat, it can cause a reflex cough to clear it. Other causes include bronchogenic carcinoma, nervousness, and smoking. Many over-the-counter products are marketed to improve environmental air factors, but there has been conflicting evidence for their effectivess.[6]

In a pediatric patient with a cough, a foreign body or object inserted or inspired into the nose or airway should be ruled out. Gastroesophageal reflux must be evaluated in children and adults with symptoms of cough.[7,8] GER is often overlooked in children. For example, if a child is beginning to prop-sit and pushes back to get out of that posture regularly, it may be because of GER irritation. This can delay developmental postures, so it is an important consideration for pediatric therapists.

A persistent cough or throat clearing might be indicative of asthma or other pulmonary diseases, but it may also be a result of GER and irritation to the upper airway. It is important to ask questions related to the patient's sleep. For example, does the person have heartburn or belching at least once a week after going to bed? Is there breathlessness at rest and nocturnal breathlessness? In a random group study in a large population of young adults, 4% were found to have GER. People with asthma and GER (9% of asthmatics had GER) had more nocturnal cough and morning phlegm with sleep-related symptoms.[9] The authors concluded that there was a strong association between asthma and GER.

Cigarette smoking is known to stop mucociliary clearance. It has been noted that for every cigarette a person smokes, the cilia are paralyzed for approximately 20 minutes. Many individuals are chain smokers and consequently must cough to provide any airway clearance. These smokers will often have significant amounts of phlegm raised first thing in the morning secondary to ciliary clearance while they slept.

Many patients with asthma find cough to be a more irritating, difficult symptom than wheezing and secretions. Yet cough is often not taken as seriously, even though it can be a life-interrupting symptom. Night cough can be a particularly difficult symptom in people with asthma and will make sleep difficult.[10] Persistent cough has also been reported following pulmonary resection. The cause seems to be unclear, but some studies have focused on the population of patients who have had a lobectomy and mediastinal lymph node resection, some of whom also had GER. These were at increased risk for continued cough, which was found to persist up to a year later. Of this group, 90% saw improvement in their coughing with medication.[11]

If a patient demonstrates retained secretions on radiography, encourage hydration (drinking water), use airway clearance mobilization techniques, and carefully evaluate the cough. Instruct the patient in controlled coughing when mucus is felt in the throat or upper airways (see Chapter 21).

Cough Associated with Eating or Drinking

If a cough is associated with eating, drinking, or taking medications, the patient's swallowing mechanism should be examined and evaluated. A barium swallow ("cookie swallow") is a fluoroscopic study in which the patient is given an opaque liquid, and a moving picture is observed to determine whether there is aspiration into the trachea. Populations commonly in need of evaluation of swallowing are patients with neurological disorders, such as those that occur with cerebrovascular accident (CVA), amyotrophic lateral sclerosis (ALS), cerebral palsy, Parkinson disease, and multiple sclerosis (MS). Patients who have tracheostomy tubes may experience difficulty in swallowing because the tube inhibits the normal movement of the larynx during swallowing. The use of a Passey-Muir valve has been found to be clinically effective in restoring a more normal swallow in patients with a tracheostomy. Older adults with chronic cough should be carefully observed and monitored, because the chronic cough may be a defense mechanism to prevent aspiration.[12] This is especially true if there are comorbidities such as a previous stroke. This list is not exhaustive; any patient who chokes when you offer fluids or who reports to you that food or water "goes down the wrong way" should be referred for evaluation of the swallowing mechanism.

Speech and language pathologists work with patients who have swallowing dysfunction (dysphagia) by helping them to learn techniques and procedures for safe swallowing. These specialists work with the patients, spouses, and parents to position patients for success, usually in a semi-Fowler sitting posture with head and neck flexion. In addition, the types and consistencies of food are evaluated. Many people have more difficulty with liquids than with puddings and other thicker consistencies. A thickening agent can be added to liquids to help patients swallow safely. Food may be ground up (pureed) if chewing is difficult. Every effort should be made to help patients eat and drink fluids successfully. However, if a patient is unable to swallow safely, alternative means of nourishment, such as feeding tubes and gastric tubes, must be used. The method can be revisited later and feeding tried again when the patient's condition improves.

Cough Pump

The cough pump is an intricate device. Mucus must be transported upward against the gravitational force and propelled cephalad by the expiratory gas flow. Generally, cough is the most effective means, because it has a large inspiration and high expiratory flow rates. Cough will clear to approximately the sixth or seventh generation of airway segments (segmental bronchi). If a patient has retained secretions, distal airway clearance techniques such as postural drainage or use of the Acapella or other device must be used to move the secretions to an area where the cough can be effective. If the patient does not have the mechanical ability to have an effective cough (as in spinal cord injury), assistive cough techniques or mechanical methods, discussed later in this chapter, will have to be employed.

Complications of Coughing

Coughing can be hazardous to the patient and should never be repeated routinely. The irritation, inflammation, and possible airway narrowing that can occur during forced exhalation may cause bronchospasm. If the cough is dry and unproductive, do not encourage frequent coughing. This is especially true for people with asthma and chronic obstructive pulmonary disease (COPD). Do not ask patients with COPD to take a deep breath before they cough. These patients do not have trouble taking in air; on the contrary, a secondary condition of COPD is increased compliance, which causes alveolar destruction and decreased elasticity of their lungs. With a patient who has COPD, ask for a mid-sized breath, which will minimize air trapping (dynamic hyperinflation). If the patient demonstrates retained secretions, first employ an airway clearance device or treatment; then use an effective and controlled technique, such as the active cycles of breathing and forced expiratory technique (FET), to mobilize the secretions.

Tussive syncope can occur when a patient has a sustained series of coughs in which the intrathoracic pressure becomes so high that venous return to the heart is impaired. The cardiac output falls, leading to dizziness and then progressing to unconsciousness. Care must be exercised, especially in patients with primary and secondary cardiovascular and pulmonary disease. These patients must learn to control their coughing to prevent untoward side effects.

Patients with chronic cough can also experience stress urinary incontinence (SUI).[13] This is often not reported to the therapist or physician because the patient is embarrassed or considers this a problem of aging rather than a condition related to the chronic cough. Such patients often do not realize that physical therapy treatment is available for SUI. This knowledge deficit has been found in adolescents and teenagers with cystic fibrosis, as well as in adults with COPD. Asking patients with chronic cough about SUI should be a part of the routine examination and evaluation. Making a referral to a pelvic floor therapist can make a difference in their quality of life as SUI is managed.

Stages of Cough

Four stages are involved in producing an effective cough.[14] The first stage requires inspiring enough air to provide the volume necessary for a forceful cough. Generally, adequate inspiratory volumes for a cough are noted to be at least 60% of the predicted vital capacity for that individual. The second stage involves the closing of the glottis (vocal folds) to prepare for the abdominal and intercostal muscles to produce positive intrathoracic pressure distal to the glottis. The third stage is the active contraction of these muscles. The fourth and final stage involves opening of the glottis and the forceful expulsion of the air. The patient usually is able to cough three to six times per expiratory effort. A minimal threshold of FEV_1 (forced expiratory volume in 1 second) of at least 60% of the patient's actual vital capacity is a good indicator of adequate muscle strength necessary for effective expulsion (Figure 22-1). Bach

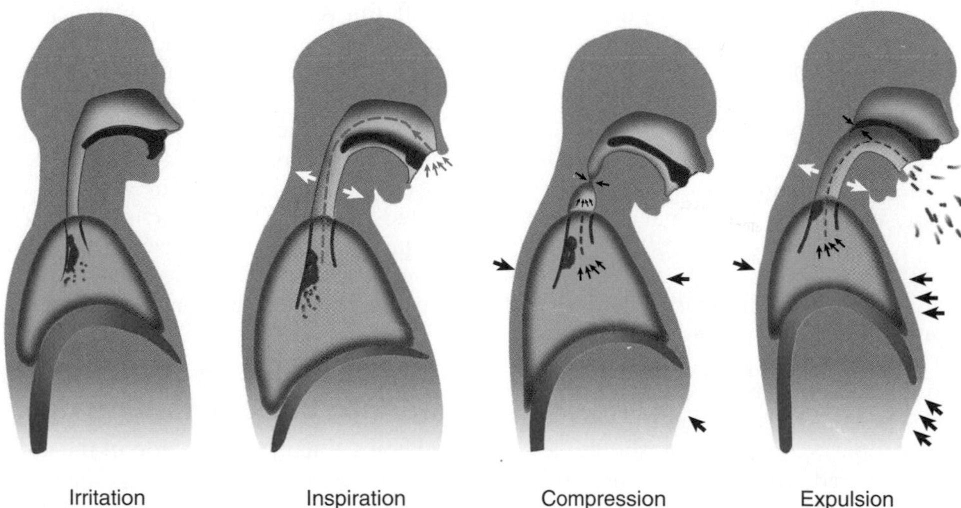

Fig. 22-1 Cough mechanics. **A,** Stage 1: adequate inspiration. **B,** Stage 2: glottal closure; stage 3: building-up of intrathoracic and intraabdominal pressure. **C,** Stage 4: glottal opening and expulsion.

and Saporito (1996)[15] established a minimal peak cough flow rate (PCFR) of 160 L/min to effectively clear secretions and to predict successful decannulation for patients with neuromuscular conditions. The use of a simple peak flow meter can help assess the cough. Drops in peak flow have been correlated in children, patients with spinal cord injury, and older adults who have a decreased ability to cough. Assessing PCFR is a simple clinical test that can objectively measure the patient's ability to provide the exhalation phase of the cough.[16-18] During a cough, alveolar, pleural, and subglottal pressures may rise as much as 200 cm H_2O.[14,19,20]

It is also important to identify the stage of the cough cycle in which the patient is having difficulty. Only then can the appropriate therapeutic intervention be directed at correcting that deficit.

Box 22-1 Positioning and Instruction to Improve Cough Effectiveness

- Position the patient for success, especially in regard to trunk alignment.
- Maximize inspiratory phase through verbal cues, positioning, and active arm movement.
- Improve hold stage through verbal cues and positioning.
- Maximize intrathoracic and intraabdominal pressures with muscle contractions, physical assist, or trunk movement.
- Instruct the patient in appropriate timing and trunk movements for expulsion.
- Make the procedure physically active on the patient's part.

Cough Evaluation

How do you assess whether a patient's cough is effective? The answer appears to be obvious: ask the patient to cough. However, the obvious answer often does not adequately analyze the functional performance of a cough, especially for a patient with neurological impairment. The clinician must first take time to prepare the patient for successful evaluation of cough. Here are guidelines for preparing the patient:

1. Do not disregard posture. Rather than simply asking the patient to cough from whatever position he or she happens to be in, ask instead, "What position do you like to be in when you feel the need to cough?" Then ask the patient to assume that posture, or assist the patient in assuming a posture as close to the preferred posture as possible. Pay close attention to the patient's choice. A patient should spontaneously choose a posture that lends itself to trunk flexion, which is necessary for effective expulsion and airway protection. A red flag, or inappropriate choice, would be a preference for coughing while supine, which involves the opposite: trunk extension and poor mechanical alignment for airway protection.
2. Now the patient is ready to demonstrate coughing. Do not make the mistake of asking a patient to "show me a cough" or he or she may simply "show you" a cough. It may not be the way the patient coughs to clear secretions. Instead, continue to set the patient up for success by asking him or her, "Can you show me how you would cough if you had secretions in your chest and you felt the need to cough them out?" With these instructions, you are asking the patient to show you something functional rather than theoretical.

Cough effectiveness can now be assessed (Box 22-1). Guidelines for objective evaluation with pulmonary function tests have been indicated previously. This section focuses on analyzing the movement patterns during all four stages of a cough. An effective cough should maximize the function of each individual stage. Thus in most patients (other than those with COPD or asthma), the clinician should see a deep inspiratory effort paired with trunk extension, a momentary hold, and then a strong cough or series of expiratory coughs on a single breath while the patient moves into trunk flexion.

Stage 1: Adequate Inspiration

Did the patient spontaneously inspire a deep breath before coughing, or did he or she cough regardless of the inspiration or expiration cycle? Did the patient spontaneously use trunk extension, an upward eye gaze, or the arms to augment the inspiratory effort? Did the patient take enough time to inspire fully before coughing? If the patient inspires adequately, he or she should be able to sustain two to six coughs per expiratory effort for a cascade effect. Neurologically impaired patients who have inadequate inspiratory efforts usually present with only one or two coughs per breath and generally produce a quieter cough.[21] If the patient cannot cough on demand (such as a young child or patient with cognitive impairment), ask the caretaker whether he or she has observed and/or heard the patient's inspiratory breath and hold before a cough. If so, how effective did the patient's process seem?

Stage 2: Glottal Closure

Did the patient hold his or her breath at the peak of inspiration before the expulsion phase, or did the patient go directly from inspiration to expiration? Did you hear a cough or a huff (a complete absence of a hold between inspiration and expiration)? If the patient intended to cough but instead produced a huff, this is an indication of insufficient glottal closure. This can result from a wide variety of situations, including glottal edema after prolonged intubation, partial or full paralysis of the vocal folds, hemiparesis of the vocal folds, or a timing or sequencing difficulty secondary to brain injuries, among other possibilities. A complete lack of glottal closure will not produce any cough sound because the vocal folds are not approximating (adducting). The huff technique may be encouraged when the patient tends to wheeze or after long-term intubation when there is vocal fold edema. However, in the "normal" population, a good hold and full cough are encouraged.

Stage 3: Building-Up of Intrathoracic and Intraabdominal Pressure

Did you see active contraction of the intercostal and abdominal muscles? Did the patient spontaneously move into trunk flexion during this phase? Did the cough have a low, resonant sound? Inadequate force is usually heard as a higher-pitched cough, often called a throaty cough. The sound is quieter overall and does not produce as many coughs per expiratory effort. It is sometimes associated with neck extension rather than flexion as the patient attempts to clear the upper airway only. The air appears to leak out rather than being propelled out of the larynx during the cough. As with inadequate lung volumes, inadequate pressure prevents the patient from coughing more than once or twice during one expiratory effort.

Stage 4: Glottal Opening and Expulsion

The timing of the opening of the glottis and the forceful expulsion of the air is directly tied into the function of the third stage. During expulsion, does the patient appear to gag before successfully allowing the air to be expelled? Does the patient seem to get stuck holding his or her breath? Deficiencies in this area are often related to brain injuries and coordination difficulties. The opposite can also occur. Some patients get stuck at the end of expulsion, especially those with severe neurological impairments or bronchospasms, and may have difficulty initiating the next inspiratory effort.

If the patient is able to follow directions and has the muscular ability and cognition to learn cough techniques, patient instruction is the next step. If the person is unable secondary to neuromuscular weakness or frailty and cannot be independent in coughing, a decision must be made about the next step to be taken to provide airway clearance of secretions. Assistive cough techniques, the CoughAssist machine, and suctioning are possible considerations; these are discussed later in this chapter.

Patient Instruction

When working with patients, especially those with primary pulmonary disease or primary disease superimposed on secondary disease (i.e., a patient with CVA), the proper patient instruction can make secretion mobilization more effective. Multiple ideas are presented here because the therapist needs a "bag of tricks." Certain techniques work well for some patients but not for others. Try several with each patient and let him or her determine what works best. Objective tests can also be used to determine the most effective intervention, such as a change in oxygen saturation, improved breath sounds via auscultation, improved expiratory flow rates, chest x-ray clearing, and a reduction in the patient's perceived work of breathing (dyspnea scale).

As mentioned previously, patients with COPD and asthma are not encouraged to take a deep breath before they cough. These patients also tend to experience expiratory wheezing when they force and prolong exhalation. This can lead to bronchospasm and respiratory distress. Patients can be taught to do the pump cough, a variation on the huff technique. A huff is often encouraged to help patients produce controlled, less stressful coughs. It may be useful when patients have been intubated with an endotracheal tube for an extended time. The vocal folds, in this case, are swollen and inflamed and will not close and form the tight seal necessary to build up the pressure for a cough. Thus patients are instructed to huff rather than cough. The huff is done with more open vocal folds, a low sound, and less effort; yet it is quite effective in mobilizing secretions, especially when combined with FET.

Pump Cough

The pump cough extends the huff technique and, clinically, is more effective. The patient is instructed to take three mid-sized huffs followed by three short, easy coughs at low lung volume, not deep breaths or deep lung volumes. Three or four sequences are performed: (1) huff, huff, huff; cough, cough, cough; (2) huff, huff, huff; cough, cough, cough; (3) huff, huff, huff; cough, cough, cough. Usually, if secretions are present, a spontaneous cough occurs, or the secretions will mobilize with the small coughs.

Series of Coughs

Another variation that decreases stress on the patient is to use a series of coughs consisting of a small breath and a small cough, then a medium breath and a medium cough, and finally a large breath and a large cough. This is a good technique to use with postoperative patients, who often become fatigued trying to cough maximally each time. For these patients, it is an effort to get air distal to the secretions in various parts of the lungs, a form of autogenic drainage.

Patients with Neuromuscular Weakness or Paralysis

For patients with transient or permanent neuromuscular weakness or paralysis, further instructions may be necessary.[20,22-25] These patients must use every physical trait to maximize the function of each stage of the cough (see Figure 22-1). Physically assisting these patients during the expulsion stage of the cough addresses only one aspect.[26,27] Care must be taken to look at all four stages to maximize the airway clearance potential of any assistive cough technique. First, the patient must be positioned for success (stage 1). The beginning of any cough requires trunk extension or inspiratory movement to maximize inhalation, whereas the expulsion stage requires trunk flexion or expiratory movement to maximize exhalation.[28] Thus for any given posture, the clinician must assess the following:

- Whether the posture allows for both trunk movements
- Whether flexion and extension are possible, which movement is more important for that particular patient, and whether that posture facilitates its occurrence
- How gravity is affecting the patient's muscle strength and function in that posture
- Whether the patient can still protect the airway in this posture

When these questions have been answered satisfactorily, the clinician is ready to instruct the patient in the act of coughing. An example may provide the best illustration of these instructions. A clinician may pick a modified sitting position for a patient with generalized weakness (e.g., incomplete spinal cord injury, developmental delay, or temporary weakness or exhaustion after a medical or surgical procedure). The patient looks slumped, so the clinician places a lumbar support (e.g., a lumbar roll, a towel, or a pillow) behind the lower back to increase trunk extension in that position. The patient is asked whether he or she is comfortable and whether he or she can swallow safely. Next, the clinician tries to maximize the first cough stage by asking the patient to take a deep breath. Observing that the patient did not appear to take in as deep a

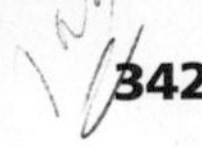

breath as the clinician thought possible, the clinician adds further instructions, such as the following:

- "Look upward while you inhale."
- "Raise both of your arms up over your head as high as you can while you inhale."
- "Squeeze your shoulders back while you inhale."
- "Straighten or extend your back while you inhale."

For patients with more limited arm function, apply appropriate ventilatory strategies detailed in Chapter 23. Very subtle movements can then be requested, such as the following:

- "Bring your arms up and out while you inhale."
- "Rotate your arms outward while you inhale."
- "Turn your forearm up while you inhale."

Although less dramatic than the larger movements described previously, these subtle motions may significantly increase the patient's inspiratory effort and provide a more active means for the patient to participate in his or her own coughing program.[29]

Stage 2 involves closing the glottis. For some patients with weakness or timing problems, a sharp loud command to "hold it" at the peak of inspiration, may be sufficient to facilitate closure. Remember to allow enough time for the patient to take in a deep inspiratory effort before being asked to "hold." Some clinicians rush the first phase by giving two instructions in quick succession, as in "Take a deep breath. Hold it." This unintentionally limits the time of the inspiratory effort. A more appropriate verbal cue would be "Take a deep breath in ... in ... in ... in ... and now hold it," allowing adequate time for the patient to inhale.

Stage 3 (building up pressure) and stage 4 (expulsion) are discussed together because their timing is interdependent. The patient now needs to move into trunk flexion, with or without the clinician's assistance, to maximize expulsion. Patients who are able to assist can be asked to do the opposite of stage 1:

- "Look down while you cough."
- "Pull both of your arms down to your hips as you cough."
- "Roll your shoulders forward while you cough."
- "Bend your trunk forward while you cough."

Likewise, patients with more limited arm function can be asked to do the following:

- "Squeeze your arms to your chest while coughing."
- "Roll your shoulders and arms inward while coughing."
- "Turn your hands down (pronation) while coughing."

In this manner the clinician has used every conceivable resource to maximize a voluntary cough. Even the weakest cough can be made more effective by applying these simple concepts:

- Position for success
- Maximize inhalation first
- Ask for a breath hold
- Encourage maximal intrathoracic and intraabdominal pressures
- Instruct the patient in appropriate timing and trunk movements for expulsion
- Make the procedure as active as possible for the patient

Objective and subjective assessments can confirm the improvement. However, even with excellent instructions, many patients with neurological disorders require a clinician's physical assistance to inhale more deeply or to exhale more forcefully because of muscle weakness or paralysis.[30]

Active Assisted Cough Techniques

If, after instruction and modification in the patient's cough, the patient still cannot produce an effective cough, then one of the following assistive cough techniques may be appropriate. However, a patient who needs some assistance to improve a cough is not excused from taking an active role in coughing. Keep the coughing process as active as possible for each patient, whether that is accomplished by adding a few verbal cues to improve overall timing or posture while the patient independently performs the cough, or whether it is accomplished by adding eye gazes for a very weak patient who cannot move the upper extremities and breathes with the assistance of a ventilator. Encourage the patient to be responsible for his or her own care by teaching the concepts involved in producing an effective cough.[31] In that manner, you will help the patient develop the problem-solving skills necessary for later modifications. Incorporate the guidelines and principles presented thus far with the specific cough techniques that follow. See Box 22-2 for a review of the techniques presented in this chapter.

Breath Stacking and Manual Chest Compression

Breath stacking is a technique that is achieved by a patient independently performing inspiration to maximal inspiratory capacity, then holding the breath and taking in 2 or 3 more breaths "on top" of the initial breath to increase vital capacity. This is followed by a cough. For a patient with neuromuscular weakness, a therapist or family member can do chest compression and assist the cough during exhalation.

In a study of patients with Duchenne muscular dystrophy, variations of breath stacking with a manual self-inflating bag were tested. One group simply used the self-inflating bag for breath stacking, whereas the other group used a combined technique of breath stacking with the bag plus manual compression for the exhalation. The combination technique proved to be most effective as measured by peak cough flow (see Figure 21-5).[32]

Manually Assisted Techniques

Costophrenic Assist

The first assistive cough technique, the costophrenic assist, can be used in any posture. After assessing the most appropriate position for the patient (most often sitting or side-lying) and

Box 22-2 Assisted Cough Techniques

Manually Assisted Techniques

1. Costophrenic assist
2. Heimlich-type or abdominal thrust assist
3. Anterior chest compression assist
4. Counter-rotation assist

Self-Assisted Techniques

1. Prone-on-elbows head-flexion self-assisted cough
2. Long-sitting self-assisted cough
3. Short-sitting self-assisted cough
4. Hands-knees rocking self-assisted cough
5. Standing self-assisted coughs

giving the patient instructions for maximizing all four coughing stages, the therapist places his or her hands on the costophrenic angles of the rib cage (Figure 22-2). At the end of the patient's next exhalation, the therapist applies a quick manual stretch down and in toward the patient's navel to facilitate a stronger diaphragmatic and intercostal muscle contraction during the succeeding inhalation. The therapist can also apply a series of repeated contractions based on proprioceptive neuromuscular facilitation (the PNF approach[33]) throughout inspiration to facilitate maximal inhalation. The patient may assist the maneuver by actively using his or her upper extremities, head and neck, eyes, trunk, or all of the above to maximize the inspiratory phase. The patient is then asked to "hold it." Just a moment before asking the patient to actively cough, the therapist applies strong pressure with his or her hands, again down and in toward the navel. In this manner the therapist is assisting both the build-up of intrathoracic pressure and the force of expiration. Of course, the patient should also actively participate by using his or her arms, trunk, or other body parts throughout the entire procedure (see Chapter 23).

This technique's obvious use would be for patients with weak or paralyzed intercostal or abdominal muscles. The therapist must remember to evaluate the effect of gravity and posture in each position for the appropriateness of this technique.[34] This technique is easy to learn and teach and can usually be used from the acute phase through the patient's rehabilitation phase, thus accounting for its popularity.

Heimlich-Type (or Abdominal Thrust) Assist

The second technique is the Heimlich-type assist, also known as the abdominal thrust assist. This method requires the therapist to place the heel of his or her hand at about the level of the patient's navel, taking care to avoid direct placement on the lower ribs (Figure 22-3). After appropriate positioning, the patient is instructed to "take in a deep breath and hold it." The therapist can then facilitate the inspiration. As the patient is instructed to cough, the therapist quickly pushes up and in, under the diaphragm with the heel of his or her hand, as in a Heimlich maneuver. The patient is instructed to assist with appropriate trunk movements as much as possible. Technically, this procedure is very effective at forcefully expelling the air,[22] as in a cough, but it can be extremely uncomfortable for the patient for several reasons:

Its concentrated area of contact

Its abrupt nature, which may elicit an undesired high neuromuscular tone response, or worse when combined with the sensory input supplied by the therapist's manual contacts

The force, which may cause gastrointestinal dysfunction such as GER

Because of its limited usefulness, the Heimlich-type, or abdominal thrust, assist should be used only when the patient does not respond to other techniques and the need to produce an effective cough is great.

The therapist can use a combination of the costophrenic and the Heimlich-type assists simultaneously when the patient is in the side-lying position. If the patient has a hemiplegic deficit or has a unilateral lung or thorax disease or trauma, emphasizing one side of the thorax over the other may be an appropriate focus during airway clearance treatments. One upper extremity is used to perform the Heimlich-type assist while the other does a unilateral costophrenic assist. In this manner, the therapist can compress simultaneously all three planes of ventilation in the lower chest. The possibilities of combining techniques and positions are numerous once the therapist understands the principles on which they were developed.

Anterior Chest Compression Assist

The third assistive cough technique is called the anterior chest compression assist because it compresses both the upper and lower anterior chest during the coughing maneuver. This is the first single technique thus far to address the compression needs of the upper and lower chest in one maneuver. The therapist puts one arm across the patient's pectoralis region to compress the upper chest; the other arm is placed parallel on the lower chest (avoiding the xiphoid process) or on the abdomen (Figure 22-4, *A*) or is placed as in the Heimlich-type

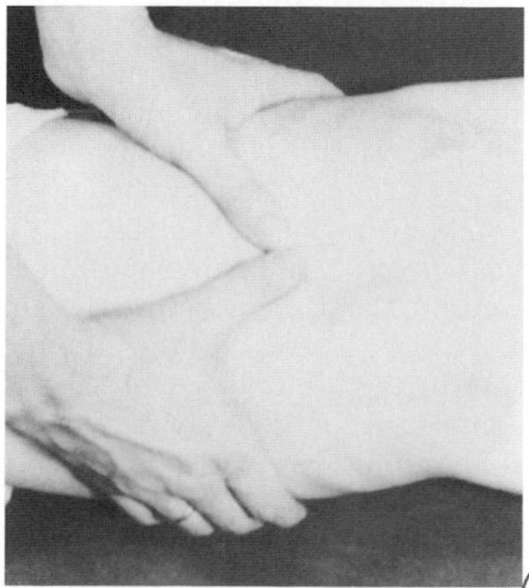

Fig. 22-2 Assisted cough techniques in supine position, costophrenic assist.

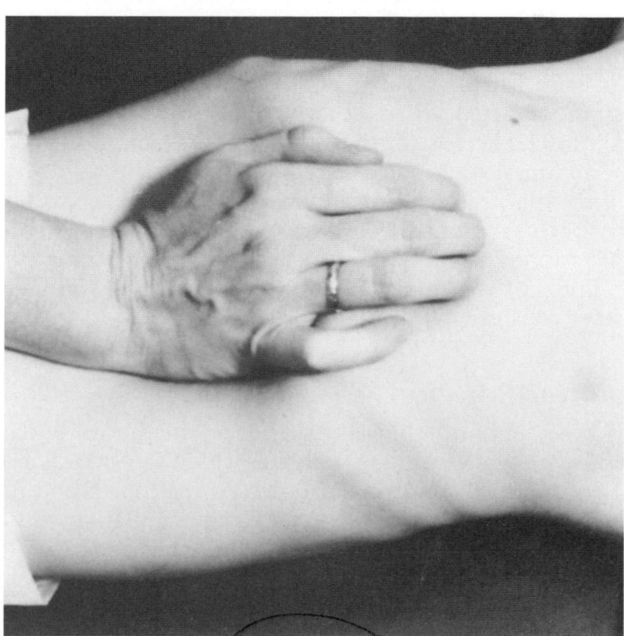

Fig. 22-3 Hand position for Heimlich-type (or abdominal thrust) assist.

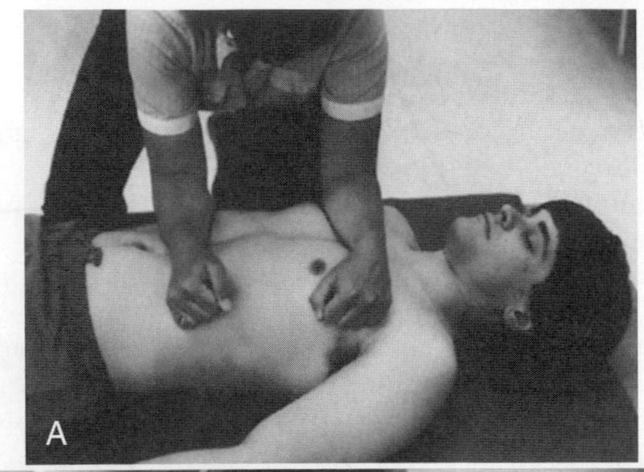

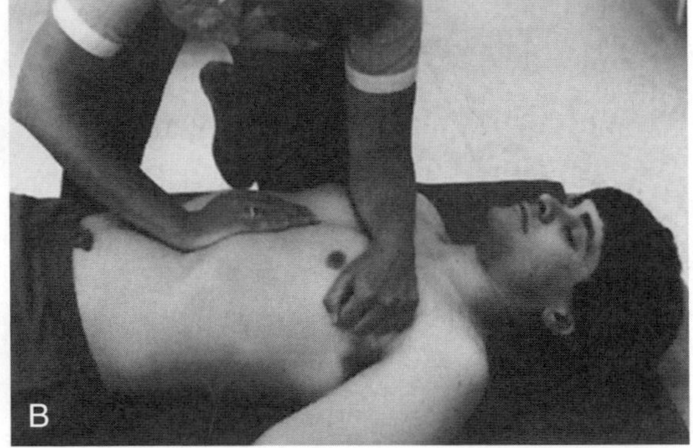

Fig. 22-4 Assistive cough techniques in supine position. **A,** Variation 1. **B,** Variation 2.

maneuver (Figure 22-4, *B*). The commands are the same as in the other techniques. Because of the direct manual contact on the chest, inspiration can be easily facilitated first, followed by a "hold." Thus the therapist can readily enhance the first two cough stages. The therapist then applies a quick force with both arms to simulate the force necessary during the expulsion phase. The directions of the force are:

1. Down and back on the upper chest
2. Up and back on the lower chest or abdominal arm

When performed together, the compression force exerted by both arms forms the letter V.

The anterior chest compression technique is more effective than the costophrenic assist for patients with very weak chest wall muscles because of the added compression of the upper anterior chest wall. These authors have found the side-lying or three-quarter supine position to be the most effective position for this technique. However, the anterior chest compression technique is not appropriate for a patient with a cavus condition of the upper anterior chest because it promotes further collapsing of the anterior chest wall.

Counter-Rotation Assist

In these authors' clinical experience, the most effective assistive-cough technique for the widest cross-section of patients with neurological disorders is the fourth and final method described: the side-lying counter-rotation assist.[18] The positioning and procedures required for the counter-rotation technique (described in detail in Chapter 23) apply for both the patient and the therapist (Figure 22-5). The therapist should recall that orthopedic precautions for the spine, rib cage, shoulder, and pelvis also apply for this technique.

The therapist begins by following the patient's breathing cycle, with his or her hands positioned over the patient's shoulder and pelvis (see Figure 22-5). The therapist then gently assists the patient in inhalation and exhalation to promote better overall ventilation. This sequence is generally repeated for three to five cycles or until the patient appears to have achieved good ventilation to all lung segments.

At this point, the patient is ready to begin the coughing phase of the procedure. The patient is asked to take in as deep a breath as possible, with the therapist assisting the patient in chest expansion (see Figure 22-5, *B*). Next, the therapist instructs the patient to "hold it" at the end of maximal inspiration. The patient is then commanded to cough out as hard as possible while the therapist quickly and forcefully compresses the chest with his or her hands in their flexion phase positions (see Figure 22-5, *A*).

The importance of following a true diagonal plane of facilitation during both the flexion and extension phases of this technique cannot be overemphasized. Failure to do so will result in the shifting of the air within the chest cavity rather than the desired forcing out of the air. This air shifting can occur to varying degrees when the upper chest and lower chest are not used together, as in all the other assistive cough techniques. When done properly, the counter-rotation assist is the only technique to rapidly close off the chest cavity in all three planes of ventilation in all areas of the chest. Unless the patient voluntarily closes his or her glottis, it is impossible to prevent the air from being forcefully expelled. However, a common mistake made by the therapist is pulling the patient back into trunk extension during the expulsion phase rather than into trunk flexion. A good rule of thumb: if you can see your patient's face when you are applying the compression force, you have pulled him or her into extension. The head and neck should stay forward and flexed so that only a facial profile can be seen.

Other effects of counter-rotation make this procedure particularly beneficial for patients with low levels of cognitive functioning:

1. The rotation component is a natural inhibitor of high tone. Thus this is the least likely of all techniques discussed so far to elicit an increase in abnormal tone during the coughing phase. In fact, the opposite usually occurs. Gentle rotation before passive coughing in a patient who is comatose can reduce high tone and frequently reduces a high respiratory rate. Both of these reduce the possibility of the patient's keeping his or her glottis closed during the expulsion phase.
2. Counter-rotation is an excellent mobilizer for a tight chest, which in itself can facilitate spontaneous deeper breaths. Tidal volumes (TVs) can therefore be increased for many patients by mobilizing the chest walls.
3. Finally, rotation can be a vestibular stimulator and may assist in arousing the patient cognitively, allowing him or her to take a more active role in the procedure.

The true beauty of the technique is the fact that no active participation on the part of the patient is required for success. Incoherent or unresponsive patients, such as patients with low functioning following a head trauma, CVA, or cerebral palsy, will still achieve good secretion clearance with this technique. The mechanics of the procedure dictate that the air within the lungs be rapidly and forcefully expelled, regardless of the patient's level of active participation. Obviously, patient

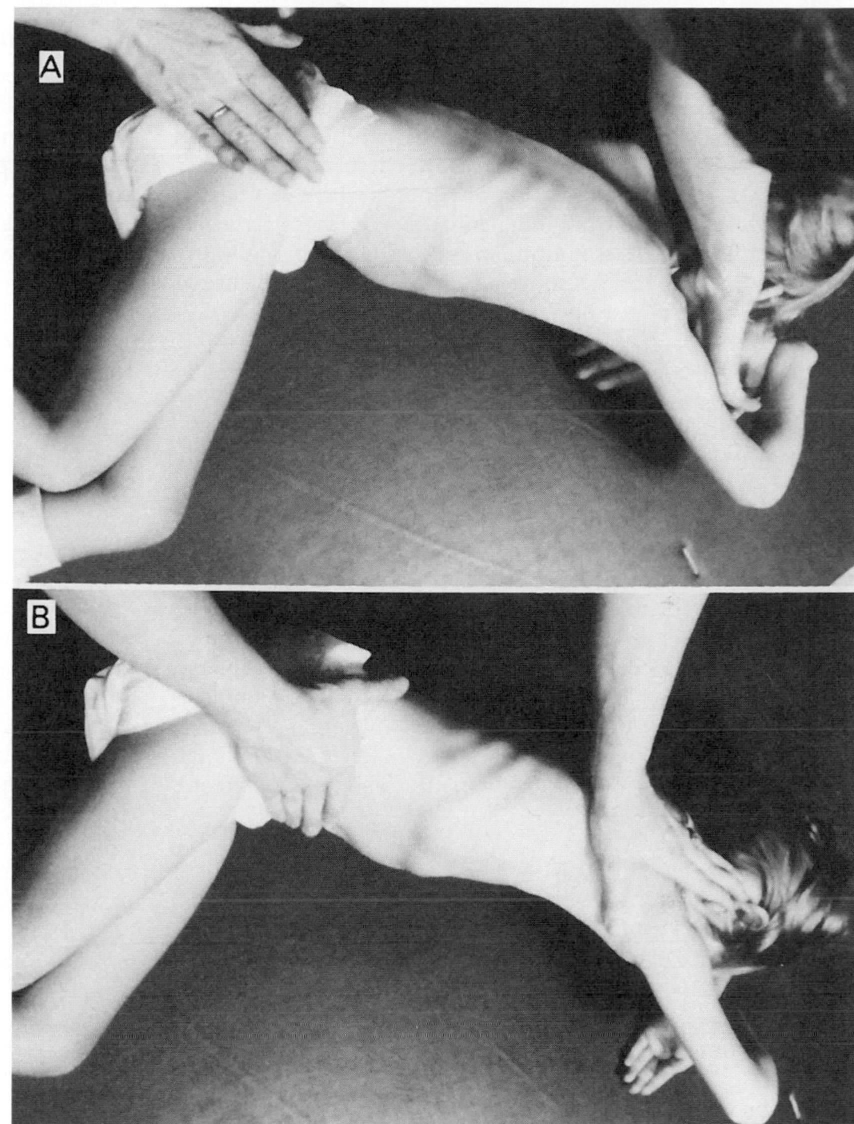

Fig. 22-5 Counter-rotation assist. **A,** Hand placement during expulsion phase. **B,** Hand placement during inspiration phase.

participation is desirable to clear secretions even more effectively and to teach the patient to eventually clear his or her own secretions, but it is not critical.

Clinical experience has demonstrated that in patients who have extremely tenacious secretions, the use of vibration may be more effective than quick chest compression during the cough itself. This prolongs the cough phase and gives the secretions time to be moved along the bronchi for successful expulsion. These patients may also require a series of three or four cough cycles before clearing most of their secretions. In general, patients from all the diagnostic groups discussed thus far, with or without good cognitive functioning, are appropriate candidates for this procedure. The majority of them find it to be the most comfortable and effective assistive means of expectorating secretions.

Self-Assisted Techniques

The coughing techniques discussed in this section are intended to be used as self-assisted procedures, so they are usually taught later in a patient's rehabilitation process. Five different techniques are presented in detail. Patients need to learn to cough in whatever position they are in for therapy or rest. Suggestions for variations are included. All self-assisted cough techniques can start out as physically assisted techniques; however, because they are more active and require greater gross motor movement, they lend themselves to self-assisted techniques.

Prone-on-Elbows, Head-Flexion Self-Assisted Cough

The prone position is not commonly used as a posture for coughing because the position itself inhibits full use of the diaphragm by preventing lower anterior chest and abdominal excursion following a neurological insult. This forces the patient to use an alternative breathing pattern that facilitates greater use of accessory muscles. Because this change in breathing patterns often occurs spontaneously, prone on elbows can be an effective posture for promoting spontaneous use of the accessory muscles during a more difficult activity (coughing). However, without the full recruitment of the diaphragm, the resultant cough will be weaker than it would be in other postures. Prone on elbows should not be the exclusive posture for a self-assisted cough. After mastering the timing of the procedure, most patients move back to another posture, usually sitting or side-lying, and to other techniques to capitalize on the functional increase in chest expansion and compression. For the population of patients who can assume a prone-on-elbows posture independently (i.e., some patients with tetraplegia), this technique may be used functionally. In this position, they can assist their own coughs when the need arises, rather than wait for someone to assist them in a position change.

The head-flexion assist requires good use of head and neck musculature, seen in patients who have sustained a spinal level injury below C4 (e.g., spinal cord injuries [SCIs], spina bifida). It can be used either as a self-assisted or a therapist-assisted procedure, using the principles of trunk extension to facilitate inspiration and trunk flexion to facilitate expiration. With the patient prone on elbows, the therapist instructs him or her to bring the head and neck up and back as far as possible, inhaling maximally (Figure 22-6, *A*). The patient is then instructed to cough out as hard as possible while throwing the head forward and down (Figure 22-6, *B*). This head-and-neck pattern can initially be assisted by the therapist to establish the desired movement pattern and gradually progressed to a resisted pattern to promote increased accessory muscle participation and to strengthen those muscle groups.

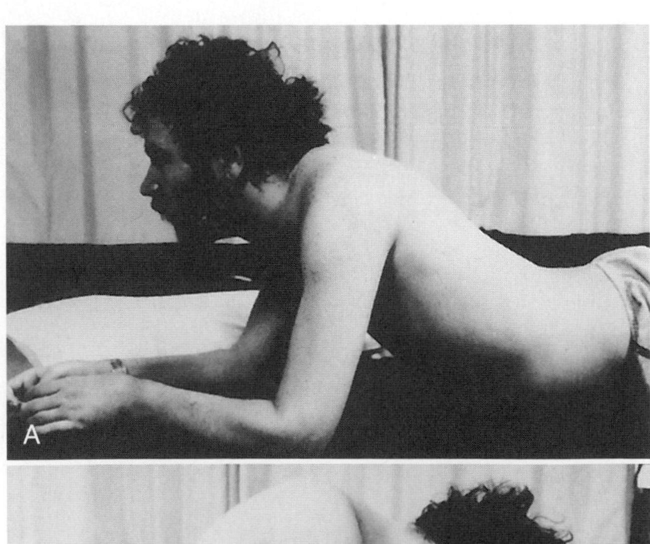

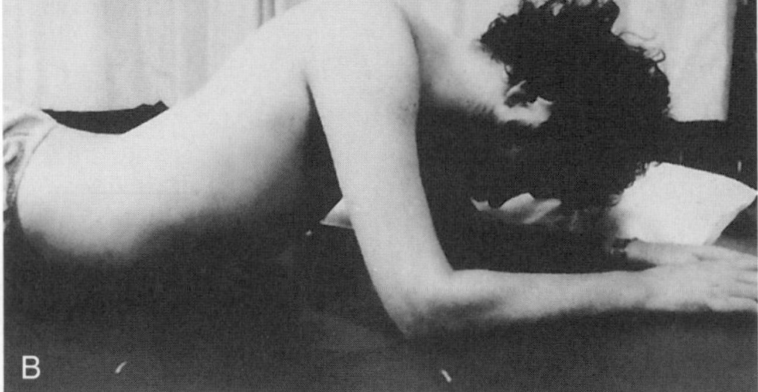

Fig. 22-6 Head-flexion assistive cough in prone-on-elbows position. **A,** Extension and inspiratory phase. **B,** Flexion and coughing phase.

Long-Sitting Self-Assisted Cough

There are two variations of this technique, one for tetraplegic patients and one for those who are paraplegic. For the tetraplegic version of the long-sitting self-assist, the patient is positioned on a mat in a long-sitting posture (legs straight out in front) and with upper extremity support. The therapist instructs the patient to extend his or her body backwards while inhaling maximally (Figure 22-7, *A*). The therapist then tells the patient to cough as the patient moves his or her upper body forward into a completely flexed posture, using shoulder internal rotation if possible (Figure 22-7, *B*). Once again, the extension aspect of the procedure is used to maximize inhalation, whereas the flexion aspect is used to maximize expiration. The self-directed chest compression occurs mainly on the superior-inferior plane of ventilation only.

The second procedure, the paraplegic version of the long-sit assist, uses the same principles as those described for the tetraplegic patient. However, paraplegic patients have active spinal extension musculature and can achieve greater trunk extension and flexion safely, thus achieving greater chest expansion before the cough and greater chest compression on a superior-inferior plane during the cough. The patient positions his or her upper extremities in a butterfly position or uses elbow retraction, depending on the level of injury (Figure 22-8, *A*). During the flexion phase, patients throw themselves onto their legs, thereby compressing both the upper and lower chest (Figure 22-8, *B*). This can be taught very successfully to patients with paraplegia, provided they have adequate trunk balance control. If the patient lacks hip flexion or is worried about bony contact or skin injury, place a pillow (or two as needed) on the legs. This will limit the hip flexion and minimize trauma from the quick thrust onto the legs.

Short-Sitting Self-Assisted Cough

A third assistive cough technique can be done with the patient sitting. The short-sitting self-assist is typically performed in a wheelchair or over the edge of a bed. The patient is instructed to place one hand over the other at the wrist and place them in his or her lap. As in the previous technique, the patient is then asked to extend the trunk backwards while inhaling maximally, followed by a strong voluntary cough. During the cough, the patient pulls his or her hands up and under the diaphragm, resembling the motion of a Heimlich maneuver (Figure 22-9). The hands mimic the abdominal muscles, which would ordinarily contract to push the intestinal contents up and under the diaphragm to aid its recoil ability. This short-sitting technique uses the diaphragm more substantially than the long-sitting procedure and is therefore generally more effective as an assistive cough. It is an effective self-assisted method for patients who have weak diaphragms or abdominal musculature. Most patients with SCI or spina bifida at C5 or below can learn this technique successfully. Patients with tetraplegia usually require trunk support and/or a seat belt from their wheelchairs to perform it independently and safely, whereas most patients with lower-level lesions resulting in paraplegia can perform it from an unsupported short-sitting position. Patients who lack good upper extremity coordination, such as many patients with Parkinson disease and multiple sclerosis (MS), cannot perform the procedure

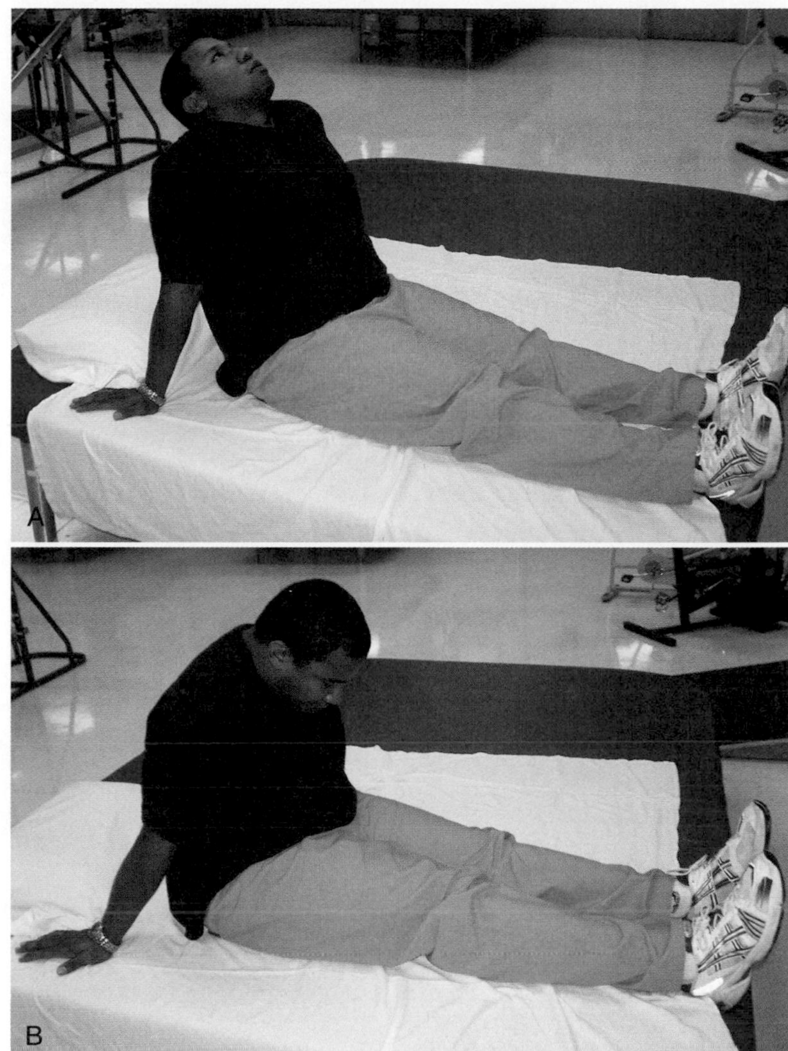

Fig. 22-7 Tetraplegic version of self-assisted cough in long-sitting position. **A,** Maximizing the inspiration phase. **B,** Maximizing the expiration, or coughing, phase. *(From Watchie J: Cardiovascular and pulmonary physical therapy, ed 2, St Louis, 2010, Saunders.)*

quickly or forcefully enough to make it effective and usually require assistance from another person.

Variations on all sitting techniques can be made readily. Clinicians are encouraged to use the concepts explained in the introduction to these cough techniques to develop techniques that work for their patients. For example, ask a patient in a wheelchair to lift his or her arms up while inhaling, hold, and then cough while throwing the arms down toward the feet or lap using maximum trunk flexion (use a seat belt for safety). Another idea is to have the patient hook one arm on a push handle of the wheelchair and move the other arm up and back (as in a pattern of shoulder flexion, abduction, and external rotation proprioceptive neuromuscular facilitation [PNF Pattern D2]);[35] make sure the patient's moving hand maximizes trunk rotation; have the patient inhale during the movement, hold, and cough while throwing the trunk and arm down toward opposite knee. When devising the most appropriate self-assisted cough for your patient, remember to look for a combination of trunk, arm, head, neck, and eye patterns that will maximize all four phases of the cough.

Hands-Knees, Rocking Self-Assisted Cough

The last assistive cough to be discussed is performed most commonly as a multipurpose activity to increase the patient's balance, strength, coordination, and functional use of breathing patterns (including quiet breathing and coughing) simultaneously. The patient assumes an all-fours position (hands-knees). He or she is then instructed to rock forward, looking up and breathing in while moving to a fully extended posture (Figure 22-10, *A*). After this, the patient is told to cough out as he or she quickly rocks backwards to the heels with a flexed head and neck (Figure 22-10, *B*). Once again, note the importance of the flexion and extension components of the cough. The rocking can be done with or without a therapist's assistance. For patients with generalized or spotty weakness throughout (e.g., some patients with SCI, head trauma, Parkinson disease, MS, cerebral palsy, or spina bifida), this method is perfect for incorporating many functional goals into a single activity. It can help prepare them for the more challenging respiratory activities they will undoubtedly face after their discharge from a rehabilitation center.

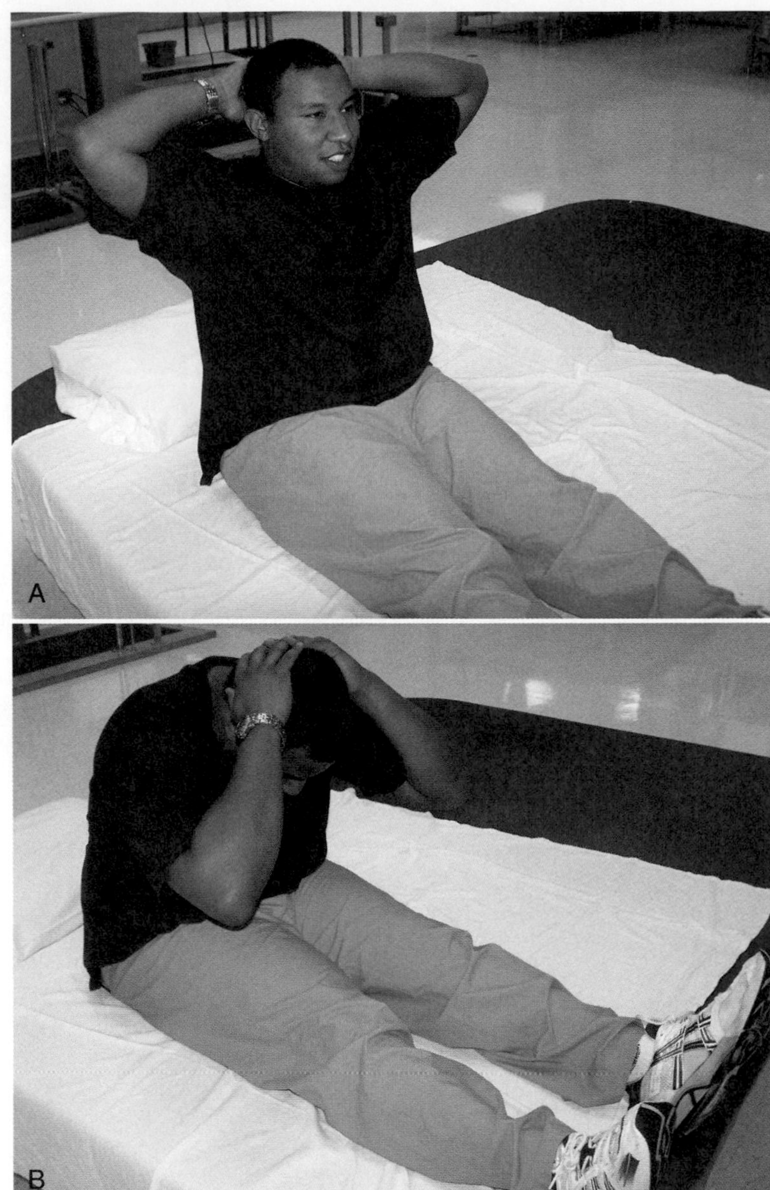

Fig. 22-8 Paraplegic version of self-assisted cough in long-sitting position. **A,** Inspiration. **B,** Expiration. *(From Watchie J: Cardiovascular and pulmonary physical therapy, ed 2, St Louis, 2010, Saunders.)*

For patients with limited lower extremity range of movement or skin concerns associated with a quick force, a pillow can be placed on the lower legs, thus restricting knee flexion and preventing direct contact of bony prominences.

Standing Self-Assisted Cough

Standing uses the same concepts as previously discussed and can be readily used for self-assisted coughs, provided the patient has adequate standing balance and upper extremity support. Any technique previously described can be modified for this posture. The number of possible combinations of trunk, head, and extremity movements during the cough maneuver is vast, so specific techniques are not detailed here.

CoughAssist Machine

As mentioned previously in the chapter, if patients are unable to be independent and assist in coughing to remove secretions, other options will be necessary. At this point, suctioning has been the most commonly used aid in secretion removal. However, it is not always tolerated well by patients. Mouth suction for oral secretions is usually appreciated and easy to use, but patients with tracheostomies and endotracheal tubes usually require more invasive—and more uncomfortable—suctioning into the trachea to remove secretions. Many patients have found a new device to be superior in comfort and in effectiveness in removing secretions; this piece of equipment, now readily available, is the CoughAssist machine.

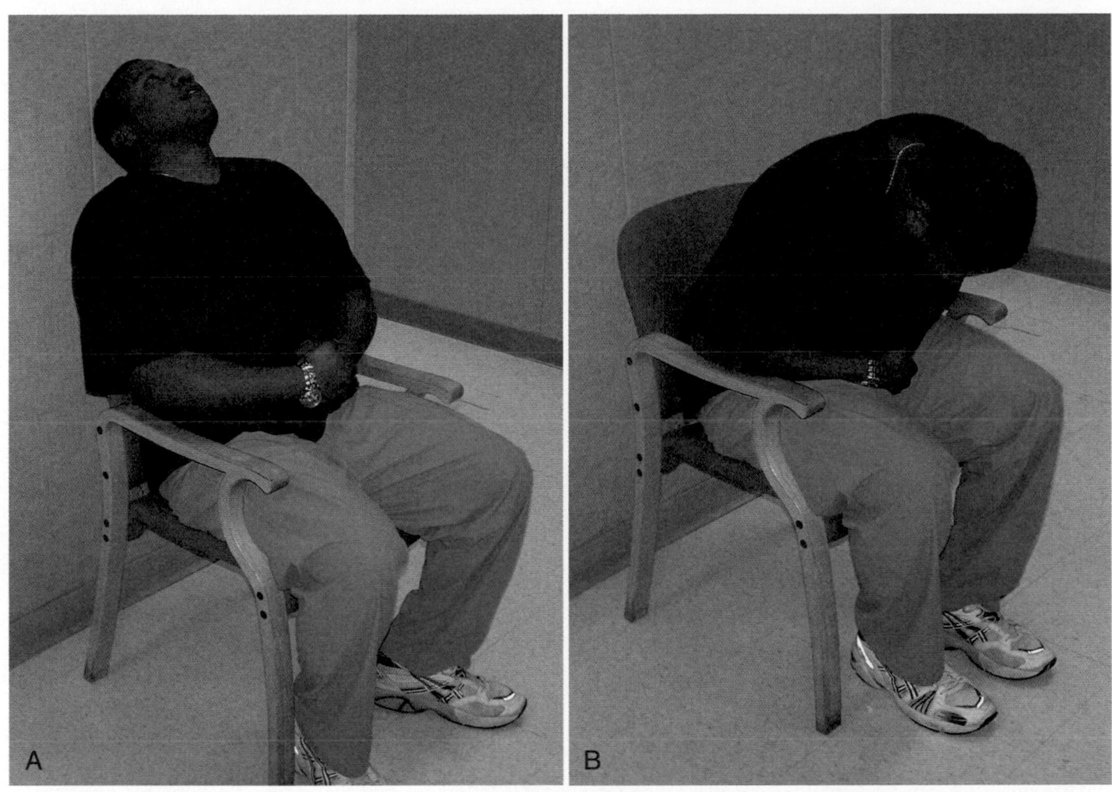

Fig. 22-9 Assisted cough in short-sitting position. **A,** Hand position for patient with good hand function. **B,** Hand position for patient with only wrist function. *(From Watchie J: Cardiovascular and pulmonary physical therapy, ed 2, St Louis, 2010, Saunders.)*

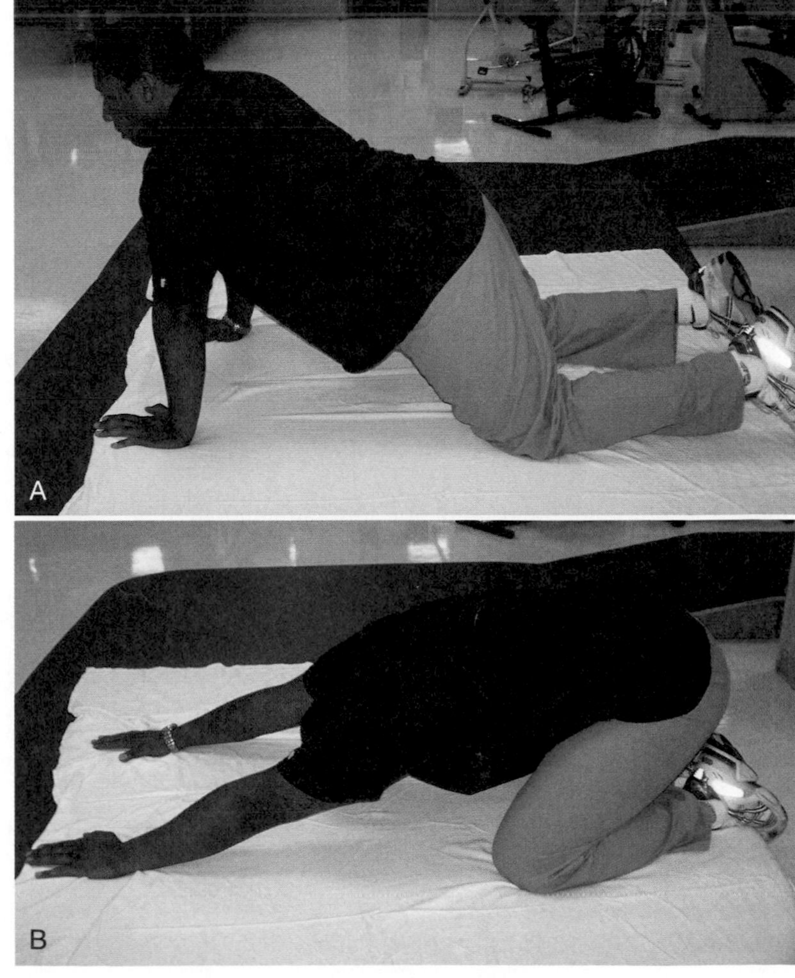

Fig. 22-10 Assisted cough in hands-knees position. **A,** Extension or inspiratory phase. **B,** Flexion or coughing phase. *(From Watchie J: Cardiovascular and pulmonary physical therapy, ed 2, St Louis, 2010, Saunders.)*

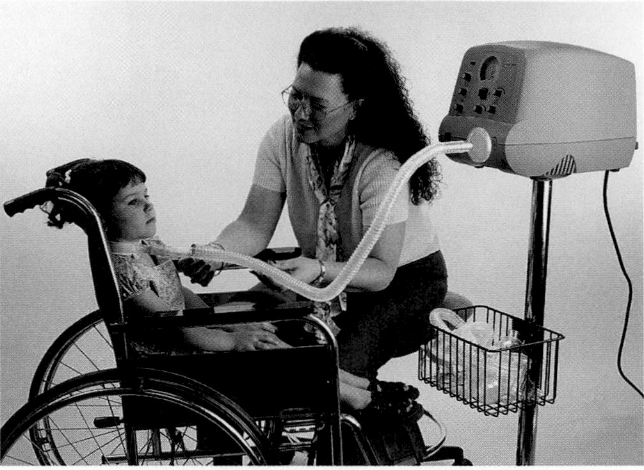

Fig. 22-11 CoughAssist machine.

The CoughAssist, previously known as the Cofflator or Mechanical Insufflator-Exsufflator (MI-E), is a noninvasive machine used for airway clearance. A positive-pressure phase (insufflation) is followed by a negative pressure phase (exsufflation), simulating a cough. This device can be used as a face mask or attached to a universal adaptor for a tracheostomy tube (Figure 22-11).

Adults and children with neuromuscular disease are susceptible to recurrent chest infections, which are a major cause of morbidity and mortality. The suggested mechanism of action of the CoughAssist machine is to improve peak cough flow.[19] In a study of 22 patients ages 10 to 56 (median age 21), spirometry and respiratory muscle strength were measured. Peak cough flows were measured with maximal coughs unassisted, then randomly with assistive coughs, noninvasive mechanical ventilation, CoughAssist machine, and exsufflation alone. All the therapeutic techniques were well tolerated and showed similar patient acceptance. However, the CoughAssist machine produced greater increases in cough pressures than did the other cough-assist techniques.[23] Considering the workload of caregivers and the availability of the CoughAssist machine, many patients with neuromuscular weakness and artificial airways could well use this as an effective adjunct in the home, as well as in other settings.

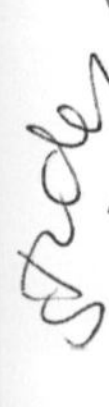

The CoughAssist machine has been used primarily in adults, but it is being used more and more in children. In a study of 62 children (median age 11.3, ranging from 3 months to 28.6 years) with neuromuscular disease and impaired cough who were seen in a pediatric respiratory clinic, it was much preferred and was considered safe, well tolerated, and effective in 90% of this population for preventing pulmonary complications.[36] In a similar study, patients with spinal cord injury also preferred the CoughAssist machine and found it effective and more comfortable than other methods for removing secretions.[37] In a direct comparison of suctioning and the CoughAssist machine for adult patients with neuromuscular impairments, Massery and colleagues found no clinically significant difference between the two mechanical interventions; however, patients preferred the CoughAssist machine 10 to 1 over suctioning.[38]

Summary

In all postures and in all techniques, for both assisted and self-assisted coughs, initial positioning and ventilatory strategies are of utmost importance to the success of the airway clearance technique. Be creative in applying the concepts in this chapter to all patient populations. Also consider the mechanical needs of patients who are not able to assist or to be independent in the secretion removal that prevents pulmonary complications. From the tiniest postural change to full-body movements and physical assists, the most effective modification exists—the therapist just needs to find it so that all patients can improve their coughing.

Review Questions

1. What are the two mechanisms of airway clearance?
2. Which patients would a therapist need to assist in their coughing?
3. How does the CoughAssist machine work, and which patients would benefit from it?
4. What is a smoker's cough, and why does it occur?
5. What are the stages of a cough?
6. When should a therapist make a referral for an evaluation of a patient's swallowing mechanism?
7. What special techniques can be taught to patients with asthma to mobilize secretions?
8. What manual techniques are most effective in patients with spinal cord injury?

References

1. Birring SS: Controversies in the evaluation and management of chronic cough. *Am J Respir Crit Care Med* 183(6):708–715, 2011 (Epub Dec 10, 2010).
2. Kardos P: Proposals for a rationale and for rational diagnosis of cough. *Pneumologie* 54:110–115, 2000.
3. Chang AB, Lasserson TJ, Gaffney J, et al. Gastroesophageal reflux treatment for prolonged non-specific cough in children and adults, Cochrane Database of Systematic Reviews, 2011, Issue 1, Art no CD004823. DOI: 00.1002/14651858.CD004823pub4.
4. Riegel B, Warmoth JE, Middaugh SJ, et al: Psychogenic cough treated with biofeedback and psychotherapy: a review and case report. *American Journal of Physical and Medical Rehabilitation* 74:155–158, 1995.
5. McGarvey LP, Edler J: Future directions in treating cough. *Otolaryngol Clin North Am* 43(1):xii, 2010.
6. Donnelly D, Everard M, Chang AB: Indoor air modification for prolonged nonspecific cough in children, Cochrane Database of Systematic Reviews, 2006, Issue 3, Art no CD005075. DO1: 10.1002/14651858.CD005075.Pub2.
7. Williams JL: Gastroesophageal reflux disease: clinical manifestations. *Gastroenterology Nursing* 26:195–200, 2003.
8. Chandra A, Moazzez R, Bartlett D, et al: A review of the atypical manifestations of gastroesophageal reflux disease. *International Journal of Clinical Practice* 58:41–48, 2004.
9. Gislason T, Janson C, Vermeire P, et al: Respiratory symptoms and nocturnal gastroesophageal reflux: a population-based study of young adults in three European countries. *Chest* 121:158–163, 2002.
10. Smith JA: Interrupting the cough reflex in asthma. *Curr Opin Allergy Clin Immunol* Feb(1):77–81, 2010.
11. Sawabata N, Maeda H, Takeda S, et al: Persistent cough following pulmonary resection: observational and empiric study of possible causes. *Annals of Thoracic Surgery* 79:289–293, 2005.
12. Termoto S, Ishii T, Yamamoto H, et al: Significance of chronic cough as a defense mechanism or a symptom in elderly patients with aspiration and aspiration pneumonia. *European Respiratory Journal* 25:210–211, 2005.
13. Jones RC, Peng A, Stoke M, et al. Mechanisms of pelvic floor muscle function and the effect of the urethra during a cough. *Eur Urol* 57(6):1101–1110, 2010 (Epub June 21, 2009).

14. Linder SH: Functional electrical stimulation to enhance cough in quadriplegia. *Chest* 103:166–169, 1993.
15. Bach JR, Saporito LR: Criteria for extubation and tracheostomy tube removal for patients with ventilatory failure. A different approach to weaning. *Chest* 110:1566–1571, 1996.
16. Clough JB, Sly PD: Association between lower respiratory tract symptoms and falls in peak expiratory flow in children. *European Respiratory Journal* 8:718–722, 1995.
17. Enright PL: Correlates of peak expiratory flow lability in elderly persons. *Chest* 120:1861–1868, 2001.
18. Massery M, Dreyer H, Borjenson A, et al: A pilot study investigating the effectiveness of assisted cough techniques and the clinical utility of a peak flow meter to measure peak cough expiratory flow in persons with spinal cord injury [abstract]. *Proceedings for the World Congress for Physical Therapy* 30, 1999.
19. Bach JR: Comparison of peak expiratory flows with manually assisted and unassisted coughing techniques. *Chest* 104:1553–1562, 1993.
20. Jaeger RJ, Turba RM, Yarkony GM, et al: Cough in spinal cord injured patients: comparison of three methods to produce cough. *Archives of Physical Medicine and Rehabilitation* 74:1358–1361, 1993.
21. Hoffman LA: Ineffective airway clearance related to neuromuscular dysfunction. *Nursing Clinics of North America* 22:151–166, 1987.
22. Braun SR, Giovannoni R, O'Connor M: Improving cough in patients with spinal cord injury. *American Journal of Physical Medicine* 63:1–10, 1984.
23. Chatwin M, Ross E, Hart N, et al: Cough augmentation with mechanical insufflation/exsufflation in patients with neuromuscular weakness. *European Respiratory Journal* 21:502–508, 2003.
24. Lahrmann H: Expiratory muscle weakness and assisted cough in ALS. *Amyotrophic Lateral Sclerosis and Other Motor Neuron Disorders* 4:49–51, 2003.
25. Sivsaothy P, Brown L, Smith IE, et al: Effect of manually assisted cough and mechanical insufflation on cough flow of normal subjects, patients with chronic obstructive pulmonary disease (COPD) and patients with respiratory muscle weakness. *Thorax* 56:438–444, 2001.
26. Fishburn MJ, Marino RJ, Dittuno JF: Atelectasis and pneumonia in acute spinal cord injury. *Archives of Physical Medicine and Rehabilitation* 71:197–200, 1990.
27. Slack RS, Shucart W: Respiratory dysfunction with traumatic injury to the central nervous system. *Clinics in Chest Medicine* 15:739–749, 1994.
28. Massery MP: What's positioning got to do with it? *Neurology Report* 18:11–14, 1994.
29. Ishii M, Matsuo Y, et al: Optimizing forced vital capacity with shoulder positioning in a mechanically-ventilated patient with amyotrophic lateral sclerosis. *Cardiopulmonary Physical Therapy Journal* 15:12–16, 2004.
30. MacLean D, Drummond C, Macpherson C, et al: Maximum expiratory airflow during chest physiotherapy on ventilated patients before and after the application of an abdominal binder. *Intensive Care Medicine* 5:396–399, 1989.
31. Estenne M, Detroyer A: Cough in tetraplegic subjects: an active process. *Annals of Internal Medicine* 12:22–28, 1990.
32. Brito MF, Moreira GA, Tufik S: Air Stacking and chest compression increase peak cough flow in patients with Duchenne muscular dystrophy, Jornal brasilero de *pneumologia* 35:973–979, October 2009.
33. Sullivan PE, Markos PD: *Clinical procedures in therapeutic exercise*, Stamford, Conn, 1996, Simon and Schuster Co.
34. Massery MP: An innovative approach to assistive cough techniques. *Topics in Acute Care Trauma Rehabilitation* 3:73–85, 1987.
35. Knott M, Voss DE: *Proprioceptive neuromuscular facilitation: patterns and techniques*, New York, 1956, Hoeber-Harper Books.
36. Miske LJ, Hickey EM, Kolb SM, et al: Use of the mechanical in-exsufflator in pediatric patients with neuromuscular disease and impaired cough. *Chest* 125:1406–1412, 2004.
37. Garstang SV, Kirschblun SC, Wood KE, Patient Preference for in –exsullation for secretion management with spinal cord injury. *J Spinal Cord Med* 23(2):80–88, 2000.
38. Massery M, Sammon K, et al: Comparing airway clearance effectiveness using a suction machine and the Cough-Assist machine for patients in acute rehabilitation [abstract]. *Cardiopulmonary Physical Therapy Journal* 14:21, 2003.

III

Chapter 23

Facilitating Ventilation Patterns and Breathing Strategies

Donna Frownfelter*

KEY TERMS

Posture/positioning
Controlled breathing
Core stability
Diaphragmatic breathing pattern
Jacobsen's progressive relaxation
Ventilatory strategies
Work of breathing

CHAPTER OUTLINE

Individuals with breathing impairments (whether primary or secondary in origin) require a variety of interventions to optimize ventilation and oxygen delivery, as well as improving functional outcomes. Some interventions are passive in nature, such as the positioning of the patient or the application of an abdominal binder for better diaphragmatic positioning. Other interventions require very active participation on the part of the therapist, patient, or both, such as in assisted-cough techniques, in glossopharyngeal breathing instruction, or in learning a more efficient breathing pattern. Ideally techniques are incorporated into the patient's total physical rehabilitation program, such as the use of ventilation strategies pairing breathing with movement. All of these diverse aspects of treatment play an important role in the development of

*With thanks to Mary Massery for previous contributions.

a successful rehabilitation program to meet the needs of patients with pulmonary impairments. No single intervention or approach is appropriate in all cases. Sound clinical judgment and experience must be exercised when applying these ideas in each person. The interventions identified in this chapter are not inclusive. They are meant to provide examples and guidelines and to stimulate the clinician's creative talents in order to incorporate the interventions into a comprehensive treatment program determined by individual needs that improve the outcomes for each patient (Box 23-1).

Positioning Concerns

All patients spend some portion of the day in a horizontal position for rest or sleep. Some who are acutely ill or medically compromised spent extended time in bed, and major emphasis must be placed on the mobilization of patients early and often to prevent immobility from exerting its negative effects on all body systems (see Chapter 18). Studies have shown that patients who are medicated and spend extended time on ventilators in the ICU have developed critical illness neuromuscular syndrome or ICU-acquired weakness. Interventions shown to help prevent this problem are physical therapy/activity and daily interruptions of sedative medication.[1,2,3] These studies validate the need for intervention to prevent untoward effects of immobility and sedation.

Despite these problems, the time spent in a horizontal position can be used as an opportunity to assist patients in passive drainage and preventing the retention of lung secretions. It can be a natural beginning in the development of a patient's long-term respiratory program (e.g., the prevention of respiratory complications in a patient with tetraplegia). Specific postural drainage positions are covered under airway clearance interventions (see Chapter 21). Using a combination of these positions and the patient's position in bed, in the hospital or at home, can help to achieve multiple goals. First, various horizontal positions can assist patients in passively clearing secretions that they may have difficulty clearing actively. Pneumonia is still the leading cause of death in patients with spinal cord injury (SCI) who are tetraplegic.[4] Second, these position changes provide for skin relief and better circulation. Finally, they assist in retarding the development of joint contractures or other musculoskeletal abnormalities. A four-position rotation (i.e., supine, prone, and side-to-side) or a modified six-position rotation (supine, three-quarter supine, side-lying, three-quarter prone on each side) is usually an effective and reasonable means of incorporating these goals into a long-term prophylactic program.

Simple adaptations may make ventilation easier in each of these postures. For example, when the patient is in the supine position, placing the patient's arms up over his or her head facilitates greater anterior upper chest expansion.[5] Likewise, positioning the pelvis in a slight posterior tilt facilitates more diaphragmatic excursion. (Detailed explanations of positioning are discussed in Chapter 42.) Observation of all precautions and contraindications to passive positioning is still warranted, and positions should be modified based on the individual need of each patient.

Just as passive positioning of the patient in bed helps to maintain airway clearance and improve ventilation potential, optimal passive positioning of the patient's skeletal frame in an upright posture (sitting, standing) helps to maximize the mechanical advantages that facilitate breathing and improve cardiovascular fluid shifts. For example, patients with SCIs resulting in tetraplegia will be unable to support their intestinal contents properly under the diaphragm to allow for maximal expansion of the chest in all three planes of ventilation (see Chapter 39). The use of an abdominal support from the iliac crest to the base of the xiphoid process provides positive-pressure support to restore intestinal positioning to an upright position (Figure 23-1). Research has documented

Box 23-1 Categories of Therapeutic Interventions Presented in this Chapter to Optimize Ventilation Patterns

1. Positioning concerns
2. Ventilatory and movement strategies
3. Manual facilitation techniques
   - Facilitating controlled breathing patterns (diaphragmatic)
   - Mobilizing the thorax
   - Facilitating upper chest breathing patterns (accessory muscles)
   - Promoting symmetrical breathing patterns (unilateral dysfunction)
   - Reducing high respiratory rates
4. Glossopharyngeal breathing
5. Enhancing phonation skills

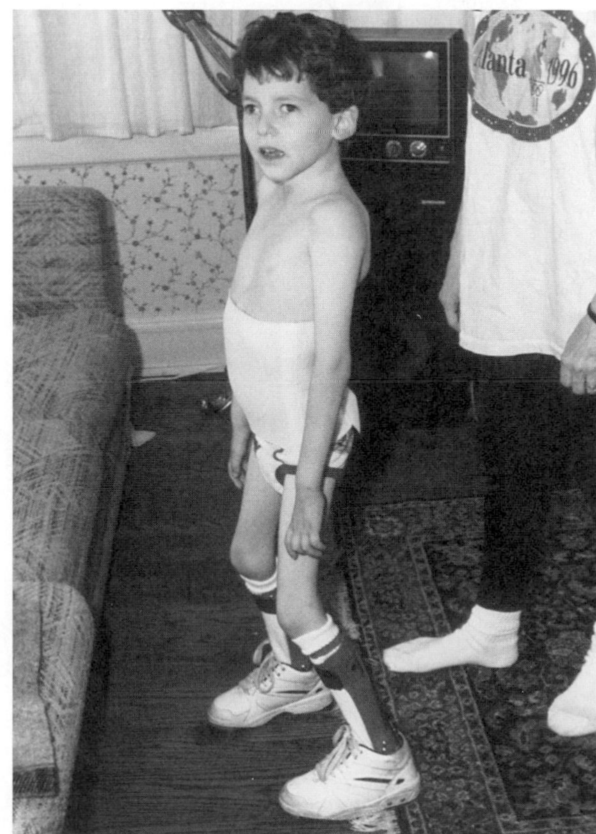

Fig. 23-1 **A,** Abdominal binder, Velcro fastener. **B,** Placement of abdominal binder.

well the significant improvements in vital capacity (VC), inspiratory capacity, and tidal volume (TV) in sitting with the use of a strong abdominal support.[6] These binders have also been used in nursing care to provide for better circulation and the prevention of hypotension.

The abdominal binder's value in cosmesis may be underrated. Many patients with neurological issues were once healthy individuals with high self-esteem who took great pride in their appearance. Many now present with protruding bellies (the anterior and inferior shift of the intestines resulting from flaccid abdominal muscles), which may be psychologically disturbing to them. Thus the use of a binder may greatly aid in the restoration of these patients' self-esteem, which should be a high-priority goal in any rehabilitation program.

A rigid type of abdominal support can be used when the vertebral column and the abdominal viscera need support. These are called body jackets or total contact thoracic lumbar sacral orthoses (TLSOs) (Figure 23-2). A TLSO is a rigid trunk support molded individually to the shape of the patient's entire trunk from the axilla down to the pubis. It is composed of two separate pieces, a front and a back, ideally with an anterior cutout in the abdomen to allow for normal diaphragmatic displacement of the viscera. In addition to these jackets, an elastic binder is applied around the abdomen to allow for

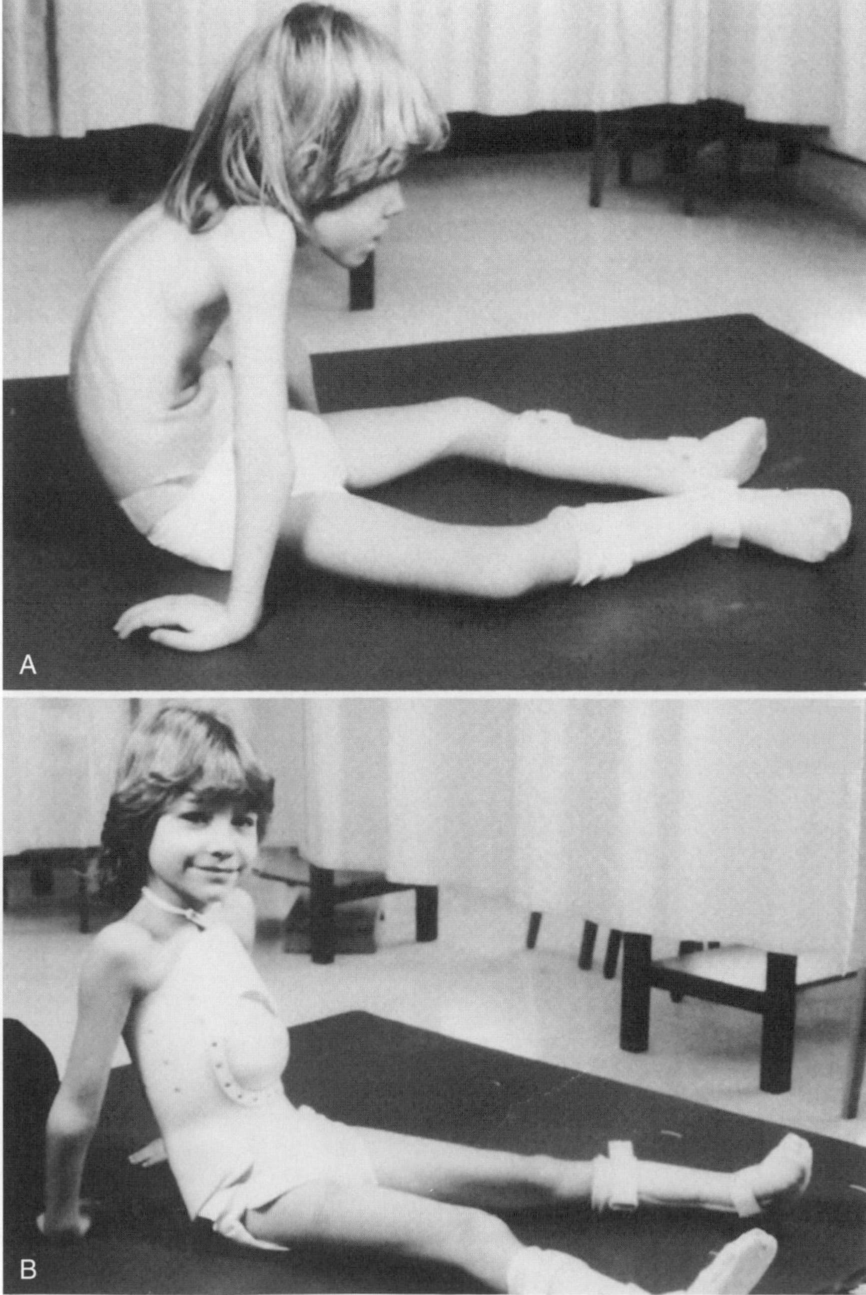

Fig. 23-2 A, Patient with C5 congenital tetraplegia, independent long-sitting. **B,** Long-sitting with body jacket support. Note the changes in head position and eye contact, hip alignment, and shoulder rotation.

diaphragmatic motion but minimize excessive displacement of the abdominal contents. This is particularly appropriate for a growing child who needs more spinal stability and for the completely flaccid patient with tetraplegia, who may also require the same support. Because head and neck positioning are so dependent on trunk positioning, a body jacket may make the difference for these patients between being dependent or independent in an upright posture. It may result in significantly better head control and eye contact and improved phonation. However, because the TLSO limits trunk movement, its usefulness for each patient must be assessed carefully.

The next consideration in passive respiratory techniques is proper wheelchair positioning. Optimal performance in ventilatory functioning, as well as many other areas of rehabilitation, depends on good alignment of the body against the force of gravity. Symmetry must be strived for through the use of a body jacket, lateral trunk supports in the wheelchair, abdominal binders, or some other means (Figure 23-3). This is especially important for patients with hemiplegia in whom habitual asymmetrical posturing leads to musculoskeletal problems later. Symmetrical breathing patterns and uniform aeration of all lung segments are augmented by careful upright positioning. Therefore everything from the type of neck and trunk support to the height and width of the arm rests to the length and type of the foot supports must be carefully analyzed for each patient.

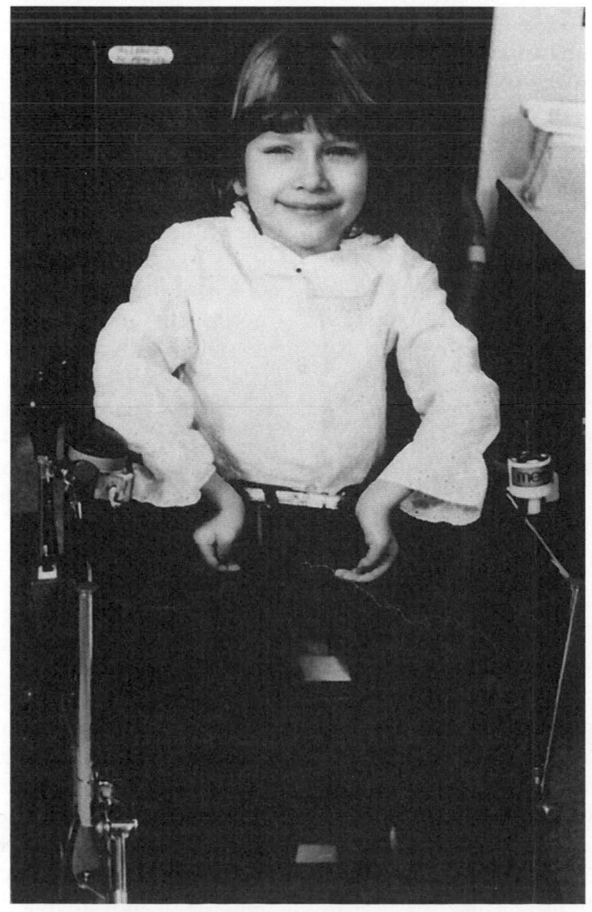

Fig. 23-3 Wheelchair alignment considerations.

Ventilatory and Movement Strategies for Improving Functional Outcomes

Observing patient movement and ventilation is inherent in the physical therapist's examination and evaluation of the patient. Patients often will hold their breath during activities. This will limit their ability to perform functional activities. When it is observed that breath holding is occurring or that the patient has dyspnea with activity, it is important to incorporate ventilatory strategies.

The patient is first positioned for successful ventilation. Then motor activities should be introduced. Interventions chosen will improve the patient's ventilatory support, or the therapist should capitalize on the patient's good ventilatory support to improve the motor activity. Using ventilatory strategies to improve motor performance or movement strategies to improve ventilation performance enables patients to achieve their functional goals sooner and have better health, including fewer respiratory complications. Generally, these simple concepts take no more than 1 to 2 additional minutes of therapy time, with no additional equipment costs other than a few extra pillows or towels. Therefore time and money are not mitigating factors. However, these ideas do require the practitioner to look carefully at the patient before beginning any treatment intervention and to ask, "Have I positioned my patient for ventilatory success?"; "Am I simply treating the patient in whatever position I found her or him in?"; and "Have I carefully chosen my verbal cues to include a ventilatory response and a functional response?" The practitioner must actively include ventilation in every activity to help the patient understand that breathing transcends all activities. Breathing is the bridge to function. A summary of the most important ventilation-movement strategies is listed in Box 23-2.

Incorporating Simple Therapy Tasks

Inspiration

After the patient has been carefully positioned for respiratory success, as described previously, begin the patient's therapy or daily-living activities. In a study looking at rhythmic pronation and supination wrist movements, inspiration and exhalation adapted and became coordinated with the arm movement (Table 23-1).[7,8] Accordingly, then, the simple task of passive

Box 23-2 Significant Ventilatory Movement Strategies

- Pair trunk extension activities with inspiration
- Pair trunk flexion activities with exhalation
- Pair shoulder flexion, abduction, and/or external rotation activities with inspiration
- Pair shoulder extension, adduction, and/or internal rotation activities with exhalation
- Pair upward eye gaze with inspiration
- Pair downward eye gaze with exhalation

Table 23-1 Anatomy of Inspiration and Expiration

	Inspiration	Expiration
Trunk	Trunk extension	Trunk flexion
Shoulders	Shoulder flexion, abduction, and external rotation movements	Shoulder extension, adduction, and internal rotation movements
Gaze	Upward eye gaze	Downward eye gaze

range of movement (ROM) can easily include the active goal of increasing ventilation by asking the patient to breathe in and look up when his or her arm is raised up into shoulder flexion. This encourages the patient to breathe in when the chest wall muscles are being stretched and the ribs are naturally opening up, causing both activities to be more successful. It also begins to teach the patient to use ventilatory strategies to optimize potential functional movement, such as in reaching up to a kitchen cabinet. Patients need to focus on avoiding breath holding and incorporating breathing during each activity.

Exhalation

Likewise, active or passive exhalation should be coordinated with the reverse upper extremity ROM pattern (i.e., the arm returning from flexion back to the patient's side). This can be done using all types of exhalation patterns, including the following:

- Passive quiet exhalation
- Forceful exhalation, as in blowing, coughing, or pursed-lips exhalation
- Vocalization patterns

Thus the therapist may ask the patient to slowly count out loud to 10 while the arm is being returned eccentrically to his or her side. The patient learns to correlate exhalation with shoulder extension while simultaneously learning a much more complex idea—that of controlling his or her rate and volume of expiration by including deliberate speech during exhalation maneuvers. Research is being done in the area of respiratory plasticity to evaluate changes with exercise and conditioning.[9,10] Clinical observation demonstrates that patients will incorporate new ventilation strategies and that these strategies become less cognitive and more based in habit as they are repeated.

In a recent study of strategies for respiratory exercise patterns with upper extremity movements in patients with chronic obstructive pulmonary disease (COPD), 15 patients were instructed in the reverse pattern. For example, with shoulder flexion they performed the activity with exhalation versus inhalation. The researchers concluded that there was less chest asynchrony and that it may be an important strategy for people with COPD to use the opposite pattern.[11] This study had only 15 patients with COPD; however, it may be noted that with ventilatory strategies, patients may try different ways of incorporating breathing. As long as patients are not breath holding, therapists should feel safe encouraging them to try techniques and see what works best for them.

To improve exhalation potential, increase the patient's relative trunk flexion alignment. While the patient is still supine and performing upper extremity ROM, ask the patient to lift his or her head and watch the hand as it returns to the side, which increases abdominal and intercostal activation. Or ask the patient to increase knee flexion, which increases posterior pelvic tilting and trunk flexion. Pairing trunk flexion with exhalation completes the trunk movement strategy for better ventilation.

Combining positioning with verbal cues for ventilation, as described in ROM activities, changes passive upper extremity ROM exercises into dynamic upper extremity ROM exercises. It encourages increased inspiratory and expiratory capacities, develops early functional motor planning strategies, and facilitates trunk mobility. In this manner the patient has the opportunity to learn from the beginning of his or her rehabilitation process that movement and breathing go hand in hand. Clinically, incorporating appropriate breathing patterns with movement early in the rehabilitation process discourages the development of Valsalva patterns or shallow breathing patterns when the motor activities become more difficult and complex. Patients who are mechanically ventilated on an assist mode or during a time of sedation interruption can accomplish this as well.

Dynamic Activities

Inhalation promotes trunk extension, exhalation promotes trunk flexion, and vice versa. This basic theme occurs naturally in all motor activities but may have ceased to become spontaneous after a neuromuscular or musculoskeletal insult. Valsalva, or breath holding, maneuvers during transitional movements, such as rolling or coming to a sitting or standing position, are often noted in these patients. By teaching them strategies that incorporate breathing into their motor plans for all motor activities, Valsalva patterns can be eliminated or minimized while simultaneously promoting better cardiovascular function.

The following activities are just a few of the common daily activities. They are typical gross motor activities, but the use of ventilatory strategies is a means of improving patients' abilities to perform them. Extrapolation of these concepts to all other motor activities should be carefully analyzed by each therapist for each individual patient, looking at the trunk patterns and type of muscle contraction that occurs in a given exercise or activity. At times there may be more than one effective ventilation strategy; there is no hard-and-fast rule. What is important is that patients breathe with the movement and not hold their breath.

Rolling

Ask patients to attempt to roll, and assess whether they tend to move with trunk extension or flexion to begin the roll. Those who roll in trunk extension patterns should be asked to breathe in while they roll and to look up. Those who roll with trunk flexion as their primary movement pattern should be instructed to roll first by inhaling, then blowing out and tucking the chin during the roll. In doing so, patients work with, not against, natural whole patterns of movements that increase the likelihood of success.

Coming Up to Sitting

Pushing up to sitting from side-lying should be evaluated in much the same manner. If patients are more effective in coming to the upright position when using trunk extension, have them inhale as they push up to sitting. Asking them to look up as they come to upright will reinforce the movement. If they are weaker and have more success in pushing up with trunk flexion, have them blow out and tuck the chin while moving. It may be helpful to allow patients to try both strategies and see which is most effective. The important consideration is that they do not hold the breath while changing the position.

Dressing

Patients often express how short of breath they become with dressing. These activities, too, can benefit from the concepts discussed here. Use of the upper extremities has been shown to involve an increase in oxygen consumption over lower extremity activities. For dressings, the recommended position is either sitting in a chair or the long-sitting position in bed for those with less trunk control (such as patients with SCI). While putting on lower extremity items such as pants, socks, and shoes in a long-sitting position, have the patient first take in a deep breath while extending his or her trunk. Then have the patient blow out, huff out, or cough while flexing the trunk to reach his or her toes. This combines the functional daily task of dressing with improving breath control, trunk control, and airway-clearance techniques.

Upper extremity dressing and upper extremity exercise can incorporate the same ideas. All movements should be coordinated with appropriate chest wall movements to maximize upper extremity tasks. Thus every time the arm is moving up above 90 degrees of shoulder flexion, the patient should be asked to breathe in, allowing for the normal shoulder/rib-cage rhythm to occur. Full shoulder flexion requires the opening of the intercostal spacing and the separation of the individual ribs.[12] Many patients with neurological impairments have lost the intrinsic mobility of the chest wall and thus may have lost some functional shoulder ROM as well. Not pairing inspiration with shoulder flexion is likely to limit the patient's shoulder ROM to approximately 140 to 150 degrees. It may also encourage Valsalva maneuvers during the activity and may cause more shoulder pain.

Coming Up to Standing

Coming up to standing requires both trunk flexion and trunk extension. Patients often use a rhythmic initiation (rocking) to begin the sit-to-stand transfer. This is a good opportunity to begin teaching breath control. Patients breathe in and then as they rock forward, they exhale; rocking backwards, they inhale as the trunk extends. There can be several cycles of rocking and breathing prior to standing before control is attained. Thus patients should initiate the forward trunk lean with exhalation and then initiate the standing phase with inhalation and trunk and neck extension. Active neck extension during assumption of standing not only facilitates greater inhalation but, along with the influence of the tonic labyrinthine reflex (TLR), also facilitates more significant contractions of the trunk and hip extensors. Clinically, this often results in a more noticeably upright posture and may make the difference between an assisted standing pivot transfer and an independent one. Returning to sitting should be accompanied by slow, controlled exhalation, such as in pursed-lips blowing or counting out loud, in order to maximize the body's controlled descent into gravity's influence.

Facilitating a Controlled Diaphragmatic Breathing Pattern

Why would a therapist want to change a patient's breathing pattern? The answer is simple—when the pattern being used is ineffective. Ordinarily, people use the pattern of breathing that is the most efficient for them. However, when the work of breathing increases and musculoskeletal, neuromuscular, or pulmonary impairment is present, abnormal patterns that are not efficient may be adopted. The patient knows that it requires hard work to breathe but often does not know how to do it with greater ease, especially during stressful situations when panic is present. The patient may spontaneously do pursed-lips breathing (PLB) but often in a forceful manner that may not relieve the dyspnea.

A healthy person uses approximately 5% of total oxygen consumption and 10% of vital capacity for the muscular work of breathing. Consequently, breathing at rest is generally perceived as effortless under normal conditions.

However, in the patients physical therapists evaluate and treat (often after surgery, respiratory disease, or dysfunction secondary to neurological insult or injury), the vital capacity may be significantly decreased and the oxygen consumption may be greatly increased because of the use of accessory muscles or the extra effort needed to breathe or cough.

Many patients with lung cancer also have COPD, which increases their postoperative complications because of impaired pulmonary function before surgery. In a study of patients with COPD who needed to undergo surgical resection for cancer, it was found that a preoperative pulmonary rehabilitation program of 10 visits over a 4-week period consisting of exercise prescription, inspiratory muscle training, and slow breathing technique improved patients' postoperative progress. The group in this program required a shorter period of time in the ICU and fewer days using a chest tube. Although this study was done with only nine patients, it has implications for improvement of postoperative success. However, in many cases, it may not be feasible to have 4 weeks of pulmonary rehabilitation before lung surgery. Some surgeons are hesitant to delay the needed surgery for pulmonary rehabilitation. A larger study would need to be conducted to demonstrate cost effectiveness, as well as the benefits and risks.[13]

Vital capacity is also affected in cases of tetraplegia, in which patients' vital capacity may be reduced to 1000 to 1500 mL from their normal 3000-mL vital capacity (50%). If the normal TV (normal volume of breathing) is 500 mL, this means that with each breath the patient would use 33% to 50% of his or her vital capacity (maximal inspiration followed by maximal exhalation). This would greatly increase the work of breathing and oxygen consumption just for normal quiet breathing. The patient would have little pulmonary reserve. This can lead to respiratory muscle fatigue. During exercise or stress, the patient would have an increased subjective feeling of shortness of breath and feel an increase in the work of breathing. In addition, patients with spinal cord injury who are smokers experience excessive vital capacity losses.[14] Commonly used terms to describe breathing patterns are listed in Box 23-3. A listing of indications for teaching controlled-breathing techniques is provided in Box 23-4.

It should be appreciated that breathing comfortably and in a controlled manner is associated with wellness and a sense of ease. Even normal individuals who are under stress and have increased work levels are more cognizant of the increase in their work of breathing. For a patient who struggles with every breath and wonders how it will be possible to get through the day, ventilatory strategies and breathing-control techniques can be the key to maximizing potential. A list of goals for teaching controlled-breathing techniques is found in Box 23-5.

Breathing control has long been used in yoga to focus and to promote meditation. This is a key to maximizing rehabilitation. Patients who cannot breathe cannot function! It is of primary importance to assess patients' breathing at rest and during exercise. People often hold their breath with exertion, especially during new activities, so it is vital to assess the cardiopulmonary and neuromuscular response to each new activity. In many rehabilitation centers and health clubs, Pilates exercise regimens have been used to help patients achieve core strength and back stabilization. Pilates is a method of physical and mental conditioning combined with body, mind, and spirit integration; it has been also used by dancers and choreographers to improve postural control, increase ease of movement, and improve their performance. The first phase of Pilates incorporates diaphragmatic breathing *before continuing with the steps* to activate the muscles of the core (multifidus, diaphragm, pelvic floor, and transverse abdominis). The belief is that when the individual has a strong core, the posture will improve and the performance of other functional activities will be improved. This is similar to our concept of teaching diaphragmatic breathing control before functional activities in people with respiratory impairments. Joseph Pilates actually used the term *contrology* to define his concepts. That is what we are striving to teach our patients—breath control, then function.[15]

Box 23-3 **Breathing Pattern Terminology**

Eupnea: Normal breathing, repeated rhythmic inspiratory-expiratory cycles

Hyperpnea: Increased breathing; usually refers to increased tidal volume with or without increased frequency

Polypnea, tachypnea: Increased frequency of breathing

Hyperventilation: Increased alveolar ventilation in relation to metabolic rate (an increase in alveolar ventilation); seen as a decrease in the arterial P_{CO_2}

Hypoventilation: Decreased alveolar ventilation in relation to metabolic rate (a decrease in alveolar ventilation); seen as an increase in P_{CO_2}

Apnea: Cessation of respiration in the resting expiratory position

Dyspnea: The patient's subjective feeling of shortness of breath

Apneusis: Cessation of respiration in the inspiratory position

Apneustic breathing: Apneusis interrupted periodically by exhalation

Cheyne-Stokes respiration: Cycles of gradually increasing tidal volume followed by gradually decreasing tidal volume (usually followed by an apneic period)

Biot respiration: Sequences of uniformly deep gasps and apnea, followed by deep gasps

Modified from Comroe JH, Jr: Physiology of respiration, *ed 2, St Louis, 1974, Mosby.*

Box 23-4 **Indications for Teaching Controlled-Breathing Techniques**

Patients with any of the following:

- Pulmonary dysfunction, either primary or secondary causes
- Pain resulting from surgery, trauma, or disease
- Apprehension or nervousness
- Bronchospasm or impending bronchospasm in asthma
- Airway clearance dysfunction
- Restriction of inspiration resulting from musculoskeletal dysfunction, such as scoliosis, kyphoscoliosis, or pectus excavatum; obesity; pregnancy; pulmonary pathology such as fibrosis; scarring resulting from radiation therapy; neurological weakness such as spinal cord injury, Parkinson disease, or myasthenia gravis
- Congestive heart failure, pulmonary edema, or pulmonary emboli
- Rib fractures
- Ventilated patients on assist control or intermittent mandatory ventilation
- Metabolic disturbances that have a compensatory respiratory response
- Debilitated or bedridden patients, who tend to have constant volume ventilation and retain secretions and are prone to pneumonia and atelectasis due to poor airway clearance

Box 23-5 **Goals of Teaching Controlled-Breathing Techniques**

- To decrease the work of breathing
- To improve alveolar ventilation
- To improve airway clearance by improving cough
- To increase strength, coordination, and efficiency of respiratory muscles
- To improve phonation and the ability to express needs and wants
- To teach the patient how to respond to and control breathing
- To assist in relaxation
- To mobilize and maintain mobility of the thorax
- To enable patients to feel self-control and confidence in managing disease or dysfunction

Considerations in Teaching Breathing Control to Patients with Primary Versus Secondary Pulmonary Dysfunction

Patients with primary lung disease, such as COPD, asthma, bronchitis, or cystic fibrosis, present a picture very different from that of patients with secondary pulmonary deficits, SCI, Parkinson disease, myasthenia gravis, or Guillain-Barré syndrome. In general, patients with primary lung disease tend to overuse their accessory muscles and greatly increase the work of breathing secondary to shortness of breath or coughing. They often complain that they have difficulty "getting the air out," which demonstrates the decreased expiratory flow rates noted on pulmonary function tests. This can lead to dynamic hyperinflation, in which patients continue to gasp and increase the respiratory rate so more air is coming in, but there is not time for the air to be exhaled. Large volumes of air can get trapped in the lungs, which causes increased feelings of shortness of breath and panic. The goal with these patients is to teach them to relax the neck and chest accessory muscles and use more diaphragmatic breathing (abdominal and lateral costal breathing) to reduce the work of breathing in combination with relaxed pursed-lips breathing and prolonged exhalation. Their treatment programs focus on energy conservation, relaxation, and pacing activity with breath control. In pulmonary rehabilitation programs, exercise is a key component. Patients learn to coordinate their breathing with their activities and find that they have less dyspnea with exertion.[16,17]

There has been controversy in the literature about the effectiveness of diaphragmatic breathing. No standardized "norms" of how to perform diaphragmatic breathing exist. However, many skilled cardiovascular and pulmonary physical therapists would consider teaching the patient with COPD how to relax the accessory muscles and use the diaphragm as an important part of the patient's pulmonary rehabilitation. Dechman reported that in a search of the literature, pursed-lips breathing was considered most effective by people with COPD and that the literature does not strongly support the use of diaphragmatic breathing in people with COPD.[18] Cahalin found there are both positive and potentially detrimental effects to diaphragmatic breathing training.[19] Each individual patient needs to be evaluated to consider whether diaphragmatic breathing may be beneficial. For example, patients with severe hyperinflation and flattened diaphragms secondarily will most likely not benefit from diaphragmatic breathing because the muscle length tension relationship is abnormal and will not result in an appropriate movement of the diaphragm. With patients who have mild to moderate COPD and are overusing the accessory muscles, diaphragmatic breathing may be very helpful; it may require less oxygen consumption, decrease the respiratory rate, and increase the tidal volume.

Patients with secondary pulmonary dysfunction, such as SCI, have a more restrictive component to inspiration. In these cases, accessory muscles may be intact, but they are not being used to facilitate deep breathing or coughing. Patients may have strong diaphragmatic breaths, but the upper chest collapses on inspiration (paradoxical breathing; see Chapter 39). The goal is to teach these patients to use the accessory muscles to balance the upper and lower chest. This facilitates an increase in vital capacity that prevents atelectasis and pneumonia by increasing the volume of ventilation and improving the cough mechanism.

The choice of appropriate ventilatory strategies is determined by the individual patient's problem. The following questions should be considered when evaluating a patient:

- Does the patient have more difficulty during inspiration or exhalation?
- Is there a normal sequence to inspiration (i.e., abdominal wall rise, then lateral costal expansion, then upper chest expansion, with a full inspiration)? Or does the chest sink and the abdomen rise on inspiration?
- Does the patient appear to be working hard to breathe? Is the patient using the accessory muscles to an extreme?
- Does the patient frequently clear the throat, have trouble coughing, or have difficulty speaking at a normal volume and for the normal length of sentences?
- Is ventilation the limiting factor in accomplishing an activity (e.g., transfer, gait, or bed mobility)?

Patients with primary pulmonary disease generally benefit from ventilatory strategies that relax the accessory muscles and facilitate relaxed diaphragmatic breathing. On the other hand, patients with secondary pulmonary dysfunction usually benefit from the balanced use of the diaphragm and accessory muscles to increase vital capacity and breath support for activities.

Pursed-Lips Breathing

Pursed-lips breathing is a strategy that is often spontaneously used by people with COPD during episodes of dyspnea. Many patients feel this breathing pattern helps to decrease their breathlessness. The effect of PLB is an increase in the time of exhalation, which results in a decrease in the end-expiratory volume and an increase in the total time of the respiratory cycle. This results in a decreased respiratory rate and increased TV. According to studies, a decrease in the Borg scale of perceived exertion also occurs when PLB is used.[20] This technique has been acknowledged by many patients with respiratory impairments as being very easy to learn and yet very effective, quick to use, and readily incorporated into their activities to reduce dyspnea.[21]

When instructing a patient in PLB, emphasis should be placed on a relaxed, slow, prolonged, controlled exhalation. Often when patients initiate PLB spontaneously, they use a forceful exhalation, which tightens the neck musculature and oral area. This builds a significant pressure that can counteract the effectiveness of the technique and the subsequent relief of dyspnea. A relaxed head, neck, and mouth are essential. If patients have difficulty relaxing the mouth, they may be encouraged to try making an *sssss*, or hissing, sound, which will still prolong exhalation and provide back pressure.

Relationship of the Diaphragm and Posture

The respiratory action of the diaphragm and other respiratory muscles is normally coordinated with the need to provide postural control of the trunk during movement of the extremities.[8] The diaphragm acts both as a muscle of respiration and as a muscle that works in providing core stability to the trunk. However, when respiratory demand increases, the diaphragm may not be able to continue to provide both of these functions.[22-27] Because the diaphragm is the primary muscle of respiration, postural control may be impaired. A complete discussion of this concept is provided in Chapter 39.

Facilitating Diaphragmatic Breathing

In the initial phases of breathing retraining, patients are taught to use the easiest intervention that facilitates diaphragmatic breathing; if it is not successful, a progression of specific facilitation and inhibition techniques will be tried. A summary of methods of facilitating diaphragmatic ventilation patterns is given in Box 23-6.

Diaphragmatic Controlled Breathing

Diaphragmatic breathing is the normal mode of ventilation. The diaphragm and intercostals are the normal muscles of quiet inspiration. When evaluating a patient's breathing pattern, the use of accessory muscles during quiet breathing should be noted; the patient with primary pulmonary disease needs to be instructed in relaxation of the accessory muscles to decrease the work of breathing. However, in a patient with a spinal cord injury or other neuromuscular disorder, these accessory muscles may assist in balancing ventilation and may also be useful in increasing vital capacity, improving the ability to cough, improving breath support for speaking, and increasing the potential for functional activities.

In general, controlled diaphragmatic breathing should be emphasized in each posture and in all therapeutic activities because carry-over of the breathing pattern from one posture to another or one activity to another is not necessarily present. If the patient is shown the pattern only when in the supine position, it may not carry over to sitting or to a sliding-board transfer, when the activity becomes more complex. A helpful sequence might be to teach the breathing pattern in side-lying, supine, sitting, and standing positions and in walking, stair climbing, and other functional activities, especially in patients with COPD. Patients with neurological impairment may require modification of the breathing pattern so that it fits well with their activity levels and capabilities.

Box 23-6 **Diaphragmatic Facilitation Techniques**

1. Relaxation technique
2. Repatterning techniques
   - Relaxed pursed-lips breathing
   - Exhalation, hold, and inhalation
3. Sniffing
4. Diaphragmatic scoop technique
5. Lateral costal facilitation technique
6. Upper chest inhibiting technique
7. Normal timing technique

Positioning Concerns

Position of Pelvis

The first step in facilitating any breathing pattern is to position the patient for ventilatory success. The details are discussed in this chapter and in Chapter 42. Often a patient's posture and pelvic position have dramatic effects on breathing. In general, a slight, relative posterior tilt of the pelvis facilitates diaphragmatic breathing, and a relative anterior tilt facilitates the opening of the anterior chest and upper chest breathing. It is helpful to see what difference a slight, relative change in pelvic position will do to a patient's ability to ventilate. This is especially true in secondary pulmonary problems related to neurological and neuromuscular dysfunction. A lumbar roll or a roll under the ischial tuberosities can facilitate an anterior pelvic tilt (see Chapter 42).

Relaxation of Upper Chest and Shoulders

Jacobsen's progressive relaxation exercises are familiar to physical therapists. Jacobsen proposed that a maximal muscle contraction would yield a maximal muscle relaxation. This technique can be applied to the upper chest and shoulders. The therapist places his or her hands on the patient's shoulder girdle. The patient is asked to shrug his or her shoulders up into the therapist's hands and hold it. "Don't let me push your shoulders down," is the therapist's command. Then, "Let your shoulders relax, let them go." The emphasis is on the relaxation phase. Verbal commands can be very important with this procedure. A strong command to "Raise your shoulders into my hands" is followed by a quiet, calmer, "Now relax and let them go," repeating quietly, "That's it, let them go, feel them relax." The addition of counter-rotation of the shoulder girdle can make this intervention more effective. Patients can learn the techniques independently and can relax their shoulders when they begin to feel tense. In addition, making shoulder circles in both directions, forward and backwards, can loosen the shoulder girdle. Sometimes the relaxation activity is all that it takes to resume a more natural pattern of breathing, and the therapist can move on to other therapeutic activities. If the patient starts to use accessory muscles again, the technique is repeated. The patient learns to feel the difference between tension and relaxation of the shoulders and can self-monitor and perform the relaxation independently.

Repatterning Technique

If a patient needs more support to gain control of breathing and is experiencing shortness of breath, a simple repatterning technique may be beneficial. An example might be a patient with asthma who has a high respiratory rate and is feeling panicky. When the patient is asked why he or she is breathing so fast, the reply will usually be, "I am not getting enough air. I can't catch my breath." The patient is asked to start with exhalation: "Try to blow out easily with your lips pursed. Don't force it; just let it come out." A helpful technique for producing a prolonged, easy exhalation is to ask the patient to visualize a candle with a flame and then imagine exhaling in a way that makes the flame flicker but not go out. Doing this allows the respiratory rate to decrease automatically. When the patient feels some control of this step, then add, "Hold your breath at the top of inspiration just for a second or two." Make sure the patient does not bear down as in a Valsalva maneuver or hold the breath longer. Last, ask the patient to take a slow breath in, hold it, and let it go out through pursed lips. Patients learn that when they are short of breath, this technique often helps them to gain control, making them feel less panicky.

Sniffing

If working toward a generalized controlled-breathing pattern does not improve the patient's ventilatory pattern adequately, a technique that more specifically addresses the need to initiate breathing from the diaphragm can be attempted. Sniffing is a simple and effective means of teaching diaphragmatic breathing.[28] Sniffing is accomplished primarily by the diaphragm. This technique can be used first, before attempting more specific diaphragmatic training with patients who are capable of attempting sniffing because of its simplicity.

As with all procedures, the most important step is the first step: position the patient appropriately to increase the likelihood of increased diaphragmatic breathing resulting from musculoskeletal alignment. This includes the following:

- Choosing a gravity-eliminated position such as side-lying or a gravity-assisted position such as a supported semi-Fowler sitting position (supported spine)
- Choosing a relatively posteriorly tilted pelvis with flexed knees
- Choosing arm flexion below 90 degrees (in relative shoulder extension, adduction, and internal rotation)
- Choosing to use a pillow or pillows under the patient's head

For each patient, choices will be different (e.g., the amount of knee flexion or the number of pillows). Find the right combination of positioning characteristics that best facilitates diaphragmatic movement for that particular patient. (For details on positioning, see Chapter 42.) In this manner the therapist sets up the patient for ventilatory success before beginning the manual or verbal technique.

Initially, ask the patient to place his or her hands on the abdomen for increased proprioceptive feedback and the relative extension, adduction, and internal rotation position of the shoulders. In a quiet voice, ask the patient to "sniff in three times." Note whether the patient demonstrates more abdominal rise or lower chest expansion or both. If so, draw attention to this fact. During exhalation, tell the patient to "let it out slowly," which helps to prolong the exhalation and slow the respiratory rate (RR) and often encourages some relaxation. Progress the training by guiding the patient to "now sniff in twice, a little deeper." Do you still see greater diaphragmatic excursion and less upper chest excursion? If so, continue by asking for "one long slow sniff." If successful, follow with "now do it more quietly," then "now do it more slowly," then "even more quietly," or "less effort," and so forth. By this time, the patient should be demonstrating an easy-onset, slower RR and a diaphragmatic pattern with relaxed shoulders.

Clinical experience has shown this technique to be highly successful with about 80% of patients who have primary pulmonary pathologies or neurological impairments. The key to success seems to stem from the relaxed tones and words that the therapist uses, which decrease anxiety and imply relaxation and not "effort." Once the pattern has been established, the patient can easily be instructed to go through the training independently, as needed. The sequence (in whole or in part) may be appropriate for patients before getting out of bed if they become anxious and demonstrate excessive upper chest breathing during this activity. For other patients, it may be appropriate before or during eating or before climbing stairs. Obviously, the application of this technique will be individualized for each patient, depending on individual impairments.

Procedure for Teaching Controlled Diaphragmatic Breathing (Scoop Technique)

Minimal patient instruction is necessary to facilitate diaphragmatic breathing using the scoop technique. It allows the patient to feel the breathing pattern; then it is brought to the patient's cognitive awareness. The patient then learns to self-cue to incorporate the breathing pattern.

The following is a suggested sequence:

1. Position the patient for success, generally side-lying in a semi-Fowler position or supine in a semi-Fowler position, with a bend in the knees to achieve a relative posterior pelvic tilt and relaxation of the abdominal muscles.
2. Place your hand on the patient's abdomen at the level of the umbilicus. Tell the patient you want to feel his or her breathing. Follow the patient's breathing pattern for a few cycles until you are in synchrony with his or her respiratory rhythm. Do not invade the patient's breathing pattern; rather, at first, follow its movement.
3. After the normal end of the patient's exhalation, give a slow stretch and "scoop" your hand up and under the anterior thorax as shown in Figure 23-4, *A*. Then ask the patient, "Now, breathe into my hand," as the slow scoop stretch is done.
4. As the scoop stretch is performed, instruct the patient to "breathe into my hand" during the inspiration. Give a scoop at the end of exhalation with each breath. The verbal command can be effectively replaced after a few respiratory cycles with the therapist's audible breathing to facilitate the ventilatory pattern.
5. After achieving some success, call the patient's attention to the awareness of the breathing pattern. For example, ask, "Can you feel how your abdomen rises as you breathe in and your ribs go up to the side?" The patient's hand can be placed on the abdomen with the therapist's hand on top. Reinforce the breathing pattern, then remove your hand and allow the patient to feel independently the ventilatory pattern (Figure 23-4, *B*).

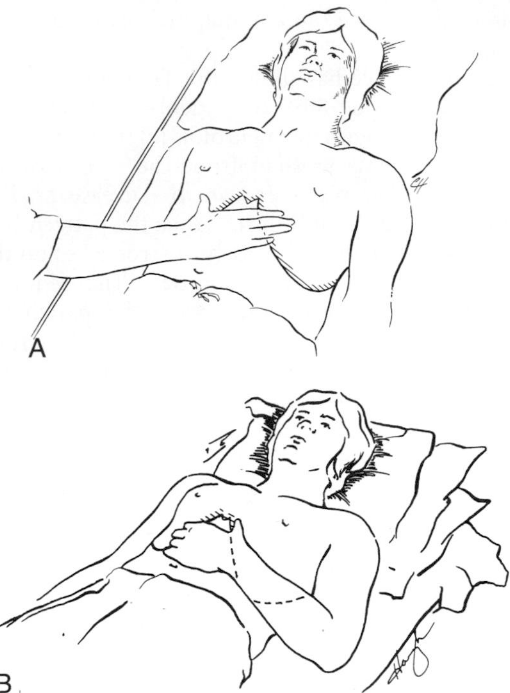

Fig. 23-4 Diaphragmatic breathing. **A,** Therapist's hand placement for diaphragmatic breathing. **B,** The patient is encouraged to continue practicing diaphragmatic breathing to become aware of his breathing pattern. This is usually the first position of the diaphragmatic breathing teaching sequence.

A few things should be taken into consideration. Don't ask patients to take too many deep breaths; they may begin to feel lightheaded because they may hyperventilate and blow off too much CO_2. The fact that they are breathing more with their diaphragms is the important consideration. Note also the position of the pelvis and trunk.

When the patient has mastered the breathing pattern in the side-lying position, try supine. Then progress to sitting (Figure 23-5, *A*), then standing (Figure 23-5, *B*), then walking (Figure 23-5, *C*) and, finally, stairs (Figure 23-5, *D*). Each position increases the difficulty in performing diaphragmatic breathing. In the side-lying or supine position, the patient is fully supported. The side-lying position is especially good for initial teaching of diaphragmatic breathing because the diaphragm is in a gravity-eliminated position. In the supine position, the patient must breathe against gravity. As he or she progresses to sitting, the patient must also provide trunk support and maintain stability against gravity, as well as relax the shoulders. In standing, the entire body must be supported, and when walking and stairs are added, the elements of breathing coordination, weight shifting, and balance increase the complexity of the activity.

Coordination of breathing for walking involves being careful not to allow the patient to hold the breath. It is important to keep inspiration and exhalation regular at a ratio of at least 1 to 1, preferably exhaling a little longer—1 to 2 or 1 to 4. In some yoga breathing techniques the exhalation is significantly longer—1 to 6, 1 to 8, or at times even longer.

In general, the preferred pattern for a patient with primary pulmonary dysfunction is as follows:

1. Have the patient pause at the base of the stairs to gain control.
2. Have the patient take a breath in and move up one step while exhaling.
3. The patient then pauses to inspire and exhales while walking up another step.
4. The patient should be encouraged to use the handrail and pace his or her movement slowly and with breath control.

A patient with neuromusculoskeletal issues who has lower extremity weakness may benefit from inspiration while ascending stairs and exhalation during descent. Going downstairs uses an eccentric muscle pattern, and exhalation is a relatively eccentric contraction of the diaphragm. Refer to the section on ventilatory and movement strategies in this chapter for additional information.

Lateral Costal Breathing

Lateral costal breathing also facilitates diaphragmatic excursion. It may be done bilaterally or unilaterally (Figure 23-6). Lower chest lateral costal expansion facilitates diaphragmatic and intercostal breathing in which the mid-chest recruits primarily intercostal activity.[29]

Upper Chest Inhibition

If all other manual facilitation interventions do not produce the desired increase in diaphragmatic breathing, inhibiting the upper chest during inhalation may be effective.

First, position the patient appropriately in a side-lying, three-quarter supine, or supine position. Begin by facilitating the diaphragm, usually with the diaphragm scoop. Slowly bring your other arm across the upper chest at about the level of the sternal angle. Leave it there for a couple of respiratory cycles without applying any pressure in order to feel the upper chest's movement.

After assessing this movement, gently allow your arm to follow the upper chest back to its resting position when the patient exhales. On the patient's next inspiratory effort, do not move your arm position. Thus your arm position will apply pressure or resistance to the expansion of the upper chest. This gentle pressure will cause postural inhibition to the anterior and superior movement of the upper chest. After each expiratory cycle, add more pressure until the patient subconsciously increases the lower chest breathing out of necessity.

When you note more diaphragmatic or lower intercostal muscle excursion, mention it to the patient. Ask the patient to try to reproduce this pattern. With your other arm, continue to facilitate the desired response, such as with the diaphragm scoop. Slowly, during each of the next series of inhalations, release your inhibition as the patient tries to maintain the improved lower chest-breathing pattern. If the patient is only partially successful, the inhibition can be partially reapplied to assist the patient. If the patient becomes anxious because the therapist's inhibition is preventing upper chest breathing, then decrease the inhibition to a comfortable level. This technique should never cause an increase in anxiety or it will only encourage more upper chest breathing rather than less. When the pressure is released on the upper chest, continue to facilitate diaphragmatic breathing and strive to have the patient do it independently.

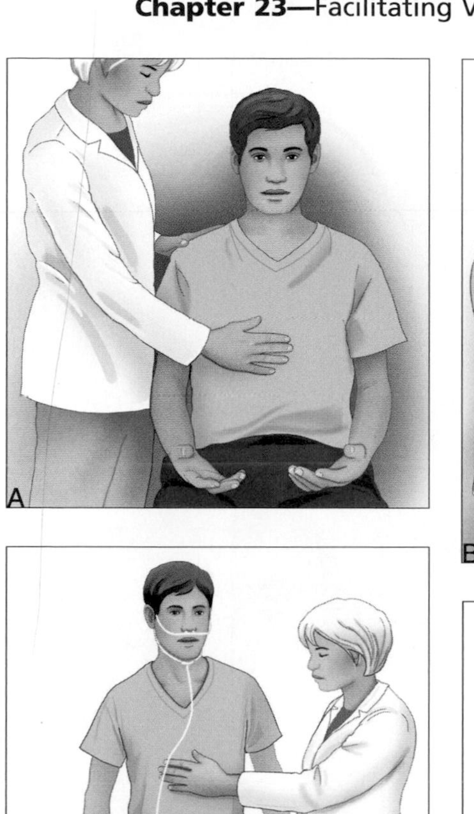
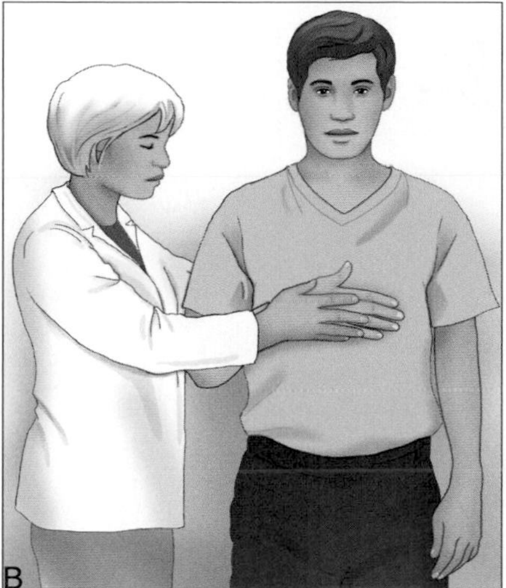
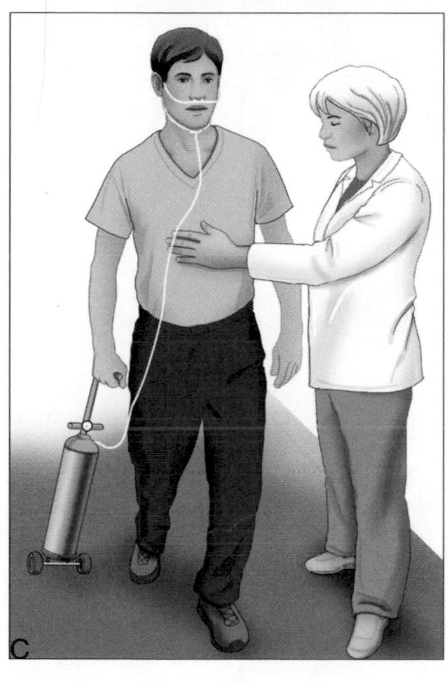
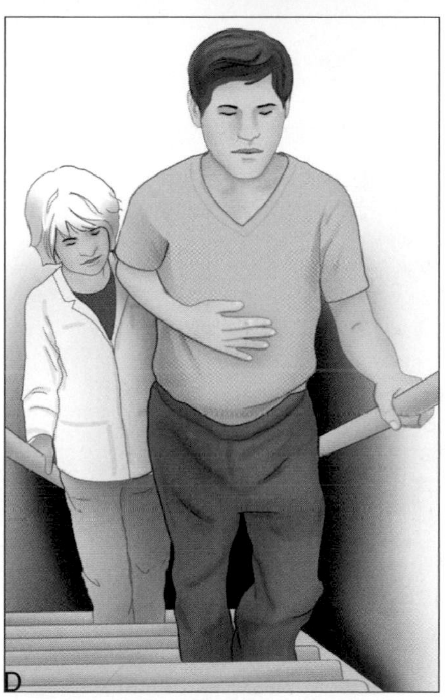

Fig. 23-5 Diaphragmatic breathing, supine. **A,** The patient advances to the sitting position for breathing retraining. Note the relaxed position of the patient's shoulders and hands. **B,** The third position in the sequence is standing. Full-length mirrors are helpful at this point. **C,** Walking is the fourth stage of retraining. The patient is encouraged to relax, control his breathing, take long steps, and slow down. **D,** Stairs are important, especially if the patient has them at home. He is instructed to pause slightly as he breathes in and to exhale as he climbs one to two steps.

Normal Timing

During normal quiet inspiration (controlled breathing), the diaphragm contracts, which is seen outwardly as a gentle rise of the abdomen. The second movement is seen as lateral costal expansion of the lower chest and, usually to a lesser extent, lower anterior chest expansion. Finally, the upper chest rises slightly, primarily in a superior-anterior plane, with less lateral expansion noted. A normal timing technique adapted from the physical therapy approach of proprioceptive neuromuscular facilitation (PNF) can help the patient work on this sequence. After the patient has learned to initiate inspiration with his or her diaphragm and lower chest wall muscles more consistently, this technique can help to put the whole sequence together. The diaphragm continues to be the primary mover, but the accessory muscles are encouraged to do what they should do, which is to assist the diaphragm for better overall ventilation.

Generally, the patient is positioned symmetrically in either a supine or a supported sitting position, with a neutral pelvic position. The therapist waits until the end of an expiratory cycle and then, using the hand placement of the diaphragm scoop, asks the patient to breathe in "here." With the other hand, the therapist moves up the chest wall to the lower sternum and touches the patient, giving instructions again to "now breathe here." Finally, the therapist uses the first hand to move up to the upper sternum (usually around the level of the sternal angle) and asks the patient to "now breathe here."

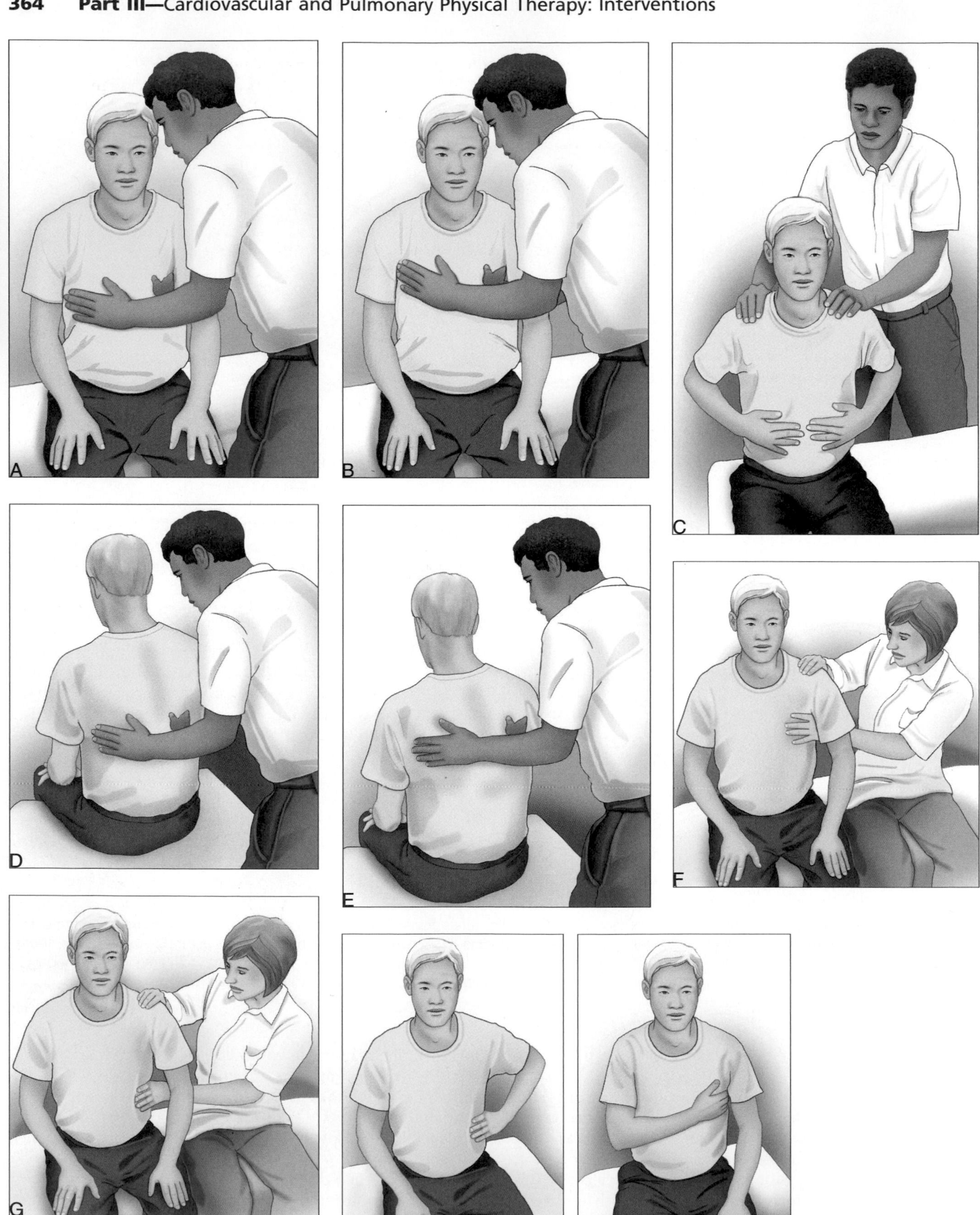

Fig. 23-6 A, Bilateral lower lobe expansion (this also facilitates diaphragmatic movement). **B,** Bilateral mid-chest expansion exercise. **C,** Self-assisted bilateral chest expansion exercise. Keep the patient's shoulders relaxed. **D,** Bilateral posterior chest expansion exercise. **E,** Bilateral posterior chest expansion exercise. **F,** Unilateral (segmental) breathing, left mid-lung field. **G,** Unilateral (segmental) breathing emphasizing the left lower lobe. Note that the patient's shoulder must remain down, with hands placed on ulnar border or palms up in his lap. **H,** The patient can perform unilateral (segmental) breathing by placing either hand on the side of the chest to be emphasized. The patient can also perform mid-chest expansion by moving the hand up.

It is important that the therapist smoothly transition from one hand to the next to assist the patient in developing a smooth motor transition from one area of the chest to the other. The manual cues provide tactile cueing rather than true motor facilitation. Because of this, the normal timing sequence is obviously a more advanced technique intended for use after success has been achieved in initial diaphragmatic training. It can address the functional need of the patient to take a quick deep breath in order to cough or a deeper breath in order to talk in longer sentences.

Mobilizing the Thorax

For some patients, controlled breathing alone may not alleviate inefficient ventilatory patterns, even with use of good positioning and appropriate ventilatory strategies. The thorax itself may be incapable of moving freely enough to allow for the adequate chest wall excursion necessary for that breathing pattern. For example, a patient with a spinal cord injury who is demonstrating an excessive diaphragmatic pattern that is unbalanced by the normal neuromuscular support of the intercostal and abdominal muscles can breathe using minimal chest wall expansion. This is often referred to as "belly breathing." It may be necessary to mobilize individual rib segments to gain the potential for chest wall expansion in all three planes of ventilation before facilitating a specific breathing pattern. If the potential for movement is not there, the breathing pattern cannot change. Likewise, a patient having primary pulmonary dysfunction and COPD, undergoing chest surgery, having chest tubes, or suffering from acute chest trauma may also find the rib cage stiff or sore and thus limited in its potential expansion. All these patients may benefit from the inclusion of rib cage mobilization in their therapy programs. The rib cage musculoskeletal limitation may be secondary to muscular atrophy or spasticity or to pain. Thus patients with either primary pulmonary dysfunction or secondary pulmonary dysfunction can benefit from the practice of chest mobilization.

It is beyond the scope of this textbook to detail all the numerous techniques involved in musculoskeletal mobilization of the thorax, but some simple techniques and suggestions for further study are presented. A summary of mobilization techniques is found in Box 23-7.

Box 23-7 Techniques to Mobilize the Thorax

- Use of towel rolls or pillows to mechanically open up the anterior or lateral chest wall
- Use of upper extremity patterns to facilitate the opening of individual rib segments
- Counter-rotation of the trunk
- Use of ventilatory-movement strategies to facilitate opening of the entire thorax
- Specific rib mobilization to free up an individual segment
- Myofascial release techniques to free up restrictive connective tissue on and around the thorax
- Soft-tissue release techniques to lengthen individual tight muscles

Once again, the therapist should note that the initial step toward achieving success is positioning. Starting with the patient in the supine position, anterior chest wall mobility can be improved by placing a vertical towel roll down the length of the thoracic spine and allowing gravity to pull the shoulders back to the bed. In this position, the anterior chest is opened up, stretching the intercostal and pectoralis muscles for easier facilitation of upper chest expansion.

In the side-lying position, the lateral aspect of the chest can be passively mobilized with gravity's assistance by placing one or more towel rolls or pillows under the lower chest (ribs 8 to 10) on the weight-bearing side. To determine an appropriate amount of side-bending, make sure that the patient's shoulder and pelvis are still in direct contact with the surface, even with the towel rolls in place. This maximizes the stretch of the chest without placing the patient in a position that is too advanced for his or her current chest wall mobility. Patients vary from tolerating only a single thin towel roll to tolerating three pillows under the lower ribs.

In both postures, active or passive stretching can be added after positioning for success. In the supine position, the patient is asked to move arms directly up over his or her head (shoulder flexion) as far as possible while watching his or her hands. Using the appropriate ventilatory strategy, the patient is also instructed to inhale during this movement. Because both full shoulder flexion and inspiration require the opening of the individual rib segments, pairing them in this gravity-assisted position promotes a greater passive chest wall stretch than either technique alone. If straight flexion is not a viable option, use a butterfly position, raising the arms up in shoulder flexion, abduction, and external rotation with elbows bent (like butterfly wings), again pairing this with voluntary maximal inspiration and upward eye gaze. Pairing inspiration and shoulder flexion maximizes the stretch on the chest and encourages better ventilatory strategies.

Ask the patient, who is in a side-lying position, to bring his or her arm up in straight flexion to maximize anterior chest expansion or to move the arm into abduction as a way of maximizing the lateral costal expansion. Pair either movement with inspiration and upward eye gaze. If upper extremity movement is not possible, passively use counter-rotation of the trunk to mobilize the chest while the patient is in the side-lying position over a towel or pillow. Continue to ask the patient to follow the movement with his or her eyes.

The same concepts can be used in upright postures, such as sitting or standing. Use a vertical towel roll along the thoracic spine, either along the back of a chair or wheelchair or along a wall. Move the patient's arms passively or actively up into the most extreme flexion or butterfly position possible. The patient will experience a more significant stretch in the anterior chest wall using the towel roll than without it. Precautions must be taken in patients with musculoskeletal problems along the spine and in patients with impaired skin tolerance.

If these general mobilization techniques do not produce enough chest wall mobility to allow freer breathing patterns to occur, more specific techniques must be considered, including the following:

- Specific rib mobilization
- Myofascial release of tight connective tissues (e.g., scar tissue secondary to areas of surgery or trauma)
- Soft tissue release in tight muscle groups (Note: Neurologically impaired patients often present with

tightness in the pectoralis, intercostal, and quadratus lumborum muscle groups, whereas orthopedically impaired patients tend to have more tightness in the neck and back muscles.)

Use the positioning and ventilatory strategies previously suggested (e.g., side-lying over a towel roll) during these specific interventions to maximize the potential gains in chest wall mobility. It is beyond the scope of this textbook to detail all the numerous techniques involved in musculoskeletal mobilization and release of the thorax. These three interventions are intended as suggestions for further study in other texts dealing primarily with musculoskeletal issues.

Facilitating Accessory Muscles in Ventilation

If the patient is still not demonstrating an optimal breathing pattern after experiencing appropriate positioning, appropriate ventilatory strategies, chest wall mobilization, and diaphragmatic retraining, specific facilitatory or inhibitory techniques should be initiated to stimulate the accessory muscles of ventilation. Specific techniques are discussed here in detail. A summary of interventions is listed in Box 23-8.

Because the diaphragm normally supplies the bulk of the inspired air during quiet breathing, diaphragmatic breathing is the preferred pattern of breathing. However, after certain neurological insults, strictly diaphragmatic breathing may not be possible or even preferred.[30] Unlike pulmonary rehabilitation programs for people with COPD or asthma, in which diaphragmatic breathing is almost always encouraged and use of accessory muscles discouraged, the restoration of independent, efficient breathing patterns for people with neurological impairment may require the regular use of accessory muscles.

Positioning continues to be the single most important aspect of all ventilatory facilitation techniques. If the patient is positioned for success, the probability of a successful response is much higher. By assessing the patient's head, upper extremity, trunk, pelvic, and lower extremity positions before every activity or technique, the therapist is empowered to use mechanical positioning and gravity to the patient's advantage rather than disadvantage. For example, a slightly posteriorly tilted pelvis tends to facilitate diaphragmatic breathing, whereas a slightly anteriorly tilted pelvis tends to facilitate upper chest breathing. Thus when the therapist is facilitating breathing with accessory muscles, the patient would be put in an advantageous posture by slightly tilting the pelvis anteriorly. In the supine position, this could be as simple as decreasing the amount of knee flexion that is present or using a small towel roll under the lumbar spine.

Box 23-8 Accessory Muscle Facilitation Techniques

1. Pectoralis facilitation
2. Sternocleidomastoid and scalenes facilitation
3. Trapezius facilitation
4. Diaphragm-inhibiting technique
   - Manual inhibition
   - Postural inhibition
5. Lateral costal facilitation
6. Serratus push-up

Pectoralis Facilitation

The pectoralis muscle group provides powerful anterior and lateral expansion of the upper chest and can substitute quite effectively for paralyzed intercostal muscles in the upper chest when trained to do so. Training usually begins in either a modified side-lying or a supine position. To increase the use of this muscle group during inspiration, the therapist should place his or her hand in the same direction as the contracting muscle fibers. Specific proprioceptive input is very important when facilitating a muscle, so make sure the hand is placed diagonally on the upper thorax (Figure 23-7).

The heel of the therapist's hand should be near the sternum and the fingers aligned up and out toward the shoulder in a diagonal pattern. The patient is asked to breathe into the therapist's hands while the therapist applies a quick manual stretch

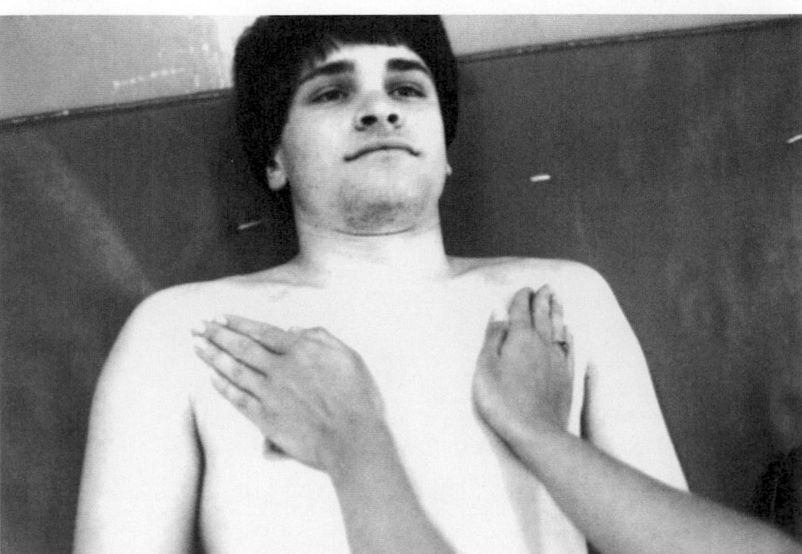

Fig. 23-7 Hand placement for facilitation of the pectoralis muscles for upper chest breathing.

(as in repeated contractions in techniques of PNF to the muscle fibers (down and in toward the sternum). This elicits the quick stretch reflex of the muscle and simultaneously provides added sensory input, which facilitates a stronger and more specific muscle contraction. To emphasize an increase in lateral expansion, facilitation should gradually be transferred from the sternal area out toward the therapist's fingertips by the patient's shoulder. The verbal cues are stronger and require more effort than the quieter verbal cues for diaphragmatic breathing.

Sternocleidomastoid and Scalene Facilitation

The same principle can be applied to the sternocleidomastoid and scalene muscles.[31] When the patient is in the supine position, the therapist need change only the angle of hand alignment to more specifically facilitate the sternocleidomastoid and scalene muscles. Turning the hands parallel to the trunk so that the fingers are pointing up toward the neck rather than pointing out toward the shoulder, the therapist applies the same quick stretch and uses the same verbal cues. The altered hand position now specifically facilitates the sternocleidomastoid and scalene muscles and secondarily influences the pectoralis muscles. The sternocleidomastoid and scalene muscles expand the chest primarily in a superior and anterior plane, whereas the pectoralis muscles expand the chest primarily in a lateral and anterior plane, thus accounting for the slight difference in the facilitation positioning.

Trapezius Facilitation

The trapezius muscle assists in superior expansion of the chest. Facilitation can be initiated in the supine or side-lying position to decrease the resistance of gravity. It can be progressed to an upright posture, in which the patient would have to work against gravity.

Placing the hands on top of the patient's shoulders, the therapist gives a quick stretch to the trapezius in a downward direction to facilitate a stronger elevation response. Repeated contractions can be added to facilitate the contraction throughout the full ROM. The shoulder-shrug motion should be paired with inhalation and upward eye gaze to maximize the facilitation response.

Inhibition of the Diaphragm

Two techniques are described to inhibit the excessive use of the diaphragm during inspiration. Ideally, the therapist is venturing to balance the use of accessory muscles—especially the intercostal, sternocleidomastoid, scalene, and trapezius muscles—with the diaphragm's contraction. This is done to prevent paradoxical movements of the chest, or worse, to prevent adverse musculoskeletal changes in the chest wall, such as pectus excavatum, which can result from muscle imbalance.

Inhibiting the diaphragm may be necessary during breathing retraining for some patients with spinal cord injuries, polio, spina bifida, developmental delays, head traumas, and cerebral palsy. The diaphragm may be too weak to produce an adequate TV or VC without the assistance of accessory muscles. In these cases the diaphragm-inhibiting technique is used to encourage the use of the accessory muscles to assist in independent voluntary ventilation. Patients learn to use their weakened diaphragm muscles in concert with intact accessory muscles. Not only does this allow for increased TV and VC, but it also may provide better aeration of all lung segments and better mobilization of the entire thorax.

An unusually strong diaphragm, acting without support from surrounding musculature, specifically the intercostals and abdominal muscles, may also need to be inhibited. For example, patients with paraplegia or lower-level tetraplegia with intact diaphragm but absent abdominal and intercostal muscles may demonstrate a paradoxical breathing pattern (see compensatory breathing patterns, Chapter 39). In this case, the accessory muscles must be encouraged to keep the diaphragm in check, attempting to avoid the development of a pectus excavatum. The goal of this breathing retraining method is to stop the paradoxical movements of the upper chest during inspiration by balancing the use of the upper and lower chest. In some cases, spastic intercostal muscles, found in some spinal cord injuries, may intercede to prevent this paradoxical movement by maintaining the upper chest's position during inspiration in spite of the negative pressure within the chest and gravity's influence on the chest. Balancing the movement of the chest should produce an increase in TV and VC potential and mobilize a greater portion of the chest.

To perform the diaphragm-inhibiting technique, the patient is positioned in a supine, semi-sitting, or side-lying position, with the top arm positioned overhead or pulled back at the waist to open up the upper chest. If the patient can tolerate it, pillows are removed from under his or her head, the pelvis tilted anteriorly, and airway safety is assessed by checking to see whether the patient can still swallow comfortably. The heel of the therapist's hand is placed lightly on the patient's abdomen at about the level of the umbilicus. No instructions are given to the patient at this point. As the patient begins to exhale a normal breath of air, the therapist gently allows the heel of his or her hand to move up and in toward the central tendon of the patient's diaphragm (see Figure 23-4). When the expiration of that breath is complete, the therapist strictly maintains the hand position in that shortened expiratory position. During the following inspiratory phase, the diaphragm will experience some gentle resistance to its inferior descent, causing inhibition to its full ROM. On the next expiration, the technique is repeated, with the therapist carefully pushing the heel of his or her hand further up and in, maintaining greater inhibition during each inspiratory phase. After two or three ventilatory cycles, a patient usually begins subconsciously to alter his or her breathing pattern to include more upper chest expansion in order to reconcile the diaphragm's transient inability to produce enough chest expansion to yield an adequate TV. The therapist should carefully observe which accessory muscles the patient spontaneously chooses. Are they used symmetrically? What is the general quality of the movement? Is the onset harsh or smooth? Does the patient appear fatigued or uncoordinated?

It is not until this point that the therapist should verbally acknowledge any alteration of the patient's breathing pattern. Without changing the hand position, the therapist tells the patient what he or she observed that is encouraging about the new breathing pattern (e.g., balance between upper and lower chest expansion or less paradoxical motion of the sternum). Then the patient is asked whether he or she notices any difference from before, bringing this breathing pattern to a conscious level. Only after some orientation to this pattern, usually no more than four to six breathing cycles in the full inhibiting pattern, should the therapist begin gradually to release the pressure being applied.

While slowly releasing pressure with each cycle of inspiration, the therapist asks the patient to try reproducing the desired pattern cognitively. It should take the same number of cycles to release the pressure as it did to apply it. This technique easily allows for gradations of inhibition, from full inhibition, when the patient is forced to use upper accessory muscles or risk becoming short of breath, to a barely proprioceptive reminder to change his or her breathing pattern. It also allows for gradation of inhibition while the patient is learning to assume control over the new breathing pattern. If, during the releasing phase of this technique, the patient begins to lose control over the new pattern, the therapist can gently reapply some pressure during the next expiratory phase to help the patient regain that control. At that point, the therapist can release or reapply pressure as necessary until the desired pattern is obtained and full release of pressure is acceptable.

This technique is particularly effective in patients who are having difficulty cognitively altering their own breathing patterns, such as small children, brain-damaged patients, or slow motor learners, because it requires no cognitive effort until success has already been achieved. Extra care must be taken to avoid initiating any applied pressure quickly because of the likelihood of eliciting unwanted abdominal contractions or spasticity[32] or eliciting a stronger diaphragmatic contraction resulting from the quick stretch reflex. The technique should never be painful. The therapist must keep his or her hand on the abdomen, not the rib cage, to properly influence the diaphragm. This technique can be progressed by changing postures, which requires greater trunk control. Can the patient still maintain the overall pattern? Can the patient breathe without paradoxical movements against gravity?

The second technique is for the more advanced patient and simply presents a physical block to diaphragmatic excursion. The patient is positioned in a prone-on-elbows position (Figure 23-8, *A*). In patients who are most severely impaired neurologically, the lower chest will be in direct contact with the surface, so lower anterior and inferior expansion is inhibited and lateral costal expansion is limited. The upper chest is positioned in extension and the upper extremities are fixed, optimizing the length-tension relationship of the anterior and superior accessory muscles for easy facilitation. In addition, anterior excursion of the upper chest is now in a gravity-assisted posture. Through the use of head and neck patterns, such as in PNF diagonals, or the use of static-dynamic activities, such as in weight shifting to one supporting limb while reaching out with the other extremity, the therapist can readily facilitate greater upper chest breathing (Figure 23-8, *B*). Therapists can use these same patterns to achieve other goals, such as increased head and neck control, increased shoulder stability, or increased upper body balance. Thus by helping patients to coordinate movement goals with ventilatory patterns, it becomes more likely that patients will incorporate these patterns functionally into their daily activities. This is the ultimate goal of any ventilatory retraining procedure.

The manual diaphragm-inhibiting technique is usually less threatening to the patient than is the prone-on-elbows inhibition technique. Prone-on-elbows position can inhibit the diaphragm so completely for neurological patients lacking spinal extensors that they become extremely short of breath. Consequently, do not position the patients in this more demanding posture until success appears likely.

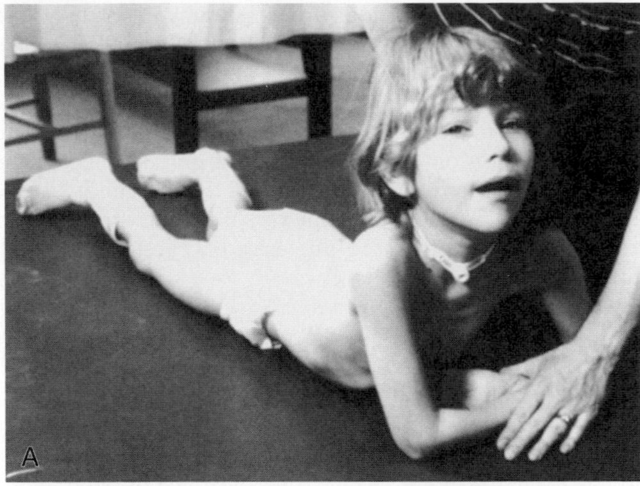

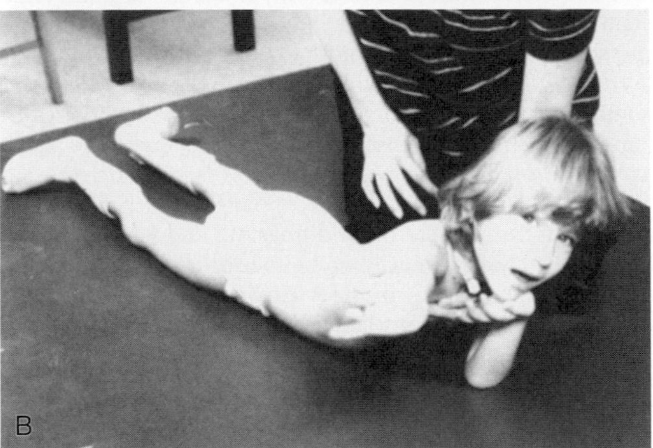

Fig. 23-8 A, Diaphragm inhibiting in prone-on-elbows position. **B,** Static-dynamic upper extremity activities in prone-on-elbows position to encourage upper chest accessory muscle participation.

Serratus Push-Up

Facilitating greater posterior chest expansion can be achieved in a prone-on-elbows position. Gravity is now assisting anterior excursion of the chest and resisting posterior excursion. To emphasize the serratus anterior muscle's role in posterior expansion, the patient is instructed to perform an upper body push-up (with or without the therapist's assistance). The serratus anterior muscle causes lateral scapular movement, thereby facilitating maximal posterior excursion of the thorax. The patient is instructed to take in a deep breath during the push-up and to exhale the air (passively or forcefully) when returning to the starting position. Forceful exhalation in this activity can be used as a forerunner to effective cough retraining. Gentle or controlled exhalation can be used to encourage greater breath support for vocalization or for eccentric trunk muscle training.

Emphasizing posterior chest expansion during inhalation is the only occasion in which inspiration should be paired with trunk flexion. In all other inspiratory situations, inspiration is paired with trunk extension and exhalation is paired with trunk flexion.

Patients with Asymmetrical Dysfunction

Patients with asymmetrical weakness need a different approach from the controlled or upper chest breathing patterns presented previously.[33] These patients need facilitation of the weaker side to promote symmetrical chest wall expansion in both the upper and lower chest. A summary of techniques is listed in Box 23-9.

Symmetrical Positioning

Symmetrical ventilatory patterns may be effortlessly achieved by altering the patient's position in each posture to maximize the chest wall's potential to move in a symmetrical pattern. This is especially true in an upright position, in which asymmetry is generally more pronounced. For example, a patient with hemiplegia may lean toward the involved side when sitting because of weakness or spasticity. Likewise, after thoracic surgery, a patient with primary pulmonary impairment may lean toward the surgical side to splint the area in order to avoid the pain caused by chest movement around the incision and the chest tubes. Both situations cause asymmetrical breathing patterns and decrease ventilation on the involved side. Improving chest wall alignment may alleviate the ventilatory deficit on the involved side. This may be achieved by the use of towel rolls or pillows to support the affected side as well as by good pain management postoperatively.

Postural Inhibition

For some patients, more aggressive positioning must be used to achieve greater chest wall excursion and ventilation on the involved side. This can be accomplished by inhibiting the chest wall movements on the uninvolved, or stronger, side. Usually, the best position in which to achieve this inhibition is side-lying. When the patient lies on his or her uninvolved side, with arms positioned below 90 degrees of shoulder flexion, lateral chest expansion into that side becomes inhibited because of the physical barrier. This forces the patient to find another way to meet his or her ventilatory needs, which indirectly facilitates chest expansion on the opposite side (the uppermost side). The therapist can then supply sensory and motor input through his or her hands to the patient's upper, middle, or lower chest on the involved or weaker side to facilitate increased ventilation on that side. Early in the rehabilitation process or soon after thoracic surgery, the patient may have difficulty performing lateral chest expansion against gravity when in a side-lying position (gravity-resisted movement). If so, place the patient in a three-quarter supine position to lessen the workload imposed by gravity. Gradually, work the patient up to a full side-lying posture to achieve the greatest strengthening benefits.

Timing for Emphasis

Another technique to promote symmetrical chest wall movements is performed in numerous postures, such as supine, sitting, or standing. The therapist places his or her hand symmetrically on the lower lateral chest wall, on the mid-chest, or on the upper anterior chest wall. At the end of exhalation, the therapist gives a quick stretch to the muscles being touched so as to facilitate a deep inspiratory effort in that area of the chest. Immediately after both sides begin to move into an inspiratory pattern, the therapist manually blocks (or inhibits) expansion of the chest on the stronger side while giving continued quick stretches to the weaker side. This facilitates greater expansion on the weak side by means of an overflow response. This technique, adapted from the PNFs timing-for-emphasis technique, uses the strength of the stronger side to facilitate movement on the weaker side. It can be applied to any area of the chest where symmetrical movements should be the norm.

Reducing Respiratory Rates

In addition to altering breathing patterns through facilitation and inhibition techniques, reducing RRs may also be necessary before arriving at an efficient breathing pattern for some patients. See Box 23-10 for a summary of techniques. Many patients with neurological impairment who have high neuromuscular tone increase their RRs to compensate for a decrease in their TVs or because of brainstem impairments that affect the respiratory centers. In addition, many patients who are anxious, such as people with asthma and those who have orthopedic or surgical conditions and are experiencing pain, may also demonstrate excessively high RRs. Attempting to restore ventilatory efficiency may require increasing TV while concurrently decreasing RR.

Box 23-9 Promoting Symmetrical Ventilatory Function for Patients with Asymmetrical Deficits

- Use of positioning to achieve more symmetrical alignment of the chest and trunk in both reclining and upright postures
- Use of postural inhibition of the stronger, or uninvolved, side to promote greater chest wall expansion on the weaker, or involved, side
- Timing-for-emphasis technique to promote active symmetrical breathing anywhere in the thorax

Box 23-10 Techniques to Reduce High Respiratory Rates

1. Previous techniques that increased tidal volume
2. Counter-rotation technique
3. Butterfly technique in sitting
   - Straight planes
   - Counter-rotation
4. Relaxed pursed-lips breathing with inspiratory and expiratory pauses

The techniques described in this chapter promote an increase in TV by improving the overall ventilatory patterns and often cause a secondary reduction in RR. Interventions such as PLB and repatterning, mobilization of the thorax, and upper chest breathing facilitation for neurologically impaired patients are often helpful in accomplishing slower, deeper, more controlled breathing.

Counter-Rotation

The technique described next has been developed specifically to promote a lower RR and improvement of chest wall mobility. The counter-rotation technique may help to reduce high neuromuscular tone and increase thoracic mobility, thus often resulting in an increase in TV and a simultaneous reduction in RR. This intervention is extremely effective for the following:

- Patients with decreased cognitive functioning after a neurological insult or after surgery
- Very young children (because verbal cues cannot be used)
- Patients with high neuromuscular tone

As described in Chapter 22, counter-rotation also can be easily adapted as a very effective assisted-cough technique. One medical contraindication for this technique, because of its rotary nature, is bony instability of the spine.

In bed or on a mat, place the patient in a side-lying position with knees bent and arms resting comfortably out in front of the head and shoulders. In this technique, the higher the upper extremities can be placed within a comfort zone, the better the result. Relaxed positioning of the patient is essential to the success of this technique, so the patient should be positioned in an open yet comfortable position. Normalizing neuromuscular tone is the first step in attempting to decrease a high RR. Patient discomfort is likely to elicit increased tone and an increased RR.

The therapist's own position is also important because it directs the force that is applied to the patient's chest. Initially, the therapist should stand behind the patient, perpendicular to the patient's trunk. If the patient is lying on the left side, the therapist places his or her left hand on the patient's shoulder and the hand on the patient's hip. The therapist then leaves the hands in place and simply follows the patient's respiratory cycle. This allows the therapist to assess the patient's subjective rate and rhythm and the patient's overall neuromuscular tone. Only after this assessment should the clinician begin the active phase of the technique. Using a PNF technique called rhythmic initiation, the patient is gently log-rolled in a small ROM in the side-lying position. The rolling is gradually increased achieving more ROM from side-lying toward prone. This progression of movement generally reduces high tone, which usually makes the second phase of the technique more effective.

During this phase, the therapist should audibly duplicate the patient's RR. As the patient moves into greater rolling ROM and begins to slow his or her RR, the therapist needs to use the patient's audible cuing as a facilitator for establishing a slower RR. Thus the therapist begins by having the patient establish the audible RR; then the therapist slowly takes over. Audible cues can be very strong facilitators of ventilatory rhythms.

The second phase requires the therapist to slowly change position. Transitioning to a diagonal posture, the therapist then stands or half-kneels behind the patient near his or her hips, turning to a diagonal position until facing the patient's head at roughly a 45-degree angle. Here the hand placement begins to get more specific. Assume again that the patient is side-lying on the left. At the beginning of the expiratory cycle, the therapist's left hand slowly glides over the patient's shoulder on the right pectoral region, with care being taken not to unintentionally use the thumb or finger tips; the right hand slowly glides back to the patient's right gluteal fossa (the hollow of the buttocks) (see Figure 22-6, *A*). The therapist can then manually compress the rib cage on all three planes of ventilation at the end of exhalation by gently pulling the shoulder back and down, while simultaneously pushing the hip up and forward. This movement promotes more complete exhalation.

When the patient begins the next inspiration, the therapist switches hand placement to capitalize on the improved potential for TV. The therapist's left hand slides back to the patient's right scapula, and the right hand slides forward just anterior to the patient's right iliac crest (see Figure 22-96, *B*). As the patient inhales, the therapist slowly stretches the chest to maximize inspiration TVs. The therapist's left hand pushes the scapula (or the thorax if the scapula is unstable) up and away from the spine, and the right hand pulls the pelvis back and down to maximize all three planes of ventilation, resulting in greater inspiration. The therapist should use the flat or heel of the hand whenever possible to avoid unintentional patient discomfort and to maximize the facilitated area.

Initially, the therapist begins and ends the respiratory cycle according to the patient's RR. However, as the patient's tone is relaxed and increased TVs are promoted by the effects of counter-rotation, the therapist gradually slows down the rate of rotation, giving the patient audible breathing cues to further facilitate a slower RR. The patient generally accommodates to a slower RR as the therapist gains more control over the patient's breathing pattern. With many patients, the results can be marked. If the patient can cognitively follow commands, he or she can be alerted to this change and encouraged to assist in voluntarily breathing at the slower rate.

The therapist can progress the technique by decreasing the manual input. The last facilitation to be removed should be the audible cues. As with the diaphragm-inhibiting technique, the therapist can reestablish control quickly if need be by simply reapplying stronger manual input. If the patient has an extremely fast RR (i.e., 50 to 60 breaths/min), the facilitation can be applied every two to three breaths to avoid fatiguing the patient or therapist.

It should be apparent that this technique need not be used exclusively for respiratory goals but rather can be incorporated into a patient's total rehabilitation program. It is a natural precursor to active rolling; it can also be used as a vestibular stimulator.

Butterfly Technique

If a patient has good motor control, an upright version of this technique may be appropriate. In unsupported sitting, stand behind or in front of the patient, depending on his or her balance needs, and ask the patient to bring the arms up into a butterfly posture (or assist the patient to bring the arms into this posture). Starting from a comfortable ROM position for that patient, begin to breathe audibly in time with the patient's

RR. When the patient inhales, raise the arms up into slightly more shoulder flexion. When the patient exhales, lower the arms slightly. Slowly begin to move in greater and greater increments of range, while breathing loudly with your patient. Through your audible breathing cues, begin to "ask" your patient to slow down the RR and take deeper slower breaths. The use of the following concurrent ventilatory strategies promotes deeper inhalations and exhalations: (1) shoulder flexion and trunk extension paired with inspiration; and (2) shoulder extension and trunk flexion paired with exhalation. Thus it becomes possible for the patient to increase TV and decrease RR.

As in the previous technique, the therapist begins by breathing loudly at the patient's respiratory rate and transitions to breathing audibly at a slower, more desirable pace. The patient picks up on this subtle cue and subconsciously reduces his or her own RR, even if unable to follow verbal commands.

This technique can be modified to encourage more intercostal and oblique abdominal muscle contractions by using a diagonal rather than a straight plane of movement. Have the patient look up and over one shoulder as he or she breathes in and brings arms up and behind the head. Then have the patient look down and away toward the opposite knee while breathing out and bringing arms down to the opposite knee (Figure 23-9).

Relaxed pursed-lips breathing can also be incorporated into the previously described techniques to reduce RR. By prolonging the expiratory phase through pursed lips, the patient secondarily decreases his or her RR automatically.

Glossopharyngeal Breathing

A small number of patients with neurological impairments require more than just promoting the use of accessory muscles or changing RR to meet basic ventilatory needs.[34] In the past decade, more people experiencing high-level SCIs (above C4) have survived the initial trauma because of advances in medical technology. The therapist in the rehabilitation setting is then faced with the difficult task of restoring quality of life. For these patients, as well as many older adult polio patients, mastery of the glossopharyngeal breathing (GPB) technique allows for greater voluntary ventilation, which many patients say improves the quality of their lives. This augmented

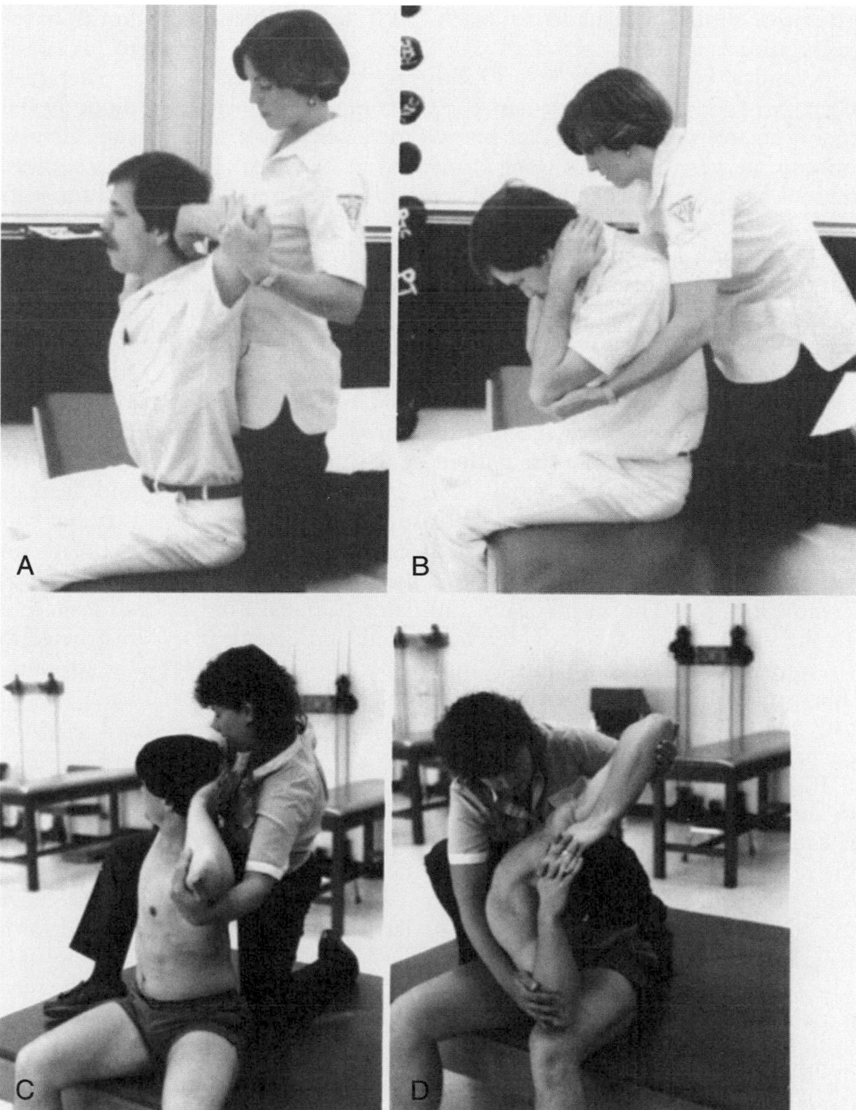

Fig. 23-9 A, Butterfly technique facilitating inspiration. **B,** Butterfly technique facilitating exhalation. **C,** Butterfly with trunk rotation facilitating inspiration. All three planes of respiration are stretched on the patient's right side. **D,** Butterfly with trunk rotation facilitating exhalation. All planes are compressed on the right side.

breathing pattern allows patients to regain some control over their lives and to regain control over their ventilation, which was lost as a result of severe neurological insult.

GPB is a technique developed in the 1950s by polio patients looking for a way to reduce their dependence on the iron lung for ventilation. It was found that by using the lips, soft palate, mouth, tongue, pharynx, and larynx, a patient could actually inhale enough air to sustain life without mechanical ventilation. Only intact cranial nerves are required. This method is sometimes referred to as "frog breathing" because it uses the principles of inspiration common to the frog. The patient learns to create a pocket of negative pressure within the buccal cavity (mouth) by maximizing that internal space, thereby causing the outside air to rush in. At that point, the patient closes off the entrance (the lips) and proceeds to force the air back and down the throat with a stroking maneuver of the tongue, pharynx, and larynx.

Research has shown consistently that use of this technique in patients who have severe neurological impairment can increase pulmonary functions significantly, especially TV and VC. If GPB is the only means of ventilation possible when a patient has been disconnected from a ventilator or phrenic nerve stimulator, mastery of this technique is critical to the patient's survival in case of mechanical or electrical failure. All attempts should be made to teach GPB to this patient population.

A clinical example may help to illustrate the usefulness of GPB. A 14-year-old male sustained a C1 complete SCI while racing in front of a train. After he was medically stable, two phrenic nerve stimulators were implanted in his chest. The patient had no unassisted means of ventilation. Neuromuscularly, the patient had limited use of one trapezius, the sternocleidomastoid, and intrinsic neck muscles. The patient and family worried that long-term nursing home placement would be inevitable because of their fear that his phrenic nerve stimulator would malfunction or a battery would wear out, causing immediate respiratory distress. The family believed it could not bear the psychological burden placed on them if the patient went home to live. GPB instruction was suggested and was begun slowly because the patient stated that he learned motor skills slowly. After a painstaking 2-month period, the patient learned to breathe without the use of his phrenic nerve stimulator for 3 to 5 minutes before becoming fatigued and hypoventilating. Within the next 1 to 2 months, he learned to breathe for up to 2 hours off of his stimulator, using GPB only. To the staff's surprise, he even learned to talk and operate his sip-and-puff wheelchair while using GPB. The patient was then successfully discharged to his home. This was not the only factor considered in his discharge planning, but it was perhaps the most significant.

Instruction in GPB takes time and concentration. It is best to start off in small time blocks of 10 to 15 minutes because it can be very fatiguing. However, for successful learning of the technique, it is also important that the patient get consistent, preferably daily, training. Once the patient has mastered the technique, practice sessions can be lengthened considerably, and the patient can be taught self-monitoring techniques. The specific goals of GPB training must be explained to the patient before the beginning of treatment in order to gain his or her support and cooperation. In addition to providing the ventilator- or stimulator-dependent patient with a TV necessary for gaining independence from mechanical assists, GPB has many other benefits. For the patient with tetraplegia who has a partially intact diaphragm (C3 to C4) or the loss of essential accessory muscles (C5 to C8), GPB can accomplish the following:

- Increase VC to produce a more effective cough
- Assist in a longer and stronger phonation effort
- Act as an internal mobilizer of the chest wall

The muscles used in this technique do not have the same internal proprioceptive, sensory, or visual feedback mechanisms as the trunk and limb muscles, so necessary adjustments in the technique are sometimes difficult to perceive. The patient cannot see his or her tongue pushing the air back or truly feel the pharynx swallowing the air into the lungs, so the therapist's external feedback system is very influential. Use of a mirror can greatly enhance the visual component of feedback. Small changes, like adjustments in posture or the suggestion of another sound to imitate, may be all that is needed for the patient to learn the stroking maneuver correctly. Success in GPB can be assessed objectively with a spirometer and a pulse oximeter. For patients incapable of breathing independently, any TV reading will indicate successful intake of air. For patients who are not ventilator dependent, a VC reading that is greater than 5% over the baseline indicates successful use of GPB. Patients with low-level tetraplegia (C5 to C8) have demonstrated increases in VC by as much as 70% to 100%.

Therapists can monitor their own successes with this technique by taking VC readings with and without GPB or by subjective analyses. Maximal inhalation, followed by three or four successful GPB strokes, will cause a feeling that the chest will burst if an attempt is made to inhale more air. Likewise, the sensation of "needing to cough" is another subjective indication of successful GPB. Conversely, a feeling of indigestion is usually indicative that air has been swallowed into the stomach instead of the lungs.

During the initial treatment session, the therapist demonstrates several times what a stroking maneuver looks like, giving the patient an idea of the motion required. The therapist continues to mimic the pattern as the patient attempts to duplicate it. This gives the patient an active model to mimic and decreases feelings of uneasiness surrounding the necessary but somewhat silly facial grimaces. If the patient is able to breathe independently, his or her ability to breath-hold and to close off the nasal passageway should be checked because air leakage is a common cause of failure. The patient is then instructed to take in a maximal inspiration before attempting the stroking maneuvers in order to eliminate the possibility of using other accessory muscles during the technique.

If possible, the patient is positioned in an upright or at least a symmetrical position. Specifically, the patient is instructed to bring the jaws down and then forward as if reaching the bottom lip up for a carrot dangling just in front and above the upper lip (Figure 23-10, *A*). Slight cervical hyperextension is necessary to allow for maximal temporal mandibular joint (TMJ) excursion. (A contraindication for this technique is a TMJ disorder.) The lips should be shaped as if they were making the sound *oop*. The patient is then told to close the mouth, reaching the bottom lip up to the top lip (Figure 23-10, *B*). The tongue and jaw are drawn back toward the throat, with the mouth and tongue formed as though saying *up* or *ell* (see Figure 23-10, *B*). The lower jaw moves in a roughly rectangular pattern. Most patients learn the stroking

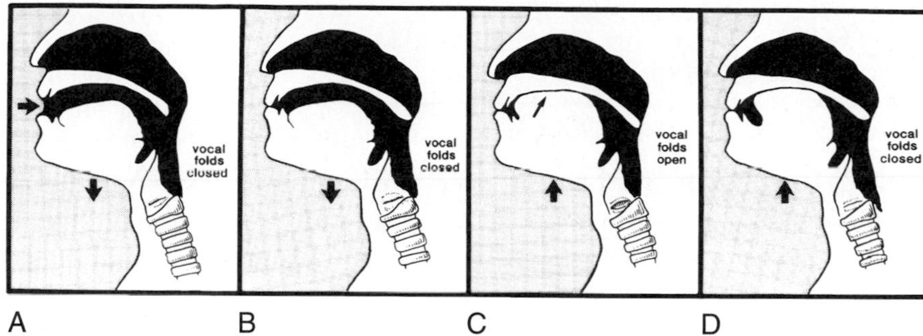

Fig. 23-10 Glossopharyngeal breathing. **A,** Mouth opened to draw in air. **B,** Jaw closed to entrap the air. **C,** Air pushed back with tongue into trachea. **D,** Vocal folds closed to prevent passive air leaks. Entire maneuver is then repeated.

Box 23-11 Common Problems in GPB Instruction

- An open nasal passage or glottis that allows the air to escape
- A feeling of indigestion, indicating that the air is being swallowed into the esophagus rather than the trachea
- Incorrect shape of the mouth as the air is being drawn in (usually not puckered enough)
- Uncoordinated backward movement of the tongue
- Inadequate jaw mobility, TMJ dysfunction, or decreased cervical ROM;
- Incorrect sounds while performing the technique, such as the word *gulp* or the sound *em*

maneuvers by making the sounds; as they become more proficient, the sounds and excessive head and neck motions diminish. Often, the students (patients) outperform the teachers (therapists) because through consistent use, they learn all of the technique's finer subtleties.

Although this technique can be broken down into several stages, as it has been here for the purpose of description, most of the literature cautions the therapist against doing so.[35] Simple, minimal instructions seem to accomplish more, perhaps because the continuity of movement is so essential to the success of the inhalation. Specific instructions can be given later if necessary.

Common problems encountered with GPB instruction can be found in Box 23-11. Avoiding any instruction for the tongue seems to produce better results. Concentrate on assisting the patient in learning the external physical movements.

Tolerance of GPB can be increased when mastery of a single stroke becomes consistent. For patients using it as an assist to their own voluntary ventilation, three to four strokes on top of a maximal inspiration is usually sufficient. Ventilator- or stimulator-dependent patients may need to use as many as 10 to 14 strokes per breath. These figures should be used only as rough guidelines. Each patient will use a slightly different technique and a different number of strokes; the only important factor is a method that works for the individual. Fatigue after long trials of GPB can be monitored effectively by an oximeter. The oxygen saturation level should stay above 90% to maintain adequate PaO_2 levels. For example, if the patient begins the GPB session with an oxygen saturation level in the upper 90s, fatigue can be monitored and anticipated by watching to see whether the oxygen level decreases. If the level begins to fall to the mid-90s and then the low 90s, you can anticipate when they will reach 90%. At that point, end the GPB training and put the patient back on the previous ventilatory support system. Pulse oximetry not only allows for accurate monitoring but also provides an objective means of monitoring progress over time. In addition, a spirometer objectively measures improvements in using GPB. It gives the patient concrete indications of success or failure in mastering the technique.

Enhancing Vocalization Skills

In contrast to procedures that assist a patient in inhalation, procedures intended to improve a patient's phonation skill must focus on elongating the expiration phase. Coughing is a gross-motor skill that relies more on force than on fine control of the ventilatory muscles for its effectiveness. Conversely, phonation requires precise, fine-motor control of these muscles and demands that the vocal folds provide a consistent air flow through the larynx. Both are expiration activities and they depend on the preceding inspiration for optimal performance; however, coughing uses concentric contractions of the expiratory muscles to force the air out, whereas quiet talking uses primarily eccentric contractions of the inspiratory muscles to slowly release the air during expiration. Because of these differences, procedures to improve coughing and phonation are different in focus. Considering the relationship between speaking and breathing and the concepts of shared respiratory control, it is notable that speaking can lead to shortness of breath and shortness of breath can alter speaking ability.[36] Previous discussions of posture and use of abdominal binders in patients with spinal cord injury should also be considered when speaking is impaired.[37] A summary of techniques is listed in Box 23-12. Coughing is covered in detail in Chapter 22.

Because the patient's TV and total inspiratory capacity are the power source for phonation, they become important concerns in a phonation program. Generally, a normal TV is adequate for conversational speech. However, larger volumes of air, thus greater inspiratory capacities, are required for singing, loud talking, or professional speaking. Therefore the breathing pattern facilitation techniques described earlier in this chapter are ideal for use before instructing the patient in better expiration control. For example, facilitating diaphragmatic and accessory-muscle breathing techniques, along with the use of quick stretches or repeated contractions, can facilitate the desired deeper inhalation.

Box 23-12 Enhancing Vocalization Skills through Increased Breath Support

1. Position to achieve a neutral chin tuck and optimal vocal fold alignment
2. Manual techniques
   - Vibration or shaking
   - Percussion or tapping
3. Eccentric resistance
   - Agonistic reversal technique
   - Functional resistance
4. Verbal techniques to refine breath support
   - Singing and whistling
   - Games
   - Wind or brass instruments
   - Stopping and starting vocalizations

Positioning Concerns

Consistent with all previous techniques, the first aspect of improving breath support for vocalization is to optimize the patient's position. The vocal folds have an ideal muscle length-tension relationship when the head is in a neutral chin tuck. In addition, an open anterior chest wall allows for the greatest potential for chest wall excursion and thus the largest VC. Use the previously described suggestions for positioning to determine whether a particular patient needs positioning to encourage a more diaphragmatic, upper chest, or unilateral breathing pattern.

Manual Techniques

Several simple techniques can be used to improve eccentric control of the diaphragm and intercostal muscles in preparation for speech. Vibration or shaking of the lower chest during expiration helps to produce a slower, more controlled recoil of the diaphragm. Why this occurs is not fully understood. It may be that the sensory and proprioceptive stimulation that the vibration or shaking provides augments the patient's concentration on those muscles, resulting in longer phonation. The patient is instructed to phonate an *ah* or *oh* sound for as long as possible. The therapist simultaneously vibrates the patient's chest with an even and gentle force throughout and slightly beyond the full expiration phase, placing his or her hands on the lateral costal borders of the thorax, the midchest, or the pectoral area, depending on which area of the chest needs the most help in controlling exhalation. This is very different from the rapid, forceful pressure that is applied to the patient's chest when promoting a deep cough. Be certain that the patient understands this important difference. Emphasize that the patient should not let air escape before vocalizing and should try to keep voice intensity consistent throughout the procedure. This will promote slow, eccentric release of the inspiratory muscles during the entire course of the vocalization. Progress can be readily monitored by timing the patient's vocalization before, during, and after this technique. About 10 to 12 seconds of vocalization at 8 to 10 syllables per breath is generally considered adequate for functional use in speech.

For a child, this technique can be modified. The child is asked to say *ah* or *oh* for as long as possible while the therapist percusses or taps lightly with his or her hands on the child's upper or lower chest so as to produce a series of staccato sounds. Usually, a child enjoys the new sound that this makes and tries repeatedly to phonate longer and louder to accentuate the different intensities. Therapeutically, this requires the child to take a deeper inhalation before vocalizing, followed by an elongated expiratory phase, both of which are necessary for functional speech. As the child becomes more adept at it, the therapist can apply more pronounced clapping over the chest, accomplishing a wider range of voice intensities and doubling as a means of percussion for postural drainage.

Eccentric Resistance Techniques

More specific facilitation can be used to increase breath support. Ideally, the patient is positioned symmetrically in a supine or supported-sitting position, allowing for maximal chest wall expansion. The patient is instructed to visualize his or her chest being pulled up toward the ceiling and held there. Next, the patient is told to vocalize slowly, trying not to let the chest "fall." Meanwhile, the therapist is applying consistent pressure to the patient's chest to try to force a quicker exhalation. The patient is told to resist this motion by trying to control and prolong expiration. As with the antagonistic reversal technique described in PNF, the therapist is resisting the patient's attempt to eccentrically contract and control the trunk muscles. This strengthens the eccentric phase of exhalation and promotes greater breath control for vocalization.

The same concept can be applied to functional tasks. Moving into gravity (i.e., coming down to sitting from a standing posture, lying down from a sitting posture, or bringing an arm down from reaching into a high cabinet) requires eccentric control of the muscles involved in the activity in order to slow the body's descent into gravity's influence. Because quiet speech uses a similar muscular contraction, teaching the patient to count out loud or otherwise vocalize when performing an overall eccentric activity usually improves both activities. For example, the patient can be instructed to reach up to a high shelf while inhaling. Then, using gravity to provide the eccentric resistance, the patient is asked to bring the arm back down to his or her lap or side while slowly counting out loud and controlling the rate of the arm's descent. The activity can be progressed several ways. The activity can include lifting something heavy off the shelf and controlling it along with the arm and trunk while lowering the object to a table or to the patient's lap. Or the postural demands of the activity can be increased. The patient could be asked to lift the same heavy object but to do so while standing, which increases the demands on the musculoskeletal system.

Verbal Techniques

Speech activities that do not require a therapist's physical assistance can be done in a group or individual setting. Singing, for instance, promotes strong and prolonged vocalization with maximal inspiration, which is a significant goal in a phonation program. Similarly, whistling or playing a kazoo or harmonica promotes long, even exhalations but is nonverbal. Both are easily incorporated into a group activity on the nursing floor, in therapy, or in the community.

Along recreational lines, games that promote controlled blowing further the refinement of motor control of the respiratory muscles. This can be accomplished by blowing bubbles (especially large ones), blowing out candles (especially trick candles), blowing a ping-pong ball through a maze, or blowing air hockey disks across the table rather than pushing them with the hand. Patients with musical inclinations should be encouraged to learn to play wind or brass instruments, in which refined breath control is mandatory for success. Obviously, the possibilities in recreational activities are endless and simply require imagination on the part of the therapist.

Further refinement of breath control for speech can be promoted by interrupting the outgoing air flow. This procedure is geared toward improving functional communication skills. Functional speech is a series of vocal stops and starts. The therapist tells the patient to take a deep breath and count out loud to 100. After a few numbers, the patient is told to "hold it" and is then told to start up where he or she left off; the therapist periodically interrupts. Because this activity requires the patient to stop and start the inhalation and exhalation phases at will in all aspects of the ventilatory cycle, it is more advanced and should be used only after some control of exhalation has been mastered.

Summary

The use of appropriate choices in positioning, together with use of an appropriate ventilatory and movement strategy for any given task, will make success in mastering that task all the more likely. If these simple, time-efficient methods of facilitation do not produce adequate ventilatory changes by themselves, it is then appropriate to add the next layer of facilitation—manual facilitation techniques. Specifically, the techniques that are described in this chapter assist in facilitating the following:

1. Greater diaphragmatic breathing patterns (or controlled breathing)
2. Increased chest wall mobility
3. Greater accessory-muscle breathing patterns (or primarily upper chest breathing)
4. More symmetrical breathing patterns (in unilateral disorders)
5. Reduction in high respiratory rates
6. Auxiliary techniques (GBP)
7. Improved phonation support

Obviously, not all techniques are appropriate for any single patient. It is up to the therapist to determine which techniques will best address a particular patient's deficits.

Positioning is vital to increasing ventilation potential and functional skills. From the beginning of the patient's respiratory program, optimizing ventilation and breath control through passive and active positioning techniques should be a priority of all health team members, not just the physical therapist. As patients progress, the clinician can and should assist them in developing better and more efficient movement strategies for higher-level activities by coordinating appropriate breathing patterns, such as trunk extension-inhalation or trunk flexion-exhalation strategies, into all activities. After these quick and easy suggestions are used, a therapist who has been exposed to numerous methods of manual facilitation and techniques to promote more effective and efficient breathing patterns can choose the most appropriate interventions. In some cases, increasing diaphragmatic breathing may be the desired outcome. In other patients, increased upper chest breathing or increased movement on one side of the chest may be more desirable. Some may benefit even more from techniques to reduce the high RR or to mobilize the thorax. For a select patient population, instruction in GPB may be necessary to support breathing without mechanical ventilatory support. Finally, the therapist can choose to use techniques to assist the patient in developing adequate breath support for vocalization and communication.

As therapists come to understand how profound the influence of effective ventilation can be on a patient's recovery from disease or trauma, they will incorporate breathing and ventilation strategies into all patient treatment. Understanding that facilitating effective ventilation goes far beyond diaphragmatic exercises, therapists can be empowered to incorporate other techniques and strategies to help their patients become healthier more quickly and to assist them in reaching their highest potential and prevent future respiratory complications.

The take-home message is that the cardiovascular and pulmonary system will be either an asset or a detriment to a patient's function. Examination and evaluation of breathing patterns and breath control will promote improved patient outcomes.

Review Questions

1. Why would a therapist want to try to change a patient's breathing pattern?
2. How can ventilatory strategies be incorporated into a treatment session?
3. When would a therapist not teach diaphragmatic breathing?
4. What is the role of relaxation in breathing control?
5. When would a therapist consider teaching the patient to use his upper chest accessory muscles more in breathing?
6. When would a unilateral breathing pattern be taught?

References

1. Schweickert WD, Hall J: ICU acquired weakness. *Chest* 131:1541–1559, 2007.
2. DeJonghe B, Lacherade JC, Durnad MC, et al: Critical illness neuromuscular syndromes. *Crit Care Clin* 23:55–69, 2007.
3. Schweickert WD, Gehlbach B, Polhman AS, et al: Daily interruption of sedative infusions and complications of critical illness in mechanically ventilated patients. *Crit Care Med* 32(6):1272–1276, 2004.
4. Schweickert WD, Pholman MC, Polhman AS, et al: A randomized trial of early physical and occupational therapy in mechanically ventilated, critically ill patients. *Lancet* 373(9678):1874–1882, 2009.
5. Beuret-Blanquart F, Boucand MH: Aging with spinal cord injury. *Annals of Readaptive Medical Physiology* 46:578–591, 2003.
6. Boaventura CD, Gastaldi AC: Effect of an abdominal binder on the efficacy of respiratory muscles in seated and supine tetraplegic patients. *Physiotherapy* 89:290–295, 2003.
7. Gandevia SC: Balancing acts: respiratory sensations, motor control and human posture. *Clinics in Experimental Pharmacology and Physiology* 29:118–121, 2002.
8. Temprado JJ, Milliex L, Grelot L, et al: A dynamic pattern analysis of coordination between breathing and rhythmic arm movements in humans. *Neuroscience Letters* 329:314–318, 2002.
9. Mitchell GS, Johnson SM: Neuroplasticity in respiratory motor control. *Journal of Applied Physiology* 94;358–374, 2003.

10. Morris KF, Baekey DM, Nuding SC, et al: Invited review: neural network plasticity in respiratory control. *Journal of Applied Physiology* 94:1242–1252, 2003.
11. Costa D, Cancerlliero KM, Ike D, et al: Strategy for respiratory exercise pattern associated with upper limb movements in COPD patients. *Clinics (San Paulo)* 66(2):299–305, 2011.
12. DeTroyer A, Kirkwood PA, Wilson TA: Respiratory action of the intercostal muscles. *J Appl Physiol* 85(2), 717–756, April 2005.
13. Benzo R, Wigle D, Novotny P, et al: Preoperative pulmonary rehabilitation before lung cancer resection: Results from two randomized studies, Lung Cancer, 2011 Jun 8 (Epub ahead of print).
14. Linn W, Spungen AM, Gong H Jr, et al: Smoking and obstructive lung dysfunction in persons with chronic spinal cord injury. *Journal of Spinal Cord Medicine* 26:28–35, 2003.
15. Dunn S: Core Contraction: Successfully integrating Pilates equipment with rehabilitation, Advance for Physical Therapy & Rehab Medicine, August 22, 2011, p. 41, 42, 51.
16. Gigliotti F, Romagnoli I, Scano G: Breathing retraining and exercise conditioning in patients with chronic obstructive pulmonary disease (COPD): a physiological approach. *Respiratory Medicine* 97:197–204, 2003.
17. Gigliotti F, Coli C, Bianchi R, et al: Exercise training improves exertional dyspnea in patients with COPD: evidence of the role of mechanical factors. *Chest* 123:1794–1802, 2003.
18. Dechman G, Wilson CR: Evidence underlying breathing retraining in people with stable chronic obstructive pulmonary disease. *Phys Ther* 84(12):1189–1197, 2004.
19. Cahalin LP, Braga M, Matsuo Y, et al: Efficacy of diaphragmatic breathing in persons with chronic obstructive pulmonary disease: a review of the literature. *J Cardiopulm Rehab* 22:7–21, 2002.
20. Bianchi R, Gigliotti F, Romagnoli I, et al: Chest wall kinematics and breathlessness during pursed lip breathing in patients with COPD. *Chest* 125:459–465, 2004.
21. Nield MA, Soo Hoo GW, Roper JM, et al: Efficacy of purse lips breathing: a breathing pattern retraining strategy for dyspnea reduction. *J Cardiopulm Rehabil Prevent* 27:237–244, 2007.
22. Hodges PW, Gandevia SC, Richardson CA: Contractions of specific abdominal muscles in postural tasks are affected by respiratory maneuvers. *Journal of Appplied Physiology* 83:753–760, 1997.
23. Hodges PW, Gandevia SC: Changes in intra-abdominal pressure during postural and respiratory activation of the human diaphragm. *Journal of Applied Physiology* 89:967–976, 2000.
24. Hodges PW, Gandevia SC: Activation of the human diaphragm during a repetitive task. *Journal of Physiology* 522:165–175, 2000.
25. Hodges PW, Heijnen I, Gandevia SC: Postural activity of the diaphragm is reduced in humans when respiratory demand increases. *Journal of Physiology* 537:999–1008, 2001.
26. Hodges PW, Gurfinkel VS, Brumagne S, et al: Coexistence of stability and mobility in postural control: evidence from postural compensation for respiration. *Experiments in Brain Research* 144:293–302, 2002.
27. Saunders S, Rath D, Hodges PW: Postural and respiratory activation of the trunk muscles changes with mode and speed of locomotion. *Gait Posture* 20:280–290, 2004.
28. Katagiri M: Neck and abdominal muscle activity during a sniff. *Respiratory Medicine* 97:1027–1035, 2003.
29. DeTroyer A, Gorman RB, Gandevia SC: Distribution of inspiratory drive to the external intercostal muscles in humans. *Journal of Physiology* 546:943–954, 2003.
30. Lissoni A, Aliverti A, Tzeng AC, et al: Kinematic analysis of patients with spinal muscular atrophy during spontaneous breathing and mechanical ventilation. *American Journal of Physical Medicine & Rehabilitation* 77:188–192, 1998.
31. Costa D: Participation of the sternocleidomastoid muscle on deep inspiration in man, an electromyographic study. *Electromyography & Clinical Neurophysiology* 34:315–320, 1994.
32. Lafffont I, Durand MC, Rech C, et al: Breathlessness associated with abdominal spastic contraction in a patient with C4 tetraplegia: a case report. *Archives of Phys Med Rehabilitation* 84:906–908, 2003.
33. Lanini B: Chest wall kinematics in patients with hemiplegia. *American Journal of Respiratory & Critical Care Medicine* 168:109–113, 2003.
34. Warren VC: Glossopharyngeal and neck accessory muscle breathing in a young adult with C2 complete tetraplegia resulting in ventilator dependency. *Physical Therapy* 82:590–600, 2002.
35. Zumwalt M, Adkins HV, Dail CW, et al: Glossopharyngeal breathing. *Physical Therapy Review* 36:455–459, 1956.
36. Bailey EF, Hoit JD: Speaking and breathing in high respiratory drive. *Journal of Speech, Language & Hearing Research* 45:89–99, 2002.
37. Hoit JD, Lohmeir H: Binding the abdomen can improve speech in men with phrenic nerve pacers. *American Journal of Speech-Language Pathology* 117:1–6, 2002.

Exercise Testing and Training: Primary Cardiovascular and Pulmonary Dysfunction

Elizabeth Dean, Donna Frownfelter, and Eduard Gappmaier

KEY TERMS

Cardiac rehabilitation
Central adaptation
Exercise testing and training principles
Lifelong health behavior change
Patient education
Peripheral adaptation
Pulmonary rehabilitation
Team work

CHAPTER OUTLINE

The principles of physical therapy practice in the management of individuals with primary cardiovascular and pulmonary conditions can be applied in formally structured programs or in one-on-one sessions. Exercise testing and training are primary components of comprehensive physical therapy management, which is detailed in Chapter 31. This chapter describes these principles. Structured cardiac and pulmonary rehabilitation programs are therapeutic multidisciplinary programs that encompass the essentials of the best physical therapy practice (Box 24-1). The distinctions among structured programs lie in the primary patient populations they serve rather than in the principles of physical therapy management, which are comparable when applied on a one-to-one basis. The general principles of comprehensive care include

Box 24-1 Definition of Cardiovascular and Pulmonary Rehabilitation

- The goal of cardiovascular and pulmonary rehabilitation is to maintain or return an individual with cardiovascular and pulmonary dysfunction to full participation in life with a high level of life satisfaction.
- Cardiovascular and pulmonary rehabilitation consists of a comprehensive interdisciplinary management program, including physical activity and exercise, education, and behavioral change designed to improve the physical and emotional status of individuals with cardiovascular and pulmonary dysfunction or their risk factors.

teamwork, patient education, exercise testing and training, long-term sustainable lifestyle change, and follow-up, and these are common across patient groups. This chapter extends the basic principles of exercise testing and training outlined in Chapter 19. The chapter highlights state-of-the-art literature and the physical therapist's central role as clinical exercise physiologist and health educator in addressing the needs of individuals with primary cardiovascular and pulmonary conditions.

The role of the physical therapist as health coach and advocate to promote lifelong health and well-being is further emphasized in the management of these patient groups. These principles are also applied when primary cardiovascular and pulmonary dysfunction is a secondary diagnosis—that is, for example, in a patient whose primary diagnosis is a frozen shoulder but who has history of ischemic heart disease or its risk factors. This underlying condition has major implications for the modification of an exercise program for the frozen shoulder in addition to implementing management to specifically address it.

Over the past decade, an extensive number of position statements, clinical practice guidelines, and consensus statements have been published to guide contemporary practice in cardiac and pulmonary rehabilitation programs. The major goal of these programs is to improve quality of life and tolerance of daily activities. An overriding objective is to institute lifelong healthy practices, including secondary prevention.[1] The application of these principles is central to the management of cardiovascular and pulmonary conditions, whether they are primary or secondary conditions. In general practice today, patients (including children) presenting to the physical therapist with musculoskeletal or neuromuscular complaints have a high probability of having underlying cardiac or pulmonary pathology, or one or more associated risk factors (see Chapter 1). Established guidelines for cardiac rehabilitation programs do not replace the expert clinical judgment of rehabilitation professionals and goal-directed, patient-centered service delivery.[2] Consistent with the World Health Organization's definition of health (see Chapter 1), both cardiac and pulmonary rehabilitation programs focus on the enhancement and maintenance of cardiovascular and pulmonary health through individualized programs designed to optimize physical, psychological, social, vocational, and emotional status overall. In addition, they promote secondary prevention through risk-factor identification and modification in an effort to prevent disease progression and the recurrence of cardiovascular and pulmonary events.[2]

A criticism of conventional cardiac and pulmonary rehabilitation programs is that they are structured with little individualization.[3] The physical therapist, who is uniquely qualified as an applied clinical exercise physiologist and health coach, needs to ensure that all components—in particular, exercise—are prescribed to meet the specific needs and comorbidities of each individual. For reference purposes, we include elements of international standards and guidelines for cardiac and pulmonary rehabilitation programs in Appendixes A and B. We caution, however, that these elements need to be tailored to an individual (based on a detailed history, assessment, and examination, and ongoing evaluation) and that such standards may change as new evidence emerges. Nonetheless, they will provide useful guidelines to physical therapists involved with setting up facilities related to cardiac and pulmonary rehabilitation.

This chapter extends the information in Chapter 31 concerning the management of chronic, primary cardiovascular and pulmonary dysfunction. In the review of the state-of-the-art literature, $\dot{V}O_{2max}$ was often reported in studies and was used to mean $\dot{V}O_{2peak}$ (see Chapter 18 for elaboration of this physiological distinction). Despite this, we have retained the term used by the original investigators in each study in our summary of these studies.

Cardiac and Pulmonary Rehabilitation: Evidence Base, Efficacy, and Practicalities

Although an interprofessional team approach is fundamental to both cardiac and pulmonary programs, individuals who regularly participate in moderate exercise experience greater control of symptoms and increased functional capacity than do those treated with drugs alone.[4] Self-management strategies learned in a pulmonary education program also contribute to perceived control of symptoms and to self-confidence.[5] This sense of control is perhaps the single best argument supporting the exploitation of noninvasive interventions for the management of chronic conditions. This component may be singularly important in determining long-term outcomes, such as reduced demands for health care and lower health care costs.[6]

The effectiveness of cardiac and pulmonary rehabilitation has been established at the highest level of evidence[2,7-19] and this is true irrespective of stage of disease.[20,21] With the aging of the population, cardiac rehabilitation has been shown to benefit octogenarians as well as younger people. Because of the issues associated with exercise testing older people, the use of a mobility index, such as the Rivermead Mobility Index, to evaluate exercise performance has been proposed even in absence of a formal exercise test.[22] Because of common lifestyle behaviors, ischemic heart disease as a primary lifestyle-related condition will remain prevalent for the foreseeable future.

These interprofessional programs have internationally recognized standards that are well described and are recommended for all patients with cardiovascular and pulmonary conditions. They specialize in patient education (including smoking cessation, nutrition and weight control, and promotion of self-management and training) that has sustained, lifelong, positive effects on cardiovascular and pulmonary status and sense of well-being.[23-26] The term *end stage* needs to be revisited, given the efficacy of rehabilitation in severely compromised individuals.[27] Considering these benefits and the enormous economic implications of keeping people healthy and out of hospitals and physicians' offices, rehabilitation can be supported as a primary intervention rather than a secondary priority after suboptimal effects of pharmacotherapy or surgery.[28]

Noninvasive cardiac and pulmonary rehabilitation is more cost-effective than medical and surgical treatments, and it offers long-term health benefits and reduced risk. However, there is a significant discrepancy between the actual provision and practice of cardiac rehabilitation and that advocated in published guidelines. These evidence-based, noninvasive, cost-effective interventions are being grossly underused, and participation rates are low.[29] Referral to cardiac rehabilitation has been reported to reflect selected groups, namely, younger age groups, those who have participated previously, those admitted to hospital with outpatient cardiac rehabilitation services, and those having a discharge diagnosis of myocardial infarction or coronary artery bypass surgery.[30,31] Significant barriers also have been reported to exist with respect to availability, referral, and utilization of these programs; payment issues are another factor.[32] Only a small proportion of individuals are referred, and of those, only a small proportion can access the programs.[33-35] Phase I inpatient cardiac rehabilitation has been reported to be a declining trend.[36] Physicians and surgeons may not have knowledge and awareness of the effectiveness of noninvasive approaches to health problems that have been managed primarily with drugs and surgery, so suitable candidates are not always referred.[37] In addition, there are psychosocial reasons for underutilization of these resources. Women are referred less commonly than men, and their drop-out rates are higher.[38,39] Thus there is a selection bias in the individuals sampled for studies of cardiac rehabilitation.[40] The participation of women is associated with insurance, level of education, bypass surgery, and transportation availability.[41] Cost containment and increasing accessibility are two primary barriers to participation in cardiac rehabilitation.[42] Low participation rates (particularly by women, minority group members, and older people) and means of increasing access have become primary areas of interest.[43]

Of the multiple facets of a cardiac rehabilitation program, different components may have different effects on individual heart health. In addition, physiological distinctions between men and women affect the incidence and manifestation of cardiovascular conditions between the two sexes and, in turn, their responses to cardiac rehabilitation. Women tend to have lower systolic blood pressure and pulse pressure than men and to have more favorable lipid and homocysteine levels.[44] However, the compliance of women's small blood vessels tends to be lower, which may reflect female sex hormones and the higher mortality rates of premenopausal women hospitalized for myocardial infarction. Women also tend to have more "silent" ischemic heart disease than men, which is more often associated with sleep disturbance in women. The results of one descriptive study also showed that women were less likely to adhere to diet and exercise modification guidelines compared with regimens for smoking cessation, medication, and stress management.[45]

Special attention needs to be paid to motivating individuals to participate in rehabilitation programs (identify facilitating factors and barriers to participation), to generalize their new skills to home activities and the community, and to continue their new lifestyle behaviors beyond formal enrollment in the program.[4] Given that education and exercise are core components of cardiac and pulmonary rehabilitation, physical therapy is uniquely positioned to implement care for individuals with cardiac or pulmonary conditions as primary or secondary diagnoses and to mobilize an interprofessional health care team for a given individual if no formal program exists. Education materials should be individualized to the learner's needs and capacities; otherwise, resources will be wasted. A marked disparity exists between the average American's reading ability (eighth grade level) and the readability levels of cardiac rehabilitation materials.[46] The large number of polysyllabic words is a primary factor.

Cardiac and pulmonary rehabilitation programs are typically conducted in formal centers in large communities. The vast majority of patients, however, do not have access to cardiac and pulmonary rehabilitation. Furthermore, long-term participation and adherence to the principles of the program have been disappointing, particularly for women.[47] The principles of these programs reflect fundamental physical therapy practice, which can be implemented on a one-to-one basis in a private practice (in a large or small community) or in a hospital that does not have a formal program in cardiac or pulmonary rehabilitation; in such settings, the outcomes are comparable to those in formal programs.[48-50] A close-to-home philosophy of care is emerging in the field of health care, including cardiac rehabilitation, in an effort to improve access to underserved people and groups.[51] When well constructed, a home-based cardiac rehabilitation program can have long-term outcomes comparable to those of a center-based program—for example, improved total cholesterol, smoking reduction, anxiety reduction, and self-reported improved physical activity and diet.[52] Patients who are stable after bypass surgery do as well (in terms of improved exercise capacity and risk reduction) in an individualized detailed home program as those participating in a supervised center-based rehabilitation program.[53]

As patients become more active, their pharmacokinetics change. Medications must be reviewed on an ongoing basis and prescriptions modified accordingly.[54] These changes reflect the long-term metabolic effects of exercise, in addition to improved health and potential weight loss. Close teamwork is needed to monitor a patient's medications and ensure that drug prescriptions are changed so that they promote weaning from medication commensurate with the benefits of noninvasive intervention, including education and exercise. Eliminating or reducing the needs for medication and pharmacological support is an important physical therapy outcome consistent with the philosophy of exploiting noninvasive care as much as possible.

Formal exercise testing and training—primary physical therapy skills—are warranted in patient diagnosis, evaluation, and exercise prescription. Early intervention with exercise for heart and lung conditions has become an established practice to counter the deleterious effects of deconditioning and the loss of cardiac and pulmonary function and to maximize remaining oxygen-transport reserve.[55]

Addressing the psychosocial components of care in cardiac and pulmonary rehabilitation is an element of the internationally accepted definition of rehabilitation. Psychosocial factors, however, constitute few, if any, aspects of the workup and assessment of an individual with heart or lung disease. A structured assessment tool to assess and monitor psychosocial factors and changes in patients with heart disease has been proposed.[56] Guidelines concerning the psychosocial component of cardiac rehabilitation are the sole focus of a position paper currently being developed in Europe. This position paper is designed to promote active psychological as well as physical well-being.[57] Given the aging of the populations of high-income countries, cardiac rehabilitation programs must pay particular attention to the needs of older adults with respect to nutrition, physical activity and exercise, program adherence, smoking cessation, psychological issues, and methods of teaching the older learner.[8] Doing so will help to reduce the high exclusion rate of this cohort of the population from cardiac rehabilitation programs.

Finally, with the advent of databases and outcome measures, projects such as the Wisconsin Society for Cardiovascular and Pulmonary Rehabilitation (WISCVPR) Web-based Outcomes Project, which focuses on outcomes for cardiac rehabilitation, are being used to develop benchmarks and further refine best practice guidelines.[58] Outcomes of pulmonary rehabilitation include quality of life, which for those with chronic lung disease, is reflected in the St George's Respiratory Questionnaire and the 36-item Short-Form Health Survey. A simple linear analog quality-of-life scale has also been shown to be valid in evaluating disease-specific, health-related quality-of-life issues in older individuals with chronic lung disease.[59] With databases and outcomes evaluation, physical therapists will be able to individualize programs to promote more immediate, more effective, and more long-lasting effects.[60] In addition, programs are being evaluated that will enhance the quality of prevention strategies initiated by health care providers through hospital-based programs for patients at risk.

Quality-improvement initiatives are becoming a focus in the literature. In 2008, one such initiative that used interactive training of hospital teams with Web-based teaching tools, enhanced adherence to prevention guidelines in hospitalized patients with cardiac disease.[61] From baseline to 1 year, this initiative reported marked improvements in smoking cessation, lipid control, blood pressure control, and cardiac rehabilitation referral. Quality-improvement initiatives for activities related to cardiac rehabilitation produce marked benefits. In addition to structured exercise, cardiac rehabilitation focuses on counseling and teaching about risk reduction in order to promote lifelong health; however, long-term studies are needed to address the issue of deterioration with respect to risk factors and lifestyle behaviors over time.[62] In 1998, a multistate outcome program for cardiovascular and pulmonary rehabilitation was shown to be feasible; it was possible to benchmark data across programs.[21] Outcomes included the SF-36 Health Survey, a patient knowledge test, and a 6-minute-walk test distance. All outcomes improved in both cardiac and pulmonary rehabilitation programs. Such outcomes are needed to systematically evaluate the effects of cardiac and pulmonary rehabilitation programs.

Although cardiac rehabilitation reduces cardiac deaths, it remains unclear whether exercise alone or the comprehensive range of interventions associated with cardiac rehabilitation is responsible.[63] The answer to this question is singularly important in refining the principles and practices of cardiac rehabilitation programs.

Studies of the efficacy of cardiac rehabilitation have been methodologically marred by selection bias: subjects tend to be low-risk, middle-aged men, whereas those who might benefit most are often excluded, namely, those who are older, at high risk, and have multiple comorbidities.[63] Those individuals who do not attend cardiac rehabilitation programs tend to be older, less aware of their cholesterol values, and less likely than attenders to believe their condition was controllable and that their lifestyle may have contributed.[64] Attention to exercise and motivational profiles has been proposed as a means of enabling rehabilitation program participants to continue with exercise.[65] Promoting self-efficacy should therefore be an important focus in tailoring cardiac rehabilitation programs. Finally, the ethnicity of program participants is rarely reported. Given the needs of the aging population, the number of people with multiple conditions, and the increasing ethnic diversity in the United States and Canada, the reports on the effects of cardiac rehabilitation, to date, have relatively limited generalizability.

As a handy reference for clinicians, key points in the assessment, evaluation, and exercise testing and prescription of patients with primary cardiovascular and pulmonary conditions are summarized in Appendix C.

Patients with Chronic Cardiac Dysfunction: Exercise Responses

Cardiac dysfunction includes a range of types of pathology, causes (acquired or congenital), and severity that may be managed medically, surgically, or in both ways (see Chapter 31 for the principles of comprehensive physical therapy management). The most common cause is ischemic heart disease and myocardial infarction. The muscle that is infarcted never recovers, so remodeling of the heart occurs, and that alters the heart's electrical functions (as shown on an electrocardiogram [ECG]) and mechanical functions (evidenced by ECG and echocardiogram). Remodeling takes place over time and with exercise. Ejection fraction (right ventricle) at rest is a poor indicator of cardiac function and exercise capacity.[66] In fact, heart failure can occur in the presence of a normal ejection fraction,[67] a form of disorder that typically occurs in women who have histories of hypertension and increased left ventricular mass.

Patients can range from being asymptomatic and having risk factors to being in severe distress and having minimal functional capacity, requiring high levels of supplemental oxygen and pharmacological support, and awaiting heart transplantation. Patients with extremely severe disease may require mechanical ventilation. To be able to classify patients' functional capacity in a semi-quantitative manner, the New York Heart Association classification of function is commonly used (see Box 31-2). Exercise is now considered an essential component in the management of individuals with stable heart failure and in those who have undergone transplantation.[68] Surgical options include keyhole surgery, open-heart surgery (e.g., coronary artery bypass surgery, valve repair, and aneurysm repair), and heart transplantation.

There is an interaction between circadian rhythms and the pathogenesis of heart rate and blood pressure variability. These rhythms are under the influence of adrenal, autonomic, hypothalamic, and pituitary activity. Thus physical exertion, sleep deprivation, emotional stress, and high-fat meals are major triggers of myocardial ischemia, angina, infarction, sudden cardiac death, and stroke, which have a higher incidence in the second quarter of the day, between 0600 and 1200.[69] Heart rate and blood pressure variation have been implicated in the pathogenesis and progression of atherosclerosis, heart failure, and thrombosis, and are independent risk factors. During this period, vitamins C and E are lower than during the rest of the day; it has been postulated that regulating the intake of these vitamins and exercising may minimize the variability of heart rate and blood pressure. Whether such regulation can then modulate cardiovascular events warrants further study.

Although dyspnea is a common limiter to exercise in cardiac failure, the other factors that contribute to exercise limitation are multiple. In addition to central hemodynamic impairments, exercise capacity is affected by impaired ventilatory control, lung function, peripheral circulation, and skeletal muscle function.[70] Exertional dyspnea has been attributed to the regulation of arterial pH during exercise.[71] Pulmonary hypertension and systemic hypotension can also limit exercise performance.[72] Explanations for these limiters include baroreceptor dysfunction, beta-receptor downregulation, abnormal vascular adaptation, and poor cardiac output in relation to elevated right ventricular afterload. The delayed $\dot{V}O_2$ responses (delayed oxygen kinetics or time constant for this variable) are associated with lactate production and early anaerobiosis.[73] Maladaptive gait changes have been ruled out as a factor influencing ventilation in patients with chronic heart failure.[74]

The physiological capacity of patients with cardiac dysfunction to adapt to exercise depends on the type and severity of impairment in the heart and in other steps in the oxygen transport pathway. Reduced alveolar-capillary membrane-diffusing capacity[75] and a ventilation to perfusion mismatch have been proposed[76] and may reflect chronically elevated pulmonary capillary pressure. A primary ventilation-perfusion mismatch defect in patients with heart failure may explain their increased ventilatory response to exercise, but this theory has been questioned.[77] Patients with severe left ventricular dysfunction enhance their aerobic capacity primarily by improving oxygen extraction at the tissue level rather than by means of central adaptation. Similarly, with aerobic exercise, these patients improve the collateralization of peripheral capillaries so as to improve blood flow to working muscles and increase nitric oxide production in the blood vessels, which mediates endothelium-dependent relaxation.[78] This effect is correlated with functional capacity. Thus evaluation of vasomotor reactivity has been proposed as a means of explaining the effects of interventions, including exercise and medications. Aortic wall elasticity modulates left ventricular function and coronary blood flow. Pulse wave velocity is a marker of arterial stiffness and is an independent predictor of $\dot{V}O_{2peak}$.[79] The exercise intolerance observed in individuals with dilated cardiomyopathy may be explained by an increase in arterial stiffness.

Although guidelines for exercise prescription have been commonly adopted for people with uncomplicated heart disease, the optimal prescription is still being refined. Moderate aerobic exercise performed alternate days for 20 to 40 minutes is generally accepted. Nonetheless, despite the general health benefits that are associated with this level of exercise, more moderate levels including brisk walking have been reported to be equally protective.[80] Such findings are important particularly for individuals who are disinclined to formally exercise at the recommended level for cardioprotection. Brisk walking is more easily integrated into daily life hence likely to be adhered to.

Individuals with Chronic Cardiac Dysfunction and Failure

The cardiac dysfunction managed by physical therapists can range from mild to severe. With increasing severity of disease, an individual's response and adaptation to exercise are altered markedly, which has major implications for exercise testing and training. Today, patients with even severe heart dysfunction may be able to participate in some level of exercise.[19] However, this needs to be done under the supervision of a competent health care team to ensure the benefits are maximized and the risks minimized.

Chronic heart failure is usually hallmarked by left ventricular dysfunction. In health, normal left stroke volume coupled with increased heart rate leads to greater cardiac output and greater metabolic demand, as during exercise. As the left ventricle becomes increasingly compromised, the individual with heart failure depends more on heart rate to increase cardiac output and peripheral oxygen extraction. Left ventricular ejection fraction during exercise is not consistently associated with resting ejection fraction,[81] even in people with objective signs of myocardial ischemia and increased heart rates during exercise. Thus the left ventricular ejection fraction at rest must be interpreted cautiously in the context of exercise and predicted exercise responses.

Determining which patients will benefit from a rehabilitation program has been the subject of debate. Goebbels and colleagues (1998)[82] reported that patients with depressed left ventricular function benefit, whereas patients whose left ventricular function has been preserved, such as may occur after myocardial infarction and coronary artery bypass surgery, tend to improve spontaneously within 3 months.[83] Proponents of selecting patients for cardiac rehabilitation however, have failed to address the past history of patients, their comorbidities, access to rehabilitation, return to work, and secondary prevention strategies to maximize their care and long-term outcomes. Noninvasive practices need to be exploited before, during, and after a myocardial event or surgery to maximize long-term gains, including reduced recurrence of the problem and need for doctor- and hospital-based care, reduced risk factors and morbidity, and prolonged quality of life. Physical therapy has a commitment to long-term outcomes, including reduced doctor- and hospital-based care, reduction or elimination of medications, and reduced probability of repeat surgeries.

Conservative management of patients with heart failure who utilize physical therapy has emerged as a major focus in the literature, in part because of the cost of surgery and an inadequate supply of organ donors. The benefits include reduction of deconditioning, including restoration of normal autonomic balance and, potentially, some primary effects on the underlying pathology.[84] Patients with chronic heart failure respond to aerobic exercise favorably, showing improvement in functional class as defined by the New York Heart Association.[85] Both $\dot{V}O_{2max}$ and anaerobic threshold improve. In addition, there is a reduction in the exaggerated ventilatory response at maximal and submaximal work rates that is usually observed in these patients. As a result, symptoms are reduced. Exercise benefits persist after patients shift from a supervised center-based to a home-based program. This finding has important practical and economic implications.

Over recent years attention has turned to exercise training of patients with cardiac failure and the role of ventilatory changes in exercise-induced dyspnea. The periodic breathing of patients with cardiovascular disease is well known clinically; however, the mechanism underlying the cycling hyperpnea and hypopnea is not clear. Fluctuations in pulmonary blood flow have been proposed as a mechanism for this periodic breathing.[86] With respect to other ventilatory correlates of heart failure, ventilatory efficiency, the ratios of $\dot{V}_E$ and $\dot{V}CO_2$, have yielded important prognostic information.[87] When used in combination with $\dot{V}O_2$ (≥15 mL/kg/min), $\dot{V}_E/\dot{V}CO_2$ (≥50 L/L) can be useful in defining a high-risk group that should be prioritized for heart transplantation.[88]

At rest, individuals with more severe heart failure have more restrictive lung pathology and impaired gas exchange.[89] During exercise, these patients have increased dead space, impaired gas exchange, and greater submaximal ventilatory responses than individuals whose disease is less severe. Exercise limitation in patients with chronic heart failure correlates with reduced FEV_1 and FVC, implicating airway resistance in the increased work of breathing in exercise intolerance.[90] In addition, an exercise-induced diffusion defect has been identified.[91] Alveolar-capillary membrane conductance has been identified as the best lung function predictor of $\dot{V}O_{2peak}$ in patients with chronic heart failure.[92] The impairment in ventilatory efficiency is associated with reduced exercise tolerance and pulmonary artery pressures.[93] Pulmonary vasoconstriction has been implicated in leading to pulmonary hypertension and alveolar hypoperfusion. Overall, exertional dyspnea observed in patients with heart failure is not the result of abnormal ventilatory function.[94]

Ventilatory exercise parameters, including $\dot{V}O_{2peak}$, $\dot{V}_E/\dot{V}O_2$, and $\dot{V}_E/\dot{V}CO_2$, are strong predictors of mortality.[95,96] $\dot{V}O_{2peak}$, however, may be underestimated, given the slowed O_2 kinetics in this population.[97] Gas exchange, therefore, should continue to be monitored throughout recovery. Submaximal respiratory gas indexes have been proposed as being more sensitive than peak $\dot{V}O_2$ for assessing functional impairment[98] and for predicting survival in ambulatory patients with chronic heart disease.[99] Nonetheless, ventilatory capacity is not likely to limit exercise performance in patients with stable chronic heart failure.[100] Ventilatory and heart rate responses are, however, strong and powerful predictors of mortality in these patients, and they are superior to the use of $\dot{V}O_{2peak}$.[101] Inspiratory capacity varies inversely with pulmonary capillary wedge pressure in individuals with chronic heart failure, and it is a strong independent predictor of functional capacity.[102]

Patients with severe chronic heart failure often have high ventilatory demands during exercise, and they have respiratory alkalosis, which is consistent with significant wasted ventilation on exertion,[103] and increased respiratory drive;[104] only a relatively small effect is attributed to ventilation-perfusion mismatch. However, increased ventilatory drive, as evidenced by the ventilatory equivalent of carbon dioxide ($\dot{V}_E/\dot{V}CO_2$), has been reported to occur infrequently.[105] Knowledge and understanding of which patients exhibit this response and which do not would be clinically useful.

Patients with severe chronic heart failure have a reduced ratio of increase in $\dot{V}O_2$ to increase in work rate during incremental exercise.[106] The reduced DO_2 due to severely compromised cardiac output is not fully compensated by an increase in oxygen extraction. These patients do tend to show improved exercise response through improved peripheral oxygen extraction. Changes in cardiac performance may reflect the Frank-Starling effect rather than changes in contractility.[107] Low cardiac output, particularly in less intense exercise, does not necessarily result in lower exercise capacity.[108] This phenomenon has been attributed to a unique mechanism that regulates arteriovenous oxygen content difference to optimize DO_2 to the tissues in patients with severe heart failure. At peak exercise, fractional oxygen extraction in the muscle is greater in patients with chronic heart failure than in healthy people in proportion to the level of the patient's impairment.[109] This observation supports the importance of peripheral adaptation to aerobic training in patients with heart failure.

Heart failure can be categorized as either diastolic or systolic; the former may be the dominant form in elderly people.[110] In stable outpatients, mortality due to diastolic failure is about half that of mortality due to systolic failure. However, when patients are hospitalized, the rates are comparable. Because of its strong prevalence among the elderly, diastolic failure exceeds systolic failure in being the cause of mortality. In diastolic failure, the Frank-Starling mechanism is impaired, causing reduced maximal cardiac output, heart rate, stroke volume, and left ventricular filling pressure. Vascular stiffness is also increased. Acute exacerbations result in pulmonary edema and are associated with hypertension, sodium intake, and lack of adherence to medication schedule. A primary goal is to reduce blood pressure, which improves symptoms and reduces exacerbations.

Exercise testing is an important means of establishing the prognosis of an individual with chronic heart failure with respect to treatment response, morbidity, and mortality. Peak $\dot{V}O_2$ pulse, ($\dot{V}O_2$/heart rate), and lean body mass adjusted for O_2 pulse are useful prognosticators.[111] Postexercise blood pressure response has shown to be a reliable and valid predictor of adverse cardiac events in individuals with dilated cardiomyopathy.[112] The postexercise blood pressure response is defined as the ratio of systolic blood pressure at 3 minutes postexercise to that at peak exercise, with a criterion of 0.79 or greater to predict complications. The 6-minute walk test has been reported not to replace $\dot{V}O_{2peak}$ as a prognosticator in individuals with advanced heart failure.[113]

Prediction of the prognosis of individuals with chronic heart failure can be improved with a two-step exercise-test protocol.[114] This test combines maximal and low-intensity exercise to improve accuracy and reproducibility. In addition, a distance of less than 300 meters walked in the 6-minute walk test (see Chapter 19) has been reported to be a useful prognostic marker of subsequent cardiac death in individuals with mild to moderate heart failure.[115] Exercise testing has also been reported to provide good prognostic value in determining postoperative outcomes (mitral and aortic regurgitation).[116] An important role for exercise testing in prognosis is emerging.

Although tests of $\dot{V}O_{2max}$ can be used to stratify patients with cardiac failure according to risk factors, these tests can be invalid as a result of premature termination by the tester or lack of motivation by the patient. Tests of anaerobic threshold may be less influenced by these factors in such a potentially compromised group.[117] Rather, the combination of a $\dot{V}O_2$ at an anaerobic threshold (gas exchange threshold) of less than 11 mL/kg/min and a $\dot{V}_E$ versus $\dot{V}CO_2$ slope of more than 34 is a better predictor of mortality at 6 months than is $\dot{V}O_{2max}$, and it may provide a guide when prioritizing patients for heart transplantation. Submaximal and endurance tests and determining the anaerobic threshold have been advocated over maximal tests for clinical evaluation of patients with heart failure because they are relatively easy to perform, are associated with less risk, and are more valid indexes of a patient's capacity for daily activity.[118,119]

Individuals with heart failure have a higher incidence of glucose intolerance compared with healthy individuals (20% lower).[120] After an aerobic exercise program, glucose uptake can increase by 25%. The mechanism of the reduction in glucose tolerance in individuals with heart failure and the remediating effects of aerobic exercise have yet to be elucidated. Whether secondary improvement in insulin sensitivity from aerobic exercise occurs in these individuals comparable to that in healthy people warrants clarification.

Body position may be an important factor to consider when exercising patients with chronic heart failure who often complain of orthopnea. However, when exercise responses in the erect and supine positions were compared in one study, no change was reported in breathlessness, and no change occurred in $\dot{V}_E/\dot{V}CO_2$. However, $\dot{V}_{Epeak}$ was greater in the upright position.[121]

Patients with chronic heart failure can benefit from aerobic training. Exercise training of patients with impaired left ventricular function is associated with improved ventilatory function.[122] In addition to improved cardiac output, long-term high-intensity exercise resulted in reduced ventilatory dead space and improved ventilatory efficiency. In men with reduced left ventricular function, high-intensity exercise (2 hours of walking daily in combination with high-intensity, monitored cycle ergometry at 70% to 80% of peak capacity for 40 minutes, four times a week for 8 weeks) has been reported to result in marked increases in $\dot{V}O_{2max}$ secondary to increased cardiac output and widening of the A-aO_2 difference.[123] No improvement in myocardial contractility tends to be observed in these patients after such an exercise program. High-intensity exercise does not impair hemodynamic status or lead to further myocardial damage. Low-intensity exercise in individuals with chronic heart failure has been shown to improve autonomic tone and reactivity to vagal and sympathetic stimulation.[124]

The effects of exercise training on pulmonary function in individuals with heart failure are becoming better understood. After training, individuals with coronary artery disease have been reported to show no change in pulmonary function, with the exception of the respiratory exchange ratio at peak exercise.[125] Also, alveolar-capillary diffusing capacity may contribute to improvement in exercise tolerance after training.[126] Pretraining pulmonary function is not correlated with improvement in exercise performance.

With aerobic exercise training, respiratory muscle endurance improves, and that contributes to improved overall exercise capacity.[127] Breathlessness is also reduced. The reverse occurs too—that is, respiratory muscle training can improve $\dot{V}O_{2peak}$, as well as respiratory muscle endurance in patients with chronic heart failure. The combination of muscle and endurance training is superior to endurance training alone in this patient cohort with respect to improved left ventricular function, $\dot{V}O_{2peak}$, and strength.[128,129]

An understanding of skeletal muscle function in individuals with chronic heart failure is important because improvements in aerobic capacity may be largely dependent on maximizing peripheral oxygen extraction. Strength training in combination with aerobic training improves walking distance in the 6-minute walk test, which is an independent prognosticator in individuals with chronic heart failure.[130] Regular endurance exercise increases oxidative enzymes in the working muscles and is associated with a shift from type II to type I fibers.[131] These skeletal muscle adaptations are independent of peripheral circulatory adaptations.

Adaptation to resistance muscle training reflects changes in the myosin heavy chain of peripheral skeletal muscle and a shift from slow aerobic to fast glycolytic and fast oxidative characteristics.[132] These findings are associated with $\dot{V}O_{2peak}$, O_{2pulse}, and tidal volume. Reduced strength of the knee flexors and extensors in patients with chronic heart failure is associated with impaired ventilatory response to exercise; thus muscle dysfunction has been proposed as a contributing factor to symptoms.[133] Improved functional outcomes, increased walking distance, and reduced muscle area with increased interstitial space after exercise training support the theory that these effects are mediated by improved capillary density and flow reserve to exercising muscle.[134]

Peripheral myopathy in individuals with chronic heart failure may contribute to exercise intolerance and training capacity.[135] Features include reduced proportion of type I fibers, shift to type II fibers, biochemical shift consistent with increased muscle fatigability, reduced mitochondrial density, and reduced capillary density.[136] However, some of these changes, such as altered capillary density, appear to be gender-specific, which may have implications for training.[137] Skeletal muscle appears to adapt to central impairment of oxygen transport in heart failure. There is histochemical and gas exchange evidence showing that physiological recovery is delayed in patients with heart failure.[138] Interestingly, markers of skeletal muscle oxygenation, including myoglobin and its derivatives, are reduced during incremental aerobic exercise to maximum, and during the recovery. As the capacity for aerobic exercise declines, patients may have greater reliance on anaerobic metabolism (but this cannot be sustained/attained in the same way), which is consistent with increasing reliance on anaerobic pathways for metabolism during exercise. Inflammatory cytokines have been implicated in the myopathy associated with heart failure.[132] However, the possibility that this outcome reflects deconditioning cannot be ruled out because patients typically are unable to achieve high exercise intensities.[139]

The recovery process in patients with heart failure has important implications for optimizing exercise training parameters and, thereby, training effects. However, further study of differences in exercise recovery characteristics between patients with heart failure and healthy people is warranted.[140,141] Evidence supports the idea that exercise intolerance in these patients is characterized by slower adaptation to acute exercise and recovery and to reduced maximal exercise capacity compared with healthy people.[142]

After angiography, positioning and mobilization have important roles after several hours of bed rest.[143] Limiting restricted mobility after cardiac catheterization to 2 hours from 6 hours has been reported to be safe, and it may limit complications.[144]

Different types of exercise stress (aerobic or resistance) have differential effects on the heart and circulation.[145] In health, for example, static exercise exerts a pressure load on the heart that can be distinguished from the normal hemodynamic response to dynamic exercise, which involves a volume load on the heart. Static exercise leads to concentric cardiac hypertrophy (left ventricular), and dynamic training is associated with eccentric hypertrophy. Static exercise can produce effects that have been associated with aerobic training. Isotonic exercise using hand weights has been reported to be associated with increases in systolic and diastolic blood pressure, rate pressure product, serum norepinephrine, and perceived exertion.[146] Pulmonary capillary wedge pressure, incidence of dysrhythmias, and ST-segment changes do not differ from rates recorded at rest. Generally, isotonic exercise is tolerated well by individuals with heart failure, and no angina or dyspnea occurs.

Low to moderately intense strength training may cause fewer cardiovascular complications than aerobic exercise training in individuals who have undergone myocardial infarction.[147] Resting blood pressure can be reduced, albeit to a lesser extent, suggesting reduced sympathetic and baroreceptor activity. In addition, lipid profiles may improve. These benefits can be observed in patients with cardiac and circulatory pathology without adverse effects. Even older, frail patients may tolerate weight training at 40% to 60% of maximal voluntary contraction. Qualitatively similar hemodynamic responses occur in response to resistance exercise, as in aerobic exercise in individuals with heart failure.[148] In general, resistance training with multiple repetitions of moderate weight produces the most beneficial effects. To ensure that a patient is able to perform optimally the activities of daily living, which require a certain degree of muscle strength, strength training is considered an integral component of a cardiac rehabilitation program.

The effect of cardiac dysfunction on regional circulation has been of interest, particularly with respect to cerebral perfusion. A recent study has shown that patients with left ventricular dysfunction can have impaired cerebral perfusion. During exercise, the adequacy of cerebral perfusion is dependent on the adequacy of cardiovascular and pulmonary function; it is compromised in patients whose cardiac output fails to increase appropriately in response to exercise.[149]

Some individuals with chronic heart failure have been reported to have sick euthyroid syndrome, in which serum-free triiodothyronine is reduced in the presence of normal free L-thyroxin and thyrotropin.[150] Sick euthyroid syndrome is a sign of poor prognosis in individuals with chronic heart failure. Exercise, however, can normalize the free triiodothyronine levels and reverse the syndrome, in turn improving exercise capacity.

Individuals with persistent life-threatening cardiac rhythms may require artificial pacemakers. Advances in this area have included biventricular pacing for individuals with systolic left ventricular failure with prolonged duration of the QRS complex. Preliminary reports suggest that these pacemakers are safe and effective.[151] Further, biventricular pacing can improve symptoms and quality of life by improving walking times and ejection fraction.[152] These effects persisted at the 6-month follow-up, and the 2-year survival rate was excellent. There are few specific guidelines for these individuals with respect to exercise testing and prescription. Similarly, there are few guidelines for individuals with automatic implantable cardioverter defibrillators.[153] Preliminary reports suggest that exercise and lifestyle recommendations are needed for individuals with pacemakers and implanted cardioverter defibrillators and that with due modification, exercise testing and training are feasible.

Ventricular dysrhythmias contribute to a significant number of deaths. Despite improved survival, this cohort of high-risk individuals may be considered inappropriate for cardiac rehabilitation. With careful patient screening and monitoring, however, some patients with ventricular dysrhythmias may safely participate in cardiac rehabilitation.[154]

Individuals after Heart Transplantation

Heart transplantation has become an accepted therapy for end-stage heart failure over the past 20 years, with its ultimate goal being the return of function and a good quality of life (see Chapter 17). Postoperatively, the resting heart rate for heart transplant recipients is higher than normal. In the early postoperative period, the peak $\dot{V}O_2$ and work rate of people who have had heart transplants are 50% of those of healthy people.[155] At ventilatory threshold, the $\dot{V}O_2$ and work rate were also 50% of normal. Peak heart rate, which increases for up to 3 minutes after peak exercise, is also significantly lower. This evidence supports the need for mandatory rehabilitation so as to maximize the benefits of this high-risk surgery, including optimizing functional work capacity, return to work, and life satisfaction.

Without training, exercise tolerance remains severely limited over the first 16 months postoperatively. This has been explained by the reduced capacity to respond to the Frank-Starling mechanism and the residual low cardiac index.[156] Rehabilitation begins preoperatively and continues for 1 year after discharge.[157] The principles of cardiac rehabilitation are applied; however, response of the denervated heart to exercise requires extended warm-up and cool-down periods and limits the maximal heart rate and $\dot{V}O_2$ that can be achieved. Reinnervation of the sympathetic nerves to the heart is associated with improved heart rate response to exercise and contractile function.[158] Hemodynamic responses to exercise are initially dependent on exogenous catecholamines rather than on the fast-responding sympathetic release from nerve endings. Systolic blood pressure is more appropriate than heart rate for assessing exercise response and recovery.[159] Anaerobiosis is achieved early. The degree to which neuroplasticity can be influenced by exercise training to promote autonomic reinnervation to the heart after transplant has yet to be established.

When compared with patients after bypass surgery in postoperative cardiac rehabilitation programs (phase II; up to 3 months postoperatively), patients with heart transplants have comparable functional outcomes.[160] However, after graduation from this program and being on a home-based program for 9 months, patients with transplants had lower $\dot{V}O_{2peak}$ and were significantly more limited at the 1-year follow-up. Thus phase I only, combined with recommendations for a home program, may be inadequate for patients after heart transplantation; they may benefit from long-term supervised training programs.

Persistently low $\dot{V}O_{2max}$ after transplant reflects in part intrinsic skeletal muscle abnormalities.[161,162] In addition to intensive aerobic exercise, resistance muscle training has an important role in countering the effects of corticosteroid-related osteoporosis and peripheral myopathy. With respect to predicting the prognosis of patients with heart failure who undergo heart transplantation, $\dot{V}O_{2peak}$ is considered a superior indicator of submaximal indexes of exercise capacity.[163]

Isometric exercise and activities requiring postural stabilization are largely avoided in people who have had heart transplants because of potential hemodynamic stress. Light isometric exercise (handgrip) attenuates increases in heart rate, blood pressure, and systemic vascular resistance. Whole-body isometric exercise also attenuates these hemodynamic variables.[164] At rest, heart rate, blood pressure, and rate pressure product are higher in individuals who have had transplants than those rates in healthy people.

Some patients who receive heart transplants have low pulmonary diffusion capacity, and this is associated with lower exercise tolerance than is found in patients who do not have this impairment.[165] Poor diffusion capacity, however, is not associated with exercise-induced hypoxemia and thus is not considered a primary contributor to impaired exercise tolerance.

Individuals with Left Ventricular Assist Devices

Left ventricular assist devices have become more common as an interim intervention for an individual awaiting heart transplant. The donor pool is small, so many individuals may not survive the wait for surgery. The Jarvik heart is a left ventricular device designed as a long-term solution for heart failure. In an initial case study describing a patient with a Jarvik heart, exercise tolerance, myocardial function, and end-organ function all improved 6 weeks after surgery.[166] The Jarvik heart shows some promise for the management of end-stage heart failure; however, its success will depend on its mechanical dependability.

Individuals with Congenital Heart Disease

Guidelines for individuals with congenital heart disease warrant development. Barriers to exercise in this cohort have been reported to be their perceived physical limitations, lack of interest, and fear.[167] Currently, guidelines are suboptimal.

Individuals with Intermittent Claudication

Intermittent claudication (IC) is the symptom of exercise-induced muscle ischemia of peripheral arterial disease. IC is a systemic complication of atherosclerosis with or without overt ischemic heart disease. The disabling pain during walking results from muscle ischemia. The risk for cardiovascular morbidity and mortality far exceeds that of severe limb ischemia or limb loss.[168] A patient with IC must be managed as a patient with heart disease as well as one with peripheral arterial disease. Conservative management is a priority and should include physical activity and exercise programs, smoking cessation, weight loss and optimal nutrition, and stress management.

Claudication symptoms may mask cardiac symptoms. In addition, a comorbidity such as arthritis can complicate the clinical picture in such a way that the underlying vascular condition is neither manifested peripherally nor centrally. During exercise testing and training, arthritis may limit the capacity of the patient who may have well been restricted by claudication pain.[169] Even in this cases, exercise training can improve exercise tolerance in the absence of improved peripheral blood flow.[169] Exercise effects include reduced submaximal heart rates and oxygen cost and reduced postexercise lactate levels. In addition, lipid profiles can be improved.

The exercise responses of patients with IC also exhibit a slowed $\dot{V}O_2$ response related to impaired muscle perfusion.[170] The associated delayed ventilatory response has been associated with the hyperemic response in the exercising muscle rather than with ischemia.

Outcome measures, including ankle-brachial index performed in a vascular laboratory to assess changes in peripheral stenoses with exercise training, are useful.[171] Ultrasound can be used to assess pulses, particularly when they are weak. Palpation of skin temperature is a crude indicator of perfusion in that skin is highly sensitive to ambient temperature. Using the back of the hand, however, and scanning bilaterally down the legs, so that skin temperature can be compared in the legs, may have some utility for identifying gross differences in blood supply.

Individuals with Anemia

The exercise responses of patients with anemia have not been well described. The capacity of the blood to transport oxygen is determined by the hemoglobin concentration and the binding characteristics of the hemoglobin. Patients who develop acute anemia are more likely to complain of dyspnea than patients who develop anemia gradually. Rather than a primary cardiac, pulmonary, or muscle compensatory mechanism, this adaptation is mediated by increased diphosphoglycerate, which decreases the affinity of hemoglobin for oxygen in the tissue. Patients with sickle cell anemia have a low $\dot{V}O_{2peak}$ and a low anaerobic threshold in the presence of a high heart rate reserve but no gas exchange abnormalities.[172] The disease is characterized by restrictive lung pathology, increased alveolar dead space, and hypoxemia.[173] Increased dead space may reflect impaired pulmonary capillary perfusion due to the sickle cells. Exercise hyperventilation is thought to be associated with increased anaerobiosis.

Individuals with Hypertension

Hypertension remains the silent killer for which effective nonpharmacological interventions are underused. Hypertension is associated with sedentary lifestyle, diet, obesity, smoking, and stress. Further, hypertension has long been linked to type 2 diabetes mellitus as well as vascular changes typically seen with aging.[174,175] Modifying one or more of these factors can reduce high blood pressure and its lethal sequelae and eliminate, or at least reduce, the need for medication. Chronic sympathetic overdrive associated with hypertension promotes left ventricular hypertrophy, cardiac dysrhythmias, and atherogenesis.[176] Further, inhibiting sympathetic overactivity may help reduce cardiovascular risk. Regular physical activity and a formal exercise program reduce the risk for hypertension or modify it. This effect is likely mediated through a decrease in total peripheral vascular resistance. African American men are particularly at risk for hypertension, and this risk can be detected by an exaggerated blood pressure response to exercise.[177] Endurance training reduces this exaggerated response and thereby may reduce the risk for developing hypertension. Along with eating a healthy low-salt diet and not smoking, exercise is a potent noninvasive intervention that can prevent, as well as control, high blood pressure. Despite the efficacy of many antihypertensive medications, potential deleterious effects of low perfusion to the vital organs with intensive blood pressure control cannot be overlooked clinically.[178]

Individuals with Type 2 Diabetes Mellitus

Type 2 diabetes mellitus is a strong risk factor for coronary artery disease and sudden cardiac death. This condition is associated with reduced baroreceptor sensitivity and heart rate variability, which are also risk factors for morbidity and mortality. Exercise training improves baroreceptor sensitivity in people with type 2 diabetes as well as glucose sensitivity, exercise tolerance, and muscle strength.[179] Prognosis may well be improved with exercise.

Type 2 diabetes mellitus results in multiple deficits to exercise capacity, both central and peripheral. Muscle blood flow may be impaired at the level of microcirculation in the absence of overt peripheral vascular disease.[180] In patients with chronic diabetes, exercise capacity is compromised by reduced oxygen delivery. A reduction in the arteriovenous oxygen difference may contribute to a reduction in $\dot{V}O_{2peak}$.[181] When smoking is controlled, individuals with diabetes mellitus who are insulin dependent and have complications have been reported not to exhibit impaired pulmonary gas exchange during exercise despite thickening of the alveolar basal lamina.[182] Individuals with non–insulin-dependent diabetes mellitus have reduced glucose transport in skeletal muscles, and this may contribute to exercise intolerance.

Diabetes mellitus is an independent risk factor for reduced left ventricular ejection fraction during exercise, as is severity of coronary artery disease.[183]

Role of Medications: Augmenters and Attenuators of Outcome

Among the factors that can confound exercise responses of patients are medications. Medications can enhance, limit, or have no effect on exercise performance. Patients with cardiovascular dysfunction, particularly those under a physical therapist's care, are likely to be taking one or more potent medications. The timing of their ingestion of these medications in relation to their performing an exercise test should be recorded in order to standardize testing procedures from one time to the next; at the very least, it is important to be aware of the confounding effects of a medication that could explain improved or worsened responses. Beta blockers are commonly taken by patients with cardiac dysfunction to improve the rhythm and contractile force of the heart. Long-term use of beta blockers causes no significant improvement in delayed heart rate recovery, which is a predictor of mortality in patients with heart failure.[184] These drugs can contribute to fatigue and exercise intolerance. Many patients are taking angiotensin-converting enzyme (ACE) inhibitors to enhance cardiac function. This classification of drug improves diffusion capacity and exercise capacity, an effect mediated through prostaglandin activity. However, this activity can be mitigated by aspirin, another drug commonly taken by patients with heart failure.[185] Thus a change in aspirin administration in combination with ACE inhibitors can worsen exercise tolerance. Captopril, a commonly prescribed ACE inhibitor, has a demonstrable beneficial effect on exercise responses in patients after myocardial infarction.[186] Ventilatory efficiency is improved, as is evidenced by a reduction in $\dot{V}_E/\dot{V}CO_2$ at submaximal workloads. Reduced perception of exertion and improved capacity to perform the activities of daily living may result from a reduction in ventilatory demand. Concurrent with physical therapy management, an inventory of the patient's medications and medication changes should be maintained and considered when conducting an exercise test or interpreting exercise test data.

Individuals with Chronic Pulmonary Dysfunction: Exercise Responses

Of individuals who participate in pulmonary rehabilitation programs, the largest proportion is made up of those with emphysema. Smoking is the primary cause of emphysematous changes in the lungs and the associated systemic complications (see Chapter 5). Patients with moderate or severe pulmonary distress may be referred to pulmonary rehabilitation. Other groups that may be referred are individuals with cystic fibrosis, asthma, interstitial lung disease, and alpha$_1$-antitrypsin deficiency. Patients with lung cancer are typically underrepresented in rehabilitation programs and warrant being targeted as a group that could benefit.

Like patients with chronic cardiac dysfunction, those with chronic pulmonary dysfunction may have a history of being managed pharmacologically or surgically. Surgical options include lung volume reduction surgery, segmentectomies, lobectomies, pneumonectomies, and lung transplantation.

Individuals with Chronic Obstructive Lung Disease

Deconditioning in patients with chronic lung disease is an anticipated consequence of the downward spiral of pathophysiological compensation for the structural and functional damage to the lungs. In individuals with severe disease, exercise intolerance may reflect limited peripheral perfusion and oxygen extraction due to the disproportionate demand on the respiratory muscles.[187] These individuals are unable to exercise at an intensity that induces a high level of aerobic conditioning, and they experience early onset of dyspnea. On experiencing dyspnea with exercise, a person with chronic obstructive pulmonary disease (COPD) reduces his or her activity level, which leads to deconditioning. With impaired aerobic capacity, anaerobic glycolysis has an increasingly important role in supporting physical activity. This leads to increased blood lactate, which needs to be buffered with bicarbonate, thereby producing additional carbon dioxide. This further increases ventilatory load and dyspnea and leads to further inactivity and deconditioning. These individuals frequently have secondary cardiac and hematological changes. The goal of physical therapy is to relieve dyspnea and increase exercise tolerance, hence, quality of life. After smoking cessation, exercise is the single best intervention for controlling dyspnea in individuals with COPD.

Exercise testing has become an established component of the workup of an individual with impaired functional capacity, including patients with chronic lung disease. Although estimating the ventilatory capacity of patients with COPD on the basis of whether a patient can climb one or two flights of stairs is no longer considered a tenable test, symptom-limited stair climbing can be used to evaluate cardiovascular and pulmonary reserve.[188] Stairs climbed in a symptom-limited stair-climbing test correlate with $\dot{V}O_{2peak}$, $\dot{V}_E$, heart rate, and respiratory rate in response to a maximal cycle ergometer test.

During acute exercise, patients with COPD have elevated heart rates and blood pressures and show increased hypoxemia and desaturation with incremental or prolonged constant work-rate exercise. Impaired exercise capacity reflects physical damage to the lungs, including impaired pulmonary vasculature[189] as well as cardiac and skeletal muscle abnormalities. Exercise capacity is marked by a disproportionate ventilatory response and differences in FEV_1, but these responses explain only a fraction of the variability in $\dot{V}O_{2max}$.[190] Variability in the ventilatory response to exercise is a primary determinant of variability in the exercise capacity of patients with COPD. In the absence of right heart failure, right ventricular end diastolic volume is highly correlated with $\dot{V}O_{2max}$ and cardiac index in patients with COPD, suggesting that right ventricular end diastolic volume compensates optimally.[191]

As in other conditions, in the management of patients with COPD, individualized training programs based on heart rate as the gas exchange threshold (anaerobic threshold), as opposed to standard protocols based on 50% of heart rate reserve, produce superior therapeutic outcomes; that is, they reduce ventilatory requirements and are safer.[192] Supervised training of individuals with COPD has been reported to have advantages over self-monitored exercise programs.[193] When two to eight programs were compared, the supervised treadmill program was superior to a community-based walking program with respect to training intensity in terms of improved $\dot{V}O_2$, $\dot{V}CO_2$, $\dot{V}_E$, and heart rate in response to moderate-intensity workloads. Research is needed to design home-based programs for selected patients in order to maximize these programs' effectiveness.

The 6-minute walk test is useful in the assessment and management of patients with COPD, for whom the test was originally developed. The discriminating capacity of the test can be increased by considering factors in addition to walking distance. Four factors based on an evaluation of 15 variables accounted for 78% of the variances in distance walked:[194]

1. Heart rate
2. Endurance
3. Impaired oxygen transport
4. Perceived exertion

Based on a walking-distance test, the effect of an exercise program can be predicted on the basis of low pretraining walking distance and higher FEV_1.[195]

Symptom-limited tests are used to estimate the effects of training on patients with COPD. In patients with low functional work capacity, objective submaximal indexes of training effects are useful. With respect to oxygen kinetics during constant work rate, the time constant of $\dot{V}O_2$ after training is reduced, and it reverts after detraining.[196] The O_2 pulse similarly increases and decreases with training and detraining, respectively, and serum lactate decreases with training and increases with detraining.

Rigorous training (80% of peak work rate, for 45 minutes, 3 times a week, for 6 weeks) results in significant training responses in individuals with severe COPD.[197] Peak work rate and exercise endurance increase. In response to constant work rate, the kinetics of O_2 uptake, CO_2 production, $\dot{V}_E$, and heart rate are reduced. Improved exercise tolerance may reflect changes in breathing pattern, specifically, increased tidal volume and reduced respiratory rate.

During the past decade, research that sought to elucidate the training responses of individuals with COPD and their adaptation to exercise has focused on peripheral muscle pathophysiology and adaptation. With refinement in exercise testing and training procedures and in measurement, changes in peripheral muscles have been found to be associated with the underlying disease. In addition, aerobic training responses reflect both central and peripheral adaptations.

Compared with healthy people matched for activity level, individuals with COPD have less muscle strength (70% to 80% of age-matched healthy people), which may be explained by deconditioning, a disease-related myopathy, or both.[198] In addition, mechanical efficiency may be impaired. Patients have large numbers of less efficient type II muscle fibers, but cross-sectional fiber area, capillarization, and mitochondrial density are comparable or reduced.[135,199] Although metabolic capacity is unchanged, differences in fiber type in COPD may explain the reduced mechanical efficiency.

Systemic factors contributing to exercise intolerance have been identified in individuals with chronic lung disease, and they appear to resemble those observed in individuals with chronic heart disease.[200] Some individuals with COPD have impaired peripheral perfusion and oxygen extraction, which may be explained by the redistribution of cardiac output from the peripheral to the respiratory muscles during increasing work rates.[187] This may be a primary exercise limiter in these patients. In a study designed to distinguish central from peripheral limitations in the exercise responses of patients with COPD, central factors rather than peripheral muscle limitations were reported to be responsible (although not wholly) for their exercise intolerance.[201] Endurance training is associated with increased skeletal muscle activity and recruitment of slow-twitch fibers.[202]

Individuals with Primary Pulmonary Hypertension

Patients with primary pulmonary hypertension have impaired exercise responses that may resemble those of patients with COPD and secondary pulmonary hypertension. During incremental exercise, the lungs become less efficient as gas exchangers because of impaired lung perfusion.[203]

Individuals after Lung Volume Reduction Surgery

Lung volume reduction surgery has become a topic of increasing interest as an invasive means of correcting the hyperinflation in the lungs of patients with COPD. A good quality of life is correlated with reduced lung hyperinflation after surgery,[204] and these improvements have been maintained for at least 18 months on follow-up.[205] A commensurate reduced work of breathing appears to facilitate performance of activities of daily living. Improvement in functional capacity after surgery has been attributed to improved breathing mechanics during exercise, as well as at rest,[206] and to improved respiratory muscle strength.[207] Specifically, higher maximum levels of tidal volume and $\dot{V}_E$ are achieved; in turn, these lead to improvements in $\dot{V}O_2$ and $\dot{V}CO_2$.

Individuals with Interstitial Lung Disease

Performing exercise testing in individuals with interstitial lung disease can elucidate the extent of the pathology and its functional consequences—diffusing capacity and alveolar arterial oxygen tension difference.[208] These patients have less ability than healthy people to recruit the pulmonary capillary bed during increased exercise stress, so they can desaturate readily.[209,210] $\dot{V}O_{2peak}$ is correlated with impairment of gas exchange and circulation, rather than with ventilatory impairment. Thus the pathophysiology of the pulmonary vasculature is considered more important than impaired ventilatory mechanics in patients with interstitial lung disease.[211] Abnormal exercise responses in individuals with pulmonary sarcoidosis may reflect subclinical right heart dysfunction.[212]

One study that examined the contribution of diffusion limitation to exercise performance in this patient group showed evidence of a ventilatory impairment that was manifested by a decrease in alveolar oxygen tension.[213] Cardiac impairment such as impaired diastolic filling may occur secondary to pulmonary fibrosis during exercise or restriction of the pleurae and thoracic cavity. Changes in gas exchange during exercise may be the most sensitive indicator of physiological limitation in patients with subclinical evidence of interstitial lung disease.[214,215] However, in terms of prognostic capability, the results of an exercise test for evaluating gas exchange do not appear to augment standard pulmonary function testing.[216]

Individuals after Lung Transplantation

Lung transplantation improves pulmonary function and quality of life in individuals such as those with cystic fibrosis. When exercise responses before and after bilateral lung transplantation are compared, exercise capacity remains low, although improved.[217] This observation has been explained on the basis of poor oxygen extraction.[218] Exercise conditioning is required in these patients postoperatively to maximize their functional capacity. However, maximum oxygen consumption may remain below that of healthy peers matched for age and gender, and anaerobiosis during exercise is achieved earlier. These responses reflect inadequate adaptation of cardiac output in these patients, as well as deconditioning.

Individuals with Asthma

There are several specific aspects to consider when testing and training individuals with exercise-induced asthma.[219] For those who are managed with medication, a low-intensity warm-up before exercise can optimize its therapeutic effect. A longer cool-down may also be beneficial. Individuals with asthma are taught to monitor their unique responses to their medication and its coordination with physical activity and exercise. They also monitor the ambient air (humidity and temperature) to anticipate the potential for bronchoconstriction and respiratory distress. With good knowledge of conditions and medication, individuals with asthma can participate in high-intensity exercise safely.

Individuals with Cystic Fibrosis

General health and wellness have become primary goals for individuals with cystic fibrosis (CF) Twenty years ago, management of people with this condition, primarily children, was based largely on passive removal of excessive secretions by means of postural drainage and vigorous percussion. Now people with cystic fibrosis are living longer, and comprehensive physical therapy management, including a regular program of exercise, is recognized as a central component of promoting general health and airway clearance.[220,221]

Although life expectancy continues to improve in people with CF, end of life usually results from respiratory infection, so exacerbations have to be prevented. With a basis of good health resulting from proper nutrition and exercise, exacerbations may occur less often and last for a shorter time. The exercise program is adjusted during these times and then ramped up afterwards. Medications, including bronchodilators, are coordinated with exercise to produce the best effects both during sessions and over the long term.[222]

Cardiac and Pulmonary Rehabilitation: Common Components

Definition, Purpose, Goals, and Outcomes

Most individuals with heart or lung disease can benefit from the principles of healthful living that underlie the philosophies of conventional cardiac and pulmonary rehabilitation programs. In comparing patients participating in these programs with nonparticipants, cardiovascular deaths are reduced by 20% and sudden death by 37% in the year after infarction.[223] Those who meet the criteria for admission and are within access of a center that offers these programs are evaluated by a multidisciplinary team that establishes the patient's short- and long-term goals and sets up an overall program that includes exercise prescription, a nutritional plan, a smoking cessation program (if required), and life-skills and stress-management instruction. These programs are patient-focused, and the health care team, including the physical therapist, serves largely as health coaches and advisers. Fundamental to that program's success is establishing an individual's readiness to change lifestyle behaviors and participate in a lifelong program of health (see Chapter 1). The health education component of the program is then targeted to shift the individual to a higher level of readiness or to engage the individual immediately in an active rehabilitation program.

The preadmission workup for cardiac rehabilitation includes a complete history and a questionnaire related to current status and health behaviors and the individual's goals (Figure 24-1). Because of the interdependence of heart and lung function, these questions are relevant to individuals being considered for admission to a pulmonary rehabilitation program, as well as to a cardiac rehabilitation program.

A key component of the assessment on admission to a cardiac or rehabilitation program is an objective assessment of the patient's risk factors, which enables risk-factor-reduction interventions to be specifically targeted and a lifelong health plan designed and implemented.

The relative benefit of structured programs as opposed to community and home-based programs is being debated. Maximizing the potential benefits of the program is key, so the program has to be optimal in terms of the individual's needs, including the setting that will produce the best short- and long-term outcomes. Exercise gains have been demonstrated in healthy middle-aged people when programs are home-based.[224] This evidence supports the idea that individuals with cardiovascular and pulmonary dysfunction who are being managed one-on-one by a physical therapist may also demonstrate benefits when the exercise program is home-based. However, further study is needed to determine the safety and effectiveness of home-based programs for candidates for cardiovascular and pulmonary rehabilitation.

The core components of cardiac and pulmonary rehabilitation programs are shown in Table 24-1; they reflect the skills and expertise of the multidisciplinary team in addressing each individual's needs in a comprehensive manner. These components include awareness of the patient's condition and health education overall, nutrition and weight control, smoking cessation, general physical activity and exercise, and stress management. Psychological support is important with respect to the patient's adjustment to his or her condition; the management of anxiety, anger, hostility, and depression; and the maximization of adherence to recommendations and guidelines related to nutrition, physical activity and exercise, smoking cessation, and a lifelong health plan. Such support is elicited from the individual's family and friends, as well as health care providers.

The exercise program focuses on improving flexibility and strength, as well as aerobic capacity, with the goals of improving the patient's health and capacity to perform the activities of daily living, thus improving quality of life. Psychosocial and end-of-life issues are also an important part of rehabilitation programs and should be addressed, particularly in individuals who are severely ill and their families.

Health education is a major component of cardiac rehabilitation and constitutes a skill in its own right. The patient requires knowledge about health and the incentive to translate this information into his or her own life. Each learner's knowledge deficits are different and learning style is unique; these should be evaluated so that health education can be properly targeted to be the right type, the right level, the right format, and delivered at the right time (see Chapter 28). Knowledge deficits need to be established so that education can be targeted specifically to meet each deficit. For instance, individuals with coronary artery disease typically have little awareness of some of the major risk factors. Generally, their knowledge about cholesterol, use of lipid-lowering medications, and achievement of cholesterol levels consistent with consensus-based guidelines is minimal.[225] Participation in structured cardiac rehabilitation programs improves

Table 24-1 Core Components of Cardiac and Pulmonary Rehabilitation

Assessment	Entrance complaint Height, weight, body mass index Education Occupation/employment Socioeconomic status Family situation Smoking history Alcohol consumption
History	Present illness (medical and surgical details of management to date) Multisystem review (e.g., cardiovascular, peripheral vascular, pulmonary, musculoskeletal, neuromuscular, gastrointestinal, endocrine, renal, liver, immune) Medication status Lab tests and investigations: blood work, ECG, x-rays and scans, exercise test Learning assessment (education level, preferred learning styles, self-efficacy, and behavioral readiness to change.
Goals	Prevention Short term Long term
Interventions	Promotion of empowerment and self-efficacy through teaching Smoking cessation Nutritional counseling (optimal nutrition, lipid management, sodium control, salt control, weight control) Hypertension management Diabetes management Psychosocial management Physical activity counseling Exercise training Work simplification and energy conservation Sleep and rest Vocational rehabilitation Recreational rehabilitation
Outcomes (monitored over the short and long term and consistent with the individual's goals)	Participation Capacity to fulfill unique life roles (e.g., parent, spouse/partner, occupation/profession, worship and spiritual life, recreation and leisure, community activities) Abilities ADLs and task-specific activities related to life roles, including work and home management
Structure and Function	Changes in physiological dependent measures consistent with goal achievements

Modified from Balady GJ, Ades PA, Comoss P, et al: Core components of cardiac rehabilitation/secondary prevention programs, A statement for healthcare professionals from the American Heart Association and the American Association of Cardiovascular and Pulmonary Rehabilitation, Circulation *102:1069-1073, 2000.*

Name:		
Birth Date and Age:		Sex:
Weight: Height:	Body Mass Index:	Waist circumference:
Summary of History	List the dates and types of the medical and surgical procedures you have had over the years.	
Medication	List the medications you are currently taking and the doses and frequencies.	
Family History	Did your father or brothers have heart disease before 55 years of age?	
	Did your mother or sisters have heart disease before 65 years of age?	
Current Status	Do you experience pain (tightness or heaviness) or angina in your chest on exercise?	
	If so, what specifically triggers it? What relieves it? How long does it take to go away?	
	Do you take medication for chest pain/angina?	
	If so, for how long? How much? What is the medication's effect?	
	Do you ever feel short of breath?	
	If so, what triggers it? What relieves it? How long does it take to go away?	
	Do you ever feel short of breath when you lie down?	
	Do you experience pain in your legs when you walk?	
	Have you had this investigated? If so, what was the diagnosis?	
	Do your ankles swell?	
	Do you have high blood pressure?	
	If so, for how long, and how has it been managed?	
	Do you have normal blood pressure now?	
	Do you take medication for high blood pressure? What medication? How much?	
	Is your blood pressure controlled now?	
	Do you have glucose intolerance?	
	Type 2 diabetes?	
	If so, for how long and how is your blood sugar controlled? Is your blood sugar within normal limits now?	
	Do you take insulin? Oral agents? What agents? How much?	
	Do you have thyroid disease?	
	If so, what, and for how long? Do you take medication for your thyroid problem? What is the medication? How much do you take?	
	Is your thyroid controlled now?	
	Do you have anemia?	
	Do you have gastrointestinal complaints?	
	If so, describe them. Are you being medically treated for them?	
	Do you have any musculoskeletal or neurologic problems?	
	If so, describe them. Are you being medically treated for them?	
	Do you have any balance problems?	
	If so, is there an explanation? Are you being medically treated for them?	
	Is your vision normal with or without corrective lenses?	
	Is your hearing normal with or without hearing aids?	
Health Behaviors	Describe your weekly food consumption in terms of whole grains, fruit and vegetables, beans and lentils, meat and fish, saturated and trans fats, refined sugar, and low fiber foods.	
	Do you have high cholesterol?	
	For how long?	
	Have you ever smoked?	
	When, how much, and for how long?	
	Do you smoke now?	
	If so, how much?	
	How much alcohol do you consume? Type, amount, and frequency:	
	What is your regular activity level (describe activity or exercise, intensity of exercise, duration, and frequency each week)?	
	How stressful is your life?	
	Identify life-event stressors.	
	Identify daily-hassle stressors.	
	What are your stress-management strategies?	
	How many hours a night do you sleep on average?	
	How many times do you wake up or get up during the night?	

Fig. 24-1 Preadmission work-up for cardiac rehabilitation.

knowledge related to heart disease, signs and symptoms, and self-management strategies. However, the learning and homework must be evaluated on each visit to determine how well the knowledge has been internalized and put into practice in daily life. Lifestyle recommendations should be suitable for application to daily living. For example, healthy food choices should be described specifically. Energy utilization should be translated into terms that are meaningful for the individual, such as 1000 kilocalories (kcal) of energy per week (although 1500 kcal/week has been identified as the threshold for reducing all-cause mortality risk[226]). People least likely to achieve the latter threshold include women, those with a body mass index of 30 or higher, and those who are 70 years of age or older. Weekly kilocalorie energy expenditure should be a component of the exercise prescription in order to ensure that maximum health benefits are achieved. The physical therapist's capacity to communicate and educate effectively will determine the long-term outcome of the program.

Many outcomes related to a sense of well-being, a health-related quality of life, sickness impact, and life satisfaction are dealt with in conjunction with physiological and clinical outcomes. The former variables are consistent with the International Classification of Function and the impact of disability on the individual, but noncardiac and nonpulmonary outcomes should also be considered.

Chronic disability is often associated with clinical depression, so management of depression alone may improve functional capacity. With respect to pulmonary disease, 45% to 63% of deaths are attributable to advanced lung disease itself.[227] Other factors that explain mortality include nutritional deficits, impaired exercise tolerance, functional performance, and social factors, including marital status. Thus nutrition and exercise are essential elements of cardiovascular and pulmonary rehabilitation. Similar findings have been reported for cardiac disease. A negative emotional state is associated with high long-term mortality. Addressing the individual's psychological status may improve functional status.[228]

Specific rehabilitation goals include the following:

- To serve as a health promotion resource for the individual, community, and health care providers
- To increase aerobic capacity and muscle strength and endurance consistent with overall health and well-being
- To improve capacity to perform the activities of daily living and maintain gainful employment
- To promote self-efficacy in healthy lifestyle behaviors for long-term health and well-being, as well as for secondary prevention
- To shift an individual to a lower risk classification
- To reduce risk for revascularization procedures, medical intervention, and physician and hospital visits
- To promote health and well-being in the patient's family and community
- To reduce direct and indirect health care costs over the short and long term

Setting and Team Members

In addition to the physical therapist, the team consists of physicians, nurses, a psychologist, a social worker, a pharmacist, and in some centers, an exercise physiologist. Typically, the physical therapist is involved with exercise testing and training, program modification and progression, and eventual discharge. Additional roles involve education and risk-factor modification. A physical therapist applies the principles and practices of cardiovascular and pulmonary rehabilitation to any patient in any setting and to patients who have cardiovascular and pulmonary dysfunction or its risk factors as a primary or secondary diagnosis or concern. The guidelines and standards for assessment and exercise testing and training must be adhered to if the best service and the best and safest outcomes are to be achieved.[229]

Components of Physical Therapy

Assessment

Central to comprehensive physical therapy management is focusing on the individual rather than on the condition. Although this chapter emphasizes exercise testing and training in individuals with primary cardiovascular and pulmonary conditions, in reality, people present with comorbidities. Thus individuals with secondary cardiovascular and pulmonary dysfunction (see Chapters 25 and 32) are likely to have a high incidence of primary cardiovascular and pulmonary dysfunction or risk for it (in comparison with the general population). For this reason, underlying risk factors and disease must be examined in all patients, irrespective of their primary presenting diagnoses.

The history, lab tests, and investigations, including scans and ECGs, and the basic assessment of an individual with cardiovascular and pulmonary dysfunction are described in Part Two, but the aspects of the assessment that warrant particular attention in exercise testing and in training individuals with cardiovascular and pulmonary dysfunction are highlighted in this section. Although the cardiovascular and pulmonary systems may be the focus of rehabilitation, a complete review of all systems is necessary to determine limitations imposed by musculoskeletal, neurological, endocrine, hematological, or other conditions. These need to be considered in both testing and training.

The assessment comprises the examination of risk factors, including profiles of the patient's nutrition intake, weight, smoking history, and stress management (including rest and sleep profiles), as well as physical activity and aerobic capacity. Before implementing any intervention, a detailed history, examination, and lab data are accumulated to provide an objective baseline. Within 6 to 8 weeks, elements of the assessment are repeated and outcome measures recorded to determine the degree to which the patient has progressed with respect to achieving short-term goals.

Predictors of long-term survival of myocardial infarction include several factors that need to be identified so that patients can be stratified according to risk. These factors include age, left ventricular ejection fraction, diabetes, hypertension, and elevated resting heart rate.[230] Attention to these factors may help to detect changes in status early and prevent adverse exercise effects by judicious modification of an exercise program. Individuals who develop late-onset heart failure have a tenfold increased risk for mortality. Glucose abnormalities (hyperglycemia and hyperinsulinemia) in those who do not have diabetes are common in individuals with heart failure (43%).[51] Further, these findings are associated with greater functional deterioration than that found in individuals with heart failure *without* glucose abnormalities. Thus knowledge of an individual's glucose tolerance is essential at baseline and over time within the rehabilitation program.

Well-being extends beyond physical health. Rehabilitation programs record and monitor outcomes related to the subjective sense of well-being, the health-related quality of life, the general quality of life, and life satisfaction. Many scales and questionnaires are available to provide outcomes and fluctuations in these variables over time.

Clinical depression is associated with ischemic heart disease in two ways. First, depression is an independent risk factor for cardiovascular disease and related increased morbidity and mortality.[231] Second, up to 45% of individuals exhibit symptoms of major depression after acute myocardial infarction. Thus individuals referred to cardiac rehabilitation need to be screened for depression, and psychotherapy, counseling, or pharmacotherapy may be indicated. Remediation of depression associated with chronic disease may augment functional capacity independent of physical rehabilitation. Depression and peak aerobic capacity have been reported to be the best independent predictors of patient-reported physical function scores in older individuals with heart disease.[232] These findings suggest a role for depression management that is independent of exercise training but augments functional capacity.

The general assessment must also include an assessment of the individual's learning style (see Chapter 1 and 28). Prochaska's Transtheoretical Model of readiness to change has important implications for rehabilitation programs that are formalized (e.g., cardiac and pulmonary rehabilitation), as well as for individual rehabilitation programs. In addition to the goal of shifting an individual into a lower risk category, another objective is to shift an individual into a higher readiness-to-change category. An individual's readiness to change health-related behavior is assessed, along with his or her intention to engage in the recommended risk-reduction behaviors, including dietary changes, physical activity and exercise, smoking cessation, and relaxation. Readiness to change may differ for each behavior. Barriers include time management, psychological adaptation, and laziness.[233] Another component of the education is the assessment of the individual's knowledge deficits regarding his or her condition.

Interventions

In addition to the exercise program, the patient may also be in a smoking-cessation program and/or a weight-loss program. During the course of management, medications may change. Detailed records of the progress of the patient in these various programs warrant monitoring so that the perceived outcome of exercise can be explained in a valid manner. Other factors such as weight loss, smoking reduction (cessation), or change in medication could explain, in whole or in part, the apparent effect of exercise.

Education

Education is the central component of cardiovascular and pulmonary rehabilitation. The patient is taught the basics of anatomy and the physiology of heart and lung health, basic nutrition, physical activity and exercise, analysis of lab tests, effects of smoking, effects of medications, and so on. In this way, the patient is empowered and, it is hoped, well motivated to be an agent of change in his or her own life. Lifestyle recommendations need to be reinforced regardless of phase of the program. One report estimated that after a coronary event, 50% of smokers resume smoking on discharge from the hospital.[234] With respect to modifying dietary habits, participants in rehabilitation programs may not understand the distinction between the benefits of eating a healthy diet versus simply cutting out certain types of foods from their diets, even after standard instruction about the role of healthy eating to their overall health.[235] Thus tailoring health education information to the needs of program participants is essential if true behavior change is to be effected over the long term.

Like exercise, education can be tailor-made to suit the learning needs of each person (see Chapter 28). Individualization of the education considers age, literacy, preferred learning style, ethnic and cultural issues, and readiness to change. Smoking cessation is the most important intervention for patients with heart disease and pulmonary disease.[236,237]

Promoting self-efficacy and perceived control are central to education strategies developed by physical therapists. Follow-up is needed, however, to ensure self-treatment is sustained over time.[238] Inadequate self-treatment behavior at follow-up suggests that new teaching and learning strategies should be developed to ensure that the quality of self-treatment is maintained.

Exercise Program

A reduction in respiratory rate in patients with chronic heart failure improves pulmonary gas exchange, reduces dyspnea, and increases exercise performance. Such improvement was reported in one study in which respiratory training in these patients involved 1 month of training to breathe at a rate of 6 breaths per minute.[239] Slowing breathing rate may have some application for patients with chronic heart failure who have impaired gas exchange and breathlessness during exercise as well as at rest.

Goals: Short Term

A distinction is made between short- and long-term goals. Short-term goals are aimed at developing and learning strategies for healthier living and reducing cardiovascular and pulmonary risk factors, particularly those that are most life-threatening. Long-term strategies are an extension of short-term goals and address the sustainability of health and fitness consistent with patients' needs, wants, and capabilities for the rest of their lives. These goals include sustained healthy diet and weight control, sustained high daily physical activity level, and aerobic exercise three times a week. In addition, if an individual is receiving medication that relates to cardiovascular dysfunction, a physical therapy outcome is to minimize, reduce, or eliminate the need for medication in the short term and long term.

Goals: Long Term

Long-term goals and outcomes are as important as the short-term physical therapy goals and outcomes. Intervention (drugs and surgery) has short-term benefits, as is evidenced by the apparently high number of repeated revascularization procedures performed, compared with the lifestyle behavioral changes inherent in physical therapy management, including education, smoking cessation, optimal nutrition, and exercise. At the point of entry into physical therapy (acute, subacute, or chronic, with cardiovascular dysfunction as a primary or secondary diagnosis), a long-term plan with goals, outcomes, and follow-ups is integral to the management plan overall (Table 24-2).

Cardiac Rehabilitation: Specific Components

Phases

Patients are referred to cardiac rehabilitation for management and secondary prevention of myocardial insufficiency and after revascularization procedures, including cardiac surgery.[240] People can also benefit if they have significant risk for disease but are asymptomatic.

The phases of cardiac rehabilitation appear in Table 24-3 (with the exception of phase I, inpatient management, which is described in Chapter 29). Phase I refers to inpatient care (medical and surgical) and the predischarge exercise test.

Phase II refers to a supervised exercise program lasting 3 to 6 months. Phase II usually takes place in a community center where the patients can be monitored during exercise and education by the rehabilitation professions can be ongoing. However, a trial of home-based phase II programs for high-risk patients after cardiac surgery produced the same results as were found in the control group, which received general guidelines to increase activity levels.[241] Further study is needed on the short- and long-term effectiveness of home-based phase II programs as opposed to center-based programs with respect to symptom recurrence, indications for revascularization procedures, and risk-factor reduction.

Phase III refers to the maintenance phase, during which the patient is responsible for exercising mostly at home. This phase lasts from 6 to 12 months.

Phase IV refers to an unsupervised community program. The patient is usually ready for this phase within 9 to 12 months. Patients may be referred to cardiac rehabilitation

Table 24-2 Comprehensive Physical Therapy Management and Lifelong Health Plan

Patient's entry point to physical therapy	A primary diagnosis of cardiovascular or pulmonary dysfunction A secondary diagnosis of cardiovascular or pulmonary dysfunction A diagnosis of cardiovascular or pulmonary dysfunction secondary to dysfunction of systems other than primary oxygen transport dysfunction (i.e., the heart, circulation, or lungs) (Chapters 6, 25, and 32)
Assessment	Readiness to change (precontemplative, contemplative, preparation, action, maintenance) Demographics, including literacy, culture, and education Learning needs and style Preventive goals and outcomes Long-term goals and outcomes Short-term goals and outcomes
Follow-up	Physical evaluation Sustained adherence to behavioral-change programs Visits to physician, clinic, hospital (details of when, why, and, if admitted to hospital, for how long) Medication changes (what, when, why, and dose or discontinued) or new medications (what, when, why, dose)

Table 24-3 Rehabilitation Phases of Cardiac and Pulmonary Rehabilitation

Phase	Cardiac Rehabilitation	Pulmonary Rehabilitation
I*		
II Under supervision in hospital, center, or community-based program or one-on-one session	6 weeks post acute episode or discharge, to 6 months Exercise retest Review of risk factors; lifestyle behaviors and changes Revision of lifestyle recommendations	≤6 weeks post acute episode or discharge, to 6 months Exercise retest Review of risk factors and lifestyle behaviors and changes Revision of lifestyle recommendations
III Under supervision in hospital, center, or community-based program or one-on-one session	6 to 12 months Exercise retest Review of risk factors and lifestyle behaviors and changes Revision of lifestyle recommendations Exit retest for recommendations for self-management phase IV	6 to 12 months Exercise retest Review of risk factors and lifestyle behaviors and changes Revision of lifestyle recommendations Exit retest for recommendations for self-management phase IV
IV Self-management	>12 months Provision for follow-up	>12 months Provision for follow-up

*Phase I is described in Chapter 29, the management of Individuals with Acute Medical Conditions.

when they are stable and not in conjunction with an acute event.

Smoking Cessation

The risk for myocardial infarction is three times higher in patients who continue to smoke after a cardiac event.[242] When patients quit, the risk for reinfarction is reduced to that of nonsmokers prior to the first infarction.

Nutrition and Weight Control

Optimal nutrition and weight control are priorities. Individuals with cardiovascular dysfunction are at risk for fluid and electrolyte imbalances and related ECG irregularities, so these aspects of nutrition need to be included. In addition, patients with chronic heart failure have some special considerations. These patients rely more on fat substrate during exercise than on carbohydrates, which may contribute to increased catecholamines and free fatty-acid levels.[243] These changes may compensate to protect muscle glycogen stores. However, given that fat metabolism is not energy-efficient, this shift may contribute to exercise intolerance.

Psychosocial Issues

Stress management and life-skills training are fundamental to rehabilitation programs in minimizing undue sympathetic arousal and impact on the cardiovascular and pulmonary systems. If indicated, help with depression control and anger and hostility management are provided by the appropriate professionals. Remediation of depression alone can enhance functional status.

Risk Reduction

Prevention and rehabilitation programs aim to reduce an individual's cardiac risk factor category. Figure 24-2 shows an example of a scale for assessing cardiac risk and identifying an individual's category of risk. Using such a scale provides

Step 1: Find your points based on your Age, Blood Pressure, LDL and HDL Cholesterol, and whether you Smoke or have Diabetes.

AGE

Age	M	F
30-34	-1	-9
35-39	0	-4
40-44	1	0
45-49	2	3
50-54	3	6
55-59	4	7
60-64	5	8
65-69	6	8
70-74	7	9

DO YOU HAVE DIABETES?

	M	F
YES	2	4
NO	0	0

CHOLESTEROL

LDL Cholesterol

	M	F
<100	-3	-2
100-129	0	0
130-159	0	0
160-189	1	2
>189	2	2

HDL Cholesterol

	M	F
<35	2	5
35-44	1	2
45-49	0	1
50-59	0	0
>59	-1	-3

DO YOU SMOKE?

	M	F
YES	2	2
NO	0	0

Blood Pressure

	M	F
<120/<80	0	-3
120-129/ 80-84	0	0
130-139/ 85-89	1	0
140-159/ 90-99	2	2
>159/>99	3	3

Fig. 24-2 Cardiac Risk Analysis: Estimate Your Risk for Developing Heart Disease in the Next 10 Years. *(Modified from The Framingham Heart Study, www.nhlbi.nih.gov/about/Framingham/index.html; and Wilson PW, D'Agostino RB, Levy D, et al: Prediction of coronary heart disease using risk factor categories, Circulation 97:1837–1847, 1998.)*

Step 2: Add up your points for Age, LDL-Cholesterol, HDL-Cholesterol, Blood Pressure, Smoking & Diabetes.

Age	
LDL-Cholesterol	
HDL-Cholesterol	
Blood Pressure	
Diabetes	
Smoking	
TOTAL POINTS	

Step 3: Find Your Risk Level Based on Your Point Total.

Total Points	<–2	–2	–1	0	1	2	3	4	5	6	7	8	9	10	11	12	13	14	15	16	≥17
% Risk Male	1	2	2	3	4	4	5	7	8	10	13	17	21	26	32	38	46	54	54	54	54
% Risk Female	1	1	2	2	2	3	3	4	5	6	7	8	9	11	12	14	16	20	22	25	30

Your **Framingham Risk** for developing Heart Disease including a Heart Attack over the next 10 years is denoted by the **%RISK Male or Female** corresponding to your **Total Points Score.**

Step 4: Compare Your Risk to Others. For comparison purposes, **Low Risk** is the risk of developing heart disease within the next 10 years for a Man or Woman of the same age with normal blood pressure and cholesterol who does not smoke or have diabetes.

COMPARATIVE RISK

MALES		
AGE	AVERAGE RISK	LOW RISK
30-34	3%	2%
35-39	5%	3%
40-44	7%	4%
45-49	11%	4%
50-54	14%	6%
55-59	16%	7%
60-64	21%	9%
65-69	25%	11%
70-74	30%	14%

FEMALES		
AGE	AVERAGE RISK	LOW RISK
30-34	<1%	<1%
35-39	1%	<1%
40-44	2%	2%
45-49	5%	3%
50-54	8%	5%
55-59	12%	7%
60-64	12%	8%
65-69	13%	8%
70-74	14%	8%

Note that there is no risk estimate for patients < 30 or older than 74 because this analysis is based on real data collected from Framingham

Fig. 24-2, cont'd

Table 24-4 Risk Stratification

Low risk	After uncomplicated myocardial infarction or bypass surgery Functional capacity below 8 METs on 3-week exercise test Asymptomatic at rest, with exercise adequate for most vocational and recreational activities No ECG evidence of ischemia, left ventricular dysfunction, or complex dysrhythmias
Intermediate risk	Functional capacity below 8 METs on 3-week exercise test Shock or congestive heart failure during recent myocardial infarction (<6 months) Inability to self-monitor heart rate Failure to adhere to exercise prescription
High risk	Severely depressed left ventricular function (ejection fraction <30%) Resting complex ventricular dysrhythmias (low-grade IV or V) Premature ventricular contractions appearing or increasing with exercise Exertional hypotension (≥15 mm Hg) Recent myocardial infarction (<6 months) complicated by serious ventricular dysrhythmias Exercise-induced ischemia of more than 2 mm ST depression Survivors of cardiac arrest

MET, Metabolic equivalents (1 MET = 3.5 mL O_2/kg of body weight/minute, which is the metabolic rate at rest).
Modified from American College of Sports Medicine: ACSM's guidelines for exercise testing and prescription, *ed 8, Philadelphia, 2010, Lippincott Williams & Wilkins.*

objective markers for risk factor modification, and evaluating the degree of risk reduction with health behavior change, an important physical therapy outcome. Table 24-4 shows the distinctions among low, intermediate, and high risk for cardiac disease.[244]

After angioplasty, bypass surgery, and medical therapy for fixed obstructions, individuals remain at risk, as judged by the proportion of patients who require further pharmacological and surgical management. Risk-reduction interventions are priorities in this cohort of individuals; they can extend survival, improve quality of life, reduce the need for further invasive procedures such as angioplasty and bypass surgery, and reduce the incidence of myocardial infarction.[245] Secondary risk reduction is as important as primary risk reduction, and it should be a routine component of both medical and surgical management.

Physical Activity and Exercise: Special Considerations

The principles and practice of exercise prescription are described in detail in Chapter 19. However, special considerations for individuals with chronic heart conditions with respect to monitoring, exercise testing, and exercise training are detailed here.

Monitoring

Assessment and monitoring considerations for the individual with heart disease are described in Part Two and Chapter 31. At the onset of the program, a baseline assessment is made of the patient's subjective sense of well-being, including health-related quality of life, impact of sickness and disability, quality of life, and life satisfaction. Related assessments are made throughout the program to observe the program's effects on these outcomes and to assess the impact of the program at its completion.

An individual with primary cardiovascular dysfunction or its risk factors requires particular attention to his or her hemodynamic status. Risk factors, however, do not necessarily predict complications during supervised exercise.[246] Serial lipid profiles, blood pressure, resting heart rate, and body weight are monitored regularly, and interventions are modified accordingly.[247] Blood pressure, however, can be abnormal in individuals with exercise-induced left ventricular systolic dysfunction, which leads to unstable hemodynamic status.[248] Blood pressure may not be a valid measure of exercise stress in such individuals. Further study is needed before exercise risk stratification guidelines can be used with any assurance to monitor supervised rehabilitation programs.

The absolute and relative changes in heart rate, blood pressure, rate pressure product, arterial saturation, and perceived exertion are particularly important. ECGs may be performed intermittently throughout exercise or continuously, as indicated. Recent evidence has questioned the conventional guideline of an ST-segment depression of greater than 1 mm in favor of a more conservative guideline, greater than 0.5 mm during or after exercise.[249] This value is associated with risk for myocardial infarction, requiring bypass surgery, and risk for cardiac mortality.

Exercise-induced silent myocardial ischemia is an important indicator of increased risk for cardiovascular disease (3.5-fold) and stroke (2.2-fold) in men when they are compared with those without silent ischemia. Other risk factors include smoking, hypercholesterolemia, hypertension, and being overweight.[250]

Recovery data are important components of the exercise testing assessment and interpretation. Delayed heart rate recovery is a predictor of mortality,[184] irrespective of angiographic evidence of disease severity.[251] Heart rate recovery is calculated as the difference in heart rate from peak exercise to that recorded at 1, 2, and 3 minutes after exercise. Women have been reported to be more susceptible to postexercise hypotension than men; an active cool-down period may offset postexercise hypotension.[252] Signs and symptoms of overexertion must be monitored (Box 24-2).

Each individual is taught to monitor his or her baseline, exercise, and recovery responses in a logbook at each visit, after the parameters have been prescribed and it is considered safe for the patient to self-monitor in the supervised setting.

Box 24-2 Signs and Symptoms of Overexertion of Particular Importance in an Individual with a Heart Condition

Signs and Symptoms During or Immediately After Exercise
- Chest pain (angina)
- Lightheadedness or confusion
- Nausea and vomiting
- Intermittent claudication
- Prolonged dyspnea (> several minutes)
- Dysrhythmia
- Inappropriate breathlessness
- Inappropriate bradycardia or tachycardia
- Inappropriate hypotension or hypertension

Delayed Effects
- Prolonged fatigue (24 hours or more)
- Insomnia
- Weight gain due to fluid retention
- Persistent ECG irregularities (e.g., PVCs and tachycardia)

PVC, Premature ventricular contraction.

Commonly, the individual is taught to record heart rate and a rating of perceived exertion. In addition, data sheets are logged with respect to stretching and warm-up, the parameters used for each day's exercise (including the aerobic exercise prescription), and the cool-down and recovery periods. Also, completion of the resistance muscle training prescription is logged.

Exercise Testing

Exercise testing is used for diagnosis, assessment of functional work capacity, assessment of the outcome of one or more interventions, including a training program, and prognosis. A poor response to exercise after percutaneous transluminal coronary angioplasty can identify restenosis.[253] The graded exercise test, or maximal stress test, is usually a short (8 to 12 minutes, ideally), progressively ramped, symptom-limited exercise test conducted on a treadmill or cycle ergometer. Several established cardiac stress test protocols, such as the Bruce and the Balke, are available. In some situations, a submaximal test is preferred because a maximal test may be risky or difficult to conduct in a valid manner because of a secondary problem. Recently, the prognostic superiority of a two-step exercise test that combines a low-intensity, steady-work-rate phase and a maximal exercise phase has been reported.[114] An exercise test may answer questions about an individual's status and thus obviate or reduce the need for more invasive and costly testing.[254]

The exercise testing protocol is designed to stress the patient's oxygen transport system—ventilation, heart, circulation, and muscles—progressively and in an integrated manner. Exercise is the single best way to assess the integrated function of these systems and their capacity for oxygen transport. For detailed evaluation and prognosis of a patient with advanced heart failure, assessment of $\dot{V}O_{2peak}$ is preferable to the use of submaximal exercise tests such as the 6-minute walk test.[113] Walking on a treadmill has been reported to have greater diagnostic sensitivity than cycling in asymptomatic men with coronary artery disease.[255]

Valid testing of functional capacity in indivi[illegible] cardiac failure is necessary because of the discordanc[illegible] results of various tests in the same individual.[256] The 6-m[illegible] walk test distance has been reported to be highly reproduc[illegible] in patients with heart failure.[257] Distance walked is somewha[illegible] correlated to the New York Heart Association functional classification and quality of life, and this correlation is stronger for individuals with mild and moderate disease severity (New York Heart Association classifications II and III).[256] Compared with more sophisticated and more invasive testing, the 6-minute walk test can serve to stratify individuals in terms of functional status, which is of therapeutic and prognostic importance.

Chapter 19 describes indications for conducting an exercise test, as well as the relative and absolute contraindications to the test. That chapter also notes the importance of maximizing test validity and reliability by adhering to strict standards for pretest conditions in the patient, including medications, testing standards, and monitoring recovery data. In addition, the chapter describes basic and advanced measures that can be taken, depending on the needs of the patient and the specific purpose of the test. In most individuals with cardiac dysfunction, an ECG is monitored continuously, along with heart rate. Blood pressure and ratings of perceived exertion and dyspnea (PE) are monitored intermittently. Additional measures are taken as indicated. For example, a patient may be limited by arthritic pain, so it is important to monitor discomfort and pain using a standardized scale (see Chapters 15 and 19). Medications must be reviewed and the time at which they were last taken must be noted in order to determine their impact on responses during the exercise test and to establish which measures will be most valid in terms of assessment of exercise response.

Potential complications that could occur during exercise in patients with heart failure must be anticipated and appropriate monitoring instituted to maximize the safety of exercise testing and training. Adverse responses include dysrhythmias and hypotension.[258]

Individuals with unexplained dyspnea are at risk for ischemia and cardiac events. Exercise echocardiography provides independently derived information that identifies patients at risk.[259] Dyspnea requires investigation in individuals with suspected or known heart disease.

Exercise testing has a role in predicting surgical outcomes. $\dot{V}O_{2peak}$ and exercise duration are good parameters for evaluating functional class and postoperative status in people who have undergone valve repairs or valvuloplasty.[116] Patients who have a $\dot{V}O_{2peak}$ of at least 19 mL/kg/min preoperatively achieve a higher functional class 1 year after surgery.

Of particular importance is identifying and recording why the test was stopped—for instance, a predetermined sign or symptom in the patient was reached, or the patient wished to discontinue. Even if the test is being conducted to determine oxygen transport capacity, the cause for termination may be a comorbidity, such as musculoskeletal strain, muscle weakness, or pain or discomfort of musculoskeletal origin.

Exercise Training

The parameters of exercise training are based on the assessment and on the short- and long-term objectives of the exercise program, and these differ for each individual. The training

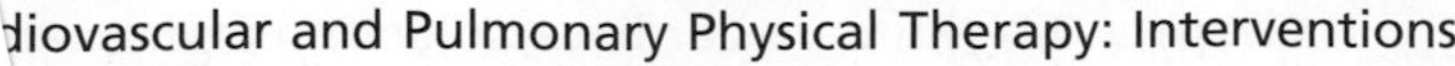

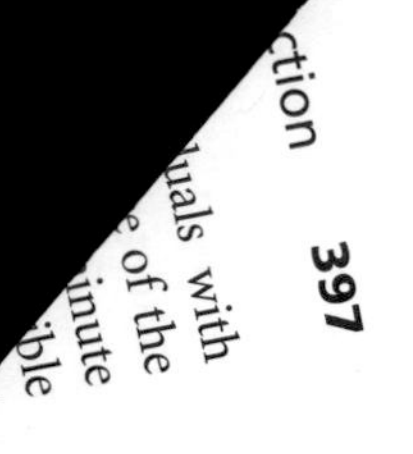

m-up defined by a work rate inter- t training zone and rest. Warm-up ect against left ventricular dysfunc- gina.[260] In a repeat test 30 minutes hold for angina and ST-segment ted to increase along with the eshold intensity has been identi- training in individuals with cardiac disease.[261] though a lower limit of 45% of $\dot{V}O_2$ reserve is commonly reported in the literature, intensities below this level cannot be ruled out, particularly in extremely deconditioned people. The absence of such a limit supports the need to consider individual differences and to prescribe exercise on an individual basis (Table 24-5).

Many types of exercise can be considered in the exercise prescription. Improvement in walking tolerance and distance is a primary goal because it is a hallmark of independence and mobility, particularly with advancing age, and it is coupled with the upright position and its associated gravitational stress. Walking has multiple physiological benefits in individuals with coronary artery disease[262] as well as in healthy people. Decisions are made based on the specificity principle. If the goal is to improve the patient's functional needs, activities that are closest to those needs are chosen. If improving aerobic fitness and maximum functional capacity is the goal, exercise that involves more limbs would be the best choice.

The use of hydrotherapy and aquacise have been prominent in Europe. Another application that has been reported to have beneficial effects on the exercise responses of individuals with chronic heart failure is thermal hydrotherapy, which involves the passive application of heat and cold.[6] A 6-week program of home-based hydrotherapy was reported to improve resting and submaximal heart rates, in addition to reducing symptoms and improving quality of life. These effects were attributed to physiological adaptations to alternating hot and cold body stimulation. Further study of this application and its mechanisms is necessary; its indications may prove to be positive in individuals challenged by even minimal amounts of exercise.

Conventionally, the exercise intensity for patients with heart disease is set at a proportion of oxygen uptake reserve or heart rate reserve, which suggests a critical threshold for training effects. However, no intensity threshold for aerobic training has been identified, so intensities below the accepted standard probably provide training stimulus, particularly for patients with low functional capacity.[261]

It has been suggested that interval training leads to more marked improvement in hemodynamics in individuals with heart failure than does steady-rate work.[263] Another suggestion is that steady-rate aerobic exercise contributes to greater well-being and quality of life. Further study is needed to examine the effects of various parameters in training protocols in this cohort.

Peak functional capacity depends on muscle strength and endurance in individuals with chronic heart failure.[264] Improvement in subjective symptoms reported in daily activities, especially dyspnea on exertion, however, depends largely on muscle endurance.

Resistance muscle training has an important role in cardiac rehabilitation programs; it allows a patient to regain lost strength, and it facilitates avocational activities and return to work soon after a cardiac event.[265] Resistance muscle training in the form of circuit weight training can be integrated into the cardiac rehabilitation program. Muscle training can be safe and therapeutic even at relatively high workloads in properly selected individuals, including older adults.[266] The hemodynamic response depends on the isometric and postural stabilization component, in addition to the load or resistance used, the muscle mass activated, the number of repetitions in the set, and the duration of each contraction, as well as the

Table 24-5 Guidelines for Exercise Prescription for Individuals with Heart Conditions

Type	Area of Focus	Intensity	Duration	Frequency
Aerobic exercise (walking, ergometry, rowing, running)	Large muscle groups	Percentage of functional capacity ($\dot{V}O_2$) based on HR, RPE, or METs 50% to 85% of HR reserve RPE 3 to 6 (0-10 scale) or 12 to 16 (18-20 scale) METs (40%-85% peak METs)	20 to 40 min continuous Three 10-min sessions per day	Less than 2 to 3 METs, short sessions several times daily 3-5 METs once daily 5-8 METs 3-5 times weekly
Resistance muscle training,* (elastic bands, cuff/hand weights, dumbbells, free weights, pulleys, weight machines)	Peripheral muscle groups	Progressively increasing loads 10% to 50% of maximum	1 to 3 sets of 8 to 15 repetitions maximum** for each muscle group	2-3 days/week

HR, Heart rate; MET, metabolic equivalent; RPE, rating of perceived exertion.

*According to American Association of Cardiovascular Pulmonary Rehabilitation (AACVPR) Guidelines for Pulmonary Rehabilitation Programs (ed 4), "to prevent soreness and minimize the risk of injury, the initial load should allow 12-15 repetitions comfortably. If 1 RM pretest is used, this load would be approximately 30-40% 1 RM for the upper body and 50-60% for hips and legs. Low-risk stratified, well-trained patients may progress to higher loads depending on program goals."

**Repetition maximum is the maximum number of times a load can be lifted before fatigue.

Modified from American College of Sports Medicine: ACSM's guidelines for exercise testing and prescription, *ed 8, Philadelphia, 2010, Lippincott Williams & Wilkins; and AACVPR:* Guidelines for Pulmonary Rehabilitation Programs, *ed 4, Champaign, Ill, 2011, Human Kinetics.*

involvement of the Valsalva maneuver. Upper-body work has been viewed conservatively as an exercise option for individuals with cardiac problems, and it warrants greater emphasis.[267] Despite caveats regarding isometric exercise for individuals with coronary artery disease, one study compared the hemodynamic responses of brief and sustained isometric exercise and dynamic exercise in individuals with heart disease and healthy people.[268] The incidence of myocardial ischemia was reported to be lower during isometric exercise than during dynamic exercise in patients at the same level of perceived exertion. The investigators postulated that isometric exercise generates high perfusion pressure in the coronary arteries and prolongs perfusion, thereby potentially protecting the myocardia from ischemia. Further study is needed to examine this hypothesis.

Lengthening (eccentric) muscle contractions and shortening (concentric) muscle contractions have distinct energetic and metabolic properties that may make one or the other better suited for certain patient populations.[269-271] Eccentric muscle contractions are associated with higher muscle tension and less metabolic demand. For low-risk individuals who have ischemic heart disease without angina, inducible ischemia, or left ventricular dysfunction, eccentric exercise can be recommended; these patients can perform high-load resistance exercise with minimal cardiovascular stress.[272]

Electrical stimulation of the quadriceps has been examined as a form of exercise for individuals with chronic heart failure.[273] Although the improvement in muscle performance and exercise capacity was comparable to that of individuals in an ergometer exercise program, the use of electrical stimulation should be considered in the overall context of the individual's needs. Active exercise has many multisystem benefits that electrical stimulation does not provide. In addition, electrical stimulation is a more passive modality than active exercise, which may be counter to the goal of self-efficacy that cardiac rehabilitation promotes.

Hydrotherapy in a home-based program has shown some interesting applications to individuals with chronic heart failure.[6] In a study of individuals with mild heart failure, an intensive 6-week program of home-based repeated brief cold stimuli appeared to improve peripheral circulation and, in turn, to improve heart-failure symptoms, heart rate response to exercise, and quality of life.

Long-Term Plan

Long-term planning, in which regular physical activity and a structured program of exercise are components, is detailed in Chapter 31 for individuals with chronic, primary cardiovascular, and pulmonary conditions.

Pulmonary Rehabilitation: Specific Components

Phases

The phases of pulmonary rehabilitation can generally be considered comparable to those of cardiac rehabilitation, although they are less well defined in terms of a formal inpatient phase after an acute episode followed by progressively less closely supervised phases (see Table 24-3). A patient with chronic lung disease is more likely to be referred when stable than in conjunction with an acute event. The first graded exercise test may be in the supervised program rather than in the hospital before discharge after an admission for acute symptoms.

Smoking Cessation

Smoking cessation is essential for the health and well-being of all people, in particular those with pulmonary disease. The physical therapist has a responsibility to address this modifiable risk as a priority of management (see Chapters 1 and 31).

Nutrition and Weight Control

The connection between nutrition and lung health has become a focus of research interest, and that research supports the role of good nutrition (in particular, the consumption of fruits, vegetables, and fish) in optimal lung health.[274,275] Diet may be an important cofactor in the development of COPD. Whether good nutrition improves damaged lungs has not been substantiated, but good nutrition improves general health and thus should be a primary recommendation when managing these patients.

Psychosocial Issues

Patients with chronic conditions have higher incidences of depression and poorer psychosocial adjustment than do individuals in the general population. Although chronically poor blood gases can affect psychological and cognitive function, the remediation of any source of depression can independently improve function. Thus depression and other psychological issues must be assessed and managed independently.

Risk Reduction

Lifestyle modification and risk factor modification are fundamental components of the pulmonary rehabilitation program; these modifications include smoking cessation, nutrition and weight control, and stress management, in conjunction with physical activity and exercise. Optimal nutrition is encouraged as a lifelong change in patients with COPD, whose nutritional status is often suboptimal.[276] Carbohydrate-rich foods, known to increase carbon dioxide production, have been targeted as a food group that should be limited in patients with COPD. Small changes in the carbohydrate constituents of diet have been reported to have a major effect on $\dot{V}CO_2$, exercise tolerance, and breathlessness.[277] Smoking cessation is essential to limit further lung damage and has the potential to reverse impaired pulmonary function, improve oxygen transport capacity, and reduce or reverse smoking-related risk factors as the period of nonsmoking lengthens. Reduction of pulmonary and cardiac risk factors in an individual with primary lung dysfunction is essential.

Physical Activity and Exercise: Special Considerations

The principles and practice of exercise prescription are described in detail in Chapter 19. However, special considerations for this patient group, with respect to monitoring, testing, and training, are detailed here.

Monitoring

The objective and subjective measures used to monitor patients with pulmonary dysfunction during exercise are comparable to those used in patients with cardiac dysfunction, because the heart and lung are interdependent. However, ventilatory parameters, such as breathing pattern, arterial saturation as gauged by pulse oximetry, and subjective sense of breathlessness, are particularly important, as are heart rate, blood pressure, and ECG readings.

Exercise Testing

The indications for and contraindications to testing are established (see Chapter 19). The goals of an exercise test are determined beforehand for each given individual. The exercise test may be selected to evaluate aerobic capacity or the strength and endurance of peripheral or respiratory muscles. The demands of upper-body work may compete with breathing demands in some patients, so upper-body work is integrated into the overall program judiciously and monitored accordingly. Upper-body strength tends to be lower than lower-body strength in patients with chronic obstructive lung conditions. Upper-body strengthening can reduce rating of perceived exertion and breathlessness and thus warrants being assessed and trained.[278]

The exercise test to assess cardiovascular and pulmonary conditioning may be maximal or submaximal and may involve a modality such as a treadmill or ergometer, depending on the device's suitability for the patient and on the best means of maximizing the test's validity and reliability. Depending on the purpose of the test, a decision is made beforehand about the patient's medications and when they are taken in relation to the timing of the test. Some patients may be tested with oxygen or purposely without oxygen, or with or without bronchodilators, depending on whether the effect of such interventions is being evaluated. It is essential to monitor dyspnea in these patients and to correlate the dyspnea rating with objective measures. Some patients may have invasive blood work done before, during, and after the test to monitor serial arterial blood gases. Pulse oximetry is routinely monitored along with heart rate and blood pressure. Some patients may require ECG monitoring. Invasive procedures such as arterial blood gas measurement are done as indicated. Respiratory muscle testing and training are based on similar principles. (Detailed descriptions appear in Chapter 26.)

Oxygen consumption studies provide a metabolic and ventilatory profile of the patient's response to progressive exercise and recovery. Submaximal and peak levels of $\dot{V}O_2$ can be examined, along with their physiological and clinical correlates. The ventilatory efficiency can be determined on the basis of the ventilatory equivalent of CO_2 (minute ventilation [$\dot{V}_E$] divided by CO_2 production [$\dot{V}CO_2$]). The limitation of oxygen consumption studies is the difficulty of ensuring a valid and reliable test. The test requires that a face mask or mouthpiece be worn, either of which can distort the patient's breathing. The patient may feel anxious when wearing such devices or may alter his or her breathing pattern because of the increased dead space in the expiratory hose.

Exercise testing can be used to diagnose exercise-limiting factors. For example, exercise testing in a patient with pulmonary fibrosis can distinguish cardiovascular and pulmonary limitations. Exercise-induced hypoxemia in this cohort has been closely related to survival.[279]

Choice of exercise testing and training modalities is determined by the indications for the test and for training. Patients with COPD show different responses to walking and to cycling.[280] Aerobic capacity in walking is less than in cycling and is associated with excessive ventilatory demand during peak exercise supported by increased ventilatory dead space, reduced ventilatory efficiency, and arterial hypoxemia. Arm ergometry is associated with greater dyssynchronous breathing than is leg work, so it may be an inappropriate modality for patients with severe disease.[281]

Low-flow oxygen is a common intervention for hypoxemia in patients with severe COPD. Although long-term oxygen therapy improves survival,[282,283] there remain many unanswered questions regarding the use of the modality and its efficacy during exercise training.[284] Further study is needed to establish its efficacy in improving exercise capacity in patients with hypoxemia, as well as without hypoxemia, and to establish the characteristics of responders versus nonresponders, which will allow for the refinement of exercise prescription in this patient cohort. A study of patients with cystic fibrosis showed that supplemental oxygen speeded recovery after a short bout of maximal exercise and preserved subsequent exercise performance.[285]

In individuals with COPD and mild exercise hypoxemia, relief of breathlessness with supplemental oxygen has been explained by a commensurate reduction in ventilatory demand and reduced blood lactate levels.[286] Short-term use of oxygen before or after exercise has not been supported.[287]

As with exercise testing of any patient, it is essential to record why an exercise test was terminated—whether it was a sign or symptom predetermined by the tester or a symptom of the patient. If it was a symptom reported by the patient, was it shortness of breath or another or unrelated cause, such as dizziness, muscle strain, plantar fasciitis, arthritic discomfort or pain, or imbalance?

Exercise Training

Training involves flexibility and strengthening, as well as aerobic exercise. Although patients learn to self-monitor and pace their exercise based on their responses, many have had long-term physical therapy and instruction in breathing control because of continued altered breathing pattern, even during ADL.[288,289] Walking in conjunction with breathing control is particularly useful for patients with pulmonary dysfunction. Pulse oximetry may have to be used to guide the training session.

Lengthening (eccentric) muscle contractions are associated with reduced energy cost, so such exercise has important therapeutic implications for individuals with poor aerobic capacity.[270] However, eccentric muscle work in the form of downhill walking or cycling on a negative-work ergometer alters breathing patterns toward a tendency to breathe rapidly and shallowly.[269,271] Thus patients require stringent monitoring when performing this type of energy-efficient exercise.

Although resistance muscle training has been receiving some attention for individuals with chronic lung disease, the prescriptive parameters for optimal benefit have yet to be defined. These parameters should become clear when the role of deconditioning as opposed to a disease-specific myopathy is better understood with respect to the reduced strength observed in these individuals.

Cardiac and Pulmonary Rehabilitation: Future Directions

The effects of cardiac and pulmonary rehabilitation have been well established on the basis of the highest levels of evidence. However, the lack of adequate access to people who would most benefit from primary prevention of heart and lung disease and from management and secondary prevention has limited the impact of these known effects for at-risk or affected individuals or for the health of the community. Health policies must be structured to enable individuals to take advantage of the resources of such programs. Physical therapists need to be well trained in the principles and practice of cardiac and pulmonary rehabilitation so that these can be applied on a one-on-one basis across areas of specialty practice. This is essential because most individuals under the care of a physical therapist have one or more risk factors. These risk factors need to be addressed, irrespective of whether the individual is presenting with cardiac or pulmonary risk factors or with a diagnosis that is primary or secondary. This knowledge is essential to ensure that physical therapy interventions are modified accordingly in patients with these conditions or their risk factors.

Based on epidemiological indicators, behavioral strategies have the greatest potential for long-term improvement in the abilities and participation of individuals with lung conditions (see Chapters 1 and 5). When effectively administered and adhered to, these interventions are not associated with the risks of invasive management, which must be minimized as much as possible commensurate with the individual's functional improvements. On the contrary, these noninvasive interventions help to ensure reduced long-term morbidity and increased health overall, thus reducing health care needs and potentially increasing individual longevity.

Finally, research is needed to establish how best to structure the principles of cardiac and pulmonary rehabilitation on an individual basis to maximize sustainable benefits for life. Some have argued for inclusion and exclusion criteria to maximize the success of the program.[290] Identifying and reducing barriers to access and participation and maximizing adherence through motivational interviewing and cognitive therapeutic interventions may maximize the impact of these services on society.

Summary

Based on state-of-the-art literature, this chapter extends the general exercise testing and training principles described in Chapter 19 to specific considerations in relation to the principles of best physical therapy practice in cardiac and pulmonary rehabilitation programs, regardless of whether delivered in a structured group format or in one-on-one sessions. Structured formal programs are often available only in large urban areas and thus have low access rates. The same principles, however, are fundamental to physical therapy practice overall and can be readily applied in a one-on-one setting in private practice or in a health care facility. These principles should be applied not only to patients with primary heart and lung conditions but also in the physical therapy management of patients being treated for musculoskeletal and neuromuscular conditions who have secondary diagnoses of chronic heart and lung conditions or who have associated risk factors. In these cases, the physical therapy program must be adapted to the requirements of these underlying conditions (or these conditions may need to be managed independently if they have not been previously identified as a priority). In this way, the patient's more serious underlying cardiovascular and pulmonary problem is addressed and the interventions, including exercise prescribed for the musculoskeletal or neuromuscular problems, are modified according to the more serious life-threatening condition. Exercise testing and training are only part of the management of individuals with chronic, primary cardiovascular and pulmonary dysfunction; the comprehensive approach to management is described in Chapter 31.

The common components of cardiac and pulmonary rehabilitation are described and then differentiated based on their distinct underlying pathophysiology and impacts on individuals. Lifelong health behavior change and reduced need for invasive care in the short term and long term are primary outcomes.

The goal of the physical therapist, who is uniquely qualified as an applied clinical exercise physiologist and health coach, is to ensure that the proper components, in particular exercise, are prescribed to meet the specific needs and comorbidities of each individual. One criticism of structured cardiac and pulmonary rehabilitation programs has been that they are overly regimented and insufficiently individualized, putting these programs at odds with contemporary principles of exercise prescription to produce optimal results. Regardless of the program type, physical therapists must prescribe exercise testing and training that will best fit the needs of each individual patient, based on a detailed multisystem assessment, and then evaluate each patient's progress accordingly.

The principles of exercise testing and training in individuals with cardiovascular and pulmonary dysfunction secondary to conditions other than primary cardiovascular and pulmonary dysfunction are described in the following chapter, Chapter 25.

Review Questions

1. Describe how the principles and practices of cardiac and pulmonary rehabilitation are included within the fundamental principles and practices of physical therapy.
2. Describe how the principles and practices of physical therapy, which include cardiac and pulmonary rehabilitation programs, can be applied in a one-on-one setting as well as in a formally structured program.
3. Describe how the goals of physical therapy management in these programs are consistent with the philosophy and framework of the WHO International Classification of Function.
4. Describe the rationale for assessing an individual's readiness to change with respect to participating in a rehabilitation program; discuss its clinical implications. Consider the limitations of this construct.
5. Describe how individuals with chronic cardiovascular conditions can adapt physiologically and psychologically to exercise.

6. Describe how individuals with chronic pulmonary conditions can adapt physiologically and psychologically to exercise.
7. Contrast and compare measurements and outcomes used for individuals with chronic cardiac conditions as opposed to those with chronic pulmonary conditions.
8. Describe the rationale for goal setting with patients at three levels: prevention, short term, and long term.
9. You have been requested to serve on a team to develop a cardiac rehabilitation program in your area. Describe how, as a physical therapist, you will contribute to this program. In particular, consider the competencies you will offer.
10. You have been requested to serve on a team to develop a pulmonary rehabilitation program in your area. Describe how, as a physical therapist, you will contribute to this program. In particular, consider the competencies you will offer.

References

1. Dafoe W, Huston P: Current trends in cardiac rehabilitation. *Canadian Medical Association Journal* 156:527–532, 1997.
2. Stone JA: Canadian guidelines for cardiac rehabilitation and cardiovascular disease prevention are available. *Journal of Cardiopulmonary Rehabilitation* 21:344–345, 2001.
3. NHS Centre for Reviews and Dissemination, University of York, effective health care: cardiac rehabilitation: 4:1–12, 1998.
4. Rosenberg H, Resnick B: Exercise intervention in patients with chronic obstructive pulmonary disease. *Geriatric Nursing* 24:90–95, 2003.
5. Klein JJ, van der Palen J, Uil SM, et al: Benefit from the inclusion of self-treatment guidelines to a self-management programme for adults with asthma. *European Respiratory Journal* 17:386–394, 2001.
6. Michalsen A, Ludtke R, Buhring M, et al: Thermal hydrotherapy improves quality of life and hemodynamic function in patients with chronic heart failure. *American Heart Journal* 46:728–733, 2003.
7. American College of Cardiology/American Heart Association Task Force on Practice Guidelines: ACC/AHA 2002 guideline update for exercise testing: Summary article. *Journal of the American College of Cardiology* 40:1531–1540, 2003.
8. Williams MA, Fleg JL, Ades PA, et al: Secondary prevention of coronary heart disease in the elderly (with an emphasis on patients ≥ 75 years of age): An American Heart Association scientific statement from the Council on Clinical Cardiology Subcommittee on Exercise, Cardiac Rehabilitation, and Prevention. *Circulation* 105:1735–1743, 2002.
9. American College of Sports Medicine: *ACSM's Resource Manual for Guidelines for Exercise Testing and Prescription*, ed 6, Philadelphia, 2009, Lippincott Williams & Wilkins.
10. American Heart Association: Exercise and physical activity in the prevention and treatment of atherosclerotic cardiovascular disease. *Circulation* 107:3109–3116, 2003.
11. European Society of Cardiology: Recommendations for exercise training in chronic heart failure patients. (2001). *European Heart Journal* 22:125–135, 2001.
12. Fabbri LM, Hurd SS: Global strategy for the diagnosis, management, and prevention of COPD 2003 update (editorial). *European Respiratory Journal* 22:1–2, 2003.
13. Global Initiative for Chronic Obstructive Pulmonary Disease: GOLD Patient Guide. May 2002. http:/www.goldcopd.com. Retrieved September 2010.
14. Global Initiative for Chronic Obstructive Pulmonary Disease: Pocket Guide to COPD Diagnosis, Management, and Prevention: A Guide for Physicians and Nurses. July 2003. http:/www.goldcopd.com; retrieved September 2010.
15. Grundy SM, Garber A, Goldberg R, et al: Lifestyle and medical management of risk factors. *Circulation* 105:153–158, 2002.
16. O'Donnell DE, Aaron S, Bourbeau J, et al: Canadian Thoracic Society recommendations for management of chronic obstructive pulmonary disease. *Canadian Respiratory Journal* 10(Suppl A):11A–65A, 2003.
17. Smith SC, Jr Blair SN, Bonow RO, et al: AHA/ACC guidelines for preventing heart attack and death in patients with atherosclerotic heart disease: 2001 update: A statement for healthcare professionals from the American Heart Association and the American College of Cardiology. *Journal of the American College of Cardiology* 38:1581–1583, 2001.
18. Suskind N, MacDonald S, Swabey T, et al: Cardiac rehabilitation and secondary prevention services in Ontario: Recommendations from a consensus panel. *Canadian Journal of Cardiology* 19:833–838, 2003.
19. Swedberg K, Hull C, Dargie H, et al: Guidelines for the diagnosis and treatment of chronic heart failure: executive summary (update 2005). The Task Force for the Diagnosis and Treatment of Chronic Heart Failure of the European Society of Cardiology. *European Heart Journal* 26:1115–1140, 2005.
20. Gerald LB, Sanderson B, Redden D, et al: Chronic obstructive pulmonary disease stage and 6-minute walk outcome. *Journal of Cardiopulmonary Rehabilitation* 21:296–299, 2001.
21. Jungbauer JS, Fuller B: Feasibility of a multi-state outcomes program for cardiopulmonary rehabilitation. *Journal of Cardiopulmonary Rehabilitation* 19:352–359, 1999.
22. Scimia F, Casadei I, Cerquetani E, et al: Functional evaluation of ultra-octogenarian patients undergoing cardiac rehabilitation: Correlation between six minute walking test and Rivermead mobility index. *Monaldi Archives of Chest Diseases* 74:159–163, 2010.
23. Botega Fde S, Cipriano Junior G, Lima FV, et al: Cardiovascular behavior during rehabilitation after coronary artery bypass grafting. *Brazilian Journal of Cardiovascular Surgery* 25:527–533, 2010.
24. Manzoni GM, Villa V, Compare A, et al: Short-term effects of a multi-disciplinary cardiac rehabilitation programme on psychological well-being, exercise capacity and weight in a sample of obese in-patients with coronary heart disease: A practice-level study. *Psychology, Health & Medicine* 16:178–189, 2011.
25. Mayou RA, Thompson DR, Clements A, et al: Guideline-based early rehabilitation after myocardial infarction. A pragmatic randomized controlled trial. *Journal of Psychosomatic Research* 52:89–95, 2002.
26. Ockene IS, Miller NH: Cigarette smoking, cardiovascular disease, and stroke: A statement for healthcare professionals from the American Heart Association. *Circulation* 96:3243–3247, 1997.
27. Roche N, Huchon GJ: Current issues in the management of chronic obstructive pulmonary diseases. *Respirology* 2:215–229, 1997.
28. Celli BR: ATS standards for the optimal management of chronic obstructive pulmonary disease. *Respiratory* 2(Suppl 1):S1–S4, 1997.
29. Campbell NC, Grimshaw JM, Ritchie LD, et al: Outpatient cardiac rehabilitation: Are the potential benefits being realized? *Journal of the Royal College of Physicians London* 30:514–519, 1996.
30. Gassner LA, Dunn S, Piller N: Aerobic exercise and the post myocardial infarction patient: A review of the literature. *Heart & Lung* 32:258–265, 2003.
31. Johnson N, Fisher J, Nagle A, et al: Factors associated with referral to outpatient cardiac rehabilitation services. *Journal of Cardiopulmonary Rehabilitation* 24:165–170, 2004.
32. Womack L: Cardiac rehabilitation secondary prevention programs. *Clinical Sports Medicine* 22:135–160, 2003.
33. Decramer M, Bartsch P, Pauwels R, et al: Management of COPD according to guidelines. A national survey among Belgian physicians. *Monaldi Archives of Chest Diseases* 59:62–80, 2003.
34. Fahy BF: Pulmonary rehabilitation for chronic obstructive pulmonary disease: A scientific and political agenda. *Respiratory Care* 49:28–36, 2004.
35. Simonds AK: Ethics and decision making in end-stage lung disease. *Thorax* 58:272–277, 2003.
36. Spencer FA, Salami B, Yarzebski J, et al: Temporal trends and associated factors of inpatient cardiac rehabilitation in patients with acute myocardial infarction: A community-wide perspective. *Journal of Cardiopulmonary Rehabilitation* 21:377–384, 2001.
37. De Busk RF: Why is cardiac rehabilitation not widely used? Western *Journal of Medicine* 156:206–208, 1992.
38. Blackburn GG, Foody JM, Sprecher DL, et al: Cardiac rehabilitation participation patterns in a large, tertiary care center: Evidence for selection bias. *Journal of Cardiopulmonary Rehabilitation* 20:189–195, 2000.

39. Halm M, Penque S, Doll N, et al: Women and cardiac rehabilitation: Referral and compliance patterns. *Journal of Cardiovascular Nursing* 13:83–92, 1999.
40. Lloyd-Williams F, Mair FS, Leitner M: Exercise training and heart failure: A systematic review of current evidence. *British Journal of General Practice* 52:47–55, 2002.
41. Missik E: Women and cardiac rehabilitation: Accessibility issues and policy recommendations. *Rehabilitation Nursing* 26:141–147, 2001.
42. Gordon NF, English CD, Contractor AS, et al: Effectiveness of three models for comprehensive cardiovascular disease risk reduction. *American Journal of Cardiology* 89:1263–1268, 2002.
43. Thomas RJ, Miller NH, Lamendola C, et al: National survey of gender differences in cardiac rehabilitation programs: patient characteristics and enrollment patterns. *Journal of Cardiopulmonary Rehabilitation* 16:402–412, 1996.
44. Winer N, Sowers JR, Weber MA: Gender differences in vascular compliance in young, healthy subjects assessed by pulse contour analysis. *Journal of Clinical Hypertension (Greenwich)* 3:145–152, 2001.
45. Gallagher R, McKinley S, Dracup K: Predictors of women's attendance at cardiac rehabilitation programs. *Progress in Cardiovascular Nursing* 18:121–126, 2003.
46. Johnson JL, Stern ED: Readability of patient education materials: A comparison of rural and urban cardiac rehabilitation sites in Minnesota. *Journal of Cardiopulmonary Rehabilitation* 24:121–127, 2004.
47. Farley RL, Wade TD, Birchmore L: Factors influencing attendance at cardiac rehabilitation among coronary heart disease patients. *European Journal of Cardiovascular Nursing* 2:205–212, 2003.
48. Ilarraza H, Myers J, Kottman W, et al: An evaluation of training responses using self-regulation in a residential rehabilitation program. *Journal of Cardiopulmonary Rehabilitation* 24:27–33, 2004.
49. Tyler DO: Activity progression in acute cardiac patients. *Journal of Cardiovascular Nursing* 12:16–32, 1997.
50. Yohannes AM, Hardy CC: Treatment of chronic obstructive pulmonary disease in older patients: A practical guide. *Drugs and Aging* 20:209–228, 2003.
51. Suskind N, McKelvie RS, Burns RJ, et al: Glucose and insulin abnormalities related to functional capacity in patients with congestive heart failure. *European Heart Journal* 21:1368–1375, 2000.
52. Jolly K, Taylor R, Lip GYH, et al: The Birmingham Rehabilitation Uptake Maximization Study (BRUM). Home based compared with hospital-based cardiac rehabilitation in a multi-ethnic population: Cost-effectiveness and patient adherence. *Heart* doi:10.1136/hrt.2007.127209, 2007.
53. Kodis J, Smith KM, Arthur HM, et al: Changes in exercise capacity and lipids after clinic versus home-based aerobic training in coronary artery bypass graft surgery patients. *Journal of Cardiopulmonary Rehabilitation* 21:31–36, 2001.
54. Persky AM, Eddington ND, Derendorf H: A review of the effects of chronic exercise and physical fitness level on resting pharmacokinetics. *International Journal of Clinical Pharmacological Therapy* 41:504–516, 2003.
55. Carter R, Nicotra B, Blevins W, et al: Altered exercise gas exchange and cardiac function in patients with mild chronic obstructive pulmonary disease. *Chest* 103:745–750, 1993.
56. Lau-Walker M: Cardiac rehabilitation: the importance of patient expectations—A practitioner survey. *Journal of Clinical Nursing* 13:177–184, 2004.
57. Sommaruga M, Tramarin R, Angelino E, et al: Guidelines on psychological interventions in cardiac rehabilitation: Methodological process. *Monaldi Archives of Chest Diseases (English abstract)* 60:40–44, 2003.
58. Vitcenda M: The Wisconsin outcomes experience: baseline outcomes of the WISCVPR Web-based Outcomes Project. *Journal of Cardiopulmonary Rehabilitation* 23:290–298, 2003.
59. Katsura H, Yamada K, Kida K: Usefulness of a linear analog scale questionnaire to measure health-related quality of life in elderly patients with chronic obstructive pulmonary disease. *Journal of the American Geriatric Society* 51:1131–1135, 2003.
60. Sanderson BK, Southard D, Oldridge N: AACVPR consensus statement. Outcomes evaluation in cardiac rehabilitation/secondary prevention programs; improving patient care and program effectiveness. *Journal of Cardiopulmonary Rehabilitation* 24:68–79, 2004.
61. LaBresh KA, Ellrodt AG, Gliklich R, et al: Get with the guidelines for cardiovascular secondary prevention: pilot results. *Archives of Internal Medicine* 164:203–209, 2004.
62. Lear SA, Ignaszewski A, Linden W, et al: A randomized controlled trial of an extensive lifestyle management intervention (ELMI) following cardiac rehabilitation: Study design and baseline data. *Current Controlled Trials in Cardiovascular Medicine* 12:9, 2002.
63. Jolliffe JA, Rees K, Taylor RS, et al: Exercise-based rehabilitation for coronary artery disease. *Cochrane Database Systematic Reviews* 1:CD001–800, 2001.
64. Cooper A, Lloyd G, Wienmanb J, et al: Why patients do not attend cardiac rehabilitation: Role of intentions and illness beliefs. *Heart* 82:234–236, 1999.
65. Sweet SN, Tulloch H, Fortier MS, et al: Patterns of motivation and ongoing exercise activity in cardiac rehabilitation settings: A 24-month exploration from the TEACH study. *Annals of Behavioral Medicine* Mar 4 [Epub ahead of print], 2011.
66. Hacker M, Stork S, Stratakis D, et al: Relationship between right ventricular ejection fraction and maximum exercise oxygen consumption: a methodological study in chronic heart failure patients. *Journal of Nuclear Cardiology* 10:644–649, 2003.
67. Klapholz M, Maurer M, Lowe AM, et al. New York Heart Failure Consortium: Hospitalization for heart failure in the presence of a normal left ventricular ejection fraction: Results of the New York Heart Failure Registry. *Journal of the American College of Cardiology* 43:1432–1438, 2004.
68. Braith RW: Exercise training in patients with CHF and heart transplant recipients. *Medicine and Science and Sports and Exercise* 30(Suppl 10):S367–S378, 1998.
69. Singh RB, Weydahl A, Otsuka K, et al: Can nutrition influence circadian rhythm and heart rate variability? Biomedical *Pharmacotherapy* 55(Suppl 1):115S–124S, 2001.
70. Harrington D, Coats AJ: Mechanisms of exercise intolerance in congestive heart failure. *Current Opinions in Cardiology* 12:224–232, 1997.
71. Koike A, Hiroe M, Taniguchi K, et al: Respiratory control during exercise in patients with cardiovascular disease. *American Review of Respiratory Disease* 147:425–429, 1993.
72. Mabee SW, Metra M, Reed DE, et al: Pulmonary hypertension and systemic hypotension as limitations to exercise in chronic heart failure. *Journal of Cardiac Failure* 1:27–33, 1994.
73. Zhang YY, Wasserman K, Sietsema KE, et al: O_2 kinetics in response to exercise: a measure of tissue anaerobiosis in heart failure. *Chest* 103:735–741, 1993.
74. Clark AL, Rafferty D, Arbuthnott K: Exercise dynamics at submaximal workloads in patients with chronic heart failure. *Journal of Cardiac Failure* 3:15–19, 1997.
75. Puri S, Baker BL, Dutka DP, et al: Reduced alveolar-capillary membrane diffusing capacity in chronic heart failure. Its pathophysiological relevance and relationship to exercise performance. *Circulation* 91:2769–2774, 1995.
76. Banning AP, Lewis NP, Northridge DB, et al: Perfusion/ventilation mismatch during exercise in chronic heart failure: An investigation of circulatory determinants. *British Heart Journal* 74:27–33, 1995.
77. Clarke AL, Volterrani M, Swan JW, et al: Ventilation-perfusion matching in chronic heart failure. *International Journal of Cardiology* 48:259–270, 1995.
78. Bellardinelli R, Perna GP: Vasomotor reactivity evaluation in cardiac rehabilitation. *Monaldi Archives of Chest Diseases* 58:79–86, 2002.
79. Bonapace S, Rossi A, Cicoira M, et al: Aortic distensibility independently affects exercise tolerance in patients with dilated cardiomyopathy. *Circulation* 107:1603–1608, 2003.
80. Manson JE, Greenland P, LaCroix AZ, et al: Walking compared with vigorous exercise for the prevention of cardiovascular events in women. *New England Journal of Medicine* 347:716–725, 2002.
81. Verberne HK, Dijkgraaf MGW, Somsen GA, et al: Stress-related variations in left ventricular function as assessed with gated myocardial perfusion SPECT. *Journal of Nuclear Cardiology* 10:456–463, 2003.
82. Goebbels U, Myers J, Dziekan G, et al: A randomized comparison of exercise training in patients with normal vs. reduced ventricular function. *Chest* 113:1387–1393, 1998.
83. Dubach P, Myers J, Dziekan G, et al: Effect of residential cardiac rehabilitation following bypass surgery. Observations in Switzerland. *Chest* 108:1434–1439, 1995.
84. Coats AJ, Adamopoulos S, Radaelli A, et al: Controlled trial of physical training in chronic heart failure. Exercise performance, hemodynamics, ventilation, and autonomic function. *Circulation* 85:2119–2131, 1992.

85. Killavuori K, Sovijarvi A, Naveri H, et al: Effect of physical training on exercise capacity and gas exchange in patients with chronic heart failure. *Chest* 110:985–991, 1996.
86. Yajima T, Koike A, Sugimoto K, et al: Mechanism of periodic breathing in patients with cardiovascular disease. *Chest* 106:142–146, 1994.
87. Tabet JY, Beauvais F, Thabut G, et al: European Journal of Cardiovascular and Preventive *Rehabilitation* 10:267–272, 2003.
88. MacGowan GA, Janosko K, Cecchetti A, et al: Exercise-related ventilatory abnormalities and survival in congestive heart failure. *American Journal of Cardiology* 79:1264–1266, 1997b.
89. Tomkiewicz-Pajak L, Podolec P, Tracz W, et al: Evaluation of the respiratory system in patients with heart failure based on spiro-ergometric exercise test parameters. *Przegl Lek* 59:568–571, 2002.
90. Witte KKA, Morice A, Clark AL, et al: Airway resistance in chronic heart failure measured by impulse oscillometry. *Journal of Cardiac Failure* 8:225–231, 2002.
91. Agostoni PG, Bussotti M, Palermo P, et al: Does lung diffusion impairment affect exercise capacity in patients with heart failure? *Heart* 88:453–459, 2002.
92. Guazzi M: Alveolar-capillary membrane dysfunction in chronic heart failure: pathophysiology and therapeutic implications. *Clinical Science (London)* 98:633–641, 2000.
93. Reindl I, Wernecke KD, Opitz C, et al: Impaired ventilatory efficiency in chronic heart failure: possible role of pulmonary vasoconstriction. *American Heart Journal* 136:778–785, 1998.
94. Russell SD, McNeer FR, Higginbotham MB: Exertional dyspnea in heart failure: a symptom unrelated to pulmonary function at rest or during exercise. Duke University Clinical Cardiology Studies (DUCCS) Exercise Group. *American Heart Journal* 135:398–405, 1998.
95. Hueslmann M, Stefenelli T, Berger R, et al: Prognostic impact of workload in patients with congestive heart failure. *American Heart Journal* 143:308–312, 2002.
96. Mejhert M, Linder-Klingsell E, Edner M, et al: Ventilatory variables are strong prognostic markers in elderly patients with heart failure. *Heart* 88:239–243, 2002.
97. Cohen-Solal A, Czitrom D, Geneves M, et al: Delayed attainment of peak oxygen consumption after the end of exercise in patients with chronic heart failure. *International Journal of Cardiology* 27:23–29, 1997.
98. MacGowan GA, Panzak G, Murali S: Exercise-related ventilatory abnormalities are more specific for functional impairment in chronic heart failure than reduction in peak exercise oxygen consumption. *Journal of Heart and Lung Transplantation* 20:1167–1173, 2001.
99. Koike A, Itoh H, Kato M, et al: Prognostic power of ventilatory responses during submaximal exercise in patients with chronic heart disease. *Chest* 121:1581–1588, 2002.
100. Clark AL, Davies LC, Francis DP, et al: Ventilatory capacity and exercise tolerance in patients with chronic stable heart failure. *European Journal of Heart Failure* 2:47–51, 2000.
101. Robbins M, Francis G, Pashkow FJ, et al: Ventilatory and heart rate responses to exercise: better predictors of heart failure mortality than peak oxygen consumption. *Circulation* 100:2411–2417, 1999.
102. Nanas S, Nanas J, Papazachou O, et al: Resting lung function and hemodynamic parameters as predictors of exercise capacity in patients with chronic heart failure. *Chest* 123:1386–1393, 2003.
103. Al-Rawas OA, Carter R, Richens D, et al: Ventilatory and gas exchange abnormalities in exercise in chronic heart failure. *European Respiratory Journal* 8:2022–2028, 1995.
104. Bellone A, Rusconi F, Frisinghelli A, et al: Gas exchange response to exercise in patients with chronic heart failure. *Monaldi Archives of Chest Diseases* 54:3–6, 1999.
105. MacGowan GA, Cecchetti A, Murali S: Ventilatory drive during exercise in congestive heart failure. *Journal of Cardiac Failure* 3:257–262, 1997a.
106. Tanabi Y, Nakagawa I, Ito E, et al: Hemodynamic basis of the reduced oxygen uptake relative to work rate during incremental exercise in patients with chronic heart failure. *International Journal of Cardiology* 83:57–62, 2002.
107. Tyberg JV, Grant DA, Kingma I, et al: Effects of positive intrathoracic pressure on pulmonary and systemic hemodynamics. *Respiratory Physiology* 119:171–179, 2000.
108. Tanehato M, Adachi H, Oshima S, et al: Improved oxygen utilization during mild exercise in heart failure. *Japanese Circulation Journal* 62:741–747, 1998.
109. Katz SD, Maskin C, Jondeau G, et al: Near-maximal fractional oxygen extraction by active skeletal muscle in patients with chronic heart failure. *Journal of Applied Physiology* 88:2138–2142, 2000.
110. Kitzman DW: Diastolic failure in the elderly. *Heart Failure Review* 7:17–27, 2002.
111. Lavie CJ, Milani RV, Mehra MR: Peak exercise oxygen pulse and prognosis in chronic heart failure. *American Journal of Cardiology* 93:588–593, 2004.
112. Kitaoka H, Hitoma N, Okawa M, et al: Prognostic significance of post-exercise blood pressure response in patients with dilated cardiomyopathy. *Journal of Cardiology*, 42:165–171, 2003.
113. Lucas C, Stevenson LW, Johnson W, et al: The 6-minute walk and peak oxygen consumption in advanced heart failure: aerobic capacity and survival. *American Heart Journal* 138:618–624, 1999.
114. Rickli H, Kiowski W, Brehm M, et al: Combining low-intensity and maximal exercise test results improves prognostic prediction in chronic heart failure. *Journal of the American College of Cardiology* 42:116–122, 2003.
115. Rostagno C, Olivo G, Comeglio M, et al: Prognostic value of 6-minute walk corridor test in patients with mild to moderate heart failure: Comparison with other methods of functional evaluation. *European Journal of Heart Failure* 5:247–252, 2003.
116. Kim HJ, Park SW, Cho BR, et al: The role of cardiopulmonary exercise test in mitral and aortic regurgitation: It can predict post-operative results. *The Korean Journal of Internal Medicine* 18:35–39, 2003.
117. Gitt AK, Wasserman K, Kilkowski C, et al: Exercise anaerobic threshold and ventilatory efficiency identify heart failure patients for high risk of early death. *Circulation* 106:3079–3084, 2002.
118. Koike A, Yajima T, Kano H, et al: Relation between oxygen uptake and carbon dioxide output during constant work rate exercise in patients with mild congestive heart failure. *American Journal of Cardiology* 77:602–605, 1996.
119. Larsen AI, Aarsland T, Kristiansen M, et al: Assessing the effect of exercise training in men with heart failure: Comparison of maximal, submaximal and endurance exercise protocols. *European Heart Journal* 22:684–692, 2001.
120. Kemppainen J, Tsuchida H, Stolen K, et al: Insulin signaling and resistance in patients with chronic heart failure. *Journal of Physiology* 550:305–315, 2003.
121. Armour W, Clark AL, McCann GP, et al: Effects of exercise position on the ventilatory responses to exercise in chronic heart failure. *International Journal of Cardiology* 66:59–63, 1998.
122. Myers J, Dziekan G, Goebbels U, et al: Influence of high-intensity exercise training on the ventilatory response to exercise in patients with reduced ventricular function. *Medicine and Science in Sports and Exercise* 31:929–937, 1999.
123. Dubach P, Myers J, Dziekan G, et al: Effect of high-intensity exercise training on central hemodynamic responses to exercise in men with reduced left ventricular function. *Journal of the American College of Cardiology* 29:1591–1598, 1997.
124. Malfatto G, Branzi G, Riva B, et al: Recovery of autonomic responsiveness with low-intensity physical training in patients with chronic heart failure. *European Journal of Heart Failure* 4:159–166, 2002.
125. Stratmann H: Effect of exercise training on multiple respiratory variables in patients with coronary artery disease: correlation with changes in exercise capacity. *Angiology* 42:948–956, 1991.
126. Guazzi M, Reina G, Tumminello G, et al: Improvement of alveolar-capillary membrane diffusing capacity with exercise training in chronic heart failure. *Journal of Applied Physiology* 97:1866–1873, 2004.
127. McConnell TR, Mandak JS, Sykes JS, et al: Exercise training for heart failure patients improves respiratory muscle endurance, exercise tolerance, breathlessness, and quality of life. *Journal of Cardiopulmonary Rehabilitation* 23:10–16, 2003.
128. Delagardelle C, Feiereisen P, Autier P, et al: Strength/endurance training versus endurance training in congestive heart failure. *Medicine and Science in Sports and Exercise* 34:1868–1872, 2002.
129. Radzewitz A, Miche E, Herrmann G, et al: Exercise and muscle strength training and their effect on quality of life in patients with chronic heart failure. *European Journal of Heart Failure* 4:627–634, 2002.
130. Hendrican MC, McKelvie RS, Smith T, et al: Functional capacity in patients with congestive heart failure. *Journal of Cardiac Failure* 6:214–219, 2000.
131. Hambrecht R, Fiehn E, Yu J, et al: Effects of endurance training on mitochondrial ultrastructure and fiber type distribution in skeletal muscle of patients with stable chronic heart failure. *Journal of the American College of Cardiology* 29:1067–1073, 1997.
132. Vescovo G, Serafini F, Dalla Libera L, et al: Skeletal muscle myosin heavy chain in heart failure: correlation between magnitude of the isozyme shift,

exercise capacity, and gas exchange measurements. *American Heart Journal* 135:130–137, 1998.
133. Clark AL, Rafferty D, Arbuthnott K: Relationship between isokinetic muscle strength and exercise capacity in chronic heart failure. *International Journal of Cardiology* 59:145–148, 1997.
134. Larsen AI, Lindal S, Aukrust P, et al: Effect of exercise training on skeletal muscle fibre characteristics in men with chronic heart failure. Correlation between muscle alterations, cytokines, and exercise capacity. *International Journal of Cardiology* 83:25–32, 2002.
135. Gosker HR, Kubat B, Schaart G, et al: Myopathological features in skeletal muscle of patients with chronic obstructive pulmonary disease. *European Respiratory Journal* 22:280–285, 2003.
136. Warburton DER, Mathur S: Skeletal muscle training in people with chronic heart failure or chronic obstructive pulmonary disease. *Physiotherapy Canada* 56:143–157, 2004.
137. Duscha BD, Annex BH, Keteyian SJ, et al: Differences in skeletal muscle between men and women with chronic heart failure. *Journal of Applied Physiology* 90:280–286, 2001.
138. Bellardinelli R, Barstow TJ, Nguyen P, et al: Skeletal muscle oxygenation and oxygen uptake kinetics following constant work rate exercise in chronic congestive heart failure. *American Journal of Cardiology* 80:1319–1324, 1997.
139. Matsui S, Tamura N, Hirakawa T, et al: Assessment of working skeletal muscle oxygenation in patients with chronic heart failure. *American Heart Journal* 129:690–695, 1995.
140. Riley M, Stanford CF, Nicholls DP: Ventilatory and heart rate responses after exercise in chronic cardiac failure. *Clinical Science (London)* 87:231–238, 1994.
141. Yamani MH, Sahgal P, Wells L, et al: Exercise intolerance in chronic heart failure is not associated with impaired recovery of muscle function or submaximal exercise performance. *Journal of the American College of Cardiology* 25:1232–1238, 1995.
142. Sietsema KE, Ben-Dov I, Zhang YY, et al: Dynamics of oxygen uptake for submaximal exercise and recovery in patients with chronic heart failure. *Chest* 105:1693–1670, 1994.
143. Pollard SD, Munks K, Wales C, et al: Position and mobilization post-angiography study (PAMPAS): A comparison of 4.5 hours and 2.5 hours bed rest. *Heart* 89:447–448, 2003.
144. Vlasic W, Almond D: Research-based practice: Reducing bed rest following cardiac catheterization. *Canadian Journal of Cardiovascular Nursing* 10:19–22, 1999.
145. Longhurst JC, Stebbins CL: The power athlete. *Cardiology Clinics* 15:413–429, 1997.
146. King ML, Dracup KA, Fonarow GC, et al: The hemodynamic effects of isotonic exercise using hand-held weights in patients with heart failure. *Journal of Heart and Lung Transplantation* 19:1209–1218, 2000.
147. Daub WD, Knapik GP, Black WR: Strength training early after myocardial infarction. *Journal of Cardiopulmonary Rehabilitation* 16:100–108, 1996.
148. Cheetham C, Green D, Collis J, et al: Effect of aerobic and resistance exercise on central hemodynamic responses in severe chronic heart failure. *Journal of Applied Physiology* 93:175–180, 2002.
149. Koike A, Itoh H, Oohara R, et al: Cerebral oxygenation during exercise in cardiac patients. *Chest* 125:182–190, 2004.
150. Psirropoulos D, Lefkos N, Boudonas G, et al: Heart failure accompanied by sick euthyroid syndrome and exercise training. *Current Opinions in Cardiology* 17:266–270, 2002.
151. Mortensen PT, Sogaard P, Mansour H, et al: Sequential biventricular pacing: evaluation of safety and efficacy. *Pacing and Clinical Electrophysiology* 27:339–345, 2004.
152. Molhoek SG, Bax JJ, Erven L, et al: American *Journal of Cardiology* 90:379–383, 2002.
153. Friedman AW, Lipman RC, Silver SJ, et al: Cardiac rehabilitation/exercise in patients with implantable cardioverter defibrillators. *Journal of the National Medical Association* 88:374–378, 1996.
154. Kelly TM: Exercise testing and training of patients with malignant ventricular arrhythmias. *Medicine and Science in Sports and Exercise* 28:53–61, 1996.
155. Chen SY, Lan C, Ko WJ, et al: Cardiorespiratory responses of heart transplantation recipients to exercise in the early postoperative period. *Journal of the Formosan Medical Association* 98:165–170, 1999.
156. Kao AC, Van Trigt P 3rd, Shaeffer-McCall GS, et al: Central and peripheral limitations to upright exercise in untrained cardiac transplant patients. *Circulation* 89:2605–2615, 1994.
157. Braith RW, Edwards DG: Exercise following heart transplantation. *Sports Medicine* 30:171–192, 2000.
158. Bengel FM, Ueberfuhr P, Schiepel N, et al: Effect of sympathetic reinnervation on cardiac performance after heart transplantation. *New England Journal of Medicine* 345:731–738, 2001.
159. Ehrman J, Keyeyian S, Fedel F, et al: Cardiovascular responses of heart transplant recipients to graded exercise testing. *Journal of Applied Physiology* 73:260–264, 1992.
160. Daida H, Squires RW, Allison TG, et al: Sequential assessment of exercise tolerance in heart transplantation compared with coronary artery bypass surgery after phase II cardiac rehabilitation. *American Journal of Cardiology* 77:696–700, 1996.
161. Gullestad L, Haywood G, Ross H, et al: Exercise capacity of heart transplant recipients: the importance of chronotropic incompetence. *Journal of Heart and Lung Transplantation* 15:1075–1083, 1996.
162. Mettauer B, Lampert E, Petitjean P, et al: Persistent exercise intolerance following cardiac transplantation despite normal oxygen transport. *International Journal of Sports Medicine* 17:277–286, 1996.
163. Pardaens K, Van Cleemput J, Vanhaecke J, et al: Peak oxygen uptake better predicts outcome than submaximal respiratory data in heart transplant candidates. *Circulation* 101:1152–1157, 2000.
164. Auerbach I, Tenebaum A, Motro M, et al: Blunted responses of Doppler-derived aortic flow parameters during whole-body heavy isometric exercise in heart transplant recipients. *Journal of Heart and Lung Transplantation* 19:1063–1070, 2000.
165. Ville N, Mercier J, Varray A, et al: Exercise tolerance in heart transplant patients with altered pulmonary diffusion capacity. *Medicine and Science in Sport and Exercise* 30:339–344, 1998.
166. Westaby S, Banning AP, Jarvik R, et al: First permanent implant of the Jarvik 2000 Heart. *Lancet* 356:900–903, 2000.
167. Swan L, Hillis WS: Exercise prescription in adults with congenital heart disease: a long way to go. *Heart* 83:685–687, 2000.
168. Schmieder FA, Comerota AJ: Intermittent claudication: magnitude of the problem, patient evaluation, and therapeutic strategies. *American Journal of Cardiology* 87:3D–13D, 2001.
169. Tan KH, Cotterrell D, Sykes K, et al: Exercise training for claudicants: changes in blood flow, cardiorespiratory status, metabolic functions, blood rheology and lipid profile. *European Journal of Vascular and Endovascular Surgery* 20:72–78, 2000.
170. Haouzi P, Hirsch JJ, Marchal F, et al: Ventilatory and gas exchange response during walking in severe peripheral vascular disease. *Respiratory Physiology* 107:181–190, 1997.
171. Olin JW, Allie DE, Belkin M, et al: ACCF/AHA Task Force on Performance Measures: ACCF/AHA/ACR/SCAI/SIR/SVM/SVN/SVS 2010 performance measures for adults with peripheral artery disease: A Report of the American College of Cardiology Foundation/American Heart Association Task Force on Performance Measures, the American College of Radiology, the Society for Cardiac Angiography and Interventions, the Society for Interventional Radiology, the Society for Vascular Medicine, the Society for Vascular Nursing, and the Society for Vascular Surgery. *Journal of Vascular Nursing* 29:23–60, 2011.
172. Callahan LA, Woods KF, Mensah GA, et al: Cardiopulmonary responses to exercise in women with sickle cell anemia. *American Journal of Respiratory and Critical Care Medicine* 165:1309–1316, 2002.
173. Pianosi P, D'Souza SJ, Esseltine DW, et al: Ventilation and gas exchange during exercise in sickle cell anemia. *American Review of Respiratory Disease* 143:226–230, 1991.
174. Hall JE, Brands MW, Zappe DH, et al: Insulin resistance, hyperinsulinemia, and hypertension: causes, consequences, or merely correlations? Proceedings of the Society for *Experimental Biology and Medicine* 208:317–329, 1995.
175. Taddei S, Virdis A, Mattei P, et al: Hypertension causes premature aging of endothelial function in humans. *Hypertension* 29:736–743, 1997.
176. Esler M, Lambert G, Jennings G: Increased regional sympathetic nervous activity in human hypertension: Causes and consequences. *Journal of Hypertension (Suppl.)* 7:S53–S57, 1990.
177. Bond V, Stephens Q, Adams RG, et al: Aerobic exercise attenuates an exaggerated exercise blood pressure response in normotensive young adult African-American men. *Blood Pressure* 11:229–234, 2002.
178. Kim YS, Davis SC, Truijen J, et al: Intensive blood pressure control affects cerebral blood blow in type 2 diabetes mellitus patients. *Hypertension*. Feb 28. [Epub ahead of print]: 2011.
179. Loimaala A, Huikuri HV, Koobi T, et al: Exercise training improves baroreflex sensitivity in type 2 diabetes. *Diabetes* 52:1837–1842, 2003.
180. Young JL, Pendergast DR, Steinbach J: Oxygen transport and peripheral microcirculation in long-term diabetes. *Proceedings of the Society of Experimental and Biological Medicine* 196:61–68, 1991.

181. Baldi JC, Aoina JL, Oxenham HC, et al: Reduced arteriovenous O_2 difference in type 2 diabetes. *Journal of Applied Physiology* 94:1033–1038, 2003.
182. Minette P, Buysschaert M, Rahier J, et al: Pulmonary gas exchange in life-long nonsmoking patients with diabetes mellitus. *Respiration* 66:20–24, 1999.
183. Yamagishi H, Yoshiyama M, Shirai N, et al: Impact of diabetes mellitus on worsening of the left ventricular ejection fraction in exercise-gated 201T1 myocardial single photon emission computed tomography in patients with coronary artery disease. *Circulation Journal* 67:839–845, 2003.
184. Racine N, Blanchet M, Ducharme A, et al: Decreased heart rate recovery after exercise in patients with congestive heart failure: Effect of beta-blocker therapy. *Journal of Cardiac Failure* 9:296–302, 2003.
185. Guazzi M, Pontone G, Agostini P: Aspirin worsens exercise performance and pulmonary gas exchange in patients with heart failure who are taking angiotensin-converting enzyme inhibitors. *American Heart Journal* 138:254–260, 1999.
186. McConnell TR, Menapace FJ, Jr Hartley LH, et al: Captopril reduces the $\dot{V}_E/\dot{V}CO_2$ ratio in myocardial infarction patients with low ejection fraction. *Chest*, 114:1289–1294, 1998.
187. Simon M, LeBlanc P, Jobin J, et al: Limitation of lower limb $\dot{V}O_2$ during cycling exercise in COPD patients. *Journal of Applied Physiology* 90:1013–1019, 2001.
188. Pollack M, Roa J, Benditt J, et al: Estimation of ventilatory reserve by stair climbing. A study in patients with chronic airflow limitation. *Chest* 104;1378–1383, 1993.
189. Fujii T, Kurihara N, Fujimoto S, et al: Role of pulmonary vascular disorder in determining exercise capacity in patients with severe chronic obstructive pulmonary disease. *Clinical Physiology* 16:521–533, 1996.
190. Bauerle O, Younes M: Role of ventilatory response to exercise in determining exercise capacity in COPD. *Journal of Applied Physiology* 79:1870–1877, 1995.
191. Keller CA, Ohar J, Ruppel G, et al: Right ventricular function in patients with severe COPD evaluated for lung transplantation. *Chest* 107:1510–1516, 1995.
192. Vallet G, Ahmaidi S, Serres I, et al: Comparison of two training programmes in chronic airway limitation patients: Standardized versus individualized protocols. *European Respiratory Journal* 10:114–122, 1997.
193. Puente-Maestu L, Sanz ML, Sanz P, et al: Effects of two types of training on pulmonary and cardiac responses to moderate exercise in patients with COPD. *European Respiratory Journal* 15:1026–1032, 2000.
194. Van Stel HF, Bogaard JM, Rijssenbeek-Nouwens LH, et al: Multivariable assessment of the 6-minute walking test in patients with chronic obstructive pulmonary disease. *American Journal of Critical Care Medicine* 163:1567–1571, 2001.
195. Zu Wallack RL, Patel K, Reardon JZ, et al: Predictors of improvement in the 12-minute walking distance following a six-week outpatient pulmonary rehabilitation program. *Chest* 99:805–808, 1991.
196. Otsuka T, Kurihara N, Fujii T, et al: Effect of exercise training and detraining on gas exchange kinetics in patients with chronic obstructive lung disease. *Clinical Physiology* 17:287–297, 1997.
197. Casaburi R, Porszasz J, Burns MR, et al: Physiologic benefits of exercise training in rehabilitation of patients with severe chronic obstructive pulmonary disease. *American Journal of Respiratory and Critical Care Medicine* 155:1541–1551, 1997.
198. Storer TW: Exercise in chronic pulmonary disease: Resistance exercise prescription. *Medicine and Science in Sport and Exercise* 33(Suppl 7):S680–S692, 2001.
199. Richardson RS, Leek BT, Gavin TP, et al: Reduced mechanical efficiency in chronic obstructive pulmonary disease but normal peak $\dot{V}O_2$ with small muscle mass contraction. *American Journal of Critical Care Medicine* 169:89–96, 2004.
200. Agusti AGN, Noguera A, Sauleda J, et al: Systemic effects of chronic obstructive pulmonary disease. *European Respiratory Journal* 21:347–360, 2003.
201. Richardson RS, Sheldon J, Poole DC, et al: Evidence of skeletal muscle metabolic reserve during whole body exercise in patients with chronic obstructive pulmonary disease. *American Journal of Respiratory and Critical Care Medicine* 159:881–885, 1999.
202. Gosselin N, Lambert K, Poulain M, et al: Endurance training improves skeletal muscle electrical activity in active COPD patients. *Muscle Nerve* 28:744–753, 2003.
203. Riley MS, Porszasz J, Engelen MP, et al: *European Journal of Applied Physiology* 83:63–70, 2000.
204. Leyenson V, Furukawa S, Kuzma AM, et al: Correlation of changes in quality of life after lung volume reduction surgery with changes in lung function, exercise, and gas exchange. *Chest* 18:728–735, 2000.
205. Cordova F, O'Brien G, Furukawa S, et al: Stability of improvements in exercise performance and quality of life following bilateral lung volume reduction surgery in severe COPD. *Chest* 112:907–915, 1997.
206. Tschernko EM, Gruber EM, Jaksch P, et al: Ventilatory mechanics and gas exchange during exercise before and after lung volume reduction surgery. *American Journal of Respiratory and Critical Care Medicine* 158:1424–1431, 1998.
207. Criner G, Cordova FC, Leyenson V, et al: Effect of lung volume reduction surgery on diaphragm strength. *American Journal of Respiratory and Critical Care Medicine* 157:1578–1585, 1998.
208. Hsia CC: Cardiopulmonary limitations to exercise in restrictive lung disease. *Medicine and Science in Sports and Exercise* 31(Suppl):S28–S32, 1999.
209. Chung F, Dean E: Pathophysiology and cardiorespiratory consequences of interstitial lung disease: Review and clinical implications. *Physical Therapy* 69:956–966, 1989.
210. Riley MS, Porszasz J, Miranda J, et al: Exhaled nitric oxide during exercise in primary pulmonary hypertension and pulmonary fibrosis. *Chest* 111:44–50, 1997.
211. Hansen JE, Wasserman K: Pathophysiology of activity limitation in patients with interstitial lung disease. *Chest* 109:1566–1576, 1996.
212. Sietsema KE, Kraft M, Ginzton L, et al: Abnormal oxygen update responses to exercise in patients with mild pulmonary sarcoidosis. *Chest* 102:838–845, 1992.
213. Heller H, Konen-Bergmann M, Overlack A, et al: Decreasing diffusion limitation on exercise in lower-graded interstitial lung disease. *Pflugers Archives* 435:762–766, 1998.
214. Medinger AE, Khouri S, Rohatgi PK: Sarcoidosis: The value of exercise testing. *Chest* 120:93–101, 2002.
215. Schwaiblmair M, Beinert T, Vogelmeier C, et al: Cardiopulmonary exercise testing following hay exposure challenge in farmer's lung. *European Respiratory Journal* 10:2360–2365, 1997.
216. Erbes R, Schalberg T, Loddenkemper R: Lung function tests in patients with idiopathic pulmonary fibrosis. Are they helpful for predicting outcome? *Chest* 111:51–57, 1997.
217. Mathur S, Reid WD, Levy RD: Exercise limitation in recipients of lung transplants. *Physical Therapy* 84:1178–1187, 2004.
218. Oelberg DA, Systrom DM, Markowitz DH, et al: Exercise performance in cystic fibrosis before and after bilateral lung transplantation. *Journal of Heart and Lung Transplantation* 17:1104–1112, 1998.
219. NHLB Institute and National Asthma Education Program Expert Panel Report. *Journal of Allergy and Clinical Immunology* 88(3):425–534, 1991.
220. Jaffe A, Bush A: Cystic fibrosis: Review of the decade. *Monaldi Archives of Chest Diseases* 56:240–247, 2001.
221. Wagener JS, Headley AA: Cystic fibrosis: Current concepts in respiratory care. *Respiratory Care* 48:234–245, 2003.
222. Weinberger M: Airways reactivity in patients with CF. *Clinical Review of Allergy and Immunology* 23:77–85, 2002.
223. Pashkow FJ: Issues in contemporary cardiac rehabilitation: A historical perspective. *Journal of the American College of Cardiology* 21:822–834, 1993.
224. Marshall P, Al-Timman J, Riley R, et al: Randomized controlled trial of home-based exercise training to evaluate cardiac functional gains. *Clinical Science (London)* 101:477–483, 2001.
225. Bairey Merz CN, Felando MN, Klein J: Cholesterol awareness and treatment in patients with coronary artery disease participating in cardiac rehabilitation. *Journal of Cardiopulmonary Rehabiliatation* 16:117–122, 1996.
226. Schairer JR, Keteyian SJ, Ehrman JK, et al: Leisure time physical activity of patients in maintenance cardiac rehabilitation. *Journal of Cardiopulmonary Rehabilitation* 23:260–265, 2003.
227. Geraldi D, Zu Wallack R: Non-pulmonary factors affecting survival in patients completing pulmonary rehabilitation. *Monaldi Archives of Chest Diseases* 56:331–335, 2001.
228. Denollet J, Brutsaert DL: Reducing emotional distress improves prognosis in coronary heart disease: 9-year mortality in a clinical trial of rehabilitation. *Circulation* 104:2018–2023, 2001.
229. Pina IL, Balady GJ, Hanson P, et al: Guidelines for clinical exercise testing laboratories. A statement for healthcare professionals from the Committee

on Exercise and Cardiac Rehabilitation, American Heart Association. *Circulation* 91:912–921, 1995.
230. Lewis EF, Moye LA, Rouleau JL, et al: Predictors of late development of heart failure in stable survivors of myocardial infarction: The CARE study. *Journal of the American College of Cardiology* 42:1446–1453, 2003.
231. Thornton LA: Depression in post-acute myocardial infarction patients. *Journal of the American Academy of Nurse Practitioners* 13:364–367, 2001.
232. Ades PA, Savage PD, Tischler MD, et al: Determinants of disability in older coronary patients. *American Heart Journal* 143:151–156, 2002.
233. Godin G, Valois P, Jobin J, et al: Prediction of intention to exercise of individuals who have suffered from coronary artery disease. *Journal of Clinical Psychology* 47:762–772, 1991.
234. Van Berkel TF, Boersma H, De Basquer D, et al: Registration and management of smoking behaviour in patients with coronary heart disease. The EUROASPIRE survey. *European Heart Journal* 20:1630–1637, 1999.
235. White S, Bissell P, Anderson C: A qualitative study of cardiac rehabilitation patients' perspectives on making dietary changes. *Journal of Human Nutrition and Diet* Feb 21 [Epub ahead of print], 2011.
236. Mokdad AH, Marks JS, Stroup DF, et al: Actual causes of death in the United States, 2000. *Journal of the American Medical Association* 291:1238–1245, 2004.
237. Pierson DJ: Translating new understanding into better care for the patient with chronic obstructive lung disease. *Respiratory Care* 49:99–109, 2004.
238. Klein JJ, van der Palen J, van den Hof S, et al: Self-treatment by adults during slow-onset exacerbations of asthma. *Patient Education and Counseling* 32(Suppl 1):S61–S66, 1997.
239. Bernardi L, Spadacini G, Bellwon J, et al: Effect of breathing rate on oxygen saturation and exercise performance in chronic heart failure. *Lancet* 351:1308–1311, 1998.
240. Pasquali SK, Alexander KP, Coombs LP, et al: Effect of cardiac rehabilitation on functional outcomes after coronary revascularlization. *American Heart Journal* 145:445–451, 2003.
241. Brosseau R, Juneau M, Sirard A, et al: Safety and feasibility of a self-monitored, home-based phase II exercise program for high risk patients after cardiac surgery. *Canadian Journal of Cardiology* 11:675–685, 1995.
242. Serrano M, Madoz E, Ezpeleta I, et al: Smoking cessation and risk of myocardial reinfarction in coronary patients: a nested case-control study. *Revue Espanole Cardiologie (English abstract)* 56:445–451, 2003.
243. Riley MS, Elborn JS, Bell N, et al: Substrate utilization during exercise in chronic cardiac failure. *Clinical Science (London)* 79:89–95, 1990.
244. American College of Sports Medicine: *ACSM's guidelines for exercise testing and prescription*, ed 8, Philadelphia, 2010, Lippincott Williams & Wilkins.
245. Smith SC Jr: The challenge of risk reduction therapy for cardiovascular disease. *American Family Physician* 55:491–500, 1997.
246. Paul-Labrador M, Vongvanich P, Merz CN: Risk stratification for exercise training in cardiac patients: Do the proposed guidelines work? *Journal of Cardiopulmonary Rehabilitation* 19:118–125, 1999.
247. Allison TG, Squires RW, Johnson BD, et al: Achieving National Cholesterol Education Program goals for low-density lipoprotein cholesterol in cardiac patients: Importance of diet, exercise, weight control, and drug therapy. *Mayo Clinic Proceedings* 74:466–473, 1999.
248. Ciampi Q, Betocchi S, Lombardi R, et al: Hemodynamic determinants of exercise-induced abnormal blood pressure response in hypertrophic cardiomyopathy. *Journal of the American College of Cardiology* 40:278–284, 2002.
249. Bodegard J, Erikssen G, Bjornholt JV, et al: Symptom-limited exercise testing, ST depressions and long-term coronary heart disease mortality in apparently healthy middle-aged men. *European Journal of Cardiovascular Prevention and Rehabilitation* 11:320–327, 2004.
250. Kurl S, Laukkanen JA, Tuomainen TP, et al: Association of exercise-induced, silent ST-segment depression with the risk of stroke and cardiovascular diseases in men. *Stroke* 34:1760–1765, 2003.
251. Vivekananthan DP, Blackstone EH, Pothier CE, et al: Heart rate recovery after exercise is a predictor of mortality, independent of the angiographic severity of coronary disease. *Journal of the American College of Cardiology* 42:831–838, 2003.
252. Carter R 3rd, Watenpaugh DE, Smith ML: Gender differences in cardiovascular regulation during recovery from exercise. *Journal of Applied Physiology* 91:1902–1907, 2001.
253. Lan C, Chen SY, Chui SF, et al: Poor functional recovery may indicate restenosis in patients after coronary angioplasty. *Archives of Physical Medicine and Rehabilitation* 84:1023–1027, 2003.
254. Mahler DA, Franco MJ: Clinical application of cardiopulmonary exercise testing. *Journal of Cardiopulmonary Rehabilitation* 16:357–365, 1996.
255. Hambrecht R, Schuler GC, Muth T, et al: Greater diagnostic sensitivity of treadmill versus cycle exercise testing of asymptomatic men with coronary artery disease. *American College of Cardiology* 70:141–146, 1992.
256. Rostagno C, Galanti G, Comeglio M, et al: Comparison of different methods of functional evaluation in patients with chronic heart failure. *European Journal of Heart Failure* 2:273–280, 2000.
257. Demers C, McKelvie RS, Negassa A, et al: Reliability, validity, and responsiveness of the six-minute walk test in patients with heart failure. *American Heart Journal* 142:698–703, 2001.
258. Hanson P: Exercise testing and training in patients with chronic heart failure. *Medicine and Science in Sports and Exercise* 26:527–537, 1994.
259. Bergeron S, Ommen SR, Bailey KR, et al: Exercise echocardiograpic findings and outcome of patients referred for evaluation of dyspnea. *Journal of the American College of Cardiology* 16:2242–2246, 2004.
260. Kelion AD, Webb TP, Gardner MA, et al: The warm-up effect protects against ischemic left ventricular dysfunction in patients with angina. *Journal of American College of Cardiology* 37:705–710, 2001.
261. Swain DP, Franklin BA: Is there a training intensity for aerobic training in cardiac patients? *Medicine and Science in Sport and Exercise* 34:1071–1075, 2002.
262. Gaenzer H, Sturm W, Neumayr G: Effects of walking on coronary artery disease in elderly men. *Circulation* 102:E16, 2000.
263. Nechwatal RM, Duck C, Gruber G: Physical training as interval or continuous training in chronic heart failure for improving function capacity, hemodynamics and quality of life: A controlled study (English abstract). *Zeitschrift fur Kardiologie* 91:328–337, 2002.
264. Suzuki K, Omiya K, Yamada S, et al: Relations between strength and endurance of leg skeletal muscle and cardiopulmonary exercise testing parameters in patients with chronic heart failure. *Journal of Cardiology* 43:59–68, 2004.
265. Verrill DE, Ribisl PM: Resistive muscle training in cardiac rehabilitation. An update. *Sports Medicine* 21:347–383, 1996.
266. Braith RW, Vincent KR: Resistance exercise in the elderly person with cardiovascular disease. *American Journal of Geriatric Cardiology* 8:63–70, 1999.
267. Kay GL: Athletic participation after myocardial revascularization. Possibilities and benefits. *Clinics in Sports Medicine* 10:371–389, 1991.
268. Li J, Zhao W, Zhou S, et al: Relationship between isometric exercise and myocardial ischemia in patients with coronary artery disease: An Echo-Doppler study. *Chinese Medical Journal (English abstract)* 113:493–497, 2000.
269. Chung F, Dean E, Ross J: Cardiopulmonary responses of middle-aged men without cardiopulmonary disease to steady-rate positive and negative work performed on a cycle ergometer. *Physical Therapy* 79:476–487, 1999.
270. Dean E: The physiology of negative work and therapeutic implications. *Physical Therapy*, 68:233–237, 1988.
271. Dean E, Ross J: Downhill walking induces rapid shallow breathing. *Pflugers Archives* 415:351–354, 1989.
272. Meyer K, Steiner R, Lastayo P, et al: Eccentric exercise in coronary patients: central hemodynamic and metabolic responses. *Medicine and Science in Sport and Exercise* 35:1076–1082, 2003.
273. Harris S, LeMaitre JP, Mackenzie G, et al: A randomized study of home-based electrical stimulation of the legs and conventional bicycle exercise training for patients with chronic heart failure. *European Heart Journal* 24:871–878, 2003.
274. Jones AYM, Dean E, Lam PKW, et al: Discordance between lung function of Chinese university students and 20-year-old established norms. *Chest* 128:1297–1303, 2005.
275. Romieu I, Trenga C: Diet and obstructive lung diseases. *Epidemiological Reviews* 23:268–287, 2001.
276. Olopade CO, Beck KC, Viggiano RW, et al: Exercise limitation and pulmonary rehabilitation in chronic obstructive lung disease. *Mayo Clinic Proceedings* 67:144–157, 1992.
277. Efthimious J, Mounsey PJ, Benson DN, et al: Effect of carbohydrate rich versus fat rich loads on gas exchange and walking performance in patients with chronic obstructive lung disease. *Thorax* 47:451–456, 1992.
278. Reis AL, Ellis B, Hawkins RW: Upper extremity exercise training in ch obstructive pulmonary disease. *Chest* 93:688–692, 1988.

279. Miki K, Maekura R, Hiraga T, et al: Impairments and prognostic factors for survival in patients with idiopathic pulmonary fibrosis. *Respiratory Medicine* 97:482–490, 2003.
280. Palange P, Forte S, Onorati P, et al: Ventilatory and metabolic adaptations to walking and cycling in patients with COPD. *Journal of Applied Physiology* 88:1715–1720, 2000.
281. Celli BR, Rassulo J, Make BJ: Dyssynchronous breathing during arm but not leg exercise in patients with chronic airflow obstruction. *The New England Journal of Medicine* 314:1485–1490, 1986.
282. Chapman KR: Therapeutic approaches to chronic obstructive pulmonary disease: An emerging consensus. *American Journal of Medicine* 100:5S–10S, 1996.
283. Wilkinson J, Rees J: Domiciliary oxygen. *British Journal of Clinical Practice* 50:151–153, 1996.
284. MacIntyre NR: Oxygen therapy and exercise response in lung disease. *Respiratory Care* 45:194–200, 2000.
285. Shah AR, Keens TG, Gozal D: Effect of supplemental oxygen on supramaximal exercise performance and recovery in cystic fibrosis. *Journal of Applied Physiology* 83:1641–1647, 1997.
286. O'Donnell DE, Bain DJ, Webb KA: Factors contributing to relief of exertional breathlessness during hyperoxia in chronic airflow limitation. *American Journal of Respiratory and Critical Care Medicine* 155:530–535, 1997.
287. Nandi K, Smith AA, Crawford A, et al: Oxygen supplementation before or after submaximal exercise in patients with chronic obstructive lung disease. *Thorax* 58:670–673, 2003.
288. Tangri S, Woolf CR: The breathing pattern in chronic obstructive lung disease during the performance of some common daily activities. *Chest* 63:126–127, 1973.
289. Thoman RL, Stroker GL, Ross JC: The efficacy of pursed-lips breathing in patients with chronic obstructive pulmonary disease. *American Review of Respiratory Disease* 93:100–106, 1966.
290. Balady GJ, Ades PA, Comoss P, et al: Core components of cardiac rehabilitation/secondary prevention programs. A statement for healthcare professionals from the American Heart Association and the American Association of Cardiovascular and Pulmonary Rehabilitation. *Circulation* 102:1069–1073, 2000.

Exercise Testing and Training: Secondary Cardiovascular and Pulmonary Dysfunction

Elizabeth Dean, Donna Frownfelter, and Eduard Gappmaier

KEY TERMS

Anorexia nervosa
Cancer
Connective tissue conditions
Diabetes
Endocrine conditions
Gastrointestinal conditions
Hematological conditions
Immunodeficiency conditions
Hepatic conditions
Musculoskeletal conditions
Neuromuscular conditions
Obesity
Renal conditions
Thyroid conditions

CHAPTER OUTLINE

This chapter extends the general principles of exercise testing and training presented in Chapter 19 and describes special considerations concerning exercise testing and training for individuals with secondary cardiovascular and pulmonary dysfunction. These special considerations are also important when managing an individual with primary cardiovascular and pulmonary dysfunction who, in addition, has cardiovascular and pulmonary dysfunction secondary to other conditions. In that case, management is modified based on the combination of comorbidities. Individuals with progressive degenerative conditions are often older and debilitated; thus the combination of problems is common. Exercise testing and training is one component of the comprehensive physical therapy management of individuals with chronic, secondary cardiovascular and pulmonary dysfunction, which is described in Chapter 32.

Secondary cardiovascular and pulmonary dysfunction refers to dysfunction of the cardiovascular and pulmonary system that is a consequence of pathology other than primary chronic heart and lung disease. Examples of such secondary conditions are described in Chapter 6. These conditions include dysfunction of the musculoskeletal, connective tissue, neurological, gastrointestinal, hepatic, renal, hematological, endocrine, and immunological systems, or some combination thereof. Nutritional disorders, specifically obesity and starvation (anorexia nervosa), also have cardiovascular and pulmonary manifestations. Conditions leading to secondary cardiovascular and pulmonary dysfunction affect one or more steps in the oxygen transport pathway in such a way that the capacity for oxygen delivery is reduced, oxygen consumption is increased, or both.[1] Often oxygen delivery is further compromised by restricted mobility. Oxygen transport limitations resulting from secondary cardiovascular and pulmonary dysfunction can present subtly, yet have significant clinical implications. Exercise has a primary role in the management of these conditions, along with the elements of comprehensive multidisciplinary prevention and long-term rehabilitation programs.

Contemporary approaches to the rehabilitation of individuals with stroke serve as a prime example of conventional practice aligning with contemporary exercise physiology principles. Over the past 20 years, stroke rehabilitation has shifted from a focus on Bobath and Brunnstrom interventions to structured exercise training. Exercise training in the management of stroke has the potential for driving brain reorganization and exploiting the property of neuroplasticity to maximize functional capacity.[2] Exercise can take advantage of the potential for neural reorganization, optimize functional capacity, and address deconditioning. A focus on endurance and strengthening exercise, task-specific training, and treadmill walking in the rehabilitation of individuals with stroke, in addition to the conventional focus on cognitive engagement, sensorimotor integration, skill acquisition, and social readjustment has been an exciting advance in the rehabilitation of people with strokes.

Another prime example of exercise testing and training being prescribed for noncardiovascular and pulmonary conditions is their inclusion as a component of prehabilitation in preparation for surgery for a range of conditions. Before orthopedic surgical procedures, for example, improvements in functional capacity have been advocated to reduce perioperative complications and speed recovery.[3] Such programs include warm-up, aerobic training, resistance training, flexibility, and daily functional activities.

As a handy reference for clinicians, key points in the assessment, evaluation, and exercise testing and prescription of patients with secondary cardiovascular and pulmonary conditions are summarized in Appendix D.

Assessment and Goals

Assessment

Knowledge of the cardiovascular and pulmonary consequences of conditions other than those of the cardiovascular and pulmonary systems enables the physical therapist to assess oxygen transport status, limitations, and risk factors in these individuals, in addition to ensuring their safety when undergoing physical activity and exercise. Such knowledge enables the physical therapist to prescribe exercise to optimize oxygen transport, maximize functional capacity and life participation, and maintain optimal long-term health.

Goals: Prevention

Many individuals with systemic conditions (see Chapter 6), the focus of this chapter, have manifestations of oxygen transport limitations or one or more risk factors. The risk factors must be identified and considered in a preventive management plan that includes exercise prescription to exploit the preventive effects of activity described in Chapters 18 and 19. Preventive goals for individuals with chronic, secondary cardiovascular and pulmonary conditions include optimizing central and peripheral adaptations to exercise, reducing biomechanical stress and strain (hence minimizing oxygen cost of exercise at submaximal work rates), optimizing fluid dynamics and hemodynamics, and optimizing lung health (e.g., alveolar ventilation, flow rates, mucociliary transport, and lymphatic drainage).

Another consideration with respect to prevention is the fact that many chronic conditions lead to deterioration over time, and this may be exacerbated further with aging and unhealthy lifestyles. Exercise training is modified over time to accommodate each individual's needs and to help offset further deterioration and associated disability. Furthermore, optimal training effects will benefit the individual's health overall and help prevent contracting illnesses whose effects may be more devastating than in the healthy population.

Mobility aids and devices may be indicated for people with progressive functional deterioration. These adjuncts are titrated to the individual's needs to avoid their overuse. Overuse can lead to loss of remaining musculoskeletal function, which must be preserved as much as possible. Thus an individual can use these adjuncts to optimize functional performance throughout the day (e.g., use a wheelchair for activities in which symptoms are anticipated, or use an ankle foot orthosis in the afternoon when the tibial anterior muscle tends to be fatigued and needs support).

Goals: Short Term

When oxygen transport limitations occur, a regimen of physical activity and exercise can be prescribed to elicit the acute effects of exercise (see Chapter 18). Prescription of exercise to elicit its acute effects has a primary role in the management of individuals during acute episodes of illness and setbacks.

Goals: Long Term

When an individual has recovered from an acute episode, or an individual requires subacute and long-term management, a regimen of physical activity and exercise can be prescribed to elicit the long-term effects of exercise described in Chapter 18. The capacity of each individual to respond to an exercise stimulus and the individual's oxygen transport reserve capacity are both assessed in detail. Knowledge of the reserve capacity is essential for optimal exercise prescription.

Individuals with Musculoskeletal Conditions

Exercise is prescribed for a broad range of conditions affecting the musculoskeletal system, with favorable outcomes and no documented deleterious effects. With increased understanding of exercise pathophysiology, physical therapists can prescribe therapeutic exercise that has the greatest benefit in terms of improved activities of daily living and life satisfaction with the least risk. Individuals with mitochondrial myopathies and nonmetabolic myopathies experience typical aerobic responses to low intensity training (i.e., improved aerobic capacity and reduced submaximal heart rate and blood lactate).[4] The extent of these training effects, however, is less in individuals with nonmetabolic myopathies compared with those who have mitochondrial myopathies. Improved aerobic capacity is associated with improved self-reported functional status and quality of life in both groups.

Osteoporosis

Exercise is central to the prevention and management of osteopenia and osteoporosis. In addition to weight-bearing exercise, relatively intense exercise promotes bone density as well as a high volume of activity.[5] Muscle stress across joints appears to be a critical component for osteogenesis; thus torsion around joints such as in racket sports is favorable provided risk for falling is minimized. Practicing tai chi may reduce bone loss in postmenopausal women and may have some role in the management of osteoporosis.[6]

Osteoarthritis

Osteoarthritis has an indirect impact on cardiovascular and pulmonary conditioning because of its effect on mobility. Aerobic exercise can improve functional aerobic capacity in individuals with osteoarthritis, but this effect is less pronounced with hydrotherapy programs.[7] In response to a fitness walking program for obese people with osteoarthritis of the knee, self-efficacy tended to improve commensurate with improved functional capacity.[8] When prescribing an increase in physical activity and exercise, the physical therapist needs to consider the person's weight (not only in terms of the general health benefits of weight loss, but also in relation to the specific need to reduce weight bearing in obese patients). Given the fact that the majority of patients undergoing lower extremity joint replacement are overweight or obese,[9] weight loss in conjunction with exercise is fundamental in the perioperative course of these patients with the expectation that some patients may avoid the need for surgery entirely. Even small amounts of weight gain have profound effects on joints and joint mechanics (hence, increased pain with exercise). In addition, most patients do not lose weight after their joint replacement surgery, so lifestyle changes need to be approached aggressively before, as well as after, surgery.[10]

Scoliosis

Individuals with idiopathic scoliosis and associated restrictive ventilatory disorder can improve pulmonary function with exercise.[11] Selected exercise can improve both vital capacity and chest wall expansion by almost 20%. The role of exercise for remediation of restrictive lung dysfunction associated with other spinal and chest wall deformities warrants further investigation. Correction of spinal defects in individuals with muscular dystrophy, for example, does not improve cardiac or pulmonary function and thus may not result in appreciably improved response to exercise.[12]

Individuals with Neuromuscular Conditions

Stroke

Because the pathoetiology of stroke involves atherosclerosis and hypertension, individuals with stroke need to be managed comparably to individuals with systemic atherosclerosis and circulatory dysfunction. Appropriate precautions must be taken when exercising these individuals or conducting other physical therapy interventions. Within weeks after a stroke, cardiorespiratory deconditioning complicates the clinical picture, along with muscle weakness, spasticity, incoordination, and abnormal gait.[13] In the subacute stage of stroke, individuals who undergo aerobic training can improve aerobic and functional abilities;[14] however, these benefits may not be reflected in the long-term by indexes such as the Frenchay Activities Index.[15,16] Although research is necessary to refine exercise testing and training procedures for individuals with stroke,[17] there is no reason to believe that these patients would not respond to aerobic conditioning to counter the deconditioning that occurs after stroke or that this intervention would not augment gait reeducation and sensorimotor integration. Evidence supports that the application of a modified treadmill training protocol, based on exercise physiology principles, can be superior to conventional approaches to the rehabilitation of people with strokes.[18]

Although individuals with physical impairment secondary to stroke present methodological challenges during exercise testing and training, submaximal oxygen consumption ($\dot{V}O$) has good agreement with maximum $\dot{V}O_2$ ($\dot{V}O_{2max}$) when the test is tightly standardized.[19] The high degree of reliability of these tests supports their use as outcome measures in this population. Metabolic assessment during short, submaximal tests, such as a five-minute walk, can provide supplemental information for evaluating gait in individuals with stroke.[20] Individuals with mild-to-moderate impairment from chronic stroke who require hand rail support on the treadmill also have been reported to have good reliability with respect to heart rate and oxygen pulse in peak-effort treadmill testing.[21] However, hand rail support is an important variable that can increase or decrease work intensity and thus must be described and recorded to facilitate comparison of exercise results across tests. Hand rail support can be described on the data sheet with respect to side or front support, one or two hands, finger support or grasp support, and heavy or light support.

Treadmill training has proven to be a useful means of improving fitness and offsetting deconditioning in individuals with stroke. Individuals with impaired gait can improve their oxygen transport reserve capacity with a regular program of treadmill walking.[22] Peak $\dot{V}O_2$ and walking workload are increased, and the energy cost associated with abnormal gait is reduced. For individuals with stroke, these changes may help to enhance functional capacity comparable to those achieved in individuals with other neurological deficits.

Treadmill training and weight support with a body harness for walking after stroke are showing promise in terms of conditioning strategy and gait reeducation.[23] Patients with severe impairments after stroke who retrain their gait with a portion of their body weight (up to 40%) supported during exercise have better outcomes after training than those who carry their full weight.[24] Older individuals and those with the most impairment show the greatest benefits. These individuals walk more symmetrically on a treadmill compared with ground walking, and they walk with less spasticity and improved movement economy.[25] Furthermore, improvement in treadmill walking speed in these individuals generalizes to balance, trunk control, functional activities, and ground locomotion.[24,26] Training at speeds comparable to an individual's normal velocity over ground is more effective than training at speeds above or below that velocity.[27] Also, when different treadmill walking protocols are compared, structured speed-dependent treadmill training, as performed in sports training, improves walking ability more than either modified progressive treadmill training or conventional gait training.[18]

Despite the compelling results of studies on partial body weight support in the rehabilitation of individuals with stroke, these and related studies often fail to address the principles of physical therapy for management of individuals with systemic atherosclerosis, which include hemodynamic monitoring and possibly electrocardiogram (ECG) screening. One exception was a study by Eng et al (2002)[28] that recommended that actual exertion (defined as a physiology measure; specifically, rate pressure product or heart rate) be measured in conjunction with walking distance in functional walk tests when testing people with stroke. When performance on several functional walk tests was compared, performance was associated with level of impairment rather than perceived exertion or intensity as measured by rate pressure product or heart rate. Thus debility may limit aerobic training capacity.

Aerobic exercise may have a preventive effect for stroke mediated by endothelium-dependent vasodilation in the cerebral arterioles.[29] Several risk factors are associated with impairment of this mechanism. Exercise stimulates the expression of endothelial nitric oxide synthase, which promotes vascular dilation and thereby exercise's potential protective and preventive effect.

Community ambulation is a meaningful outcome for people with stroke.[30] A discrepancy exists, however, between mobility outcomes on standardized measures of community-based individuals and the extent to which they actually get out in the community. Gait velocity is an important variable in determining community ambulation capacity.

Resistance muscle training has been of interest as a component of physical therapy management of individuals with stroke. Strength training augments the benefits of aerobic exercise with respect to functional strength[31] without reinforcing abnormal movement patterns.[32] One study, however, reported no difference between leg exercise training programs with and without resistance.[33] Inadequate exercise prescription to explain the absence of an effect of resistance training cannot be ruled out.

When prescribing exercise for individuals with stroke, it must be remembered that stroke results from a hemodynamic insult—usually high blood pressure. Aerobic exercise and resistance muscle training elicit unique hemodynamic responses; thus the hemodynamic status of individuals with stroke must be assessed in the initial baseline review, considered carefully in the exercise prescription, and assessed in the outcomes of these programs. If blood pressure is being pharmacologically managed, then an objective of exercise will be to augment oxygen transport efficiency and normalize blood pressure. Medications must be followed so that these can be reduced or withdrawn in response to an overall effect of a comprehensive exercise and management program.

Spinal Cord Injury

Spinal cord injury (SCI) can afflict anyone at any age and is certainly a risk in older adults because of the higher probability of falls. Most often, however, SCI results from trauma incurred in young adulthood, and it is more prevalent in men. Depending on the level of the injury, individuals with SCI have altered hemodynamic response to exercise and positional stress. Life expectancy has increased in recent decades for these individuals, which correspondingly has increased their incidence of cardiac risk factors and disease.[34] An active lifestyle and regular exercise are imperative to ensure that these risk factors and related cardiac morbidity are reduced. Heart rate is highly correlated with respiratory minute volume, $\dot{V}O_2$, and workload, which enables exercise to be prescribed in a predictable manner for this group. Exercise capacity is a function of the capacity of the patient to increase heart rate.[35] Significant aerobic gains in peak $\dot{V}O_2$ and work rate peak result from aerobic exercise in combination with functional electrical stimulation of the lower extremity muscles performed, on average, twice a week. Recovery times also improve with training.

Individuals with SCI have a higher heart rate and lower stroke volume during exercise compared with individuals without SCI.[36] Cardiac output is lower at rest. Peak exercise responses are greater for those without SCI with the exception of heart rate. Despite higher heart rates for a given workload, stroke volume and cardiac output are lower. An intact autonomic nervous system is necessary for a large increase in cardiac output and blood flow to working muscles. Thus, depending on the level of the lesion, the heart and peripheral circulation and their capacity to respond to increased work demand are affected.[37] Assessment of autonomic nervous system status is key in exercise testing and training individuals with SCI.[38]

Arm ergometry can be used to test the aerobic capacity of individuals with SCI. Because of the small muscle mass of the arms compared with the legs, the pressure of contracting upper extremity muscles over blood vessels, and the need for postural stabilization, hemodynamic responses are disproportionately elevated compared with the same work intensity performed by the legs. With training, $\dot{V}O_2$ on-off kinetics, but not heart rate, is accelerated in individuals with SCI.[39] Cardiac output during exercise also tends to be lower for these individuals. Thus $\dot{V}O_2$ kinetics may be a prime limiter of exercise capacity in people with SCI, which could contribute to their lower anaerobic threshold with deconditioning.

Wheelchair athletes with SCI show cardiovascular adaptation to exercise. Echocardiographic evidence shows an increase in left ventricular volume compared with individuals without SCI, but this adaptation is less than in healthy runners.[40] Both long-term arm and leg exercise produce morphometric changes in cardiac mass and volume; however, these changes are less pronounced in wheelchair athletes compared with runners. Also, submaximal heart rates are greater for the wheelchair athletes than for runners.

Movement economy varies depending on how a specific activity is performed mechanically. Wheelchair propulsion is more mechanically and energetically efficient, using a pumping motion rather than the traditional semicircular motion.[41] This has implications for energy conservation and minimization of upper extremity overload in individuals with SCI and for optimizing energy-efficient wheelchair design.

Movement economy (i.e., energy cost in relation to workload) is a concern in managing individuals with physical deformity related to musculoskeletal impairments because of the increased energy cost associated with physical activity of tasks and exercise in general. The degree to which spasticity contributes to increased energy cost is unclear. In individuals with acquired brain injury, for example, $\dot{V}O_2$ increases with exercise in a predictable, linear manner, although energy cost does not increase disproportionately with spasticity.[42]

Finally, unlike able-bodied individuals, those with SCI do not show comparable cardiac adaptation. The typical left ventricular enlargement is not observed,[43] suggesting that peripheral factors are responsible for conditioning with training in this cohort.

Chronic Effects of Poliomyelitis

The last poliomyelitis epidemic in the United States occurred in the 1950s. Individuals who had poliomyelitis as children at that time are now older adults. The delayed effects of having lived for years with poliomyelitis and its associating limitations may begin to manifest with or without postpolio syndrome (PPS). The chronic effects of poliomyelitis affect functional capacity, exercise tolerance, and cardiovascular and pulmonary risk. About 50% of individuals who had poliomyelitis develop PPS. The principles for prescribing exercise are distinct for those survivors of poliomyelitis, with or without PPS.[44,45]

PPS is hallmarked by new fatigue, muscle weakness, and pain.[46] In addition, survivors of poliomyelitis with PPS may experience exercise intolerance, choking and swallowing dysfunction, temperature sensitivity, and psychological problems. Patients who did not have ventilatory involvement at onset, as well as those who had bulbar involvement at disease onset, may have impaired pulmonary function with PPS. During exercise, ventilatory involvement may be evidenced by impaired blood gases that are not apparent at rest.[47] This has been proposed as a mechanism for delaying diaphragmatic fatigue. In addition to the chronic effects of poliomyelitis, survivors of poliomyelitis are also afflicted with the same health challenges faced by their peers who have no history of poliomyelitis. This clinical picture may be further superimposed with weight gain and reduced activity, hence, deconditioning, which is associated with aging in Western cultures.

Overuse abuse has been proposed as a mechanism of the delayed-onset effects of poliomyelitis.[48] Injudicious prescription of strengthening or aerobic exercise can be deleterious to the patient because it contributes to the overuse abuse of affected, as well as unaffected, muscle.[45] A reduced motor unit pool has less capacity to recover with prolonged demands, and this pool is further reduced with advancing years. With a prescribed program of rest and activity that augments muscle and endurance capacity without contributing to the patient's symptoms, an individual can show improved tolerance to activities of daily living.[44]

Because of the overuse abuse phenomenon associated with PPS, an injudicious exercise program (aerobic or muscle strengthening) can lead to further overuse and progressive deterioration.[49] Thus reserve capacity for exercise is assessed based on a detailed assessment so that overuse is not worsened.

An exercise test can be used to assess conditioning and movement economy, which are distinct entities.[46] Modified aerobic training can be prescribed within the limits of subjective complaints of fatigue and discomfort/pain rather than with conventional indexes of exercise intensity (i.e., heart rate and blood pressure). Although conventional submaximal indexes of conditioning may not be apparent after several weeks of training, walking tolerance at subthreshold levels (measured by walking duration) may improve, along with movement economy.[46] Thus some patients with a history of poliomyelitis can respond favorably to a modified walking program.

Individuals with postural malalignment experience biomechanical stress over joints during ambulation, which in turn can contribute to increased energy cost.[50] An individual's overall energy cost must be considered when prescribing exercise. Activities normally associated with low energy cost for an individual with normal posture and muscle strength can have significantly higher metabolic demand in an individual with postural deformity, limb length discrepancy, and strength asymmetry. Because fatigue and pain are symptoms associated with PPS, these subjective parameters must be monitored before, during, and between exercise sessions to monitor immediate and delayed effects and capacity to recover after exercise. In this way deleterious exercise workloads may be minimized. Overall, objective measures of walking performance are reported to be associated with subjective reports of functional capacity.[51]

New muscle weakness is a marker of PPS. Modified strengthening programs may benefit individuals whose muscles are weak from overuse whereas conventional muscle strengthening programs are indicated for muscles weakened by deconditioning.[45] This distinction, that is, muscles that are weak and fatigued from overuse vs. muscles weak from deconditioning, is critical in the physical therapy management of this population. Stronger muscles may help improve peripheral extraction of oxygen at the peripheral level and thus contribute to an aerobic training effect and improved endurance.

Down Syndrome

Down syndrome is an example of a condition marked by mental as well as physical challenges. People with the syndrome vary widely with respect to the severity of the condition and their functional capacity, which ranges from living totally independently and being gainfully employed to being somewhat dependent in these domains. Many individuals with the syndrome benefit from physical therapy that includes a lifelong exercise program, usually commencing in childhood during growth and development. Longevity has improved as a result of improved detection and management of heart defects and prevention of respiratory complications. With greater life expectancy, individuals with the syndrome encounter many of the same acute and chronic conditions that individuals without the syndrome encounter over their lifetime, such as the diseases associated with higher civilization. Cardiac defects and sleep apnea are more common in persons with Down syndrome than in the general population.[52] These conditions may affect exercise capacity; thus exercise and monitoring must be individualized to each person's unique needs. Obesity and deconditioning can further complicate the clinical presentation. Communication style must be adapted with respect to the exercise prescription and health maintenance program. Optimal health is necessary to maximize function and long-term self-care. A caregiver may need to be involved to promote a sustained program of regular physical activity and exercise.

Individuals with Connective Tissue Conditions

The exercise limitations of individuals with connective tissue conditions result in part from the restrictive component of lung dysfunction associated with these conditions. These individuals may have normal chest x-ray and conventional pulmonary function yet have histochemical abnormalities of their lungs (e.g., shrinking lung associated with scleroderma).

Resting data are limited in predicting responses to activities of daily living and exercise. Thus exercise testing is a primary tool to assess pulmonary function dynamically and thereby unmask abnormalities that can compromise daily function.[53] Women with systemic lupus erythematosus (SLE) have a several-fold increase in incidence of heart disease over other women, corresponding to an increased number of cardiac risk factors.[54] In addition, hypertension and diabetes are also more prevalent in this group.

Individuals with Rheumatoid Conditions

Individuals with rheumatoid arthritis (RA) have a higher incidence of cardiovascular disease and related mortality. Despite normal left ventricular systolic function, left ventricular diastolic function is impaired without clinical evidence of cardiovascular disease, which may place this group at risk.[55] At maximal exercise, heart rate, systolic blood pressure, and peak $\dot{V}O_2$ are comparable for individuals with RA and healthy people.

Contemporary approaches to the management of people with RA include exercise prescription for strength, endurance, and emotional well-being.[56] Joint inflammation may be reduced with judiciously prescribed exercise.

Individuals with Gastrointestinal Conditions

Conditions such as irritable bowel syndrome and Crohn's disease are characterized by disturbed homeostasis related to gut motility and function. Because these conditions are chronic and medical care is noncurative, physical deconditioning and debility are common. Few studies have examined the acute or chronic effects of exercise in this population, so specific guidelines for testing and training are lacking. One study examined the effects of moderately intense exercise (60% of $\dot{V}O_{2max}$ for 1 hour) on gastrointestinal function in individuals with Crohn's disease who were in remission.[57] The conventional measures of gastrointestinal function were unchanged. It may be necessary to observe caution because of oxygen metabolite production and potential zinc deficiency. Individuals with gastrointestinal conditions have nutritional deficits that must be considered when placing increased metabolic demands on energy substrate stores. The capacity of these individuals to respond to exercise appropriately will fluctuate with exacerbations and remissions of their conditions. It is hoped that with improved health and functional capacity, the duration between exacerbations will be increased, the severity of exacerbations will be reduced, and speed of recovery will be increased.

Individuals with Hepatic Conditions

The exercise responses of individuals with hepatopulmonary syndrome (HPS) are not well understood, which has hampered attempts to define guidelines for mobilization and exercise testing and training. One study, however, has shown that individuals with HPS have markedly reduced aerobic capacity and exercise-induced hypoxemia that exceeds the limitations of patients with liver disease but without the syndrome.[58] Hypoxemia and increased ventilatory dead space at peak exercise support impairment in the pulmonary circulation.

Exercise capacity and maximum oxygen consumption are impaired by cirrhosis. This can be explained by an associated cirrhotic cardiomyopathy. Myocardial thickening and ventricular stiffness lead to decreased diastolic function and inotropic and chronotropic incompetence when the oxygen transport system is stressed during exercise.[59]

Individuals with Renal Conditions

Limitation of mitochondrial oxidative capacity has been ruled out as a limiter of exercise capacity in patients with chronic renal failure.[60] Muscle oxygen conductance, however, is low.

Exercise has a role in the management of individuals undergoing hemodialysis. One study examined the role that normalizing hemoglobin has on exercise response of these individuals.[61] Although both young and old subjects showed evidence of improved oxygen transport and exercise tolerance, exercise responses were not normalized completely. Further, impaired potassium regulation appeared related to hemoglobin concentration and was thought to contribute to exercise limitation.

Patients with end-stage renal disease can also benefit from exercise. Minimally, deconditioning may be prevented, but alternatively, functional status will be improved. An ideal exercise program should have both aerobic exercise and resistance muscle training components, and the prescription for both should be designed to minimize cardiovascular and musculoskeletal risks. Exercise is initiated at a low level to ensure the exercise responses are normal and the patient responds favorably before progression of the prescription. With respect to exercising patients who are severely ill, the consequences of not exercising must be considered.[62] Regular physical activity, particularly when the patient is relatively stable and well, must be encouraged. This ensures that the patient is as well as possible when a change in his or her condition occurs, which in turn speeds recovery and minimizes associated challenges to aerobic and strength status.

Erythropoietin therapy in the management of patients with chronic renal failure fails to augment peak $\dot{V}O_2$ as much as might be predicted from a corresponding increase in hemoglobin.[63] Lactate differences may explain abnormal muscle oxygen transport and reduced exercise tolerance in these patients. Erythropoietin-mediated increases in hemoglobin, however, reduce the respiratory exchange ratio at submaximal exercise (comparable to activities of daily living), reflecting a decrease in anaerobic metabolism and reduced exercise stress.[64]

Chronic renal insufficiency is strongly associated with exercise induced ischemia in individuals with atherosclerosis. The greater the severity of atherosclerosis in these individuals with chronic renal insufficiency, the greater their cardiovascular risk.[65]

Frequent exercise for patients with renal disease has been proposed as a means of maximizing effective use of their anemia-imposed reduced oxygen delivery capacity.[66]

Individuals with Hematological Conditions

Sickle cell anemia is a common hematological condition in the United States with a high prevalence in the African American population. Patients with sickle cell disease have reduced hemoglobin and oxygen transport capacity. On maximal exercise testing and endurance testing, they have lower exercise tolerance; however, their responses relative to deconditioned individuals without sickle cell anemia are generally comparable.[67] Thus exercise performance of these individuals must be interpreted in this context.

Individuals with Endocrine Conditions

Individuals with diabetes warrant special consideration with respect to exercise testing and training. Exercise imposes demands on energy substrates and their utilization. Blood glucose abnormalities associated with diabetes necessitate monitoring blood glucose fluctuations before, during, and after exercise. The physical therapist must ensure that the individual eats appropriate foods and at appropriate times in relation to physical activity and exercise. Obesity management is fundamental to the goals of an exercise program as well as normalizing blood glucose metabolism.

Autonomic neuropathies, myopathies, and angiopathies contribute to abnormal exercise responses. Acute exercise responses (e.g., heart rate and blood pressure) may be blunted, as may subjective response to exercise. People with diabetes have a higher incidence of silent ischemia. Heart rate and blood pressure may be less valid indexes of workload. Peripheral vascular disease may result from the direct effect of diabetes, as well as vascular occlusive disease, which is accelerated in individuals with diabetes compared with those who do not have this condition. Altered glucose transfer may also interfere with normal exercise responses. Weight control and nutrition are important to optimize training responses. The capacity to exhibit an optimal training response depends on disease severity, management of the disease, and complications (HbA_{1c} provides an index of potential complications). Limb perfusion and skin perfusion are monitored before and after exercise. Well fitting, smooth, clean socks must be worn at all times.

Special considerations include monitoring blood glucose before, during, and after exercise (immediate and delayed), at least initially when prescribing exercise for a person with diabetes. Exercise is postponed if blood glucose is extremely high and in the presence of ketone bodies. Daily regular exercise is recommended to maintain health and optimal blood glucose regulation. Intensity should be mild to moderate for a given individual.[68] Exercise is judiciously timed with the intake of both foods of optimal glycemic index for the person's needs and insulin or oral agents, as indicated. With improved glucose tolerance and insulin sensitivity and a long-term aerobic exercise program, the need for insulin or oral agents will be affected. The need for these will be eliminated, ideally, or at least reduced.

Individuals with thyroid disease warrant close monitoring. Those who are hypothyroid will be more easily fatigued. Their medical management requires close monitoring to ensure that their condition is normalized as much as possible. If it is, these individuals should have generally normal exercise responses. Those with hyperthyroidism will have high resting heart rates and blood pressure and exaggerated exercise responses.

Individuals with Immunodeficiency Conditions

The pharmaceutical drugs that have been developed to improve the survival of individuals with human immunodeficiency virus (HIV) and acquired immune deficiency syndrome (AIDS) (e.g., highly active antiretroviral therapy [HAART]) can impair oxygen transport, hence reducing functional capacity. At peak exercise, heart rate has been reported to be lower and stroke volume higher in individuals with HIV taking HAART when compared with individuals with HIV not taking the drug.[69] The a-vO_2 difference was lower at peak exercise for those on the drug. HAART is a primary contributor to decreased muscle oxygen extraction-utilization in individuals infected with HIV. The physical therapist must be highly knowledgeable about the combined response of exercise and the potent medications used to control the disease in these individuals. This is important in order to build on an individual's exercise reserve capacity when health is best, as well as to maintain health and social participation. It is hoped that with improved health and conditioning, morbidity and its severity are reduced.

Immunodeficiency has been implicated in chronic fatigue syndrome (CFS). This syndrome, currently of unknown etiology, appears to run its course over time. Guidelines for exercise testing, particularly maximal testing and training, have been uncertain. In one study individuals with CFS were exercise-tested to the maximal extent. Exercise responses were comparable to individuals with reduced conditioning without CFS, supporting the theory that the physiological responses of individuals with CFS were not abnormal and that exercise testing resulted in no harmful or deleterious effects.[70]

Individuals with Cancer

The physical capacity of cancer survivors and their capacity to respond to exercise conditioning vary depending on the primary type of cancer, the presence of metastases, chemotherapy and radiation therapy and their schedule of administration, and other morbidity.[71] Mind-body considerations, including the psychological, cognitive, and physiological (immune) interface of the patient's presentation and related outcomes, are emphasized. Given that cancer is a leading cause of morbidity and premature mortality and that many cancer survivors can expect to die with the condition rather than *from* it as a result of advances in cancer management, the role of exercise has been a focus of attention over the past decade or so. The goals have been to improve health and conditioning, potentially augment remission and reduce progression through immunity stimulation, and reduce the negative effects of the potent treatments that are often administered. Muscle weakness and fatigue are primary complaints of patients with cancer. These complaints are likely related to the body's attempt to heal itself and in response to the potent treatments, as well as the overall deconditioning associated with illness.[72,73]

General guidelines for exercise testing and prescription include resistance training in conjunction with aerobic exercise.[71] Exercise provides both psychological and physical benefits in enabling an individual to thrive when living with cancer. The parameters of the exercise program may vary depending on a patient's response to potent radiation and chemotherapy (i.e., reducing the intensity and frequency or temporarily discontinuing the program). The role of exercise in improving the health and well-being of people with cancer and in attenuating the negative effects of potent treatments has been a hotbed of research in recent years. Significant advances can be expected in refining exercise testing and training parameters in the near future.

Individuals with Nutrition-Related Conditions

Obesity

In preparation for exercise prescription, the individual who is obese requires a comprehensive multisystem assessment to establish all factors that may limit exercise tolerance. These individuals require high volumes of physical activity and exercise (see the physical activity and exercise pyramid in Chapter 1) in conjunction with a nutritious dietary program. Introducing more exercise, however, must be done gradually so that it is as enjoyable as possible and also less likely to cause musculoskeletal strain and injury. Biomechanics change with weight loss, and exercise becomes biomechanically less stressful and better tolerated.

Prescriptive parameters for optimal weight loss remain a matter of debate with respect to prolonged, low-intensity aerobic exercise versus short, high-intensity exercise. Moderate intensities of effort, however, have been reported to be more effective at mobilizing fat, whereas heavy exercise promotes energy expenditure after exercise.[2] The critical factor is the number of calories expended, and burning calories is best achieved with a regularly active lifestyle supplemented with additional formal exercise sessions. Lower-intensity exercise may be favored to avoid musculoskeletal strain or for psychological and motivational reasons. Aerobic training increases lipid oxidation during exercise in fasting conditions.[74] Such a regimen maintains glucose homeostasis and facilitates fat oxidation. Additional benefits of endurance training for individuals who are obese include reduced cholesterol and insulin concentrations in the blood.

Some individuals may benefit from a structured program (see Chapter 32) and the social support of others in the program.

Anorexia Nervosa

The malnutrition and weight loss due to catabolism associated with anorexia nervosa predisposes individuals with the condition to deconditioning and impaired oxygen transport reserve capacity. Such capacity is vital to optimally respond and adapt to exercise and the physical demands of daily life in the short and the long term.[75] Fluid and electrolyte imbalance can complicate the clinical picture and is the primary cause of death in extreme cases. Although quantitatively abnormal, responses to exercise may be appropriate in the absence of abnormal myocardial performance. Exercise is prescribed in conjunction with an optimal nutritional plan so that further catabolism is not precipitated.

Summary

This chapter extends the general exercise testing and training principles covered in Chapter 19 and describes special considerations for exercise testing and training individuals with cardiovascular and pulmonary dysfunction secondary to conditions other than primary chronic heart and lung disease. Exercise testing and training is one component of a comprehensive physical therapy management program that is described in Chapter 32.

Conditions that can lead to secondary cardiovascular and pulmonary dysfunction include dysfunction of the musculoskeletal, connective tissue, neurological, gastrointestinal, hepatic, renal, hematological, endocrine, and immunological systems, or some combination thereof. Nutritional disorders, specifically obesity and starvation (anorexia nervosa), also have cardiovascular and pulmonary manifestations. Exercise has a primary role in the management of these conditions, along with the elements of a comprehensive multidisciplinary prevention and rehabilitation program. Knowledge of the potential cardiovascular and pulmonary consequences of conditions other than primary cardiovascular and pulmonary disease is essential to prescribe mobilization and exercise safely and therapeutically for individuals with these conditions to maintain their health and well-being (capacity for activity and participation in life with least physiological risk). Individuals with these conditions are often managed by physical therapists. Thus the cardiovascular and pulmonary manifestations must be considered with respect to physical activity recommendations and the prescription of optimal and safe exercise programs.

Individuals with the potential for cardiovascular and pulmonary dysfunction secondary to noncardiovascular and pulmonary conditions are at significant health risk. Even minor illnesses can have a major impact on their functional capacity. Further, many of these conditions have a progressive degenerative component. This, coupled with aging, can result in what may seem to be a sudden functional decline. Thus oxygen transport of these individuals can benefit from the general health benefits of a lifelong program that includes an exercise program modified based on changes in their condition. Finally, individuals with chronic, secondary cardiovascular and pulmonary conditions likely have underlying risk factors for primary cardiovascular and pulmonary conditions comparable to the general population, if not to a greater extent. Thus both types of pathoetiology must be considered when evaluating limitations in life participation and related activities and their remediation, as well as when evaluating preventive measures for lifelong health and well-being.

Review Questions

1. Describe how chronic, secondary cardiovascular and pulmonary dysfunction associated with the following conditions can limit a person's participation in life and associated activities in the absence of chronic, primary cardiovascular and pulmonary conditions.
    1. Musculoskeletal (osteoporosis and osteoarthritis)
    2. Connective tissue (systemic lupus erythematosus, scleroderma) and autoimmune conditions (rheumatoid arthritis)
    3. Neurological (stroke, spinal cord injury, chronic effects of poliomyelitis)
    4. Gastrointestinal
    5. Hepatic
    6. Renal
    7. Hematological
    8. Endocrine
    9. Immunological
    10. Obesity
    11. Anorexia nervosa
2. Describe special considerations for exercise testing and training of individuals with the conditions listed in question 1.

References

1. Dean E: Oxygen transport deficits in systemic disease and implications for physical therapy. *Physical Therapy* 77:187–202, 1997.
2. Shepherd RB: Exercise and training to optimize functional motor performance in stroke: Driving neural reorganization? *Neural Plasticity* 8:121–129, 2001.
3. Ditmyer MM, Topp R, Pifer M: Prehabilitation in preparation for orthopedic surgery. *Orthopedic Nursing* 21:43–51, 2002.
4. Taivassalo T, De Stefano N, Chen J, et al: Short-term aerobic training response in chronic myopathies. *Muscle Nerve* 22:1239–1243, 1999.
5. Shephard RJ: Absolute versus relative intensity of physical activity in a dose response context. *Medicine and Science in Sports and Exercise* 33(Suppl 6):S400–S418, 2001.
6. Qin L, Au S, Choy W, et al: Regular Tai Chi Chuan exercise may retard bone loss in postmenopausal women: A case-controlled study. *Archives of Physical Medicine and Rehabilitation* 83:1355–1359, 2002.
7. Escalante Y, García-Hermoso A, Saavedra JM: Effects of exercise on functional aerobic capacity in lower limb osteoarthritis: A systematic review. *Journal of Science in Medicine and Sport Nov 24* [Epub ahead of print], 2010.
8. Schlenk EA, Lias JL, Sereika SM, et al: Improving physical activity and function in overweight and obese older adults with osteoarthritis of the knee: A feasibility study. *Rehabilitation Nursing* 36:32–42, 2010.
9. Cluett J: Joint pain and obesity, 2009. www.About.com, Guide Updated January 07, 2009; retrieved March 2011.
10. Cluett J: Will joint replacement help me lose weight? 2010. www.About.com, Guide Updated September 07, 2010; retrieved March 2011.
11. Weiss H: The effect of an exercise program on vital capacity and rib mobility in patients with idiopathic scoliosis. *Spine* 16:88–93, 1991.
12. Roberto R, Fritz A, Hagar Y, et al: The natural history of cardiac and pulmonary function decline in patients with Duchenne muscular dystrophy. *Spine Feb 1* [Epub ahead of print], 2011.
13. Kelly JO, Kilbreath SL, Davis GM, et al: Cardiorespiratory fitness and walking ability in subacute stroke patients. *Archives of Physical Medicine and Rehabilitation* 84:1780–1785, 2003.
14. Katz-Leurer M, Shochina M, Carmeli E, et al: The influence of early aerobic training on the functional capacity in patients with cerebrovascular accident at the subacute stage. *Archives of Physical Medicine and Rehabilitation* 84:1609–1614, 2003.
15. Katz-Leurer M, Carmeli E, Shochina M: The effect of early aerobic training on independence six months post stroke. *Clinical Rehabilitation* 17:735–741, 2003.
16. Meek C, Pollack A, Potter J, et al: A systematic review of exercise trials post stroke. *Clinical Rehabilitation* 17:6–13, 2003.
17. Saunders DH, Greig CA, Young A, et al: Physical fitness training for stroke patients. Cochrane Database Systematic Reviews 1, CD003316, 2004.
18. Pohl M, Mehrholz J, Ritschel C, et al: Speed-dependent treadmill training in ambulatory hemiparetic stroke patients: a randomized controlled trial. *Stroke* 33:553–558, 2002.
19. Eng JJ, Dawson AS, Chu KS: Submaximal exercise in persons with stroke: Test-retest reliability and concurrent validity with maximal oxygen consumption. *Archives of Physical Medicine and Rehabilitation* 85:113–118, 2004.
20. Teixeira da Cunha-Filho I, Henson H, Qureshy H, et al: Differential responses to measures of gait performance among healthy and neurologically impaired individuals. *Archives of Physical Medicine and Rehabilitation* 84:1774–1779, 2003.
21. Dubrovolny CL, Ivey FM, Rogers MA, et al: Reliability of treadmill exercise testing in older patients with chronic hemiparetic stroke. *Archives of Physical Medicine and Rehabilitation* 84:1308–1312, 2003.
22. Macko RF, Smith GV, Dobrovolny CL, et al: Treadmill training improves fitness reserve in chronic stroke patients. *Archives of Physical Medicine and Rehabilitation* 82:879–884, 2001.
23. Moseley AM, Stark A, Cameron ID, et al: Treadmill training and body weight support for walking after stroke. *Stroke* 34:3006, 2003.
24. Barbeau H, Visintin M: Optimal outcomes obtained with body-weight support combined with treadmill training in stroke subjects. *Archives of Physical Medicine and Rehabilitation* 84:1458–1465, 2003.
25. Hesse S, Werner C, von Frankenberg S, et al: Treadmill training with partial body weight support after stroke. *Physical Medicine Rehabilitation Clinics of North America* 14(Suppl 1):S111–S123, 2003.
26. Mudge S, Rochester L, Recordon A: The effect of treadmill training on gait, balance and trunk control in a hemiplegic subject: A single system design. *Disability and Rehabilitation* 25:1000–1007, 2003.
27. Sullivan KJ, Knowlton BJ, Dobkin BH: Step training with body weight support: Effect of treadmill speed and practice paradigms on poststroke locomotor recovery. *Archives of Physical Medicine and Rehabilitation* 83:683–691, 2002.
28. Eng JJ, Chu KS, Dawson AS, et al: Functional walk tests in individuals with stroke: Relation to perceived exertion and myocardial exertion. *Stroke* 33:756–761, 2002.
29. McCarty MF: Up-regulation of endothelial nitric oxide activity as a central strategy for prevention of ischemic stroke: Just say NO to stroke. *Medical Hypotheses* 55:386–403, 2000.
30. Lord SE, McPherson K, McNaughton HK, et al: Community ambulation after stroke: How important and obtainable is it and what measures appear predictive? *Archives of Physical Medicine and Rehabilitation* 85:234–239, 2004.
31. Carr M, Jones J: Physiologic effects of exercise on stroke survivors. *Topics in Stroke Rehabilitation* 9:57–64, 2003.
32. Riolo L, Fisher K: Is there evidence that strength training could help improve muscle function and other outcomes without reinforcing abnormal movement patterns or increasing reflex activity in a man who has had a stroke? *Physical Therapy* 83:844–851, 2003.
33. Moreland JD, Goldsmith CH, Huijbregts MP, et al: Progressive resistance strengthening exercises after stroke: a single-blind randomized controlled trial. *Archives of Physical Medicine and Rehabilitation* 84:1433–1440, 2003.
34. Vidal J, Javierre C, Segura R, et al: Physiologic adaptations to exercise in people with spinal cord injury. *Journal of Physiology and Biochemistry* 59:11–18, 2003.
35. Barstow TJ, Scremin AM, Mutton DL, et al: Changes in gas exchange kinetics with training in patients with spinal cord injury. *Medicine and Science in Sports and Exercise* 28:1221–1228, 1996.
36. Jacobs PL, Mahoney ET, Robbins A, et al: Hypokinetic circulation in persons with paraplegia. *Medicine and Science in Sports and Exercise* 34:1401–1407, 2002.
37. Dela F, Mohr T, Jensen CM, et al: Cardiovascular control during exercise: Insights from spinal cord-injured humans. *Circulation* 107:2127–2133, 2003.

38. Mills PB, Krassioukov A: Autonomic function as a missing piece of the classification of Paralympic athletes with spinal cord injury. *Spinal Cord Mar 1.* [Epub ahead of print], 2011.
39. Fukuoka Y, Endo M, Kagawa H, et al: Kinetics and steady-state of $\dot{V}O_2$ responses to arm exercise in trained spinal cord injured humans. *Spinal Cord* 40:631–638, 2002.
40. Price DT, Davidoff R, Balady GJ: Comparison of cardiovascular adaptations to long-term arm and leg exercise in wheelchair athletes versus long-distance runners. *American Journal of Cardiology* 85:996–1001, 2000.
41. de Groot S, Veeger HE, Hollander AP, et al: Effect of wheelchair stroke pattern on mechanical efficiency. *American Journal of Physical Medicine and Rehabilitation* 83:640–649, 2004.
42. Dawes H, Bateman A, Culpan J, et al: The effect of increasing effort on movement economy during incremental cycling exercise in individuals early after acquired brain injury. *Clinical Rehabilitation* 17:528–534, 2003.
43. Gates PE, Campbell IG, George KP: Absence of training-specific cardiac adaptation in paraplegic athletes. *Medicine and Science in Sports and Exercise* 34:1699–1704, 2002.
44. Dean E, Dallimore D: Physical therapy in the management of chronic poliomyelitis and postpolio syndrome. In Silver JK, Gawne AC, editors, (2004): *Postpolio syndrome*, Philadelphia, 2004, Hanley & Belfus.
45. Dean E, Dallimore D: Muscle function and training of individuals with the chronic effects of poliomyelitis with and without postpolio syndrome. *Physiotherapy Canada* 57:1–14, 2005.
46. Dean E, Ross J: Effect of modified aerobic training on movement energetics in polio survivor. *Orthopedics* 14:1243–1246, 1991.
47. Weinberg J, Borg J, Bevegard S, et al: Respiratory response to exercise in postpolio patients with severe inspiratory muscle dysfunction. *Archives of Physical Medicine and Rehabilitation* 80:1095–1100, 1999.
48. Perry J, Barnes G, Gronley JK: The postpolio syndrome: An overuse phenomenon. *Clinical Orthopedics* 233:145–162, 1988.
49. Dean E, Ross J, MacIntyre D: A rejoinder to "Exercise programs for patients with post-polio syndrome: A case report"—a short communication. *Physical Therapy* 69:695–699, 1989.
50. Dean E, Ross J: Movement energetics of individuals with a history of poliomyelitis. *Archives of Physical Medicine and Rehabilitation* 74:478–483, 1993.
51. Noonan V, Dean E, Dallimore M: Are objective measures of disability related to self-reports in individuals with the late effects of poliomyelitis? A validation study. *Archives of Physical Medicine and Rehabilitation* 81:1422–1427, 2000.
52. Bosch JJ: Health maintenance throughout the life span for individuals with Down syndrome. *Journal of the American Academy of Nurse Practitioners* 15:5–17, 2003.
53. Schwaiblmair M, Behr J, Fruhmann G: Cardiorespiratory responses to incremental exercise in patients with systemic sclerosis. *Chest* 110:1520–1525, 1996.
54. Bruce IN, Urowitz MB, Gladman DD, et al: Risk factors for coronary heart disease in women with systemic lupus erythematosus: The Toronto Risk Factor Study. *Arthritis and Rheumatism* 48:3159–3167, 2003.
55. Mustonen J, Laakso M, Hirvonen T, et al: Abnormalities in left ventricular diastolic function in male patients with rheumatoid arthritis without clinically evident cardiovascular disease. *European Journal of Clinical Investigation* 23:246–253, 1993.
56. Forrest G, Rynes RI: Exercise for rheumatoid arthritis. *Contemporary Internal Medicine* 6:23–28, 1994.
57. D'Inca R, Varnier M, Mestriner C, et al: Effect of moderate exercise on Crohn's disease patients in remission. *Italian Journal of Gastroenterology and Hepatology* 31:205–210, 1999.
58. Epstein SK, Zilberberg MD, Jacoby C, et al: Response to symptom-limited exercise in patients with hepatopulmonary syndrome. *Chest* 114:736–741, 1998.
59. Wong F, Girgrah N, Graba J, et al: The cardiac response to exercise in cirrhosis. *Gut* 2001;49:268–275, 2001.
60. Sala E, Noyszewski EA, Campistol JM, et al: Impaired muscle oxygen transfer in patients with chronic renal failure. *American Journal of Physiology. Regulatory, Integrative and Comparative Physiology* 280:R1240–R1248, 2001.
61. McMahon LP, McKenna MJ, Sangkabutra T, et al: Physical performance and associated electrolyte changes after haemoglobin normalization: A comparative study in haemodialysis patients. *Nephrology, Dialysis, and Transplant* 14:1182–1187, 1999.
62. Copley JB, Lindberg JS: The risks of exercise. *Advances in Renal Replacement Therapy* 6:165–171, 1999.
63. Marrades RM, Roca J, Campistol JM, et al: Effects of erythropoietin on muscle O_2 transport during exercise in patients with chronic renal failure. *Journal of Clinical Investigation* 97:2092–2100, 1996.
64. Lundin AP, Akerman MJ, Chesler RM, et al: Exercise in hemodialysis patients after treatment with recombinant human erythropoietin. *Nephron* 58:315–319, 1991.
65. Ix JH, Shlipak MG, Liu HH, et al: Association between renal insufficiency and inducible ischemia in patients with coronary artery disease: the heart and soul study. *Journal of the American Society for Nephrology* 14:3233–3238, 2003.
66. Williams C: Haemoglobin—Is more better? *Nephrology, Dialysis, Transplantation* 10(Suppl 2):48–55, 1995.
67. Oyono-Enguelle S, LeGallais D, Lonsdorfer A, et al: Cardiorespiratory and metabolic responses to exercise in HbSC sickle cell patients. *Medicine and Science in Sports and Exercise* 32:725–731, 2000.
68. American College of Sports Medicine, Thompson WR, Gordon NF, Pescatello LS: *ACSM's guidelines for exercise testing and prescription*, ed 8, Philadelphia, 2010, Wolters Kluwer Health/Lippincott Williams & Wilkins.
69. Cade WT, Fantry LE, Nabar SR, et al: A comparison of Qt and a-vO_2 in individuals with HIV taking and not taking HAART. *Medicine and Science in Sports and Exercise* 35:1108–1117, 2003.
70. Mullis R, Campbell IT, Wearden AJ, et al: Prediction of peak oxygen uptake in chronic fatigue syndrome. *British Journal of Sports Medicine* 33:352–356, 1999.
71. Salmon PG, Swank AM: Exercise-based disease management guidelines for individuals with cancer: Potential application in a high-risk mid-southern state. *Journal of Exercise Physiology (online)* 5:1–10, 2002.
72. Carlos Dimeo F: Effects of exercise on cancer-related fatigue. *Cancer* 92:1657–1743, 2001.
73. Baracos VE: Management of muscle wasting in cancer-associated cachexia. Understanding gained from experimental studies. *Cancer* 92(Suppl 6):1669–1677, 2001.
74. Thalamus C, Stich V, Riviere D, et al: Effects of a longitudinal training program on responses to exercise in overweight men. *Obesity Research* 11:247–256, 2003.
75. Rowland T, Koenigs L, Miller N: Myocardial performance during maximal exercise in adolescents with anorexia nervosa. *Journal of Sports Medicine and Physical Fitness* 43:202–208, 2003.

Chapter 26 III

Respiratory Muscle Training

Rik Gosselink and Simone Dal Corso

KEY TERMS

Asthma
Chronic heart failure
Chronic obstructive pulmonary disease
Cystic fibrosis
Neuromuscular conditions
Quadriplegia
Respiratory muscle testing
Weaning failure

CHAPTER OUTLINE

The capacity of the respiratory muscle pump is vital for the movement of air to the level of gas exchange in the respiratory system. Impairment of the respiratory pump compromises ventilation, gas exchange, and tissue respiration. The respiratory muscles drive ventilation. In conditions where the load on the respiratory muscles is increased or the capacity of the respiratory muscles is decreased, muscle weakness can occur. Breathing pattern (i.e., rapid shallow breathing) adapts, however, to help counter respiratory muscle fatigue.[1] Although this adaptation decreases the effectiveness of gas exchange, a breathing pattern with a lower tidal volume and higher breathing rate helps minimize respiratory muscle fatigue.

Although the adaptation in breathing pattern affects the effectiveness of gas exchange, prevention of muscle fatigue and respiratory arrest requires modification of the breathing pattern (i.e., there is a decrease in tidal volume and an increase in breathing rate). Figure 26-1 illustrates this adaptation in patients at risk for respiratory failure. Respiratory muscle weakness increases the relative load for breathing (inspiratory pressure/maximum inspiratory pressure [PI/PI_{max}] ratio, see Figure 26-1), and this can lead to clinical consequences such as dyspnea, impaired exercise performance, ineffective coughing, respiratory insufficiency, weaning failure, and death. Dysfunction of the respiratory muscles is observed in several conditions such as chronic obstructive pulmonary disease, asthma, cystic fibrosis, neuromuscular disease including spinal cord injury, congestive heart failure, and critical illness. This chapter describes the clinical relevance of respiratory muscle weakness, the assessment and testing of respiratory muscle function, and the application and effectiveness of respiratory muscle training for the conditions above and its role in weaning some patients from mechanical ventilation.

Respiratory Muscle Assessment

Respiratory Muscle Strength Testing

Clinically, respiratory muscle strength is measured as PI_{max} and maximum expiratory pressure (PE_{max}). These pressures are measured using a small cylinder that fits in the patient's mouth with a circular mouthpiece (Figure 26-2). A small leak in the cylinder (2 mm diameter and 15 mm length) prevents high pressures that could be caused by the contraction of the cheek muscles.[2] Standardizing the lung volume at which the pressures are measured is crucial.[3] To prevent chest wall and lung recoil pressures from contributing to the pressure generated by the inspiratory muscles, measurements are recorded at functional residual capacity (FRC). This lung volume, however, is difficult to standardize. In clinical practice, PI_{max} is measured from residual volume, whereas PE_{max} is measured at total lung capacity (TLC). At least five repetitions should be performed. Respiratory muscle testing is described in detail in the American Thoracic Society/European Respiratory Society position statement (2002).[4]

Several groups of investigators have published norms for PI_{max} and PE_{max} (Table 26-1).[2,7,8] Regardless of the norms used,

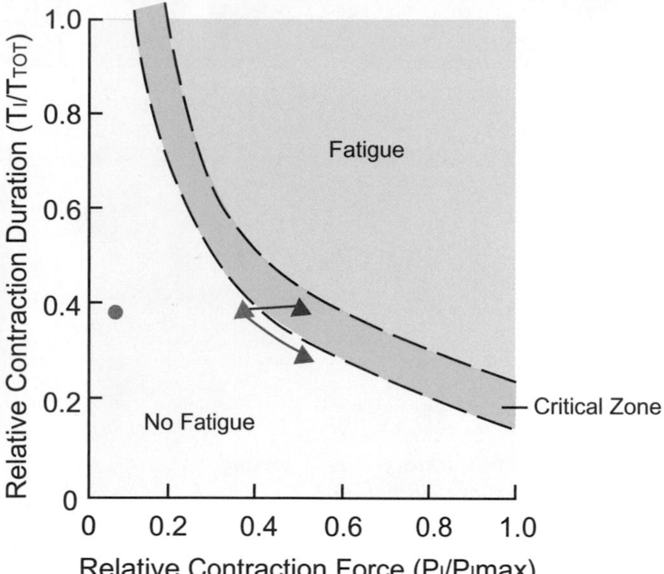

Fig. 26-1 The relationship between relative contraction force (PI/PI_{max}) and relative contraction duration (TI/T_{TOT}) in a healthy subject (d) and a patient with COPD (m). The hatched area represents the critical zone in which fatigue develops. With progressive mechanical loading (e.g., exercise and acute exacerbation), the patient with COPD needs to increase PI and, therefore, might fall into the fatiguing zone (*dashed arrow*). This is generally avoided by a concomitant reduction in the duration of inspiration, TI/T_{TOT} (*solid arrow*). This results in a decrease in tidal volume and a consequent increase in respiratory rate to maintain constant minute ventilation. Interventions aimed at reducing the load on the inspiratory muscles (PI) or increasing the maximum capacity of the inspiratory muscles (PI_{max}) reduce the relative contraction force of the inspiratory muscles. This prevents muscle fatigue and, thus, respiratory insufficiency. *(Modified from Bellemare F, Grassino A: Effect of pressure and timing of contraction on human diaphragm fatigue,* J Applied Physiol *53:1190-1195, 1982).*

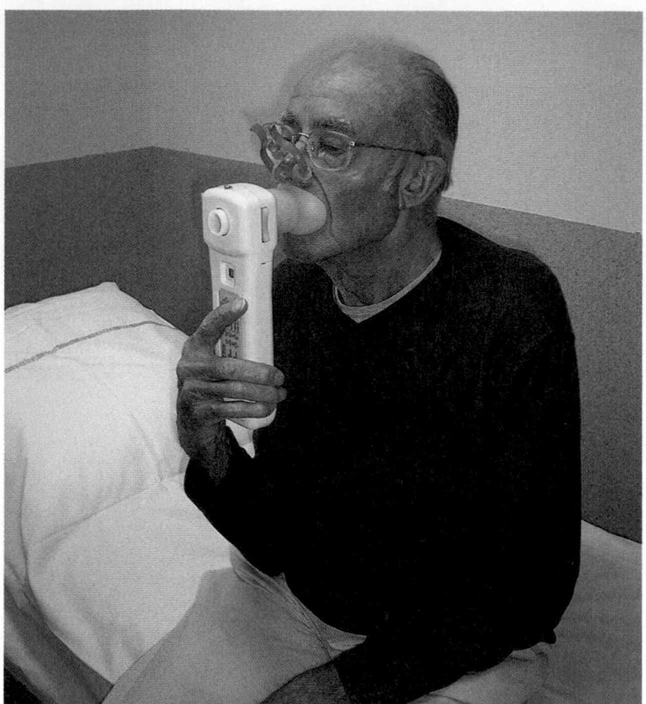

Fig. 26-2 Assessment of respiratory muscle strength with measurement of mouth pressure.

Table 26-1 Reference Values for Maximal Inspiratory and Expiratory Mouth Pressures in Healthy Adults

Reference		PI_{max} (cm H_2O)	PE_{max} (cm H_2O)
Black and Hyatt (1969)[2]	M	124 ± 22	233 ± 42
	F	87 ± 16	152 ± 27
Rinqvist (1966)[5]	M	130 ± 32	237 ± 46
	F	98 ± 25	165 ± 30
Leech et al (1983)[6]	M	114 ± 36	154 ± 82
	F	71 ± 27	94 ± 33
Rochester and Arora (1983)[7]	M	127 ± 28	216 ± 41
	F	91 ± 25	138 ± 39
Wilson et al (1984)[8]	M	106 ± 31	148 ± 17
	F	73 ± 22	93 ± 17
Vincken et al (1987)[9]	M	105 ± 25	140 ± 38
	F	71 ± 23	89 ± 24
Bruschi et al (1992)[10]	M	120 ± 37	140 ± 30
	F	84 ± 30	95 ± 20

M, Male; F, female.

the standard deviation is typically large. Therefore weakness is not easy to define.[11] Inspiratory weakness is defined as a PI_{max} lower than 50% of predicted[12] in the presence of clinical signs (e.g., dyspnea, impaired cough, and orthopnea) consistent with reduced respiratory muscle strength. Other methods, such as the sniff maneuver, have been developed as tools to quantify global respiratory muscle function.[13] The results of the sniff maneuver have been reported to be highly reliable in children with neuromuscular disease. More invasive methods such as electric or magnetic diaphragm stimulation can provide more accurate and detailed information on diaphragmatic function[14] and are useful in the diagnosis of diaphragmatic paresis. For most clinical applications, however, the assessment of inspiratory and expiratory mouth pressures is sufficient.

Respiratory Muscle Endurance Testing

Several tests for assessing respiratory muscle endurance capacity have been described. Most commonly the patient breathes against a submaximal inspiratory load (60% to 75% PI_{max}) for as long as possible.[15,16] This test can detect changes in inspiratory muscle endurance after training. Incremental threshold loading, breathing against an incremental load (approximately 5 cm H_2O) every 2 minutes, is also reproducible.[17] The highest load that can be sustained for two minutes is termed the *sustainable pressure* and is expressed as a percentage of the maximal load.[17,18] Healthy people can usually sustain 70% of the PI_{max} for 2 minutes.[18] Johnson and colleagues[17] reported large intra-individual variations in this percentage, which tends to decrease with age. The sustainable pressure has been shown to be less than the maximal inspiratory and expiratory pressures in individuals with chronic obstructive pulmonary disease (COPD).[19] A third method[20-22] is a repetitive maximal inspiratory or expiratory maneuver performed against an occluded airway with a well-defined contraction duration (10 seconds) and relaxation time (5 seconds). The relative decline in maximal pressure after 18 contractions is a measure of the endurance capacity of the respiratory muscles.

Respiratory Muscle Training Methods

Comparable to muscle training of the peripheral skeletal muscles, training of the respiratory muscles aims to improve specific characteristics of inspiratory or expiratory muscle contraction force, endurance, or velocity (Table 26-2).[23-25]

Inspiratory Muscle Training

Because the inspiratory muscles are mainly involved in repetitive contractions with low intensity, training strategies emphasize enhancing inspiratory muscle endurance. Two types of training (i.e. threshold loading [Figure 26-3] and normocapnic hyperpnea [NCH] [Figure 26-4]) are currently practiced. During NCH, the patient is asked to breathe at a high proportion (>60%) of the maximal voluntary ventilation for 15 to 20 minutes.[23,26] In the past, the equipment used for this type of training was complicated, but recently a simpler, partial rebreathing system has been developed.[27]

During inspiratory resistive breathing the patient inhales through a mouthpiece with an adapter fitted with an adjustable diameter. This resistance is flow-dependent. Adequate training intensity is achieved only with feedback of the target pressure if flow and pressure are tightly coupled.[28] Recently, a flow-independent resistance has been developed, the so-called threshold loading valve, a valve that opens at a critical pressure.[29,30] Training intensity varies across studies, from as high as maximal sustained inspiratory (Müller) maneuvers[31] to 50% to 80% PI_{max}[16,32-34] to a low intensity of 30% PI_{max}.[34-37] All these studies carefully controlled the target pressure or the threshold loading during training.[30] Threshold loading has the advantage of being independent of inspiratory flow rate[30] but requires a build-up of negative pressure before flow is initiated; hence it is inertive in nature. The fact that threshold loading enhances velocity of inspiratory muscle shortening[38]

Table 26-2 Training Modalities for Inspiratory Muscle Resistive Training (IMT) and Respiratory Muscle Endurance Training (RMET)

	IMT	RMET (Voluntary Isocapnic Hyperpnea)
Type	Strength	Endurance
Duration	15 minutes, twice daily,	30 minutes, 6-12 weeks
Frequency	5-7x per week	5x per week
Intensity	30-50%PImax with individual incremental load, weekly control of load/technique	V_E = 50-60% MVV, breathing frequency 50-60/min

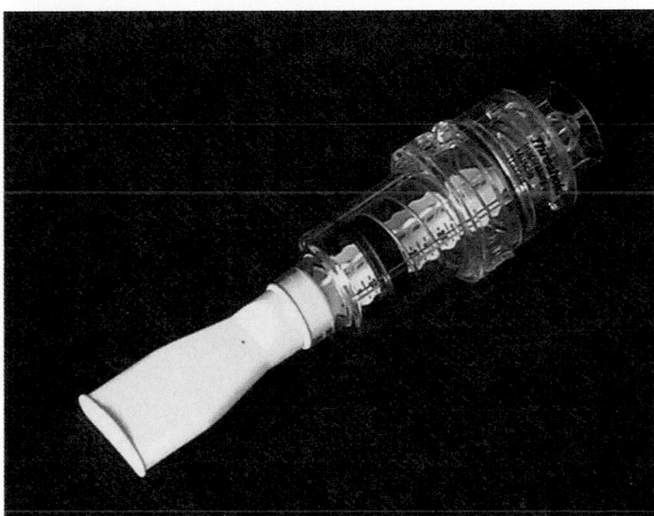

Fig. 26-3 Threshold loading device.

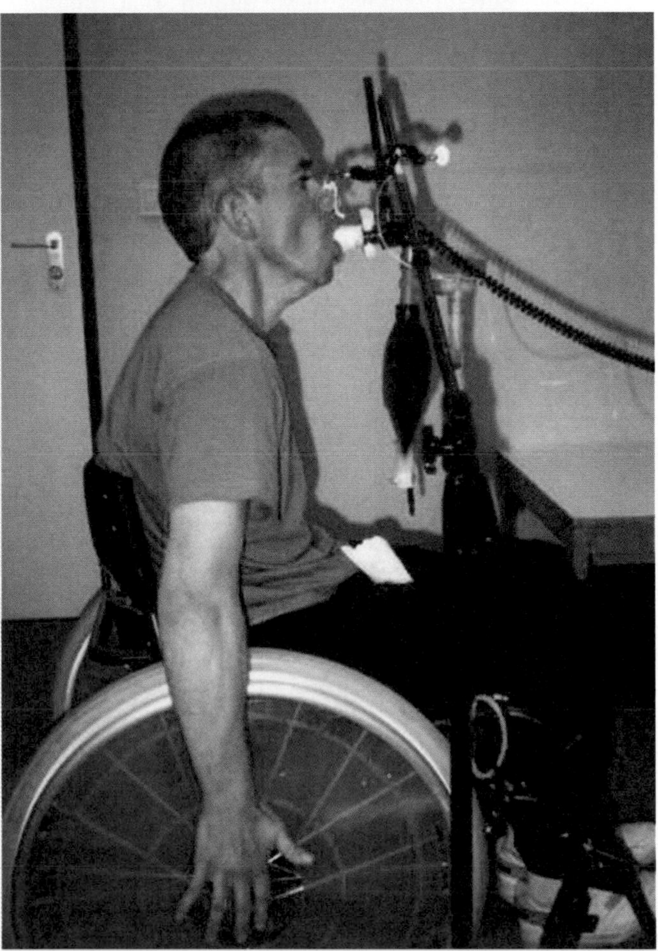

Fig. 26-4 Normocapnic hyperpnea equipment.

could provide additional benefit because this shortens inspiratory time and increases time for exhalation and relaxation. Increased relaxation time may prevent the development of muscle fatigue in patients who are at risk. In addition, shortening inspiratory time will increase expiratory time, thus reducing dynamic hyperinflation, which is an important advantage in patients with COPD.

Expiratory Muscle Training

Explosive expiratory maneuvers and low-intensity contractions of the abdominal muscles are similar to those involved in coughing, the Valsalva maneuver, and exercise. Consequently, training parameters for expiratory muscle training can be either high-intensity strength training or moderate- to low-intensity endurance training. An example of the parameters for endurance expiratory muscle training is 30 minutes of continuous training at 15% to 45% of PE_{max}.[39] An example of strength training parameters is 15 Valsalva maneuvers at 60% of PE_{max}.[40] Both training programs can be implemented using expiratory resistance at the mouth, such as threshold loading.[40,41]

Respiratory Muscle Training in Health

Diaphragm fatigue can occur during sustained high-intensity exercise.[42,43] Several studies have shown that unloading respiratory muscles (by using low-density gas mixtures or mechanical ventilation) can lead to an increase in exercise performance.[44,45] In athletes, heavy (but not moderate) respiratory muscle work has an impact on whole body exercise performance by affecting limb blood flow and limb muscle fatigue during heavy exercise.[46,47] One mechanism to explain these improvements in exercise performance is the "respiratory muscle metaboreflex" (Figure 26-5).[47] Therefore a rational basis exists for improving the strength and endurance of the respiratory muscles in order to improve exercise performance. In 14 competitive rowers, inspiratory muscle training (IMT) significantly improved PI_{max} and performance on a 5000-meter trial compared with a placebo control group.[48] A small but significant decrease in swimming time needed to cover 100 meters and 200 meters was observed after 6 weeks of IMT compared with a placebo control group.[49] After following 5 weeks of respiratory muscle endurance training (RMET), nine competitive cyclists had a 25 seconds (+2%) improvement on an 8-km trial. No differences were founded in peak work rate or maximal exercise capacity ($\dot{V}O_{2max}$).[50] Leddy and colleagues (2007)[51] reported a 4% decrease in time on a 4-mile run after 4 weeks of RMET. All these small improvements in exercise performance are also practical and relevant since small differences in athletes' performance can be the difference between winning and losing a race. On the other hand, several studies in endurance athletes observed no differences in maximal exercise capacity, other than an increase in respiratory muscle strength and endurance.[52,53]

An overview of the literature shows important methodological limitations of the available studies, such as a low number of study participants, no comparison with a (randomized) control group, and exercise performance outcomes that are less sensitive (maximal exercise capacity instead of a

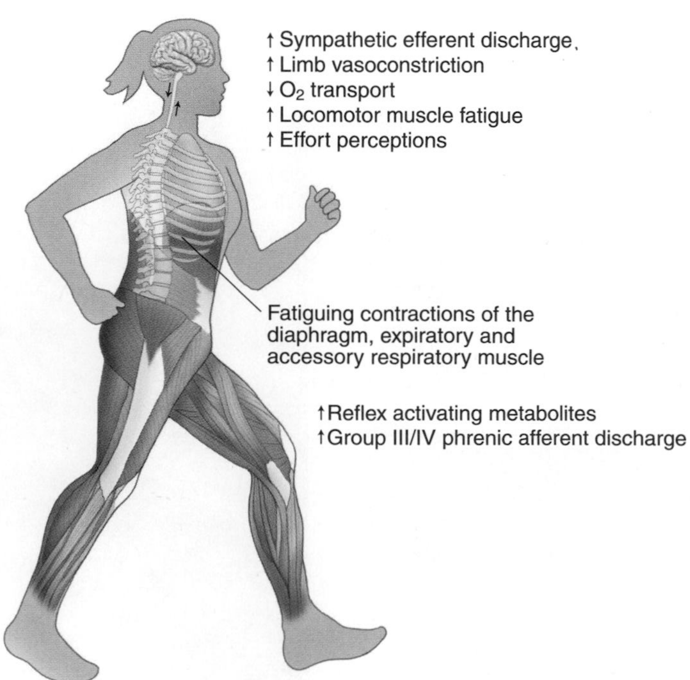

Fig. 26-5 Effects of high respiratory muscle work of breathing on exercise performance. (Qlimb = limb muscle perfusion). *(From Romer LM, Polkey MI: Exercise-induced respiratory muscle fatigue: Implications for performance, J Appl Physiol 104:879-888, 2008.)*

time trial). Based on our current understanding and available studies, we conclude that the capacity to meet high ventilatory demands improves with respiratory muscle training in healthy people and this can be associated with an improvement in exercise performance. Future studies are needed to confirm the beneficial effects of respiratory muscle training on exercise performance in health.

Respiratory Muscle Training in Disease

Chronic Obstructive Pulmonary Disease

Respiratory muscle weakness is often observed in patients with chronic obstructive pulmonary disease (COPD).[54-58] Adaptation of the diaphragm results in greater fatigue resistance and improved muscle function.[59,60] The diaphragm is remodeled in part by the transformation of fast fiber types to slow fiber types.[61,62] Despite these adaptations, both functional inspiratory muscle strength[55] and endurance[56] remain compromised in patients with COPD and contribute to hypercapnia,[63] dyspnea,[64,65] nocturnal oxygen desaturation,[33] and reduced walking distance.[66] During exercise, patients with COPD use a larger proportion of their maximal inspiratory pressure than healthy people.[67] This pattern of breathing is closely related to dyspnea during exercise[67] and may induce respiratory muscle fatigue and probably limits exercise capacity.

Another mechanism involved in the potential role of respiratory muscles in exercise limitation is the respiratory muscle metaboreflex (see Figure 26-5). Inspiratory muscles should become more fatigue-resistant by increasing their work capacity and should consume a smaller fraction of the total cardiac output during exercise, which in turn, should be available for the working muscles during exercise. In patients with COPD, diaphragmatic fatigue after exercise has been observed in only a small number of patients.[11,68] However, this might be related to the insufficient length of the exercise protocols and the absence of inspiratory muscle weakness in the subjects evaluated. Improved limb muscle blood flow after IMT has been observed in patients with chronic heart failure[69-71] but has not yet been studied in patients with COPD. Reductions in dynamic hyperinflation and dyspnea during exercise after IMT have also been proposed as mechanisms linking inspiratory muscle capacity to whole body endurance capacity; thus further study is needed.[72]

Compelling evidence suggests that breathing against an inspiratory load increases both maximal inspiratory pressure[16,28,32-37,73] and endurance of the inspiratory muscles.[28,33,34,73] Respiratory muscle training has been reported to produce hypertrophy of predominantly type I and IIA fibers in the diaphragms of hamsters.[74,75] The proportion of type I fibers and size of type II fibers in the external intercostals after IMT has been recently reported to increase in a study of patients with COPD.[76] Dyspnea[36,37,77] and nocturnal desaturation time[33] also decreased, while exercise performance tended to improve (Table 26-3).[78,79] In addition to exercise training, IMT can improve exercise capacity more than exercise training alone.[16,32,35,37] Based on systematic reviews with meta-analyses, IMT can improve inspiratory muscle strength and endurance, functional exercise capacity, and quality of life while also decreasing dyspnea.[78,79] The addition of IMT to a general exercise training program improved PI_{max} and tended to improve the exercise performance of patients with inspiratory muscle weakness (PI_{max} < 60 cm H_2O).[78,79] Long-term effects were shown for exercise performance and dyspnea in patients with COPD who continued performing their training program three times per week at high training intensity (60% PI_{max}).[80] NCH was applied in one randomized controlled trial and resulted in enhanced respiratory muscle endurance and exercise capacity as well as quality of life in patients with COPD.[26] Inspiratory muscle endurance training was shown to be less effective than respiratory muscle strength training.[79]

In conclusion, well-controlled inspiratory muscle training for people with inspiratory muscle weakness secondary to COPD can improve inspiratory muscle function, and it can lead to further improvement in exercise capacity, as well as decreased dyspnea and nocturnal desaturation time. Training intensity, however, should be at least 30% of the maximal inspiratory pressure and training duration for 30 minutes per day.

Table 26-3 Effect Size of Inspiratory Muscle Training Based on Meta-Analysis (n = 32)

	Effect size	P value
PI_{max} (cm H_2O)	13	.001
Endurance (s)	261	.001
Endurance (cm H_2O)	13	.001
6MWD (m)	32	.001
MVV (L)	3	.37
$\dot{V}O_{2max}$ (mL/kg/min)	1,3	.06
CRDQ score (points)	3,8	.007
Dyspnea (Borg)	−0.9	.001
Dyspnea (TDI)	+2.8	.001

PI_{max}, Maximal inspiratory pressure; 6MWD, 6-minute walk distance; MVV, maximal voluntary ventilation; $\dot{V}O_{2max}$, maximal oxygen uptake capacity; CRDQ, chronic respiratory disease questionnaire; Borg, scale of breathlessness; TDI, total dyspnea index.

From Gosselink R, De Vos J, van den Heuvel SP, et al: Impact of inspiratory muscle training in patients with COPD: What is the evidence? Eur Respir J *2011;37:416-425, 2011.*

Asthma

Respiratory muscle weakness is not frequently observed in patients with asthma.[80-82] Although some studies report a moderate reduction in inspiratory muscle strength,[81] other studies have not found inspiratory muscle strength to be affected.[20,56] Inspiratory muscle endurance has been shown to be increased in people with asthma[20] but reduced in those who are steroid dependent.[56] In patients with asthma, dyspnea has been observed to be greater in women than in men, resulting in their greater need for beta-2 agonists. This may reflect sex differences in inspiratory muscle strength.[80] IMT has been studied in people with asthma, and evidence from randomized trials supports that, in addition to improvements in inspiratory muscle strength, dyspnea and beta-2 agonist use was reduced in those with high dyspnea and high use of beta-2 agonists,[83] especially among women.[80] A Cochrane review, however, concluded that the evidence supporting a role for IMT for people with asthma was inconclusive.[84]

Cystic Fibrosis

Reports on the inspiratory muscle strength in people with cystic fibrosis (CF) have also been contradictory. Some have shown that inspiratory muscle strength is decreased,[85-88] whereas others have shown that it is normal[89,90] and others have shown it is supranormal.[91-93] The discrepancy across studies can be attributed to methodological inconsistencies such as age, degree of pulmonary dysfunction, nutritional status, and the assessment of PI_{max}. Severity of disease, nutritional depletion, and systemic inflammation have been considered contributors to respiratory muscle weakness in people with CF.[94] On the other hand, normal or supranormal PI_{max} in the CF population can be explained by the chronic increase of respiratory workload due to the combination of progressive airflow obstruction, hyperinflation, and airway resistance, which could produce a training effect.[89,95-97]

Given the similarities in abnormal lung mechanics for people with CF and with COPD, the rationale to indicate IMT for patients with CF is based on the benefits observed with this intervention in patients with COPD. There are few reports on IMT in patients with CF.[91,95,96,98,99] The modalities of IMT used in these patients are similar to those described for other patients with chronic obstructive diseases such as COPD and asthma. Early studies described the use of the NCH[98] and inspiratory resistive training[91] modalities. Recent studies, however, have used threshold loading.[95,96,99] As yet, there is no consensus by experts regarding the optimal training intensity for patients with CF. Even though training at low intensity (40% PI_{max}) improves inspiratory endurance,[95] high-intensity training (80% PI_{max}) can further augment inspiratory muscle function, pulmonary function, and exercise capacity.[96]

Recently, two meta-analyses have been published about the effects of inspiratory muscle training in patients with CF.[100,101] Both systematic reviews point out a scarcity of randomized controlled trials and a huge difference among inspiratory muscle training protocols. Therefore evidence is weak supporting IMT as a means of improving inspiratory muscle function in children, adolescents, and adults with CF. In addition, the benefit of IMT on dyspnea, exercise capacity, and quality of life for these populations remains unclear.

Quadriplegia

Several studies have reported that inspiratory or expiratory muscle training is a means of enhancing inspiratory or expiratory muscle function in individuals with quadriplegia, reducing dyspnea, and improving exercise performance.[102-105] In one systematic review, the investigators concluded that respiratory muscle training (RMT) tended to improve expiratory muscle strength, vital capacity, and residual volume. Insufficient data were available to make conclusions concerning the effects of RMT on inspiratory muscle strength, respiratory muscle endurance, quality of life, exercise performance, and respiratory complications.[105] A randomized controlled trial showed that NCH training in patients with spinal cord injury improved respiratory muscle strength and endurance. Further, respiratory complications occurred less frequently after training.[105]

Neurological and Neuromuscular Disease

Independent of the site of the pathology (e.g., the central nervous system, peripheral nerves, neuromuscular junction, and/or muscles themselves), respiratory muscle weakness associated with other factors (e.g., pulmonary dysfunction and immobility) plays a role in increasing the risk for ventilatory failure and respiratory complications, hence, morbidity and mortality.

The mechanisms underlying respiratory muscle dysfunction in patients with neuromuscular disease (NMD) are complex and dependent on the particular disease and its stage. In patients with amyotrophic lateral sclerosis (ALS), involvement of inspiratory muscle weakness is prominent and underlies ventilatory insufficiency and symptoms, while expiratory muscle weakness is mainly present in symptomatic patients and affects cough.[106] Progressive respiratory muscle weakness has been described in Duchenne muscular dystrophy (DMD). A recent study has confirmed a progressive impairment of the diaphragm compensated by an increase in the contribution of the ribcage to tidal volume.[107] Patients with Parkinson syndrome can exhibit respiratory muscle weakness even if the severity is mild, but the syndrome is less associated with dyspnea.[108] The weakness is associated with impaired exercise performance while quality of life and daily living activities appear unaffected.[109] Respiratory muscle function is affected in patients with acute ischemic stroke but it is not related to dyspnea.[110] Diaphragm contractility is affected on the contralateral side, which may be related to an increased incidence of pneumonia.[111] In addition, acute ischemic stroke has been related to expiratory muscle weakness and reduced peak flow rate, which may determine cough inefficiency.[112] Besides diminished respiratory strength and endurance, patients with generalized myasthenia gravis are more dyspneic than are control subjects.[113]

The indications for IMT in NMD are based on the benefits of strengthening the respiratory muscles, which may delay pulmonary complications and the onset of respiratory failure.[114] Studies have reported improved respiratory muscle function after IMT in various types of NMD.[115-117] Inspiratory muscle training (60% of sniff nasal inspiratory pressure, for 10 minutes, 3 times a day, 7 days a week, for 12 weeks) resulted in strengthening of the inspiratory muscles and also delayed the decline in respiratory function in patients with ALS.[118] Because of controversy about the benefits of respiratory muscle training in patients with DMD, either improvement or insignificant changes in respiratory muscle function, a recent statement of American Thoracic Society does not completely recommend this intervention for these patients.[4]

In studies that reported improvement in respiratory muscle function, the inspiratory resistance adjustments varied from 30%[117] to 70%-80% PI_{max}[119] and the period of training from 6 weeks to 24 months. An additional benefit was reduced perception of respiratory load, which could translate into reduced dyspnea.[117] In patients with Parkinson syndrome, IMT increased both strength and endurance of the respiratory muscles and reduced the perception of dyspnea.[120] One study has described the benefits of expiratory muscle training for patients with Parkinson disease.[121] An improvement in voluntary cough and swallowing was observed after training the expiratory muscles, which consisted of five sets of five breaths against 75% PE_{max} for 4 weeks. However, whether these benefits can prevent aspiration in these patients remains unclear. In patients with subacute stroke, IMT improved respiratory muscle function, exercise capacity, and quality of life.[122] In summary, the protocol consisted of two 15-minute sessions, starting with a load of 40% PI_{max} and going up to 60% PI_{max} (threshold loading) for six times a week for 6 weeks. Patients with myasthenia gravis have showed improvement in respiratory muscle function and also in dyspnea symptoms after inspiratory[123,124] and inspiratory plus expiratory muscle training.[125] For patients with multiple sclerosis, IMT has been recommended by Klefbeck and colleagues (2003)[126] as an additional intervention to physical training. In that study, patients breathed daily for 30 times through an inspiratory resistance of 40%-60% PI_{max} imposed by the threshold loading over a 10-week period. Although inspiratory muscle function is commonly affected in neuromuscular diseases, expiratory muscle strength is preferentially impaired in patients with multiple sclerosis[40] and it is inversely related to their disability status;[127] thus EMT has been shown to be beneficial for patients with multiple sclerosis.[40,128]

An association exists between training intensity and improvement of respiratory muscle capacity.[116] Patients with NMD who have more than 25% of predicted pulmonary function can respond to training.[31,117] Patients with severe impairment of ventilatory function, however, may show less improvement in respiratory strength because they are less able to achieve the critical training intensity, respiratory muscle weakness may predispose their muscle to damage rather than benefit from training, and their muscle mass may be insufficient. In the long term, the progression of most neuromuscular diseases affecting muscle probably impedes an optimal training effect.

Inspiratory and expiratory training enhances the respiratory muscle performance in patients with NMD. The transfer of these gains to increased cough effectiveness, reduced respiratory infection, and delayed ventilatory failure warrant detailed study.

Chronic Heart Failure

Although impairment of cardiac function is the principal factor associated with reduced functional capacity in people with chronic heart failure (CHF), abnormal respiratory muscle function plays an important role in premature exercise termination and contributes to sensory consequences, especially breathlessness on exertion. Exertional dyspnea can result from respiratory muscle weakness, increased respiratory muscles activity, or both.[64]

Reduced respiratory muscle strength in patients with CHF has been shown both with volitional[129-131] and nonvolitional (twitch transdiaphragmatic pressure)[132] measurements. Changes in pulmonary function secondary to ventricular dysfunction, increased left ventricular size, chronic pulmonary congestion, reduced lung compliance, and increased airway resistance[133] result in an altered breathing pattern in which patients breathe near residual volume at rest and experience limitations related to expiratory flow with minimal exercise.[134] Therefore the ventilatory muscles are subjected to increased work of breathing (WOB),[133,135] which may lead to respiratory muscle fatigue. As a positive consequence of the high WOB in people with heart failure, however, the diaphragm exhibits a predominance of slow myosin heavy chain isoforms with an increase in oxidative enzymes and a decrease in glycolytic capacity.[136] These adaptations are similar to those observed after endurance training of the limb muscles in healthy people. These observations are consistent with the well-preserved endurance of the inspiratory muscles when expressed as a function of endurance time, as well as the inspiratory muscle load-to-capacity ratio in patients with CHF.[137]

The effects of inspiratory muscle training in patients with CHF have been well documented.[44,70,138-144] No consensus exists in the literature related to types of training, intensity, and duration of IMT, which may explain the range in responses of patients with CHF to IMT. Based on the literature, the usual intensity is at least 30% of PI_{max},[44,70,138,142,144] but an intensity of 60% of PI_{max}[143] has also been used. Although some studies used IMT three times per week,[138,139,141,143] others trained the patients either six[140] or seven times per week.[70,144] The duration of each session varied between 10 and 30 minutes, and sessions were performed over 6 to 12 weeks.

IMT for people who have CHF increases inspiratory strength[44,70,138-140,142-144] and endurance,[138,140-143] increases maximal exercise capacity as reflected by improved exercise duration[141] or oxygen consumption,[70,142,143] increases submaximal exercise capacity evaluated by the 12-minute walking test[140] and 6-minute walking distance,[70,138,140-143] and improves both dyspnea[139-143] and quality of life.[70,143] Recently, IMT has been reported to improve oxygen uptake efficiency in patients with CHF and inspiratory muscle weakness (PI_{max} < 70% of predicted).[145] In addition, 4 weeks of IMT led to an improvement of limb blood flow during exercise.[69] It has been speculated that IMT reduces inspiratory muscle overload and, in turn, peripheral muscle vasoconstriction, a contributor to exercise limitation in these patients.[146]

Based on its capacity to improve respiratory muscle performance and exercise capacity, IMT can be considered an additional tool that is safe and effective in the comprehensive management of respiratory muscle dysfunction in patients with CHF.

Weaning Failure

The majority (75% to 80%) of patients who are mechanically ventilated can be weaned to breathe spontaneously without difficulty.[147] Patients who experience difficulty weaning have poorer prognoses, including increased mortality and prolonged intensive care unit (ICU) stay and rehabilitation. Several factors contribute to weaning failure, such as the underlying disease, age, muscle weakness, malnutrition, hypoxemia and hypercapnia, and medications (e.g., corticosteroids and muscle relaxants). The method of weaning affects the outcome.[147] Current expert opinion supports that familiarity and skill are the most important determinants of the choice of weaning. The specific method seems less important. Weaning based on bedside assessment and the use of standardized protocols is effective. Daily screening of respiratory function and trials of spontaneous breathing result in shortening of the period of mechanical ventilation, thus reducing the complications and costs associated with an ICU stay.[148-152]

A spontaneous breathing trial can be used to assess readiness for extubation with the performance of serial measures such as tidal volume, respiratory rate, maximal inspiratory airway pressure, and the rapid shallow breathing index.[153] Early detection of worsening clinical signs such as distress, airway obstruction, and paradoxical chest wall motion, ensures that serious problems are prevented. Airway patency and protection (i.e., an effective cough mechanism) should be assessed before the commencement of weaning. Peak cough flow is a useful parameter to predict successful weaning in patients with neuromuscular disease or spinal cord injury when extubation is anticipated.[154] A rating of "airway care score" has been developed based on the quality of the patient's cough during airway suctioning, the absence of excessive secretions, and the frequency of airway suctioning.[150] These therapist-driven protocols are action plans based on consensus and expert opinion. Physical therapists contribute to the assessment and treatment of patients who have difficulty being weaned from mechanical ventilation. Noninvasive ventilation can facilitate weaning,[155] prevent postextubation failure in patients at risk,[156] and reduce ICU costs.[157] In addition, there is accumulating evidence that weaning problems are associated with failure of the respiratory muscles to resume ventilation.[158] Inspiratory muscle training might be beneficial in patients who fail to wean. Uncontrolled trials of inspiratory muscle training (IMT, threshold loading; see Figure 26-3) observed an improvement in inspiratory muscle function and a reduction in duration of mechanical ventilation and weaning time.[159-162] Interim analysis of a randomized controlled trial comparing inspiratory muscle training at moderate intensity ($\approx$50% PI_{max}) with sham training in patients with weaning failure showed that a larger proportion of the training group (76%) could be weaned compared with the sham group (35%).[163] The addition of IMT in the management of acute critically ill patients from the beginning of mechanical ventilation neither reduced weaning time nor the reintubation rate.[164]

Biofeedback of the pattern of breathing to the patient can also enhance the weaning process of patients receiving long-term mechanical ventilation.[165] Voice and touch may be used to augment weaning success either by stimulation to improve ventilatory drive or by reducing anxiety.[166] Environmental influences, such as ambulating with a portable ventilator, have been shown to benefit attitudes and outlooks in long-term ventilator-dependent patients.[167]

Summary

Respiratory muscle weakness and fatigue have been identified in a variety of conditions and associated with clinically important symptoms such as dyspnea, impaired cough, exercise impairment, respiratory insufficiency, and weaning failure; and survival. Respiratory muscle training is a treatment option for weak respiratory muscles seen in a range of conditions. However, its indications, contraindications, and the specific criteria that determine the type of testing and training, intensity of training, and potential side effects warrant elucidation. Regardless, tools have emerged that are enabling physical therapists to identify and assess the severity of respiratory muscle weakness and thereby intervene in a timely and effective manner.

Review Questions

1. Define respiratory muscle weakness and explain how it is measured. How does it clinically manifest?
2. Distinguish respiratory muscle weakness from respiratory muscle fatigue.
3. How are respiratory muscle strength and endurance related to exercise capacity, and how is exercise capacity related to respiratory muscle strength and endurance?
4. Describe current concepts and principles related to respiratory muscle strength testing.
5. Describe how respiratory muscle endurance testing differs from respiratory muscle strength training. What are the training implications?
6. Distinguish between inspiratory and expiratory muscle training, how they are assessed, and how their different training programs are prescribed.
7. Explain what the differences in inspiratory and expiratory muscle strength and endurance indicate about individuals with each of the following conditions: asthma, cystic fibrosis, quadriplegia, and chronic heart failure.
8. How might respiratory muscle training augment weaning? How would the indications be established?
9. What remains to be elucidated in the area of respiratory muscle testing and training?

References

1. Bellemare F, Grassino A: Effect of pressure and timing of contraction on human diaphragm fatigue. *Journal of Applied Physiology* 53:1190–1195, 1982.
2. Black LF, Hyatt RE: Maximal respiratory pressures: Normal values and relationship to age and sex. *American Review of Respiratory Disease* 99:696–702, 1969.
3. Coast JR, Weise SD: Lung volume changes and maximal inspiratory pressure. *Journal of Cardiopulmonary Rehabilitation* 10:461–464, 1990.
4. American Thoracic Society/European Respiratory Society: ATS/ERS Statement on respiratory muscle testing. *American Journal of Respiratory Critical Care Medicine* 166:518–624, 2002.
5. Rinqvist T: The ventilatory capacity in healthy adults: an analysis of causal factors with special reference to the respiratory forces. *Scand Journal of Clinical Laboratory Investigation* 18(Suppl):1–111, 1966.
6. Leech JA, Ghezzo H, Stevens D, et al: Respiratory pressures and function in young adults. *American Review of Respiratory Disease* 128:17–23, 1983.
7. Rochester D Arora NS: Respiratory muscle failure. *The Medical Clinics of North America* 67:573–598, 1983.
8. Wilson DO, Cooke NT, Edwards RHT, et al: Predicted normal values for maximal respiratory pressures in Caucasian adults and children. *Thorax* 39:535–538, 1984.
9. Vincken W, Ghezzo H, Cosio MG: Maximal static respiratory pressures in adults: Normal values and their relationship to determinants of respiratory function. *Bulletin of European Physiopathology of Respiration* 23:435–439, 1987.
10. Bruschi C Cerveri I, Zoia MC: Reference values of maximal respiratory mouth pressures: A population-based study. *American Review of Respiratory Disease* 146:790–793, 1992.
11. Polkey MI, Kyroussis D, Keilty SE, et al: Exhaustive treadmill exercise does not reduce twitch transdiaphragmatic pressure in patients with COPD. *American Journal of Respiratory Critical Care Medicine* 152:959–964, 1995.
12. DeVito E, Grassino A: Respiratory muscle fatigue. Rationale for diagnostic tests. In Roussos C. editors: *The thorax*, ed 2, New York, 1995, Marcel Dekker Inc.
13. Koulouris N, Mulvey DA, Laroche CM, et al: The measurement of inspiratory muscle strength by sniff esophageal, nasopharyngeal, and mouth pressures. *American Review of Respiratory Disease* 139:641–646, 1989.

14. Yan S, Gauthier AP, Similowski T, et al: Evaluation of human contractility using mouth pressure twitches. *American Review of Respiratory Disease* 145:1064–1069, 1992.
15. Rochester DF: Tests of respiratory muscle function. *Clinical Chest Medicine* 9:249–261, 1988.
16. Wanke T, Formanek D, Lahrmann H, et al: The effects of combined inspiratory muscle and cycle ergometer training on exercise performance in patients with COPD. *European Respiratory Journal* 7:2205–2211, 1994.
17. Johnson PH, Cowley AJ, Kinnear WJ: Incremental threshold loading: A standard protocol and establishment of a reference range in naive normal subjects. *European Respiratory Journal* 10:2868–2871, 1997.
18. Martyn JB, Moreno RH, Pare PD, et al: Measurement of inspiratory muscle performance with incremental threshold loading. *American Review of Respiratory Disease* 135:919–923, 1987.
19. Van't Hul AJ, Chadwick-Straver RVM, Wagenaar RC, et al: Inspiratory muscle endurance is reduced more than maximal respiratory pressures in COPD patients. *European Respiratory Journal* 10:168S, 1997.
20. McKenzie DK, Gandevia SC: Strength and endurance of inspiratory, expiratory, and limb muscles in asthma. *American Review of Respiratory Disease* 134:999–1004, 1986.
21. McKenzie DK, Gandevia SC: Influence of muscle length on human inspiratory and limb muscle endurance. *Respiratory Physiology* 67:171–182, 1987.
22. Gandevia SC, McKenzie DK, Neering IR: Endurance capacity of respiratory and limb muscles. *Respiratory Physiology* 53:47–61, 1983.
23. Leith DE, Bradley ME: Ventilatory muscle strength and endurance training. *Journal of Applied Physiology* 41:508–516, 1976.
24. Tzelepis GE, Vega DL, Cohen ME, et al: Pressure-flow specificity of inspiratory muscle training. *Journal of Applied Physiology* 77:795–801, 1994.
25. Tzelepis GE, Vega DL, Cohen ME, et al: Lung volume specificity of inspiratory muscle training. *Journal of Applied Physiology* 77:789–794, 1994.
26. Scherer TA, Spengler C, Owassapian D, et al: Respiratory muscle endurance training in chronic obstructive pulmonary disease. Impact on exercise capacity, dyspnea, and quality of life. *American Journal of Respiratory Critical Care Medicine* 162:1709–1714, 2000.
27. Boutellier U, Piwko P: The respiratory system as an exercise limiting factor in normal sedentary subjects. *European Journal of Applied Physiology* 64:145–152, 1992.
28. Belman MJ, Shadmehr R: Targeted resistive ventilatory muscle training in chronic pulmonary disease. *Journal of Applied Physiology* 65:2726–2735, 1988.
29. Nickerson BC, Keens TG: Measuring ventilatory muscle endurance in humans as sustainable inspiratory pressure. *Journal of Applied Physiology* 52:768–772, 1982.
30. Gosselink R, Wagenaar RC, Decramer M: The reliability of a commercially available threshold loading device. *Thorax* 51:601–605, 1996.
31. Wanke T, Toifl K, Merkle M, et al: Inspiratory muscle training in patients with Duchenne muscular dystrophy. *Chest* 105:475–482, 1994.
32. Dekhuijzen PN Folgering HT, van Herwaarden CL: Target-flow inspiratory muscle training during pulmonary rehabilitation in patients with COPD. *Chest* 99:128–133, 1991.
33. Heijdra YF, Dekhuijzen PN, van Herwaarden CL, et al: Nocturnal saturation improves by target-flow inspiratory muscle training in patients with COPD. *American Journal of Respiratory Critical Care Medicine* 153:260–265, 1996.
34. Preusser BA, Winningham ML, Clanton TL: High versus low intensity inspiratory muscle interval training in patients with COPD. *Chest* 106:110–117, 1994.
35. Larson JL, Kim MJ, Sharp JT, et al: Inspiratory muscle training with a pressure threshold breathing device in patients with chronic obstructive pulmonary disease. *American Review of Respiratory Disease* 138:689–696, 1988.
36. Lisboa C, Munoz V, Beroiza T, et al: Inspiratory muscle training in chronic airflow limitation: Comparison of two different training loads with a threshold device. *European Respiratory Journal* 7:1266–1274, 1994.
37. Lisboa C, Villafranca C, Leiva A, et al: Inspiratory muscle training in chronic airflow limitation: Effect on exercise performance. *European Respiratory Journal* 10:537–542, 1997.
38. Villafranca C, Borzone G, Leiva A, et al: Effect of inspiratory muscle training with intermediate load on inspiratory power output in COPD. *European Respiratory Journal* 11:28–33, 1998.
39. Weiner P, Magadle R, Beckerman M, et al: Comparison of specific expiratory, inspiratory, and combined muscle training programs in COPD. *Chest* 124:1357–1364, 2003.
40. Gosselink R, Kovacs L, Decramer M: Respiratory muscle involvement in multiple sclerosis. *European Respiratory Journal* 13:449–454, 1999.
41. Weiner P, Magadle R, Beckerman M, et al: Specific expiratory muscle training in COPD. *Chest* 124:468–473, 2003.
42. Johnson BD, Babcock MA, Suman OE, et al: Exercise-induced diaphragmatic fatigue in healthy humans. *Journal of Physiology* 460:385–405, 1993.
43. Babcock MA, Pegelow DF, McClaran SR, et al: Contribution of diaphragmatic power output to exercise-induced diaphragm fatigue. *Journal of Applied Physiology* 78:1710–1719, 1995.
44. Johnson PH, Cowley AJ, Kinnear WJ: A randomized controlled trial of inspiratory muscle training in stable chronic heart failure. *European Heart Journal* 19:1249–1253, 1998.
45. Harms CA, Wetter TJ, St Croix CM, et al: Effects of respiratory muscle work on exercise performance. *J Appl Physiol* 89:131–138, 2000.
46. Harms CA, Babcock MA, McClaran SR, et al: Respiratory muscle work compromises leg blood flow during maximal exercise. *J Appl Physiol* 82:1573–1583, 1997.
47. Dempsey JA, Sheel AW, St Croix CM, et al: Respiratory influences on sympathetic vasomotor outflow in humans. *Respir Physiol Neurobiol.* 130:3–20, 2002.
48. Volianitis S, McConnell AK, Koutedakis Y, et al: The influence of prior activity upon inspiratory muscle strength in rowers and non-rowers. *Int J Sports Med* 20:542–547, 1999.
49. Kilding AE, Brown S, McConnell AK:: Inspiratory muscle training improves 100 and 200 m swimming performance. *Eur J Appl Physiol* 108:505–511, 2010.
50. Sonetti DA, Wetter TJ, Pegelow DF, et al: Effects of respiratory muscle training versus placebo on endurance exercise performance. *Respiratory Physiology* 127:185–199, 2001.
51. Leddy JJA, Limprasertkul S, Patel F, et al: Isocapnic hyperpnea training improves performance in competitive male runners. *Eur J Appl Physiol* 99:665–676, 2007.
52. Williams JS, Wongsathikun J, Boon SN, et al: Inspiratory muscle training fails to improve endurance capacity in athletes. *Med Sci Sports Exerc* 34:1194–1198, 2002.
53. Inbar OP, Weiner Y, Azgad A, et al: Specific inspiratory muscle training in well-trained endurance athletes. *Med Sci Sports Exerc* 32:1233–1237, 2000.
54. Decramer M, Demedts M, Rochette F, et al: Maximal transrespiratory pressures in obstructive lung disease. *Bulletin European Physiopathological Respiration* 16:479–490, 1980.
55. Rochester DF, Braun NMT: Determinants of maximal inspiratory pressure in chronic obstructive pulmonary disease. *American Review of Respiratory Disease* 132:42–47, 1985.
56. Perez T, Becquart LA, Stach B, et al: Inspiratory muscle strength and endurance in steroid-dependent asthma. *American Journal of Respiratory Critical Care Medicine* 153:610–615, 1996.
57. Polkey MI, Green M, Moxham J: Measurement of respiratory muscle strength. *Thorax* 50:1131–1135, 1995.
58. Polkey MI, Kyroussis D, Hamnegard CH, et al: Diaphragm strength in chronic obstructive pulmonary disease. *American Journal of Respiratory Critical Care Medicine* 154:1310–1317, 1996.
59. Levine S, Kaiser L, Leferovich J, et al: Cellular adaptations in the diaphragm in chronic obstructive pulmonary disease. *New England Journal of Medicine* 337:1799–1806, 1997.
60. Orozco-Levi M, Gea J, Lloreta JL, et al: Subcellular adaptation of the human diaphragm in chronic obstructive pulmonary disease. *European Respiratory Journal* 13:371–378, 1999.
61. Levine S, Nguyen T, Kaiser LR, et al: Human diaphragm remodeling associated with chronic obstructive pulmonary disease: clinical implications. *American Journal of Respiratory Critical Care Medicine* 168:706–713, 2003.
62. Levine S, Gregory C, Nguyen T, et al: Bioenergetic adaptation of individual human diaphragmatic myofibers to severe COPD. *Journal of Applied Physiology* 92:1205–1213, 2002.
63. Begin P, Grassino A: Inspiratory muscle dysfunction and chronic hypercapnia in chronic obstructive pulmonary disease. *American Review of Respiratory Disease* 143:905–912, 1991.
64. Killian KJ, Jones NL: Respiratory muscles and dyspnea. *Clinics in Chest Medicine* 9:237–248, 1988.
65. Hamilton N, Killian KJ, Summers E, et al: Muscle strength, symptom intensity, and exercise capacity in patients with cardiorespiratory

disorders. *American Journal of Respiratory Critical Care Medicine* 152:2021–2031, 1995.
66. Gosselink R, Troosters T, Decramer M: Peripheral muscle weakness contributes to exercise limitation in COPD. *American Journal of Respiratory Critical Care Medicine* 153:976–980, 1996.
67. O'Donnell DE, Bertley JC, Chau LK, et al: Qualitative aspects of exertional breathlessness in chronic airflow limitation: pathophysiologic mechanisms. *American Journal of Respiratory Critical Care Medicine* 155:109–115, 1997.
68. Mador MJ, Kufel TJ, Pineda LA, et al: Diaphragmatic fatigue and high-intensity exercise in patients with chronic obstructive pulmonary disease. *Am J Respir Crit Care Med.* 161:118–123, 2000.
69. Chiappa GR, Roseguini BT, Vieira PJC, et al: Inspiratory muscle training improves blood flow to resting and exercising limbs in patients with chronic heart failure. *J Am Coll Cardiol* 51:1663–1671, 2008.
70. Dall'Ago P, Chiappa GR, Guths H, et al: Inspiratory muscle training in patients with heart failure and inspiratory muscle weakness: a randomized trial. *J Am Coll Cardiol* 47:757–763, 2006.
71. Winkelmann ER, Chiappa GR, Lima CO, et al: Addition of inspiratory muscle training to aerobic training improves cardiorespiratory responses to exercise in patients with heart failure and inspiratory muscle weakness. *Am Heart J* 158:768–767, 2009.
72. Petrovic MI, Werner M, Reiter W, et al: Effects of inspiratory muscle training on dynamic hyperinflation in patients with COPD. *Eur Respir J* 34:678s, 2009.
73. Patessio A, Rampulla C, Fracchia C, et al: Relationship between the perception of breathlessness and inspiratory resistive loading: a report on a clinical trial. *European Respiratory Journal* 7:587S-591S, 1989.
74. Bisschop A, Gayan-Ramirez G, Rollier H, et al: Intermittent inspiratory muscle training induces fiber hypertrophy in rat diaphragm. *American Journal of Respiratory Critical Care Medicine* 155:1583–1589, 1997.
75. Rollier H, Bisschop A, Gayan-Ramirez G, et al: Low load inspiratory muscle training increases diaphragmatic fiber dimensions in rats. *American Journal of Respiratory Critical Care Medicine* 157:833–839, 1998.
76. Ramirez-Sarmiento A, Orozco-Levi M, Guell R, et al: Inspiratory muscle training in patients with chronic obstructive pulmonary disease: structural adaptation and physiologic outcomes. *American Journal of Respiratory Critical Care Medicine* 166:1491–1497, 2002.
77. Harver A, Mahler DA, Daubenspeck JA: Targeted inspiratory muscle training improves respiratory muscle function and reduces dyspnea in patients with chronic obstructive pulmonary disease. *Annals of Internal Medicine* 111:117–124, 1989.
78. Lotters F, van Tol B, Kwakkel G et al: Effects of controlled inspiratory muscle training in patients with COPD: A meta-analysis. *European Respiratory Journal* 20:570–576, 2002.
79. Gosselink R, deVos J, van den Heuvel SP, et al: Impact of Inspiratory Muscle Training in patients with COPD: What is the evidence? *Eur Respir J* 2011;37:416–425, 2011.
80. Weiner P, Magadle R, Massarwa F, et al: Influence of gender and inspiratory muscle training on the perception of dyspnea in patients with asthma. *Chest* 122:197–201, 2002.
81. DeBruin PF, Ueki J, Watson A, et al: Size and strength of the respiratory and quadriceps muscles in patients with chronic asthma. *European Respiratory Journal* 10:59–64, 1997.
82. Lavietes MH, Grocela JA, Maniatis T, et al: Inspiratory muscle strength in asthma. *Chest* 93:1043–1048, 1988.
83. Weiner P, Berar-Yanay N, Davidovich A, et al: Specific inspiratory muscle training in patients with mild asthma with high consumption of inhaled beta$_2$-agonists. *Chest* 117:722–727, 2000.
84. Ram FS, Wellington ER, Barnes NC: Inspiratory muscle training for asthma. Cochrane Database Syst Rev CD003792, 2003.
85. Pradal U, Polese G, Braggion C, et al: Determinants of maximal transdiaphragmatic pressure in adults with cystic fibrosis. *American Journal of Respiratory Critical Care Medicine* 150:167–173, 1994.
86. Szeinberg A, England S, Mindorff C, et al: Maximal inspiratory and expiratory pressures are reduced in hyperinflated, malnourished, young adult male patients with cystic fibrosis. *American Review of Respiratory Disease* 132:766–769, 1985.
87. Mier A, Redington A, Brophy C, et al: Respiratory muscle function in cystic fibrosis. *Thorax* 45:750–752, 1990.
88. Lands L, Desmond KJ, Demizio D, et al: The effects of nutritional status and hyperinflation on respiratory muscle strength in children and young adults. *American Review of Respiratory Disease* 141:1506–1509, 1990.
89. Lands LC, Heigenhauser GJF, Jones NL: Respiratory and peripheral muscle function in cystic fibrosis. *American Review of Respiratory Disease* 147: 865–869, 1993.
90. Hanning RM, Blimkie CJ, Bar-Or O, et al: Relationships among nutritional status and skeletal and respiratory muscle function in cystic fibrosis: Does early dietary supplementation make a difference? *American Journal of Clinical Nutrition* 57:580–587, 1993.
91. Asher MI, Pardy RL, Coates AL, et al: The effects of inspiratory muscle training in patients with cystic fibrosis. *American Review of Respiratory Disease* 126:855–859, 1982.
92. O'Neill S, Leahy F, Pasterkamp H, et al: The effects of chronic hyperinflation, nutritional status, and posture on respiratory muscle strength in cystic fibrosis. *American Review of Respiratory Disease* 128:1051–1054, 1983.
93. Marks J, Pasterkamp H, Tal A, et al: Relationship between respiratory muscle strength, nutritional status, and lung volume in cystic fibrosis and asthma. *American Review of Respiratory Disease* 133:414–417, 1986.
94. Pinet C, Cassart M, Scillia P, et al: Function and bulk of respiratory and limb muscles in patients with cystic fibrosis. *Am J Respir Crit Care Med* 168:989–994, 2003.
95. De Jong W, van Aalderen WM, Kraan J, et al: Inspiratory muscle training in patients with cystic fibrosis. *Respiratory Medicine* 95:31–36, 2001.
96. Enright S, Chatham K, Ionescu AA, et al: Inspiratory muscle training improves lung function and exercise capacity in adults with cystic fibrosis. *Chest* 126:405–411, 2004.
97. Dufresene V, Knoop C, Van Muylem A, et al: Effect of systemic inflammation on inspiratory and limb muscle strength and bulk in cystic fibrosis. *Am J Respir Crit Care Med* 80:153–158, 2009.
98. Keens TG, Krastins IRB, Wannamaker EM, et al: Ventilatory muscle endurance training in normal subjects and patients with cystic fibrosis. *American Review of Respiratory Disease* 116:853–860, 1977.
99. Sawyer EH, Clanton TL: Improved pulmonary function and exercise tolerance with inspiratory muscle conditioning in children with cystic fibrosis. *Chest* 104:1490–1497, 1993.
100. Houston BW, Mills N, Solis-Moya A: Inspiratory muscle training for cystic fibrosis. *Cochrane Database Syst Rev CD006112, 2008.*
101. Reid WD, Geddes EL, O'Brien K, et al: Effects of inspiratory muscle training in cystic fibrosis: A systematic review. *Clin Rehabil* 22:1003–1013, 2008.
102. Uijl SG, Houtman S, Folgering HT, et al: Training of the respiratory muscles in individuals with tetraplegia. *Paraplegia* 37:575–579, 1999.
103. Liauw MY, Lin MC, Cheng PT, et al: Resistive inspiratory muscle training: Its effectiveness in patients with acute complete cervical cord injury. *Archives of Physical Medical Rehabilitation* 81:752–756, 2000.
104. Estenne M, Knoop C, Vanvaerenbergh J, et al: The effect of pectoralis muscle training in tetraplegic subjects. *American Review of Respiratory Disease* 139:1218–1222, 1989.
105. Van Houtte SY, Vanlandewijck C, Kiekens CM, et al: Patients with acute spinal cord injury benefit from normocapnic hyperpnea training. *J Rehabil Med* 40:119–125, 2008.
106. Polkey MI, Lyall RA, Green M, et al: Expiratory muscle function in amyotrophic lateral sclerosis. *American Journal of Respiratory Critical Care Medicine* 158:734–741, 1998.
107. Lo Mauro A, D'Angelo MG, Romei M, et al: Abdominal volume contribution to tidal volume as an early indicator of respiratory impairment in Duchenne muscular dystrophy. *Eur Respir J* 35:1118–1125, 2010.
108. Weiner P, Inzelberg R, Davidovich A, et al: Respiratory muscle performance and the perception of dyspnea in Parkinson's disease. *Canadian Journal of Neurological Science* 29:68–72, 2002.
109. Haas BM, Trew M, Castle PC: Effects of respiratory muscle weakness on daily living function, quality of life, activity levels, and exercise capacity in mild to moderate Parkinson's disease. *American Journal of Physical Medical Rehabilitation* 83:601–607, 2004.
110. Lanini B, Gigliotti F, Coli C, et al: Dissociation between respiratory effort and dyspnoea in a subset of patients with stroke. *Clinical Science (London)* 103:467–473, 2002.
111. Urban PP, Morgenstern M, Brause K, et al: Distribution and course of cortico-respiratory projections for voluntary activation in man. A transcranial magnetic stimulation study in healthy subjects and patients with cerebral ischemia. *Journal of Neurology* 249:735–744, 2002.
112. Harraf F, Ward K, Man W, et al: Transcranial magnetic stimulation study of expiratory muscle weakness in acute ischemic stroke. *Neurology* 71(24):2000–2007, 2008.

113. Keenan SP, Alexander D, Road JD, et al: Ventilatory muscle strength and endurance in myasthenia gravis. *Eur Respir J* 8:1130–1135, 1995.
114. McCool FD, Tzelepis GE: Inspiratory muscle training in patients with neuromuscular disease. *Physical Therapy* 75:1006–1014, 1995.
115. DiMarco AF, Kelling JS: The effects of inspiratory resistive training on respiratory muscle function in patients with muscular dystrophy. *Muscle Nerve* 8:284–290, 1985.
116. Winkler G, Zifko U, Nader A, et al: Dose-dependent effects of inspiratory muscle training in neuromuscular disorders. *Muscle Nerve* 23:1257–1260, 2000.
117. Gozal D, Thiriet P: Respiratory muscle training in neuromuscular disease: long-term effects on strength and load perception. *Medical Science of Sports Exercise* 31:1522–1527, 1999.
118. Cheah BC, Boland RA, Brodaty NE, et al: Inspirational-inspiratory muscle training in amyotrophic lateral sclerosis. *Amyotroph Lateral Scler* 10(5–6):384–392, 2009.
119. Koessler W, Wanke T, Winkler G, et al: 2 Years' experience with inspiratory muscle training in patients with neuromuscular disorders. *Chest* 120:765–769, 2001.
120. Inzelberg R, Peleg N, Nisipeanu P, et al: Inspiratory muscle training and the perception of dyspnea in Parkinson's disease. *Can J Neurol Sci* 32(2):213–217, 2005.
121. Pitts T, Bolser D, Rosenbek J, et al: Impact of expiratory muscle strength training on voluntary cough and swallow function in Parkinson disease. *Chest* 135:1301–1308, 2009.
122. Sutbeyaz ST, Keseoglu F, Inan L, et al: Respiratory muscle training improves cardiopulmonary function and exercise tolerante in subjects with subacute stroke. *Clin Rehabil* 24:240–250, 2010.
123. Fregonezi GAF, Resqueti VR, Güel R, et al: Effects of 8-week, interval-based inspiratory muscle training and breathing retraining in patients with generalized myasthenia gravis. *Chest* 128:1524–1530, 2005.
124. Rassler B, Hallebach G, Kalischewski P, et al: The effect of respiratory muscle endurance training in patients with myasthenia gravis. *Neuromuscul Disord* 17(5):385–391, 2007.
125. Weiner P, Gross D, Meiner Z, et al: Respiratory muscle training in patients with moderate to severe myasthenia gravis. *Can J Neurol Sci* 25(3):236–241, 1998.
126. Klefbeck B, Nedjad JH: Effect of inspiratory muscle training in patients with multiple sclerosis. *Arch Phys Med Rehabil* 84:994–999, 2003.
127. Aiello M, Rampello A, Granella F, et al: Cough efficacy is related to the disability status in patients with multiple sclerosis. *Respiration* 76:311–316, 2008.
128. Chiara T, Martin AD, Davenport PW, et al: Expiratory muscle strength training in persons with multiple sclerosis having mild to moderate disability: Effect on maximal expiratory pressure, pulmonary function, and maximal voluntary cough. *Arch Phys Med Rehabil* 87:468–473, 2006.
129. Ambrosino N, Opasich C, Crotti P, et al: Breathing pattern, ventilatory drive and respiratory muscle strength in patients with chronic heart failure. *European Respiratory Journal* 7:17–22, 1994.
130. Hammond MD, Bauer KA, Sharp JT, et al: Respiratory muscle strength in congestive heart failure. *Chest* 98:1091–1094, 1990.
131. McParland C, Krishnan B, Wang Y, et al: Inspiratory muscle weakness and dyspnea in chronic heart failure. *American Review of Respiratory Disease* 146:467–472, 1992.
132. Hughes PD, Polkey MI, Harrus ML, et al: Diaphragm strength in chronic heart failure. *American Journal of Respiratory Critical Care Medicine* 160:529–534, 1999.
133. Evans SA, Watson L, Cowley AJ, et al: Static lung compliance in chronic heart failure: relation with dyspnoea and exercise capacity. *Thorax* 50:245–248, 1995.
134. Johnson BD, Weisman IM, Zeballos RJ, et al: Emerging concepts in the evaluation of ventilatory limitation during exercise: The exercise tidal flow-volume loop. *Chest* 116:488–503, 1999.
135. Clark A, Coats A: The mechanisms underlying the increased ventilatory response to exercise in chronic stable heart failure. *European Heart Journal* 13:1698–1708, 1992.
136. Tikunov B, Levine S, Mancini D: Chronic congestive heart failure elicits adaptations of endurance exercise in diaphragmatic muscle. *Circulation* 95:910–916, 1997.
137. Hart N, Kearney MT, Pride NB, et al: Inspiratory muscle load and capacity in chronic heart failure. *Thorax* 59:477–482, 2004.
138. Mancini DM, Henson D, La Manca J, et al: Benefit of selective respiratory muscle training on exercise capacity in patients with chronic congestive heart failure. *Circulation* 91:320–329, 1995.
139. Cahalin LP, Semigran MJ, Dec GW: Inspiratory muscle training in patients with chronic heart failure awaiting cardiac transplantation: Results of a pilot clinical trial. *Physical Therapy* 77:830–838, 1997.
140. Weiner P, Waizman J, Magadle R, et al: The effect of specific inspiratory muscle training on the sensation of dyspnea and exercise tolerance in patients with congestive heart failure. *Clinical Cardiology* 22:727–732, 1999.
141. Darnley GM, Gray AC, McClure SJ, et al: Effects of resistive breathing on exercise capacity and diaphragm function in patients with ischaemic heart disease. *European Journal of Heart Failure* 1:297–300, 1999.
142. Martinez A, Lisboa C, Jalil J, et al: Selective training of respiratory muscles in patients with chronic heart failure. *Revista medica de Chile* 129:133–139, 2001.
143. Laoutaris I, Dritsas A, Brown MD, et al: Inspiratory muscle training using an incremental endurance test alleviates dyspnea and improves functional status in patients with chronic heart failure. *European Journal of Cardiovascular Prevention and Rehabilitation* 11:489–496, 2004.
144. Padula CA, Yeaw E, Mistry S: A home-based nurse-coached inspiratory muscle training intervention in heart failure. *Appl Nurs Res*; 22:18–25, 2009.
145. Stein R, Chiappa GR, Güths H, et al: Inspiratory muscle training improves oxygen uptake efficiency slope in patients with chronic heart failure. *J Cardiopulmonar Rehabil Prev* 29(6):392–395, 2009.
146. Duscha BD, Schulze PE, Robbins JL, et al: Implications of chronic heart failure on peripheral vasculature and skeletal muscle before and after exercise training. *Heart Fail Rev* 13:21–37, 2008.
147. Nava S, Rubini F: Noninvasive mechanical ventilation to facilitate weaning from mechanical ventilation. In Hill NS, Levy M, editors: *Ventilator management strategies for critical care*, New York, 2001, Marcel Dekker.
148. Cohen IL, Bari N, Strosberg MA, et al: Reduction of duration and cost of mechanical ventilation in an intensive care unit by use of a ventilatory management team. *Critical Care Medicine* 19:1278–1284, 1991.
149. Horst HM, Mouro D, Hall-Jenssens RA, et al: Decrease in ventilation time with a standardized weaning process. *Archives of Surgery* 133:483–488, 1998.
150. Ely EW, Baker AM, Dunagan DP, et al: Effect on the duration of mechanical ventilation of identifying patients capable of breathing spontaneously. *New England Journal of Medicine* 335:1864–1869, 1996.
151. Kollef MH, Shapiro SD, Silver P, et al: A randomized, controlled trial of protocol-directed versus physician-directed weaning from mechanical ventilation. *Critical Care Medicine* 25:567–574, 1997.
152. Nava S, Evangelisti I, Rampulla C, et al: Human and financial costs of noninvasive mechanical ventilation in patients affected by COPD and acute respiratory failure. *Chest* 111:1631–1638, 1997.
153. Yang KL, Tobin MJ: A prospective study of indexes predicting the outcome of trials of weaning from mechanical ventilation. *N Engl J Med* 234:1445–1450, 1991.
154. Bach JR, Saporito LR: Criteria for extubation and tracheostomy tube removal for patients with ventilatory failure. A different approach to weaning. *Chest* 110:1566–1571, 1996.
155. Nava SN, Ambrosino E, Clini M, et al: Noninvasive mechanical ventilation in the weaning of patients with respiratory failure due to chronic obstructive pulmonary disease. A randomized, controlled trial. *Ann Intern Med* 128:721–728, 1998.
156. Nava SC, Gregoretti F, Fanfulla E, et al: Noninvasive ventilation to prevent respiratory failure after extubation in high-risk patients. *Crit Care Med* 33:2465–2470, 2005.
157. Stoller JK, Mascha EJ, Kester L, et al: Randomized controlled trial of physician-directed versus respiratory therapy consult service-directed respiratory care to adult non-ICU inpatients. *Am J Respir Crit Care Med* 158:1068–1075, 1998.
158. Vassilakopoulos T, Zakynthinos S, Roussos C: The tension-time index and the frequency/tidal volume ratio are the major pathophysiologic determinants of weaning failure and success. *Am J Respir Crit Care Med* 158:378–385, 1998.
159. Aldrich TK, Karpe JP, Uhrlass RM, et al: Weaning from mechanical ventilation: Adjunctive use of inspiratory muscle resistive training. *Critical Care Medicine* 17:143–147, 1989.
160. Aldrich TK, Uhrlass RM: Weaning from mechanical ventilation: Successful use of modified inspiratory resistive training in muscular dystrophy. *Critical Care Medicine* 15:247–249, 1987.
161. Martin AD, Davenport PD, Franceschi AC, et al: Use of inspiratory muscle strength training to facilitate ventilator weaning: a series of 10 consecutive patients. *Chest* 122:192–196, 2002.

162. Sprague SS, Hopkins PD: Use of inspiratory strength training to wean six patients who were ventilator-dependent. *Physical Therapy* 83:171–181, 2003.
163. Martin D, Davenport PW, Gonzalez-Rothi J, et al: Inspiratory muscle strength training improves outcome in failure to wean patients. *Eur Respir J* 28:369s, 2006.
164. Caruso P, Denari SD, Ruiz SA, et al: Inspiratory muscle training is ineffective in mechanically ventilated critically ill patients. *Clinics* 60:479–484, 2005.
165. Holliday JE, Hyers TM: The reduction of weaning time from mechanical ventilation using tidal volume and relaxation biofeedback. *American Review of Respiratory Disease* 141:1214–1220, 1990.
166. Hall JB, Wood LD: Liberation of the patient from mechanical ventilation. *JAMA* 257:1621–1628, 1987.
167. Esteban A, Alia I, Ibanez J, et al: Modes of mechanical ventilation and weaning. A national survey of Spanish hospitals. The Spanish Lung Failure Collaborative Group. *Chest* 106:1188–1193, 1994.

Complementary Therapies as Cardiovascular and Pulmonary Physical Therapy Interventions

Meryl I. Cohen and Carol M. Davis

KEY TERMS

- Alternative therapy
- Chronic obstructive pulmonary disease
- Complementary therapy
- Congestive heart failure
- Coronary artery disease
- Coronary care unit
- Energy-based therapy
- Holistic approach
- Integrative medicine
- Mind/body therapy

CHAPTER OUTLINE

What does the literature say about a possible role for complementary and alternative therapies in helping to achieve common therapeutic goals for patients with cardiac, pulmonary, and/or vascular pathology? Believe it or not, there is a wealth of literature available, with some articles reflecting greater scientific rigor than others. Cardiovascular and pulmonary pathology is highly correlated with increased stress, and many complementary therapies are designed specifically to help people modify stress-related behaviors.

What Are Complementary Therapies?

Complementary therapies are often viewed as holistic, mind/body, or energy-based therapies, and they are categorized and referred to in a variety of different ways. Some other common names include alternative therapies, alternative medicine, and integrative therapies. Complementary therapies are used by physical therapists to complement (usually not to replace) traditional therapies from the allopathic model of health care and are considered energy-based therapies that stress the importance of vibration or energy flow, both in the application of the intervention and in the response by the patient.

The goal of most of these therapies is to "unblock" obstructed body energy so that the body can heal itself.[1] It is hypothesized that homeostasis, balance, and self-regulation (the highly advanced ability of the body/mind to supply optimum conditions for metabolism, such as proper pH, body temperature, etc.) result from the unrestricted flow of body energy, along with molecules from breathing, fluid, and nutrition.[2,3] A system out of balance becomes vulnerable to early mortality. A system in balance becomes resistant to inflammation. Some suggest that inflammation is the foundation of all diseases and disorders.[4] Two large studies, one in men and one in women, demonstrated that higher levels of C-reactive protein correlate with a higher risk for heart attack and stroke and treatments that reduce C-reactive protein level reduce heart disease risk.[5,6] Therefore complementary therapies are used to facilitate the flow of body energy (or chi) and thus help the body restore balance and return to a healthier state.

Examples of Complementary and Alternative Therapies

The following are examples of complementary and alternative therapies that have been found to be useful in health care. A list and brief description of these therapies can be found in Appendix E.

Manual Therapies

Manual therapies, also known as body work, include myofascial release, craniosacral therapy, Rosen method, Rolfing, Hellerwork, soma, neuromuscular therapy, massage, and osteopathic and chiropractic medicine. The manual therapies involve the use of hands on the body/mind surface to stimulate bioelectromagnetic force. How this occurs remains a mystery. Research by Hunt and others is currently being conducted to measure energy flow from the body.[7-9] Perhaps both mechanical and energetic forces stimulate response from the tissue in several ways. It has been hypothesized that mechanical force may be transformed into a chemical response within the collagen of the myofascia, causing a flow of the polyglycoid layer of the collagen by way of a piezoelectric effect.[10] For patients with cardiovascular and pulmonary pathology, the manual therapies can assist in opening up the ribcage and vertebral spine to allow increased ventilation and better posture, thereby supporting cardiorespiratory health.

Mind/Body Interventions

Mind/body intervention include psychotherapies, support groups, meditation, imagery, hypnosis, dance and music therapy, art therapy, prayer, neurolinguistic psychology, biofeedback, yoga, Pilates, and tai chi. These interventions are examples of how movement and verbal and nonverbal communication with the mind/body can open up new pathways for thought and thereby unblock potentially blocked energy flow or chi. Likewise, with the new understandings of epigenetics (see discussion below), the energy (or vibration) of one's perception or belief drives DNA function, either for means of growth or for means of protection/survival.[2,3] These interventions are quite prevalent in the treatment of cardiorespiratory and pulmonary disorders. Stress is positively affected when the person is aware of thoughts and habits that affect the mind/body in a negative way. These interventions put the patient back in control of negative behaviors, and focusing on the breath is often an integral part of furthering relaxation.

Movement Awareness Interventions

Movement awareness interventions include Feldenkrais method, the Alexander technique, and the Trager approach. It is postulated that movement awareness interventions help people bring to consciousness the way in which they tend to move habitually so that they can practice new ways of moving and holding themselves posturally, thus freeing up blocked energy that gets trapped in fascia and soft tissue as a result of maintaining habitual postures. Those people who walk with protracted scapulae and forward heads are revealing fascial restrictions around the thoracic inlet, lungs, and mediastinum. It is hypothesized that tight fascia, revealed in extremes of posture, restricts blood flow and nerve conduction critical to the maintenance of healthy heart tissue.

Energy Work

TRADITIONAL CHINESE MEDICINE

Traditional Chinese medicine includes acupuncture, acupressure, reflexology, and qi gong. These approaches within the system of traditional Chinese medicine focus on enhancing the flow of chi along body pathways or meridians, but the concept of meridians and energy flow is just one part of this complex, centuries-old system of health care. The acupuncture or acupressure or reflexology point is a specific point where access to the flow of chi on a meridian is most available. One analogy is that an acupuncture point is to a flow of chi as a subway entrance is to the train tracks below the surface.

BIOELECTROMAGNETICS

Bioelectromagnetics include thermal applications of magnets and nonionizing radiation such as radiofrequency hyperthermia laser and pulsed electromagnetic field therapy. Credible research exists on the effects of electromagnetic energy for wound healing and bone repair. *Biomicroelectromagnetics* is the term applied to the energy that seems to emanate from the hands of people who have been accepted as healers.[8] Ultrasound and diathermy have been used in physical therapy for decades as deep heat mechanisms, and although there is not a clear understanding of the mechanism of action, it undoubtedly involves a stimulation of energy flow; therefore this therapeutic approach falls in the bioelectromagnetic category. The use of magnets in physical therapy is quite controversial, but there are some very compelling results from case studies that make it important to include in this category.

PERSONAL TRANSMISSION OF HEALING ENERGY

Methods of personal transmission of healing energy include Reiki, noncontact therapeutic touch, and distant healing prayer. The practitioner goes through a period of training in order to learn how to focus attention and intention on transmitting the universal life force for healing and well-being, either through touch (Reiki), manipulation of bioenergy fields (noncontact therapeutic touch), or focusing the mind for distant healing effects (intercessory prayer and Reiki).

Herbal Approaches

Naturopathy and homeopathy represent the use of plants and animal substances to fight off disease and the use of wise nutrition to combat illness. Naturopathy, like osteopathic medicine, represents an entire system of health care that uses homeopathy, osteopathy, proper nutrition, and other means to bring about healing. Naturopathic physicians complete 4 years of medical school. Homeopathy involves the use of minute chemicals in diluted solution to resolve chemical imbalances in the body. Proper nutrition has long been associated with cardiac and pulmonary health, especially in Dean Ornish's plan for healing from cardiac pathology.[11]

Mind/Body Link

Mind/body health care has brought about a way of linking the traditional linear research methods with the more contemporary, complementary, and alternative health care practices. The influence of the mind on the body was first introduced in the Western hemisphere by Herbert Benson, a well-known Harvard cardiologist, through his research on Tibetan monks who were able to control their autonomic nervous system to the extent that they could lower their body temperatures and respiration rates and enter a wakeful, hypometabolic physiological state by will.[12] This information shocked the Western world, and Benson presented his data most dramatically by videotaping the actual sessions of the monks taking control of their bodies with their minds.

The proof that the mind and body are inextricably linked has since been well documented in various studies. Indeed, there is a basic science devoted to the study of the effect of the mind on the body: *psychoneuroimmunology*, a term that Ader and Cohen are credited with creating. Studies have shown that the mind affects the immune system by way of the autonomic nervous system and by way of the "fluid" nervous system, or the nonadrenergic and noncholinergic nervous system.[13]

Candice Pert has clearly articulated the physiological functioning of the fluid nervous system, which manifests by way of the effects of thought on the neurotransmitters, the neuropeptides, and the steroids of the body.[14] The neurotransmitters and the neuropeptides communicate with most of the cells of the body. This science has been termed *psychoneuroendocrinology*. It is no longer correct to assume that the mind resides only in the cranium or the brain. In truth, the mind has been shown to reside in every cell in the body. According to Pert and others, the science clearly reveals that all cells have memory.[14] The biochemistry of psychoneuroendocrinology reflects a flow that is different from that of microelectropotentials or the exchange of energy from the hands of the therapist, but which illustrates, nonetheless, that the mind and the body are inseparable and the mind communicates with every cell of the body.

Complementary and alternative therapies are energy-based therapies that require an understanding that there is such a phenomenon as vital flow of energy in the body and that the natural state of the body is to be healthy.[15] Cells are constantly in a state of flux, with old cells dying off and new cells being created continuously. But the body/mind persists in continuously working toward fighting off disease and healing cells whose loss would threaten the thriving of the entire system. With this awareness, illness is understood as an aberration set up by an imbalance caused by restriction in flows. The body has many energies, or vibrations, and the ways that we can observe energy at work in the body are varied. For example, electrocardiograms, electroencephalograms, and electromyograms all measure the energy output from various body organs. The piezoelectric effect, another energy phenomenon, enables osteoblastic activity, which keeps our bones strong. Mechanical energy in gravity is transformed to chemical energy to allow the osteoblasts to deposit calcium appropriately in our skeleton. But now we understand that perhaps the most powerful of the many vibrations our cellular receptors respond to is the vibration of perception.

The science of epigenetics posits that the genes in our cells respond to vibrational signals. For the cells to function, receptors on the surface of the cell wall must respond to the vibration to which they are attuned, resulting in a cascade of actions that lead to the DNA ordering the appropriate protein chain linkage to result in the needed function.[2,14] Basic to the understanding of the mind and body being inseparably linked is the fact that one of the most powerful vibrations that cells respond to is the vibration of perception or belief.[2,14] The more a person perceives threat, stress, or danger, the more there is a resulting vibration to which cells respond with an autonomic fight or flight response—the hypothalamic-pituitary-adrenal (HPA) axis.[16] It has been long understood that chronic stress contributes to pathology in the cardiovascular and pulmonary systems. The DNA of cells is responding in a "digital" (on-or-off) way either to signals vibrating for growth needs or signals vibrating for protection needs. When protection needs take over, blood is shunted to life-sustaining viscera and to the extremities for flight or fight. Thus some organs are not being nourished in a health-producing manner. Over time, immune system function is also diminished and this can lead to inflammation and disease of the heart and lungs.[17] A system out of balance becomes vulnerable to early mortality. A system in balance becomes resistant to inflammation. As stated previously, some suggest that inflammation is the foundation of all diseases and disorders.[4]

Biomicroelectro-potentials, or the subtle energies in electromagnetic fields that emanate from the hands of "healers," are currently being researched.[8,18] It is believed that complementary and alternative therapies have an effect on patients by way of the energy that emanates from the healer's hands. This energy is of a frequency of 0.3 to 30 Hz, which is usually centered around 8 to 10 Hz.[19,20]

As we move into this new century, many researchers and practitioners in health care are seriously exploring and publishing studies that reveal new ways of viewing reality. What we know about quantum physics and systems theory, combined with what we have observed and experienced in terms of the inadequacies of traditional allopathic medicine in overcoming chronic illness and autoimmune disease and the growing tendency of patients and clients to seek out complementary and alternative therapies, situates us well into a paradigm shift, a revolution in the linear and materialistic view of reality. A common perspective is that current medicine falls short because it is designed on the infectious disease model, or mechanistic model, in which it is hoped that a single drug or intervention will be able to cure and save lives.

Most current diseases, especially the chronic diseases that affect people, do not lend themselves to single-purpose cures. Chronic illness is most adequately addressed when the patient is involved in the healing process as an active partner, when the patient is willing to make certain lifestyle changes to eliminate choices that interfere with wellness, and when illness is perceived by patients and practitioners not as a simple biophysiological event but as a system or contextual event. We are all consciously and unconsciously influenced by a variety of systems that we are embedded within and that mandate our reactions to inflammation and illness. No two people react to illness in the exact same way, and no two people heal from illness in the exact same way. Practically any physical therapist or health care professional will admit that how a person thinks or perceives has an enormous amount to do with how he or she responds to health and illness. A vast range of systems affect all of us at any given time—just a few examples are our birth order, our identity, how we feel about ourselves and our family members, how well we enjoy our work and our recreation, how meaningful our relationships are, what the weather is like, who won the Super Bowl, and what we ate for breakfast.[21]

Traditional Therapies Applied from a Holistic Approach—Intention

Patients with cardiovascular and pulmonary complications often present with comorbidities of acute and chronic diseases that challenge our available interventions. The application of energy medicine or holistic approaches in treating these patients is becoming more commonplace. Indeed, many traditional therapies can be applied from a holistic approach. For instance, in working with patients with cardiovascular and pulmonary pathology, treatments such as massage, exercise, and relaxation can be approached by a therapist in a traditional manner in which the intention is a mechanical, linear effect, or it can be approached in a holistic or mind/body manner in which the intention is to attempt to influence the flow of vital energy. When massage and exercise are offered as treatments from a holistic perspective, the idea is to enhance the flow of body energy and bring about homeostasis.

Researchers confirm the importance of hope and faith in one's physician and practitioners, including physical therapists.[22] It has been established that a patient's belief that the practitioner has hope for the patient's recovery seems to help, but exactly how this facilitates healing remains unclear. It seems to be related to the concept of intention and the effects of consciousness and nonlocal mind.[22]

To ignore the positive effect of therapeutic presence is to neglect a powerful intervention. How practitioners interact with their patients, not just what they *do*, is vitally important.[1] Time and again, patients mention that a critical factor in their healing response was the positive effect of being truly listened to by their care provider. Now research is finally documenting the effects of positive intention and the therapeutic exchange of energy.[22]

The Problem of Scientific Evidence

Should physical therapists use complementary therapies that have shown good clinical results but have not been proven scientifically to be efficacious? The answer is yes, but not a simple yes. At the foundation of this issue are two ethical questions. What right do we, as professionals, have to subject patients to treatments that have not been proven to be efficacious by way of scientific evidence? Conversely, what right do we have to deny patients holistic treatments that have been shown for centuries to benefit patients and have a negligible chance of causing harm? Physical therapy has a long history of using therapeutic agents for the good of patients without any science to explain efficacy or mechanism of action. And now that we are finally doing this important research on ultrasound, heat, exercise, and electrical modalities, we can apply this knowledge to complementary therapies such as tai chi, yoga, transcendental meditation, and craniosacral therapy.

Some contradictions inevitably arise when we attempt to apply traditional scientific principles to the study of complementary therapies. Reductionist science tries to show evidence of cause and effect by reducing the experimental variables (ideally, to just one) and by reducing all possible outcomes in order to eliminate the effects of chance (or other causes) on the evidence that is collected. However, unlike single cells or molecules, human beings and their illnesses do not lend themselves to being reduced in such a manner. People are whole systems of interacting needs and functions (physical, intellectual, emotional, spiritual, and social) that cannot be fully understood by separation from one another or by reduction. Systems theory, from the life sciences, is foundational to holistic or complementary therapies and states that the whole can never be fully understood by reducing it to its parts, because the whole is always more than the sum of the parts. How the parts interact with one another is critical to understanding the whole. Reductionism tries to control for this confounding variable.

Complementary therapies such as tai chi, acupuncture, biofeedback, meditation, cognitive behavioral therapy, music therapy, hypnosis, electrical stimulation, prayer and distant healing efforts, yoga, and qi gong have been shown to be effective in the relief of pain and anxiety and in the improvement of balance by way of the randomized controlled trial (RCT).[23] Literature reviews of mind/body therapies in the treatment of musculoskeletal disorders with implications for older adults have been conducted.[24,25] Still, the fact remains that many complementary therapies, especially those manual therapies designed to assist in the release of fascial restrictions in order to restore the flow of the body's self-regulating energy, do not lend themselves to study by the RCT because energy itself cannot be measured or seen. Only the results of energy can be measured (heat, work, movement, etc.), and we cannot yet validate what results occur from what intervention, except by way of anecdote and measuring the effects of treatment on impairments and function. However, scientists such as Valerie Hunt, James Oschman, Gary Schwartz, Linda Russek, Candace Pert, and others are busy working out the biochemical, quantum physics, and systems theories that postulate physiological and biochemical mechanisms of action, which will allow us to hypothesize basic cellular energy theory.[10,26-28] This basic cellular energetic theory can then be tested to describe the evidence that we need. If we can hypothesize a basic mechanism of action of myofascial release, for example, then we can examine whether that action does indeed take place in the way that the theory postulates. However, we will never be able to *see* energy, any more, for instance, than we can see velocity.

Demonstration of efficacy and safety is paramount to professional care. But is this goal actually achievable to the satisfaction of the scientific community? Not as long as reductionism remains the gold standard in the search for reality. In 1997, the Council on Scientific Affairs of the American Medical Association suggested that "physicians should evaluate the scientific perspectives of unconventional theories for treatment and practice, looking particularly at potential utility, safety and efficacy of these [holistic] modalities."[23]

Holistic approaches should not be exempt from careful study. In addition to randomized trials, complementary therapies must be researched by way of case studies, single case designs, and other methods of systematic examination of intervention and results. And as we build the body of evidence justifying the positive benefits of the restored flow of healing energy that help the body/mind self-regulate and heal itself, we may just come to realize that complementary therapies have done more to restore healing to health care than had been anticipated. What follows is a review of the evidence of how complementary therapies influence normal cardiovascular and pulmonary responses and the effect that they have on patients with cardiovascular and pulmonary conditions.

Use of Specific Complementary Therapy Interventions in Cardiovascular and Pulmonary Conditions

As described throughout Part III of this book, the goal of physical therapy intervention is to improve the efficiency of the oxygen transport and gas exchange systems. The decision to use a specific complementary therapy and integrate it into more traditional cardiovascular and pulmonary treatments is often dependent on the practitioner's familiarity with the intervention. Rehabilitation practitioners without specialized training in a complementary therapeutic intervention frequently do not realize that they are already incorporating components of complementary therapies in established, traditional therapeutic interventions. Patient education, including behavioral and biofeedback techniques used to alter breathing patterns and reduce sympathetic nervous system stimulation, are forms of mind/body therapies. These interventions have been studied extensively, reported in the literature, and are widely used and accepted in clinical practice.[29-31]

Physical therapy practitioners with expertise in a specific complementary intervention may decide to focus their treatment on cardiovascular and pulmonary impairments. Tai chi and yoga are mind/body therapies that emphasize coordinated breathing with movement. These interventions may be used as the primary approach to treat the impairment, or they may complement traditional physical therapy. The body of evidence addressing the usefulness of these interventions in improving oxygen transport has expanded in both quantity and quality in recent years.[32-36]

Other interventions that have not been subjected to rigorous, scientific study may still be worthy of clinical application. For example, the Alexander technique, which emphasizes posture and movement, intuitively suggests an improvement in oxygen transport. An improvement in posture optimizes muscle function, thoracic cage efficiency, and hence oxygen transport; however, there is limited research published on this technique in relation to the cardiovascular and pulmonary systems.[37]

The increasing consumer demand for complementary and alternative medical (CAM) therapies has occurred despite the lack of rigorous or acceptable scientific investigation into many of them. In an attempt to protect the general public from unethical and unsafe practices, the National Heart, Lung, and Blood Institute and the National Center for Complementary and Alternative Medicine (NCCAM) have proposed that large-scale clinical trials be performed to determine standards of practice and safety standards.[38] NCCAM proposed initiatives to support research and the development of specialized centers to study cardiovascular disease and also reported a 96% increase in funding for these initiatives in 2005.[39,40] It is important for all health care practitioners to become familiar with some of the more popular CAM therapies, recognize that our patients are using them, and be especially aware of the effects of these therapies on the cardiovascular and pulmonary systems.

The following section reviews the normal cardiovascular and pulmonary responses to various CAM interventions in healthy individuals. A presentation of the evidence for using specific complementary and alternative medicine therapies to treat major cardiovascular and cardiovascular and pulmonary pathologies follows. A discussion of naturopathic and homeopathic therapies is outside the scope of this chapter. Breathing exercises will be discussed in relation to a specific CAM therapy. Traditional breathing exercises (e.g. diaphragmatic, pursed-lip, etc.) are addressed elsewhere in this book.

Cardiovascular and Pulmonary Responses to Complementary and Alternative Medical Therapies

Tai Chi

Tai chi is one of the most well-studied mind/body therapies. During sessions of the many forms of tai chi (see Appendix E), cardiovascular responses have been documented in novices as well as in master practitioners. In several of these studies, responses have been compared to cardiovascular and pulmonary responses observed in other forms of exercise (e.g. bicycle ergometry and treadmill ambulation). Most investigations are small and have methodological shortcomings. A brief sampling of the results of several studies addressing the cardiovascular and pulmonary responses found during tai chi practice can be found in Table 27-1. In general, in these studies of healthy individuals, gender and experience level do not seem to influence the responses. It is reasonable to conclude that tai chi is a low- to moderate-intensity exercise that emphasizes the oxygen transport system. Investigators generally conclude that tai chi is a safe activity for healthy individuals. Prescreening for mind/body interventions is recommended, however, just as would be expected for any other exercise intervention.[37]

Several authors have investigated the cardiovascular and pulmonary benefits of a prolonged program of tai chi. In contrast to the studies reported in Table 27-1, several others demonstrate that experienced tai chi chuan practitioners achieve significantly higher maximum oxygen consumption ($\dot{V}O_{2max}$) levels than do sedentary subjects.[46-52] These authors conclude that tai chi is a form of aerobic exercise, it has benefits for health-related fitness, and it may slow the decline in cardiorespiratory fitness in older, healthy individuals.

In a small study (n = 32), Wang and colleagues (2002)[34] studied endothelium-dependent dilation in skin vasculature in healthy, older (69.9 ± 1.5 years), male tai chi practitioners and a control group. Their results demonstrate that when compared with older sedentary men (67.0 ± 1.0 years), long-time, experienced practitioners of tai chi have more favorable arterial and venous hemodynamics. In some cases these vascular findings were comparable to a group of younger, healthy, sedentary men (23.5 ± 0.68 years).

Young and colleagues (1999)[53] compared the effects of aerobic exercise and tai chi on blood pressure responses in

Table 27-1 Cardiovascular and Pulmonary Responses Found During Continuous Tai Chi Exercise

Study Authors	Tai Chi Form	Sample Characteristics and Methods	Cardiovascular and Pulmonary Responses
Schneider, 1991[41]	Wing chun (WG) Tai chi chuan (TCC)	Experienced practitioners $\dot{V}O_{2max}$ measured on treadmill	TCC: 36.4% $\dot{V}O_{2max}$, 59.8% HR_{max}, $\dot{V}_E/\dot{V}O_2$ 21.7 WG: 52.4% $\dot{V}O_{2max}$, 70.5% HR_{max}, $\dot{V}_E/\dot{V}O_2$ 24.2
Lan, 2001[42]	Yang tai chi chuan	15 men Age 26-56 years Experienced practitioners (>1 year) $\dot{V}O_2$ measured on cycle ergometer	TCC: 58% HR_{max} (max on cycle was 186 ± 8), 55% $\dot{V}O_{2max}$ (max on cycle was 39.1 ± 7.7)
Brown, 1989[43]	Tai chi chuan (long form Yang style, Cloud H)	6 men Experienced practitioners $\dot{V}O_2$ measured on cycle ergometer	TCC: Vf 11.3, $\dot{V}_E/\dot{V}O_2$ 23.47, V_D/V_T 20% Cycle: Vf 15.7, $\dot{V}_E/\dot{V}O_2$ 27.41, V_D/V_T 27% Cardiac output, stroke volume, and HR were not significantly different between TCC and ergometry at the same $\dot{V}O_2$
Fontana, 2000[44]	Tai chi in slow and fast movements in sitting and standing	26 healthy adults Age 21-50 years Convenience sample Novice and experienced practitioners	METs: Sitting 1.5 ± 0 .2, Slow standing 2.3 ± 0.3, Fast standing 2.6 ± 0.5, Breathing exercises 3-3.6, 43%-49% predicted HR_{max}
Chao, 2002[45]	Tai-chi/qi-gong (54 motions divided into 3 sets)	47 adults Age 32-76 years Experienced practitioners (mean 3.6 ± 2.6 years)	50% $\dot{V}O_{2max}$ in older adults (≥65 years) 60% $\dot{V}O_{2max}$ in women Each motion ± 3 METs

$\dot{V}O_{2max}$, Maximum oxygen uptake (in L/min or mL/kg/min); $\dot{V}_E/\dot{V}O_2$, ventilatory equivalent for oxygen; *Vf,* ventilatory frequency in breaths per minute; V_D/V_T, ratio of dead space ventilation to tidal volume; *METs,* metabolic equivalents (1 MET = 3.5 mL of oxygen/kilogram/weight).

older individuals (79% women). In this RCT of 62 sedentary older adults (66.7 ± 5.2 years), subjects participated in 12 weeks of either aerobic exercise or tai chi. Baseline systolic blood pressure (BP) was 130 to 159 mm Hg. Subjects were not on antihypertensive medication, and results indicated similar statistically significant reductions in systolic BP occurred in both intervention groups. Of note, the aerobic exercise group demonstrated a significant increase in predicted $\dot{V}O_{2max}$, whereas the tai chi group did not. The authors concluded that both light- and moderate-intensity exercise programs can have an important effect on systolic blood pressure. Thornton and colleagues (2004)[54] found similar reductions in BP in normotensive sedentary women, ages 33 to 55 years. In contrast, Chen and colleagues (2006)[55] found no reduction in BP in older adult residents of long-term care facilities when they participated in a 6-month simplified tai chi program. Their program was customized for deconditioned subjects, and the authors concluded that the lack of significant changes in BP was due to the very low intensity of the exercise.

Yoga

Another popular mind/body intervention is yoga. The cardiovascular responses to several types of yoga in healthy children and adults have been investigated.[56-59] General conclusions are difficult to make, given the weaknesses of the studies and the different characteristics of the types of yoga studied. Table 27-2 lists cardiovascular and pulmonary responses before and after a single yoga session or a period of yoga practice. Overall it appears that those forms of yoga that primarily involve meditation show minimal changes in cardiovascular and pulmonary parameters when compared with those forms that include stimulation phases.

Other Mind/Body Therapies

Although social support is not typically considered a mind/body therapy, part of the success of many of the CAM interventions has been attributed to group interactions or those interactions between subject and practitioner. In a review of 81 studies, Uchino and colleagues (1996)[66] investigated the benefits of social support on the cardiovascular, endocrine, and immune systems. Social support includes individual, family, or group interactions. There is strong evidence correlating a decrease in cardiovascular reactivity in healthy individuals when social support is increased.

Manual Therapies/Body Work Therapies

There is a paucity of literature addressing cardiovascular and pulmonary responses to body work interventions in healthy individuals. One study of therapeutic massage demonstrated statistically significant reductions in cardiovascular parameters after a 3-day intervention of slow-stroke back massage on individuals in a rehabilitation setting.[67] Twenty-four adults (age range 52 to 88 years) underwent daily intervention. Statistically significant decreases in systolic and diastolic BP were noted each day; this was true for heart rate (HR) and respiratory rate (RR) only on days 1 and 3. Subjects also reported improved perception and less anxiety.

Cottingham and colleagues (1988b)[68] investigated the effects of the Rolf method of soft tissue mobilization on parasympathetic nervous system (PNS) tone in 32 young, healthy men. This RCT compared a group that performed 45 minutes of Rolfing with pelvic mobilization (pelvic lift) with a control group that received a 45-minute durational touch without Rolfing (pelvic lift intervention). At baseline all subjects had

Table 27-2 Cardiovascular and Pulmonary Responses to Yoga Practices in Healthy Individuals

Study Authors	Type of Yoga	Sample Characteristics and Methods	Cardiovascular and Pulmonary Responses
Telles, 1993[60]	Brahmakumaris Raja yoga meditation	18 males Age 20-52 years (34.1 ± 8.1) Experienced practitioners Subjects served as own control in sessions of random thinking	Yoga: HR increased compared with baseline and control Yoga and control: no difference in measures of autonomic function
Schell, 1994[61]	Hatha yoga	Experienced practitioners Control group volunteers	Yoga: HR decreased during practice compared with controls Yoga and control: no difference in BP or endocrine measures
Ray, 2001[62]	Hatha yoga	40 men Age 19-23 years $\dot{V}O_{2max}$ measured on cycle ergometer Both yoga and conventional physical exercise groups performed 1 hour of activity every morning for 6 months	Yoga: $\dot{V}O_{2max}$ increased from baseline; perception of exertion decreased from baseline Conventional physical exercise: $\dot{V}O_2$ increased from baseline; no change in perception of exertion (no information was given regarding differences between group outcomes)
Telles, 2000[63]	Cyclic meditation (calming and stimulating) Shavasana (calming)	40 male volunteers Age 27 ± 5.7 years Experienced practitioners Measurements taken before and after yoga session	CM: $\dot{V}O_2$ decreased 32.1%, RR rate decreased 18%, TV decreased 28.8% SH: $\dot{V}O_2$ decreased 10.1%, RR decreased 15.2%, TV decreased 15.9% Results were significantly different from baseline and decreases were significantly greater in CM than SH
Knowles, 2003[64]	Asanas (yoga poses) Pranayama (breathing exercises)	Single case study Age 42 years Healthy male Performed 6 days per week for 10 weeks 5 poses and 2 breathing exercises	Vital capacity: increased 9% Chest circumference measures: increased in all regions Chest flexibility measures: increased in forward bending
Haggins, 2007[65]	Hatha yoga	20 practitioners with <1 year yoga experience Age 31 ± 8.3 years 18 females 30 min sitting, 56 min beginner yoga, 10 min TM walking at 2-3 mph	Measurements taken at rest and after yoga, 2 mph TM and 3 mph TM Measures included $\dot{V}O_2$, HR, %MHR, METs, kcal/min Metabolic cost of yoga comparable to TM walking at 2 mph

$\dot{V}O_2$, Oxygen consumption (mL/min); *RR*, respiratory rate (breath rate); *TV*, tidal volume (breath volume), *CM*, cyclic meditation; *SH*, shavasana; *TM*, treadmill; *HR*, heart rate; *%MHR*, percent maximum heart rate.

an anterior pelvic tilt. PNS tone was measured before, immediately after, and 24 hours after intervention. Results demonstrated a significant increase in PNS tone and decreased standing pelvic tilt angle in the intervention group. Earlier, Cottingham and colleagues (1988a)[69] demonstrated an increase in PNS tone with the pelvic lift technique unrelated to the durational touch used simultaneously in the technique. The authors concluded that this intervention of soft tissue pelvic manipulation (i.e., durational touch plus pelvic lift) can help individuals with muscle dysfunction and conditions associated with reduced PNS activity and increased sympathetic nervous system activity. Reduced PNS and increased SNS can be representative of deconditioning.

In a small study of 12 children and adults, investigators attempted to examine the reliability of craniosacral intervention interpretation among three expert practitioners of craniosacral therapy.[70] They also investigated the relationship of the craniosacral rate to HR and BP of subject and practitioner. Results demonstrated no interrater reliability among the three practitioners. Results also demonstrated no relationship between HR and BP and the craniosacral rates. Although this study did not attempt to report on the effects of craniosacral therapy on cardiovascular parameters, the results do shed light on potential considerations for future study design.

Green and colleagues (2004)[71] conducted a rigorous review of the evidence for using craniosacral therapy. Nine of the 34 studies reviewed looked at whether movement of cranial bones was possible, and 10 of the 34 studies looked at whether cerebrospinal fluid moves rhythmically. The authors concluded that evidence supports the belief that there is a cranial "pulse" or rhythm that is separate from the cardiac or respiratory rhythms.

Energy Work Interventions

A few studies addressing the cardiovascular and pulmonary responses to energy work in healthy subjects have been conducted. Some of these are summarized in Table 27-3. In most cases, methodological weaknesses limit generalizations about the results. Studies of Reiki demonstrate trends toward increased relaxation and improved immune system markers.[74-76] In a study of qi-training, the authors provide a

Table 27-3 Cardiovascular and Pulmonary Responses to Energy Work in Healthy Individuals

Study Authors	Energy Work	Sample Characteristics and Methods	Cardiovascular and Pulmonary Responses
Hinman, 2002[72]	Magnets Negative polarity Positive polarity	Double-blind RCT 75 adults, 25 in each group Age 21-57 years Measurements at rest, 1, 5, 10, 15 minutes on magnet mattress and 5 min after exposure	BP and HR responses were not significantly different between positive polarity, negative polarity, and control groups
Martel, 2002[73]	Magnets	Prospective RCT 20 healthy men Age 25 ± 2 years Magnets worn for 30 min on 2 separate occasions Measurements at 10, 20, 30 min	Forearm blood flow responses were not significantly different from placebo
Wardell, 2001[74]	Reiki	Convenience sample 23 healthy subjects Age 29-55 years Treatment consisted of 30 min of Reiki by expert practitioner Measurements before, during, and after session	Pretreatment to posttreatment: significant decrease in anxiety, BP; trend to decrease in EMG (muscle tension) and salivary cortisol; significant increase in salivary IgA; trend to increase galvanic skin temperature, indicating relaxation
Wetzel, 1989[75]	Reiki	48 healthy individuals (plus 10 controls) Monitored over 24 hours	Pretreatment to posttreatment: significant improvement in hemoglobin and hematocrit
Olson, 2003[76]	Reiki	24 subjects with cancer pain Treated 1.5 hours with Reiki or 1.5 hours of rest for 4 consecutive days	Significant decrease in HR, DBP, on day 1 Significant decrease in pain on days 1 and 3 Trend to decrease in DBP on day 3 Significant increase in psychological quality of life from day 1 to day 7 No change in SBP or RR days 1-4
Lee, 2000[77]	Qi-training (3 stages): Sound 10 min Motion 10 min Meditation 10 min	12 healthy volunteers Age 19-37 years 1 hour per day, 6 times per week 1.3 ± 0.2 years of training	After 10 min: significant decrease in SBP and RPP, trend in decrease HR, RR After 60 min: significant decrease in HR, SBP, RR, and RPP from baseline

RCT, Randomized control trial; *DBP*, diastolic BP; *SBP*, systolic BP; *RPP*, rate-pressure product.

detailed description of the intervention facilitating replication of the study with a larger sample.[77] The two studies investigating responses to magnets demonstrate no significant differences from control.[72,73] Of interest, in a study investigating the safety of prosthetic mini-magnets in individuals with cardiac pacemakers, the authors found no electrocardiographic changes in 9 of 12 subjects. When the magnets were moved at least 1 cm away from the pacemaker implant, the changes in the other 3 subjects no longer existed.[78]

In a well-written and well-designed paper, investigators reported on the effects of acupuncture on autonomic nervous system (ANS) function.[79] Twelve healthy volunteers, six men and six women, ages 23 to 48 years, underwent randomized needle insertion into three distinct acupuncture sites. Measures of ANS function were monitored during the 25-minute intervention period and for the 60 minutes after intervention at each insertion site. An interesting combination of results was found, depending on the needle insertion site. Stimulation of the ear site resulted in increased PNS activity during both the needle insertion and the poststimulation periods. Stimulation of the skin over the left thenar muscle resulted in increased sympathetic nervous system (SNS) and PNS activity during both measurement periods. Stimulation of the right thenar muscle resulted in an increase in SNS and PNS activity during the poststimulation period, but no changes were seen during the needle insertion period. These results begin to shed light on which acupuncture interventions may be cardiosuppressive and possibly account for the calmness and relaxation often reported after treatment. Delayed responses may have a therapeutic effect as well.

In a controversial study by Rosa and colleagues (1998),[80] the investigators failed to demonstrate that those practitioners of noncontact therapeutic touch were able to perceive a "human energy field." Significant limitations to the study have been noted, including experimenter bias, inconsistent conclusions, and incomplete statistical analysis.[81] Although this study does not address cardiovascular and pulmonary responses to therapeutic touch, it does provoke discussion about the difficulties of conducting research on this intervention.

A study by Haas and colleagues (1986)[82] is worthy of mention in this discussion of energy interventions. These authors were able to demonstrate the ability of musical rhythm to "pace" respirations. In a sample of 20 healthy volunteers (half of whom were musically trained), breathing rhythms were correlated with metronome and tapping rhythms. This ability of musical rhythms to entrain respiration may have potential benefits in managing stress-induced respiratory patterns.

Risk Factors for Coronary Artery Disease

Numerous complementary therapies have been studied and shown efficacious in the management of known risk factors for coronary artery disease (CAD).[83-85] Specifically, interventions addressing psychological stress and hypertension have been extensively examined.

Stress Reduction

First studied in the late 1970s and early 1980s, the benefits of meditation and the "relaxation response" have been recognized by Benson and colleagues (1977).[86] They postulated that when properly applied, these interventions facilitated downregulation of the SNS and upregulation of the PNS.

During 15 to 30 minutes of practicing the relaxation response, changes in cardiovascular and pulmonary parameters have been noted. These include a decrease in RR and oxygen consumption ($\dot{V}O_2$) and an increase in cardiac output (CO) without a concurrent increase in BP, reflecting a reduction in peripheral vascular resistance. In addition, skilled practitioners of the relaxation response demonstrate a decrease in $\dot{V}O_2$ at a constant workload during treadmill activity.[87]

In an important paper addressing the impact of psychological factors on the development of cardiovascular disease, researchers related CAD to depression, anxiety, personality factors and character traits, social isolation, and chronic life stress.[88] Several authors have addressed behavioral interventions effective in the management of these psychosocial stresses.

In a comprehensive metaanalysis of 70 articles, the treatment of trait anxiety with transcendental meditation (TM), progressive relaxation, relaxation response, and electromyographic (EMG) biofeedback were reviewed. Sources for the reviewed articles included journals, dissertations, and books. All interventions had a positive effect on self-reports or physiological measures of anxiety. Transcendental meditation had the strongest effect of the four interventions studied. In general, subjects who received more frequent interventions initially and who were followed the longest received the most benefit. It was recommended that future studies measure performance outcomes and that subjects be closely followed in an attempt to reduce loss due to attrition.[89]

Miller and colleagues (1995)[90] reported on 22 subjects with anxiety disorders who participated in a noncontrolled clinical trial. Subjects were trained in mindfulness meditation, participated in a once-a-week group program for 8 weeks, and were followed-up for 3 years. Significant reductions in medications and counseling requirements were noted. The authors concluded that "mindfulness training … may be able to provide medical patients suffering from anxiety with a set of tools for achieving effective long-term non-pharmacological self-regulation … and be used as a complement to more conventional medical interventions."[90] Conversely, Astin (2003)[30] reported an increase in anxiety levels in 17% to 31% of subjects practicing relaxation interventions and an increase in anxiety levels in up to 53.8% of subjects practicing TM. No negative medical consequences were reported as a result of the increased anxiety levels. Several causes for this negative response were postulated, including subjects' fear of losing control, general restlessness, intrusive thoughts, and feelings of vulnerability.

Several small, noncontrolled clinical studies examining the effects of TM on blood levels related to cardiovascular disease have been reported. Infante and colleagues (2001)[91] measured plasma catecholamine levels (epinephrine, norepinephrine, and dopamine) in 19 skilled practitioners of TM. Resting values were compared with catecholamine levels in nonmatched controls. Results demonstrated lower values in the skilled practitioners when compared with the controls. The authors concluded TM may have been responsible for the lower catecholamine levels and consequent downregulation of the SNS. Similarly, Schneider and colleagues (1998)[92] concluded that TM may have been responsible for lower serum lipid peroxide levels found in 18 practitioners of TM compared with higher levels found in 23 nonmatched, nonpracticing control subjects. Lipid peroxide has been implicated in the pathophysiology of atherosclerosis.

Cognitive approaches to the reduction of stress have been subjected to clinical study. McCrone and colleagues (2001)[93] compared the effectiveness of psychoeducational interventions on 33 male subjects with risk factors for CAD. In addition to nutrition counseling and exercise training, educational sessions addressing cardiovascular disease, risk factors, and stress reduction were offered to 25 participants. These subjects were also trained to use specific skills to improve their responses to stress and were given audiotapes to practice progressive muscle relaxation. Eight subjects in the nonrandomized control group received weight management counseling and health education only and did not participate in any discussions related to stress management. All subjects, ranging in age from 57 to 79 years, participated in the interventions for 6 months. Although both groups showed improvements in risk factor profiles, improvement was greater in the group trained in stress management interventions. Significant improvements were noted in BP, lipid profile, obesity indices, and fitness level.

In spite of a positive theoretical basis for the use of CAM therapies in stress management, many interventions have not been subjected to systematic investigation. Table 27-4 summarizes the effects of tai chi, Feldenkrais method, yoga, and therapeutic massage in stress management. Although these four studies have significant methodological weaknesses, the number of subjects participating in each study is formidable. These initial attempts at providing efficacy of the respective intervention help suggest a launching ground for future study.

Hypertension

There is a significant body of literature that addresses the benefits of CAM interventions in the management of hypertension (HTN). The majority of the larger studies address mind/body interventions, with most demonstrating positive effects on BP. In 1999 the Canadian Hypertension Society and the Heart and Stroke Foundation of Canada published guidelines recommending "individualized cognitive behavior modification to reduce the negative effects of stress."[98]

Eisenberg and colleagues (1993)[99] performed a metaanalysis addressing the effectiveness of cognitive behavioral therapies on HTN. Interventions accepted in this review were biofeedback, meditation, the relaxation response, progressive relaxation techniques, and stress management interventions such as imagery. They collected more than 800 published papers; however, because of methodological problems in the majority

Table 27-4 Effect of Selected CAM Therapies in Stress Management in Healthy Individuals

Study Authors	CAM Therapy	Sample Characteristics and Methods	Outcomes
Jin, 1992[94]	Tai chi	48 male and 48 female Experienced practitioners Subjected to mental stress before intervention Randomized to 4 groups (tai chi, brisk walking, meditation, neutral reading) Measurements before and after intervention	Pretreatment to posttreatment: significant decrease in salivary cortisol levels; improved mood states; reduction in HR, BP, for tai chi were similar to walking at 6 km/h
Kolt, 2000[95]	Feldenkrais	54 volunteers College age Followed-up for 2 weeks Randomized to 3 groups Reduction maintained 1 day later (Feldenkrais, relaxation, or control) Measurements taken 4 times (baseline, before fourth session, after fourth session, 1 day after fourth session)	Feldenkrais and relaxation groups: significantly reduced anxiety scores in females after fourth session when compared with anxiety scores before fourth session and to controls
Hanley, 2003[96]	Therapeutic massage	69 subjects Randomized to 3 groups (6 sessions of therapeutic massage, 6 sessions of relaxation tape used in surgery, relaxation tape to use at home)	Pretreatment to posttreatment: significant improvements in sleep scale and index of well-being scores in all 3 groups; strong patient preference for therapeutic massage
Kalayil, 1989[97]	Yoga meditation and progressive relaxation	80 middle-grade students Randomly assigned to 4 groups (YM, PR, reading control, and catnap)	At baseline all 4 groups were similar in HR and state anxiety Results included: YM and PR decreased state anxiety, headaches, and general tension; YM decreased HR; catnap decreased headache when compared with reading control

YM, Yoga meditation; *PR*, progressive relaxation.

of papers, their limited inclusion criteria of adult subjects with diastolic BP of 90 to 114 mm Hg, lack of randomized control design, weak description of the study, and poor reporting of BP values, only 26 studies were entered for detail review. Results of this comprehensive analysis of 1264 patients indicated superior outcomes in the group receiving cognitive intervention techniques when compared with controls. No one intervention demonstrated more favorable outcomes than any other. In addition, when control groups were subjected to a placebo intervention (i.e., sham biofeedback), no significant differences in outcomes were noted. This is consistent with the belief that an intervention effect is inherent in the concept of placebo.[31]

In two RCTs of African American subjects, investigators examined the effects of stress reduction approaches on HTN. In one study, 111 males and females with mean BP of 147/92 mm Hg and mean age of 67 years were randomized to a 3-month trial of TM and progressive muscle relaxation (PMR) or a lifestyle modification education control program.[100] Results demonstrated that TM had a greater effect at lowering both systolic and diastolic BP than did PMR and that both intervention groups demonstrated a significantly greater impact on BP reduction than did the control group. In a small but well-designed study, Barnes and colleagues (2001)[101] recruited 34 African American adolescents (ages 15 to 18 years) with high-normal BP (>85th and <95th percentile for age and sex, respectively. After randomization, 17 subjects participated in 2 months of daily, 15-minutes sessions of TM. The control group attended seven weekly, 1-hour lessons on health education. Measures of cardiovascular function were collected at rest and during performance of a stressful activity (at baseline and again at the end of the intervention period). Although no significant changes were noted in resting values, results indicated that individuals in the TM group responded more favorably to stressor activities. Blood pressure increased appropriately during the activity in both groups; however, the degree of elevation was reduced in the TM group when compared with controls.

Reduction in antihypertensive medication requirements has been reported when mind/body therapies are added to the management regimen of HTN. In an RCT, Shapiro and colleagues (1997)[102] studied 39 individuals with medically treated HTN. Subjects trained in cognitive behavior therapies (i.e. PMR, biofeedback, deep diaphragmatic breathing, and imagery) showed a 73% reduction of BP medication requirements during the study follow-up period compared with a 35% reduction in the control group. In addition, 55% of subjects in the intervention group were completely free of medication compared with only 30% of subjects in the control group. The reduction in BP levels was consistent across clinical, ambulatory, and home settings.

Yucha and colleagues (2004)[103] reviewed 20 RCTs investigating the effects of biofeedback on HTN. Several forms of biofeedback, including thermal, EMG, and electrodermal, resulted in reductions in blood pressure when the intervention was combined with related cognitive therapy and relaxation training. When biofeedback was the sole intervention, significant reductions in BP were not demonstrated. Wang and colleagues (2004)[104] performed a systematic review of the effects of tai chi on chronic conditions, including HTN. They reported on four moderate-sized studies: two randomized controlled trials and two nonrandomized controlled trials. Outcomes of all four studies indicated significant reduction in BP in older individuals and in those recovering from acute MI.

In addition to the mind/body therapies discussed above, several additional studies investigating the effects of select CAM therapies in individuals with HTN are summarized in Table 27-5. Although the evidence presented in these studies is weak, these investigations provide valuable insights to consider when structuring future research protocols. Several review articles addressing effects of other interventions are summarized in Table 27-6. In general, the results of these investigations assist in providing evidence for the benefit of the intervention in the management of HTN. In one review, Levin and Vanderpool (1989)[110] consider the beneficial effects of religious commitment and affiliation in the management of HTN. Possible explanations offered for lower blood pressure in individuals with HTN include the psychosocial effects of membership in an organized religious community, the inherent health promotion behaviors and preferences often supported by religious traditions, and the psychodynamics of religious rites, faith, and belief systems.

In the review articles of the effects of qi gong in HTN, authors acknowledge significant methodological weaknesses in many of the studies reviewed.[111,112] Some of the reported weaknesses include selection biases, lack of randomization, noncompliance with the intervention, concerns regarding BP measurement reliability, and the differences among the many styles of qi gong , which were not typically considered. Two review articles on the effects of tai chi on HTN are included in Table 27-6. Significant improvement in BP was reported in the eight studies reviewed by Yeh and colleagues (2008).[113] Lee and colleagues (2010)[114] found conflicting results in their review; they attributed their inconsistent outcomes to inadequate baseline BP testing in all four of the studies reviewed (one study was common to both of these reviews). Finally, Kim and colleagues (2010)[115] presented a thorough review of 20 articles on the effects of acupuncture on HTN. They acknowledged that 17 of the 20 studies were poor quality and concluded that further "rigorously designed studies" are needed.[115] Of note, no significant adverse reactions were documented in any of the tai chi or acupuncture articles reviewed.

Cardiovascular Conditions

Much of the pathophysiological basis for applying CAM therapies to cardiovascular conditions rests in the relationship between the cardiovascular system and the ANS.[116] Stimulation of the ANS, specifically the SNS, can cause both an increase in circulating levels of catecholamines and damage to endothelial cells lining arterial walls. Often triggered by psychological factors, the resulting increase in metabolic and myocardial oxygen demand has a negative impact on the oxygen transport system.[88] Interventions that can reduce or reverse these responses to SNS stimulation have a potential positive effect on cardiovascular conditions. Recently, a

Table 27-5 Effect of Selected CAM Therapies in the Management of HTN

Study Authors	CAM Therapy	Sample Characteristics and Methods	Outcomes
Paran, 1996[105]	Biofeedback	38 patients (15 white-coat HTN; 23 essential HTN) Random assignment Biofeedback given 1 time per week for 4 weeks	Pretreatment to posttreatment: both groups had statistically significant reductions in BP in the clinic; white-coat HTN had significantly lower SBP and DBP at home than essential HTN
Patel, 1975[106]	Yoga (and biofeedback), "psychophysical relaxation exercise"	40 patients with HTN Followed-up for 9-12 months 20 received intervention; 20 remained as controls	Statistically significant reductions in BP and anti-HTN medication requirements in intervention group
Brownstein, 1989[107]	Yoga relaxation	Case report Age 46 years Male History of mild essential HTN 6-week program	Discontinuation of anti-HTN medications; normalization of DBP; return to full flight status (aviator in U.S. Air Force)
Zucker, 1997[108]	Qi gong (breathing, meditation, movement)	22 patients with HTN (15 in intervention group, 7 control) Intervention classes 2 times per week for 8 weeks	Pretreatment to posttreatment: significant decreases in SBP, DBP, MAP, RR in intervention group; significant increases in QOL in intervention group
McCraty 2003[109]	Stress reduction (Inner Quality Management) Biofeedback	32 information technology employees with HTN Mean age 46, 9 females; Intervention (I): three sessions totaling 16 hours over 2 weeks followed by home program with optional review session at 2 months and follow-up measures at 3 months	Both control (C) and I reduced BP; reduction in I was significantly greater than C; 3 in I were able to reduce or terminate BP medications Compared with C, I showed significant increase in well-being and work satisfaction, and decrease in stress symptoms, depression, phobic anxiety Reduced BP was correlated with reduced stress symptoms

MAP, Mean arterial blood pressure; *QOL*, quality of life.

Table 27-6 **Select CAM Therapies and their Effects on HTN: Summary of Review Papers**

Study Authors	CAM Therapy	Number of Articles Reviewed	Outcome Variables	Outcome
Levin, 1989[110]	Religion*: RC, RA	20	SBP, DPB, HTN, heart disease mortality, HTN-related mortality, history of HTN	RC: 19 studies demonstrate intervention is associated with lower BP or lower rates of HTN; 5 studies demonstrate protective effects of intervention RA: significantly lower rates of HTN-related morbidity and mortality in highly devout, behaviorally strict groups (e.g., Mormons, Buddhists, Seventh-Day Adventists, clergy)
Sancier, 1999[111]; Mayer, 1999[112]	Qi gong	30	BP, measures of blood flow, CHF, acute MI, stroke, total mortality rate	Decreased stroke and mortality; decreased anti-HTN medication requirements
Yeh 2008[113]	Tai chi	8	SBP, DBP, compliance, medications	Tai chi groups demonstrated significant reductions in BP, higher compliance with home program, and more effective BP control
Lee 2010[114]	Tai chi, >60 years old	4	BP	Two reviews reported significant reduction in BP in tai chi group when compared with control or wellness education program Two reviews reported no reduction in BP compared with resistance training, usual activity or aerobic exercise
Kim 2010[115]	Acupuncture, traditional meridian needle insertion points	20	BP	Significant reductions in BP in both high- and low-quality studies; duration of reduction in BP was variable amongst studies; magnitude of BP reduction was greater when acupuncture, rather than sham treatment, was used in conjunction with anti-HTN medications

RC, Religious commitment; *RA*, religious affiliation.

*Measures of religion include religious attendance, church membership, religious affiliation, ethnic traditions within Judaism, monastic orders, clergy status, religious education, and subjective religiosity.

number of authors have looked at the impact of various CAM interventions on heart rate variability (HRV).[117-121] The variability in R-R intervals between normal sinus rhythm cardiac cycles reflects the balance of SNS and PNS cardiac control. Low HRV has been associated with disease, whereas high HRV tends to indicate cardiovascular health and improved prognosis. In addition, *patterns* of HRV appear to reflect alterations in emotions and have been used to further demonstrate cardiovascular physiological responses to CAM interventions.[122]

Coronary Artery Disease

Beneficial effects of CAM interventions in the use of CAD management are documented throughout the published literature.[29,30,32,123-125] Although significant methodological problems are apparent in many papers, numerous large, well-designed studies can be found. Much of the evidence supporting the use of these interventions in individuals with CAD demonstrates improvement in exercise tolerance, reduction of ischemia, and reduction of anxiety and depression. Mind/body techniques, including cognitive behavioral interventions, yoga, tai chi, guided imagery, and music therapy, have been successfully used in patients with CAD. The benefits of energy work, including distant healing prayer and qi gong, in patients with CAD have been reported.

In 1959, Friedman and Rosenman[126] first documented the relationship between certain emotional behaviors and the prevalence of CAD.[127] They defined the type A behavior pattern as "an emotional syndrome characterized by a continuously harrying sense of time urgency and easily aroused free-floating hostility."[127] In subsequent decades, the study of interventions aimed at modifying the behavior of individuals with type A behavior pattern and CAD was undertaken.

In a large study of post-myocardial infarction (MI) patients with type A behavior, 1013 subjects were randomized into three groups.[127] Of the total, 270 subjects received group cardiac counseling, 592 subjects received both cardiac counseling and type A behavioral counseling, and the remaining 151 individuals did not receive any counseling. Subjects were followed for 4½ years to determine the impact of type A behavior counseling on recurrent coronary events (both nonfatal infarctions and cardiac deaths). Cardiac counseling sessions consisted of 90-minute group meetings during which diet, exercise, medications, cardiovascular pathophysiology, and possible surgical procedures were discussed. Type A behavioral counseling sessions included progressive muscle relaxation, as well as specific psychotherapeutic interventions. Results indicated statistically significant reductions in recurrence rates of cardiac events in both intervention groups, with a greater reduction in the rate of recurrent events in those subjects who received both forms of counseling.

In a landmark study of 48 patients with known CAD, Ornish and colleagues (1990)[11] analyzed the number of coronary artery lesions detected at angiography before and after a year-long lifestyle intervention. In addition to a low-fat vegetarian diet, smoking cessation, and a moderate exercise program, subjects participated in a stress management training program of guided imagery. At the end of the year, the 28 subjects in the intervention group demonstrated statistically significant fewer coronary lesions than the 20 subjects in the usual-care control group. The regression in coronary atherosclerosis was attributed to the comprehensive lifestyle changes, brought about without the assistance of lipid-lowering medications. Clinical reports of angina were reduced as well.

Upon recognition of the impact of emotions on the recurrence rate of cardiac events in individuals with CAD, behavioral interventions became routine therapies in cardiac care.[33] Dusseldorp and colleagues (1999)[128] published a metaanalysis of the results of 37 studies investigating the effects of psychoeducational programs on patients with known CAD. All studies were conducted between 1974 and 1997 and were categorized according to stress management (SM) and health education (HE) interventions. Interventions used included various combinations of education, cognitive-behavioral therapies, relaxation, imaging, and emotional support. A number of studies included SM and HE interventions in combination with standard exercise training programs typically found in traditional cardiac rehabilitation programs. Results from studies administering either SM or HE intervention suggested a 34% reduction in fatal cardiac events and a 29% reduction in recurrent MI. The authors concluded that although psychoeducational therapies should be encouraged in cardiac rehabilitation programs, future research focusing on specific SM or HE interventions is warranted. In another metaanalysis addressing the effects of psychosocial interventions in subjects with CAD, Linden and colleagues (1996)[129] reviewed 23 studies of 2024 patients and 1156 control subjects. In addition to the typical education component of cardiac rehabilitation programs, almost half of the studies included in this analysis involved some form of CAM treatment as an intervention. These included relaxation, breathing relaxation, and music therapy. Just as in the aforementioned metaanalysis, the benefits of adding a psychosocial component to these cardiac rehabilitation programs significantly reduced morbidity and mortality and psychological distress.

In 2000, in a scientific statement presented by the American Heart Association and the American Association of Cardiovascular and Pulmonary Rehabilitation, psychosocial management was identified as a "core component of cardiac rehabilitation/secondary prevention programs."[130] Suggested interventions included "individual and/or small group education and counseling regarding adjustment to coronary heart disease, stress management, and health-related lifestyle change ... supportive rehabilitation environment and community resources to enhance patient's and family's level of social support."[130]

The relationship between mental stress and myocardial ischemia in men with CAD has been well studied. Investigators have found an increased likelihood of having mental–stress-induced ischemia in individuals who experience daily life ischemia.[131] Individuals with chronic anxiety and depression also exhibit more episodes of myocardial ischemia than those without documented anxiety and depression.[132] In a 5-year, nonrandomized controlled study of 94 men with documented mental–stress-induced ischemia, researchers reported on the usefulness of a stress management program.[133,134] In addition to educational classes, the intervention group received instruction aimed at reducing the physiological effects of stress. This included instruction in progressive muscle relaxation and individual sessions of EMG biofeedback. Outcomes of recurrent cardiac events were significantly reduced in the stress management group when compared with the control group at 1-, 2-, and 5-year follow-up. Overall reductions in hostility and clinical depression were also reported as statistically and clinically significant. The 5-year financial burden, including hospitalization and physician costs, was also significantly less in the stress management group. Similar results were reported by Zamarra and colleagues (1996)[135] in a small, nonrandomized controlled study of the effects of an 8-month trial of TM. At follow-up bicycle exercise testing, participants demonstrated increases in exercise duration and maximal workload achieved and a delay in the onset of ST depression. In an early paper, Benson and colleagues (1975)[136] reported on the beneficial effects of the relaxation response in reducing the number of premature ventricular contractions (PVC) in individuals with stable CAD. Subjects in this report practiced the relaxation response for 20 minutes, twice a day. Frequency of PVCs was documented by Holter monitor at baseline and again after 4 weeks.

In a thorough review Villagomeza (2006)[137] explored the impact of spirituality in patients with heart disease. Twenty-six studies were discussed and included patients with acute MI, coronary artery bypass graft surgery, congestive heart failure, and heart transplant. Definitions of spirituality were listed for all articles reviewed. Most studies were descriptive or observational, and most measurement instruments were interview- and questionnaire-based; several studies used physiological and performance-based measurements. The author did not focus any conclusions on the effects of "spirituality" on heart disease but rather addressed a framework from which spirituality could be more easily studied. Irrespective of the definition of spirituality used in the 26 reviewed papers, the impact on outcomes appeared favorable.

Several studies have demonstrated no or limited improvements in cardiovascular outcomes with the intervention of specific behavioral therapies. In a large (n = 2328) RCT of early post-MI intervention, investigators reported limited benefit of psychological counseling.[138] In this 2-year follow-up study, patients with acute MI returned within 28 days of the acute event to participate in 7 weeks of outpatient counseling, including PMR and skills to reduce stress. Subjects in the intervention group experienced significantly fewer episodes of angina; however, mortality, clinical complications, and clinical sequelae of CAD did not differ between groups. The authors concluded that the intervention was conducted too soon after the cardiac event, possibly accounting for the reduced treatment effect. In a study of patients participating in a phase II cardiac rehabilitation program, progressive muscle relaxation and guided imagery interventions failed to result in beneficial outcomes.[139] Although there were methodological limitations

Table 27-7 Effect of Selected Mind/Body Therapies in CAD

Study Authors	MBT Therapy	Sample Characteristics and Methods	Outcomes
Manchanda, 2000[140]	Yoga	Prospective RCCT 42 men with CAD 2 groups Intervention: yoga, RF control, diet control, moderate exercise Control: RF control, AHA step 1 diet control	Yoga group: (compared with controls) significant decrease in number of anginal episodes per week; improved exercise capacity; decreased body weight, total cholesterol, LDL cholesterol, triglycerides; fewer revascularization procedures; more lesion regression and less lesion progression (angiographic findings); improved functional class, symptomatic status, and RF profile
Friedlander, 1986[141]	Religion (Orthodox Jewish)	Had first MI: 454 men (51% secular) 85 women (50% secular) Healthy, no CAD: 295 men (21% secular) 391 women (16% secular)	Higher risk for first MI if: older, smoker, less education; European born; secular, men and women; results persisted 2-3 months after acute event
Strawbridge, 1997[142]	Religion	5286 survey respondents Followed-up for 28 years Analyzed for association between attendance at religious services and mortality	Frequent attenders compared with infrequent attenders: lower mortality rates; results were stronger for females; improved health practices (stop smoking, increase exercising, increase social contacts, stay married)
Chang, 2010[143]	Tai Chi	54 patients with CAD; 22 did 90 min tai chi 1x/week for 6 months 32 patients usual care Modified Bruce TM at baseline and 6 months	Improved RPP and RPP reserve in tai chi group compared with usual care
Park, 2010[144]	Tai Chi	85 adults with CAD (50 males); 53-75 years (mean 66 years); measures at baseline and 6 months 33 received tai chi (1x/week for 60 min) and education nutrition (1 hr /month) stress management (1 hr/month) 19 received tai chi only 33 received usual care	Tai chi is safe for population Tai chi with education significantly improved cardiovascular risk factors (BP, lipids), QOL, BMI when compared with tai chi–only group

MBT, Mind/body therapy; *RCCT*, randomized control clinical trial; *RF*, risk factors; *AHA*, American Heart Association; TM, treadmill; *RPP*, rate-pressure product; *QOL*, quality of life; *BMI*, body mass index.

in this paper, the authors similarly concluded the timing of the interventions may have contributed to the absence of benefit.

Results of the effects of selected mind/body therapies in CAD are summarized in Table 27-7. Manchanda and colleagues (2000)[140] investigated the effects of yoga on numerous cardiovascular measures. Although improved outcomes were documented in the intervention group when compared with controls, the demonstrated benefits may be due to the moderate exercise component of the intervention and not necessarily the yoga component.

Tai chi practice has been recommended as a therapeutic intervention in balance disorders and fall prevention in older adults.[25,145,146] Its potential benefits as replacement for or as an adjunct therapy in cardiac rehabilitation programs have been suggested as well.[143,144,147] In an interesting commentary in 1992, Ng stated that tai chi "has many similarities with … walking exercise—the most recommended aerobic exercise for coronary artery disease."[148] Further clinical study is warranted to provide evidence of the benefit of tai chi in the population with CAD.

Two papers addressed the use of several mind/body and manual therapies to assist with anxiety reduction in patients undergoing cardiac catheterization. McCaffrey and colleagues (2005)[149] reported on the use of music therapy, massage, guided imagery, and therapeutic touch. These interventions were performed within the hour before the diagnostic procedure. Outcomes demonstrated reduction in BP, HR, and worry, along with improved mood, in the intervention group when compared with the control group. In another study, using a visual analogue scale, authors demonstrated that "PalmTherapy" was effective in reducing anxiety levels before the procedure. PalmTherapy is an intervention that uses continuous pressure on various points in the hand.[150]

There is minimal evidence available investigating the effects of energy work on patients with CAD. Several studies compared acupuncture to sham acupuncture in individuals with angina.[151] Although no significant differences were noted in the number of anginal episodes or nitroglycerin use, the use of sham acupuncture has been questioned. As noted earlier, not all practitioners agree on proper needle location; hence what one practitioner thinks is an active acupuncture site may be considered a sham site to another practitioner. An interesting review of the effects of acupuncture on cardiac dysrhythmias was recently published.[152] The authors considered the ineffectiveness of antiarrhythmic drugs in managing certain dysrhythmias and aimed to examine the impact of acupuncture on reducing these abnormal cardiac rhythms. They reported on eight studies; seven were case studies or case series, and one was a randomized controlled trial. A total of 150 subjects participated in the eight studies, and the mean age was 54 years. Male and female participants were included, and dysrhythmias, although diverse, were primarily supraventricular tachycardia, sinus bradycardia, and ventricular extrasystoles. All participants received antiarrhythmic medications in addition to acupuncture. Treatments ranged between 1 day and 6 months, and between 1 and 50 sessions; each session lasted an average of 20 minutes. The primary outcome measured in all studies was the frequency of dysrhythmia presentation or conversion to normal sinus rhythm. Between 87% and 100% of participants demonstrated improvement; no dropouts or adverse effects were reported. There were significant methodological weaknesses in many of the studies, which led the authors to conclude that future large, rigorous trials are warranted.

Another role for CAM therapies that address stress reduction in patients with CAD is based on the relationship between chronic stress and reduced immune system function. Individuals with depressed immune systems are more vulnerable to inflammatory processes, the latter recently implicated in CAD.[153-155]

Cardiac Surgery

The Complementary Care Center (CCC) at Columbia-Presbyterian Medical Center is a "multifaceted program dedicated to evaluating and researching the effects of new modalities in health care."[156] Since 1995, practitioners at this center have been evaluating and researching the effects of various types of CAM therapies. One area of intervention involves patients having cardiac surgery. Upon initial evaluation, these patients are offered several options to help with recovery and healing. Some of these modalities include meditation, music therapy, yoga, massage, and therapeutic touch. Audiotapes can be used at various times in the perioperative period, including 5 to 10 days preoperatively, intraoperatively, immediately postoperatively, and during the recuperation phase. Therapeutic touch has been offered on the day of surgery and on postoperative days 2 and 3. Group yoga classes are offered to those patients who are medically stable as early as the third postoperative day. In addition, patients are encouraged to contact a religious leader of their choice. Continuation of these therapies is offered to the patient after hospital discharge. Patients can choose to attend sessions at the center or at a more convenient site.

The innovative approach used at the CCC resonates with the philosophy of increasing the patient's participation in his or her health and healing. Liu and colleagues (2000)[157] have reported on the use of CAM therapies in 376 consecutive patients undergoing cardiac surgery. Patients were surveyed before surgery, and 75% reported using CAM therapies. When prayer and vitamins were excluded, 44% reported using CAM therapies. Seventy-two percent of subjects were male, 76% were white, and 59% were well educated. No differences in overall CAM use were found among sex, age, race, or education level. The authors did offer an important recommendation. They noted that only 17% of patients had discussed their use of CAM therapies with their physicians, and 48% of patients did not want to discuss the topic at all. Since the frequency of CAM use found in this sample was consistent with the frequency of CAM use reported in the general population, the authors reinforced the importance of questioning patients about their use of CAM therapies.[158]

Evidence supporting the use of selected CAM therapies perioperatively is found in Table 27-8. Although methods were not always comprehensive in these studies, all demonstrated improvement in cardiovascular outcomes. In the study by Barnason and colleagues (1995)[160] the authors concluded that effects of the music therapy on outcomes were consistent with a relaxation response, and in the study by Garbossa (2009),[162] authors concluded that education and instruction in hospital routine significantly reduced preoperative anxiety when compared with control subjects.

In another small but clinically important study, Miller and Perry (1990)[163] examined the benefit of a deep-breathing relaxation technique on pain tolerance in patients undergoing cardiac surgery. On the evening before surgery, 15 subjects were taught a slow, rhythmic, deep-breathing relaxation technique in addition to traditional preoperative instruction. The remaining 14 subjects only received the traditional preoperative instruction. All subjects were visited by the investigators on the day of surgery and on postoperative day 1 for conversation; however, only subjects in the intervention group were encouraged to perform the relaxation technique. Patients in the relaxation group had significant decreases in systolic and diastolic BP, HR, RR, and self-report of pain (on visual descriptor scale) when compared with controls. The authors concluded that "relaxation techniques may interrupt the pain-anxiety cycle" and that, although there were methodological problems with their study, this "may be an effective non-narcotic, noninvasive pain-relieving modality after" cardiac surgery. Additional study of the relaxation response has demonstrated a reduction in postoperative arrhythmias, as well as reduced tension and anger in patients undergoing cardiac surgery.[32]

Congestive Heart Failure

There are a limited number of published investigations on the effects of CAM therapies in patients with congestive heart failure (CHF). Results of several papers are summarized in Table 27-9. It is of interest that two of these papers used several interventions to achieve improved outcomes. This may be of value, given the multiplicity of systems affected in CHF. Unfortunately, the degree of ventricular impairment was not documented in these studies. In addition, care must be taken when interpreting results of single case studies of patients with cardiac disease. The placebo effect evoked by the investigator's enthusiasm and expectation of success has been well studied in this population.[169,170] Symptomatic and objective improvements have been documented in angina outcomes related to pharmacological interventions and after sham cardiac surgical procedures.

Two studies listed in Table 27-9 discuss the impact of tai chi on patients with CHF.[167,168] The authors of both studies concluded that tai chi is a safe and effective adjunct in the usual

Table 27-8 **Effects of Selected CAM Therapies on Outcomes of Cardiovascular Surgery**

Study Authors	CAM Therapy	Sample Characteristics and Method	Outcome
Lan, 1999[159]	Tai chi	Prospective, 1-year program, 20 patients >3 months since CABG Age 53-64 years All males Tai chi group: 20 min w/up, 24 min tai chi, 10 min c/d; daily program Control group: walking program 10 min w/up, 30 min walking, 10 min c/d; 3 times per week $\dot{V}O_{2max}$ measured on cycle ergometer	Tai chi: increased $\dot{V}O_{2max}$; increased compliance with attendance
Barnason, 1995[160]	Music therapy	Prospective, random, repeated measures 96 subjects underwent elective CABG Age 37-84 years 65% male Three groups (music therapy, music-video therapy, rest group) 30-minute intervention on postoperative days 2 and 3 (inpatient)	Music therapy: improved mood; decreased heart rate; decreased SBP or DBP
Oxman, 1995[161]	Social support Religion	232 patients 21 deaths within 6 months of elective open heart surgery	Predictors of mortality: history of previous cardiac surgery; greater impairment in presurgery ADL; older age; lack of participation in social or community groups; absence of strength and comfort from religion
Garbossa, 2009[162]	Cognitive	51 patients undergoing CABG were randomized; 24 educated on CABG procedure preoperatively regarding what to expect; 27 received usual care	Preoperative anxiety was reduced in educated group compared with usual care No effect on length of stay in hospital

CABG, Coronary artery bypass graft surgery; *w/up*, warm-up; *c/d*, cool down; *ADL*, activities of daily living.

management of patients with CHF. Authors suggest large randomized controlled trials are warranted for this population. Finally, a pilot study involving the impact of "HeartMath" on patients with CHF was reported.[117] HeartMath includes a psychoeducational intervention that addresses "positive emotion refocusing and emotional restructuring."[109] Authors acknowledged that this intervention warrants further exploration; however, they concluded that improvements in emotional well-being carry over to improvements in functional capacity in patients with CHF.

Patients in the Coronary Care Unit

In two interesting, detailed, and well-designed studies, investigators examined the effects of intercessory prayer (praying for others) on outcomes of patients admitted to a coronary care unit.[171,172] With only slight differences in design, Harris and colleagues attempted to replicate the results that Byrd demonstrated a decade earlier. Both studies were large, randomized, controlled, blinded trials (Byrd with 393 subjects, Harris with 990 subjects). Patients were admitted to the coronary care unit (CCU) with a wide variety of diagnoses in both studies. In addition to common cardiac diagnoses, patients had conditions such as pneumonia, chronic obstructive lung disease, diabetes mellitus, renal failure, sepsis, liver disease, and gastrointestinal bleeding. Patients were monitored for new problems, new diagnoses, and new therapeutic interventions that occurred after hospital admission through discharge. This information contributed to the scoring systems used by investigators to determine distinctions between recovery rates and severity of complications during hospitalization. Intercessors in the Byrd study were "born again" Christian individuals, while intercessors in the Harris study represented a variety of Christian traditions, including 35% nondenominational, 27% Episcopalian, and Protestant or Roman Catholic observers. In the original study, Byrd assigned three to seven intercessors to each patient in the intervention group. Intercessors were asked to pray daily (until hospital discharge) for the individual's rapid recovery and prevention of complications, as well as contribute other prayers they believed would be beneficial to the patient. They were provided the patient's first name, diagnosis, general condition, and pertinent updated information. Harris and colleagues randomly assigned a five-member team to pray for each patient. Intercessors were not given any information about the patient. They were asked to pray daily for 28 days for a "speedy recovery with no complications" and anything else the intercessor believed appropriate. Results from both studies demonstrated statistically significant better outcomes in patients who were prayed for when compared with those not prayed for. Although in both studies the length of hospital stay was not significantly different between control and intervention groups, the CCU course severity scores were significantly different between control and intervention groups. Control subjects in the Byrd study required more frequent ventilatory assistance, antibiotics, and diuretics than subjects in the intervention group. Control subjects in the study by Harris and colleagues received higher scores on a scale quantifying severity of clinical outcomes from excellent to catastrophic than did subjects in the intervention group.

Table 27-9 **Effects of Selected CAM Therapies in CHF**

Study Authors	CAM Therapy	Sample Method and Characteristics	Outcome
Moser, 1997[164]	Skin-temperature biofeedback Relaxation Guided imagery	40 patients with advanced CHF Randomized to intervention (BFR) or control (C) BFR included 1 session of skin-temperature biofeedback, guided imagery of hand warmth, and progressive muscle relaxation C group underwent measurement session but no intervention	Baseline: comparable measurements between groups When comparing BFR with C, BFR showed: increased skin temperature in finger and foot; increased cardiac output; decreased systemic vascular resistance; decreased RR No changes in oxygen consumption or catecholamines were found in either group
Bernardi, 1998[165]	Complete yoga breathing	15 patients with CHF; 11 healthy volunteer controls (C) CHF patients were randomized to intervention (YB) or rest (R) YB included reduction of RR through controlled breathing (CB) and altered breathing pattern within each breath to include diaphragm, lower chest, then upper chest in inspiration and expiration, 1 hour per day for 1 month Measurements at baseline, end of 1 month and 1 month after completion Maximum symptom-limited cycle ergometer exercise test	Baseline: Sa_{O_2} was lower during spontaneous breathing (SB) in CHF compared with C; Sa_{O_2} instability was higher during SB in CHF compared with C At 1 month: Sa_{O_2} decreased during SB in YB compared with R, and approximated C during CB R results compared with YB: decreased sensation of dyspnea; decreased SB rate 13.4 ± 1.5 to 7.6 ± 1.9 bpm; Sa_{O_2} (%) increased 92.5 ± 0.3 to 93.2 ± 0.4; $\dot{V}o_{2max}$ increased 13.9 to 15.9 ± 0.8; maximum cycle workload increased 92 ± 6 to 100 ± 4 watts
Shinnick, 2002[166]	Meditation Acupuncture Qi gong	Case report 97-year-old terminally ill male Utilized interventions PRN	Qi gong used to increase body temperature Acupuncture to help sleep and improve appetite Meditation increased peacefulness, lucidity, and ability to control breathing
Luskin 2002[117]	Psychoeducational biofeedback (HeartMath, HM)	Pilot study; 33 patients, NYHA Class 1-3; mean age 66 years 8-week intervention (HM) or control (C) HM received 10 hours training over 10 weeks and home program ≥5x/day	When compared with C, HM decreased 22% perceived stress (C increased 7%) and decreased 34% depression (C increased 13%); HM significantly improved mental health and vitality on SF 36; HM increased 14% on 6 MWT (C decreased 2%)
Yeh G 2004[167]	Tai Chi	30 patients; NHYA Class 1-4; EF <40% (mean 23% ± 7%); mean age 64; 19 males Tai chi (TC) group received 1 hour tai chi 2x/week and usual care for 12 weeks, control (C) group received usual care Measurements were taken at baseline and at 12 weeks	Compared with C, TC group improved QOL, increased distance on 6MWT, decreased serum BNP; there was a trend to increase $\dot{V}o_{2peak}$
Barrow 2007[168]	Tai Chi Chuan and Chi Kung	52 patients; NYHA 2-3; mean age 68.9; 42 males Patients were randomized to receive 55 minutes of tai chi (TC) 2x/week or standard care (C), for 16 weeks	No difference was found in the Incremental Shuttle Walk Test between groups; significant improvement was found in TC group in symptom scores and reduction in depression scores

Sa_{O_2}, Oxygen saturation; *bpm*, breaths per minute; *PRN*, whenever needed; *6MWT*, 6 minute walk test; *$\dot{V}o_{2peak}$*, peak oxygen uptake; *QOL*, quality of life; *BNP*, brain naturietic peptide

The basis of this therapeutic effect of distance healing remained unexplained by the authors. The outcomes provided by these two randomized controlled clinical trials, however, warrant continued exploration into the possible benefits of intercessory prayer in medical outcomes. McCullough and colleagues (2000)[173] reported data from 42 publications in a metaanalysis examining the association of religious involvement to all-cause mortality. Their results resonate with those of the Byrd and Harris studies, and they concluded, from sampling more than 126,000 participants, that religious involvement was significantly associated with lower mortality rates. Similarly, they recommend that "elucidating the nature of this robust but poorly understood association could be a fruitful topic for future research at the interface of psychology and health."[173]

Music has been used as a method to induce relaxation in patients in the CCU. Bolwerk (1990)[174] presented 17 patients (11 males) with music therapy within the first 48 hours of CCU admission after experiencing an acute MI. Eighteen control patients (16 males) were given usual care. Anxiety levels were monitored in both groups within 48 hours of hospital admission and again 3 days later. Both groups were similar at baseline. Those patients in the intervention group received 3 consecutive days of 22 minutes of "relaxing, calming" music. At repeat testing, significantly greater reductions in anxiety scores were found in those individuals who received music therapy compared with the control group. Although there were significant limitations in the design of the study, the authors concluded that the repetitive nature of music can reduce anxiety in patients experiencing an acute MI.

Pulmonary Conditions

The basis for using CAM therapies in the management of individuals with cardiovascular and pulmonary disease is twofold. In addition to focusing treatment goals on the reduction of SNS stimulation and metabolic demands, CAM therapies also alter the mechanics of the musculoskeletal pump of the thorax. As addressed earlier in Part III of this book, improvements in thoracic mobility and movement efficiency contribute to reduced metabolic demands and improved oxygen transport.

Asthma

Numerous factors have been implicated as causative agents of asthma. In addition to respiratory infection and allergens, emotional stress has been identified as a trigger. Generalized panic symptoms have been found to be both a cause of asthma as well as a response to an exacerbation of asthma. Panic and anxiety states correlate with hyperventilation, a symptom closely related to a hyperactive respiratory drive. A heightened respiratory drive is not always favorable in individuals with known asthma because it can further challenge airways that are already bronchoconstricted.[81] Hyperventilation itself may exacerbate asthma because the rapid movement of cooler and dryer air into the airways can trigger further bronchoconstriction.

Repressive coping styles have also been associated with asthma morbidity.[81] Individuals with this behavior pattern typically ignore their symptoms, including dyspnea, and fail to seek timely health care. These individuals tend to have relatively high levels of endogenous opioids, neurochemicals that can depress unpleasant sensations. Consequently, these substances may limit an individual's ability to recognize early signs of bronchoconstriction. Additional evidence suggests that reduced immune system responsiveness in the setting of chronic emotional stress heightens inflammatory and infective processes, both of which are implicated in asthma exacerbation.

Numerous CAM therapies have been studied in attempts to reverse a number of these factors associated with asthma morbidity. Many of these studies have methodological shortcomings; however, several are well designed and provide insights into possible mechanisms of intervention efficacy. It is reported that between 4% and 79% of adults with asthma and between 33% and 89% of children with asthma use CAM therapies as part of their disease management regimen.[175] Relaxation therapy has been widely investigated; however, the results are inconsistent.[176,177] In a metaanalysis of six studies on the effects of relaxation training in children with emotionally triggered asthma, McQuaid and Nassau (1999)[178] concluded that "relaxation training is probably a most efficacious intervention" in this population. They noted concern regarding methods used in the articles reviewed and noted that only three of the studies reviewed in this analysis used appropriate controls, and only one examined maintenance of posttreatment effect. Although statistical significance was achieved in these investigations, the reduction of symptoms was less than 10% of baseline values, leading the authors to believe that the changes would not be clinically significant. Lehrer (1998)[81] also concluded that relaxation therapy may only be effective with specific asthma patients. His results indicate significant improvement in asthma exacerbation in individuals with emotionally triggered events when relaxation interventions are used. He noted worsening of symptoms when they were acute, however, and concluded that "relaxation training may provide protection from emotionally induced asthma"[81] when symptoms are chronic. Some theories regarding the failure of relaxation therapy to benefit individuals with asthma relate to its effect on the ANS. Evidence demonstrates that relaxation therapy downregulates the beta receptors of the SNS and thus reduces bronchodilation, an unfavorable outcome for individuals with asthma.

In a metaanalysis of 31 studies published between 1972 and 1993, Devine reported on the effects of psychoeducational care on adults with asthma. Psychoeducational interventions were defined as "education, behavioral skill development, cognitive therapy, and/or nonbehavioral support/counseling."[179] The author concluded that, despite methodological flaws primarily due to small numbers of subjects, education and relaxation-based behavioral interventions demonstrated improvement in clinical measures of pulmonary function. These measures included peak expiratory flow rate (PEFR), functional status, regimen compliance, use of medications, psychological well-being, and ability to use an inhaler properly. Similarly, a review of 12 well-designed studies investigating the effects of limited asthma education (information only) demonstrated a significant improvement in perceived asthma symptoms and reduced visits to the emergency department in adults with asthma.[180] In a controlled study of 35 children ages 5 to 6 years, researchers investigated the effects of a 6-month psychoeducational program that included guided imagery on several clinical and immunological outcomes associated with asthma control.[181] In addition to education classes and workshops for parents, daily instruction was given to the children to imagine visual images of unobstructed airways, mast cells, and immunoglobulin E (IgE) suppression. The results demonstrated significant reductions in the number of asthmatic episodes requiring medical attention and reduced bronchodilator requirements in the intervention group when compared with the control group. Spirometric values, specifically forced expiratory volume in 1 second (FEV_1), improved in the intervention group despite reduction in bronchodilator use. In addition, markers associated with immune system function (specific IgE levels, leukocyte surface markers, B cells) demonstrated improved efficiency. Conversely, a review of eight clinical trials investigating the effects of a limited asthma education program on more than 1400 children with asthma failed to demonstrate any reduction in emergency department visits or hospital admissions.[182] It appears that the addition of a guided imagery program to an asthma education program improves outcomes in children.

In a well-designed RCT of the effects of guided imagery on a group of adult patients with asthma, outcome measures failed to reveal statistically significant differences between intervention and control groups.[183] Measures of FEV_1, anxiety, depression, quality-of-life scales, and the number of visits to the emergency department were not different between groups.

Those subjects who practiced mental imagery, however, demonstrated statistically significant decreases in medication usage and reported feeling more power and control in their ability to change the course of their disease. Authors stressed the pilot nature of this study and concluded that if a larger sample was studied, more significant outcomes may have been achieved because there were trends favoring the mental imagery group in all outcome measures.

Preliminary study of the effects of the Alexander technique on measures of pulmonary function warrants further investigation.[184-186] To date, no controlled studies investigating the effects of this technique on individuals with asthma have been published. Although performing artists (musicians, singers, actors) with or without asthma reportedly benefit from this intervention, systematic study is lacking. Austin and Ausubel (1992)[184] documented improved pulmonary function measures in 10 healthy adults after 20 private sessions of therapy with the Alexander technique. No such improvement was found in 10 healthy adults in an untreated matched control group. Significant increases were demonstrated in PEFR, maximum voluntary ventilation (MVV), maximal inspiratory pressure (MIP), and maximal expiratory mouth pressure (MEP).

Both EMG and thermal biofeedback interventions have been studied in the management of asthma. Several of these interventions have been aimed at increasing HR. It has been postulated that by increasing HR, the accompanying increase in beta SNS activity produces increased bronchodilation. The few studies investigating this intervention have not been able to validate this theory due to design flaws.[81] Other trials of biofeedback have focused on general muscle relaxation and facial muscle relaxation. In a comprehensive review, McQuaid and Nassau (1999)[178] concluded that studies investigating biofeedback with general muscle relaxation demonstrate similar results as those trials using relaxation without biofeedback. These results are inconclusive and conflicting in individuals with asthma. Similarly, Ritz and colleagues (2004)[187] recently concluded in their review that studies addressing the use of biofeedback in the treatment of asthma were of poor quality and limited their ability to recommend this intervention. There is, however, strong evidence supporting the use of EMG biofeedback on the frontalis muscle of children with asthma.[178,188] Tension in this muscle has been correlated with increased airway resistance, presumably a consequence of a trigeminal-vagal reflex. Well-designed, carefully detailed studies examining reduced tension in facial muscles have demonstrated improvements in clinical measures of pulmonary function, including PEFR and asthma severity.[188]

The effects of yoga on asthma have been investigated by several authors. A summary of selected studies is found in Table 27-10. Results of these studies are still insufficient to draw sound conclusions. These initial trials, however, provide reasonable evidence supporting the use of yoga as complementary in the management of asthma. Although a discussion of breathing techniques is outside the scope of this chapter, there is evidence suggesting the value of certain interventions in asthma management.[193] Yoga breathing overlaps with some of these breathing exercises (e.g. slow, deep breathing mimics pranayama yoga exercise). In addition, Wronski (2008)[194] offered a preliminary discussion of the benefits of Pilates breathing in children with asthma.

Writing about emotionally traumatic events has been shown to have physical and psychological benefits. Smyth and colleagues (1999)[195] studied 58 adults with asthma (mean age 41 years). Subjects were randomized to an intervention group that was instructed to write about the most stressful event in their lives, while the control group wrote about an emotionally neutral event. Subjects were instructed to write for 20

Table 27-10 Effect of Yoga on Asthma

Study Authors	Type of Yoga	Sample Characteristics and Method	Outcomes
Tandon, 1978[189]	Yogic breathing exercises and posture	22 patients with severe chronic airway obstruction Matching groups of 11 subjects Yoga group (YG) and control group (CG) followed-up monthly for 9 months; CG received physiotherapy breathing	Compared with CG, the YG showed: significant increase in maximum work by 60.55 kpm; symptomatic improvement
Jain, 1991[190]	Yoga	46 young individuals with asthma Age 11-18 years All had history of childhood asthma Subjects acted as their own controls	Compared with baseline, significant increase in pulmonary function and exercise capacity At 2-year follow-up, reduced symptoms and drug requirements
Vedanthan, 1998[191]	Slow breathing (pranayama) Postures (asanas) Meditation	Adults with asthma Age 19-52 years 17 volunteers randomly divided into yoga (YG) and nonyoga groups (NYG) YG practiced 3 times per week for 16 weeks Both groups maintained daily symptom and medication diaries; AM and PM PEFR; weekly spirometry and questionnaires	Compared with NYG, the YG showed: significant degree of relaxation and positive attitude; better yoga exercise tolerance; trend towards decreased use of beta adrenergic inhalers; no difference in pulmonary function measures
Sodhi, 2009[192]	Yoga breathing	128 patients with mostly mild asthma randomized into 2 groups, 8 weeks of yoga training (YT) or control (C); PFT performed at baseline, 4 and 8 weeks	YT group increased % predicted PEFR, FEV_1, FVC, FEF_{25-75}, FEV_1/FVC when compared with C

minutes, on three consecutive days. At a 2-week follow-up, mean FEV_1 in the intervention group increased significantly from 63.9% of predicted values to 76.3% of predicted values. These statistically significant improvements were maintained at 2- and 4-month follow-up testing. No changes in FEV_1 were noted in the control group. Although the results of this study are complicated by the inclusion of subjects with rheumatoid arthritis, the authors offer strong preliminary evidence for the value of this writing intervention.

Most of the CAM therapies discussed thus far in the management of asthma have been mind/body techniques. Although there is a paucity of publications addressing the effects of body work on asthma, the effects of manual therapy on asthma have been reviewed.[196,197] In general, the methodological differences between all studies and the shortcomings of each individual study preclude any strong recommendation supporting the use of manual therapy in the treatment of asthma. Two of the studies reported on chiropractic manipulation as compared with sham maneuvers, and a third compared massage therapy with a relaxation control group. Significant improvement in measures of lung function was found in the massage therapy study. Two studies found no differences between intervention and control groups when chest physiotherapy was compared with placebo and when footzone (reflexology) therapy was compared with a no-treatment control group.

Acupuncture, a form of energy work, has been discussed extensively in the management of asthma. Several review studies and metaanalyses have been published addressing the effects of acupuncture on various outcomes related to asthma.[198-201] Inclusion criteria for an article to be reviewed in one of these publications consisted of randomized control design and measurement of objective pulmonary function outcomes, most often FEV_1. Significant disagreement exists among investigators regarding details of acupuncture interventions, including proper location of needles, depth of needle penetration, and frequency and duration of treatment.[202-205] There is general agreement, however, that strong evidence exists to support the *process* of inserting acupuncture needles into individuals with asthma. Medici and colleagues[204] have demonstrated that whether or not the actual point of needle insertion is considered proper is unessential. They successfully demonstrated that regardless of the site of needle insertion, certain physiological responses occur with acupuncture that improve pulmonary function in patients with asthma. They offer several possible rationales for the improvement—a direct physiological release of substances in response to the invasiveness of inserting the needles into the body, a physiological response triggered by the interaction between practitioner and subject (including the intention of the practitioner to heal the subject), or some other unknown, as yet undefined, factor. Hence most investigators conclude that more research is necessary to understand the complexities of acupuncture as an intervention and how it can best be prescribed in the treatment of asthma. It is important to note here that although very rare, there have been a few reports of pneumothorax and cardiac tamponade occurring consequent to needle insertion in the thorax.[206]

Preliminary evidence exists that qi gong may be an effective adjunct to medical management of asthma.[111] When pharmacological intervention is combined with qi gong, reported benefits include symptom reduction, improved immune system function, decreased sick leave and hospitalization days, decreased emergency department visits, and decreased antibiotic requirements for bronchial infections. These effects could result in a reduction in asthma-related morbidity and a substantial cost savings.

Chronic Obstructive Pulmonary Diseases

Pulmonary rehabilitation programs have been traditionally used as adjuncts to pharmacological management of chronic obstructive pulmonary disease (COPD). These programs generally consist of exercise training and a variety of educational and supportive interventions. Strong evidence has been shown to support pulmonary rehabilitation interventions in improving outcomes in patients with COPD.[207-211] These outcomes include reduced perception of dyspnea, increased work tolerance, and increased physical conditioning. Results, however, are inconsistent with regard to improvements in pulmonary function measures.

Devine and Pearcy (1996)[179] performed a metaanalysis of 65 studies investigating the effects of psychoeducational therapies in adults with COPD. For purposes of their analysis, they included education, exercise, and/or psychosocial support as psychoeducational therapies. Most of the articles were found in journals (66%) and dissertations (29%) and were published between 1954 and 1994. Of the studies, 34% were RCTs, 54% included a control group, and 15% had a placebo-type control. Data were included on 3642 individuals, with 72% reported as having COPD, 25% reported as having COPD or asthma, and 3% as having COPD, asthma, or other chronic pulmonary disease. Subjects ranged in age between 43 and 70 years, 81% of the studies had more men than women, and 19% had men only. Almost half of the studies were conducted in an outpatient setting, and about one-fourth were conducted in the inpatient hospital setting. The remaining studies involved various settings, including home.

Although the results of Devine and Pearcy's analysis revealed significant benefits of various interventions, the authors noted methodological weaknesses in many of the studies, including no mention of the duration of intervention in almost half of them. Statistically significant benefits of the various interventions are listed in Table 27-11. In general, education-only interventions were of benefit in improving the subject's knowledge of psychomotor skills. Relaxation-type interventions were effective in improving dyspnea and psychological well-being. An overwhelming benefit of pulmonary rehabilitation interventions was demonstrated in many studies. All of the pulmonary rehabilitation programs included in this analysis had education and large-muscle exercise components; 75% had breathing retraining; 57% had relaxation training; 54% had physical therapy; 43% had psychosocial support; 40% had occupational therapy; 29% had nutritional education; and 18% had vocational counseling. Although the results of this analysis begin to shed light on the benefits of individual interventions, more research is warranted. Recognition of the contribution of each of the specific CAM therapies offered within the umbrella of pulmonary rehabilitation may be difficult. This is consistent with Devine and Pearcy's conclusion that further research efforts to break down interventions within pulmonary rehabilitation may not be clinically wise, given the complex needs of these patients.

In a recent review of psychological interventions for individuals with cystic fibrosis (CF), Glasscoe and Quittner

Table 27-11 **Effect of Various Psychoeducational Interventions on Outcomes in Individuals with COPD**

Outcome Variable and Measurement	Number of Studies	Statistically Significant Beneficial Interventions	Nonstatistically Beneficial Interventions
Psychological well-being (e.g., anxiety, mood questionnaires)	26	Relaxation-type therapy Pulmonary rehabilitation	Education only
Endurance (e.g., time/distance able to exercise)	16	Pulmonary rehabilitation	Education
Oxygen uptake ($\dot{V}O_{2max}$)	8	Vigorous exercise (e.g., 60 minutes of supervised exercise 3 times per week for 9 weeks)	Mild exercise (e.g., 10 minutes of exercise 3 times per day)*
Functional status (e.g., sickness impact profile)	—	Pulmonary rehabilitation Breathing exercise and large muscle exercises	Education only
Dyspnea (visual analogue scales)	—	Pulmonary rehabilitation Progressive muscle relaxation	Guided imagery
Pulmonary function (static volumes and FEV_1)	—	Static volumes improved Pulmonary rehabilitation	FEV_1 no change Education only relaxation/imagery Pulmonary rehabilitation
Knowledge of psychomotor skills (e.g., accurate inhaler use)	—	Education only	
Adherence (self-reports, provider assessed compliance)	—	Pulmonary rehabilitation	Education only
Utilization of health care (e.g., ED visits, hospitalizations and LOS)	—	Pulmonary rehabilitation	Education only

ED, Emergency department; *LOS*, length of stay.

*Significant negative effect.

Based on data from Devine EC, Pearcy J: Meta-analysis of the effects of psychoeducational care in adults with chronic obstructive pulmonary disease, Patient Education and Counseling *29:167–178, 1996.*

(2009)[212] found 13 randomized controlled trials studying 529 pooled participants. Interventions were primarily behavioral or educational and focused on promoting improved quality of life and knowledge for effective disease management. Patients and family members demonstrated improvement in emotional and knowledge-based outcomes; no consistent lung function measurement outcomes were noted.

Intuitively, yoga would seem a beneficial adjunct to the medical management of COPD. Components of yoga include slow breathing, or pranayama, and body positions, or asanas. At times meditation is included as well. Unfortunately, investigation of the effects of yoga on COPD is in its infancy and is still mostly anecdotal.[213] The reports include improved perceptions of dyspnea and decreased anxiety.

Similarly, singing therapy would appear to benefit individuals with breathing impairments. Irons (2010a; 2010b)[214,215] performed two appropriate literature reviews to study this: one to determine the effects of singing therapy on individuals with bronchiectasis, and one on individuals with CF. No studies were found for either population. Alternatively, music therapy, used primarily for relaxation, has been found effective as a complement to chest physical therapy in toddlers with CF[216] and in adults with infectious lung diseases.[217] In a recent review, Huth (2005)[218] reported on the benefits of massage therapy in the same populations. Individuals with CF and those with chronic lung disease demonstrated reduction in anxiety and improved measures of pulmonary function after 2 to 4 weeks of a 20-minute intervention. Further research is needed because these studies were small and had numerous methodological limitations.

Lung Cancer

Two large and thorough reviews recently reported on noninvasive interventions used for patients with lung cancer.[219,220] Only randomized controlled trials were included, and several of the studies analyzed were common to both reviews. Sola (2009)[220] categorized studies into six groups according to intervention, including the use of treatments for breathlessness, structured nursing support programs, nutritional intervention, psychotherapeutic interventions, exercise, and reflexology. Primary outcome measures were well-being and quality of life. Measures of pulmonary function were not reported; measures of functional activity were reported in two studies. All studies reported significant improvement in well-being or in quality of life in the intervention groups when compared with controls. When breathlessness was the primary outcome measure, all studies also reported significant improvement in the intervention group when compared with controls.[219] Interventions for breathlessness included individualized counseling and psychosocial support, breathing control training, relaxation and anxiety management, and activity pacing. The authors of both reviews recommended caregiver training for this population given the many components of intervention required to effectively tailor a noninvasive program for each individual. They also suggested large, well-designed, higher-quality studies in the future.

Summary

This chapter has several purposes: (1) to introduce the reader to complementary therapies in general, (2) to define several of the common complementary therapies found in rehabilitation and then examine the literature on the effects of these therapies on the normal cardiovascular and pulmonary systems, and (3) to discuss the efficacy of the use of these complementary therapies with patients with cardiovascular and pulmonary pathologies. The quality of evidence found in the literature is inconsistent, with designs representing the entire research spectrum, from individual case studies to large and well-designed RCTs. The most sophisticated studies found were those investigating the efficacy of tai chi, yoga, acupuncture, intercessory prayer, and psychoeducational group work on various cardiovascular and pulmonary conditions, including CAD, CHF, cardiac surgery, COPD, asthma, and HTN.

Given the widespread presence of cardiovascular and pulmonary illness in our society and the fact that people are using complementary therapies, it is essential that therapists be adequately prepared to understand, administer, and correctly interpret responses to these interventions and that they strive to conduct and publish the required research to establish efficacy.

Review Questions

1. Describe the cardiovascular and pulmonary responses to mind/body therapies in healthy individuals and discuss how these responses may be helpful or harmful to patients with cardiac or pulmonary diseases.
2. Identify three CAM therapies that include components of traditional physical therapy (e.g., yoga, tai chi, biofeedback, massage, Alexander method) and compare and contrast goals of the CAM therapies with goals of traditional physical therapy relative to the cardiovascular and pulmonary systems.
3. Choose three forms of energy work therapies and discuss their (possible) effects on the cardiovascular and pulmonary systems.
4. Design a study investigating the effects of one energy work intervention and one manual therapy/body work intervention on cardiovascular and pulmonary responses in individuals with cardiac or pulmonary disease.
5. Choose a cardiovascular and pulmonary diagnosis and describe how you would plan a program using CAM therapies to help treat a patient with the diagnosis.

References

1. Davis CM, editor: *Complementary therapies in rehabilitation. Evidence for efficacy in therapy, prevention and wellness*, ed 2. Thorofare, NJ, 2009, SLACK, Inc.
2. Lipton BH: *The biology of belief*, Santa Rosa, Calif, 2005, Elite Books.
3. Waterland RA, Jirtle RL: Transposable elements: targets for early nutritional effects on epigenetic gene regulation. *Molecular and Cell Biology* 23(15):5293–5300, 2003.
4. Oschman JL: Breakthrough in subtle energies and energy medicine. *Bridges* 16:5–9, 2003.
5. Ridker PM, Cushman M, Stampfer MJ, et al: Inflammation, aspirin, and the risk of cardiovascular disease in apparently healthy men. *New England Journal of Medicine* 336:973–979, 1997.
6. Ridker PM, Hennekens CH, Buring JE, et al: C-Reactive protein and other markers of inflammation in the prediction of cardiovascular disease in women. *New England Journal of Medicine* 342:836–843, 2000.
7. Hunt V: *Infinite mind: The science of the human vibrations of consciousness*, Malibu, CA, 1989, Malibu Publishing Co.
8. Rubik B: Energy medicine and the unifying concept of information. *Alternative Therapies in Health and Medicine* 1:34–39, 1995.
9. Oschman JL: Charge transfer in the living matrix. *J. Bodywork and Movement Therapies* 13:215–228, 2009.
10. Oschman JL: *Energy medicine: The scientific basis*, New York, 2000, Churchill Livingstone.
11. Ornish D, Brown SE, Billings JH, et al: Can lifestyle changes reverse coronary heart disease? *Lancet* 336:129–133, 1990.
12. Wallace RK, Benson H, Wilson AF: A wakeful hypometabolic physiologic state. *American Journal of Physiology* 221:795–799, 1971.
13. Ader R, Cohen N: The influence of conditioning on immune responses. In Ader R, Felten D.L, Cohen N, editors: *Psychoneuroimmunology*, ed 2, San Diego, 1991, Academic Press.
14. Pert C: *Molecules of emotion*, New York, 1997, Scribner.
15. Kaptchuk TJ: Historical context of the concept of vitalism in complementary and alternative medicine. In Micozzi MS, editor: *Fundamentals of complementary and alternative medicine*, New York, 1996, Churchill Livingstone.
16. Holden C: Future brightening for depression treatments. *Science* 302:810–813, 2003.
17. Kopp MS, Rethelyi J: Where psychology meets physiology: chronic stress and premature mortality: The Central-Eastern European health paradox. *Brain Research Bulletin* 62:351–367, 2004.
18. Waechter RL, Sergio L: Manipulation of the electromagnetic spectrum via fields projected from human hands: A Qi energy connection? *Subtle Energies and Energy Medicine* 13:233–250, 2004.
19. Zimmerman J: Laying on of hands healing and therapeutic touch: A testable theory. *BEMI Currents, Journal of the Bio-Electro-Magnetics Institute* 2:8–17, 1990.
20. Seto A, Kusaka C, Nakazato S, et al: Detection of extraordinary large bio-magnetic field strength from human hands. *Acupuncture and Electro-therapeutics Research International Journal* 17:75–94, 1992.
21. Mehl-Madrona L: Connectivity and healing: Some hypotheses about the phenomenon and how to study it. *Advances in Mind Body Medicine* 21:12–28, 2005.
22. Jonas WB, Crawford CC: Science and spiritual healing: a critical review of spiritual healing, "energy medicine" and intentionality. *Alternative Therapy* 9:56–61, 2003.
23. Luskin FM, Newell KA, Griffith M, et al: A review of mind/body therapies in the treatment of musculoskeletal disorders with implications for the elderly. *Alternative Therapies* 6:46–56, 2000.
24. Spencer JW, Jacobs JJ, editors: *Complementary and alternative medicine: An evidence based approach*, St Louis, 1999, Mosby.
25. Wolf SL, Barnhart HX, Ellison GL, et al: The effect of tai chi chuan and computerized balance training on postural stability in older subjects. *Physical Therapy* 77:371–383, 1997.
26. Hunt V: *Infinite mind—the science of the human vibrations of consciousness*, Malibu, CA, 1989, Malibu Publishing Co.
27. Schwartz G, Russek L: Dynamical energy systems and modern physics: Fostering the science and spirit of complementary and alternative medicine. *Alternative Therapies* 3:46–56, 1997.
28. Pert CB, Ruff MR, Weber RJ, et al: Neuropeptides and their receptors: A psychosomatic network. *Journal of Immunology* 35(Suppl 2):820s–826s, 1985.
29. Leskowitz E, Marcozi M: *Complimentary and alternative medicine in rehabilitation*, New York, 2003, Churchill Livingstone.
30. Astin JA, Shapiro SL, Eisenberg DM, et al: Mind-body medicine: State of the science, implications for practice. *Journal of the American Board of Family Practice* 16:131–147, 2003.
31. Spencer JW, Jacobs JJ, editors: *Complementary and alternative medicine: An evidence-based approach*, ed 2, St. Louis, 2003, Mosby.
32. Luskin FM, Newell KA, Griffith M, et al: A review of mind-body therapies in the treatment of cardiovascular disease. Part I: Implications for the elderly. *Alternative Therapy Health Medicine* 4:46–61, 1998.
33. Levy JK: Standard and alternative adjunctive treatments in cardiac rehabilitation. *Texas Heart Institute Journal* 20:198–212, 1993.

34. Wang JS, Lan C, Chen SY, et al: Tai chi chuan training is associated with enhanced endothelium-dependent dilation in skin vasculature of healthy older men. *Journal of American Geriatrics Society* 50:1024–1030, 2002.
35. Mamtani R, Mamtani R: Ayurveda and yoga in cardiovascular diseases. *Cardiology in Review* 13(3):155–162, 2005.
36. Cheng TO: Tai chi: The Chinese ancient wisdom of an ideal exercise for cardiac patients. *International Journal of Cardiology* 117:293–295, 2007.
37. Ives JC, Sosnoff J: Beyond the mind-body exercise hype. *The Physician and Sportsmedicine* 28:67–83, 2000.
38. Lin MC, Nahin R, Gershwin E, et al: State of complementary and alternative medicine in cardiovascular, lung, and blood research. *Circulation* 103:2038–2041, 2001.
39. Wong SS, Nahin RL: National Center for Complementary and Alternative Medicine Perspectives for Complementary and Alternative Medicine Research in Cardiovascular Diseases. *Cardiology in Review* 11(2):94–98, 2003.
40. Nahin RL: Identifying and pursuing research priorities at the National Center for Complementary and Alternative Medicine. *The FASEB Journal* 19:1209–1215, 2005.
41. Schneider D, Leung R: Metabolic and cardiorespiratory responses to the performance of wing chun and tai chi chuan exercises. *International Journal of Sports Medicine* 12:319–323, 1991.
42. Lan C, Chen SY, Lai JS, et al: Heart rate responses and oxygen consumption during tai chi chuan practice. *American Journal of Chinese Medicine* 29:403–410, 2001.
43. Brown DD, Mucci WG, Hetzler RK, et al: Cardiovascular and ventilatory responses during formalized tai chi chuan exercise. *Research Quarterly for Exercise and Sport* 60:246–250, 1989.
44. Fontana JA: The energy costs of a modified form of tai chi exercise. *Nursing Research* 49:91–96, 2000.
45. Chao YF, Chen SY, Lan C, et al: The cardiorespiratory response and energy expenditure of tai-chi-qui-gong. *American Journal of Chinese Medicine* 30:451–462, 2002.
46. Jin P: Changes in heart rate noradrenaline, cortisol and mood during tai chi. *Journal of Psychosomatic Research* 33:197–206, 1989.
47. Lai JS, Wong MK, Lan C, et al: Cardiorespiratory responses of tai chi chuan practitioners and sedentary subjects during cycle ergometry. *Journal of the Formosan Medical Association Taiwan Ti Zhi* 92:894–899, 1993.
48. Lai JS, Lan C, Wong MK, et al: Two-year trends in cardiorespiratory function among older tai chi chuan practitioners and sedentary subjects. *Journal of American Geriatrics Society* 43:1222–1227, 1995.
49. Lan C, Lai JS, Wong MK, et al: Cardiorespiratory function, flexibility, and body composition among geriatric tai chi chuan practitioners. *Archives of Physical Medical Rehabilitation* 77:612–616, 1996.
50. Lan C, Lai JS, Chen SY, et al: 12-month tai chi training in the elderly: its effect on health fitness. *Medicine and Science in Sports and Exercise* 30:345–351, 1998.
51. Thomas GN, Hong AWL, Tomlinson B, et al: Effects of Tai chi and resistance training on cardiovascular risk factors in elderly Chinese subjects: a 12-month longitudinal, randomized, controlled intervention study. *Clinical Endocrinology* 63:663–669, 2005.
52. Hui SSC, Woo J, Kwok T: Evaluation of energy expenditure and cardiovascular health effects from Tai Chi and walking exercise. *Hong Kong Medical Journal* 15(1) Suppl Feb 2, 2009.
53. Young DR, Appel LJ, Jee SH, et al: The effects of aerobic exercise and tai chi on blood pressure in older people: Results of a randomized trails. *Journal of American Geriatrics Society* 47:277–284, 1999.
54. Thornton EW, Sykes KS, Tang WK: Health benefits of tai chi exercise: Improved balance and blood pressure in middle-aged women. *Health Promotion International* 19(1):33–38, 2004.
55. Chen K-M, Lin J-N, Lin, H-S, et al: The effects of a simplified tai-chi exercise program (STEP) on the physical health of older adults living in long-term care facilities: A single group design with multiple time points. *International Journal of Nursing Studies.* Doi:10.1016/j.ijnurstu.2006.11.008. 2006.
56. Raub JA: Psychophysiologic effects of Hatha Yoga on musculoskeletal and cardiopulmonary function: A literature review. *The Journal of Alternative and Complementary Medicine* 8(6):797–812, 2002.
57. Jayasinghe SR: Yoga in cardiac health (A review). *European Journal of Cardiovascular Prevention and Rehabilitation* 11:369–375, 2004.
58. Galantino ML, Galbavy R, Quinn L: Therapeutic effects of yoga for children: a systematic review of the literature. *Pediatric Physical Therapy* 20:66–80, 2008.
59. Birdee GS, Yeh GY, Wayne PM, et al: Clinical applications of yoga for the pediatric populations: a systematic review. *Academae Pediatrics* 9(4):212–220, 2009.
60. Telles S, Desiraju T: Autonomic changes in Brahmakumaris Raja yoga meditation. *International Journal of Psychophysiology* 15:147–152, 1993.
61. Schell FJ, Allilio B, Schonecke OW: Physiological and psychological effects of hatha-yoga exercise in healthy women. *International Journal of Psychosomatics* 41:46–52, 1994.
62. Ray US, Sinha B, Tomer OS, et al: Aerobic capacity and perceived exertion after practice of hatha yoga exercises. *Indian Journal of Medical Research* 114:215–221, 2001.
63. Telles S, Reddy SK, Nagendra HR: Oxygen consumption and respiration following two yoga relaxation techniques. *Applied Psychophysiology and Biofeedback* 25:221–227, 2000.
64. Knowles C, Hamilton K: Effects of yoga poses and breathing exercises on vital capacity in a healthy middle-aged man. *Cardiopulmonary Physical Therapy* 14:25, 2003.
65. Haggins M, Moore W, Rundle A: Does practicing hatha yoga satisfy recommendations for intensity of physical activity which improves and maintains health and cardiovascular fitness? *BMC Complementary and Alternative Medicine.* 7:40–49, 2007.
66. Uchino BN, Cacioppo JT, Kiecolt-Glaser JK: The relationship between social support and physiological processes: a review with emphasis on underlying mechanisms and implications for health. *Psychological Bulletin* 119:488–531, 1996.
67. Holland B, Pokorny ME: Slow stroke back massage: its effect on patients in a rehabilitation setting. *Rehabilitation Nursing* 26:182–186, 2001.
68. Cottingham JT, Porges SW, Richmond K: Shifts in pelvic inclination angle and parasympathetic tone produced by Rolfing soft tissue manipulation. *Physical Therapy* 68:1364–1370, 1988b.
69. Cottingham JT, Porges SW, Lyon T: Effects of soft tissue mobilization (Rolfing pelvic lift) on parasympathetic tone in two age groups. *Physical Therapy* 68:352–356, 1988a.
70. Wirth-Pattullo V, Hayes KW, Echternach JL, et al: Interrater reliability of craniosacral rate measurements and their relationship with subjects' and examiners' heart and respiratory rate measurements. *Physical Therapy* 74:16–29, 1994.
71. Green C, Martin CW, Bassett K, et al: A systematic review and critical appraisal on the scientific evidence in craniosacral therapy. *Database of Abstracts of Reviews of Effectiveness* 2:2004.
72. Hinman MR: Comparative effect of positive and negative static magnetic fields on heart rate and blood pressure in healthy adults. *Clinical Rehabilitation* 16:669–674, 2002.
73. Martel GF, Andrews SC, Roseboom CG: Comparison of static and placebo magnets on resting forearm blood flow in young, healthy men. *Journal of Orthopaedic and Sports Physical Therapy* 32:518–524, 2002.
74. Wardell DW, Engebretson J: Biological correlates of Reiki touch healing. *Journal of Advanced Nursing* 33:439–445, 2001.
75. Wetzel W: Reiki healing: A physiologic perspective. *Journal of Holistic Nursing* 7:47–54, 1989.
76. Olson K, Hanson J, Michaud M: A phase II trial of Reiki for the management of pain in advanced cancer patients. *Journal of Pain and Symptom Management* 26:990–997, 2003.
77. Lee MS, Kim BG, Huh HJ, et al: Effect of qi-training on blood pressure, heart rate and respiration rate. *Clinical Physiology* 20:173–176, 2000.
78. Hiller H, Weissberg N, Horowitz G, et al: The safety of dental mini-magnets in patients with permanent cardiac pacemakers. *Journal of Prosthetic Dentistry* 74:420–421, 1995.
79. Haker E, Egekvist H, Bjerring P: Effect of sensory stimulation (acupuncture) on sympathetic and parasympathetic activities in healthy subjects. *Journal of the Autonomic Nervous System* 79:52–59, 2000.
80. Rosa L, Rosa E, Sarner L, et al: A close look at therapeutic touch. *Journal of the American Medical Association* 279:1005–1010, 1998.
81. Lehrer PM: Emotionally triggered asthma: A review of research literature and some hypotheses for self-regulation therapies. *Applied Psychology and Biofeedback* 23:13–41, 1998.
82. Haas F, Distenfeld S, Axen K: Effects of perceived musical rhythm on respiratory pattern. *Journal of Applied Physiology* 61:1185–1191, 1986.
83. Taylor-Pilliae RE, Haskell WL, Froelicher ES: Hemodynamic responses to a community-based tai chi exercise intervention in ethnic Chinese adults with cardiovascular disease risk factors. *European Journal of Cardiovascular Nursing* 5:165–174, 2006.
84. Yeh GY, Wang C, Wayne PM, et al: Tai chi exercise for patients with cardiovascular conditions and risk factors: A systematic review. *Journal of Cardiopulmonary Rehabilitation Prevention* 29(3):152–160, 2009.
85. Pratt C: Alternative Prevention and Treatment of Cardiovascular Disease. *Primary Care Clinics Office Practice* 37:325–337, 2010 Part I.

86. Benson H, Kotch JB, Crassweller KD: The relaxation response: A bridge between psychiatry and medicine. *Medical Clinics of North America* 61:929–938, 1977.
87. Schiller AD: Meditation. In Lescowitz E, Marcozi M, editor: *Complementary and alternative medicine in rehabilitation*, New York, 2003, Churchill Livingstone.
88. Rozanski A, Blumenthal JA, Kaplan J: Impact of psychological factors on the pathogenesis of cardiovascular disease and implications for therapy. *Circulation* 99:2192–2217, 1999.
89. Eppley KR, Abrams AI, Shear J: Differential effects of relaxation techniques on trait anxiety: A meta-analysis. *Journal of Clinical Psychology* 45:957–974, 1989.
90. Miller JJ, Fletcher K, Kabat-Zinn J: Three-year follow-up and clinical implications of a mindfulness meditation-based stress reduction intervention in the treatment of anxiety disorders. *General Hospital Psychiatry* 17:192–200, 1995.
91. Infante JR, Torres-Avisbal M, Pinel P, et al: Catecholamine levels in practitioners of the transcendental meditation technique. *Physiology and Behavior* 72:141–146, 2001.
92. Schneider RH, Nidich SI, Salerno JW, et al: Lower lipid peroxide levels in practitioners of the transcendental meditation program. *Psychosomatic Medicine* 60:38–41, 1998.
93. McCrone SH, Brendle D, Barton K: A multibehavioral intervention to decrease cardiovascular disease risk factors in older men. *American Association of Critical-Care Nurses* 12:5–16, 2001.
94. Jin P: Efficacy of tai chi, brisk walking, meditation, and reading in reducing mental and emotional stress. *Journal of Psychosomatic Research* 36:361–370, 1992.
95. Kolt GS, McConville JC: The effects of a Feldenkrais(tm) awareness through movement program on state anxiety. *Journal of Bodywork and Movement Therapies* 4:216–220, 2000.
96. Hanley J, Stirling P, Brown C: Randomized controlled trial of therapeutic massage in the management of stress. *British Journal of General Practice* 53:20–25, 2003.
97. Kalayil JA: A controlled comparison of progressive relaxation and yoga meditation as methods to relieve stress in middle grade school children. *Dissertation Abstracts International* 49:3626, 1989.
98. Spence JD, Barnett PA, Linden W, et al: Recommendations on stress management. *Canadian Medical Association Journal* 160:S46-S50, 1999.
99. Eisenberg DM, Delbanco TL, Berkey CS, et al: Cognitive behavioral techniques for hypertension. *Annals of Internal Medicine* 118:964–972, 1993.
100. Schneider RH, Staggers F, Alexander CN, et al: A randomized controlled trail of stress reduction for hypertension in older African Americans. *Hypertension* 26:820. 1995.
101. Barnes VA, Treiber FA, Davis H: Impact of transcendental meditation on cardiovascular function at rest and during acute stress in adolescents with high normal blood pressure. *Journal of Psychosomatic Research* 51:597–605, 2001.
102. Shapiro D, Hui KK, Oakley ME, et al: Reduction in drug requirements for hypertension by means of a cognitive-behavioral intervention. *American Journal of Hypertension* 10:9–17, 1997.
103. Yucha CB, Clark L, Smith M, et al: The effect of biofeedback in hypertension (structured abstract). *Database of Abstracts of Reviews of Effectiveness* 2, 2004.
104. Wang C, Collet JP, Lau J: The effect of tai chi on health outcomes in patients with chronic conditions. *Archives of Internal Medicine* 164:493–501, 2004.
105. Paran E, Amir M, Yaniv N: Evaluating the response of mild hypertensives to biofeedback-assisted relaxation using a mental stress test. *Journal of Behavior Therapy and Experimental Psychiatry* 27:157–167, 1996.
106. Patel C: 12-month follow-up of yoga and biofeedback in the management of hypertension. *Lancet* 1:62–64, 1975.
107. Brownstein AH, Dembert ML: Treatment of essential hypertension with yoga relaxation therapy in a USAF aviator: A case report. *Aviation, Space, and Environment Medicine* 60:684–687, 1989.
108. Zucker PB: The effects of qi gong on resting systemic blood pressure and quality of life in hypertensive adults. *Cardiopulmonary Physical Therapy* 8:24, 1997.
109. McCraty R, Atkinson M, Tomasino D: Impact of a workplace stress reduction program on blood pressure and emotional health in hypertensive employees. *The Journal of Alternative and Complementary Medicine* 9(3):355–369, 2003.
110. Levin JS, Vanderpool HY: Is religion therapeutically significant for hypertension? *Social Science Medicine* 29:69–78, 1989.
111. Sancier KM: Therapeutic benefits of qigong exercises in combination with drugs. *The Journal of Alternative and Complementary Medicine* 5:383–389, 1999.
112. Mayer M: Qigong and hypertension: a critique of research. *The Journal of Alternative and Complementary Medicine* 5:371–382, 1999.
113. Yeh FY, Wang C, Wayne PM, et al: The effect of tai chi exercise on blood pressure: A systematic review. *Preventive Cardiology* 11:82–89, 2008.
114. Lee MS, Lee E-N, Kim J-I, et al: Tai chi for lowering resting blood pressure in the elderly: A systematic review. *Journal of Evaluation in Clinical Practice* 16:818–824, 2010.
115. Kim L-W, Zhu J: Acupuncture for essential hypertension. *Alternative Therapies* 16(2):18–29, 2010.
116. Haskell WL, Luskin FM, Marvasti FF: Atheroscleortic vascular disease. In Spencer J, Jacobs J, editors: *Complementary and alternative medicine: An evidence-based approach*, ed 2, St. Louis, 2003, Mosby.
117. Luskin F, Reitz M, Newell K, et al: A controlled pilot study of stress management training of elderly patients with congestive heart failure. *Preventive Cardiology* 5(4):168–176, 2002.
118. Kranitz L, Lehrer P: Biofeedback applications in the treatment of cardiovascular diseases. *Cardiology in Review* 12(3):177–181, 2004.
119. Walton KG, Schneider RH, Nidich S: Review of controlled research on the transcendental meditation program and cardiovascular disease. *Cardiology in Review* 12(5):262–266, 2004.
120. Moravec CS: Biofeedback therapy in cardiovascular disease: Rationale and research overview. *Cleveland Clinic Journal of Medicine* 75(Suppl 2):S35–S38, 2008.
121. Nolan RP, Jong P, Barry-Bianchi SM, et al: Effects of drug, biobehavioral and exercise therapies on heart rate variability in coronary artery disease: a systematic review. *European Journal Cardiovascular Prevention and Rehabilitation* 15:386–396.
122. McCraty R: Coherence: Bridging personal, social, and global health. *Alternative Therapies* 16(4):10–24, 2010.
123. Arthur HM, Patterson C, Stone J: The role of complementary and alternative therapies in cardiac rehabilitation: A systematic evaluation. *European Journal Cardiovascular Prevention and Rehabilitation* 13(1):3–9, 2006.
124. Yeh GY, Davis RB, Phillips RS: Use of complementary therapies in patients with cardiovascular disease. *American Journal of Cardiology* 98:673–680, 2006.
125. Pratt C: Alternative prevention and treatment of cardiovascular disease. *Primary Care Clinics Office Practice* 37:339–366, 2010 Part II.
126. Friedman M, Rosenman RH: Association of specific overt behavior pattern with blood and cardiovascular findings. *Journal of the American Medical Association* 169:1286, 1959.
127. Friedman M, Thoresen CE, Gill JJ, et al: Alteration of type A behavior and its effect on cardiac recurrence in post myocardial infarction patients: Summary results of the recurrent coronary prevention project. *American Heart Journal* 112:653–665, 1986.
128. Dusseldorp E, van Elderen T, Maes S, et al: A meta-analysis of psychoeducational programs for coronary heart disease patients. *Health Psychology* 18:506–519, 1999.
129. Linden W, Stossel C, Maurice J: Psychosocial interventions for patients with coronary artery disease. *Archives of Internal Medicine* 156:745–752, 1996.
130. Balady GJ, Ades PA, Comoss P, et al: Core components of cardiac rehabilitation/secondary prevention programs: A statement for healthcare professionals from the American Heart Association and the American Association of Cardiovascular and Pulmonary Rehabilitation. *Circulation* 102:1069–1073, 2000.
131. Stone PH, Krantz DS, McMahon RP, et al: Relationship among mental stress-induced ischemia and ischemia during daily life and during exercise: The psychophysiologic investigations of myocardial ischemia study. *Journal of the American College of Cardiology* 33:1476–1484, 1999.
132. Sullivan MD, LaCroix AZ, Spertus JA, et al: Five-year prospective study of the effects of anxiety and depression in patients with coronary artery disease. *American Journal of Cardiology* 86:1135–1138, 2000.
133. Blumenthal JA, Jiang W, Babyak MA, et al: Stress management and exercise training in cardiac patients with myocardial ischemia. *Archives of Internal Medicine* 157:2113–2223, 1997.
134. Blumenthal JA, Babyak M, Wei J, et al: Usefulness of psychosocial treatment of mental stress-induced myocardial ischemia in men. *American Journal of Cardiology* 89:164–168, 2002.
135. Zamarra JW, Schneider RH, Besseghini I, et al: Usefulness of the transcendental meditation program in the treatment of patients with coronary artery disease. *American Journal of Cardiology* 77:867–870, 1996.

136. Benson H, Alexander S, Feldman CL: Decreased premature ventricular contractions through use of the relaxation response in patients with stable ischemic heart-disease. *Lancet* 306:380–382, 1975.
137. Villagomeza LR: Mending broken hearts. The role of spirituality in cardiac illness: A research synthesis, 1991-2004. *Holistic Nursing Practice* 20(4):169–186, 2006.
138. Jones DA, West RR: Psychological rehabilitation after myocardial infarction: Multicentre randomized controlled trail. *British Medical Journal* 313:1517–1521, 1996.
139. Collins JA, Rice VH: Effects of relaxation in phase II cardiac rehabilitation: Replication and extension. *Journal of Acute and Critical Care* 26:31–44, 1997.
140. Manchanda SC, Narang R, Reddy KS, et al: Retardation of coronary atherosclerosis with yoga lifestyle intervention. *Journal of the Association of Physicians of India* 48:687–694, 2000.
141. Friedlander Y, Kark JD, Stein Y: Religious orthodoxy and myocardial infarction in Jerusalem: A case control study. *International Journal of Cardiology* 10:33–41, 1986.
142. Strawbridge WJ, Cohen RD, Shema SJ, et al: Frequent attendance at religious services and mortality over 28 years. *American Journal of Public Health* 87:957–961, 1997.
143. Chang RY, Koo M, Kan KM, et al: Effects of tai chi rehabilitation on heart rate responses in patients with coronary artery disease. *American Journal of Chinese Medicine* 38(3):461–472, 2010.
144. Park IS, Song R, Oh KO, et al: Managing cardiovascular risks with tai chi in people with coronary artery disease. *Journal of Advanced Nursing* 66(2):282–292, 2009.
145. Lee KM: The use of tai chi for improving the health status of older adults. GeriNotes: Section on Geriatrics. *American Physical Therapy Association* 11:9–14, 2004.
146. Wayne PM, Krebs DE, Wolf SL, et al: Can tai chi improve vestibulopathic postural control? *Archives of Physical Medical Rehabilitation* 85:142–152, 2004.
147. Taylor-Piliae RE: Tai chi as an adjunct to cardiac rehabilitation exercise training. *Journal of Cardiopulmonary Rehabilitation* 23:90–96, 2003.
148. Ng RK: Cardiopulmonary exercise: A recently discovered secret of tai chi. *Hawaii Medical Journal* 51:216–217, 1992.
149. McCaffrey R, Taylor N: Effective anxiety treatment prior to diagnostic cardiac catheterization. *Holistic Nursing Practice* 19(2):70–73, 2005.
150. Blaer Y, Jafari J, Podberezsky A, et al: Single-blind and double-blind randomized controlled trials of PalmTherapy, an alternative medical approach for anxiety before cardiac catheterization. *eCAM* 5(1):103–105, 2008. doi:10.1093/ecam/nel 111
151. Heidenreich PA, McDonald KM, Hastie T, et al. An evaluation of beta-blockers, calcium antagonists, nitrates, and alternative therapies for stable angina. *Agency for Healthcare Research and Quality*, 1999. Publication # 00-E003, November 1999.
152. VanWormer AM, Lindquist R, Sendelbach SE: The effects of acupuncture on cardiac arrhythmias: A literature review. *Heart Lung* 37:425–431, 2008.
153. Ross R: Atherosclerosis: An inflammatory disease. *New England Journal of Medicine* 340:115–126, 1999.
154. Ridker PM, Rifai N, Rose L, et al: Comparison of C-reactive protein and low-density lipoprotein cholesterol levels in the prediction of first cardiovascular events. *New England Journal of Medicine* 347:1557–1565, 2002.
155. Ehrenstein MR, Jury EC, Mauri C: Statins for atherosclerosis: As good as it gets? *New England Journal of Medicine* 352:73–75, 2005.
156. Whitworth J, Burkhardt A, Oz M: Complementary therapy and cardiac surgery. *Journal of Cardiovascular Nursing* 12:87–94, 1998.
157. Liu EH, Tuner LM, Lin SX, et al: Use of alternative medicine by patients undergoing cardiac surgery. *Journal of Thoracic Cardiovascular Surgery* 120:335–341, 2000.
158. Eisenberg DM, Kessler RC, Van Rompay MI, et al: Perceptions about complementary therapies relative to conventional therapies among adults who use both: Results from a national survey. *Annals of Internal Medicine* 135:344–351, 2001.
159. Lan C, Ssu-Yuan C, Lai JS, et al: The effect of tai chi on cardiorespiratory function in patients with coronary artery bypass surgery. *Medicine and Science in Sports and Exercise* 31:634–638, 1999.
160. Barnason S, Zimmerman L, Nieveen J: The effects of music interventions on anxiety in the patient after coronary artery bypass grafting. *Heart and Lung Journal of Acute and Critical Care* 24:124–132, 1995.
161. Oxman TE, Freeman DH, Manheimer ED: Lack of social participation or religious strength and comfort as risk factors for death after cardiac surgery in the elderly. *Psychosomatic Medicine* 57:5–15, 1995.
162. Garbossa A, Maldaner E, Mortari DM, et al: Effects of physiotherapeutic instructions on anxiety of CABG patients. *Reviews Brasil Circulation Cardiovascular* 24(3):359–366, 2009.
163. Miller KM, Perry PA: Relaxation technique and postoperative pain in patients undergoing cardiac surgery. *Pain Management* 19:136–146, 1990.
164. Moser DK, Dracup K, Woo MA, et al: Voluntary control of vascular tone by using skin-temperature biofeedback-relaxation in patients with advanced heart failure. *Alternative Therapy Health Medicine* 3:51–59, 1997.
165. Bernardi L, Spadacini G, Bellwon J, et al: Effect of breathing rate on oxygen saturation and exercise performance in chronic heart failure. *Lancet* 351:1308–1311, 1998.
166. Shinnick P, Freed S: A case study of the synchronization of human energy in an acute condition of chronic heart disease through complementary treatment. *Subtle Energies and Energy Medicine* 13:209–232, 2002.
167. Yeh GY, Wood MJ, Lorell BH, et al: Effects of tai chi mind-body movement therapy on functional status and exercise capacity in patients with chronic heart failure: A randomized controlled trial. *American Journal of Medicine* 117:51–548, 2004.
168. Barrow DE, Bedford A, Ives G, et al: An evaluation of the effects of tai chi chuan and chi kung training in patients with symptomatic heart failure: A randomised controlled pilot study. *Postgraduate Medicine* 83:717–721, 2007.
169. Benson H, McCallie DP: Angina pectoris and the placebo effect. *The New England Journal of Medicine* 300:1424–1429, 1979.
170. Bienenfeld L, Frishman W, Glasser SP: The placebo effect in cardiovascular disease. *American Heart Journal* 132:1207–1221, 1996.
171. Byrd RC: Positive therapeutic effects of intercessory prayer in a coronary care unit population. *Southern Medical Journal* 81:826–829, 1988.
172. Harris WS, Gowda M, Kolb JW, et al: A randomized, controlled trial of the effects of remote, intercessory prayer on outcomes in patients admitted to the coronary care unit. *Archives of Internal Medicine* 159:2273–2278, 1999.
173. McCullough ME, Hoyt WT, Larson DB, et al: Religious involvement and mortality: A meta-analytic review. *Health Psychology* 19:211–222, 2000.
174. Bolwerk CAL: Effects of relaxing music on state anxiety in myocardial infarction patients. *Critical Care Nursing Quarterly* 13(2):63–72, 1990.
175. Slader CA, Reddel HK, Jenkins CR, et al: Complementary and alternative medicine usein asthma: Who is using what? *Respirology* 11:373–387, 2006.
176 Ritz T: Relaxation therapy in adult asthma: Is there new evidence for its effectiveness? *Behavior Modification* 25:640–665, 2001.
177. Huntley A, White AR, Ernst E: Relaxation therapies for asthma: A systematic review. *Thorax* 57:127–131, 2002.
178. McQuaid EL, Nassau JH: Empirically supported treatments of disease-related symptoms in pediatric psychology: Asthma, diabetes, and cancer. *Journal of Pediatric Psychology* 24.305–328, 1999.
179. Devine EC, Pearcy J: Meta-analysis of the effects of psychoeducational care in adults with chronic obstructive pulmonary disease. *Patient Education and Counseling* 29:167–178, 1996.
180. Gibson PG, Powell H, Coughlan J, et al: Limited (information only) patient education programs for adults with asthma. *Cochrane Database Systematic Reviews* 2:CD001005. 2004.
181. Castes M, Hagel I, Palenque M, et al: Immunological changes associated with clinical improvement of asthmatic children subjected to psychosocial intervention. *Brain, Behavior, and Immunity* 13:1–13, 1999.
182. Haby MM, Waters E, Robertson CF, et al: Interventions for educating children who have attended the emergency room for asthma. *Cochrane Database of Systematic Reviews* 1:CD001290. 2001.
183. Epstein GN, Halper JP, Barrett EAM, et al: A pilot study of mind-body changes in adults with asthma who practice mental imagery. *Alternative Therapies* 10:66–71, 2004.
184. Austin JH, Ausubel P: Enhanced respiratory muscular function in normal adults after lessons in proprioceptive musculoskeletal education without success. *Chest* 102:486–490, 1992.
185. Dennis J, Cates C: Alexander technique for chronic asthma. *The Cochrane Library* 2:CD000995. 2004.
186. Dennis JA, Cates CJ: Alexander technique for chronic asthma (review). *The Cochrane Library*, Issue 4 2008.
187. Ritz T, Dahme B, Roth WT: Behavioral interventions in asthma biofeedback techniques, *Journal of Psychosomatic Research* 56:711–720, 2004.
188. Kotses H, Harver A, Segreto J, et al: Long-term effects of biofeedback-induced facial relaxation on measures of asthma severity in children. *Biofeedback and Self-Regulation* 16:1–21, 1991.
189. Tandon MK: Adjunct treatment with yoga in chronic severe airways obstruction. *Thorax* 33:514–517, 1978.
190. Jain SC, Rai L, Valecha A, et al: Effect of yoga training on exercise tolerance in adolescents with childhood asthma. *Journal of Asthma* 28:437–442, 1991.

191. Vendanthan PK, Kesavalu LN, Murthy KC, et al: Clinical study of yoga techniques in university students with asthma: a controlled study. *Allergy and Asthma Proceedings* 19:3–9, 1998.
192. Sodhi C, Singh S, Dandona PK: A study of the effect of yoga training on pulmonary functions in patients with bronchial asthma. *Indian Journal of Physiology and Pharmacology* 53(2):169–174, 2009.
193. Ernst E: Breathing techniques: Adjunctive treatment modalities for asthma? A systematic review. *European Respiratory Journal* 15:969–972, 2000.
194. Wronski W Nowak M: Pilates breathing exercise method as a form of pneumological rehabilitation in children and youths with bronchial asthma. *Przegl Lek* 65 (Suppl 2):9–11, 2008.
195. Smyth JM, Stone AA, Hurewitz A, et al: Effects of writing about stressful experiences on symptom reduction in patients with asthma or rheumatoid arthritis. *Journal of the American Medical Association* 282:1304–1309, 1999.
196. Hondras MA, Linde K, Jones AP: *Manual therapy for asthma (Cochrane Review). The Cochrane Library 2*, Chichester, UK, 2004, John Wiley & Sons, Ltd.
197. Hondras MA, Linde K, Jones AP: Manual therapy for asthma (review). *Cochrane Database of Systematic Reviews*, 2009. Issue 2. Art. No.: CD001002. DOI: 10.1002/14651858.CD001002.pub2.
198. Jadad AR, Moher M, Browman GP, et al: Systematic reviews and meta-analyses on treatment of asthma: Critical evaluation. *British Medical Journal* 320:537–540, 2000.
199. Martin J, Donaldson ANA, Villarroel R, et al: Efficacy of acupuncture in asthma: Systematic review and meta-analysis of published data from 11 randomized controlled trials. *European Respiratory Journal* 20:846–852, 2002.
200. McCarney RW, Linde K, Lasserson TJ: Homeopathy for chronic asthma (Cochrane Review). *The Cochrane Library* 2:CD000353. 2004.
201. McCarney RW, Brinkhaus B, Lasserson TJ, et al: Acupuncture for chronic asthma (review). *Cochrane Database of Systematic Reviews*, 2009. Issue 3. Art. No.: CD000008. DOI: 10.1002/14651858.CD000008.pub2.
202. Biernacki W, Peake MD: Acupuncture in treatment of stable asthma. *Respiratory Medicine* 92:1143–1145, 1998.
203. Birch S: Acupuncture and bronchial asthma: A long-term randomized study. *The Journal of Alternative and Complementary Medicine* 8:751–754, 2002.
204. Medici TC, Grebski E, Wu J, et al: Acupuncture and bronchial asthma: A long-term randomized study of the effects of real versus sham acupuncture compared to controls in patients with bronchial asthma. *The Journal of Alternative and Complementary Medicine* 8:737–750, 2002.
205. Shapira MY, Berkman N, Ben-David G, et al: Short-term acupuncture therapy is of no benefit in patients with moderate persistent asthma. *Chest* 121:1396–1400, 2002.
206. Niggemann B, Gruber C: Side-effects of complementary and alternative medicine. *Allergy* 58:707–716, 2003.
207. Ries AL: Position paper of the American Association of Cardiovascular and Pulmonary Rehabilitation: Scientific basis for pulmonary rehabilitation. *Journal of Cardiopulmonary Rehabilitation* 10:418–444, 1990.
208. Troosters T, Casaburi R, Gosselink R, et al: Pulmonary rehabilitation in chronic obstructive pulmonary disease. *American Journal of Respiratory and Critical Care Medicine*. Jul 1;172(1):19–38, 2005.
209. Nici L, Donner C, Wouters et al: American Thoracic Society / European Society Statement on Pulmonary Rehabilitation. *American Journal of Respiratory and Critical Care Medicine* 173:1390–1413, 2006.
210. Nici L, Limberg T, Hilling L, et al: Clinical competency guidelines for pulmonary rehabilitation professionals: American Association of Cardiovascular and Pulmonary Rehabilitation position statement. *Journal of Cardiovascular and Pulmonary Rehabilitation Prevention*. 27(6):355–358, 2007.
211. Ries AL, Bauldoff F, Carlin B, et al: Pulmonary rehabilitation: Joint ACCP/AACVPR evidence-based clinical practice guidelines. *Chest* 131(suppl):4S–42S, 2007.
212. Glasscoe CA, Quittner AL: Psychological interventions for people with cystic fibrosis and their families (review). *Cochrane Database of Systematic Reviews*, 2009. Issue 3. Art. No.: CD003148. DOI: 10.1002/14651858.CD003148.pub2.
213. Crawford J: Yoga holds potential as COPD therapy. *ADVANCE for Physical Therapists & PT Assistants*. August 2. p 55, 2004.
214. Irons JY, Kenny DT, Chang AB: Singing for children and adults with bronchiectasis (review). *Cochrane Database of Systematic Reviews*, 2010a. Issue 2. Art. No.: CD007729. DOI: 10.1002/14651858.CD007729.pub2.
215. Irons JY, Kenny DT, Chang AB: Singing for children and adults with cystic fibrosis (review). *Cochrane Database of Systematic Reviews*, 2010b. Issue 5. Art. No.: CD008036. DOI: 10.1002/14651858.CD008036.pub2.
216. Grasso MC, Button BM, Allison DJ, et al: Benefits of music therapy as an adjunct to chest physiotherapy in infants and toddlers with cystic fibrosis. *Pediatric Pulmonology* 29:371–381, 2000.
217. Roux FH, Bouic PJD, Bester MM: The effect of Bach's Magnificat on emotions, immune, and endocrine parameters during physiotherapy treatment of patients with infectious lung conditions. *Journal of Music Therapy* 44(2):156, 2007.
218. Huth MM, Zink KA, VanHorn NR: The effects of massage therapy in improving outcomes for youth with cystic fibrosis: An evidence review. *Pediatric Nursing* 31(4):328–332, 2005.
219. Zhao I, Yates P: Non-pharmacological interventions for breathlessness management in patients with lung cancer: A systematic review. *Palliative Medicine* 22:693–701, 2008.
220. Sola I, Thompson EM, Subirana Casacuberta M, et al: Non-invasive interventions for improving well-being and quality of life in patients with lung cancer (review). *Cochrane Database of Systematic Reviews*, 2009. Issue 1, Art. No: CD004282. DOI: 10.1002/14651858.CD004282.pub3.

Chapter 28

III

Patient Education

Kelly Hawthorne, Katherine Ennis, and Alexandra J. Sciaky

KEY TERMS

Education
Effectiveness
Health behaviors
Health consequences
Health literacy
Learning theory
Methods
Needs assessment
Resources
Wellness

CHAPTER OUTLINE

According to the *Guide to Physical Therapist Practice,* patient/client-related instruction is one of the three major components of physical therapist intervention.[1] In cardiovascular and pulmonary physical therapy, choosing an effective procedural intervention is based on the physiological evaluation of the patient. Similarly, choosing effective patient instruction or education methods is based on the learning needs assessment of the patient.[2] The overall goal of patient education is for the patient to practice health behaviors that promote health, well-being, and independence in self-care. Cardiovascular and pulmonary patient education can pose a significant challenge to the physical therapist. Patient education interventions can range from teaching a hospitalized patient about cardiac risk factor modification to designing a series of community-based exercise classes for children with asthma. Meeting this challenge is important because the benefits of patient education include reduced health-care costs, reduced disability, enhanced patient decision making, improved patient knowledge, and increased quality of life. In addition, physical therapists share with other health-care providers the responsibility of ensuring that patients have the opportunity to make informed choices in their care. Unless effective patient education is implemented, this opportunity will be lost.

The overall objective of this chapter is to provide the clinician with an understanding of the principles and practice of effective patient education. To meet this objective, patient education is defined and pertinent learning theories are presented, supported by examples of how they relate to cardiovascular and pulmonary patient education. The learning needs assessment of the patient is explained, followed by a description of patient education methods and materials. Because the effectiveness of patient education efforts is important to evaluate, methods to determine effectiveness are addressed. Finally, interprofessional considerations and educational resources are discussed.

Defining Patient Education

Physical therapists believe that patient education is an important part of patient care.[3] The teaching role of the physical therapist has been reported as highly valued by patients as well.[4] According to the Consumer and Patient Health Information Section of the Medical Library Association (1996),[5] patient education is "a planned activity, initiated by a health professional, whose aim is to impart knowledge, attitudes and skills with the specific goal of changing behavior, increasing compliance with therapy and, thereby, improving health."[5]

Several factors make patient education unique when compared with other types of teaching. The patient may have limited or no access to teaching because of financial and/or geographical barriers to health care. The learner may lack a sense of well-being because of signs and symptoms of an acute illness, making learning more difficult. The relationship between the teacher and the learner in patient education may be perceived as hierarchical—a medical authority figure instructing a lay person. The learner's emotional status may be fearful or anxious, depending on the medical situation. Superimposed time constraints, such as length of hospital stay or length of clinic appointment, may have a direct impact on patient education. The physical therapist and the patient may be from different cultures. Furthermore, the learner may have limited health literacy. Any of these factors may pose barriers to learning. In addition, the patient's family dynamics may be altered as family members try to cope with the patient's illness or disability. The physical therapist's responsibility extends to determining readiness and ability to learn and including the family in the education process.

Objectives

The overall objective of patient education is to effect a durable cognitive improvement that results in a positive change in an individual's or group's health behavior. In most cases the physical therapist must embark on a process to meet this objective in the course of procedural interventions. The education process consists of assessing the learning needs of the patient, identifying measurable, realistic objectives, planning and implementing the patient education program, and finally, evaluating its effectiveness. Specific examples of patient education learning objectives are listed in Box 28-1.

Achieving these objectives will lead to the achievement of a host of documented benefits of patient education. These include reduced length of hospital stay,[6] reduced patient anxiety,[7] improved health-related knowledge,[8] increased quality of life,[9] and improved response and adherence to medical treatment.[10] Patient education has also been shown to empower patients to take more active roles in their health care.[11] Patients who are educated partners in their care are able to be smart consumers in the health-care system and adapt more readily to the changes in their lifestyles that result from illness. Educated patients learn and understand the health consequences of their behaviors and choices.

Box 28-1 Patient Education Objectives

1. Enhanced patient-clinician rapport
2. Increased knowledge of health disorder/condition
3. Increased adherence to physical therapy treatment plan
4. Decreased health-care costs
5. Increased self-efficacy
6. Increased ability to make informed health-care choices
7. Improved patient outcomes (such as quality of life, mobility, etc.)

Learning Theory: Concepts Pertinent to Cardiopulmonary Patient Education

Behavioral scientists of the 20th century developed a variety of learning theories and models that attempt to explain the complexities of human behavior. Subsequent models have emerged that specifically address health behavior. Although a comprehensive discussion of these models is beyond the scope of this chapter, a list of references for further reading may be found at the end of this chapter (see Bibliography). The discussion of the three theoretical concepts that follows is designed to provide the clinician with a rationale for patient education practice in terms of its basis in learning theory. The concepts are social-cognitive theory, the health-belief model, and the behavior-modification approach.

The social-cognitive theory as developed by Bandura (1986)[12] posits that human behavior can be explained and predicted using the following key regulators: incentives, outcome expectations, and efficacy expectations. For example, a myocardial infarction patient perceives value in following the exercise program (incentive). Patients with this incentive will attempt to exercise if they believe that their current sedentary lifestyle poses a threat to health. These patients also believe exercise will reduce that threat (outcome expectation) and that they are personally capable of performing the exercise program (efficacy expectation). Outcome and efficacy expectations directly relate to patients' beliefs about their capabilities and the relationship of their behaviors to successful outcomes. In essence, then, behavior is influenced by perceptions that create expectations for similar outcomes over time.

To function competently in a given environment requires a belief in one's ability to attain a certain level of performance. Bandura terms this self-efficacy.[13] He argues that perceived self-efficacy influences all aspects of behavior, including learning new skills and inhibiting or stopping current behaviors. Self-efficacy has the following four primary determinants:

1. Performance accomplishments, which is the strongest determinant and refers to "acting out" the desired behavior and mastering the task, resulting in increased self-efficacy
2. Vicarious experience, which involves learning through observing the actions of others, especially actions with clear, rewarding outcomes
3. Verbal persuasion
4. One's physiological state as it relates to the perceived ability to perform a given task

For example, a pulmonary rehabilitation program increases a patient's self-efficacy when the patient successfully completes multiple exercise sessions (performance accomplishments), learns how to deal with dyspnea by consulting fellow program graduates (vicarious experience), receives counseling on energy conservation techniques from the staff (verbal persuasion), and notes that oxygen saturation measured 95% before exercising (physiological state).

The health-belief model, developed in the early 1950s, theorizes that patients are likely to take a health action in the following situations: they believe they are at risk for illness; they believe that the disease poses a serious threat to their lives should they contract it; they desire to avoid illness and believe that certain actions will prevent or reduce the severity of the illness; and they believe that taking the health action is less threatening than the illness itself.[14] This model was originally developed in an attempt to understand why large numbers of people failed to accept preventative care or screening tests for early disease detection. Subsequent studies have used the model to analyze compliance with regimes for hypertension, asthma, and diabetes.[15] The health-belief model conveys that in the context of health behavior some stimulus or "cue to action" is necessary to initiate the decision-making process. These cues can be internal (i.e., a productive cough) or external (i.e., instructional video on pulmonary hygiene techniques). Once the behavior commences, it is understood that many demographic, structural, personal, and social elements are capable of influencing the behavior. In addition, perceived barriers (i.e., unpleasant side effects) may limit or prevent undertaking the recommended behavior.

The behavior-modification approach has its roots in operant-learning theory and consists of techniques that manipulate environmental rewards and punishments in relationship to a specified behavior.[16] The theme of this approach is that an individual's behavior can gradually be shaped to meet a set objective. According to Becker (1990),[17] the behavior-modification approach frequently follows a general plan: "identify the problem; describe the problem in behavioral terms; select a target behavior that is measurable; identify the antecedents and consequences of the behavior; set behavioral objectives; devise and implement a behavior change program; and evaluate the program."[17] This plan is similar to the patient/client management model[1] that physical therapists use to achieve optimal patient care outcomes. The physical therapist examines the patient, describes the problem(s) in functional terms (evaluation and diagnosis), sets short-term and long-term functional goals, designs a plan of care to meet those goals (prognosis), implements the plan (intervention), and reevaluates the patient. These similarities may facilitate the use of the behavioral-modification approach by physical therapists.

Health-care contracts can be useful in implementing the behavior-modification approach. An example of such a contract may be seen in Box 28-2. The contract should be realistic, measurable, and renewable.[18] Specific goals, time frames, behaviors, and contingencies are written in the contract. The clinician and patient discuss and then sign the contract. Positive and negative reinforcements are used to facilitate the desired behaviors in the patient. Ideally, once the contract expires, the patient feels competent and is able to continue the desired behaviors without the external reinforcements.

Box 28-2 **Health Care Contract**

Date:

Contract goal: [specific outcome to be attained]

I, [Client's Name], agree to [Detailed description of required behaviors, time, and frequency limitations] in return for [Positive reinforcements contingent on completion of required behaviors; timing and mode of delivery of reinforcements].

I, [Provider's Name], agree to [Detailed description of required behaviors, time, and frequency limitations].

(Optional) I, [Significant Other's Name], agree to [Detailed description of required behaviors, time, and frequency limitations].

(Optional) Aversive consequences: [Negative reinforcements for failure to meet minimum contract requirements].

We will review the terms of this agreement and will make desired modifications, on [date]. We hereby agree to abide by the terms of the contract describe above.

Signed: [Client]

Signed: [Significant Other, if relevant]

Signed: [Provider]

Contract effective from [Date] to [Date].

From Janz NK, Becker MH, Hartman PE: Contingency contracting to enhance patient compliance: A review, Patient Education Counseling *5:165–178, 1984.*

Needs-Based Approach to Patient Education

The most important aspect of planning for patient education is assessing the learner. The process of patient education requires assessment of the total patient and family, including an understanding of the psychosocial, socioeconomic, educational, vocational, and cultural qualities of the patient and family unit.[19] Assessing educational needs of the patient allows the physical therapist to determine what the patient needs to know to meet the desired cognitive and behavioral teaching objectives. This assessment also increases patient-teacher rapport and allows the physical therapist to individualize the learning experience.

Learning Needs Assessment

Tools

The American Physical Therapy Association's Commission on Accreditation of Physical Therapy Education in their Normative Model of Physical Therapist Professional Education: Version 2004[20] requires that the graduate physical therapist be able to "effectively educate others using culturally appropriate teaching methods that are commensurate with the needs of the learner."[20] Learning needs can be assessed in a variety of ways. These include patient and family interviews, questionnaires and surveys, written tests, and observation of patient performance.[21] Interviews allow the physical therapist to ask questions directed at determining the patient's view of the illness, including associated beliefs and attitudes. Questionnaires and surveys can be used in conjunction with the interview to document the patient's responses to specific questions about his or her condition. Open-ended questions such as "What are the major problems your illness has caused for you and your family?" elicit more information than a multiple-choice format. Written tests can be helpful in determining what patients already know when the tests are given, before any teaching. These tests can also identify problems with reading, comprehension skill, and health literacy. Observing patients as they perform a skill, such as diaphragmatic breathing, reveals whether the patient can demonstrate the correct technique. The physical therapist can also pose questions to the patient during the demonstration to determine whether the patient knows the rationale for the exercise.

Areas to Assess

The learning needs assessment encompasses the following five major areas: perceptual, cognitive, motor, affective, and environmental (Box 28-3). By addressing these five areas, the physical therapist will obtain an accurate picture of the patient's learning abilities, knowledge level, performance skills, attitudes, and cultural influences.

The perceptual area encompasses the learner's ability to receive information via the senses. If the learner's sight, hearing, or sense of touch is impaired, the instructor may need to make modifications so that the information can be received by the learner. The comprehension of symbols, such as numbers, words, or pictures, also needs to be assessed in the perceptual area. The instructor needs to know what meaning the learner attributes to the symbols that will be used in the education program to ensure clarity.

The cognitive area addresses the learner's knowledge and problem-solving skills. The instructor needs to know how much the learner already knows and what needs to be learned. The instructor also needs to know if the learner has any problems with memory. Short- or long-term memory deficits may require that the instructor integrate a prompting system into the education plan.

The patient's fine- and gross-motor skills and functional mobility are covered in the motor area. The instructor needs to be aware of the physiological changes in the patient that affect abilities to perform activities necessary for a given education program. For example, if patients who are wheelchair users are interested in attending a support group, the physical therapist would ensure that it is being held in a room that is wheelchair accessible.

The affective area comprises the learner's attitudes, beliefs, and readiness to learn. Identifying the learner's value-belief system will assist the instructor in determining what is important to the learner and facilitating motivation. The patient's perception of wellness may vary from the absence of disease to an enhanced healthy state. What the instructor feels is important to learn may not be what the patient feels is important to learn. Identifying what the patient values early on will prevent instructor (and patient) frustration later.

Cultural influences and personal and societal resources are included in the environmental area. It is important for the instructor to be aware of the patient's lifestyle, religion, traditions, roles, and primary language in order to individualize the patient's learning experience. Presence or absence of the patient's resources may affect consistency in, and access to, patient education.

All five of these areas can be addressed with the use of a learning needs assessment survey (Box 28-4). By using a survey in combination with the physical therapy patient evaluation, the therapist can gather all the necessary information to create an optimal patient education experience. The survey in Box 28-4 consists of three parts, which can be adapted to any patient care setting. In the pediatric setting, some of the questions could be asked of the parent(s) or rephrased to address school-age children. Part I primarily assesses the patient's perception of the illness or disability and its impact on the patient's life. Part II lists a wide variety of teaching methods and asks the patient to indicate which methods he or she personally feels are most useful. Part III identifies specific topics about which the patient would like to know more. This part is also helpful in alerting the therapist that referrals to other members of the interprofessional health-care team may be required. For example, if the patient selects "I would like to know more about what I should eat," the therapist would make a referral to the dietitian. Patients' answers provide clues to learning style preferences that work best for them and can often provide clues to health literacy issues.

Box 28-3 Learning Needs Assessment Areas

Perceptual
- Ability to receive input (vision, hearing, and touch)
- Comprehension of symbols (figures, numbers, words, and pictures)

Cognitive
- Knowledge and analytical skills
- Memory

Motor
- Fine- and gross-motor skills
- Physical adaptations and responses to illness or stimuli

Affective
Attitudes
Value-belief system
Motivation (readiness to learn)
Perception of overall wellness
Environmental
Personal and societal resources
Amount of instructor contact and setting
Cultural influences (language, traditions, roles, religion, and lifestyle)

Health Literacy

Certain barriers, such as limited health literacy, can alter the effectiveness of patient education and rehabilitation interventions, such as promoting lifestyle behavior changes.[22,23] Health literacy can be described as a person's ability to comprehend health information and use that information to make informed decisions about his or her health and medical care.[24] Specifically, the patient needs these skills when reading consent forms, prescription drug information, food labels, rehabilitation instructions, and appointment slips or when filling out a health insurance form or reviewing a health care bill.[25-27] Health literacy is required to read a peak flow meter, to understand body mass index (BMI), and to recognize whethera blood pressure reading is considered high.[28] Signs of limited health literacy can be found in Box 28-5. Limited health literacy increases the risk for hospitalization, the overall cost of health care, and mortality rates. Studies have shown that patients with limited health literacy are more likely to report difficulties with activities of daily living (ADLs) and instrumental activities of daily living (IADLs) as a result of poor or diminished physical health and pain that interferes with normal work activities.[29] Those with limited health literacy also have higher rates of diabetes, hypertension, obesity, depressive symptoms, and physical limitations. Older adults with limited health literacy also may demonstrate a higher incidence of heart failure, arthritis, and multiple health conditions, and they tend to have a greater need for complex medical

Box 28-4 Learning Needs Assessment Survey

Your physical therapist would like to help you learn what you need to know to function as independently as possible and manage your illness/disability. Please answer the following questions.

Part I

Name:

Please describe your illness and/or disability here:

1. Do you have any problems seeing or hearing?
2. Do you have any body areas that are numb (can't feel)?
3. How long have you had this illness/disability?
4. What problems has it caused you?
5. Are you able to care for yourself at home?
6. Are you responsible for the care of any others at home?
7. Do you have someone at home to help you? If so, whom?
8. What questions or concerns do you have?
9. Do you practice a religion? If so, which?
10. What language(s) do you understand best?
11. How much education/schooling have you had?
12. What is your occupation?

Part II

There are many different ways to learn. Please read the list of ways to learn below and circle the ones that help you learn best.

Reading
Listening to lectures
Watching demonstrations
Using interactive videos or computer programs
Attending seminars
Practicing a skill or doing a simulation
Taking written tests
Group discussion
Reflecting by myself
Playing games
Role playing
Computer/Internet activities
Other

Part III

I would like to know more about (check all that apply to you):

___ How to clear mucus from my lungs
___ What causes heart disease
___ How to avoid shortness of breath
___ What I should eat
___ Exercise
___ My medications
___ Monitoring myself
___ Planning my social life and/or work life
___ What to do if I have chest pain
___ Planning for sexual intimacy
___ What causes lung disease
___ Coping with my feelings
___ How to stay well
___ How to quit smoking
___ How to sleep better
___ How to access community resources

Other things I would like to know:

The three most important things I need to know are:

Box 28-5 Signs of Limited Health Literacy

Incompletely or inaccurately completed registration or intake forms
Frequently missed appointment times
Inability to name medications or explain purpose of medications or difficulty in taking medications correctly
Lack of follow-through with referrals to other health-care providers
Lack of follow-through with home exercise programs or illness/disease management strategies

From Weiss BD: Health literacy and patient safety: Help patients understand. Manual for clinicians, ed 2, Chicago, Ill, 2007, American Medical Association and AMA Foundation. Available at: http://www.amaassn.org/ama1/pub/upload/mm/367/healthlitclinicians.pdf

management.[29,30] Patients with limited health literacy have less knowledge about hypertension, diabetes, and asthma.[25] Inadequate health literacy skills are key factors in the exacerbation of heart failure.[31]

Health literacy is also linked to improved compliance with a physical therapy plan of care and ultimately leads to better health and medical care outcomes.[32] Current cardiovascular and pulmonary research demonstrates that patients with adequate health literacy are more likely to keep records of their blood glucose test results[33] and demonstrate improved medication compliance with a diagnosis of cardiovascular disease.[34] Patients with chronic obstructive pulmonary disease (COPD) who receive and understand self-management education have decreased hospital admissions.[35] Although outside the scope of this chapter, certain formal assessment tools can be used to determine an adult patient's health literacy level (Table 28-1).

Interpretation of Findings

The next important step after gathering information with the learning needs assessment survey is to interpret the findings. The physical therapist looks at the answer to each item on the survey and uses that information in the process of designing the content and method for teaching that patient. Primary and secondary prevention can be integrated into the content to promote overall wellness. Interpretation of the survey findings means applying the patient's current health concerns, learning abilities, and knowledge deficits to future learning activities. By identifying the patient's needs, the physical therapist is able to make informed choices in the planning and implementation of each patient's education experience.

Formulation and Prioritization of Goals

As physical therapists set intervention goals for their patients, they should include educational goals. Intervention goals usually describe functional outcomes (e.g., "The patient will perform a stand-and-pivot transfer from bed to chair, independently"), and they are written in behavioral terms. Educational goals should also be written in behavioral terms. For example, "Mr. J will safely perform percussion and postural drainage to Mrs. J's right lower lobe." The stated behavior

Table 28-1 Health Literacy Screening and Assessment Tools

Test	Characteristics	Advantages	Disadvantages
Rapid Estimate of Adult Literacy in Medicine (REALM)	Consists of 66 items Used to measure how well patients read words frequently encountered in medical settings Score divides health literacy skills into four categories of grade-equivalent reading levels	Takes 3-4 minutes to administer	Inability of the test to distinguish reading levels beyond ninth grade Test does not measure understanding of the words Test is only available in English
Test of Functional Health Literacy in Adults (TOFHLA)	"Gold standard" of health literacy testing Consists of a 50-item reading comprehension section and 17-item numeric ability test Scores patients in three different categories consisting of adequate, marginal, or inadequate health literacy	Available in English and Spanish and 14-point font Measures a wide range of reading levels and measures comprehension skills	Takes 22 minutes to administer
Test of Functional Health Literacy in Adults, short version (S-TOFHLA)	Shortened version of TOFHLA Consists of two prose passages to assess reading comprehension Scores patients in three different categories: adequate, marginal, or inadequate health literacy Useful in identifying patients with very limited reading ability	Takes 7 minutes to administer Available in English and Spanish and 14-point font	Measures only reading comprehension
Short Assessment of Health Literacy for Spanish-Speaking Adults (SAHLSA)	Based on the REALM Measures health literacy in patients who speak Spanish Consists of 50 words, each with a correct and incorrect meaning A score between 0 and 37 indicates inadequate health literacy	Takes 5 minutes to administer	
Newest Vital Sign (NVS)	A six-question assessment based on an ice cream nutrition label Assesses literacy and numeracy	Takes 3-5 minutes to administer Available in English and Spanish Has high sensitivity for detecting limited health literacy	
Single-Item Literacy Screener (SILS)	Question asks, "How often do you need to have someone help you when you read instructions, pamphlets, or other written material?" Respondents choose one of these responses: 1-Never, 2-Rarely, 3-Sometimes, 4-Often, or 5-Always A score of 2 or greater is considered positive	Takes less than 1 minute to administer	

From Cutilli CC: Do your patients understand? OrthopNurs *24(5):372–377, 2005; Davis TC, Long SW, Jackson RH, et al: Rapid estimate of adult literacy in medicine: A shortened screening instrument,* Fam Med *25(6):391–395, 1993; Mancuso JM: Assessment and measurement of health literacy: An integrative review of the literature,* Nurs Health Sci *11:77–89, 2009; Parker RM, Baker DW, Williams MV, et al: The test of functional health literacy in adults: Anew instrument for measuring patients' literacy skills,* J Gen Int Med *10(10):537–541, 1995; Baker DW, Williams MV, Parker RM, et al: Development of a brief test to measure functional health literacy,* Patient Educ Couns *38(1):33–42, 1999; Lee SY, Bender DE, Ruiz RE, et al: Development of an easy-to-use Spanish health literacy test,* Health Serv Res *41(4 Pt 1):1392–1412, 2006; Weiss BD, Mays MZ, Martz W, et al: Quick assessment of literacy in primary care: The newest vital sign,* Ann Fam Med *3:514–522, 2005; Pfizer: The newest vital sign: Anew health literacy assessment tool for health care providers. Available at:* http://www.pfizerhealthliteracy.com/physicians-providers/NewestVitalSign.aspx; *and Morris NS, MacLean CD, Chew LD, et al: The single-item literacy screener: Evaluation of a brief instrument to identify limited reading ability,* BMC Fam Pract *7(1):21, 2006.*

must be observable and measurable. Motor skills can be observed, knowledge skills can be tested, and safety can be documented.

Prioritizing the patient's educational goals in conjunction with other intervention goals enhances the therapist's efficiency. Referring again to the learning needs assessment survey (see Box 28-4) to determine what knowledge is important to the patient will guide the therapist in creating the most appropriate prioritization of goals. Simplicity is usually best. Overwhelming patients with a huge list of items to be accomplished may discourage them before they even start. If the patient's learning needs are great, start by breaking down the list of goals into smaller groups. Choose the most important goals and try to accomplish those first. If you run into a series of failures, tackle the next group. Build on each success the patient experiences.

Educational Methods

Method Selection

In addition to considering the level of health literacy of the patient and the caregiver, using the learning needs assessment survey (see Box 28-4) will allow the clinician to choose education methods that will facilitate optimal learning in a given patient or group. The patient(s) can self-select the available learning methods that have the greatest learning potential. A combination of methods may be necessary to achieve the educational goals that have been set. If a patient is not sure which methods to indicate, the therapist can base the choice on the other information provided in the survey (e.g., sensory deficits, health literacy level, or type of information desired).

One way to determine learning styles without completing a survey is to ask patients (or their caregiver) about any hobbies and how they became proficient with the hobby. For example, did they read about it, watch a video, or take a class to learn about the hobby?[32] Surveys generally require regular updates to ensure that all of the offered methods are listed and that any discontinued methods are removed from the list. In addition, the physical therapist should assess potential learning materials for readability, age-appropriateness, accuracy of content, intended audience, and clarity.[19] Recently, even the American Diabetes Association (ADA) and the American Heart Association (AHA) had their written materials reviewed for things such as reading level, word usage, clear and specific behavioral recommendations, etc.[36] Please see Box 28-6 for guidelines for creating patient education materials, as well as Box 28-7 for resources for developing and assessing readability of printed patient education materials.

Advantages and Disadvantages

Each education method has its own advantages and disadvantages. Table 28-2 lists the key advantages and disadvantages of 13 education methods. The table is designed to assist the physical therapist in determining the settings and populations in which the methods will be most useful. However, this is not a comprehensive list. In fact, some health education challenges require truly innovative approaches.

In Boston, Massachusetts, for example, community healthcare providers were faced with a dilemma. The incidence of acquired immune deficiency syndrome (AIDS) among women of color was increasing. Latino, African-American, and Haitian women were not receiving vital information about how to prevent the transmission of the human immunodeficiency virus (HIV). These communities were largely distrustful of the healthcare establishment and were not mobilized to stop the spread of HIV. How could they be reached? The Boston Women's AIDS Information Project (BWAIP) trained lay women to educate other women in the places where they congregate, such as beauty salons. Informational brochures, condoms, and posters were distributed in a number of beauty salons in communities where women were at highest risk for contracting HIV. Lay and professional educators gave presentations, showed videos, and answered questions from the staff and patrons of these establishments, thus empowering them to disarm myths about AIDS, to encourage other women to make appropriate behavior changes, and to make referrals to neighborhood health centers for testing and evaluation.

Another area of education that may require a unique approach is teaching young children about their bodies and health. In 1993, members of the interdisciplinary team caring for children with cystic fibrosis (CF) at Texas Children's Hospital in Houston held a CF Education Day for the children and their parents. The children ranged in age from 7 to 11 years. To teach them about anatomy, a special anatomy apron was fabricated. The apron had life-sized removable organs made of stuffed fabric. The children took turns wearing the apron

Box 28-6 Guidelines for Creating Printed Patient Education Materials

- Avoid using unfamiliar words. Use plain language. Use only monosyllabic or disyllabic words in short sentences.
- Keep line length between 40 and 50 characters.
- Use large fonts (at least 14 points). Avoid using italics, all capital letters, or fancy script text.
- Use layouts with substantial amounts of white (blank) space.
- Focus materials on desired behaviors rather than on medical facts.
- Avoid using blue, green, or lavender because older adults may have more difficulty differentiating these colors.
- Use more than one form of communication to clarify written concepts, such as pictures that are culturally sensitive and personally relevant.

From Vanderhoff M: Patient education and health literacy, PT *13(9):42–46, 2005; National Work Group on Literacy and Health: Communicating with patients who have limited literacy skills: Report of the National Work Group on Literacy and Health,* J Fam Pract *46:168–176, 1998; Chang M, Kelly A. Patient education: addressing cultural diversity and health literacy issues.* Urologic Nursing. *2007; 27 (5): 411–417; and U.S. Department of Health and Human Services: Quick guide to health literacy. Office of Disease Promotion and Health Promotion.Available at:* http://www.health.gov/communication/literacy/quickguide/quickguide.pdf.

Box 28-7 Resources for Developing and Assessing Readability of Printed Patient Education Materials

- Federal Plain Language Guidelines
- Clear & Simple: Developing Effective Print Materials for Low-Literate Readers
- Quick Guide to Health Literacy
- Quick Guide to Health Literacy and Older Adults
- Beyond the Brochure: Alternative Approaches to Effective Health Communication
- An Author's Guide—Substitute Word List
- How to Write Low-Literacy Materials
- An Author's Guide—SMOG Readability Formulas
- The Fry Testing Readability Formula
- Fry Readability Graph
- In Other Words ... Assessing Readability: Rules for Playing the Numbers Game
- Writing for a Changing World: Reaching Low-Literacy Audiences with Print Material

Table 28-2 **Comparison Chart for Education Methods (Adults and Children Unless Otherwise Noted)**

Type	Advantages	Disadvantages
Reading	Patient can refer back to material. Low effort for instructor.	Requires instructor follow-up for comprehension.
Lecture	Time-efficient for instructor. Cost-efficient.	Low interaction. May pacify rather than engage.
Demonstration	Adds sensory data to learning. Allows for problem solving and modification.	Instructor needs proficiency in the skill being taught.
Video	Access to restricted areas. Portrays events that are infrequent, costly, and difficult to reproduce. Portable.	Noninteractive. May pacify rather than engage. Requires costly electronic equipment. Difficult to control quality.
Audiotape	Portable. Useful for sight-impaired learner.	Requires electronic equipment.
Group discussion	Effective use of instructor time. Enlarges pool of real-life experiences. Nonthreatening to some learners. Mutual support possible.	Not as much individual attention given. Group may be hard to control (e.g., too talkative, shy, hostile). Strong facilitator skills needed.
Clubs, camps, and retreats	Draws on community and individual resources. Needs less professional input and time.	Same as above. Some risk for perpetuating myths and false information.
Individual instruction	Instructor can tailor learning to student's needs and desires. More one-on-one time.	Inefficient use of instructor time. Limited pool of experience on which to draw.
Games and directed activities	Helpful for children. Reduces anxiety. Uses repetition. Fun. Unexpected experiences can lead to new understandings or insights.	May be difficult to schedule space and find participants.
Computer programs	Interactive, self-paced. Large information capacity. Time-efficient for instructor.	Expensive. Special equipment and space needed. May require expert help.
Seminars and workshops	Diversity of instructors and formats. Pool of experts and community resources. Can tailor content broadly or narrowly.	Expensive. May cause scheduling and space problems.
Role-playing	Allows trial runs, problem-solving, simulated experiences.	Threatening to some. Can be time-consuming. Instructor needs to be skilled in techniques and in dealing with effects on participants.
Oral and written tests	Can provide instructor with evidence of what learner needs to be taught and what has been learned.	Literacy and supplies required, if written. May be time-consuming.

and learned to identify and locate the organs by removing and replacing the apron's heart, lungs, intestines, and pancreas.

By evaluating the advantages and disadvantages of available education methods, the physical therapist can choose the methods that are most effective and use them to his or her best advantage. Consideration must be given to cost, equipment, scheduling, labor, time, site, flexibility, and reusability. For example, digitally recorded or videotaped presentations may be easy for the instructor to schedule, present, and reuse, but they can be costly to purchase and they require expensive equipment for viewing.

Content

The specific content of patient education materials and programs should be determined by the needs of the individual or group being taught. There are, however, topics common to many cardiovascular and pulmonary education efforts. These topics are listed in Box 28-8. The physical therapist can use these topics as a checklist to explore the content covered (or to be covered) in a given cardiopulmonary education experience. Although physical therapists may not be responsible for teaching on all these topics, they should be familiar with all the topics taught by the healthcare team. Educational materials on all of these topics have already been developed by a variety of healthcare providers, educators, and organizations and may be available for use by physical therapists (see Interprofessional Considerations and Resources, later in this chapter).

Determination of Effectiveness

Determining the effectiveness of patient education efforts involves evaluating what the patient learned, as well as how the teacher taught. Sometimes patients learn in spite of educational efforts. Physical therapists need to examine their effectiveness at teaching and strive to improve their teaching skills just as they strive to improve their other clinical skills. Being able to communicate ideas and receive meaningful feedback from patients from diverse racial, ethnic, vocational, religious, and generational backgrounds is crucial for physical therapists. Formal or informal surveys of patients and families who have participated in education efforts can provide the physical therapist with information on teaching effectiveness from the patient and family perspective.

Physical therapists are responsible for evaluating and documenting the results of their patients' education activities.

Box 28-8 Cardiovascular and Pulmonary Patient Education Content

Health promotion/wellness
Smoking cessation
Infection control
Risk-factor awareness and modification
Benefits and effects of pleasurable activity
Resumption of sexual activity
Normal cardiovascular and pulmonary anatomy and physiology, oxygen transport
Cardiovascular and pulmonary disease process
Airway clearance techniques and suctioning
Energy conservation and pacing techniques
Stress management: awareness of anxiety and depression and relaxation training
Resumption of school activities (children)
Instructions geared for parents of children with cardiovascular and pulmonary conditions
Cardiopulmonary resuscitation (CPR), basic life support
Heart rate, blood pressure, and dyspnea self-monitoring
Nutrition
Medications (schedules, actions, and side effects)
Use of oxygen and other respiratory equipment
Medical procedures (cardiac catheterization, bronchoscopy, cardiopulmonary transplantation)
Community resources
Emergency procedures
Problem-solving techniques
Sleep management skills

From Kunik ME, Veazey C, Cully JA, et al: COPD Education and cognitive behavioral therapy group treatment for clinically significant symptoms of depression and anxiety in COPD patients: A randomized controlled trial, Psychol Med *38, 385–396, 2008.*

Observing a patient or caregiver perform a skill (such as paced breathing) will give the physical therapist the opportunity to determine whether the patient or caregiver has learned and properly performed the skill. Once the physical therapist has observed the skill being properly performed or when the patient or caregiver has "taught back" the skill, the therapist can document it as such in the medical record. The amount of supervision and equipment required, if any, should also be included in the documentation.

Presenting information in visual form, for example, using pictorial aids and videos, has been recommended[37] for patients diagnosed with COPD who are identified as having limited health literacy. For patients undergoing cardiac catheterization, an interactive, computer-based information program is suggested.[38] Patient education for patients with coronary heart disease should be "multi-faceted and interprofessional."[39]

Teacher-Learner Relationship

According to Locke (1986),[40] the primary step to understanding others is an awareness of one's self. Acknowledging one's own personal values, interests, and biases will significantly increase one's sensitivity toward others. The skilled teacher is aware of his or her own communication style and its limitations and can convey the desire to help despite those limitations.

The teacher-learner relationship that develops between physical therapist and patient is largely the result of communication between the two in the context of culture. Communication is a two-way process consisting of verbal and nonverbal messages. The interpretation of these messages depends on the cultural cues operating in the educational setting. Fairchild (1970)[41] defines culture as all social behavior, such as customs, techniques, beliefs, organizations, and regard for material objects, including behaviors transmitted by way of symbols. According to Locke (1992), "the primary mode of transmission of culture is language, which enables people to learn, experience, and share their traditions and customs."[42] In addition, culture can be expressed or experienced via economic and political practices, art, and religion. Health care and medicine have their own cultures. To meet the needs of culturally diverse populations and engage in positive, productive relationships, physical therapists must operate from a framework of cross-cultural understanding. This understanding and knowledge can then be reflected in patient education efforts.

For example, in a large, urban, acute care hospital, two physical therapy staff members were working together to treat an older adult Jewish woman who was critically ill. The clinicians worked carefully to reposition the woman without disturbing the many tubes and lines that were present. Later the woman expressed that she did not want to have two physical therapy clinicians working with her at the same time. She confided to the nurse that it felt it was too much like the Jewish ritual washing of the body after death, which is traditionally performed by two people. This interpretation of the therapy surprised the physical therapy staff members who had treated the woman, because although they were also Jewish, this thought never occurred to them. The next time the clinicians went to see the woman, they explained why it was necessary for both of them to be present during the treatment. They also encouraged the woman to have other supportive people present and to play her favorite recorded music during the therapy session.

Communication

Patients with cardiovascular and pulmonary diseases, such as congestive heart failure, are not always comfortable communicating with health-care professionals or questioning the physician's decisions. In *Circulation* (2009),[43] the American Heart Association's publication, health-care professionals are encouraged to avoid using medical jargon and phrases (such as "echo," "stress test," and "ECG"), because these terms may confuse patients. Instead, health care providers should explain in plain terms the action steps they want a patient to take.[43] In 2011, the Heart Failure Society of America described a five-step process for clinicians working with patients who have heart failure,[44] culminating in encouraging patients' use of the "Ask Me 3" questions:[45]

1. What is my main problem?
2. What do I need to do?
3. Why is it important for me to do this?

Physical therapists can use the communication strategies outlined in Box 28-9 to create an effective educational experience to fit the individual learner's needs. These guidelines can

Box 28-9 Communication Strategies

Avoid talking down to the patient.
Use active listening; ask open-ended questions.
Avoid jargon; minimize information about anatomy and physiology.
Use simple sentence structure and plain language.
Speak slowly; use analogies.
Introduce no more than four main messages per session.
Stress concrete, specific action steps the patient should take.
Create an environment conducive to patients asking questions.
Ensure understanding of information through regular review, patient demonstration, and repetition. Use the "teach back" method and have patients restate the information in their own words.
Give directed feedback to correct errors until full understanding is achieved.

From Vanderhoff M: Patient education and health literacy, PT *13(9):31,42, 2005; Weiss BD: Health literacy and patient safety: Help patients understand. Manual for clinicians, ed 2, Chicago, Ill, 2007, American Medical Association and AMA Foundation. Available at:* http://www.ama-assn.org/ama1/pub/upload/mm/367/healthlitclinicians.pdf; *U.S. Department of Health and Human Services: Quick guide to health literacy. Available at:* http://www.health.gov/communication/literacy/quickguide/quickguide.pdf; *Chang M, Kelly A. Patient education: addressing cultural diversity and health literacy issues.* Urologic Nursing. *2007; 27 (5): 411–417; Oates D, Paasche-Orlow M. Health literacy: communication strategies to improve patient comprehension of cardiovascular health.* Circulation. *2009; 119:1049–1051; and Hironaka LK, Paasche-Orlow MK: The implications of health literacy on patient-provider communication,* Arch Dis Childhood *93:428–432, 2008.*

be tailored to a variety of patient populations with differing levels of health literacy.

Patient Adherence

The effectiveness of physical therapy treatment, or of any medical treatment, depends on the patient following the health-care provider's recommendations (adherence). Unfortunately, there is often a gap between what the patient is asked to do and what the patient actually does. This gap, or nonadherence, has an incidence rate estimated to be between 18% and 35%.[46,47] Factors affecting patient adherence include knowledge about the illness and its expected course, complexity of the recommendations, convenience, availability of support system, financial resources, the patient's beliefs, and the effectiveness of patient education, especially for pulmonary patients.[48]

Patient education can improve adherence when the information explains what behaviors are expected, when they should be performed, and what to do if problems arise. Plans for patient education sessions should strive to avoid or remove barriers to patient adherence. These efforts include simplifying and individualizing treatment regimens, fostering collaborative teacher-learner relationships, enlisting family support, making use of interdisciplinary and community resources, and providing continuity of care.[49] By using an approach that integrates these efforts, the physical therapist can optimize patient adherence to the prescribed physical therapy program.

Interprofessional Considerations and Resources

The interprofessional health-care team has evolved as the complexity and number of available medical treatments has grown. Physical therapists are trained to function as part of an interprofessional team and are responsible for learning the areas of responsibility and expertise covered by each member of their team. The team concerned with cardiovascular and pulmonary care consists of licensed and nonlicensed health-care providers and may include any or all of the following:

Physician
Nurse
Physical therapist
Occupational therapist
Exercise physiologist
Dietitian
Laboratory technologist
Pharmacist
Social worker
Chaplain or pastoral care associate
Clinical psychologist
Speech/language pathologist
Vocational rehabilitation counselor
Home-care personnel
Respiratory therapist
Equipment vendors
Insurance company representative

All of the above providers may not be present on every team, but their services should be available for patients who need them. By understanding what services and patient education materials are provided by each discipline, the physical therapist can reinforce previously presented concepts and avoid giving conflicting information. This also allows the physical therapist to make referrals to the appropriate discipline when other knowledge deficits are identified.

Interprofessional team members can also provide the physical therapist with important patient feedback and information. Teaching methods found to be successful with a given patient by the nurse, for example, could be communicated to the physical therapist. The therapist can then use similar methods with that patient for physical therapy education objectives. Communication between team members is enhanced by regular team meetings or rounds and by having an electronic medical record to document completed patient education experience.

Health-related organizations can also be rich resources for patient education information. The American Heart Association and the American Lung Association, for example, offer many cardiovascular and pulmonary materials to health-care providers for little or no cost. State public health and local community service agencies may also be sources for printed or audiovisual materials. The U.S. Department of Health and Human Services has numerous divisions and institutes that address health education and research. Cardiovascular and pulmonary publications can be obtained from the Federal Consumer Information Center, Washington, DC (or at www.hhs.gov).

Community organizations such as YMCA, YWCA, and the American Red Cross offer a wealth of health education materials and classes. Many of these agencies also have catalogs of their educational offerings, which can be obtained by calling

Box 28-10 Sources of Easy-to-Read Health Education Material

- American Heart Association
- American Cancer Society
- American Diabetes Association
- American Dietetic Association
- National Cancer Institute
- National Heart Lung and Blood Institute
- APTA—Move Forward—Information for Consumers
- MedlinePlus

their local offices. Local public, medical, and hospital libraries are also useful for seeking out available health education materials. Many Chambers of Commerce keep lists of local support groups or clubs, such as Breather's Club or Heartbeats. Regional state colleges or universities have departments dedicated to health education and may have cardiovascular and pulmonary materials to share. Please refer to Box 28-10 for a list of trusted online sources of patient information.

Summary

This chapter defines patient education and describes selected learning theories as they relate to cardiovascular and pulmonary patient education. The evaluation of the patient's learning needs is emphasized, and the advantages and disadvantages of a variety of educational methods are discussed. The role of the teacher-learner relationship and patient adherence are explained in reference to the determination of patient education and treatment effectiveness. Finally, interprofessional health-care team interactions and resources for patient education materials are considered.

Review Questions

1. Discuss the benefits of patient education, including the impact on health-care costs and the patient's perception of wellness.
2. Contrast and compare a variety of teaching methods used in patient education.
3. Explain the rationale for patient education using concepts of adult learning theories or models.
4. Describe the aspects of planning for patient education.
5. Discuss the components of a learning needs assessment survey and ways to modify it for specific patient populations.
6. Critique a variety of written patient education materials using criteria specific to patients with cardiovascular and pulmonary conditions.
7. Explain how to determine the effectiveness of patient education activities from both the patient's and the physical therapist's point of view.
8. Discuss the components of a health literacy assessment and ways to modify interventions for those with limited health literacy.

References

1. American Physical Therapy Association: Guide to physical therapist practice, ed 2. *Physical Therapy* 81:9–744, 2001.
2. Rankin SH, Stallings KD: *Patient education: issues, principles and practices*, ed 2, Philadelphia, 1990, JB Lippincott.
3. Chase L, Elkins JA, Readinger J, et al: Perceptions of physical therapists toward patient education. *Physical Therapy* 73:787–795, 1993.
4. Grannis CJ: The ideal physical therapist as perceived by the elderly patient. *Physical Therapy* 61:479–486, 1981.
5. The Consumer and Patient Health Information Section of the Medical Library Association *Bull Med Libr Assoc* 84(2):238–239, 1996. http://caphis.mlanet.org/chis/librarian.html. Accessed September, 2011.
6. Devine E, Cook T: A meta-analysis of effects of psychoeducational interventions on length of post surgical hospital stay. *Nursing Research* 32:333–339, 1983.
7. O'Rourke A, Levin B, Whitecross S, et al: The effects of physical exercise training and cardiac education on levels of anxiety and depression in the rehabilitation of coronary artery bypass graft patients. *Int Disabil Stud. July-Sep* 12(3):104–106, 1990.
8. Rowland L, Dickinson ET, Newman P, et al: Look After Your Heart Programme: impact on health status, exercise knowledge, attitudes and behavior of retired women in England. *Journal of Epidemiology and Community Health* 48:123–128, 1994.
9. Manzetti JD, Hoffman LA, Sereika SM, et al: Exercise, education, and quality of life in lung transplant candidates. *Journal of Heart and Lung Transplantation* 13:297–305, 1994.
10. Mazzuca S: Does patient education in chronic disease have therapeutic value? *Journal of Chronic Disease* 35:521–529, 1982.
11. Smith CE: Nurses' increasing responsibility for patient education. In Smith CE, editor: *Patient education: nurses in partnership with other health professionals*, Orlando, 1987, Grune& Stratton.
12. Bandura A: *Foundations of thought and action: a social cognitive theory*, Englewood Cliffs, NJ, 1986, Prentice-Hall.
13. Bandura A: Self-efficacy: toward a unifying theory of behavioral change. *Psychological Review* 84:191–215, 1977.
14. Roenstock IM: Historical origins of the health belief model. *Health Education Monographs* 2:328–335, 1974.
15. Becker MH, Janz NK: The health belief model applied to understanding diabetes regimen compliance. *Diabetes Education* 11:41–47, 1985.
16. Redman BK: *The process of patient education*, St Louis, 1993, Mosby.
17. Becker MH: Theoretical models of adherence and strategies of improving adherence. In Shumaker SA, Schron ER, Ockene JK, editors: *The handbook of health behavior change*, New York, 1990, Springer Publishing.
18. Herje PA: Hows and whys of patient contracting. *Nursing Education* 5:30–34, 1980.
19. Nemshick MT: Designing educational interventions for patients and families. In O'Rourke A, Lewin B, Whitcross S, et al: (1990). The effects of physical exercise training and cardiac education on levels of anxiety and depression in the rehabilitation of CABG patients, *International Disability Studies* 12:104–106, 1997.
20. Commission of Accreditation of Physical Therapy Education: *Evaluative criteria for accreditation of education programs for the preparation of physical therapists*, Alexandria, Va, 2004, American Physical Therapy Association.
21. Haggard A: *Handbook of patient education*, Rockville, Md, 1989, Aspen Publishers.
22. Bass PF, 3rd, Wilson JF, Griffith CH, et al: Residents' ability to identify patients with poor literacy skills. *Academic Medicine: Journal of the Association of American Medical Colleges* 77(10):1039–1041, 2002.
23. Zorn M, Allen MP, Horowitz AM, compilers: *Understanding health literacy and its barriers [bibliography on the Internet]*, Bethesda, Md, 2004, National Library of Medicine. Available at: http://www.nlm.nih.gov/pubs/cbm/healthliteracybarriers.html.
24. Ishikawa H, Yano E: Patient health literacy and participation in the health-care process. *Health Expectations* 11:113–122, 2008.
25. White S, Chen J, Atchison R: Relationship of preventive health practices and health literacy: a national study. *American Journal of Health Behaviors* 32(3):227–242, 2008.
26. Bennett IM, Chen J, Soroui JS, et al: The contribution of health literacy to disparities in self-rated health status and preventive health behaviors in older adults. *Annals of Family Medicine* 7:204–211, 2009.
27. Cutilli CC: Health literacy in geriatric patients: an integrative review of the literature. *Orthopedic Nursing* 26(1):43–48, 2007.
28. Kutner M Greenberg E, Jin Y, et al: *The Health Literacy of America's Adults:Results from the 2003 National Assessment of Adult Literacy (NCES*

2006-483). U.S. Department of Education, Washington, DC, 2006, National Center for Education Statistics.
29. Wolf MS, Gazmararian JA, Baker DW: Health literacy and functional health status among older adults. *Archives of Internal Medicine* 165:1946–1952, 2005.
30. Sudore RL, Mehta KM, Simonsick EM, et al: Limited health literacy in older people and disparities in health and healthcare access. *Journal of the American Geriatrics Society* 54:770–776, 2006.
31. Murray MD, Tu W, Wu J, et al: Factors associated with exacerbation of heart failure include treatment adherence and health literacy skills. *Clin Pharmacol Ther* 85(6):651–658, 2009.
32. Chang M, Kelly AE: Patient education: addressing cultural diversity and health literacy issues. *Urologic Nursing* 27(5):411–417, 2007.
33. Mbaezue N, Mayberry R, Gazmararian J, et al: The impact of health literacy on self-monitoring of blood glucose in patients with diabetes receiving care in an inner-city hospital. *J Natl Med Assoc.* 102(1):5–9, 2010.
34. Safeer R, Cook C, Keenan J: The impact of health literacy on cardiovascular disease. *Vascular Health and Risk Management* 2(4) 457–464, 2006.
35. Effing T, Monninkhof EEM, van der Valk PP, et al: Self-management education for patients with chronic obstructive pulmonary disease. *Cochrane Database of Systematic Reviews* 2007, Issue 4. Art. No.:CD002990. DOI:10.1002/14651858.CD002990.pub2.
36. Hill-Briggs F, Smith A: Evaluation of diabetes and cardiovascular disease print patient education materials for use with low-health literate populations. *Diabetes Care* 31:667–671, 2008.
37. Roberts N, Ghassi R, Patridge M: Health literacy in COPD. *International Journal of COPD* 3(4):499–507, 2008.
38. Tait A, Voepel-Lewis T, Moscucci M, et al: Patient comprehension of an interactive, computer-based information program for cardiac catheterization. *Arch Intern Med* 169(20):1907–1914, 2009.
39. Brown J, Clark A, Dalal H, et al: Patient education in the contemporary management of coronary heart disease. *Cochrane Database of Systematic Reviews* 2010, Issue 12. Art. No.: CD008895. DOI: 10.1002/14651858. CD008895
40. Locke DC: Cross-cultural counseling issues. In Palmo AJ, Weikel WJ, editors: *Foundations of mental health counseling*, Springfield, IL, 1986, Charles C. Thomas.
41. Fairchild HP, editor: *Dictionary of sociology and related sciences*, Totowa, NJ, 1970, Rowan & Allanheld.
42. Locke DC: *Increasing multicultural understanding: a comprehensive model*, Newberry Park, 1992, Sage Publications.
43. Oates DJ, Paasche-Orlow MK: Health literacy: communication strategies to improve patient comprehension of cardiovascular health. *Circulation* 119:1049–1051, 2009.
44. Evangelista L, Rasmusson K, Laramee A, et al: Health literacy and the patients with heart failure—implications for patient care and research: A consensus statement of the Heart Failure Society of America. *J Card Fail* 16(1):9–16, 2010.
45. Ask Me 3. Available at: http://www.npsf.org/askme3.
46. Banzer JA: Results of cardiac rehabilitation in patients with diabetes mellitus. *American Journal of Cardiology* 93:81–84, 2004.
47. Pasternak RC: Understanding physician and consumer attitudes concerning cholesterol management: results from the National Lipid Association surveys. *American Journal of Cardiology* 94:9F-15F, 2004.
48. Reid J, Jamieson A, Bond J, et al: A pilot study of the incidence of post-thoracotomy pulmonary complications and the effectiveness of pre-thoracotomy physiotherapy patient education. *Physiother Can.* 62:66–74, 2010.
49. Meichenbaum D, Turk DC: *Facilitating treatment adherence: a practitioner's guidebook*, New York, 1987, Plenum Press.

Bibliography

Ajzen I: From intentions to actions: a theory of planned behavior. In Kuhl J, Beekman J, editors: *Action control: from cognition to behavior*, New York, 1985, Springer-Verlag.

Bandura A: *Social learning theory*, Englewood Cliffs, NJ, 1977, Prentice-Hall.

Eraker SA, Becker MH, Strecher VJ, et al: Smoking behavior, cessation techniques and the health decision model. *American Journal of Medicine* 78:817–825, 1985.

Fabrega H: Toward a model of illness behavior. *Medical Care* 11:470–484, 1973.

Janz NK, Becker MH: The health belief model: a decade later. *Health Education Quarterly* 11:1–47, 1984.

Leventhal H, Meyer D, Gutman M: The role of theory in the study of compliance to high blood pressure regimens. In Haynes RC, Mattson ME, Engebretson TO, Jr, editors: *Patient compliance to prescribed antihypertensive medication regimes: a report to the National Heart, Lung, and Blood Institute, (NIH Publication No. 81-2102)*, Washington, DC, 1980, U.S. Department of Health and Human Services.

Lorig K: *Patient education. A practical approach*, ed 2, Thousand Oaks, Calif, 2000, Sage Publications.

Shepard KF, Jensen GM, editors: *Handbook of teaching for physical therapists*, Newton, Mass, 2002, Butterworth-Heinemann.

Marlatt GA, Gordon JR, editors: *Relapse prevention: maintenance strategies in addictive behavior change*, New York, 1985, Guilford.

Stetchen VJ, Devellis BM, Becker MH, et al: The role of self-efficacy in achieving health behavior change. *Health Education Quarterly* 13:73–92, 1986.

Part IV

Cardiovascular and Pulmonary Physical Therapy: Acute Conditions

PART IV OUTLINE

IV

Chapter 29

Individuals with Acute Medical Conditions

Elizabeth Dean

KEY TERMS

Asthma
Atelectasis
Bronchiolitis
Bronchitis
Chronic airflow limitation
Cystic fibrosis
Hypertension
Interstitial pulmonary fibrosis
Pneumonia
Stable angina
Stable myocardial infarction
Tuberculosis

CHAPTER OUTLINE

This chapter describes the physical therapy management of individuals with primary, acute dysfunction of the cardiovascular and pulmonary systems. Such dysfunction may limit participation in life and its related activities in the short- or long-term. Further, such dysfunction can constitute life threat in the absence of limitations to life participation and quality of life (e.g., hypertension and dysrhythmias). Management principles for people with several types of common acute medical conditions are described. Although medical conditions are usually classified as either primary pulmonary disease or primary cardiovascular disease, the heart and lungs work synergistically to effect gas exchange and cardiac output and in series with the peripheral vascular circulation to effect tissue perfusion.[1,2] Thus impairment of one organ system invariably has implications for the function of the other. Threat to or impairment of oxygen transport has implications for all other organ systems; thus a multisystem approach is essential for overall management (see Chapters 1 and 5). The primary, acute pulmonary conditions that are presented in this chapter include atelectasis, pneumonia, bronchitis, bronchiolitis, acute exacerbations of chronic airflow limitation, asthma, cystic fibrosis, interstitial pulmonary fibrosis, and tuberculosis. For further epidemiological and pathophysiological detail on these conditions, refer to Mason and colleagues (2010)[3] and West[4] (2007). The primary, acute cardiovascular conditions presented include hypertension, medically stable angina, and uncomplicated myocardial infarction. For further details on these conditions, refer to Sokolow and Cheitlin[5] (2004), Fauci and colleagues[6] (2008), and Woods and colleagues[7] (2009).

The pathophysiology underlying the medical management of each condition extends the pathophysiology content of Chapter 5 and, in turn, provides a basis for each condition's physical therapy management. The management principles presented are not intended to serve as treatment prescriptions for any particular patient. The treatment priorities presented are based on the underlying pathology, as well as the potential complexity of its manifestation for a patient. Without discussion of a specific patient and knowledge of other clinically relevant factors (i.e., the effects of restricted mobility, recumbency, and the effects of extrinsic and intrinsic factors on the patient's presentation including sociocultural context; see Chapter 17); however, the specific parameters of the treatment prescription cannot be completely established. Integration of patient-specific information is essential for treatment to be specific and maximally effective. Chapter 31 extends the principles involved with the management of many of the acute medical conditions described in this chapter, detailing their subacute and chronic stages.

Cardiovascular Pathology

Hypertension

Pathophysiology and Medical Management

Essential hypertension, the "silent killer" (of unknown etiology), is the most common type of hypertension (90% of all reported cases). Although salt sensitivity has been implicated in hypertension in African Americans and increased rennin production in the Hispanic population,[8] salt consumption is a serious health concern in the North American population. Widespread campaigns are being aimed at reducing salt consumption in the pediatric as well as adult population.[9] Reducing consumption by one-third is estimated to reduce the prevalence of hypertension substantially.

Generally, hypertension is classified as mild, moderate, or severe. It is generally managed pharmacologically with vasodilators (i.e., afterload reducers), diuretics (i.e., volume reducers), and beta-blocking agents (i.e., inotropic agents). Despite a primarily pharmacological orientation to the management of hypertension, a high proportion of individuals with hypertension still have high blood pressure and are at increased risk for its deadly complications. Hypertension is a significant health care concern in that the condition is frequently associated with heart disease, stroke, and renal dysfunction and failure.[10] Thus its consequences can be dire. As described in Chapter 1, hypertension often occurs in the presence of obesity and diabetes, which complicates the clinical picture further.

Pharmacological management may have a role in the control of hypertension, given its serious consequences and the necessity of maintaining blood pressure within acceptable limits. Like all medication, its effects must be monitored closely to ensure that the desired outcomes are being achieved. The following decisions must be made:

1. To what degree does pharmacological intervention appear warranted, given the patient's severity of hypertension and overall clinical picture?
2. To what degree could the hypertension be managed with nonpharmacological interventions?
3. To what degree could pharmacological and nonpharmacological interventions be used concurrently? What type of schedule might be anticipated to wean the patient off medication with time or at least minimize it?

Principles of Physical Therapy Management

Physical therapists treat patients with hypertension as a primary or secondary diagnosis. If it is a secondary diagnosis, it is important that the diagnosis is not overlooked. What the physical therapist can do for the hypertension may be clinically more significant than management of the primary diagnosis for which the patient is referred. As with many other lifestyle-related conditions, antihypertensive medication may be perceived by the patient as addressing the problem, whereas in many instances, it only addresses the effect. Lifestyle changes are necessary to normalize blood pressure with the goal of eliminating the need for blood pressure medication.[11]

Exercise therapy can be an effective intervention for the management of hypertension with the primary goal of eliminating the need for medication.[12] Secondarily, physical therapy with a focus on exercise and health education, including smoking cessation and basic nutritional counseling, is aimed at reducing the need for medication or its potency. The foundation of management in a patient with hypertension is a lifestyle review and recommendations in consultation with the patient. Recommendations include nutrition, weight control, exercise, smoking cessation, and stress management.[13] Medical management may include beta blockers and diuretics to reduce plasma volume or other antihypertensive medication. A prescription of regular aerobic exercise may control hypertension.[14] The prescription is based on a consideration of the patient's coexistent problems and general health status. If obesity is a concurrent problem, an exercise program is prescribed to address both concerns.

More frequently, physical therapists treat patients whose hypertension is a secondary condition. Thus, whether the patient is being treated for osteoarthritis, stroke, or cardiovascular and pulmonary dysfunction, treatment is modified accordingly. An exercise prescription includes generalized aerobic exercise at an intensity that is optimally therapeutic and not associated with any excessive or untoward hemodynamic responses.

Patients with labile hypertension are the most difficult patients for whom to prescribe an exercise program because of the irregularity of their blood pressure responses. The intensity is modified at each session to accommodate these variations. Because beta blockers and other medications blunt heart rate responses to exercise, the exercise prescription parameters are defined on the basis of some other objective hemodynamic response or on subjective responses (e.g., the Borg scale of perceived exertion).

The benefits of a modified aerobic exercise prescription include elimination of medication, reduction of medication, and improved pharmacological control on the same dose of medication. In addition, the patient derives all the other multisystem health benefits of exercise. A program of aerobic exercise should be carried out in conjunction with other lifestyle changes associated with blood pressure control (e.g., nutrition, weight control, stress reduction, and smoking cessation program). Medications should be monitored by the physician during the training program. In addition to exercise having a direct effect on controlling hypertension, the effect of exercise on overall metabolism may alter the absorption and degradation of the medications, which in turn can reduce the prescriptive requirements of that medication. Those types of exercise that are associated with a disproportionate hemodynamic challenge (e.g., static movements and stabilizing postures) are not usually indicated. Rather, aerobic exercise that is rhythmic, involves the large muscles of the legs and possibly the arms, and is performed frequently is indicated. Physical therapy outcomes include reduction or elimination of antihypertensive medication with self-monitoring and optimal lifestyle management.

A patient who is being managed acutely with high blood pressure may benefit from relaxation strategies, breathing control, and stress management. Further, complementary therapies, as described in Chapter 27 may have an important role. For noninvasive physical therapy management of hypertension, see Chapter 31.

Angina

Pathophysiology and Medical Management

Angina refers to pain resulting from ischemia of the myocardium and often precedes myocardial infarction. Coronary artery disease is the primary cause of myocardial infarction and is among the leading causes of death in the Western world. Lifestyle factors, including high-fat diet, stress, and low activity levels, contribute to atherosclerosis and fat deposition within the coronary blood vessels. When these deposits narrow or totally occlude the vessel lumen, blood flow is restricted or totally obstructed. As the heart continues to demand oxygen and nutrients in order to work properly, blood supply must be increased. If one or more of the myocardial blood vessels is stenosed, insufficient blood reaches the working myocardial fibers, and ischemia and pain result. The classic description of anginal pain is retrosternal, vice-like, gripping pain radiating to the left side and down the arm and up into the neck; however, anginal pain may occur bilaterally anywhere above the umbilicus. Furthermore, patients vary considerably with respect to the degree to which the severity of the pain correlates with the degree of myocardial ischemia and infarction. Thus even apparently minimal chest pain may be associated with significant ischemia, and its clinical significance should not be minimized. Approximately 10% to 15% of individuals who have a myocardial infarction do not report chest pain. Chest pain can also be blunted in individuals with diabetes as a result of the autonomic neuropathy.

Principles of Physical Therapy Management

The management of patients with ischemic heart disease who are hemodynamically unstable and require intensive monitoring to assess and to monitor physical therapy treatment is described in Chapter 34. This section addresses management of the patient with a cardiac medical condition who is stable and uncomplicated. Physical therapists must be knowledgeable and proficient in management of the patient with cardiac conditions because these patients are referred with cardiac disease as a primary or secondary problem. With respect to heart disease being a secondary diagnosis, patients often come to the physical therapist for the management of an orthopedic complaint with a history of angina, frank myocardial infarction, or hypertension. The principles for physical therapy in management of patients with acute ischemic heart disease are presented within the principles of phase I cardiac rehabilitation (Table 29-1). Because physical therapy invariably involves physically stressing a patient either with therapeutic exercise or with the application of a therapeutic modality, the physical therapist must address the following questions when managing a patient with ischemic heart disease and its risk factors:

1. Does the patient's cardiac status preclude treatment? Why?
2. Is additional information about the patient necessary before physical therapy assessment and treatment? What information?
3. How should treatment be modified? Why?
4. Is the patient using antianginal medication appropriately? Is the prescription current? Does the patient have the antianginal medication present at all times?
5. Are there other medications that may influence the patient's cardiovascular and pulmonary status and response to treatment? What are they? How might the patient's responses to treatment, particularly exercise, be affected?
6. What physiological parameters should be monitored before, during, and after treatment?
7. What is the patient's knowledge about his or her condition? Can the patient clearly identify what triggers the angina and what makes it worse and better? What lifestyle changes have been made? What should be reinforced and what education is necessary?

Table 29-1 Phase I of Cardiac and Pulmonary Rehabilitation (Inpatient, <7 to 10 days)*

Cardiac Rehabilitation	Pulmonary Rehabilitation
After anginal attack, myocardial infarction, operative procedures including bypass surgery and valve surgery	After acute exacerbation or thoracic surgery (e.g., admission lung resection)
Optimize oxygen transport by directing treatment to the underlying limitations of structure and function (impairments)	Optimize oxygen transport by directing treatment to the underlying limitations of structure and function (impairments)
Risk factors assessment	Risk factor assessment
Assessment of knowledge deficits and learning style	Assessment of knowledge deficits and learning style
Readiness to change assessment	Readiness to change assessment
Predischarge submaximal exercise test	Predischarge submaximal exercise test
Discharge lifestyle recommendations: ▪ Smoking cessation ▪ Nutrition and weight control ▪ Physical activity and exercise ▪ Stress management	Discharge lifestyle recommendations: ▪ Smoking cessation ▪ Nutrition and weight control ▪ Physical activity and exercise ▪ Stress management
Plan for follow-up	Plan for follow-up

*Phases II, III, and IV are related to subacute and chronic care (see Chapter 31).

Modified from Piotrowicz R, Wolszakiewicz J: Cardiac rehabilitation following myocardial infarction. *Cardiology Journal* 15:481–487, 2008.

A key consideration in the management of any person with cardiovascular dysfunction is minimizing myocardial strain. Thus mobilization and exercise prescription must incorporate appropriate warm-up, steady-rate, cool-down, and recovery phases, and the type of exercise should be rhythmic and involve the legs (i.e., areas of large muscle mass) and possibly the arms as well. Initially, low-intensity activity that restricts the heart rate to no more than 20 beats above resting heart rate may be indicated to minimize the work of the heart without immobilizing the patient completely. Ejection fraction is not necessarily a good indicator of exercise tolerance because these variables are not well correlated. Upper-extremity work alone is more hemodynamically demanding than lower extremity work and thus is prescribed cautiously, if at all, at least in the early stage. Exercise or physical activity involving sustained static postures and isometric muscle contraction are contraindicated. Breathing should be coordinated with activity such that breath holding and straining are avoided.

An individual with a history of angina, regardless of whether he or she is taking antianginal medications, must be hemodynamically monitored (i.e., heart rate, blood pressure, rate pressure product, and subjective responses; ECG monitoring may also be indicated).

Individuals prone to angina may exhibit symptoms in certain body positions.[15,16] Usually, this reflects an increased workload and increased work of the heart. Recumbent positions increase the mechanical work of the heart by increasing central blood volume.[17] These patients are not encouraged to lie flat. Instead, the head of bed is elevated 10 to 15 degrees. Side-lying positions, particularly left side-lying, increase the work of the heart by compressing the heart and impeding ventricular filling and ejection. Patients with impaired oxygen transport and without prior cardiac disease may exhibit myocardial stress and ischemia in these body positions. Thus patients with impaired or threatened oxygenation must be monitored closely, particularly during turning and activities in which oxygen demand is increased—at these times, oxygen delivery must be increased correspondingly.

The use of medication to minimize the risk for angina and ischemic heart disease warrants review. The need for statins, commonly prescribed lipid-lowering medications, can be reduced through optimal lifestyle choices in many patients. One inherent danger of such a drug, however, in addition to its well documented side effects, is that patients may become complacent, believing that the drug will offset the need to make necessary lifestyle changes. More important, lifestyle changes largely address the cause of the problem, whereas medication such as statins only address an effect. The principles of the physical therapy management of patients with stabilized angina include health education, risk factor reduction, and a long-term health program (see Chapters 24 and 31).

Uncomplicated Myocardial Infarction

Pathophysiology and Medical Management

Myocardial infarction, commonly referred to as a heart attack, refers to insufficient myocardial perfusion resulting in a macroscopic area of damage and necrosis of the heart. Infarction results most frequently from narrowing and occlusion of the coronary blood vessels secondary to atherosclerosis. Other causes include occlusion secondary to a thrombus or embolus, reduced blood pressure, or coronary vasospasm. Angina, or ischemic chest pain, often precedes or accompanies a myocardial infarction. Infarctions vary in severity from being silent (i.e., having no characteristic signs and symptoms and thus going undetected) to being fatal. Most infarctions, when detected, require some hospitalization and monitoring to ensure that the infarction is not evolving further and that the patient is medically stable and in no danger. Chapter 34 describes the management of patients with complicated myocardial dysfunction who are admitted to a coronary care unit. This section focuses on the patient with mild heart disease, the patient with cardiac dysfunction who is discharged from hospital, the patient who has a history of ischemic heart disease, and the patient who is hospitalized for a condition other than heart disease but develops and is being managed for myocardial ischemia. Judicious movement and body positioning are essential elements in the management of the patient with myocardial infarction.[18] Because these interventions can place significant demands on cardiovascular and pulmonary function and oxygen transport, they must be prescribed specifically by physical therapists with considerable knowledge and expertise in the area.

Principles of Physical Therapy Management

Table 29-1 shows the primary components of care in the acute phase of management (phase I of cardiac rehabilitation). Physical therapy constitutes a prime hemodynamic stress secondary to exercise and gravitational stress secondary to mobilization/exercise and body position changes. Thus it is essential to establish the adequacy of the patient's cardiovascular and pulmonary system to effect oxygen transport during and between treatments. The optimal treatment prescription is based on the patient's overall signs and symptoms of coronary insufficiency and hemodynamic instability. The physical therapist must be knowledgeable in detecting inadequate myocardial tissue perfusion and in reducing and preventing myocardial tissue damage. In addition, acute or chronic impaired heart pump function leads to reduced cardiac output and systemic tissue perfusion. Clinical manifestations include reduced mentation, reduced renal function, fatigue, malaise, and moist, cool, and cyanotic skin.

Regardless of whether the patient is being treated in the hospital (in a general ward or in the physical therapy department within the hospital) or in the private physical therapy clinic, the patient must be hemodynamically monitored. Minimally, heart rate and blood pressure must be taken before, during, and after treatment, along with a subjective rating of anginal chest pain. ECG monitoring is usually continuous in the early stages of the infarction. The object of treatment is to have the patient remain below his or her anginal threshold so that anginal pain is avoided. Breathlessness or rating of perceived exertion may also be used. The rate pressure product (RPP) (i.e., the product of heart rate and systolic blood pressure) is highly correlated with myocardial oxygen uptake and work. Previous stress tests will establish the RPP at which angina occurs, and the intensity of the exercise dose should be set at 65% to 80% of this threshold. Patients on beta-blockers have a blunted hemodynamic response to exercise, particularly heart rate responses. In such cases, use of ratings of perceived exertion to define the upper and lower limits of an acceptable mobilization stimulus may be indicated.

In some cases, patients have labile angina (i.e., the onset of angina does not occur reliably at a given RPP). This patient and the patient who reports angina at rest are at higher risk, and appropriate precautions must be taken. First, the patient must be assessed to establish that treatment is not precluded (see pertinent questions to be answered before treating a patient with angina). Second, monitoring is essential and may include ECG monitoring. Third, treatments are prescribed below symptom threshold, which is usually consistent with a low exercise intensity in these patients. Comparable with any patient experiencing low functional work capacity, exercise prescribed on an interval schedule enables the patient to achieve a greater volume of work.

When selecting body positions for the patient with a myocardial infarction, the therapist selects those that will minimize the work of breathing and of the heart.[19] Significant central fluid shifts are minimized by encouraging the upright position as much as possible to reduce the work of the heart[20] and by raising the head of the bed 10 to 15 degrees when the patient is recumbent. Patients with elevated intracardiac pressures are less susceptible to orthostatism (see Chapter 20).

Similar to the management of the patient who has a history of angina, the therapist should avoid body positions, static postures, activities, and respiratory maneuvers associated with increased hemodynamic strain (e.g., breath holding).

Relaxation is central in the management of the cardiac patient who is prone to being anxious and apprehensive. Furthermore, such patients have a high prevalence of sleep-disordered breathing,[21] so a sleep assessment is warranted. Relaxation interventions that can be suggested include autogenic relaxation, progressive relaxation, Benson's relaxation response procedures, biofeedback, and meditation. Also, the patient needs to identify and minimize stress triggers and effective, individual-specific, nonpharmacological relaxants. Relaxation training with or without pharmacological support can be integrated into treatment.[7] Patients with ischemic heart disease are often apprehensive and anxious about the intensity of physical activity they can undertake. Thus performing physical activity and exercise while monitored and under the supervision of a physical therapist is often reassuring and gives the patient confidence to perform activity when unsupervised.

The quality and quantity of the patient's sleep and a profile of sleep-wake periods should be reviewed to ensure he or she is deriving maximal benefit. Rapid-eye-movement sleep with bursts of sympathetic activity during the early hours of the morning may constitute a period of increased risk for the patient with cardiac dysfunction.

Appropriate safety precautions must be taken in all settings where physical therapists practice, given that most physical therapy interventions physically stress patients and that coronary symptoms can occur regardless of whether the patient has a known underlying ischemic heart disease. In addition, because the overall U.S. population is aging, physical therapists are treating a growing number of older persons who are known to have a higher prevalence of cardiovascular conditions. In addition, young adults are presenting with symptoms and signs of cardiovascular conditions.

Optimal lifestyle habits and a lifelong health plan are central to maximizing recovery and improving an individual's long-term prognosis. Good nutrition and hydration, good sleep habits, stress management, smoking cessation, and regular physical exercise are all salient to comprehensive physical therapy management (see Chapters 24 and 31). As in the management of patients with other lifestyle-related conditions, the physical therapist needs to reinforce public health policy and health promotion guidelines regarding healthy lifestyle choices, including avoidance of inactivity and regular physical activity.[22]

Pulmonary Pathology

Atelectasis

Pathophysiology and Medical Management

Atelectasis refers to partial collapse of lung parenchyma. The pathophysiological mechanisms contributing to atelectasis are multiple (Table 29-2). These mechanisms include physical compression of the lung tissue (e.g., resulting from increased pleural fluid, pus, pneumothorax, compression during thoracic surgery, or adjacent areas of lung collapse) or obstruction of an airway (e.g., due to secretions or tumor) with subsequent reabsorption of oxygen from the trapped air by the pulmonary capillaries resulting in a collapse of the lung tissue distal to the obstruction (i.e., reabsorption atelectasis).

There are two primary types of atelectasis: microatelectasis and segmental and lobar atelectasis. Microatelectasis is characterized by a diffuse area of lung units that are perfused but not ventilated, leading to a right-to-left shunt. Ill and hospitalized patients who are deprived of being regularly upright and moving have reduced lung volumes and are prone to breathing at low lung volumes, which leads to microatelectasis. Thus such patients require prophylactic measures to avoid the effects of atelectasis on oxygen transport and gas exchange. When the conditions for normal lung inflation are removed, alveolar collapse occurs instantly.

Microatelectasis is associated with reduced lung compliance because of reduced lung expansion. Patients who are mechanically ventilated are prone to microatelectasis because the normal mechanics of breathing are violated. This may be explained in part by restricted mobility, recumbency, and reduced arousal, in addition to reduced functional residual capacity (FRC). Positive end-expiratory pressure (PEEP) is routinely added to minimize these effects. High ventilator system pressure is required to counter reduced lung compliance, which indicates that atelectatic lung tissue it not readily re-expandable.

Microatelectasis is not diagnosed readily with chest x-ray but can be established in conjunction with clinical findings. Nonetheless, microatelectasis can be anticipated in every ill and hospitalized patient whose normal respiratory mechanics are disrupted, particularly in recumbent, relatively immobile patients. These effects are further exacerbated in patients who are smokers, older, overweight, sedated, have abdominal masses, spinal deformities, or chest wall asymmetry, or some combination of these factors.

Commensurate with its distribution, atelectasis presents with reduced chest wall movement and reduced breath sounds over the involved area. A chest x-ray shows increased density over the involved areas with a shift of the trachea and mediastinum toward the collapsed lung tissue. The patient may be tachypneic and cyanotic because of shunting. Segmental atelectasis results from progression of microatelectasis and obstruction of airways with reabsorption of gas in the distal lung units of a bronchopulmonary segment or lobe.

The patient who depends on a mechanical ventilator to breathe is predisposed to atelectasis because of an unnatural, monotonous breathing pattern, restricted movement, and abnormal and prolonged recumbent body positions. These factors contribute to reduced mucociliary transport, abnormal distribution of pulmonary mucus, and the accumulation of mucus in the dependent lung fields. Furthermore, production of mucus may be increased as a result of tracheostomy or the presence of an endotracheal tube. Mucociliary clearance is further compromised by reduced ciliary activity resulting from high concentrations of oxygen, medication, and loss of an effective cough due to an artificial airway.

The effect of atelectasis on oxygen transport reflects its type and distribution. Hypoxemia, right-to-left shunt, reduced lung compliance, and increased work of breathing are common

Table 29-2 Pathophysiological Mechanisms Contributing to Atelectasis

Central Mechanisms	Breathing at low lung volumes (e.g., when in pain or after certain medications) Inability to generate adequate inspiratory pressure and volume Central disruption of breathing centers controlling normal periodic and rhythmic breathing pattern
Extramural Mechanisms	Chest wall deformity Asymmetry of intrathoracic structures Respiratory muscle weakness (e.g., neuromuscular disease) Phrenic nerve inhibition (e.g., secondary to upper abdominal or cardiovascular thoracic surgery) Compression of lung parenchyma secondary to pleural fluid accumulation, blood, plasma, and pus Compression of lung parenchyma during surgery Reduced lung expansion secondary to reduced movement Compression of lung parenchyma secondary to static body positioning Compression of lung parenchyma secondary to prolonged static body positioning Mechanical ventilation Increased alveolar surface tension
Mural Mechanisms	Airway narrowing secondary to increased bronchial smooth muscle tone Calcification or altered anatomical integrity of airways Edema of the bronchial wall and epithelium
Intramural Mechanisms	Impaired mucociliary transport Increased pulmonary secretions Inspissated pulmonary secretions Altered distribution of pulmonary secretions Mucus plug
Space-Occupying Lesions	Exudative and transudative fluid in the lung parenchyma Foreign-body aspiration Inflammation
Other Factors	Increased compliance and dynamic airway compression secondary to age-related changes to the lung Increased time constants because of increased airway resistance, reduced compliance, or both Splinting or casting of chest wall restricting normal three-dimensional chest wall movement Pain and altered breathing pattern Medications including narcotics, sedatives, and relaxants Supplemental oxygen

clinical manifestations. An increased temperature reflects inflammation or infection and not atelectasis per se.

Principles of Physical Therapy Management

Because it can develop instantaneously when respiratory mechanics are disrupted, microatelectasis should be anticipated and prevented. Those factors that contribute to atelectasis for a given patient are countered accordingly with aggressive prophylactic management. Many of the causes of atelectasis outlined in Table 29-2 can be readily reversed. The assessment includes a detailed analysis of the underlying cause(s) and mechanism(s) so that these can be addressed directly for a given patient.

Atelectasis is always treated aggressively because it has the potential to worsen, develop into a severe clinical manifestation, and lead to pneumonia. In turn, overwhelming pneumonia can precipitate acute respiratory distress syndrome (Chapter 36), which is associated with considerably poorer outcomes. Based on long-standing physiological evidence, treatment continues to be primarily directed at reversing the underlying contributing mechanisms whenever possible. For example, atelectasis resulting from restricted mobility is remediated with mobilization. Atelectasis resulting from prolonged static positioning and monotonous tidal ventilation is managed with mobilization, manipulating body position to increase alveolar volume of the atelectatic area, manipulating body position to optimize alveolar ventilation, or some combination of these interventions. Atelectasis arising from reduced arousal is managed by minimizing the causative factors contributing to reduced arousal coupled with frequent sessions of mobilization and the upright position to stimulate arousal, promote greater tidal volumes and alveolar ventilation, increase zone 2 (area of optimal ventilation and perfusion matching), increase FRC, and minimize closing volume. Most often in a given patient, atelectasis results from a combination of these factors, thus necessitating a multipronged approach in its management.

Breathing control and coughing maneuvers augment the cardiovascular and pulmonary physiological effects of mobilization and body positioning. Coordinating these interventions distributes ventilation more uniformly rather than directing gas to already open alveoli, which overdistends these units. The distribution of ventilation has long been known to be altered primarily by body positioning rather than deep breathing.[23] Sustained maximal inspiratory efforts may augment alveolar ventilation; however, the parameters necessary for such efforts to be maximally therapeutic remain to be elucidated.

If impaired mucociliary transport or excessive secretions are obstructing airways and contributing to atelectasis, mobilization of pulmonary secretions is the goal. Mobilization and a physiological stir-up regimen[24] are instituted as soon as possible for multiple reasons in patients who are acutely ill to augment oxygen transport and minimize reduction in aerobic capacity (Chapter 18). In the event of excessive secretions, mobilization may need to be more vigorous to stimulate eucapnic deep breaths and inspiratory efforts and, hence, effective coughs. Stir-up, coined 70 years ago by Dripps and Waters[25] aptly describes the clinical role of physiologically perturbing a patient to reduce risk and improve outcomes.

Pneumonia

Pathophysiology and Medical Management

Pneumonia is a common complication and cause of morbidity and mortality in the hospitalized patient, particularly in the very young and very old. Comparable to other types of infections, pneumonia results when the normal defense mechanisms fail and, in this case, inadequately protect the lungs from infection, particularly where atelectasis has developed. Infiltrates secondary to pneumonia may result from areas of atelectasis as well as contribute to further atelectasis.

As air is inspired through the nasal passages, it is cleansed of particulate matter by filtration (cilia sweep it to the nasopharynx), impaction (irregular contour of the chamber causing particles to rain out), swelling of hygroscopic droplet nuclei (which are either filtered or become impacted), and defense factors located in the mucous blanket, such as immunoglobulins (IgA), lysozymes, polymorphonuclear leukocytes, and specific antibodies. Particles that escape one of these defense mechanisms in the nasopharynx may be prevented from entering the lower airways of the larynx. The mucosa of the larynx is sensitive to chemical irritation or mechanical deformation and responds by eliciting the cough reflex. The high velocities created by the cough are sufficient to clear several branches of the tracheobronchial tree of particulate matter. The cough reflex is frequently absent or depressed in patients who are unconscious from drug overdose, epilepsy, alcohol ingestion, or head injury. Patients with artificial airways are more susceptible to infection because the normal defense mechanisms are bypassed, causing organisms to be deposited directly in the lower airways. In the lower airways, the cough mechanism is rendered ineffective by endotracheal tubes, which prevent approximation of the vocal cords, and by tracheostomy tubes, which cause air to bypass the cords altogether.

The trachea and the tracheobronchial tree to the level of the respiratory bronchioles are protected by the cough reflex, filtration (again by cilia, which transport particles to the pharynx), impaction, and chemical factors (IgA). Below the level of the respiratory bronchioles, the cough reflex is ineffective and filtration and transportation of particles by cilia cannot occur because cilia are absent. The alveolar macrophages play an important role in protecting these airways from particulate matter. Macrophages ingest organisms and transport them to the lymphatic system or higher in the tracheobronchial tree, where cilia can sweep them to the pharynx. This process of phagocytosis can be slowed or stopped by hypoxia, alcohol ingestion, air pollutants, corticosteroids, immunosuppressant agents, starvation, cigarette smoke, and even supplemental oxygen.

Routes of Infection

A patient who has impaired or ineffective defense mechanisms of the respiratory tract becomes susceptible to a variety of organisms. The major routes of infection include airborne organisms, circulation, contiguous infection, and aspiration. In the past 20 years, hospitalized patients whose immunity is compromised are susceptible to superbug infections, which necessitates aggressive medical management and isolation techniques.[26]

Viral Pneumonias

Most respiratory viral infections are contracted by droplets from the respiratory tracts of infected persons. These viruses are responsible for interstitial pneumonias, tracheobronchitis, bronchiolitis, and the common cold. The ciliated cells of the respiratory tract are the most frequent site of infection. They become paralyzed and degenerate, with areas of necrosis and desquamation. The mucociliary blanket becomes interrupted because destruction of the cilia leaves a thin layer of nonciliated basal replacement cells. Inflammatory responses cause exudation of fluid and erythrocytes in both the alveolar septae and the airways. Congestion and edema become predominant with the formation of intraalveolar hyaline membranes. These changes in the normal mucosal structure and cilia increase the susceptibility of the involved lung to superimposed bacterial infections. This is the most common complication associated with viral infections and is usually responsible for the fatalities that occur.

The patient with viral pneumonia presents with fever, dyspnea, loss of appetite, and a persistent, nonproductive cough. On auscultation, normal breath sounds are heard throughout both lung fields with scattered inspiratory crackles. X-ray changes range from minor infiltrates to severe bilateral involvement. Consolidation and pleural effusions occur less frequently. Secondary bacterial infections occur frequently, causing patients to develop productive coughs.

Influenza may lead to viral pneumonia in 1% to 5% of cases. Influenza includes acute viral respiratory tract infection and is characterized by a sudden onset of headache, myalgia, and fever. The route of infection is by inhalation of airborne particles from an infected person. The incubation period is 24 to 72 hours.

Pulmonary lesions include edema of the respiratory epithelium with necrosis and hemorrhage. At the alveolar level, interstitial edema, proliferation of type I cells, hemorrhage, and an increased number of macrophages are seen. In patients with pneumonia, secondary bacterial infections are frequent and are the cause of most fatalities.

Medical management of viral infections is supportive and preventive. Patients should receive vaccines whenever possible to build up antibodies against specific viruses. Once the patient has contracted the organism, treatment becomes supportive, with rest, salicylates, and high fluid intake being the main treatment priorities. Patients who become more acutely ill with viral pneumonia should be on a vigorous preventative program to lessen the possibility of bacterial infection. Recovery also depends on good nutrition, hydration, sleep, rest, and reduced stress.

PRINCIPLES OF PHYSICAL THERAPY MANAGEMENT

Patients may respond to mobilization coordinated with breathing control exercises and positional rotation for enhancing alveolar ventilation, mucociliary transport, and gas exchange overall.[27] Extreme body positions have long been known to enhance alveolar volume and ventilation as well as ventilation and perfusion matching.[28-31] Vigorous treatment should be initiated at the first sign of a superimposed bacterial infection, which is often accompanied by a productive cough. The appropriate devices should be prescribed at this time (e.g., ultrasonic or medication nebulizers to loosen secretions). Postural drainage may be indicated in addition to mobilization for airway clearance. Treatments, particularly mobilization, must be paced to avoid unduly tiring the patient or increasing oxygen demand beyond the patient's capacity to adequately deliver oxygen. Increasing oxygen demands excessively may compromise the patient's gas exchange. Patient education is also fundamental to the treatment that is to be instituted between treatments (i.e., mobilization and positional rotation coordinated with breathing control and coughing maneuvers).

The goal of cardiovascular and pulmonary physical therapy in the management of viral pneumonia is to augment alveolar ventilation, increase perfusion, increase diffusion, and improve ventilation and perfusion matching, thereby reducing the threat to oxygen transport and gas exchange. Treatments are prescribed to optimize oxygen transport and gas exchange, minimize fatigue and lethargy, and help reduce further infection risk.

Bacterial Pneumonia

Bacterial pneumonia causes the largest number of deaths per year by an infective agent and is a major cause of death, particularly in young patients and older adults. The patient presents with an abrupt onset of a severe illness characterized by fever, tachypnea, dyspnea, hypoxemia, tachycardia, and a cough that produces bloody or purulent sputum. The clinical findings depend on the organism involved and the extent of the pneumonia in the lungs. The infective process may resolve with medications, aerosols, and physical therapy, or it may spread to contiguous areas, causing pleural effusion and empyema.

Bacterial pneumonia can occur as either primary or secondary infections. Primary pneumonias arise in otherwise healthy individuals and are usually pneumococcal in origin. Secondary pneumonias occur when the patient's defense system becomes ineffective.

Pneumococcal pneumonia is caused by pneumococcal bacteria, a gram-positive organism. It occurs most frequently in the winter months in adults, often males, between 15 and 40 years of age. Patients present clinically with abrupt illness characterized by fever, cough, purulent or rust-colored sputum, and pleuritic chest pain over the affected lung field. Physical examination may reveal decreased expansion of the chest over the affected area and muscle splinting. On auscultation, there may be bronchial breath sounds (indicating consolidation), decreased or absent breath sounds, and wheezes or crackles over the affected lung. Chest x-rays may show atelectasis, infiltrates, and consolidation.

There are four stages associated with bacterial infection of lung tissue: engorgement, red hepatization, gray hepatization, and resolution. The engorgement stage occurs within the first few days of infection and is characterized by vascular engorgement, serous exudation, and evidence of bacteria colonization. Red hepatization occurs within 2 to 4 days as a result of diapedesis of the red blood cells. The alveoli are full of polymorphonuclear leukocytes, fibrin, and red blood cells. The organism continues to multiply within the fluid exudate. Areas of consolidation become evident. Gray hepatization occurs within 4 to 8 days and is characterized by evidence of abundant fibrin, decreased polymorphonuclear leukocytes, and dead bacteria. Consolidation continues to be a problem in this stage. Resolution occurs after 8 days as areas of consolidation begin to resolve. Many macrophages are seen, and evidence of enzymatic digestion of exudate is present. The affected tissue becomes softer with large amounts of grayish-red fluid present within the alveoli. This process continues for 2 to 3 weeks with the lung gradually assuming a more normal appearance.

Pleural involvement occurs frequently, with the pleural spaces filling with the same type of fluid seen within the alveoli. Resolution is slower because there are few surfaces available for phagocytosis. Complications that may occur in patients with pneumococcal involvement include empyema, superinfections (occur when large numbers of new organisms invade the lung), abscesses, atelectasis, and delayed resolution (defined as taking more than 4 weeks to resolve).

Treatment of pneumococcal pneumonia includes the use of antibiotics. Thoracentesis is performed when pleural fluid is present. The patient should also receive ultrasonic nebulization and physical therapy. If severe, supplemental oxygen therapy may be indicated.

Staphylococcal pneumonia is caused by a gram-positive organism. It rarely occurs in the healthy adult but is a frequent cause of pneumonia in children, infants, and patients with chronic lung diseases, especially carcinoma, tuberculosis, and cystic fibrosis. Clinically, the patient's manifestations are similar to those seen in the patient with pneumococcal pneumonia. Some differences appear in the chest x-ray (e.g., patchy areas of infiltrate). Consolidation occurs infrequently in this type of pneumonia. Pleural effusions, empyema, abscesses, bronchopleural fistulas, and pneumatoceles (subpleural cyst-like structures) often occur. Treatment includes medication, rest, increased fluid intake, ultrasonic nebulization or medication nebulizers, and aggressive physical therapy.

Streptococcal pneumonia is caused by a gram-positive organism, *Streptococcus pyogenes*. It occurs most frequently in very young, very old, or debilitated patients. The clinical picture is very similar to that of staphylococcal pneumonia. Again, consolidation is rare and chest x-rays usually show one or more areas of patchy infiltrates. Complications are rare, but empyema does occasionally occur. Treatment for this organism is the same as that for pneumococcal pneumonia.

Haemophilus influenzae pneumonia is caused by a gram-negative organism and occurs primarily in children as bronchiolitis and in adults who have chronic bronchitis. The clinical picture is the same as for the other bacterial pneumonias, with numerous areas of infiltration evident on x-ray. On auscultation, breath sounds are generally good, with crackles heard at the end of inspiration. Treatment of this pneumonia includes antibiotics, oxygen, ultrasonic nebulization, and physical therapy.

Other gram-negative organisms causing pneumonia include *Escherichia coli* and *Pseudomonas aeruginosa*. These are seen most frequently in patients with underlying disease, especially pulmonary disease, and in those who are debilitated. These organisms are frequently the cause of superinfections in individuals who have received massive doses of broad-spectrum antibiotics. Clinically, these patients present with cough, fever, and dyspnea. On auscultation, crackles, bronchial breathing, and diminished or absent breath sounds can be noted. X-ray changes frequently show bibasilar infiltrates, with the amount of involvement being widely variable. As for other bacterial pneumonias, treatment includes medications, ultrasonic nebulization, and physical therapy.

Principles of Physical Therapy Management

The goals of management of bacterial pneumonia include reversing alveolar hypoventilation, increasing perfusion, reducing right-to-left shunt, increasing ventilation and perfusion matching, minimizing the effects of impaired mucociliary transport, minimizing the effects of increased mucous production, and optimizing lymphatic drainage of the lungs. Bacterial pneumonia is frequently associated with increased mucus production. With respect to airway clearance, management focuses on augmenting mucociliary clearance overall, reducing excess mucus accumulation, and reducing mucus stasis. The role of traditional manual physical therapy techniques remains equivocal in the management of adults with pneumonia.[32] Patients are often mobile and should be encouraged to be so to promote lung expansion, augment flow rates, stimulate deep tidal volumes (breaths), and augment mucociliary transport and lymphatic drainage.[27,33,34] The oxygen demands of mobilization and exercise, however, must be within the patient's capacity to delivery oxygen. These interventions are prescribed such that they avoid jeopardizing this balance and unduly fatiguing the patient. Deep breathing and effective coughing are important maneuvers for clearing airways with special attention to the avoidance of airway closure. Prescriptive body positioning can be used to optimize ventilation and perfusion matching,[29,35-37] which may be more uniform in the prone position[38] (see Chapter 20). A secondary goal is offsetting aerobic deconditioning from this episode of acute illness, particularly in older adults or patients who are debilitated with chronic conditions.

Acute Exacerbation of Chronic Bronchitis

Pathophysiology and Medical Management

Chronic bronchitis is a common condition in smokers and is characterized by a cough that produces sputum for at least 3 months overall and recurs for 2 consecutive years. Pathological changes include increased size of the tracheobronchial mucous glands and goblet cell hyperplasia. Mucous cell metaplasia of bronchial epithelium results in a decreased number of cilia. Ciliary dysfunction and disruption of the continuity of the mucous blanket are common. In the peripheral airways, bronchiolitis, bronchiolar narrowing, and increased amounts of mucus are observed.

Chronic bronchitis results from long-term irritation of the tracheobronchial tree. The most common cause of irritation is cigarette smoking. Inhaled smoke stimulates the goblet cells and mucous glands to secrete excessive mucus. Smoke also inhibits ciliary action. The hypersecretion of mucus, ciliary damage, and dyskinesis lead to impaired mucus transport and a chronic productive cough. The fact that smokers secrete an abnormal amount of mucus increases the risk for respiratory infections and increases the length of the recovery time from these infections. Although smoking is the most common cause of chronic bronchitis, other factors that have been implicated are air pollution, certain occupational environments, and recurrent bronchial infections.

Although many patients with chronic bronchitis have a high partial pressure of carbon dioxide on arterial blood ($Paco_2$), the pH is normalized by renal retention of bicarbonate. Over the long term, the bone marrow produces more red blood cells, leading to polycythemia. The work of the heart is increased as a result of higher blood viscosity. Long-term hypoxemia leads to increased pulmonary artery pressure and right ventricular hypertrophy.

Patients with chronic bronchitis have tenacious, purulent sputum that is difficult to expectorate. In an exacerbation (usually caused by inflammation or infection or both), these patients produce even more sputum, which tends to be retained and to stagnate. Retained secretions obstruct airways, thus air flow, and reduce alveolar volume. The resulting ventilation and perfusion inequality increases hypoxemia, carbon dioxide (CO_2) retention, accessory muscle use, metabolic demand, and breathing rate. Partial arterial oxygen tension (Pao_2) is further reduced, and $Paco_2$ tends to increase. Hypoxemia and acidemia increase pulmonary vasoconstriction, which increases pulmonary artery pressure and predisposes the patient to right heart dysfunction or failure over time.

A patient with an acute exacerbation of chronic bronchitis tends to have the following characteristics: (1) The patient is often stocky in build and dusky in color. (2) The patient exhibits significant use of accessory muscles of respiration and has audible wheezing or wheezing that is audible on auscultation. (3) Intercostal or sternal retraction of the chest wall may be noted. (4) Edema in the extremities, particularly around the ankles, and neck vein distention reflect decompensated right heart failure. (5) The patient may report that breathing difficulty began with increased amounts of secretions (with a change in their normal color), which is often difficult to expectorate, and increased cough productivity. (6) Pao_2 is reduced, $Paco_2$ increased, and pH reduced. Pulmonary function tests indicate reduced vital capacity, forced expiratory volume in 1 second (FEV_1), maximum voluntary ventilation, and diffusing capacity, as well as increased FRC and residual volume. Debility and deconditioning contribute to suboptimal health, accentuated symptoms, and compromised function.

Principles of Physical Therapy Management

During an exacerbation requiring hospitalization, patients with chronic bronchitis are usually treated with intravenous fluids, antibiotics, bronchodilators, and low-flow supplemental oxygen. Diuretics and digitalis are often given to treat associated right heart failure. Airway clearance interventions are selected (i.e., mobilization, body positioning, and possibly postural drainage). These interventions are coordinated with breathing control and coughing maneuvers to facilitate secretion removal and optimize coughing and expectoration while minimizing dynamic airway compression and alveolar collapse. During recovery, exercise is increased with supplemental oxygen as needed. These patients need to avoid exposure to bronchial irritants (e.g., cigarette smoking, second-hand smoke, and air pollutants) and be adequately hydrated to thin secretions to facilitate mucociliary transport and expectoration.

Patients with chronic bronchitis can benefit from a comprehensive rehabilitation program designed for patients with chronic pulmonary disease, and such a program is best initiated within 1 month of an exacerbation.[39] Even modest exercise has long been known to improve walking capacity and subjective well-being.[40] Components of acute management are shown in Table 29-1 and are comparable to cardiac rehabilitation phase I. Specific details of exercise prescription in the management of chronic obstructive pulmonary disease and of a comprehensive pulmonary rehabilitation program are described in Chapters 24 and 31. Maximizing health and risk factor reduction are principal goals to minimize further pulmonary pathological changes and damage including irreversible emphysema. High-priority strategies include targeted education, smoking cessation, and nutritional and exercise counseling. Individuals who do not have access to such formal structured pulmonary programs (the majority of people), can be managed by the physical therapist, who applies the same principles of practice on an individual basis.

Bronchiolitis

Pathophysiology and Medical Management

Bronchiolitis results from peripheral airway inflammation. Although bronchiolitis is more often seen in babies and small children because of the small caliber of their airways (Chapter 37), adults may be afflicted with this condition, often secondary to some other condition. In severe bronchiolitis, the exudate in the peripheral airways becomes organized into a connective tissue plug extending into the peripheral airway. The inflammatory process resembles that in other tissues (i.e., an inflammatory stage followed by a proliferative healing stage). Such inflammation is associated with vascular congestion, increased vascular permeability, formation of exudate, mucus hypersecretion, shedding of the epithelium, and narrowing of the bronchioles. Fluid is exuded out of the circulation onto the alveolar surfaces, replacing the surfactant. This, in turn, increases the surface tension and promotes airway closure. The secretion production associated with airway irritants and inflammation results from the excess mucus production in combination with the inflammatory exudate, consisting of fluid protein and cells of the exudate. The underlying pathophysiological cascade contributes to both a restrictive and an obstructive component of pulmonary limitation. Airway obstruction results if these exudative substances are not removed. The airway epithelium has the capacity to repair and reline the lumen. A rapid turnover of cells may contribute to cell sloughing and further airway obstruction and a thickened basement membrane. The obstruction associated with bronchiolitis leads to ventilation and perfusion abnormalities and diffusion defect. Clinically, the patient presents with a productive cough. Obliterative bronchiolitis has been reported to be the most significant long-term complication of heart-lung transplantation.[3] Medical management is directed at inflammation control with medications, fluid management, and oxygen administration if necessary. Prevention of infection is a priority.

Principles of Physical Therapy Management

The principal pathophysiological deficits of bronchiolitis include ventilation and perfusion inequality and a diffusion defect. These deficits result from secretions produced by inflammation and increased mucus production and from atelectasis of adjacent alveoli. Physical therapy promotes mucociliary transport and the removal of secretions and mucus to central airways, promotes alveolar expansion and ventilation, optimizes ventilation and perfusion matching and gas exchange, and reduces the risk for infection.

Bronchiolitis is common in babies and young children. The effects of inflammation and obstruction in small children are always serious because the anatomical and physiological components of the cardiovascular and pulmonary systems are smaller, respiratory muscle tone is less well developed, the anatomical configuration of the chest wall is cylindrical, breathing is less efficient under 2 years of age, spontaneous movement and body positioning are more restricted (infants in particular spend more time in non-upright positions), and children are at greater risk for infection (see Chapter 37).

Acute Exacerbation of Chronic Airflow Limitation

Pathophysiology and Medical Management

Chronic airflow limitation (chronic obstructive lung disease) is a leading cause of preventable death from smoking. There are two principal types of emphysema: centrilobular and panlobular. Both types can coexist; however, centrilobular emphysema is 20 times more common than panlobular emphysema. Centrilobular emphysema is characterized by destruction of respiratory bronchioles (see Figure 5-1), as well as edema, inflammation, and thickened bronchiolar walls. These changes are more common and more marked in the upper lung fields. This form of emphysema is found more often in men than women, is rare in nonsmokers, and is common among individuals with chronic bronchitis. Panlobular emphysema is characterized by destructive enlargement of the alveoli distal to the terminal bronchioles (see Figure 5-1). This type of emphysema is also found in individuals with alpha$_1$ antitrypsin deficiency. Airway obstruction in these individuals is caused by loss of elastic recoil or radial traction on the bronchioles. When individuals with normal lungs inhale, the airways are stretched open by the enlarging elastic lung, and during exhalation the airways are narrowed as a result of the decreasing stretch of the lung. The lungs of individuals with panlobular emphysema, however, have decreased elasticity because of disruption and destruction of surrounding alveolar walls. In turn, this leaves the bronchioles unsupported and vulnerable to collapse during exhalation. This form of emphysema can be local or diffuse. Lesions are more common in the bases than the apices and tend to be more prevalent in older adults.

Bullae, emphysematous spaces larger than 1 cm in diameter, may be found in patients with emphysema (see Figure 5-2). They appear to develop from an obstruction of the conducting airways that permits the flow of air into the alveoli during inspiration but does not allow air to flow out during expiration. This causes the alveoli to become hyperinflated and eventually leads to destruction of the alveolar walls with a resultant enlarged air space in the lung parenchyma. These bullae can be more than 10 cm in diameter and, by compression, can compromise the function of the remaining lung tissue (see Figure 5-3). If this happens, surgical intervention to remove the bulla is often necessary. Pneumothorax, a serious complication, can result from the rupture of bullae.

Both types of emphysema can lead to chronic chest wall changes. The loss of elastic recoil of the lung parenchyma disturbs the balance between the normal lung elastic recoil pulling the chest wall in and the natural mechanical tendency of the chest wall to spring out. This balance is essential in maintaining normal FRC (i.e., the air in the lungs at the end of a normal tidal breath). Because the residual volume of the lungs is increased, FRC is correspondingly increased. This increase is not functional, however, because it reflects increased dead space. These patients are still prone to dynamic airway compression and airway closure because of the loss of the normal elastic recoil of the lung parenchyma (i.e., increased compliance). This contributes to uneven distribution of ventilation and decreased diffusing capacity. The pressure volume curve is shifted and ventilation is less efficient.

With loss of elastic recoil and the normal tethering of the alveoli keeping them patent, the chest wall tends to expand outward, thereby contributing to the hyperinflated chest associated with the patient with chronic airflow limitation. The alveolar units are structurally less uniform and the distribution of ventilation becomes even less homogeneous. Inspiratory and expiratory times of the alveolar units also become heterogeneous. The alveoli require long inspiratory filling times (i.e., long time constants). For this reason, the patient with chronic airflow limitation adopts a characteristic breathing pattern in which inspiration and expiration tend to be prolonged. On expiration, the patient may spontaneously adopt a pursed-lip breathing pattern, which is believed to augment alveolar patency and promote collateral ventilation and gas exchange in the lungs by creating positive back pressures. In addition, the patient may expire actively to compensate for the loss of the passive elastic recoil that normally empties the lungs at end tidal volume. Overall, the work of breathing is increased. As the lungs become more chronically hyperinflated, the chest wall becomes increasingly barrel-shaped and rigid. Loss of both the normal shape of the chest wall and the bucket and pump handle motions further compromises efficient respiratory mechanics and breathing.

The most common complaint of the patient with emphysema is dyspnea. Physically, these individuals appear thin and have an increased anteroposterior chest wall diameter. Depending on disease severity, they breathe using the accessory muscles of inspiration (Chapter 5). These patients may be observed leaning forward, resting their forearms on their knees, or sitting with their arms extended at their sides, pushing down against the bed or chair to elevate their shoulders and improve the effectiveness of the accessory muscles of inspiration.

Patients with emphysema have increased respiratory work to maintain relatively normal blood gases. On auscultation, decreased breath sounds can be noted throughout most or all of the lung fields. Radiologically, the emphysema patient has overinflated lungs, flattened hemidiaphragms, and a small, elongated heart (see Figure 5-4). Pulmonary function tests show a decreased vital capacity, FEV_1, maximum voluntary ventilation, and a greatly reduced diffusing capacity. The total lung capacity, the residual volume, and the FRC are increased. Arterial blood gases reflect a mildly or moderately lowered PaO_2, a normal or slightly raised $PaCO_2$, and a normal pH. Patients with emphysema, unlike patients with chronic bronchitis, tend to develop cardiac insufficiency with progression of the condition, leading to failure at the end stage of the disease. At this stage, cardiac hypertrophy may be evident.

Hypoxemia leads to hypoxic pulmonary vasoconstriction, which shunts blood from under-ventilated to better-ventilated areas of the lung. The afterload against which the right heart has to pump is increased. This elevates pulmonary vascular resistance and pulmonary artery blood pressure (i.e., pulmonary hypertension). Over the long term, the right heart hypertrophies to work against this increased resistance and eventually may fail (right ventricular failure). Heart enlargement secondary to any cause alters the electrical conduction pattern, affecting electromechanical coupling and cardiac output. The altered size and heart position within the chest wall can be detected by ECG changes, as well as by echocardiogram.

Treatment of emphysema that requires hospitalization often includes intravenous fluids, antibiotics, and low-flow supplemental oxygen. Some patients require bronchodilators, diuretics, and digitalis. Patients with chronic airflow limitation can adapt to high $PaCO_2$ levels and thus can become dependent on their hypoxic drives to breathe. Therefore low-flow supplemental oxygen is administered to these patients to avoid abolishing their O_2-dependent drive to breathe.

The incidence of emphysema increases with age. It is most often found in patients with chronic bronchitis and is more prevalent in smokers than nonsmokers. There appears to be a hereditary factor. Severe panlobular emphysema can develop in patients with an $alpha_1$ antitrypsin deficiency relatively early in life, even though they never smoked. Repeated lower respiratory tract infections may also play a role in the pathology of emphysema.

Chronic bronchitis and emphysema are marked by a progressive loss of lung function and corresponding cardiac dysfunction. Death rates reported by various studies depend on the methods of selection of patients, types of diagnostic tests, and other criteria. In general, the death rates 5 years after diagnosis are 20% to 55%. The 5-year survival rates based on FEV_1 have been reported to be 80% in patients with a FEV_1 greater than 1.2 L, 60% in patients with an FEV_1 close to 1 L, and 40% for patients with an FEV_1 less than 0.75 L. If these flow rates, however, are found in patients with complications of resting tachycardia, chronic hypercapnia, and a severely impaired diffusing capacity, the survival rates are reduced by 25%. Other factors that have been associated with a poor prognosis are right ventricular failure, weight loss, radiological evidence of emphysema, a dyspneic onset, polycythemia, and Hoover's sign (inward movement of the ribs on inspiration). The most frequent causes of death in patients with airflow limitation are congestive heart failure (secondary to right ventricular failure), respiratory failure, pneumonia, bronchiolitis, and pulmonary embolism.

As emphysema becomes chronic, the hemidiaphragms become more horizontally positioned, placing the muscle fibers at a less efficient position on their length tension curve.[41] When the muscle fibers of respiration are mechanically disadvantaged, the work of breathing is increased, thereby also increasing energy demands and oxygen cost. Respiratory muscle weakness and fatigue are serious complications of chronic lung disease that predispose the patient to respiratory muscle failure (Chapters 26 and 34).

The net effects of the pathological changes on gas exchange are hypoxemia, hypercapnia, and reduced pH consistent with respiratory acidosis. Long-term respiratory insufficiency leads to chronically impaired oxygen transport and gas exchange. To compensate for hypercapnia, production of bicarbonate is increased to buffer retained CO_2 (i.e., compensated respiratory acidosis). Red blood cell production (i.e., polycythemia) is increased, raising the oxygen-carrying capacity of the blood. The negative effect of polycythemia, however, is increased viscosity of the blood, leading to increased risk for circulatory stasis, thromboses, and increased work of the heart.

Principles of Physical Therapy Management

Standards of practice for chronic obstructive lung disease have been well documented globally.[42,43] Priorities are minimizing exacerbations and reducing overuse of antibiotics.[44] Physical therapy has a primary role in helping to prevent this condition and its sequelae (including premature death), as well as in managing it without drugs and surgery as much as possible.

The patient with emphysema is prone to chronic pulmonary infections and respiratory insufficiency. The clinical picture is hallmarked by alveolar collapse and destruction, ventilation and perfusion mismatch, and diffusion defect. These defects result in impaired or threatened oxygen transport if the physiological compensations are unable to maintain adequate blood gases. Shortness of breath is exacerbated, and breathing is labored. Increased work of breathing reflects airway obstruction and inefficiency of respiratory mechanics and the respiratory muscles. Because of long-term airway disease, mucociliary transport is disrupted. Therefore in the presence of a pulmonary infection and increased production of pulmonary secretions, secretion removal can be a major problem for the patient.

Table 29-1 shows the primary components of care in the acute phase of management, which can be compared with acute cardiac care (phase I of cardiac rehabilitation). Specific treatments are prescribed for the patient based on the specific clinical findings (i.e., the type and severity of the cardiovascular and pulmonary dysfunction and the presence of infection). Therefore treatments include mobilization coordinated with breathing control and coughing maneuvers, which are effective in enhancing alveolar ventilation, mobilizing secretions, and facilitating ventilation and perfusion matching. Body positioning can be prescribed to alter the distribution of ventilation, to aid mucociliary transport, and to remove pulmonary secretions. Although "pure" emphysema is typically dry, postural drainage positions can facilitate the removal of pulmonary secretions from specific bronchopulmonary segments if indicated. In any given body position, alveolar volume is augmented in the uppermost lung fields and alveolar ventilation is augmented in the lowermost lung fields. The type and extent of pathology determine the degree of benefit these physiological effects will have on oxygen transport.

In addition, body positioning is essential to optimize respiratory mechanics and enhance pulmonary gas exchange, thereby reducing the work of breathing and the work of the heart. The assessment defines the parameters of the treatment prescription that will be effective in relieving the work of breathing and the work of the heart. This information is essential not only for prescribing beneficial positions but also for avoiding deleterious positions. A sitting, leaned-forward position will assist ventilation secondary to the gravitational effects of the upright position on cardiovascular and pulmonary function. If the arms are supported, this position stabilizes the upper chest wall and rib cage, thereby facilitating inspiration. Some patients, in respiratory distress and with horizontally positioned hemidiaphragms, benefit from recumbent positions in which the hemidiaphragms are elevated within the chest wall by the viscera falling against the underside of the hemidiaphragms in this position (i.e., viscerodiaphragmatic breathing).[45] The muscle fibers of the diaphragm are mechanically placed in a more favorable position with respect to their length-tension characteristics. This effect may further be augmented in the head-down position in some patients.[46] Other patients, however, cannot tolerate recumbent positions; in fact, respiratory distress may be increased. If optimal treatment outcome has not been achieved with mobilization and body positioning coordinated with breathing control and coughing maneuvers, conventional physical therapy procedures may offer additional benefit in some patients (e.g., postural drainage and manual techniques if a refractory purulent infective process is present).

Because of the tendency toward dynamic airway compression resulting from the highly compliant airways of individuals with emphysema, open-glottis coughing maneuvers are indicated. Specific outcome measures are recorded before, during, and after treatment to assess short- and long-term treatment effects. In addition, between-treatment maneuvers are central to maximizing overall treatment effectiveness. Conveying information effectively and specifically to the patient, nursing staff, and perhaps family members is therefore crucial to achieving a maximal treatment outcome.

As with the individual who has chronic bronchitis, people with chronic airflow limitation due to emphysema should be prescribed a lifelong health program that includes smoking cessation, basic nutritional counseling, and exercise counseling (see Chapters 24 and 31). Based on the assessment, the physical therapist makes a decision with respect to whether professional counseling may augment outcomes (e.g., smoking cessation counselor), whether the patient may benefit from pharmacological support for smoking cessation, and whether the general practitioner needs to be consulted. A decision is also made as to whether a professional nutritionist should be involved. Improved aerobic conditioning can reduce the frequency and severity of subsequent acute exacerbations.[47] Quality of life is associated with fewer clinical signs and symptoms.[48]

Acute Exacerbation of Asthma

Pathophysiology and Medical Management

Asthma is a condition characterized by an increased responsiveness of bronchial smooth muscle to various stimuli and is manifested by widespread narrowing of the airways that changes in severity either spontaneously or as a result of treatment. During an asthma attack, the lumen of the airways is narrowed or occluded by a combination of bronchial smooth muscle spasm, inflammation of the mucosa, and an overproduction of viscous, tenacious mucus.

Asthma that begins in patients under the age of 35 years is usually allergic or extrinsic. These asthma attacks are precipitated when an individual comes into contact with a given substance to which he or she is sensitive, such as pollens or household dust (see Table 29-1). Patients with asthma can be allergic to a number of substances rather than only one or two.

If a patient's first asthma attack occurs after the age of 35, often there is evidence of chronic airway obstruction with intermittent episodes of acute bronchospasm. These individuals, whose attacks are not triggered by specific substances, are referred to as having nonallergic or intrinsic asthma (Table 29-3). Chronic bronchitis is commonly found in this group, and this is the type of asthma most often seen in the hospital setting.

The patient with asthma presents with the following picture during an attack. Lung volumes and expiratory flow rates are reduced, and the distribution of ventilation is less homogeneous.[24] The patient has a rapid rate of breathing and uses the accessory respiratory muscles (see Figure 5-6). The expiratory phase of breathing is prolonged, with audible wheezing. The patient may cough frequently, but unproductively, and may complain of tightness in the chest. Radiologically, the lungs may appear hyperinflated or show small atelectatic areas (reabsorption atelectasis). Early in the attack arterial blood gases reflect slight hypoxemia and a low P_{CO_2} (from hyperventilation). If the attack progresses, the P_{O_2} continues to fall as the P_{CO_2} increases above normal. As obstruction becomes severe, deterioration of the patient is evidenced by a high CO_2, a low P_{O_2}, and a pH of less than 7.3.

Patients who are hospitalized are treated with intravenous fluids, bronchodilators, supplemental oxygen, and corticosteroids. Breathing control in the acute attack relaxes the patient, helps manage the attack more effectively, and provides a means of helping to reduce subsequent attacks. Airway clearance procedures may have a role if the cough becomes productive. Patients should avoid bronchial irritants and substances that worsen or induce significant bronchospasm or an attack.

An asthmatic attack that persists for several hours and is unresponsive to medical management is referred to as status asthmaticus. This condition constitutes a medical emergency, necessitating admission to the intensive care unit (see Chapter 34).

Table 29-3 Factors That Precipitate Asthmatic Symptoms

General Precipitating Factor	Specific Examples of Triggers
Allergic or extrinsic asthma	Pollen (especially ragweed) Animals Feathers Molds Household dust Food
Nonallergic or intrinsic asthma	Inhaled irritants Cigarette smoke Dust Pollution Chemicals
Ambient environment	High humidity Cold air
Respiratory infections	Common cold Bacterial bronchitis
Drugs	Aspirin
Emotions	Stress Excitement
Exercise	Continuous aerobic Continuous aerobic in cool environment

Principles of Physical Therapy Management

The hallmark of an acute exacerbation of asthma is bronchospasm, an increased responsiveness of airway smooth muscle to various stimuli (i.e., reversible airway obstruction). Although bronchospasm can be a feature of chronic bronchitis and emphysema, the primary cause of airway obstruction in these conditions results from anatomical and physiological changes that are not usually reversible.

Table 29-1 shows the primary components of care in the acute phase of management, which are comparable to acute cardiac care (phase I of cardiac rehabilitation). Physical therapy is directed at improving gas exchange without aggravating bronchospasm and other symptoms and reversing these when possible. In one systematic review, the role of breathing exercises for people with acute asthma was not substantiated.[49] Thus relaxing the patient's overbreathing by whatever method works best is recommended. Patients experiencing an acute asthmatic attack may reduce their respiratory rate with a CO_2 rebreathing bag; the benefits may be augmented by reducing a hyperventilatory response with optimal positioning.[50] Overall oxygen demand, including that associated with an increased work of breathing, needs to be reduced during an exacerbation of asthma. This may require reduced activity, body positioning that improves breathing efficiency, judicious rest and sleep periods, altered diet or restricted diet, adequate hydration, maintenance of a thermoneutral environment, rest, reduced arousal, reduced social interaction and excitement, and reduced environmental stimulation. Although general relaxation does not directly relax bronchial smooth muscle, it will assist breathing control, reduce arousal and metabolic demands, and promote more efficient breathing.

Airway narrowing and obstruction is a hallmark of this condition secondary to increased bronchial smooth muscle tone and airway edema. Even small amounts of pulmonary secretions can obstruct the lumen of narrowed airways, which leads to reabsorption atelectasis distal to the site of obstruction, impaired gas exchange, and reduced Pa_{O_2}. Thus mucociliary transport is a priority. Mucous clearance can be further impeded by the addition of serous fluid to pulmonary mucus, resulting from airway irritation and inflammation. Cilia are less effective at clearing mucoserous fluid compared with mucus alone. In addition, sheets of ciliated epithelium are shed into the bronchial lumen, further contributing to the stasis of secretions. Thus optimizing the mobilization of secretions and their removal is a priority even in the presence of scant secretions. Interventions that optimize mucociliary transport are selected to minimize exacerbating bronchospasm and further increases in airway resistance.

The primary goals in the management of asthma include reducing airway narrowing, improving alveolar ventilation, reducing the work and energy cost of breathing, reducing hypoxemia or minimizing its threat, and optimizing lung compliance.

Treatment outcome is assessed with indices of oxygen transport overall and of the function of the individual steps in the pathway.[51] Bedside spirometry, including peak expiratory flow rate, is a sensitive indicator of ensuing compromise in oxygen transport. Some patients use a peak expiratory flow rate meter at home to detect such changes and as an early indicator of the need for medical attention.

Individuals with asthma can often learn to control their condition effectively with optimal health education and an overall lifelong health program (see Chapters 24 and 31).

Acute Exacerbation of Cystic Fibrosis

Pathophysiology and Medical Management

Cystic fibrosis (CF) is a complex multisystem disorder transmitted by an autosomal-recessive gene that affects the exocrine glands. CF involves all of the major organ systems in the body and is characterized by increased electrolyte content of the sweat, chronic airflow limitation, ventilation inhomogeneity, and pancreatic insufficiency. Definitive diagnosis of CF includes positive family history, clinical symptoms of poor digestion, growth or recurrent pulmonary infection, and most important, a positive sweat chloride test. Survival has increased dramatically since 1940 when survival was reported to be approximately 2 years. Thus, although CF is congenital and manifests in childhood, this condition has now become an adult disorder. Adult patients with CF often have an upper lobe infiltrate, with evidence of atelectasis and bronchiectasis, and chronic staphylococcal infections. The beat frequency of the cilia is often slowed to approximately 3 mm per minute, compared with 20 mm per minute in age-matched, healthy, control subjects.[52] Patients can be categorized into three general groups: those with no significant pulmonary signs, those with pulmonary signs and occasional cough and sputum, and those with pulmonary signs and constant cough and sputum. Those patients in the last group tend to have significantly impaired pulmonary function test results, reduced diffusing capacity, and increased hemoptysis, particularly in the presence of an abnormal chest x-ray and hyperinflation. Airway hyperreactivity appears to be variable.

Peripheral airways are often abnormal either anatomically or functionally because of mucus plugging. The lungs of patients with CF may be excessively stiff at maximal lung capacity, with a loss of elastic recoil at low lung volumes. Regional ventilation is nonuniform and contributes to ventilation and perfusion mismatch and hypoxemia.[24]

The chronic pulmonary limitation in CF is related to increased secretion of abnormally viscous mucus, impaired mucociliary transport resulting in airway obstruction, bronchiectasis, hyperinflation, infection, and impaired regional ventilatory function, leading to impaired ventilation and perfusion matching and gas exchange. Radiologically, changes are most pronounced in the upper lobes, especially the right upper lobe.

Principles of Physical Therapy Management

Prophylactic cardiovascular and pulmonary physical therapy, including facilitation of mucociliary transport and maximizing alveolar ventilation, in conjunction with the judicious use of antibiotics, provides effective measures for controlling or slowing the effects of bronchial and bronchiolar obstruction. Involvement of the patient and caregivers in chronic care in the long term is particularly important. Understanding the pathology and course of CF is essential to modify treatment prescription during exacerbations and remissions of the disease.

Table 29-1 shows the primary components of care in the acute phase of management, which can be compared generally with acute cardiac care (phase I of cardiac rehabilitation). The clinical deficits related to oxygen transport include impaired mucociliary transport, increased mucus production, increased difficulty clearing mucus, impaired ventilation and perfusion matching, right-to-left shunt, a diffusion defect, respiratory muscle weakness or fatigue, and reduced cardiovascular and pulmonary conditioning. The increased production of mucus and the difficulty removing mucus increase the risk for bacterial colonization and chronic respiratory infections. These manifestations of CF are worsened with recumbency. Significant postural hypoxemia has been reported in patients with CF when moving from sitting to a supine position.[53] Thus the object of treatment is to optimize oxygen transport and pulmonary gas exchange. Given the pathophysiological deficits in an acute exacerbation of CF, the specific goals are to enhance mucociliary transport, promote airway clearance, optimize alveolar ventilation and therefore gas exchange, maximize the efficiency of oxygen transport overall, and prevent and minimize infection.

Although the degree to which patients with chronic lung conditions, and in particular CF, can respond to aerobic training may be limited, it is essential that their capacity to transport oxygen overall is optimized to compensate for deficits in specific steps of the oxygen transport pathway.[54] Deconditioning severely impairs oxygen transport. Improved aerobic capacity and cardiovascular and pulmonary conditioning are central in the management of patients with CF. Prescriptive aerobic exercise enhances the efficiency of oxygen transport overall by reducing airway resistance by mobilizing secretions, improving the homogeneity of ventilation in the lungs and therefore ventilation and perfusion matching, optimizing oxygen extraction at the tissue level, and increasing respiratory muscle endurance.[55] If optimal conditioning is maintained, oxygen transport is not as compromised during acute exacerbations given the improved efficiency of oxygen transport overall. These effects will be lost, however, as the patient deconditions secondary to restricted mobility and recumbency during the acute episode. Thus it is important that mobility is minimally restricted during an exacerbation (based on the clinical assessment and morbidity) and that exercise conditioning is a mainstay of management between exacerbations. An important additional effect of long-term exercise, which has particular importance for patients with CF, is improved immunity.[56] This may minimize the risk for infection and perhaps minimize the severity of an infection once acquired. Patients with CF can have an abnormal hemodynamic response to exercise and myocardial adaptation; thus appropriate cardiac assessment and monitoring is indicated.[57]

In severe exacerbations the patient is extremely stressed physiologically and has significantly increased oxygen consumption because of the increased work of breathing and for the heart. In addition, the patient is prone to arterial desaturation. Thus minimizing undue oxygen demand and fatigue guides the selection of treatment interventions and their parameters in conjunction with stringent monitoring. These patients become hypoxemic and distressed readily. Treatment interventions are selected based on the assessment and the patient's ability to tolerate the treatment and derive optimal benefit. Gradual, paced, low-intensity mobilization and frequent body positioning enhance mucociliary transport and airway clearance and maximize the efficiency of the steps in the oxygen transport pathway. Postural drainage can offer additional benefit in these patients if further clearance is required. The addition of manual techniques may be indicated; however, stringent monitoring must be carried out given their potential deleterious effects on gas exchange.[58]

Forced coughing and expiratory techniques can contribute to airway closure, whereas huffing and other forms of modified coughing with an open glottis minimize airway closure and can be more effective in removing secretions that have accumulated centrally without compromising ventilation and gas exchange. Forceful coughing, in which the glottis closes, contributes to airway closure and thus should be avoided, particularly in patients with elevated pulmonary artery pressure, because of the concomitant increase in intrathoracic pressure and strain on the heart and lungs. Patients with CF have severe paroxysms of coughing. This significantly increases intrathoracic pressure, which in turn impedes venous return and cardiac output. Although coughing is an essential mechanism for mucociliary clearance in these patients, the untoward cardiac effects must be minimized.

Over the past decade, other interventions aimed at secretion clearance in the treatment of patients with CF have included autogenic drainage, the use of the positive expiratory pressure (PEP) mask, and the Flutter valve.[2,59] One study of patients with CF hospitalized for acute exacerbations compared the short-term efficacy of three regimens: postural drainage (PD), positive expiratory pressure physiotherapy (PEP), and high-frequency chest compression (HFCC) physical therapy.[60] The authors reported no change in lung function or in sputum production when the number of coughs was considered.

Autogenic drainage is based on the theory that the equal pressure point is shifted along the airways by altering the lung volume at which the patient breathes. The patient initially breathes slowly and deliberately at low lung volumes, then at mid and high lung volumes. Breathing at low lung volumes is believed to loosen secretions from the walls of the airways. This is followed by breathing at mid lung volumes, which is believed to help localize and collect the secretions. Finally, breathing at high lung volumes is believed to centralize and facilitate the removal of the secretions with coughing. Thus autogenic drainage may enhance the effectiveness of the patient's cough by manipulating lung volumes and flow rates and controlling coughing to avoid unproductive coughing and wasteful expenditure of energy. The patient is coached by the physical therapist to breathe slowly and deliberately at the volumes set by the therapist, who gauges the patient's ventilatory effort and work by placing his or her hands around the patient's chest. The patient is not encouraged to breathe below end-expiratory volume and is encouraged to suppress coughing until the expelling phase (i.e., the phase during which the patient is breathing at high lung volumes).

Autogenic drainage may be a useful adjunct for facilitating airway clearance in patients with CF. It is a procedure that patients may use independently and can be applied relatively unobtrusively. It helps optimize the patient's coughing efforts and minimizes the potential for airway closure in these patients. This procedure is designed to minimize exhaustive, metabolically costly coughing and preserve energy to expectorate most effectively.[61]

The PEP mask and Flutter® valve device are believed to reduce airway closure in conjunction with exercise, thus optimizing alveolar ventilation and enhancing mucociliary clearance in patients with CF.[62] Individuals with CF can often learn to control their condition effectively with optimal health education and overall lifelong health program (see Chapters 24 and 31).

Acute Exacerbation of Interstitial Pulmonary Fibrosis

Pathophysiology and Medical Management

Interstitial lung disease has been associated with various occupations and the inhalation of inorganic and organic dusts. Conditions associated with the inhalation of inorganic dusts include silicosis, asbestosis, berylliosis, and talc or coal pneumoconiosis. These conditions are most often seen in miners, welders, and construction workers. Workers exposed to organic material, such as fungal spores and plant fibers, may develop a serious pulmonary reaction known as extrinsic allergic alveolitis. Generally, interstitial lung disease is characterized by inflammation of the lung parenchyma, which may resolve completely or progress to fibrosis. Interstitial pulmonary fibrosis results from the deposition of connective tissue after repeated bouts of infection. The pathophysiological deficits are commensurate with morphological changes of interstitial infiltration and fibrosis, intraalveolar exudate, and alveolar replacement (see Figure 5-12). Lung compliance and lung volumes are reduced, expiratory flow at mid lung volume is increased (stiff, inelastic lungs), diffusing capacity is reduced, and hypoxemia can be present in the absence of hypercapnia. The chest x-ray of a patient with interstitial pulmonary fibrosis secondary to sarcoidosis is shown in Figure 5-12. Other changes include increased resting heart rate, pulmonary hypertension, impaired gas exchange, and shortness of breath during exercise, as well as at rest in some cases. Symptoms can be reversed by removing the worker from the exposure through change of employment, modification of the materials handling process, or use of protective clothing and masks. Repeated exposure to these organic dusts may result in irreversible interstitial fibrosis.

Reaction to fumes and gases can also lead to chronic restrictive patterns of lung disease. Individuals exposed to plastics being heated at high temperatures are also exposed to gases that are toxic to the respiratory system. Chronic pathological changes and impaired gas exchange can result.

Medical management is directed at reducing inflammation, reducing pulmonary hypertension, and increasing arterial oxygenation. Pharmacological management may include corticosteroids for inflammation, immunosuppressive agents, and oxygen therapy. Removing the patient from the work environment contributing to interstitial pulmonary fibrosis is essential in managing the disease and its long-term consequences.

Principles of Physical Therapy Management

The primary clinical manifestations of an acute exacerbation of interstitial pulmonary fibrosis reflect an acute or chronic problem, usually resulting from an inflammatory episode, pulmonary infection, or both. The mechanisms responsible include reduced alveolar ventilation, an inflammatory process and its manifestations, potential airway obstruction, increased work of breathing, and in severe cases, increased work of the heart. These patients are susceptible to desaturation during exercise and thus need to be monitored closely.

Table 29-1 shows the primary components of care in the acute phase of management, which are similar to those of acute cardiac care (phase I of cardiac rehabilitation). In mild cases mobilization increases the homogeneity of ventilation and ventilation and perfusion matching. Between treatments and in the management of the severely affected patient, body positioning is used to reduce the work of breathing and arousal, maximize alveolar ventilation, maximize ventilation and perfusion matching, and optimize coughing.

Patients with moderate-to-severe interstitial lung disease may desaturate during sleep and readily desaturate on physical exertion.[63] Thus they warrant close monitoring during and between treatments. Increased pulmonary vascular resistance secondary to hypoxic vasoconstriction contributes to increased work of the right heart and potential cardiac insufficiency.

General debility and deconditioning warrant an exercise program that can optimize the conditioning and function of all of the steps in the oxygen transport pathway.[64] Individuals with interstitial pulmonary fibrosis require health education and an overall health program to help manage their symptoms (see Chapters 24 and 31).

Tuberculosis

Pathophysiology and Medical Management

Although the incidence of tuberculosis, a lifelong disease, has declined significantly over the past several decades, this disease has been experiencing a resurgence in the industrialized world in recent decades. This may reflect declining sanitation and health standards in some segments of the population and immigration patterns.

Most infections result from inhalation of airborne tubercle bacilli, which triggers an inflammatory response. This response includes flooding of the affected area with fluid leukocytes and later macrophages. The area becomes consolidated; pathologically, the condition is considered a tuberculous pneumonia. The infiltrating macrophages become localized and fused, resulting in the characteristic tubercle. Within 2 to 4 weeks the central part of the lesion necroses. Tuberculosis is associated primarily with pulmonary infection that is comparable with other infectious pneumonias. Tuberculosis, however, is distinct in that it may affect other parts of the body. Symptoms include fatigue, fever, reduced appetite, weight loss, night sweats, hemoptysis, and a cough with small amounts of nonpurulent sputum with pulmonary involvement. The course of the disease is variable. Some lesions heal promptly, whereas other patients experience progression and ensuing death. Other systems that can be involved include brain and meninges, kidney, reproductive, and bone. In some individuals the disease appears to remit, whereas in others tuberculosis progresses to affect other organ systems or previously dormant foci can be reactivated.

The effects of tuberculosis on pulmonary function are variable, depending on the extent and type of lesions. Lesions may involve the lung parenchyma, the bronchi, the pleurae, and chest wall. Parenchymal involvement can reduce lung volumes, leading to hypoventilation of perfused lung units. Significant disease leads to impaired arterial blood gases, whereas areas of unaffected lung may adequately compensate in milder cases. If fibrosis has occurred, lung compliance will be correspondingly reduced. Airflow resistance may be increased from narrowing or distortion of the bronchioles because of fibrosis. Pleural involvement may result in effusions, empyema, pleural fibrosis, and spontaneous pneumothorax. Unlike parenchymal damage, small amounts of pleural restriction can produce significant changes in pulmonary function. Clinically, patients with significant pleural involvement have significant restrictive disease and correspondingly low lung volumes. The work and energy cost of breathing are markedly increased. Shortness of breath is a common complaint. Comparable with an interstitial pulmonary fibrosis patient, the patient adopts a rapid, shallow breathing pattern to reduce the high cost of elastic work of breathing. Thus the dead space tends to be hyperventilated and alveolar hypoventilation results.

In addition to alveolar hypoventilation, lung tissue and pulmonary vascular damage impairs ventilation and perfusion matching and diffusing capacity. In severe cases, hypoxemia and hypercapnia are present. Chronic adaptation includes polycythemia and hypervolemia. Right heart failure may ensue.

The lungs become shrunken and geometrically distorted because of fibrotic changes in the lungs. These changes can lead to kinking and obstruction of the pulmonary blood vessels and maldistribution of pulmonary blood flow, which further compromises ventilation and perfusion matching.

Tuberculosis may be associated with an obstructive component. An increase in airflow resistance comparable with emphysema can be present. This obstruction results from chronic infection, mucosal edema, retained secretions, and bronchospasm.

Antibiotics can be effective in managing the disease well enough to avoid hospitalization. If detected early, the prognosis is favorable, provided the patient adheres to the medication schedule and the bacilli do not become resistant to the medications. Surgery may be indicated to resect lung segments that are chronically involved. The extent and severity of the disease determines the course of recovery.

Maintenance of good general health is particularly important in the management, control, and prevention of tuberculosis (e.g., sanitation, balanced diet, sleep, regular exercise, and stress control). Finally, smoking has been attributed to a disproportionate number of deaths due to pulmonary tuberculosis, thus smoking cessation education and counseling is essential.[65]

Principles of Physical Therapy Management

Although the acute presentation of tuberculosis is comparable with acute pneumonia (refer to pneumonia section), there are some important differences with respect to physical therapy management.[66] First, tuberculosis is particularly infectious; thus special precautions should be taken by the physical therapist to prevent its spread during its infectious stage. Second, patients may be prone to fatigue; treatments should be selected to promote improved oxygen transport without exceeding the patient's capacity to deliver oxygen and without contributing to excessive fatigue. Stimulation of the oxygen transport system with exercise is necessary to avoid the deleterious effects of deconditioning and further compromise of oxygen transport. The patient warrants being monitored closely.

There are few evidence-based guidelines to inform physical therapy management of a patient with pulmonary tuberculosis. The effects of medication, however, are likely to be enhanced with a healthy diet, exercise, and rest. Based on extent and rate of recovery, regular, moderate-intensity exercise every other day for 30 minutes is the eventual goal. Initially, however, performing simple activities such as brisk walking outdoors can help eliminate the bacteria. For patients whose symptoms have largely subsided, stationary biking or resistance training can augment health. Maintaining a program of maximal health and regular exercise is essential.

Summary

Primary, acute medical conditions that affect the cardiovascular and pulmonary systems can have an impact on an individual's participation in life and its composite physical activities. However, serious limitations of structure and function (impairments) may be present that do not affect life participation and yet are life threatening. Both categories must be managed by the physical therapist. In this chapter, principles are presented for the management of individuals with common acute medical conditions including primary lung dysfunction (e.g., atelectasis, pneumonia, bronchitis, bronchiolitis, acute exacerbations of chronic airflow limitation, asthma, cystic fibrosis, interstitial pulmonary fibrosis, and tuberculosis) and primary cardiovascular dysfunction (e.g., hypertension, uncomplicated angina, and myocardial infarction). The focus of the chapter is the pathophysiology underlying these disorders, along with the mechanisms by which they threaten or impair an individual's heart-lung interaction and oxygen transport. Thus the bases for the principles of physical therapy are described rather than specific treatment prescriptions, which necessitate consideration of particular cases. Treatment prescription is based on the effects (and the underlying pathology) of restricted mobility, recumbency, extrinsic factors, and intrinsic factors on an individual's oxygen transport status. Management is directed at the underlying pathophysiological mechanisms resulting from these four factors wherever possible, secondarily to symptom reduction. To prioritize treatments, the most physiological interventions are exploited foremost because these address multiple steps in the oxygen transport pathway. Less physiological interventions (i.e., conventional cardiovascular and pulmonary physical therapy) are instituted after the most physiological interventions have been exploited or are instituted in conjunction with these. The challenge of clinical problem solving is determining the optimal treatment prescription for a given individual that will effect the best outcomes with respect to oxygen transport and eventual sustained return to full participation in life with the least risk in the shortest period of time.

Review Questions

1. Describe how acute limitations of structure and function of the cardiovascular and pulmonary systems can affect an individual's participation in life and related activities (i.e., from no relationship to potentially extensive relationship). Discuss the role of physical therapy in both circumstances, i.e., no relationship and extensive relationship of these variables.
2. Describe the primary cardiovascular and pulmonary pathophysiology and how a patient is likely to present clinically with the following acute conditions: atelectasis, pneumonia, bronchitis, bronchiolitis, acute exacerbations of chronic airflow limitation, asthma, cystic fibrosis, interstitial pulmonary fibrosis, tuberculosis, hypertension, stable angina, and stable myocardial infarction.
3. Relate physical therapy management and treatment interventions for patients with each of the acute conditions listed in question 2 to the underlying pathophysiology. Provide the rationale for your choices.

References

1. Dantzker DR: Oxygen transport and utilization. *Respiratory Care* 33:874–880, 1988.
2. Pryor JA, Prasad SA: *Physiotherapy for respiratory and cardiac problems: Adults and paediatrics*, ed 4, Edinburgh, 2008, Churchill Livingstone/Elsevier.
3. Mason RJ, Broaddus VC, Martin T, et al: *Murray and Nadel's Textbook of Respiratory Medicine*, ed 5, Philadelphia, 2010, Elsevier.
4. West JB: *Pulmonary pathophysiology: The essentials*, ed 7, Philadelphia, 2007, Lippincott Williams & Wilkins.
5. Sokolow M, Cheitlin MD: *Clinical cardiology*, ed 7, Stamford, 2004, Appleton & Lange.
6. Fauci A, Kasper DL, Longo D, et al: *Harrison's principles of internal medicine, (Vol 2)*, ed 17, Boston, 2008, McGraw Hill.
7. Woods SL, Froehlicher ESS, Motzer SA: *Cardiac nursing*, ed 6, Philadelphia, 2009, Lippincott Williams & Wilkins.
8. Kramer H, Han C, Post W, et al: Racial/ethnic differences in hypertension and hypertension treatment and control in the multi-ethnic study of atherosclerosis (MESA). *American Journal of Hypertension* 17:963–970, 2004.
9. National Institutes of Health: *Average blood pressure on the rise among American children/teenagers*, Washington, DC, 2004, U.S. Department of Health and Human Services.
10. Mayo Clinic: High blood pressure dangers: Hypertension's effects on your body. www.mayoclinic.com/health/high-blood-pressure/HI00062; Retrieved January 2011, 2011.
11. Dean E, Lomi C, Bruno S, et al: Addressing the common pathway underlying hypertension and diabetes in people who are obese: The ultimate knowledge translation gap. *International Journal of Hypertension* (In press), 2011.
12. Kokkinos PF, Narayan P, Papademetriou V: Exercise as hypertension therapy. *Cardiology Clinics* 19:507–516, 2001.
13. Dean E, editors: Physical therapy in the 21st century: A paradigm shift and implications. *Physiotherapy Theory and Practice* 25:327–462, 2009.
14. Froelicher VF, Myers JN: *Exercise and the heart: Clinical concepts*, ed 4, Philadelphia, 2000, Elsevier.
15. Langou RA, Wolfson S, Olson EG, et al: Effects of orthostatic postural changes on myocardial oxygen demands. *American Journal of Cardiology* 39:418–421, 1977.

16. Prakash R, Parmley WW, Dikshit K, et al: Hemodynamic effects of postural changes in patients with acute myocardial infarction. *Chest* 64:7–9, 1973.
17. Kaneko K, Milic-Emili J, Dolovich MB, et al: Regional distribution of ventilation and perfusion as a function of body position. *Journal of Applied Physiology* 21:767–777, 1966.
18. Harrison TR: The abuse of rest as a therapeutic measure for patients with cardiovascular disease. *Journal of the American Medical Association* 125:1075–1077, 1944.
19. Sonnenblick EH, Ross J Jr, Braunwald E: Oxygen consumption of the heart. Newer concepts of its multifactorial determination. *American Journal of Cardiology* 22:328–336, 1968.
20. Levine SA, Lown B: "Armchair" treatment of acute coronary thrombosis. *Journal of the American Medical Association* 148:1365–1369, 1952.
21. Sharma S, Parker AT: Prevalence of obstructive sleep apnea in patient population undergoing cardiac rehabilitation. *Journal of Cardiopulmonary Rehabilitation Prevention*. Jan 13. [Epub ahead of print], 2011.
22. Fletcher GF, Balady G, Blair SN, et al: Statement on exercise: benefits and recommendations for physical activity programs for all Americans. A Statement for Health Professionals by the Committee on Exercise and Cardiac Rehabilitation of the Council on Clinical Cardiology, American Heart Association. *Circulation* 94:857–862, 1996.
23. Roussos CS, Fixley M, Geriest J, et al: Voluntary factors influencing the distribution of inspired gas. *American Review of Respiratory Disease* 116:457–467, 1977.
24. Ross J, Dean E: Integrating physiological principles into the comprehensive management of cardiopulmonary dysfunction. *Physical Therapy* 69:255–259, 1989.
25. Dripps RD, Waters RM: Nursing care of the surgical patient. 1. The "stir-up." *American Journal of Nursing* 41:23–34, 1941.
26. Lindsay JA, Holden MTG: Staphylococcus aureus: superbug, super genome? *Trends in Microbiology* 12:378–385, 2004.
27. Orlava OE: Therapeutic physical culture in the complex treatment of pneumonia. *Physical Therapy Review* 39:153–160, 1959.
28. Dean E: Effect of body position on pulmonary function. *Physical Therapy* 65:613–618, 1985.
29. Douglas WW, Rehder K, Beynen FM, et al: Improved oxygenation in patients with acute respiratory failure: the prone position. *American Review of Respiratory Disease* 115:559–566, 1977.
30. Grimby G: Aspects of lung expansion in relation to pulmonary physiotherapy. *American Review of Respiratory Disease* 110:145–153, 1974.
31. Piehl MA, Brown RS: Use of extreme position changes in acute respiratory failure. *Critical Care Medicine* 4:13–14, 1976.
32. Yang M, Yuping Y, Yin X, et al: Chest physiotherapy for pneumonia in adults. *Cochrane Database Systematic Reviews* 2:CD006338, 2010.
33. Dean E, Ross J: Oxygen transport. The basis for contemporary cardiopulmonary physical therapy and its optimization with body positioning and mobilization. *Physical Therapy Practice* 1:34–44, 1992.
34. Wolff RK, Dolovich MB, Obminski G, et al: Effects of exercise and eucapnic hyperventilation on bronchial clearance in man. *Journal of Applied Physiology* 43:46–50, 1977.
35. Clauss RH, Scalabrini BY, Ray RF, et al: Effects of changing body position upon improved ventilation-perfusion relationships. *Circulation* 37(Suppl 4):214–217, 1968.
36. Hasani A, Pavia D, Agnew JE, et al: The effect of unproductive coughing/FET on regional mucus movement in the human lungs. *Respiratory Medicine* 85:23–26, 1991.
37. Zack MB, Pontoppidan H, Kazemi H: The effect of lateral positions on gas exchange in pulmonary disease. *American Review of Respiratory Disease* 110:149–153, 1974.
38. Mure M, Domino KB, Lindahl SGE, et al: Regional ventilation-perfusion distribution is more uniform in the prone position. *Journal of Applied Physiology* 88:1076–1083, 2000.
39. Marciniuk DD, Brooks D, Butcher S, et al: Optimizing pulmonary rehabilitation in chronic obstructive pulmonary disease—practical issues: A Canadian Thoracic Society Clinical Practice Guideline. *Canadian Respiratory Journal* 17:159–168, 2010.
40. Sinclair DJ, Ingram CG: Controlled trial of supervised exercise training in chronic bronchitis. *British Medical Journal* 280:519–521, 1980.
41. Druz WS, Sharp JT: Electrical and mechanical activity of the diaphragm accompanying body position in severe chronic obstructive pulmonary disease. *American Review of Respiratory Disease* 125:275–280, 1982.
42. Celli BR, MacNee W, Agusti A, et al: Standards for the diagnosis and treatment of patients with COPD: a summary of the ATS/ERS position paper. *European Respiratory Journal* 23:932–946, 2004.
43. Pauwels RA, Buist S, Calverley PMA, et al. on behalf of the GOLD Scientific Committee: Global Strategy for the Diagnosis, Management, and Prevention of Chronic Obstructive Pulmonary Disease. NHLBI/WHO Global Initiative for Chronic Obstructive Lung Disease (GOLD) Workshop Summary. *American Journal of Respiratory and Critical Care Medicine* 163:1256–1276, 2001.
44. White AJ, Gompertz S, Stockley RA: Chronic obstructive pulmonary disease. 6: The aetiology of exacerbations of chronic obstructive pulmonary disease. *Thorax* 58:73–80, 2003.
45. Barach AL: Chronic obstructive lung disease: postural relief of dyspnea. *Archives of Physical Medicine and Rehabilitation* 55:494–504, 1974.
46. Barach AL, Beck GJ: Ventilatory effects of head-down position in pulmonary emphysema. *American Journal of Medicine* 16:55–60, 1954.
47. Güell R, Casan P, Belda J, et al: Long-term effects of outpatient rehabilitation of COPD: A randomized trial. *Chest* 117:976–983, 2000.
48. Seemungal TAR, Donaldson GC, Paul EA, et al: Effect of exacerbation on Quality of life in patients with chronic obstructive pulmonary disease. *American Journal of Respiratory and Critical Care Medicine* 157:1418–1422, 1998.
49. Holloway E, Ram FS: Breathing exercises for asthma. *Cochrane Database Systematic Reviews* 2000;(3):CD001277, 2003.
50. Duggan M, Kavanagh BP: Atelectasis in the perioperative patient. *Current Opinions in Anaesthesiology* 20:37–42, 2007.
51. Epstein CD, Henning RJ: Oxygen transport variables in the identification and treatment of tissue hypoxia. *Heart and Lung* 22:328–348, 1993.
52. Wood RE, Wanner A, Hirsch J, et al: Tracheal mucociliary transport in patients with cystic fibrosis and its stimulation by terbutaline. *American Review of Respiratory Disease* 111:733–738, 1975.
53. Stokes DC, Wohl MEB, Khaw KT, et al: Postural hypoxemia in cystic fibrosis. *Chest* 87:785–789, 1985.
54. Dean E, Ross J: Integrating current literature in the management of cystic fibrosis: a rejoinder. *Physiotherapy Canada* 41:46–47, 1989.
55. Keens TG, Krastins IRB, Wannamaker EM, et al: Ventilatory muscle endurance training in normal subjects and patients with cystic fibrosis. *American Review of Respiratory Disease* 116:853–860, 1977.
56. Pyne DB: Regulation of neutrophil function during exercise. *Sports Medicine* 17:245–258, 1994.
57. Hull JH, Ansley L, Bolton CE, et al: The effect of exercise on large artery haemodynamics in cystic fibrosis. *Journal of Cystic Fibrosis* 2011 Jan 8. [Epub ahead of print], 2011.
58. Kirilloff LH, Owens GR, Rogers RM, et al: Does chest physical therapy work? *Chest* 88:436–444, 1985.
59. Pryor JA: *Respiratory care*, Edinburgh, 1993, Churchill Livingstone.
60. Braggion C, Cappelletti LM, Cornacchia M, et al: Short-term effects of three chest physiotherapy regimens in patients hospitalized for pulmonary exacerbations of cystic fibrosis: A cross-over randomized study. *Pediatric Pulmonology* 19:16–22, 1995.
61. McIlwaine M: Chest physical therapy, breathing techniques and exercise in children with CF. *Paediatric Respiratory Reviews* 8:8–16, 2007.
62. International Physiotherapy Group for Cystic Fibrosis: Physiotherapy for people with cystic fibrosis: from infant to adult [homepage on the internet]: 2009. www.cfww.org/docs/ipg-cf/bluebook/bluebooklet2009websiteversion.pdf. Accessed September 2011.
63. Chung F, Dean E: Pathophysiology and cardiorespiratory consequences of interstitial lung disease-review and clinical implications. *Physical Therapy* 69:956–966, 1989.
64. Holland A, Hill C: Physical training for interstitial lung disease. *Cochrane Database Systematic Reviews* 4:CD006322, 2008.
65. World Health Organization: Exercise 27: Proportion of TB deaths due to smoking. Retrieved January 2011, 2005.
66. Levchenko GI: [Physiotherapy in the treatment of pulmonary tuberculosis]. *Voen Med Zh* 323(5):49–51, 112, 2002 May, [Article in Russian].

IV

Chapter 30

Individuals with Acute Surgical Conditions

Elizabeth Dean

KEY TERMS

Analgesia (nonpharmacological)
Anesthesia
Cardiovascular surgery
Medications
Risk factor identification
Sedation
Surgery
Thoracic surgery

CHAPTER OUTLINE

The overall success of surgery is not measured according to its technical success alone. Rather, surgical success is based on the following:

- The patient's complete return to full participation in life and the capacity to perform its requisite activities
- Avoidance of recurrence of the problem for which the individual's surgery was indicated
- Reduced subsequent doctor- and hospital-based care and need for medication
- Lifelong health

The physical therapist is involved at all stages of perioperative care as indicated (before, during, and after surgery) and has a primary role in identifying individuals at risk of perioperative complications and preventing those complications as well as ensuring true surgical success as defined previously. A high proportion of surgery is needed for lifestyle-related conditions (e.g., ischemic heart disease, smoking-related conditions, hypertension and stroke, type 2 diabetes mellitus, and obesity). Given the prevalence of these conditions and their risk factors (which necessitate elective surgeries and contribute to their complications and delayed recovery), physical therapists need to lead in developing preoperative preparation programs that include health education (initiating or supporting smoking cessation and optimal nutrition), weight reduction, and judiciously prescribed exercise programs. The healthier that people are, the less likely that they will need surgery for non-accidental reasons. Furthermore, recovery from surgery for any reason will be augmented if the person is healthier; complications will be fewer, and rate of recovery will be improved. In turn, hospital stay will be reduced and the likelihood of recurrence of the initial problem may be also reduced.

The decision as to whether and to what extent physical therapy is indicated is based on the individual's need rather than strictly on his or her condition. The patient's condition is one factor that can determine perioperative risk, operative course, and long-term outcomes. Factors other than the primary indication for surgery, however, can have a more important effect on perioperative course and outcomes. Because of this, the preoperative assessment determines who requires physical therapy management and who does not. Physical therapy prevents complications and addresses oxygen transport threats and deficits. In the long term, physical therapy helps ensure that the individual returns to the highest level of living and regains or surpasses premorbid presurgical functional status. In cases in which the underlying condition can recur, a prime physical therapy objective is to minimize this possibility. Surgical outcomes, based on the physical therapy perspective within the International Classification of Functioning, Disability and Health,[1] are shown in Box 30-1.

The purpose of this chapter is to review the identification of surgical risk in a given individual and the management of patients with cardiovascular and pulmonary risk factors and dysfunction secondary to acute surgical conditions. Surgery today has become more extreme in two ways. First, minimally invasive surgery has shortened the operative period, hastened discharge, and reduced risk.[2] Second, with advances in instrumentation, monitoring, and anesthesia, more invasive, prolonged, and risky surgery is being performed with improved chances of survival.

The cardiovascular and pulmonary effects of anesthesia and surgery are described. The two types of surgery that have the greatest impact on cardiovascular and pulmonary function, namely thoracic and cardiovascular surgery, are highlighted. These surgeries are particularly invasive and lengthy, often require heavy and prolonged anesthesia and sedation, are typically performed on older people whose health status may be poor, and are generally associated with increased risk. Thus they warrant intensive perioperative physical therapy. Patients are assessed with respect to their presurgical and surgical hemodynamic and oxygen transport status to establish oxygen transport capacity and the degree to which increased metabolic demands associated with the perisurgical conditions as well as interventions can be met. In particular, cardiac output and oxygen delivery (DO_2) will increase to compensate for these increased metabolic demands. Increased metabolic demands, however, are dependent on age, severity of illness, type of surgery, comorbidity, and complications.[3] Furthermore, people who are overweight or obese, a common lifestyle-related condition, are more likely to require surgery. Obesity can reduce arterial oxygen tensions and the compliance of the respiratory system irrespective of the tidal volume or respiratory rate.[4] A detailed analysis of these factors can identify risks, expedite early intervention such as mobilization, and increase survival.

The four categories of factors that threaten or impair oxygen transport are described in Chapter 17. These factors include the underlying pathology, restricted mobility and recumbency, extrinsic factors related to the patient's care, and intrinsic factors related to the patient. This chapter examines in detail the effects of surgery, including the effects of anesthesia and other medications on oxygen transport as well as the impact of the underlying condition, restricted mobility and recumbency, and factors associated with the patient on an individual's status postoperatively. These are described in a format to facilitate assessment and ongoing evaluation.

Treatment principles are presented. These are not intended, however, to be a treatment prescription for a particular patient. The effects of anesthesia and surgery must be considered in addition to the underlying pathology and the effects of restricted mobility, body position, and intrinsic and extrinsic factors (see Chapter 17). All these factors must be considered and integrated in prescribing treatment and defining the specific parameters of the prescription. Such integration is essential for treatment to be targeted to the underlying problems and to be maximally effective.

Box 30-1 Surgical Outcomes and their Components Related to Physical Therapy

Perioperative Goals
- Prevent perioperative complications (i.e., oxygen transport, musculoskeletal, neuromuscular, endocrine, gastrointestinal, renal, immunological, skin, and psychological)
- Remediate oxygen transport limitations (limitations of structure and function)
- Minimize the need for invasive intervention including mechanical ventilatory support and supplemental oxygen, if these are required
- Encourage patient empowerment vis-à-vis self-efficacy
- Conduct patient education and assessment of whether educational goals were met or warrant modification
- Educate team regarding physical therapy goals and how medical, surgical, and nursing roles can augment noninvasive physical therapy outcomes
- Minimize hospital stay
- Achieve seamless transition to the community
- Follow up in the community

Long-Term Goals
- Return of the individual to full participation in life and composite activities[1]
- Sustained lifelong health
- Patient empowerment vis-à-vis self-efficacy
- Patient education and assessment of whether education goals were met or warrant modification
- Avoidance of recurrence of the original problem
- Reduction of postoperative doctor- and hospital-based care
- Reduced health care costs
- Reduced burden of disease (suffering and cost) to the individual, family, community, and society

Perioperative Course

Surgery and Its Cardiovascular and Pulmonary Consequences

Factors that place a patient at risk can contribute to perioperative cardiovascular and pulmonary dysfunction if preventive strategies fail (Box 30-2). Cardiovascular and pulmonary complications are the major cause of perioperative morbidity and mortality, particularly in patients undergoing thoracic or cardiovascular surgery.[5] The physical therapist must establish the risk factors based on premorbid health assessment including age, smoking habits, nutrition, weight, regular physical activity and fitness, sleep, and stress, as well as cardiac dysfunction, lung dysfunction, musculoskeletal dysfunction, neuromuscular dysfunction, and endocrine dysfunction—in particular, type 2 diabetes mellitus.[6]

Physical therapy has a role in preparing patients for surgery some weeks in advance—a service that is not being fully exploited in health care. Maximizing a patient's health will lead to fewer complications, will shorten hospital stay, and will hasten recovery and return to full participation in daily life. Interventions can include health education, including initiating or supporting smoking cessation. Smoking cessation or smoking reduction by at least 50% has been shown to improve the outcomes after hip and knee replacements.[7] Comparable benefits could be expected for other types of surgery,

Box 30-2 Surgical Factors that Contribute to Perioperative Cardiopulmonary Risk and Dysfunction

- Type of surgery
- Surgical procedures
- Anesthetics (general, with or without intubation, or regional) and sedation and reduced arousal
- Muscle-relaxant agents and neuromuscular blockade
- Supplemental oxygen and humidification
- Static body position assumed
- Duration of surgery and static body positioning
- Incisions
- Use of the cardiopulmonary bypass machine (CBM)
- Use of the extracorporeal membrane exchanger (ECMO)
- Dressings and binders
- Splints and fixation devices
- Lines and leads
- Monitoring devices
- Chest tube placement and number
- Catheters
- Perioperative anxiety, discomfort, and pain
- Perioperative pain control management
- Perioperative fluid balance management
- Perioperative blood and plasma transfusions

particularly cardiovascular and thoracic procedures. Optimizing nutrition and prescribing an exercise program, even if modified because of the patient's underlying condition, can augment oxygen transport. Thus, when oxygen transport is unavoidably compromised by anesthesia and surgery, the patient has greater reserve capacity.

People who are overweight and obese have direct, serious weight-related morbidity including hypertension, type 2 diabetes mellitus, lipid-related heart conditions, and sleep apnea. In addition, people who require joint replacement surgery because of arthropathy secondary to irreversible joint damage are more likely to be overweight.[8] Thus, overweight and obesity constitute major complications during surgery and recovery. Given their prevalence, overweight and obesity warrant being addressed by physical therapists in every patient, whether surgical or medical (see Chapters 1 and 6). Furthermore, body mass index as well as weight-to-hip ratio and age have been reported to be significant predictors for type 2 diabetes mellitus and hypertension, which further complicates the clinical presentation and management of surgical patients who are overweight or obese.[9]

Early surgery for hip fracture in older adults has not been shown unequivocally to result in improved outcomes—that is, reduced complications (pneumonia and bed sores), earlier recovery, and reduced mortality.[10] It is likely that clinically some patients may benefit whereas others may benefit from some delay. Irrespective, the outcomes of physical therapy will be enhanced in either situation if instituted in a timely manner. Studies are needed to establish the degree to which physical therapy including lifestyle behavior change (weight loss in particular) may avert surgery all together, or appropriately delay it. In some patients, early surgery may be preferable. In this case, some finite period of time in which a course of physical therapy could be instituted prior to surgery, could augment surgical outcomes.

Anesthesia and Supplemental Oxygen

Anesthesia results in depression of breathing. Thoracic respiratory excursion is reduced. The tone and pattern of contraction of the respiratory muscles, particularly the diaphragm and the intercostal muscles, change, which contributes to many secondary cardiovascular and pulmonary effects observed after surgery. The loss of end-expiratory diaphragmatic tone causes the diaphragm to ascend into the chest by 2 cm during anesthesia with or without paralysis.[11] Reductions in functional residual capacity (FRC) are correlated with this change and with altered chest wall configuration and increased thoracic blood volume.[12,13] One of the most pervasive and predictable clinical effects observed in the postoperative period is alveolar collapse. Total lung capacity, FRC, and residual volume are decreased. The FRC is reduced in the supine position compared with the erect sitting position[14,15] and is further reduced with the induction of anesthesia. Anesthesia, however, fails to reduce FRC in the sitting position.

The consequences of reduced FRC with anesthesia and surgery have major implications for postoperative complications and the course of recovery. Airway closure occurs with anesthesia, and this likely contributes to intrapulmonary shunting. Compression atelectasis of the dependent (lowermost) lung fields occurs during surgery.[16] In addition, compression atelectasis occurs when lung tissue and surrounding structures are being physically manipulated by the surgeon. Although reduced airway caliber in areas of low lung volume can be offset by the airway-dilating effect of many inhaled anesthetics, airway resistance is increased by obstruction of the breathing circuits, valves, and tracheal tubes. The airways may also be obstructed with foreign matter such as blood and secretions, or from bronchospasm caused by irritation. Because of the decrease in FRC, lung compliance is decreased and the work of breathing is increased. Hypoxemia secondary to transpulmonary shunting is usually maximal within 72 hours after surgery and may not be completely resolved for several days. Persistent reduction in FRC after surgery delays the restoration of the normal alveolar-arterial oxygen gradient.

Anesthesia and tissue dissection contribute to major changes in lung volume, mechanics, and gas exchange. The extent and duration of these changes increase with the magnitude of the operative procedure and degree of anesthesia required. Tissue oxygenation can be threatened during the intraoperative period, and the relationship between oxygen consumption ($\dot{V}O_2$) and delivery (DO_2) compromised.[17] Mismatch between $\dot{V}O_2$ and DO_2 is associated with a complicated clinical course and prolonged intensive care unit stay in the absence of conventional indicators such as low ejection fraction and longer cardiovascular and pulmonary bypass time.[18] Oxygen extraction increases to compensate for reduced DO_2. Early optimization of the ratio of $\dot{V}O_2$ and DO_2 is indicated to reduce perioperative morbidity and mortality.

The fraction of inspired oxygen (FIO_2) depends on the mode of oxygen administration. Low-flow nasal oxygen reduces hypoxemia in the absence of hypercapnia and marked transpulmonary shunting in the postoperative patient. Low oxygen flows and low FIO_2 tend to be delivered via nasal cannula whereas higher flows can deliver higher FiO_2 via oxygen masks and masks with reservoir bags. FiO_2 and the body position of the patient at the time a blood sample is taken must always be considered when arterial blood gas values are interpreted. The FiO_2 is selected to provide adequate oxygenation with the lowest oxygen concentration possible.

After surgery the normal pattern of breathing is disrupted. Shallow, monotonous tidal ventilation without normal occasional, spontaneous deep breaths causes alveolar collapse within an hour.[15] Unless resolved within a few hours, atelectasis becomes increasingly resistant to reinflation. This complication is exacerbated in patients receiving narcotics.

Tachypnea and tachycardia are commonly observed, with gross atelectasis secondary to hypoventilation. Breath sounds are decreased at the bases, and the coarse wheezes associated with mucus obstructing airflow can be heard on auscultation. Left lower lobe atelectasis is common after cardiac surgery.

Immediate Postoperative Period

After surgery the patient is detained in the recovery room until vital signs have stabilized, there is no apparent internal or external bleeding, and the patient is responding to his or her name. Patients recovering from minor surgery are usually transferred to a ward once discharged from the recovery room. A patient is transferred to the intensive care unit after surgery if complications arose during surgery, if the patient cannot be readily stabilized and requires close monitoring, or if the patient had more serious surgery such as cranial, cardiovascular thoracic, or emergency surgery such as that resulting from multiple trauma (see Chapter 35).

Rest during the postoperative period needs to be prescribed as carefully as treatment because rest is the time for healing, repair, and restoration. Sleep deprivation impairs recovery and healing. Sleep at night is biologically more restorative than daytime sleep. Thus daytime and nighttime cues are given to restore the patient's circadian rhythms. Although injudicious and excessive recumbency, bed rest, and prolonged periods in any given body position are deleterious, special attention is given to maximizing the periods of high-quality rest and sleep and minimizing disruption of nighttime sleep. Appropriate rests are interspersed within each treatment according to the patient's needs to avoid reaching suboptimal, suprathreshold physiological states. Suprathreshold states are associated with an inappropriate balance between DO_2 and VO_2 such that the patient's condition becomes compromised (e.g., hemodynamically unstable, cardiovascular and pulmonary distress is precipitated, or both).

Pharmacological Considerations

Common pharmacological agents prescribed for patients perioperatively are described in Chapter 45. Physical therapists need a thorough knowledge of these when managing the surgical patient so management can be optimized.

Several factors are particularly important in managing surgical patients because these factors can affect the patients' sensitivity to narcotic analgesics such as morphine.[19,20] There is considerable intersubject response variability to these agents. Older patients, for example, can be expected to be more sensitive to narcotics. Diverse multisystem pathology has a marked effect on the degradation, absorption, biotransformation, and excretion of morphine. Exaggerated effects of morphine have been reported when administered in conjunction with other agents such as other narcotic analgesics, phenothiazines, tranquilizers, or sedative-hypnotics; in addition, such exaggerated effects have been reported in patients with respiratory depression, hypotension, and sedation and in patients who are unconscious. Situations in which exaggerated drug effects have been reported are commonly encountered in the intensive care setting and can result in unpredictable responses. Finally, the physical dependence and abuse potential of these agents cannot be ignored.

The physical therapist must be familiar with the patient's medications and the indications, side effects, and contraindications of each. The physical therapist can determine to what extent oxygen transport may be compromised by medication effects and whether some recommendation must be made to minimize untoward drug effects on arousal or some other factor that negatively affects oxygen transport and gas exchange. For example, although narcotics are excellent analgesics, they have widespread systemic effects including reduced arousal, cardiovascular and pulmonary depression, gastrointestinal depression, and muscle relaxation, all of which can compromise oxygen transport. Thus, consideration must be given regarding whether other forms of analgesia including non pharmacological interventions can be used. In managing the needs of a patient experiencing postoperative pain, the following questions should be considered:

- Have nonpharmacological means of analgesia been exploited?
- If pharmacological analgesia is indicated, could analgesics other than narcotics be used?
- Can the dose of narcotic be reduced so that satisfactory pain control can be achieved in combination with nonpharmacological interventions?

The administration of narcotics has important implications for physical therapy. These powerful analgesics are often the medications of choice for major pain relief and comfort. Their secondary effects, however, which include reduced arousal and monotonous tidal ventilation, are primary physical therapy concerns. Narcotics interfere with a patient's ability to cooperate with treatment. If narcotics impair the patient's ability to participate in treatment, analgesia with a less systemic effect is indicated. Patient-controlled analgesia (PCA) is an effective means of having the patient regulate the amount of analgesia he or she is receiving.[21] Patients have been reported to administer less medication to themselves than nurses assessing their analgesia needs. Intravenous administration prolongs the peak-effect time of analgesics and therefore helps the patient tolerate longer, more intense treatments. Oversedation must be avoided if the patient is to derive maximal benefit from cardiovascular and pulmonary physical therapy treatments.

Physical therapists have available to them a range of noninvasive pain control interventions that should be considered in the acute surgical ward as well as in postsurgical follow-up in the outpatient clinic. These include relaxation strategies, deep breathing, body positioning, physical support, coordination of treatments, and electrotherapy. Transcutaneous electrical nerve stimulation (TENS), for example, can be a useful adjunct in the management of postoperative pain in some patients. Pain control with TENS may enable the patient to participate more fully in mobilization, deep breathing, and coughing. Research is needed, however, to evaluate this technique in the management of acute pain and define the prescription parameters necessary to produce an optimal therapeutic effect for a given patient. The role of nonpharmacological means of managing acute pain in place of or in conjunction with pharmacological means warrants greater exploitation clinically to produce the best analgesia with the least side effects and risks. Nonpharmacological analgesia enables patients to participate more fully in physical therapy treatments in the absence of the untoward side effects often associated with drug administration.

Prevention of Complications

Special attention in the postoperative period is given to the prevention or management of cardiovascular and pulmonary complications associated with reduced arousal, surgical pain, and restriction of lung capacity and secondary to dressings, binders, and diminished ability to cooperate, move spontaneously, and hyperventilate the lungs periodically. Patients are prone to aspiration in the immediate postoperative period, particularly while the sedation and anesthetic agents are wearing off. This risk is further increased if an artificial airway is required, or if an artificial airway is needed and mechanical ventilation is instituted. Postextubation atelectasis must be anticipated and avoided. To minimize this risk, patients are asked not to eat or drink fluids the day before surgery.

Endotracheal intubation and mechanical ventilation are indicated if blood gas values fail to improve with conservative management. See Chapter 33 for treatment priorities for a patient during mechanical ventilation and the course of weaning.

A complication of thoracic and upper abdominal surgery is irritation or compression trauma of the phrenic nerve. This complication may be more common than expected. Inhibition of the phrenic nerve impairs the contraction of the affected hemidiaphragm, causing it to ascend into the thorax and contribute to atelectasis on that side. This inhibition may last for several days.

The patient's body position is changed frequently in the initial postoperative period. The patient is usually encouraged to change his or her body position frequently, transfer, sit in a chair, and ambulate as soon as possible after surgery. The importance of frequent postural changes and early ambulation in the initial postoperative period are stressed. Early ambulation is a priority in the management of all surgical patients unless contraindicated.

Factors Determining Surgical Response and Outcomes

A patient's response to and outcome after surgery as well as potential complications depend on multiple factors (see Box 30-2). The type of surgery determines the degree of invasiveness, type or types of anesthetics and sedatives, type and level of respiratory support, static body position assumed during surgery, approximate duration of the surgery and period of anesthesia, incisions, dressings, lines, leads, catheters, monitoring devices, chest tubes, type and degree of pain that can be expected, and necessity for and type of pain control after surgery.

Pathophysiology

The type and severity of underlying cardiovascular and pulmonary dysfunction increase a patient's risk of compromised oxygen transport and gas exchange perioperatively.

Restricted Mobility and Recumbency

Surgery imposes two nonphysiological states on the patient that significantly affect oxygen transport:

- Restricted mobility
- Recumbency, specifically a prolonged period of static positioning with the patient breathing at monotonous tidal volumes

Extrinsic Factors

Surgery and related factors are the primary extrinsic factors contributing to cardiovascular and pulmonary dysfunction in the perioperative period.

Intrinsic Factors

Intrinsic factors that contribute to cardiovascular and pulmonary dysfunction in the surgical patient include a patient's premorbid status (e.g., preexisting cardiovascular and pulmonary, renal, endocrine, and hematological pathology). In addition, lifestyle factors are significant (i.e., preoperative conditioning level, nutrition, hydration, stress levels, weight, and smoking history).

Preoperative Assessment And Preparation For Surgery

To minimize risk, reduce perioperative morbidity and mortality, maximize healing, and shorten postoperative recovery, patients need to be in the best physical and medical condition before anesthesia and surgery. In the case of elective surgery, patients often can be prescribed aerobic training (prescribed to meet the individual's needs and capacity), smoking cessation, and weight-control programs beforehand. A preparatory preoperative role for physical therapy warrants greater attention and is currently underused in terms of improving the perioperative course and achieving optimal, sustainable surgical outcomes.

Preoperative physical therapy management includes the preoperative assessment and education; the primary components are shown in Box 30-3. During this time the physical therapist has an opportunity to develop rapport with the patient. The assessment establishes the risk of complications and prolonged hospital stay and the type and extent of perioperative physical therapy required. Postoperative neurological syndromes are common. Ongoing assessment helps ensure that these are identified and addressed early.[22] The assessment establishes what the postoperative priorities will be; however, these are modified based on the postoperative assessment. The surgical procedures are described and the effects of surgery and anesthesia and sedation on gas exchange are reviewed so that the patient understands the importance of being actively involved in physical therapy, both during and between treatments after surgery.

There are no strict guidelines about which patients should receive perioperative physical therapy. Rather, the need for physical therapy should be made on a case-by-case basis, with the degree of the physical therapist's involvement determined on the basis of the patient's need. Although nonthoracic surgeries are generally associated with few cardiovascular and pulmonary complications (e.g., surgery of the extremities or lower abdomen), patients with preexisting cardiovascular and pulmonary pathology, hematological or neuromuscular pathology, or musculoskeletal pathology of the chest wall are at greater risk even in these relatively low-risk types of surgeries. In addition, patients are at additional risk if they are older or younger, smoke, or are overweight or pregnant. Thus each surgical patient must be assessed individually to establish the degree of relative risk during surgery and the necessity of perioperative physical therapy. In this way perioperative complications can be anticipated and avoided or reduced, which is preferable to managing complications once they have developed. The cardiovascular and pulmonary assessment is particularly important in the older individual, and early mobilization is critical postoperatively.

Even though a patient may have had minimally invasive surgery and an uneventful perioperative course, the physical therapist still may have a critical role in helping to achieve long-term surgical outcomes. Recurrence is possible, particularly if surgery was related to lifestyle factors. The physical therapist can take maximal advantage of contact with the patient and be actively involved in developing a program of sustained, lifelong health.

The importance of a thorough preoperative assessment and teaching by the physical therapist cannot be overstated. The components of preoperative assessment and teaching are summarized in Box 30-3. In cases of elective surgery, preoperative teaching includes a general description of the surgery to be performed, the effect of anesthesia and surgery on cardiovascular and pulmonary function, and the systemic effects of restricted mobility and recumbency. The lines, leads, and catheters usually associated with the surgery are explained. The patient is instructed in breathing control maneuvers, supported coughing, chest wall mobility exercises, mobility exercises for the limbs (e.g., hip and knee and foot and ankle exercises), turning in bed, sitting up, transferring, chair sitting, and walking erect postoperatively. In addition, the patient is taught methods of maximizing comfort with body positioning and supporting the surgical incision. If the bed has controls the patient can manipulate, he or she is taught how to make bed adjustments as required. The postoperative course is explained in general terms so the patient can anticipate this period. If the patient is well informed preoperatively, he or she will be better oriented and capable of cooperating when he or she wakes from the anesthesia.

Preoperative teaching is a central component of physical therapy management of the surgical patient. Such teaching establishes rapport with the physical therapist, who informs the patient about what to expect before and after surgery. In addition to reviewing the surgical procedures, the physical therapist reviews, and has the patient perform, deep breathing and supported coughing maneuvers, relaxation, bed mobility, positioning, transfers, and mobilization. Preoperative teaching reduces the patient's anxiety and encourages the patient to be as active as possible in his or her recovery. Preoperative teaching reduces postoperative complications and the length of the hospital stay. High-risk patients benefit from preoperative teaching, and their cooperation is more easily solicited after the surgery. Understanding the patient's perception of his or her condition, the surgery, expectations, and self-efficacy are also central to postoperative recovery.

Box 30-3 Objectives of the Preoperative Physical Therapy Assessment and Teaching

- Develop rapport with patient
- Assess cognitive status, capacity to cooperate, language and communication skills, and cultural and ethnic beliefs and attitudes toward surgery and care
- Assess the patient and estimate degree of surgical risk (e.g., age, smoking, previous cardiopulmonary dysfunction, neuromuscular dysfunction, musculoskeletal deformity, obesity, substance abuse, pregnancy, nutritional status, hydration status, and pain and discomfort)
- Describe the general preoperative, intraoperative, and postoperative course
- Review specific surgical procedures relevant to physical therapy (e.g., anesthesia, type of surgery, body position during surgery, airway, mechanical ventilation, duration, incisions, infusions, drainage systems, chest tubes, and recovery room)
- Provide the rationale for, describe, demonstrate, and have the patient practice and provide feedback on the following breathing control maneuvers: maximal inspiratory hold, supported coughing maneuvers, relaxation, bed mobility and positioning, transfers, and mobilization
- For patients at risk of postoperative cardiopulmonary dysfunction and complications, review the use of the incentive spirometer and conventional airway clearance interventions (e.g., postural drainage and manual techniques, if indicated)
- Ask for any questions

The physical therapist may be consulted by the surgeon to help make a poor-risk patient into a better-risk patient. Patients with upper–respiratory tract infections before surgery may have their surgeries postponed, depending on the type and extent of surgery to be performed, level of anesthesia indicated, and other medical conditions including cardiovascular and pulmonary disease, age, and smoking history. Patients with preoperative lower–respiratory tract infections constitute a greater operative risk; hence these patients often have their surgeries postponed until the infection has resolved. Patients with chronic cardiovascular and pulmonary diseases require a prolonged period of preoperative physical therapy in preparation for surgery. Elective surgery is not usually considered during an exacerbation of chronic lung disease. Even minor surgery may be potentially hazardous for the patient with previous lung disease. The adverse effects of total anesthesia on these patients are magnified because of their reduced pulmonary reserve capacity. Smoking should be discontinued for as long as possible before surgery. The patient is placed on an exercise conditioning program, a regimen of bronchial hygiene, oxygen if necessary, and prophylactic antibiotics. Even patients with extremely low functional work capacity can enhance the efficiency of the steps in the oxygen transport pathway (see Chapters 18 and 19) with a modified aerobic exercise conditioning program. This preoperative preparation may take one to several weeks, depending on the patient and the indications for surgery. Patients who are overweight can reduce their risk of perioperative complications by losing weight. Body mass is a major determinant of lung function, respiratory mechanics, and oxygenation during anesthesia,[23] and adverse effects on these can lead to major surgical complications and problems during recovery.

Preoperative inspiratory muscle training has gained renewed interest as a means of preserving respiratory muscle function postoperatively and reducing postoperative pulmonary complications. Although maximal inspiratory pressure can be preserved,[24,25] studies are needed to show that this intervention augments outcomes over and above the benefits of an exercise program before surgery. Furthermore, a narrowly focused intervention such as inspiratory muscle training may overlook the benefits of a more holistic preoperative preparation program. Such training needs to be prescribed judiciously.

Postoperative Management

Goals

The goals of postoperative physical therapy management related to oxygen transport appear in Box 30-4. The patient is mobilized in a systematic sequence that progresses from supine to turning in bed to sitting over the bed to standing to sitting in a chair to walking (Table 30-1). Some patients progress through these steps quickly, whereas others take longer. The rate at which patients are progressed depends on their responses. Pain medications are coordinated as needed with treatments to maximize treatment effectiveness. This progressive sequence is comparable to that of phase I of cardiac rehabilitation, the inpatient phase for surgical as well as medical patients, and includes education, counseling, and treatment as indicated. These goals are addressed between as well as during treatments. The patient is instructed in mobilization and body positioning coordinated with deep breathing and supported coughing maneuvers between treatment sessions, and these

Box 30-4 Goals of Postoperative Physical Therapy Related to Oxygen Transport

- Maximize arousal
- Control anxiety and pain
- Maximize alveolar volume
- Optimize alveolar ventilation
- Optimize perfusion
- Maximize lung volumes and capacities, especially functional residual capacity
- Minimize closing volume
- Minimize intrapulmonary shunting
- Optimize lung compliance
- Optimize mucociliary transport
- Optimize clearance of mucus
- Optimize ventilation and perfusion matching and gas exchange
- Maximize expiratory flow rates
- Maximize chest tube drainage
- Optimize fluid balance systemically (renal function)
- Optimize lung water balance and distribution
- Promote optimal lymphatic draining
- Minimize third spacing and collection of fluid
- Minimize the risk of aspiration
- Minimize undue work of breathing
- Minimize undue work of the heart
- Maximize chest wall mobility and movement in three planes
- Optimize body and posture alignment when sitting, standing, walking, and recumbent
- Optimize circulatory status and tissue perfusion
- Optimize peripheral blood flow and velocity
- Optimize muscle pump action
- Minimize effects of central fluid shifts with recumbency
- Maintain fluid-volume regulating mechanisms
- Minimize pain nonpharmacologically and coordinate with the patient's pain medications as indicated
- Maximize cardiopulmonary endurance
- Optimize relaxation and sleep
- Provide instruction to patient regarding between-treatment 'treatment'

Table 30-1 Template for Progressing Mobilization in Surgical Patients

Level	Date	Activity	Bathroom	Bathing
1		Confined to bed Assessment Body positioning	Portable toilet when possible	Personal care by nurse May wash hands and feet
2		Sit up in chair for 20 minutes, three times per day	Use portable toilet	May wash in bed (not legs, back, or feet)
3		Sit up in chair as much as possible		Bathe at bedside
4			Walk to bathroom	Bathe at sink (sitting)
5		Walk around room as able		Bathe at sink
6		Short walks in hall two or three times per day		
7		Walk in halls as able		Take shower (sitting) or tub bath
8		Walk one flight of stairs with assistance		
9		Discharge		

Adapted from Makrides L: *Cardiac rehabilitation manual,* Halifax, Nova Scotia, Canada, 1997, Cardiac Prevention Research Centre, Dalhousie University.

interventions should be performed hourly during waking hours.[26,27] Such a regimen has been reported to result in favorable outcomes for invasive abdominal surgery.[28]

In addition to the primary treatment goals related to oxygen transport, other postoperative goals include the following:

1. Maximize the patient's ability to perform activities of daily living.
2. Maintain or increase general muscle strength and endurance.
3. Maximize muscle and soft tissue length and ligament integrity.
4. Maintain normal arousal and neurological function.
5. Reduce anxiety and stress.
6. Maintain skin integrity.
7. Maintain normal cognitive function to avoid disorientation and hospital-related psychoses.
8. Prescribe secondary prevention.

These goals are achieved with the prescription of mobilization and its constituent mobility exercises including hip and knee flexion and extension exercises and foot and ankle exercises. These exercises are performed hourly regardless of whether the patient is sitting in the chair or resting in bed.

Finally, there are important preventive goals (e.g., minimizing the effects of restricted mobility and recumbency on all organ systems) (see Chapters 19 and 20). Of particular concern in the surgical patient is the risk of thromboemboli and pulmonary emboli and the risk of pressure points and skin breakdown. Thus mobilization and regular activation of the muscle pumps to minimize circulatory stasis and frequent body-position changes are essential to reduce risks, which can have serious consequences for the patient's recovery. Compression stockings are often put on the patient after surgery. These are not removed, except for cleaning and redistributing pressure, until the patient is consistently up and about. These stockings facilitate venous return and increase blood flow and velocity, thereby minimizing the risk of thrombus formation. Should thrombus formation be suspected, it may be necessary to attach an intermittent compression device to the legs to simulate muscle pump action.

With the exception of patients undergoing thoracic or cardiovascular surgery, patients are usually extubated before leaving the operating room or recovery area. Provided no complications develop, most other patients do not require an airway. Patients undergoing major thoracic surgery or cardiovascular surgery remain intubated and mechanically ventilated from several hours to 24 hours after surgery to minimize the work of breathing and hence the work of the heart required to meet the metabolic demands of respiration. These patients are informed that artificial airway and mechanical ventilation enables them to breathe more efficiently initially. A patient is also informed that he or she will not be able to speak while the airway is in place and may have a sore throat after its removal.

Patients are usually aroused and repositioned before leaving the operating room, although this is seldom remembered by patients. Not recalling the immediate postoperative course is common. Patients are likely to be receiving some form of pharmacological analgesia (e.g., morphine). If blood was required intraoperatively, whole blood, packed cells, or plasma may still be infused in the immediate postoperative period or for a longer period of time. Saline or other solutions are also infused for regulation of fluid balance until the patient is able to drink and eat normally. Once vital signs have stabilized, wounds are stable and not draining, and the patient is reasonably alert, he or she is transferred to the ward. The patient is retained in the recovery area should further monitoring be required. If complications develop and oxygen transport and gas exchange are threatened, the patient may be transferred to the intensive care unit.

The physical therapist may be consulted to assess and treat the patient as soon as he or she leaves the operating room or while in the recovery room. Most frequently the physical therapist sees the patient once he or she has been transferred to the ward and has been settled. The first 24 hours are critical.

The risk of cardiovascular and pulmonary complications is greatest during the perioperative period and diminishes as the patient becomes increasingly upright and mobile. Atelectasis and aspiration after extubation are major risks for the patient who has been intubated. The goal immediately after extubation is to promote optimal alveolar ventilation, maximize lung volumes and capacities (especially FRC), minimize closing volumes, and maximize expiratory flow rates and hence cough effectiveness. Areas most susceptible to atelectasis are those that may have been physically compressed during surgery (e.g., the left lower lobe of the cardiovascular surgical patient and areas adjacent to a lobectomy or segmentectomy area).

Surgery constitutes a major insult to the body. After the trauma of surgery, anesthesia, sedation, fluid loss, incisions, and the increased energy requirements for healing and repair, patients can be expected to be lethargic and challenging to arouse. The relaxed state induced by anesthesia, sedation, and narcotics increases the risk of aspiration. This risk is exacerbated further in some patients by nausea and vomiting associated with anesthesia and narcotics. Moving and positioning the patient upright whenever possible and interacting with the patient stimulate the reticular activating system, making the patient more responsive and aroused. The increased metabolic demands that this requires, along with increased catecholamine release, helps overcome the residual effects of anesthesia, sedation, and muscle relaxants and their threat to oxygen transport, provided the demands are not beyond the capacity of the oxygen transport system to deliver oxygen.

Alternatively, some patients are restless and agitated after the effects of anesthesia have worn off. Hypoxemia can lead to restlessness and agitation. Thus it is important that these patients not be inappropriately sedated. This compounds their need for treatment while making them less able to cooperate with treatment simultaneously.[29,30]

At the outset of any treatment the patient needs to be aroused as much as possible to cooperate fully and derive the maximum benefit from treatment. The physical therapist interacts continuously with the patient to arouse him or her fully, maintain arousal, stimulate normal cognitive function and orientation, and elicit feedback from the patient to assess his or her response to treatment. Narcotics depress respiratory status and arousal, and these effects are accentuated in patients whose metabolic states have been disrupted with illness and in older persons. Thus the physical therapist must be vigilant in detecting untoward residual effects of narcotics in the surgical patient. Balancing sedation and analgesia with the needs of having the patient arousable and alert warrants good communication among the team members.

Early Postoperative Physical Therapy

Rationale

The role of perioperative physical therapy has been debated. Some argue that the nursing staff can assume responsibility for the prevention of postoperative complications, particularly in patients who have undergone minimally invasive and short surgeries. The assessment and goals of the physical therapist, however, are unique and are not duplicated by the medical or nursing staff or respiratory therapist.

Physical therapists identify threats to oxygen transport as well as its limitations and prevent and remediate these by prescribing and exploiting noninvasive interventions. Furthermore, the physical therapist considers multiple factors that threaten the long-term health and function of the patient after discharge. The physical therapist has a primary commitment to returning the patient to full participation in the community and prolonged, sustained health. A decision to institute physical therapy for a given patient is not based on the type of surgery alone. Rather it is determined through a systemic assessment of age, weight, fitness, smoking status, comorbidities, anxiety and stress, and external factors related to the patient's potential response to anesthesia and surgery.

To sustain alveolar inflation and normal FRC postoperatively, mobilization and body positioning coordinated with breathing control and supported coughing must be carried out frequently (i.e., every 1 to 2 hours) to maintain optimal alveolar volume and distribution of ventilation. Maximal inspiratory maneuvers are coordinated with mobilization and body positioning at least every hour as tolerated. Maximal inspiratory maneuvers alone, however, are unlikely to be effective because the inspiratory pressure may be insufficient to inflate atelectatic alveoli. Rather, patent alveoli will tend to be overexpanded. Mobilization and body positioning will directly alter the intrapleural pressure gradient and thereby optimize alveolar expansion. In patients who are obese and anesthetized and paralyzed, the prone position increases FRC, lung compliance, and oxygenation.[23,31] Being prone may have some postoperative role in some patients who are obese, but the hazards of recumbent positions must be weighed against the benefits of being upright.

Normal passive expiratory efforts to end tidal volume are encouraged, and maximal or forced expiratory efforts are usually avoided to prevent airway closure and potential increase of atelectasis. Huffing (glottis open) rather than coughing (glottis closed) also minimizes airway closure. With huffing there is less risk of bronchospasm than with coughing, in which the glottis is closed, transpulmonary pressure is increased, and a compressive phase is involved. If indicated, coughing maneuvers are most effective in the sitting or slightly leaned-forward position, in which lung volumes and forced expiratory flow are maximized and the respiratory muscles are at a mechanical advantage with respect to the length-tension characteristics of the muscle fibers. Airway closure is position-dependent (see Chapter 20); therefore the degree of expiration encouraged by the physical therapist should be based on the patient's body position. Airway closure is potentiated in patients who are older, smoke, or are obese and in patients who are in horizontal as opposed to upright body positions.

Mobilization and body positioning coordinated with breathing control and supported coughing maneuvers offer the greatest benefit to oxygen transport in the postoperative patient. Specific benefits are described in Chapters 18, 19 and 20. They include maximizing FRC, reducing closing volume, maximizing expiratory flow rates, promoting mucociliary transport, promoting airway clearance, optimizing lymphatic drainage, minimizing the effects of increased thoracic blood volume, maintaining fluid-volume regulating mechanisms, and minimizing the work of breathing and of the heart. Sustained maximal inspiration is one intervention that promotes alveolar expansion. Each deep breath is performed to maximal inspiration (i.e., to total lung capacity) with a 3- to 5-second breath hold. This maneuver may reduce pulmonary complications by promoting alveolar inflation and gas exchange. The patient is encouraged to repeat this maneuver several times hourly; frequently during mobilization; and before, during, and after body-position changes.

Although the benefits of incentive spirometry (Figure 30-1) postoperatively are equivocal at least after thoracic surgery,[32] it may be useful in patients who are resistant or unable to cooperate fully with maximal inspiratory efforts or be adequately mobilized. Postoperative hypoxemia may be reduced with this technique, which uses the principle of sustained inspiration using a feedback device (either flow or volume feedback) to achieve maximal inflating pressure in the alveoli and maximal inhaled volume. Spirometers with a volume-controlled device, however, may improve diaphragmatic excursion more than flow-dependent devices.[33] With proper instruction, the incentive spirometer can be used independently by the patient, which can be an advantage. This technique ensures that each inspiration is physiologically optimal and is reproduced precisely from one inspiration to the next. Patients who are surgical risks may benefit from being taught how to use the incentive spirometer preoperatively by the physical therapist in order to promote better inflation of the lungs with incentive spirometry postoperatively. However, use of a spirometer does not replace being upright and moving as

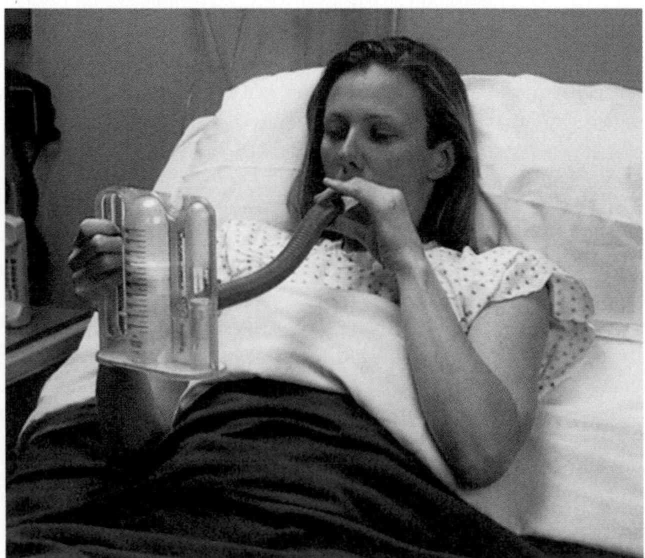

Fig. 30-1 Incentive spirometers. (From Harkreader H, Hogan MA, Thobaben M: *Fundamentals of nursing: Caring and clinical judgment*, ed 3. St. Louis, 2007, Saunders.)

much as possible. The patient continues with a regimen of breathing control and coughing maneuvers in conjunction with being upright and moving until full mobility and activities of daily living are resumed.

The application of intermittent positive pressure breathing (IPPB) appears to be less effective for the postoperative patient than previously believed. The details of this modality are described in Chapter 43.

Exercise testing echocardiography performed early after coronary bypass surgery can identify individuals who are high risk and would benefit from intensive secondary prevention as a particular focus in a cardiac rehabilitation program.[34] Early exercise training improves autonomic nervous system function in addition to aerobic and functional capacity.[35]

Getting the Surgical Patient "Upright and Moving"

Mobilization in the upright position coordinated with breathing control and supported coughing maneuvers is encouraged immediately after the patient is first aroused after surgery, unless contraindicated, to help reverse and mitigate reduced arousal, atelectasis, FRC, and impaired mucociliary transport associated with surgery. Mobilization augments cardiovascular and pulmonary function (see Chapters 18 and 20), particularly when the patient is upright.[36,37] These beneficial effects are enhanced by improved three-dimensional chest wall motion, improved gut motility, and reduced intraabdominal pressure. Extremity movement during ambulation increases alveolar ventilation, enhances ventilation and perfusion matching by increasing zone two of the lungs, and optimizes diffusing capacity through stimulating dilatation and recruitment of alveolar capillaries. The upright position ensures that the spine is erect, upper body musculature is relaxed, and the chest wall is symmetrical. Slouching and leaning, particularly to the affected side, reduce alveolar ventilation and contribute to uneven distribution of ventilation and areas of atelectasis.[38,39] In addition, if this abnormal posture is maintained, mucociliary transport of the area is impaired and mucus collects and stagnates, increasing the risk of bacterial colonization and infection. Symmetrical posture is monitored at all times (i.e., during ambulation, sitting at bedside, bed mobility exercises, sitting up in bed, and lying in bed). Slouching and favoring the affected side will lead to cardiovascular and pulmonary complications and possibly musculoskeletal complications in the short and long term.

Mobilization and active exercise in upright postures whenever possible are prescribed based on the need to enhance multiple steps in the oxygen transport pathway. The priority is to perform as much activity as possible out of bed and upright (i.e., ambulation, transferring, sitting upright in a chair, and chair exercises with or without hand weights or exercise bands). When in bed, similar devices can be used, including a monkey bar to facilitate moving in bed for patients other than cardiovascular thoracic patients (e.g., the orthopedic patient with extremity fractures and traction). In addition, the use of the monkey bar is beneficial to perform repetitive bouts of exercises that maintain upper-extremity strength and some general endurance capacity, relieve pressure and stiffness, and facilitate frequent turning. Cycle pedals can be adapted to chairs for recumbent exercise in bed, if necessary. Patients whose positioning is restricted with fixation and traction devices require hand, wrist, or ankle weights, and possibly pulleys and other devices, to maintain muscle strength and power. Movements performed with moderately heavy weights for multiple sets (e.g., three sets of 10 repetitions) develop muscle strength. Movements performed with lighter weights for multiple sets (e.g., five to 10 sets of 10 repetitions) tend to develop endurance and aerobic capacity. Because of the restrictions imposed by these devices, maintaining joint range is essential (i.e., of the neck, spinal column, and chest wall, as well as the extremities). The rotation component of joint movement is readily compromised; thus this must be an integral component of joint range-of-motion exercises. Proprioceptive neuromuscular facilitation (PNF) movements of the extremities can be beneficial. PNF movements of the chest wall can be coordinated with breathing control and supported coughing maneuvers. Upper body and trunk mobility and strengthening are important goals, particularly in the patient with chest wall incisions. The prescription is progressed gradually in the patient with a chest wall incision, particularly in the patient with a median sternotomy who is usually restricted to unresisted, upper-extremity mobility exercises in the first several weeks.

Prescription of body positioning is essential in the management of the patient postsurgically for two reasons. First, without direction, the patient will tend to assume a deleterious body position (i.e., maintaining a restricted number of body positions that favor the affected side for prolonged periods of time with minimal movement and "stirring up"). Therefore once the effects of mobilization have been exploited in a given treatment session, body positions that continue to enhance oxygen transport for a given patient and discourage excessive time in deleterious body positions are prescribed for "between-treatment" times. When not ambulating, patients are encouraged to assume a wide range of body positions (e.g., semiprone) between treatments, as frequently as possible (i.e., at least every 1 to 2 hours).[40-43]

Thoracic and Cardiovascular Surgery

Thoracic Surgery

Thoracic surgery refers to surgery that necessitates opening the chest wall. By convention this term excludes specialized cardiovascular surgery (i.e., surgery of the heart and great vessels). Thoracic surgery is commonly performed for lung resections secondary to cancer (e.g., pneumonectomy, lobectomy, segmentectomy, and wedge resection). In addition, thoracic surgery is performed to remove an irreversibly damaged area of lung tissue secondary to bronchiectasis, benign tumors, fungal infections, and tuberculosis.

The most common incisions are posterolateral thoracotomy and median sternotomy. The posterolateral thoracotomy procedure requires the patient to assume the side-lying position with the involved side uppermost for the duration of the surgery. The uppermost arm is fully flexed anteriorly. The incision is made through an intercostal space, corresponding to the location of the lesion to be excised. The muscles incised include the latissimus dorsi, serratus anterior, external and internal intercostals laterally, and trapezius and rhomboid posteriorly.

At the conclusion of the surgery, chest tubes are placed to evacuate air and fluid from the pleural space by means of an underwater chest tube drainage system. The chest tube and drainage system resolve the pneumothorax created by reestablishing negative pressure in the pleural space and help to reinflate the remaining atelectatic lung tissue. After thoracic surgery, two chest tubes are usually inserted, one at the apex of the lung to evacuate air and one at the base of the lung to drain serosanguineous fluid. The therapist should become familiar with the various drainage systems, how drainage can be facilitated with mobilization and body positioning coordinated with breathing control and supported coughing maneuvers, and certain precautions that must be observed to avoid impairing drainage or disconnecting the tubing. Physical therapy for patients undergoing thoracic surgery has been reported to be cost-effective when a primary component of an interprofessional patient care management strategy[44] as well as when administered prophylactically.[45]

Provided the chest tubes are not kinked, there is no contraindication to lying on the side of the chest tubes. Lying on this side, which is usually the side of the surgery and incision, is typically avoided by the patient. Consistent with the adage down with the good lung, a patient prefers to lie on the nonsurgical side. Prolonged periods in any position, however, particularly lying on the unaffected side, places these lung fields at risk. To minimize the risk of positional complications and hypoxemia, the patient is encouraged to turn to both sides. The specific positions and the duration of time spent within each, however, are based on a comprehensive assessment of the patient's condition and the indications and contraindications for each body position.

Patients may appear to splint themselves, thereby restricting chest wall motion, to avoid pain when moving and deep breathing. They also may resist maximal inspiratory efforts when coughing. Although pain likely contributes to breathing at low lung volumes and ineffective coughing, phrenic nerve inhibition in patients with thoracic and upper abdominal surgeries is likely a more important factor restricting lung expansion. Being upright and moving is associated with increased FRC and tidal volume. Although modalities such as incentive spirometry may have a role in improving lung function in some high risk patients, generally it does not enhance recovery after thoracic surgery.[32]

Postoperative complaints of pain are both musculoskeletal and pleural in origin. The large number of muscles incised, particularly in the posterolateral thoracotomy incision, combined with the operative position, contribute to the patient's complaints of chest wall pain, shoulder soreness, and restricted movement. Deep breathing and coughing maneuvers may be associated with considerable discomfort after surgery. Pain is accentuated by apprehension and anxiety. Therefore treatments are coordinated with relaxation, noninvasive pain control modalities, and pain medication schedules to elicit the full cooperation of the patient.

Cardiovascular Surgery

Cardiovascular surgery is specialized thoracic surgery involving the heart and great vessels, most commonly for lifestyle-related ischemic heart disease. Even for individuals over 90 years of age, outcomes can be favorable.[46]

Because the flow of blood through the cardiovascular and pulmonary system is interrupted, the patient is placed on a cardiovascular and pulmonary bypass machine or on a machine called an *extracorporeal membrane oxygenator.* Cardiovascular surgery is most commonly performed for coronary artery bypass grafting, valve replacements, and aneurysm repairs. Because patients acquire an oxygen debt during the bypass procedure, high oxygen demands are present postsurgically.[47]

After bypass surgery, patients in whom the saphenous vein is excised for graft material have the added complication of surgery and wound healing in one leg. Mobility exercises on that leg are often restricted until there is no risk of bleeding or interference with healing. Comparable with the thoracic surgical patient, a cardiovascular patient leaves the operating room with various monitoring lines and leads, intravenous fluid infusion apparatus, possible blood or plasma infusion devices, a Swan-Ganz catheter (see Chapter 16), a central venous pressure line, an arterial line, a Foley catheter, and oxygen cannulas.

The preoperative preparation and teaching and the postoperative physical therapy management are intensive. Because of the invasiveness of cardiovascular surgery, patients are usually treated postoperatively in a specialized intensive care unit (see Chapter 33). The preoperative and postoperative physical therapy management of patients in the intensive care unit is a specialized area and is described in Chapters 34, 35 and 36.

Providing the patient with information about what to expect during the perioperative course relieves fear and anxiety. In addition, relaxation procedures can be useful. Patients must be reassured that their incisions and suture lines will not be disrupted with movement and physical therapy and that supported coughing and supporting themselves when moving will maximize comfort. Until the patient's condition has stabilized, the patient's mobility is restricted to low-intensity mobilization to promote its benefits on gas exchange and reduce metabolic demands and body positioning to optimize alveolar ventilation coordinated with deep breathing and supported coughing maneuvers. Although breathing exercises have been shown not to augment the benefits of body positioning and mobilization in patients after cardiac surgery,[48] synchronizing breathing control with these interventions will ensure that the secretions stimulated with changing body position and moving are removed. Conventional airway clearance interventions (e.g., postural drainage and manual techniques) may be prescribed in the presence of excessive secretions or difficulty in mobilizing secretions and in the event of productive hydrostatic pneumonia. One systematic review concluded that so-called "prophylactic respiratory physiotherapy" after cardiac surgery was unsubstantiated.[49] Critical components of contemporary physical therapy in the management of patients after cardiac surgery, however, include body positioning and early mobilization, which were not included as key words. The systematic review limited physical therapy simply to breathing exercises and nonspecific chest physiotherapy, which is not consistent with contemporary practice.

Patients undergoing cardiovascular surgery are transferred from the cardiovascular intensive care unit to the ward as quickly as possible. From the ward, these patients should be referred to a physical therapist and a cardiac rehabilitation program in the community for continuity of care and to maximize the functional gains resulting from the surgery. Established performance measures can be useful to streamline care and to help the patient sustain healthy living and medication adherence as needed.[50]

From the hospital to the community, exercise is prescribed progressively to maximize oxygen transport at each step of the rehabilitation period (i.e., acute, before and immediately after discharge, and in the long term). The conditioning effects of exercise enable the patient to resume various activities of daily living commensurate with an increasing oxygen transport system capacity. Activities involving straining and isometric contractions are avoided. Weight lifting may be introduced in a long-term rehabilitation program, but the weights must not be sufficient to cause strain. Patients with median sternotomy incisions are usually prohibited from using their arms to support themselves when sitting or driving and during activities that may strain the incision site for several weeks or more.

Finally, comparable to high-risk patients undergoing thoracic surgery, preoperative inspiratory muscle training has been examined in the management of high-risk patients undergoing cardiovascular surgery, in whom it has been shown to improve surgical outcomes.[51] Gven the benefits of an exercise program before surgery as well as early mobilization, inspiratory muscle training needs to be shown to augment the benefits of these established interventions. Given the multisystem benefits of exercise before and after surgery, inspiratory muscle training is not an alternative.

Summary

Optimal surgical outcome is a team effort that extends beyond the technical success of the surgery. It is based on the return of the individual to full participation in life and long-term health, including no recurrence of the patient's problem and reduced need for biomedical care and drugs in the short and long term; these also are primary physical therapy outcomes. This chapter reviews the principles of perioperative physical therapy management in individuals slated for surgery with a view to maximizing both short- and long-term outcomes. The physical therapy has a key role in risk factor identification and early intervention. Although risk is increased with more invasive and prolonged surgeries, this should not be assumed. Even minor surgery with an apparently uneventful immediate postoperative period can have an untoward outcome because of underlying risk factors. Indication for physical therapy is based on risk factors rather than condition or type of surgery. Given the prevalence of lifestyle-related conditions and their risk factors (e.g., ischemic heart disease, smoking-related conditions, hypertension and stroke, type 2 diabetes mellitus and obesity) that both necessitate elective surgeries and contribute to their complications and delayed recovery, physical therapists need to lead in developing preoperative preparation programs that include health education (initiating or supporting smoking cessation and optimal nutrition), weight reduction, and judiciously prescribed exercise programs.

Teamwork is the essence of successful surgical outcomes. The physical therapist is highly involved from assessment of the patient preoperatively with respect to anticipated necessity of treatment afterward based on a detailed assessment of perioperative risks, to treatment postoperatively, to, most important, postdischarge follow-up to ensure function is regained and the benefits of surgical and related management are sustained over the long term. Physical therapy intervention for the surgical patient is based on indications for that individual rather than the type of surgery.

The four categories of factors contributing to or threatening oxygen transport were described in Chapter 17 and are evaluated in the preoperative and postoperative assessments. These factors include pathology, restricted mobility and recumbency, extrinsic factors related to the patient's care, and intrinsic factors related to the patient. This chapter examines in detail those factors related to surgery and anesthesia in particular, and the impact of underlying disease, restricted mobility, recumbency, and intrinsic factors on the effects of surgery and anesthesia. The role of the physical therapist, an integral member of the surgical team, is to ensure optimal long-term outcomes well beyond the technical success of the surgery, particularly in individuals who have undergone cardiovascular and thoracic surgery. A prime physical therapy outcome in patients who have undergone thoracic or cardiovascular surgery is prevention of both recurrence of the patient's problem and repeated surgery.

Surgery and its physiological effects are described. Special reference is made to two specialized types of surgery that unfortunately have become all too common—namely, thoracic and cardiovascular surgery. These have the greatest impact on cardiovascular and pulmonary function.

Review Questions

1. Describe what is meant by "surgical outcome is a team effort."
2. Given the prevalence of lifestyle-related conditions and their risk factors, describe the role of physical therapists in the 21st century with respect to their role in preparing patients for elective surgery.
3. Why is it that the decision for the physical therapist to treat a patient postoperatively cannot be made based on the type of surgery alone?
4. Describe the physiological effects of surgery including the specific surgical procedure; type, depth, and duration of anesthesia; sedation; types of respiratory support; static body position assumed during surgery; length of surgery; number and type of invasive perioperative procedures; and incisions.
5. Describe surgical risk factors. Why are detection of these of primary importance in the physical therapy assessment and management of the surgical patient?
6. Relate cardiovascular and pulmonary physical therapy management and treatment interventions to the underlying pathophysiology associated with surgery and those factors listed in Question 3, and provide the rationale for your choice.
7. Differentiate the role of physical therapists on the surgical team from the role of the medical and surgical staff and the nursing staff, specifically in terms of their unique noninvasive perspective and related clinical competencies.
8. Describe the role of physical therapy follow-up in the management of the patient who has had surgery, including return to the community.

References

1. World Health Organization International Classification of Functioning Disability and Health: www.who.int/classifications/icf/wha-en.pdf. Received September 2010, 2001.
2. Toomasian JM, Peters WS, Siegel LC, et al: Extracorporeal circulation for post-access cardiac surgery. *Perfusion* 12:83–91, 1997.
3. Shoemaker WC, Appel PL, Kram HB: Hemodynamic and oxygen transport responses in survivors and nonsurvivors of high-risk surgery. *Crit Care Med* 21:977–990, 1993.
4. Sprung J, Whalley DG, Falcone T, et al: The effects of tidal volume and respiratory rate on oxygenation and respiratory mechanics during laparoscopy in morbidly obese patients. *Anesth Analg* 97:268–274, 2003.
5. Kertai MD, Poldermans D, Bax JJ, et al: Cardiac risk and perioperative management. *J Cardiovasc Surg* 44:431–435, 2003.
6. Hashimoto J, Suzuki T, Nakahara T, et al: Preoperative risk stratification using stress myocardial perfusion scintigraphy with electrocardiographic gating. *J Nucl Med* 44:385–390, 2003.
7. Møller AM, Villebro N, Pedersen T, et al: Effect of preoperative smoking intervention on postoperative complications: a randomised clinical trial. *Lancet* 359:114–117, 2002.
8. Wendelboe AM, Hegmann KT, Biggs JJ, et al: Relationships between body mass indices and surgical replacements of knee and hip joints. *Am J Prev Med* 25:290–295, 2003.
9. Mason EE, Renquist K, Jiang D: Predictors of two obesity complications: diabetes and hypertension. *Obes Surg* 2:231–237, 2002.
10. Simunovic N, Devereaux PJ, Bhandari M: Surgery for hip fractures: Does surgical delay affect outcomes? *Ind J Orthop* 45(1):27–32, 2011.
11. Froese AB, Bryan AC: Effects of anesthesia and paralysis on diaphragmatic mechanics in man. *Anesthesiology* 41:242–255, 1974.
12. Hedenstierna G, Standberg A, Brismar B, et al: Functional residual capacity, thoracoabdominal dimensions and central blood volume during general anesthesia with muscle paralysis and mechanical ventilation. *Anesthesiology* 62:247–254, 1985.
13. Hedenstierna G, Tokics L, Strandberg A, et al: Correlation of gas exchange impairment to development of atelectasis during anaesthesia and muscle paralysis. *Acta Anaesthesiol Scand* 30:183–191, 1986.
14. Behrakis PK, Baydur A, Jaeger MJ, Milic-Emili J: Lung mechanics in sitting and horizontal body positions. *Chest* 83:643–646, 1983.
15. Lumb AB, Pearl RG: *Nunn's Applied respiratory physiology*, ed 6, Philadelphia, 2005, Butterworth Heinemann.
16. Duggan M, Kavanagh BP: Atelectasis in the perioperative patient. *Curr Opin Anaesthesiol* 20:37–42, 2007.
17. Lugo G, Arizpe D, Dominguez G, et al: Relationship between oxygen consumption and oxygen delivery during anesthesia in high-risk surgical patients. *Crit Care Med* 21:64–69, 1993.
18. Polonen P, Hippelainen M, Takala R, et al: Relationship between intra- and postoperative oxygen transport and prolonged intensive care after cardiac surgery: a prospective study. *Acta Anaesthesiol Scand* 41:810–817, 1997.
19. Brunton LL, Chabner BA, Knollmann BC, editors: *Goodman and Gilman's The pharmacological basis of therapeutics*, ed 12, New York, 2010, McGraw-Hill Companies.
20. Malamed SF: *Sedation. A guide to patient management*, ed 5, Philadelphia, 2010, Elsevier.
21. Wuhrman E, Cooney MF, Dunwood CJ, et al: Patient controlled analgesia (PCA). *Pain Manag Nurs* 7:134–147, 2006.
22. Weinstein CS, Woodard WJ, DeSilva RA: Late neurocognitive changes from neurological damage following coronary bypass surgery. *Behav Med* 24:131–137, 1998.
23. Pelosi P, Croci M, Ravagnan I, et al: The effects of body mass on lung volumes, respiratory mechanics, and gas exchange, during general anesthesia. *Anesth Analg* 87:654–660, 1998.
24. Dronkers J, Veldman A, Hober E, et al: Prevention of pulmonary complications after upper abdominal surgery by preoperative intensive inspiratory muscle training: a randomized controlled pilot study. *Clin Rehabil* 22:134–142, 2008.
25. Kulkarni SR, Fletcher E, McConnell AK, et al: Pre-operative inspiratory muscle training preserves postoperative inspiratory muscle strength following major abdominal surgery—a randomised pilot study. *Ann R Coll Surg Engl* 92:700–707, 2010.
26. Blomqvist CG, Stone HL: Cardiovascular adjustments to gravitational stress. In Bohr DF, Somlyo AP, Sparks HV Jr, editors: *Handbook of physiology, section 2: the cardiovascular system*, vol 2. Bethesda, Md., 1980, American Physiological Society.
27. Orlava OE: Therapeutic physical culture in the complex treatment of pneumonia. *Phys Ther Rev* 39:153–160, 1959.
28. Fagevik Olsén M, Hahn I, Nordren S, et al: Randomized controlled trial of prophylactic chest physiotherapy in major abdominal surgery. *Br J Surg* 84:1535–1538, 1997.
29. Dripps RD, Waters RM: Nursing care of the surgical patient. 1. The "stir-up." *Am J Nurs* 41:530–534, 1941.
30. Ross J, Dean E: Integrating physiological principles into the comprehensive management of cardiopulmonary dysfunction. *Phys Ther* 69:255–259, 1989.
31. Pelosi P, Croci M, Calappi E, et al: Prone positioning improves pulmonary function in obese patients during general anesthesia. *Anesth Analg* 83:578–583, 1996.
32. Gosselink R, Schrever K, Cops P, et al: Incentive spirometry does not enhance recovery after thoracic surgery. *Crit Care Med* 28:679–683, 2000.
33. Yamaguti WP, Sakamoto ET, Panazzolo D, et al: Diaphragmatic mobility in healthy subjects during incentive spirometry with a flow-oriented device and with a volume-oriented device. *J Bras Pneumol* 36:738–745, 2010.
34. Sellier P, Chatellier G, D'Agrosa-Boiteux MC, et al: Use of non-invasive cardiac investigations to predict clinical endpoints after coronary artery bypass surgery in coronary artery disease patients: results from the prognosis and evaluation of risk in the coronary operated patient (PERISCOP) study. *Eur Heart J* 24:916–926, 2003.
35. Takeyama J, Itoh H, Kato M, et al: Effects of physical training on the recovery of the autonomic nervous activity during exercise after coronary artery bypass grafting: effects of physical training after CABG. *Jpn Circ J* 64:809–813, 2000.
36. Levine SA, Lown B: 'Armchair' treatment of acute coronary thrombosis. *JAMA* 148:1365–1369, 1952.
37. Lewis FR: Management of atelectasis and pneumonia. *Surg Clin North Am* 60:1391–1401, 1980.
38. Don HF, Craig DB, Wahba WM, et al: The measurement of gas trapped in the lungs at functional residual capacity and the effects of posture. *Anesthesiology* 35:582–590, 1971.
39. Glaister DH: The effect of posture on the distribution of ventilation and blood flow in the normal lung. *Clin Sci* 33:391–398, 1967.
40. Dean E: Effect of body position on pulmonary function. *Phys Ther* 65:613–618, 1985.
41. Douglas WW, Rehder K, Beynen FM, et al: Improved oxygenation in patients with acute respiratory failure: the prone position. *Am Rev Respir Dis* 115:559–566, 1977.
42. Piehl MA, Brown RS: Use of extreme position changes in acute respiratory failure. *Crit Care Med* 4:13–14, 1976.
43. Remolina C, Khan AU, Santiago TV, et al: Positional hypoxemia in unilateral lung disease. *N Engl J Med* 304:523–525, 1981.
44. Wright CD, Wain JC, Grillo HC, et al: Pulmonary lobectomy patient care pathway: A model to control cost and maintain quality. *Ann Thorac Surg* 64:299–302, 1997.
45. Varela G, Ballesteros G, Jiménez MF, et al: Cost-effectiveness analysis of prophylactic respiratory physiotherapy in pulmonary lobectomy. *Eur J Cardiothorac Surg* 29:2216–2220, 2006.
46. Bacchetta MD, Ko W, Girardi LN, et al: Outcomes of cardiac surgery in nonagenarians: a 10-year experience. *Ann Thorac Surg* 75:1215–1220, 2003.
47. Utoh J, Moriyama S, Okamoto K, et al: The effects of cardiopulmonary bypass on postoperative oxygen metabolism. *Surg Today* 29:28–33, 1999.
48. Brasher PA, McClelland KH, Denehy L, et al: Does removal of deep breathing exercises from a physiotherapy program including pre-operative education and early mobilization after cardiac surgery alter patient outcomes? *Aust J Physiother* 49:165–173, 2003.
49. Pasquina P, Walder B: Prophylactic respiratory physiotherapy after cardiac surgery: systematic review. *BMJ* 327:1379–1385, 2003.
50. Thomas RJ, King M, Lui K, et al: AACVPR/ACC/AHA 2007 Performance Measures on Cardiac Rehabilitation for Referral to and Delivery of Cardiac Rehabilitation/Secondary Prevention Services. Cardiovascular Nurses Association, and the Society of Thoracic Surgeons. *J Am Coll Cardiol* 50:1400–1433, 2007.
51. Hulzebos EH, Helders PJ, Favié NJ, et al: Preoperative intensive inspiratory muscle training to prevent postoperative pulmonary complications in high-risk patients undergoing CABG surgery. A randomized clinical trial. *JAMA* 296:1851–1857, 2006.

Part V

Cardiovascular and Pulmonary Physical Therapy: Chronic Conditions

PART V OUTLINE

V

Chapter 31

Individuals with Chronic Primary Cardiovascular and Pulmonary Dysfunction

Elizabeth Dean and Donna Frownfelter

KEY TERMS

Angina
Asthma
Bronchiectasis
Chronic airflow limitation
Cystic fibrosis
Diabetes
Interstitial pulmonary fibrosis
Lung cancer
Myocardial infarction
Peripheral vascular disease
Valvular heart disease

CHAPTER OUTLINE

This chapter reviews the pathophysiology and medical management in relation to the comprehensive physical therapy management of individuals with chronic primary cardiovascular and pulmonary pathology. Exercise testing and training are major components of the comprehensive physical therapy management of individuals with chronic primary cardiovascular and pulmonary conditions, and this topic is presented in detail in Chapter 24.

Because the heart and lungs are interdependent and function as a single unit, primary lung or heart disease must be considered with respect to the other organ and in the context of oxygen transport overall.[1,2] Despite a plethora of research and numerous official position statements and clinical practice guidelines, the definition and diagnoses of chronic heart disease and chronic lung disease and their management remain inconsistent in practice.[3] Although there is consensus regarding the effectiveness of both cardiac and pulmonary rehabilitation,[4] this inconsistent practice is associated with the underuse, overuse, and misuse of therapies regardless of their established effectiveness.

Although there is no clear line between obstructive and restrictive patterns of lung disease, the distinction is based on the primary underlying pathophysiological problems. The primary conditions that are discussed include obstructive lung disease (i.e., chronic airflow limitation, asthma, bronchiectasis, and cystic fibrosis) and restrictive lung disease (i.e., interstitial pulmonary fibrosis). Lung cancer, which has the characteristics of both obstructive and restrictive patterns of pathology, is also presented.

The long-term physical therapy management of people with heart disease is then presented, with special attention given to angina, myocardial infarction, and heart valve disease. Chronic vascular conditions including peripheral vascular disease (PVD), hypertension, and type 2 diabetes mellitus with its associated angiopathies are also presented.

The principles of the physical therapy management of people with various chronic primary cardiovascular and pulmonary conditions are presented rather than treatment prescriptions, which cannot be discussed without consideration of a specific patient (see Case Study Guide to accompany the text on-line). In this context, the general goals of the long-term management of people with each condition are presented, followed by the essential monitoring required and the primary interventions for maximizing cardiovascular and pulmonary function and oxygen transport. The selection of interventions for any given patient is based on the physiological hierarchy. The most physiological interventions are exploited first, followed by less physiological interventions and those whose effectiveness is less well documented (see Chapter 17).

The principles outlined in this chapter also apply to the individual who has a secondary diagnosis of one or more chronic primary cardiovascular and pulmonary conditions. These principles can be used to modify physical therapy management prescribed for some other condition or indicate the need for special monitoring.

A template of care is shown in Table 31-1. Although there are many commonalities of physical therapy management across patients, only a detailed knowledge of each specific patient, in terms of his or her underlying pathologies and other factors, will lead to the optimal management plan and treatment prescriptions.

Table 31-1 **Template of Principles of Comprehensive Physical Therapy Management for Chronic Primary Cardiovascular and Pulmonary Dysfunction**

Levels of the International Classification of Function, Disability and Health	Related Objective of Therapeutic Goals
Participation	Life participation (capacity to fulfill life's roles) Empowerment and self-efficacy
Activities	Self-care Ambulation Home management Employment Vocational activities
Structure and Function	Impairments of structure and function of oxygen transport and related factors (see Chapter 2)
Level of Goal	Examples of Focus of Physical Therapy Management
Prevention	Preserve oxygen transport function and prevent threat to this system Assess readiness to change health behavior
Short-term	Identify and treat limitations of structure and function of the oxygen transport system (associated with the greatest risk of future morbidity and mortality) Identify other factors that impair participation and activity (see Chapters 1 and 17)
Long-term	Develop a lifelong health plan Achieve maintenance stage of readiness to change (see Chapter 1) Develop plan for follow-up

Individuals with Primary Cardiovascular Disease

Angina

Pathophysiology and Medical Management

Angina pectoris refers to pain resulting from reduced blood flow to the myocardium. Even though it is usually elicited during exercise, angina may be triggered by stress or in severe cases may occur at rest. Atherosclerosis of one or more of the coronary arteries is the principal cause. Coronary vasospasm is a less common cause of angina. The pathophysiology of angina is described in detail in Chapter 5. A history of angina necessitates further examination to establish the severity of the coronary artery occlusion. Individuals with manifestations of heart disease are categorized according to their limitation during physical activity based on the New York Heart Association (NYHA) Functional Classification (Table 31-2).

If angina is severe and refractory to medical management, the patient is scheduled for coronary bypass surgery (Chapters 29 and 30) to restore normal coronary blood flow. The acute and long-term management of the surgical cardiac patient is presented in Chapter 30. In less severe cases, angina is managed conservatively with medications (e.g., sublingual nitroglycerin, nitroglycerin patch, education, and physical therapy). After the patient's condition has stabilized, a graded exercise tolerance test may be conducted under supervision in a cardiac stress testing facility where 12-lead electrocardiogram (ECG) monitoring can be performed. The exercise intensity at which the patient exhibits angina (i.e., the anginal threshold) can be quantified and serve as the basis for the prescription of physical activity and exercise.

Principles of Physical Therapy Management

Patients may be referred to physical therapy with a history of angina as a primary or secondary problem. Regardless, angina is managed with the same care and vigilance because it can be a life-threatening condition either way. A patient for whom antianginal medication is prescribed must have the medication present. The medication must not have expired and must be within visible access during treatment. The physical therapist should examine the medication before treatment to ensure that the expiratory date has not passed and to take responsibility for positioning the medication near the patient

Table 31-2 **New York Heart Association Functional Classification**

Classification	Characteristics
I	No symptoms and no limitation in ordinary physical activity.
II	Mild symptoms and slight limitation during ordinary physical activity.
III	Marked limitation in activity as a result of symptoms, even during less-than-ordinary activity. Comfortable only at rest.
IV	Severe limitations. Experiences symptoms even while at rest.

for access to it should the patient develop angina during treatment.

The goals of long-term management of the patient with angina include the following:

- Maximize the patient's quality of life, general health, and well-being through maximizing physiological reserve capacity
- Educate regarding heart disease, self-management, nutrition, weight control, smoking reduction and cessation, anger and stress management, disease prevention, risk factors, medications and their use, physical activity, and exercise
- Maximize aerobic capacity and efficiency of oxygen transport of all steps in the pathway
- Optimize physical endurance and exercise capacity
- Optimize general muscle strength and thereby peripheral oxygen extraction
- Design comprehensive lifelong health and rehabilitation programs with the patient

Patient monitoring includes hemodynamic monitoring (i.e., heart rate, blood pressure, rate-pressure product, and dyspnea). Subjective responses to treatment, particularly exercise, should also be recorded (e.g., Borg's rating of perceived exertion). Signs of chest pain, dyspnea, anxiety, lightheadedness, dizziness, disorientation, discoordination, cyanosis, coughing, and chest sound changes (i.e., a gallop) must be monitored. Angina is not an acceptable symptom under any circumstance. Should it occur, treatment is immediately discontinued and emergency measures instituted as indicated. Treatments will be safer and more precisely prescribed with continuous ECG monitoring. Without ECG monitoring, treatments must be conservative. If there is any doubt at any time concerning the hemodynamic stability of a patient and his or her ability to tolerate treatment safely, the patient should be referred to a general practitioner or cardiologist for clearance before being treated.

Medication that is necessary to maximize treatment response is administered before treatment. Knowledge of the type of medication, its administration route, and time to as well as duration of peak efficacy is essential if treatment is to be maximally effective.

For the long-term management of patients with angina, interventions include some combination of education, aerobic exercises, strengthening exercises, chest wall mobility exercises, relaxation, activity pacing, and energy conservation. Education includes information about heart disease and risk factors (i.e., smoking, diet, stress, weight, alcohol, coffee, and being physically active in hot environments) and appropriate preventative strategies (i.e., smoking reduction and cessation, low-fat diet, reduced alcohol consumption, exercise, relaxation, activity pacing, and stress management).

Patients with angina are at risk of having an infarction; therefore vigilance and stringent monitoring are necessary to detect angina or frank myocardial infarction. These patients are potentially hemodynamically unstable; thus their hemodynamic responses before, during, and after treatment, particularly aerobic and strengthening exercises, should be monitored and recorded. Minimally, heart rate, blood pressure, and rate-pressure product should be recorded, along with the patient's subjective responses to treatment. Heavy lifting, static exercise, straining, the Valsalva maneuver, and heavy, repetitive upper-extremity work are avoided during physical activity and exercise. These activities are associated with a disproportionate hemodynamic response. Physical activity and aerobic exercise are prescribed at a target heart rate or perceived exertion ranges that are below the anginal threshold based on a graded exercise tolerance test (see Chapters 19 and 24). Peak exercise tests in patients with cardiac dysfunction that may elicit angina or ST-segment changes are performed in a cardiac stress testing laboratory, usually under the supervision of a cardiologist unless in a specialized facility where physical therapists perform such testing.

The body position in which aerobic exercise is performed is important in patients with heart disease. Positions of recumbency increase the volume of fluid shifted from the periphery to the central circulation. This increases venous return and the work of the heart. Therefore upright body positions have long been known to minimize cardiac work during exercise in these patients and during rest after exercise.[5,6]

Sexual dysfunction is common in individuals with systemic atherosclerosis owing in part to underlying pathology (dyslipidemia, vascular insufficiency, and diabetes), medication, and the psychological impact of heart disease.[7] In terms of energy demands, those of sexual activity are comparable to those of other daily activities (e.g., walking 1 mile on the level). Optimizing health in general with diet and exercise can contribute to regression of atherosclerosis and improved peripheral circulation. Breathing control, body positioning, and energy conservation strategies such as exercising at a high energy time of day may also help minimize symptoms. Also, patients should be advised to avoid sexual activity within an hour of eating, and even then not to consume a heavy meal.

Myocardial Infarction

Pathophysiology and Medical Management

Angina frequently precedes frank myocardial ischemia and infarction. Myocardial ischemia is reversible, whereas infarction denotes myocardial injury and cell death (i.e., necrosis). Injured myocardial cells either recover or die during the healing period. Thus minimizing further damage and maximizing the healing during this 6-week period is critical. Myocardial infarctions can range from being silent and unnoticed by the patient to being life-threatening. They can occur anywhere in the myocardium but occur primarily in the ventricles (in the left more frequently than in the right ventricle). The greater the severity, the greater the risk of ventricular insufficiency, acute pulmonary edema, and left ventricular failure. Because myocardial ischemia and infarction impair the pumping action of the heart and thus cardiac output, patients tend to be hypoxemic and in need of oxygen. Even after the oxygen has been discontinued and the myocardium has healed, the patient may continue to be vulnerable hemodynamically. The myocardium will have some scarring that will affect both the electrical excitability (producing dysrhythmias) and the mechanical function of the heart. In addition, the patient may continue to have low-normal arterial blood gases. Hypoxemia is lethal in that it triggers dysrhythmias and predisposes tissues to hypoxia. Thus hypoxemia must be avoided. After myocardial infarction, patients are usually discharged home on several medications (e.g., nitroglycerin, calcium antagonists, beta blockers, and diuretics). Depending on the severity of involvement, patients usually continue to require one or more of these medications over the long term. The need for oxygen is usually short term and restricted to the patient's hospital stay.

The patient's ECG will be important for determining the parameters of exercise, the level of monitoring required, and education. Dysrhythmias are described in Chapter 4, and basic ECG reading is presented in Chapter 12. Ventricular dysrhythmias can be lethal. Occasional premature ventricular contractions must be monitored to ensure that their frequency remains low and that coupling does not occur. Atrial fibrillation is considered a relatively serious dysrhythmia. It is associated with a high incidence of coronary disease, stroke, and overall mortality.[8] Medication or a pacemaker may be necessary.

Central sleep-disordered breathing is highly prevalent in individuals with left ventricular dysfunction and is associated with abnormal cardiac autonomic control and increased dysrhythmias.[9] Although sleep-disordered breathing may not be related to the severity of hemodynamic dysfunction, loss of recuperative sleep will affect functional capacity as well as capacity and motivation to participate in an exercise program and be physically active.

Health-related quality of life reported by individuals with chronic heart failure is associated with function and exercise capacity, not with ejection fraction.[10] Health-related quality of life should be an outcome measure for all individuals managed for heart failure because it provides important supplemental information that is independent of physiological indices of cardiac function and the NYHA classification of function (see Table 31-2).

Nonpharmacological approaches to the management of individuals with heart failure are an essential component to the overall management of the condition.[11] These measures are incorporated into an individualized program of health behavior change, and include the following:

- Promote adherence to the recommendations
- Maintain an adequate diet
- Maintain a normal weight
- Avoid added sodium (salt and preservatives)
- Maintain optimal blood cholesterol and triglyceride levels
- Maintain normal blood sugar
- Maintain normal blood pressure
- Restrict fluid in the presence of congestive heart failure
- Avoid smoking
- Exercise regularly
- Restrict alcohol use to a moderate amount, if any
- Receive flu and pneumococcal vaccinations

All patients with cardiovascular risk factors can benefit from cardiac rehabilitation. After a cardiac event, patients are typically discharged with drugs, the prospect of surgery, and rather infrequently with referral to an individual physical therapist or one who is a member of the cardiac rehabilitation team. There is a high incidence of recurrence and repeated surgery with further associated mortality and burden of disease. The physical therapist as a noninvasive practitioner has a primary responsibility to help avoid recurrence of symptoms and repeated surgeries. This is consistent with the physical therapist's overriding objective of reducing the need for invasive care (i.e., drugs and surgery) and developing a sustainable, lifelong health plan with the patient.

Risk factor modification is a major goal. A marker of inflammation such as C-reactive protein along with appropriate lipid testing findings may be a more discriminating risk factor than lipid profiling alone.[12] Refining the risk factor definition on the basis of C-reactive protein level will help target management (e.g., indicate necessity for intensified exercise programs, weight loss, and smoking cessation).

Principles of Physical Therapy Management

After discharge from the hospital, many patients who have had a myocardial infarction see a physical therapist either privately or through a cardiac rehabilitation program. Patients may remain on a supervised rehabilitation program, including an exercise program, for 6 to 12 months in a specialized center (see Chapter 24).

Regardless of the setting, physical therapy includes education, psychosocial support, and a supervised setting for exercising safely and developing confidence during physical exertion. In addition, an exercise program is specifically prescribed for the patient to enhance oxygen transport (i.e., delivery, uptake, and utilization at the tissue level), thereby minimizing the metabolic demand on the heart.

Depression is a common symptom reported by individuals with coronary artery disease and is associated with increased morbidity and mortality. Individuals with depressive symptoms are more likely to exhibit myocardial ischemia during mental stress testing and during activities of daily living.[13] Myocardial ischemia induced by mental stress may be a mechanism by which depression increases the risk of morbidity and mortality in individuals with coronary artery disease. Although aggressive type A individuals are thought to have an increased incidence of heart disease compared with passive type B personalities, anger and hostility have been identified as the toxic negative emotions most implicated in morbidity and mortality related to heart disease.[14]

A graded exercise tolerance test is conducted before the patient leaves the hospital or when he or she is enrolled in an exercise program. The time between the exercise test and the exercise prescription and implementation of the exercise program should be minimal. Peak (formerly referred to as *maximal*) exercise tests are conducted in the presence of a cardiologist (unless in a specialized facility where physical therapists may do such testing) and provide the optimal basis for an exercise prescription. Submaximal exercise tests can be conducted by the physical therapist and can provide the basis for an exercise program; however, the prescription should be conservative compared with the prescription based on the peak exercise test. The principles and practice of exercise testing are described in Chapters 19, 24, and 25. Such testing is both an art and an exacting science and should be carried out in a rigidly standardized manner to ensure the test results are maximally valid, reliable, and useful.

As with the patient with angina and no overt infarction, the following caution must be adhered to with the patient who has a history of myocardial infarction. A patient for whom antianginal medication is prescribed must have the medication present. The medication must not have expired and must be within visible access during treatment. The physical therapist should examine the medication before treatment to ensure that the expiratory date has not passed and take responsibility for positioning the medication near the patient for access to it should the patient develop angina during treatment.

The goals of long-term management of the patient with myocardial infarction include the following:

- Maximize the patient's quality of life, general health, capacity to return to work, and well-being through maximizing physiological reserve capacity
- Educate regarding myocardial infarction, self-management, nutrition, weight control, smoking reduction and cessation, relaxation and stress management, risk factors, disease prevention, medications, lifestyle, activities of daily living, and avoidance of static exercise, straining, and the Valsalva maneuver
- Maximize aerobic capacity and efficiency of oxygen transport
- Reduce the work of the heart
- Optimize physical endurance and exercise capacity
- Optimize general muscle strength and thereby peripheral oxygen extraction
- Design comprehensive lifelong health and rehabilitation programs with the patient

Patient monitoring includes hemodynamic monitoring (i.e., heart rate, blood pressure, and rate-pressure product). Subjective responses to treatment, particularly exercise, should also be recorded (e.g., Borg's rating of perceived exertion). Angina is not an acceptable symptom under any circumstance. Should it occur, treatment is immediately discontinued and emergency measures instituted. Treatments will be safer and more precisely prescribed with continuous ECG monitoring. Without ECG monitoring, treatments must be conservative. If there is any doubt at any time about the hemodynamic stability of a patient and his or her ability to tolerate treatment safely, the patient should be referred to a general practitioner for clearance before being treated.

Medication that is needed to maximize treatment response is administered before treatment (e.g., antidysrhythmic agents). Knowledge of the type of medication, its administration route, and time to and duration of peak efficacy is essential if treatment is to be maximally efficacious.

The primary interventions for maximizing cardiovascular and pulmonary function and oxygen transport in patients with myocardial infarction include some combination of education, aerobic exercise, strengthening exercises, chest wall mobility exercises, body positioning, breathing control and coughing maneuvers, relaxation, activity pacing, and energy conservation. An ergonomic assessment of both work and home environments may be indicated to minimize myocardial strain.

Education focuses on teaching the basic pathophysiology of heart disease, its risk factors, and prevention. Health promotion practices are advocated (e.g., smoking reduction and cessation, good nutrition, weight control, hydration, high-quality rest, and sleep periods). In addition, types of physical activity that impose undue myocardial strain, increase intrathoracic pressure, and restrict venous return and cardiac output, such as heaving lifting, straining, or the Valsalva maneuver, are avoided. The patient is taught to monitor and practice vigilance in monitoring his or her own condition (e.g., new signs of infarction). These patients are potentially hemodynamically unstable and thus their hemodynamic responses before, during, and after treatments, particularly exercise, should be monitored and recorded (i.e., heart rate, blood pressure, and rate-pressure product should be taken, along with their subjective responses to treatment).

Peak exercise tests in cardiac patients that may elicit angina or ST-segment changes are performed in a cardiac stress testing laboratory under the supervision of a cardiologist. The parameters of the exercise prescription are set based on a peak exercise test. Intensity is set within a heart rate, oxygen consumption, and exertion range (e.g., 70% to 85% of the anginal threshold) (see Chapter 19).

Aerobic exercise of large muscle groups rather than small muscle groups (e.g., arm ergometry) is selected to minimize the increased hemodynamic demand and strain and the increased work of the heart associated with working smaller, upper-body muscles. Hot and humid conditions also place additional stress on the heart; therefore exercising under these conditions should be avoided.

As with patients with angina, the body position in which aerobic exercise is performed by patients with myocardial infarction is important. Positions of recumbency increase the volume of fluid shifted from the periphery to the central circulation. This increases venous return and the work of the heart. Therefore upright body positions are selected for these patients to minimize cardiac work during exercise and during rest after exercise.[5,6,15]

Valve Disease

Pathophysiology and Medical Management

Valve dysfunction is either congenital or acquired and may require treatment as a primary condition or be present as a secondary condition. Any of the heart and pulmonary valves may be affected. Rheumatic fever was a common cause of rheumatic heart disease and in particular mitral valve insufficiency. Interconnecting lymphatic vessels between the tonsils and the heart are thought to be responsible. Calcification of valves that impairs opening and closing is another example of an acquired valve dysfunction.

Clinically, patients with valve disease may demonstrate exertional dyspnea, excessive fatigue, palpitations, fluid retention, and orthopnea. These signs and symptoms are often relieved when exertion is discontinued. Aerobic exercise, however, has been shown to reduce the symptoms of prolapsed valve.[16] Anxiety has been reported to decrease general well-being. If effectively managed, however, reduced anxiety can improve or reduce chest pain, fatigue, and dizziness.

Prophylactic antibiotics against endocarditis are administered to most patients with significant valvular involvement and in mild disease before procedures such as dental work.

Principles of Physical Therapy Management

The goals of long-term management of the patient with valvular heart disease include the following:

- Maximize the patient's quality of life, general health, and well-being through maximizing physiological reserve capacity
- Educate regarding cardiac valvular disease, self-management, nutrition, weight control, smoking reduction and cessation, relaxation and stress management, cardiac risk factors, disease prevention, medications, lifestyle, activities of daily living, and avoidance of static exercise, straining, and the Valsalva maneuver
- Maximize aerobic capacity and efficiency of oxygen transport

- Optimize physical endurance and exercise capacity
- Reduce the work of the heart
- Optimize general muscle strength and thereby peripheral oxygen extraction
- Design comprehensive lifelong health and rehabilitation programs with the patient

Physical therapists are involved in the management of patients with valve defects with regard to both the medical aspects, either as a primary or secondary problem, and surgical aspects. After surgery these patients progress well; the principles of their management are presented in Chapter 30. With respect to the medical management of valve defects, the goal is to optimize oxygen transport in the patient for whom surgery is not indicated either because the defect is not sufficiently severe or because the patient cannot or refuses to undergo surgery. Although the mechanical defect cannot be improved, oxygen transport may be improved in some patients with judicious exercise prescription. The parameters of the exercise prescription are usually moderate in that inappropriate exercise doses can further disrupt the inappropriate balance between oxygen demand and supply and thus further exacerbate symptoms. In addition, there is the potential for further valvular dysfunction if the myocardium is mechanically strained.

The goal of the aerobic exercise prescription is to identify the exercise dose that will optimize the efficiency of other steps in the oxygen transport pathway such that the available oxygen delivered to the peripheral tissues is maximally used without constituting a significant mechanical strain on the heart. Maximizing work output over time is the goal. Thus, the severely compromised patient will perform a greater volume of functional work over time with short, frequent sessions of exercise rather than longer, less-frequent sessions.

If the valve defect is a secondary problem, the physical therapist must assess the severity of the defect and its functional consequences. The following questions must be addressed:

1. Does the defect preclude treatment?
2. Does the defect require that treatment be modified? If so, how?
3. What special precautions should be taken?
4. What signs and symptoms would indicate the patient is distressed?
5. What parameters should be monitored?
6. Is the patient taking medications as prescribed? How might these medications alter the patient's response to treatment?
7. Is there any evidence of heart failure? If so, what will the effects of exercise be?
8. If there is no evidence of heart failure at rest, what is the chance that insufficiency will develop with exercise?

Comparable with management of the patient with a history of angina with or without a history of myocardial infarction, body positions, activities, and respiratory maneuvers that are associated with increased hemodynamic strain are avoided.

Medication that is necessary to maximize treatment response is administered before treatment. Knowledge of the type of medication, its administration route, and time to and duration of peak efficacy is essential if treatment is to be maximally effective.

Patients with valve disease are potentially hemodynamically unstable; thus their hemodynamic responses before, during, and after treatments, particularly exercise, should be monitored and recorded. Monitoring includes hemodynamic monitoring (i.e., heart rate, blood pressure, and rate-pressure product). Subjective responses to treatment (e.g., rating of perceived exertion) should also be recorded. Signs of dyspnea, chest pain, lightheadedness, dizziness, disorientation, discoordination, cyanosis, coughing, and chest sound changes (i.e., a gallop) must be monitored. Treatments will be safer and more precisely prescribed with continuous ECG monitoring. Without ECG monitoring, treatments must be conservative. If there is any doubt about the hemodynamic stability of a patient and his or her ability to tolerate treatment safely, the patient should be referred to his or her general practitioner for clearance before being treated.

The primary interventions for maximizing cardiovascular and pulmonary function and oxygen transport in patients with cardiac defects include some combination of education, aerobic exercise, strengthening exercises, chest wall mobility exercises, body positioning, breathing control, coughing maneuvers, relaxation, activity pacing, and energy conservation. An ergonomic assessment of both work and home environments may be indicated to minimize myocardial strain.

Exercise prescription for patients with valvular heart disease is modified to ensure that the energy demand is commensurate with oxygen supply. Otherwise excessive oxygen demand will worsen the patient's response to physical activity and lead to further distress and possibly to reduced functional capacity. Aerobic exercise of large muscle groups rather than small muscle groups (e.g., arm ergometry) is selected to minimize the increased hemodynamic demand and strain and the increased work of the heart associated with working smaller, upper-body muscles. As for other types of cardiac conditions, exercising in hot and humid conditions should be avoided.

The body position in which aerobic exercise is performed is important in patients with heart disease. Positions of recumbency increase the volume of fluid shifted from the periphery to the central circulation. This increases venous return and the work of the heart. Therefore upright body positions are selected for these patients to minimize cardiac work during exercise and during rest after exercise.[5,6]

Peripheral Vascular Disease

Pathophysiology and Medical Management

Peripheral vascular disease refers to diseases of the arteries and the veins. Peripheral arterial disease results primarily from atherosclerosis and occlusion of the peripheral arteries (e.g., thoracic aorta, femoral artery, and popliteal artery).[17] The diagnosis may be overlooked until serious limb ischemia is evident.[18] Diabetes mellitus, which can result in microangiopathy and autonomic polyneuropathy, is another important cause of PVD in the lower extremities. Venous disease results in phlebitis, venous stasis, and thromboembolus and leads to valvular incompetence of the veins of the legs.

Arterial occlusion results in reduced blood flow to the extremities and hence reduced segmental blood pressure distal to the occlusion (i.e., lower ankle-brachial index). In mild cases of arterial stenosis the patient may be asymptomatic because considerable stenosis has to occur before there is significant reduction in peripheral blood flow. If atherosclerosis develops gradually, collateral circulation may develop sufficiently to offset progressive vessel narrowing. Clinically the patient reports limb pain on exercise, coldness in the affected leg, and possibly numbness. The characteristic limb pain results from ischemia and is referred to as *intermittent claudication.* Mild to moderately severe cases are managed conservatively. Pain at rest is suggestive of severe stenosis and significant reduction of blood flow to the limb. Significantly reduced blood flow leads to ischemic color changes, skin breakdown, ulceration, and eventually gangrene. Bypass surgery is performed to revascularize a threatened limb. In severe cases in which gangrene has developed, amputation of the limb is indicated. The severity of PVD is a significant predictor of cardiovascular mortality. Individuals with PVD show a systemic endothelial dysfunction and an increase in the serum concentration of white blood cells, endothelin, and C-reactive protein that may trigger acute coronary syndromes.

Individuals with intermittent claudication can have a marked decrease in exercise tolerance and thus can benefit from aerobic exercise, which may stimulate the development of collateral blood vessels around the stenosed vessel. This condition can severely restrict mobility, which reduces function in addition to aerobic capacity and efficient oxygen transport overall.

Individuals with PVD from diffuse systemic atherosclerosis can be expected to have stenosis of the coronary arteries even though they may be asymptomatic. These individuals are monitored as stringently as if they had overt ischemic heart disease.

Venous insufficiency can lead to thromboemboli, skin lesions, and poorly healing ulcers of the lower extremities. Furthermore, the risk of infection and slow healing is increased.

Individuals with PVD secondary to diabetes mellitus have accelerated atherosclerosis compared with age-matched individuals without diabetes. Diabetes affects the macrocirculation and microcirculation; thus wounds must be prevented, particularly in the lower legs and feet, and managed aggressively should they occur. These individuals may be at risk for lower extremity lesions because of autonomic neuropathy and angiopathy. To restore insulin sensitivity and promote weight loss, activity levels must be significantly increased, and a formal exercise program instituted. Weight-bearing activities are safe for individuals with poor sensation in the feet and do not increase the risk of reulceration.[19]

Principles of Physical Therapy Management

It should be assumed that individuals with peripheral arterial disease have coronary and cerebral arterial disease necessitating aggressive risk factor management to reduce the risk of myocardial infarction, stroke, and death.[20] Primary interventions include smoking cessation; treatment of hypertension, glucose intolerance, and diabetes; and management of low-density lipoprotein cholesterol.

The goals of long-term management of the patient with PVD secondary to atherosclerosis include the following:

- Maximize the patient's quality of life, general health, and well-being through maximizing physiological reserve capacity
- Educate regarding atherosclerosis, heart disease, and other sequelae, self-management, nutrition, weight control, smoking reduction and cessation, risk factors, disease prevention, medications, lifestyle, activities of daily living, and avoidance of static exercise, straining, and the Valsalva maneuver
- If impaired peripheral perfusion of the limbs is present, educate regarding self-assessment of the skin; sock type, care, and cleanliness; shoe fitting; and wound care if indicated
- Maximize aerobic capacity and efficiency of oxygen transport
- Optimize the work of the heart
- Optimize physical endurance and exercise capacity
- Optimize general muscle strength and thereby peripheral oxygen extraction
- Design comprehensive lifelong health and rehabilitation programs with the patient

The goals of long-term management of the patient with PVD secondary to diabetes mellitus must incorporate both the principles for the management of the patient with PVD secondary to atherosclerosis and secondary to diabetes mellitus.

Patient monitoring includes hemodynamic monitoring (i.e., heart rate, blood pressure, and rate-pressure product). Subjective responses to treatment, particularly exercise, should also be recorded (e.g., pain scale and Borg's rating of perceived exertion). These patients have an increased risk of angina. Angina is not an acceptable symptom under any circumstance. Thus, before undertaking a therapeutic exercise program, patients should be cleared by their physicians or cardiologists. Individuals with diabetes are potentially hemodynamically unstable; thus their hemodynamic responses before, during, and after treatment, particularly exercise, should be monitored and recorded (i.e., heart rate, blood pressure, and rate-pressure product should be taken), along with their subjective responses to exercise (e.g., pain and perceived exertion). If there is any doubt at any time about the hemodynamic stability of a patient and his or her ability to tolerate treatment safely, the patient should be referred to a general practitioner for clearance to begin or continue treatment.

Medication that is needed to maximize treatment response is administered before treatment. Knowledge of the type of medication, its administration route, and time to and duration of peak efficacy is essential if treatment is to be maximally effective.

The primary interventions for maximizing cardiovascular and pulmonary function and oxygen transport in patients with PVD secondary to atherosclerosis include some combination of education, aerobic exercises, strengthening exercises, relaxation, activity pacing, and energy conservation. Exercise, in particular walking, is an important component of management to ameliorate symptoms and improve functional capacity and quality of life.[18,21] Pharmacotherapy may help relieve symptoms in the short term, whereas exercise benefits are likely to be long term in terms of addressing systemic atherosclerosis. An ergonomic assessment of both work and home environments may be indicated to minimize myocardial strain.

Individuals with PVD may underestimate their increased risk of cardiovascular disease[22]; thus education focuses on teaching the basic pathophysiology of atherosclerosis, its risk factors, prevention, and reversal. Health promotion practices are advocated (e.g., smoking reduction and cessation, nutrition, weight control, and regular physical activity and exercise). In addition, types of physical activity that impose undue myocardial strain, increase intrathoracic pressure, and restrict venous return and cardiac output, such as heavy lifting, straining, or the Valsalva maneuver, are avoided. The patient is taught to practice vigilance in monitoring for signs and symptoms of vascular insufficiency in the affected limb and intermittent claudication. Any sign of skin redness in the feet should be monitored closely. In the patient with diabetes, any threat of skin breakdown requires medical attention and discontinuation of exercise until medical clearance has been obtained. Patients with peripheral artery disease are taught to take special care of their feet before and after exercise. The feet and footwear should be kept clean. The inner surfaces of shoes and socks should be smooth.

During peak exercise tests, patients with PVD secondary to atherosclerosis have an increased risk of angina or ST-segment changes. Such tests therefore should be performed in a peripheral vascular laboratory or cardiac stress testing laboratory under the supervision of a peripheral vascular specialist or cardiologist. The parameters of the exercise prescription are based on a peak exercise test. Walking is the activity or exercise of choice because this activity is most severely limited by intermittent claudication, which has implications for function. Intensity of the training stimulus is based on pain rating in conjunction with hemodynamic and other subjective responses. The patient walks at a comfortable, even cadence within his or her pain tolerance (objectively defined on the pain scale) so that limping and gait deviation are minimized.

The body position in which aerobic exercise is performed is important in patients with PVD. Positions of recumbency eliminate the vertical gravitational gradient. This gradient increases blood pressure in the lower extremities. Therefore the claudication threshold is lowered in recumbent positions. Recumbent positions also increase venous return and the work of the heart. Therefore upright body positions are selected for these patients to maximize blood pressure in the lower extremities and to minimize cardiac work during exercise and during rest after exercise.[5]

The management of venous stasis and disease requires patient involvement to promote healthy lifestyle (exercise and smoking cessation). Compression garments may help to facilitate venous return. Good foot and skin care and shoes that fit well are essential. The patient is taught to assess the skin of the lower extremities daily for signs of skin breakdown and abrasions. Because of impaired peripheral perfusion, skin lesions can occur quickly and then may be resistant to healing and at increased risk of infection.

Hypertension

Pathophysiology and Medical Management

Systemic hypertension or high blood pressure is a serious condition. Most patients experience no symptoms; thus adherence to medication regimens is often poor. Approximately 90% of hypertension is termed *essential hypertension* (i.e., no known cause). Hypertension predisposes a patient to stroke, myocardial infarction, renal dysfunction and failure, hemorrhage, and infarction of other vital organs. Blood pressure tends to increase with age. With the aging of the population, the incidence of hypertension is increasing. Increased blood pressure results from increased peripheral vascular resistance; therefore medications are prescribed that reduce myocardial afterload and peripheral vascular resistance. Hypertension and antihypertensive medication are risk factors for type 2 diabetes mellitus.[23] Therefore avoiding a patient's need for medication or at least reducing it is a singularly important physical therapy outcome.

There are other serious consequences of chronic high blood pressure. Patients with existing cardiovascular disease (i.e., hypertension) are at risk for multisystemic manifestations that must be assessed, e.g., signs and symptoms of cerebrovascular and renal impairments. In addition, this population tends to be older, and older populations are known to have a higher prevalence of cardiac dysrhythmias. Thus such patients' cardiac status, including ECG history, should be obtained.

Pulmonary hypertension may occur in the absence of primary cardiac disease. So-called "primary pulmonary hypertension" is often associated with altered resting lung function. Abnormal lung mechanics and diffusing capacity are directly associated with disease severity and may contribute to the dyspnea and fatigue reported by individuals with primary pulmonary hypertension.[24]

Principles of Physical Therapy Management

Physical therapy contributes to increased metabolic demands and therefore imposes a hemodynamic load resulting in increased heart rate and blood pressure. The assessment should document the history of hypertension, its medical management, and the patient's response. Regardless of the condition being treated, the hypertensive patient's blood pressure must be monitored accurately and treatment modified accordingly.[25] Blood pressure medications, however, are known to attenuate hemodynamic responses to exercise (Chapter 44); thus blood pressure as an index of hemodynamic status may be limited in some individuals.

Interventions for the physical therapy management of hypertension are cause specific. Lifestyle factors are exploited to help reduce blood pressure and optimize long-term health. A program of aerobic exercise can effectively reduce high blood pressure in some patients. The parameters of the exercise prescription necessary to control hypertension include an aerobic type of exercise that is rhythmic and involves large muscle groups, an intensity of 60% to 75% of the patient's age-predicted maximal heart rate, 60 to 90 minutes' duration, and performance of the exercise five to seven times weekly for 3 months to achieve an optimal effect. The exercise intensity should be equivalent to a perceived exertion rating of 3 to 5 on the Borg scale (the patient is able to speak while exercising without gasping), provided that blood pressure does not increase excessively. Only modest exercise intensities are prescribed if the patient has extremely high resting blood pressure to ensure that blood pressure does not rise excessively and is not maintained at a high level for a prolonged period. If the patient's hypertension responds to the exercise regimen, exercise must be included in the patient's lifestyle in order for the effects to be maintained. In addition to exercise, many patients lose weight, adopt healthier lifestyle habits, and learn stress management and coping skills concurrently. When exercise is combined with a weight loss program, both resting and stress-induced blood pressures are reduced. The resulting hemodynamic profile resembles that of successful control with pharmacotherapy.[26]

Elderly individuals with hypertension may exhibit hypotension for almost 24 hours after exercise, along with lower cardiac output, stroke volume, and left ventricular end diastolic volume.[27] Thus such individuals should be examined for this effect, and exercise should be modified accordingly.

The goals of long-term management of the patient with hypertension include the following:

- Maximize the patient's quality of life, general health, and well-being through maximizing physiological reserve capacity
- Educate regarding hypertension, self-management, nutrition, weight control, smoking reduction and cessation, relaxation and stress management, risk factors, lifestyle factors, disease prevention, and medications and their applications and side effects
- Maximize aerobic capacity and efficiency of oxygen transport
- Optimize physical endurance and exercise capacity
- Optimize general muscle strength and thereby peripheral oxygen extraction
- With the effects of lifestyle changes (physical activity, weight loss, nutrition, smoking cessation, and potentially stress management), medication must be weaned correspondingly
- Design comprehensive, lifelong health and rehabilitation programs with the patient

Patient monitoring includes hemodynamic monitoring (i.e., heart rate, blood pressure, and rate-pressure product). Subjective responses to treatment, particularly exercise, should also be recorded. Signs of dyspnea, headache, lightheadedness, dizziness, disorientation, discoordination, cyanosis, coughing, and chest sound changes (i.e., a gallop) must be monitored. Blood pressure responses that fail to increase with increasing work load and power output may be indicative of congestive heart failure.

Treatments will be safer and more precisely prescribed with continuous ECG monitoring. Without ECG monitoring, treatments must be conservative. If there is any doubt about the hemodynamic stability of a patient and his or her ability to tolerate treatment safely, the patient should be referred to a general practitioner or cardiologist for clearance before being treated.

Medication that is necessary to maximize treatment response is administered before treatment (i.e., hypertension medications). Knowledge of the type of medication, its administration route, and time to and duration of peak effectiveness is essential if treatment is to be maximally effective. A primary goal of noninvasive approaches to blood pressure control is to eliminate or minimize medication. The physical therapist monitors the blood pressure closely within and between visits. The patient is taught to log morning blood pressures at home and to log medication. A close working relationship is needed with the patient's invasive practitioner during weaning of the medication.

The primary interventions in the long-term management of hypertension include education, aerobic exercise, general body strengthening, range-of-motion exercises, body mechanics, relaxation, stress management, pacing, and energy conservation. The patient is instructed in self-monitoring blood pressure as well as recording his or her blood pressure, those factors associated with both high and low pressures, and blood pressure changes that occur after medication has been taken. Such monitoring enables the patient to self-manage his or her hypertension and thereby reduces, if not entirely eliminates, need for medication. Patients, however, should alter their medications only with their physicians' approval. Physical therapists work closely with both hypertensive patients and physicians.

Systemic blood pressure responses to dynamic exercise are greater for upper-extremity than lower-extremity work.[28] Thus exercise prescription includes aerobic exercise of the large muscle groups. Avoiding small muscle group work avoids increases in peripheral vascular resistance and hence hemodynamic work, as well as the increased exertion, strain, and work of the heart experienced with upper-extremity work. Exercise is also performed in erect and upright positions rather than recumbent positions to minimize the increased work of the heart secondary to central fluid shifts that occur when the patient is lying in recumbent positions.

Self-monitoring is an important responsibility of the individual with hypertension, given the need to establish valid measures on which interventions are based and modified.[25] The most valid blood pressures are recorded by a well-trained individual with a reliable and accurate automatic blood pressure measurement system. The physical therapist can calibrate the home unit against a sphygmomanometer in the clinic or hospital. The individual is advised to measure his or her blood pressure first thing in the morning and record it.

Type 2 Diabetes Mellitus and Metabolic Syndrome

Pathophysiology and Medical Management

Type 2 diabetes mellitus is a condition associated with impaired insulin metabolism that can result in serious long-term multisystem consequences.[29] The disease is classified as either insulin-dependent or non–insulin-dependent diabetes mellitus. Insulin is the carrier responsible for transporting glucose into the cells to undergo oxidation. Juvenile-onset diabetes is frequently the insulin-dependent type, whereas adult-onset diabetes often is the non–insulin-dependent type. The underlying pathophysiology of juvenile- and adult-onset diabetes, however, is distinct. Juvenile-onset (type 1) diabetes results from an inadequate number of islets of Langerhans in the pancreas, which are responsible for insulin production. Adult-onset (type 2) diabetes, on the other hand, results from reduced insulin sensitivity. In Western industrialized countries, adult-onset diabetes is associated with obesity, inactivity, poor diet, and stress. In addition, medications can contribute to blood sugar disturbances. The sequelae of type 2 diabetes mellitus that frequently result from poor regulation and management of the disease include angiopathy, peripheral neuropathy, autonomic neuropathy, gastrointestinal paresis, visual disturbance, and renal dysfunction.[30]

Individuals with type 2 diabetes mellitus have an accelerated rate of atherosclerotic changes in the vasculature compared with age- and sex-matched individuals without diabetes. These individuals are also prone to PVD secondary to microangiopathy, macroangiopathy, and autonomic neuropathy. People with type 2 diabetes mellitus constitute a significant proportion of patients with PVD who require surgical amputation of affected limbs as a consequence of peripheral ischemia. Muscle infarction is a less common but clinically important complication of longstanding diabetes.[31] Muscle infarction manifests with pain and swelling over the affected area and at times a palpable mass and elevated creatine kinase levels. The symptoms resolve with conservative management including analgesics and relative immobility of the affected muscle.

Abnormalities of blood sugar metabolism can also be observed in individuals without diabetes. Diabetogenic factors, such as restricted mobility and stress, lead to glucose intolerance and insulin oversecretion.[32,33] In the individual without diabetes, these effects can be tolerated over the short term. These factors, however, may result in a critical situation for the individual with diabetes.

Metabolic syndrome is increasingly common and includes central obesity, low high-density-lipoprotein cholesterol, hypertension, and often insulin resistance and hypertriglyceridemia.[34]

Principles of Physical Therapy Management

Patients with type 2 diabetes mellitus may be referred to a physical therapist for several reasons. First, a newly diagnosed diabetic patient may be referred so that the physical therapist can expose the patient to a quantified exercise stimulus under supervised conditions and thereby help refine the prescription of insulin. Second, a patient may be referred for an exercise prescription to help minimize the insulin dose or avoid insulin administration entirely, depending on disease type and severity and the patient's response. Third but most frequently, patients are seen by a physical therapist for the treatment of some other condition and also report type 2 diabetes mellitus in their histories. A history of type 2 diabetes mellitus must be considered in the treatment of a patient who is referred for any reason to either improve or at least not contribute to abnormal blood glucose levels and late complications.

Patients with type 2 diabetes mellitus are treated cautiously. Exercise increases metabolic demand commensurate with intensity and hence cellular demand for glucose.[35] Usually insulin administration is increased in preparation for exercise. Many active individuals who have type 2 diabetes mellitus are closely attuned to their dietary and insulin needs, which permits them to be as physically active as people without diabetes. Individuals with type 2 diabetes mellitus seen by physical therapists, however, are often labile and less well managed. Thus a readily available sugar source must be nearby for insulin regulation when a person with diabetes exercises or when the physical therapist exercises a patient with type 2 diabetes mellitus on an ergometer after anterior cruciate ligament repair.

In addition, people with type 2 diabetes mellitus may have hemodynamic disturbances because of an autonomic neuropathy and may exhibit impaired fluid-volume regulation during exercise.[30] Patients may experience postural hypotension and become dizzy and lightheaded. In addition, diabetic patients may require a longer cool-down period to adjust hemodynamically after exercise.

Hypoglycemia or low blood sugar is one of the most common complications of type 2 diabetes mellitus. This condition results from excess administration of insulin or oral hypoglycemic agent, insufficient food in relation to insulin dose, or an abnormal increase in physical activity or exercise. Hyperglycemia is common in patients who are obese and have adult-onset diabetes. High insulin levels are associated with a higher risk of coronary artery disease. Myocardial infarction and stroke are common causes of death. Another complication is cardiac hypertrophy secondary to hypertension and cardiomyopathy, which predisposes the patient to congestive heart failure. The incidence of PVD is also increased in diabetic patients.

The goals of the long-term management of type 2 diabetes mellitus and metabolic syndrome include the following:

- Maximize the patient's quality of life, general health, and well-being through maximizing physiological reserve capacity
- Educate regarding type 2 diabetes mellitus or metabolic syndrome, self-management, nutrition (good nutrition with optimal lipid and triglyceride dietary control), weight control, blood sugar regulation and its management (i.e., the balance among nutrition, diet, exercise, stress, and insulin requirements), medications, smoking reduction or cessation, relaxation, stress management, and foot care, if necessary, in conjunction with hygiene and infection control
- Maximize aerobic capacity and efficiency of oxygen transport
- Optimize physical endurance and exercise capacity
- Optimize general muscle strength and thus peripheral oxygen extraction
- With the effects of lifestyle changes (physical activity, weight loss, nutrition, smoking cessation, and, potentially, stress management), medication must be weaned correspondingly
- Design comprehensive lifelong health and rehabilitation programs with the patient

Monitoring includes signs and symptoms of hypoglycemia (e.g., lightheadedness, weakness, fatigue, disorientation, and glucose tolerance test results) or hyperglycemia (e.g., glucose tolerance test results).

Hemodynamic responses (i.e., heart rate, blood pressure, and rate-pressure product) provide an index of the intensity of an exercise stimulus; however, these responses may be attenuated in the diabetic patient because of the autonomic neuropathy (both parasympathetic and sympathetic neuropathies).

Subjective responses to exercise, including the rating of perceived exertion, may be more valid indicators of exercise intensity than hemodynamic responses in the person with type 2 diabetes mellitus. The patient is taught to be vigilant in monitoring for signs and symptoms of vascular insufficiency in the affected limb. Any sign of skin redness in the feet should be monitored closely. In individuals with type 2 diabetes mellitus, any threat of skin breakdown requires medical attention and discontinuation of exercise until medical clearance has been obtained. Healing is considerably delayed in the so-called "diabetic foot." Without appropriate attention, infection and potential necrosis can ensue. Individuals with peripheral autonomic neuropathy are taught to monitor their footwear and socks diligently, to ensure the inner surfaces are clean and smooth before each exercise session, and to check for areas of redness or abrasion on their feet after exercise.

Medication that is necessary to maximize treatment response is administered before treatment (e.g., insulin or oral hypoglycemic agents). Knowledge of the type of medication, its administration route, and time to and duration of peak efficacy is essential if treatment is to be maximally effective. With lifestyle changes, including physical activity and weight loss, the physical therapist works closely with the invasive practitioner to monitor medication and the patient's changing requirements consistent with the medication weaning process.

The primary interventions in the long-term management of type 2 diabetes mellitus include education, maintenance of a log of diet and insulin regimens, activity and exercise, aerobic exercise, strengthening exercises, relaxation, stress management, activity pacing, and energy conservation.[36] It may be necessary to consult a nutritionist to assist with promoting lifelong change.

Generally there are no contraindications to patients with type 2 diabetes mellitus being physically active and participating in an exercise program. Daily exercise is advocated for insulin-dependent and non–insulin-dependent diabetic patients to optimize glucose control. The exercise prescription parameters are set at 40% to 85% of peak functional work capacity.[35] If the patient is exercising daily, the exercise parameters are set at the lower end of this range. If the exercise sessions are less frequent (e.g., in the case of an individual with non–insulin-dependent diabetes whose blood glucose is well maintained and whose weight is acceptable), exercise intensity is set at the higher end of this range.

The risk of hypoglycemia can be reduced by observing the following precautions: frequently monitor blood glucose, decrease the insulin dose (in consultation with the physician) or increase carbohydrate intake before exercise, avoid injecting insulin into areas that are active during exercise, avoid exercise during peak insulin activity, consume carbohydrates before, during, and after prolonged aerobic activity, and be knowledgeable about the signs and symptoms of hypoglycemia.[35]

Individuals with Primary Pulmonary Disease: Obstructive Patterns

Chronic Airflow Limitation

Chronic airflow limitation is a descriptive term that refers to those disorders that previously were termed *chronic obstructive pulmonary disease* (COPD) (e.g., chronic bronchitis, emphysema, bronchiectasis, and cystic fibrosis). Although there may be a reversible component, airflow obstruction associated with these disorders is largely irreversible. The pathophysiology of these conditions is reviewed in Chapter 5, and special considerations with respect to exercise testing and training are detailed in Chapter 24.

Bates[37] described the syndrome of chronic airflow limitation as being caused by four external factors, mediated by four primary tissue responses, and modified by four physiological responses. The principal external causative factors include inhaled irritants, allergens, infections, and climate. The four principal tissue responses include large and small airway changes, airway hyperreactivity, bronchiolar damage, and alveolar destruction. The principal physiological responses include a reversible increased airway reactivity component, pulmonary vascular response to alveolar hypoventilation, control of breathing response to ventilation-perfusion imbalance and hypoxemia, and tissue defenses against elastase. Decline in pulmonary function and rate of development of the syndrome depend on the combination of causative factors and individual responses.

Management of chronic lung disease should be an integrated and comprehensive program that depends on teamwork, good communication, an approach focused on the individual, and his or her adherence to health recommendations.[3] Because of the primary contribution of lifestyle to most cases of heart and lung conditions, there is a long but variable latency before clinical signs and symptoms manifest.[38] Therefore advocating healthy lifestyles and working with each individual to embrace such a lifestyle as health insurance will ultimately reduce the burden of the diseases of civilization.

Chronic Bronchitis

Pathophysiology and Medical Management

Chronic bronchitis is usually associated with a history of smoking and is defined as mucous hypersecretion and cough producing sputum for 3 months or more over a 2-year period.[39] Over the first few years of smoking, reversible airway changes occur. Over 10 to 15 years of smoking, mucous hypersecretion and chronic bronchitis become apparent. After 25 to 35 years of smoking, irreversible airway damage and chronic disability occur. Smoking is the major cause of emphysema and lung cancer.

The patient with chronic bronchitis is prone to infection and repeated periods of morbidity. Deterioration of aerobic capacity and functional capacity is related to the severity of the condition. Nutrition and hydration may be impaired, particularly in severe cases, because of neglect and the excessive energy cost of activities of daily living. Sleep may be irregular; thus the patient's symptoms are worsened (e.g., reduced endurance, fatigue, and lethargy) because of lack of normal physiological restoration from sleep.

The natural history of chronic bronchitis related to smoking includes mucous hypersecretion, reduction in forced expiratory volume in 1 second (FEV_1), and increased heterogeneity of the distributions of ventilation, perfusion, ventilation-perfusion matching, and diffusion.[40,41] General debility and deconditioning ensue.

Smoking contributes to increased mucus production in the small airways, increased mucus in the large airways, respiratory bronchiolitis, reduced elastic recoil, increased airway reactivity, and vascular changes.[37] These changes lead to nonuniformity of time constants in the lung, with consequent inhomogeneous distribution of inspired gas and premature small airway closure, and to nonuniformity of ventilation, perfusion, and diffusion distributions. Although variable among smokers, pulmonary function changes generally correspond to the amount smoked and duration of smoking history. Over time the pulmonary function profile becomes increasingly consistent with chronic airflow limitation (i.e., reduced FEV_1 and reduced FEV_1/forced vital capacity); however, these are late indicators of pulmonary changes. Signs of uneven distribution of ventilation and increased closing volumes, indicative of small airway involvement, are early pulmonary function changes in smokers. Exercise diffusing capacity is reduced, which explains in part the reduced maximal volume of oxygen use of smokers. Dynamic compliance with breathing frequency is also reduced. Residual volume is increased as a percent of total lung capacity (TLC). Tracheal mucous velocity is reduced, and secretion clearance is impaired. Any patient with a smoking history, regardless of a diagnosis, has some degree of chronic airflow limitation, which must be considered when these patients receive medical or surgical care, as well as physical therapy.

The cardiac manifestations of chronic bronchitis stem from airway obstruction, secretion accumulation and reduced capacity to expectorate effectively, polycythemia, low arterial oxygen tension, and cardiovascular and pulmonary deconditioning. Increased airway resistance secondary to obstruction increases oxygen demand and hence the work of breathing. This increased demand is superimposed on an oxygen transport system that is already compromised. The cardiovascular system attempts to compensate for chronically reduced arterial oxygen tension by increasing cardiac output (i.e., stroke volume and heart rate). As blood gases deteriorate, the production of red blood cells increases (i.e., polycythemia) to enhance the oxygen-carrying capacity of the blood. Polycythemia increases the viscosity of the blood, however, and in turn, the work of the heart to pump blood to the pulmonary and systemic circulations. Furthermore, viscous blood is prone to circulatory stasis and clotting.

Low arterial oxygen tension leads to hypoxic pulmonary vasoconstriction and increased pulmonary vascular resistance (i.e., pulmonary hypertension). This also increases the work of the right side of the heart in terms of ejecting blood to the lungs. Chronic overwork of the right ventricle leads to hypertrophy, insufficiency, and eventual failure of the right heart (cor pulmonale). Chronically reduced arterial oxygen can increase the demand on the left side of the heart to maintain cardiac output. Similar to right-sided failure, the left side of the heart may become hypertrophied and over time may fail.

The increased intrathoracic pressures generated during chronic coughing reduce venous return, cardiac output, and coronary perfusion and increase blood pressure. These effects exert additional myocardial strain, lead to arterial desaturation, and increase the potential for cardiac dysrhythmias.

The complications of chronic bronchitis are exacerbated by cardiovascular and pulmonary deconditioning. Despite the pathology, the efficiency of oxygen transport along the steps in the pathway is suboptimal. This reduced efficiency results in an overall increase in the oxygen demands of the patient, who is unable to adequately supply oxygen.

Pharmacological support in the long-term management of chronic bronchitis includes bronchodilators (e.g., oral, metered-dose inhalant, inhaled powdered, or aerosol), corticosteroids (e.g., oral or inhaled), expectorants, antibiotics, inotropic agents (e.g., digitalis), beta blockers, antidysrhythmic agents, and diuretics. Patients with chronic lung disease must be monitored closely during exercise because of the potential cardiac effects of disease and medications (e.g., beta-blocker agents attenuate the normal hemodynamic responses to exercise; bronchodilators, such as albuterol (Ventolin), elicit tachycardia).

Principles of Physical Therapy Management

Based on a comprehensive patient assessment, the goals of long-term management for the patient with chronic bronchitis may include the following:

- Maximize the patient's quality of life, general health, and well-being through maximizing his or her physiological reserve capacity
- Assess lifestyle-related health risk factors
- As indicated, address multisystem conditions that affect presenting signs and symptoms (regarding comorbidity, see Chapters 6, 13, 25, and 32)
- Educate the patient about chronic bronchitis; self-management; effects of smoking, nutrition, weight control, smoking reduction or cessation, stress management, and other lifestyle factors; medications; infection control, and role of a long-term rehabilitation program
- Facilitate mucociliary transport
- Optimize secretion clearance
- Optimize alveolar ventilation
- Optimize lung volumes and capacities and flow rates
- Optimize ventilation and perfusion matching and gas exchange
- Reduce the work of breathing
- Reduce the work of the heart
- Maximize aerobic capacity and efficiency of oxygen transport
- Optimize physical endurance and exercise capacity
- Optimize general muscle strength and thereby peripheral oxygen extraction
- Design comprehensive lifelong health and rehabilitation programs with the patient

Patients are monitored for dyspnea, respiratory distress, symptomatic breathing pattern (depth and frequency), arterial desaturation, cyanosis (delayed sign of desaturation); as well as heart rate, blood pressure, and rate-pressure product are monitored. Patients with cardiac dysfunction or low arterial oxygen tensions require ECG monitoring, particularly during exercise. If supplemental oxygen is used, the fraction of inspired oxygen (FiO_2) administered is recorded. Subjectively, breathlessness is assessed using a modified version of the Borg scale of perceived exertion.

Medication that is needed to maximize treatment response (e.g., bronchodilators) is administered before treatment. Knowledge of the type of medication, its administration route, and time to and duration of peak effectiveness is essential if treatment is to be maximally effective.

The primary interventions for maximizing cardiovascular and pulmonary function and oxygen transport in patients with chronic bronchitis include some combination of education, aerobic exercise, strengthening exercise, chest wall mobility exercise, range-of-motion exercises, body positioning, breathing control and coughing maneuvers, airway clearance interventions, relaxation, activity pacing, and energy conservation. An ergonomic assessment of the patient's work and home environments may be indicated to minimize oxygen demand and energy expenditure in these settings.

The use of supplemental oxygen depends on the severity of the disease. Some patients have no need for supplemental oxygen, some need it only during exercise, and some patients require continuous oxygen with proportionately more delivered during activity and exercise compared with rest. Supplemental oxygen is not usually required until lung damage becomes extreme (i.e., the morphological changes are consistent with the irreversible changes associated with emphysema).

Education is a principal focus of the long-term management of the patient with chronic bronchitis. Education includes the reinforcement of preventive health practices (e.g., smoking reduction and cessation, cold and flu prevention, flu shots, aerobic exercise, strengthening exercises, nutrition, weight control, hydration, pacing of activities, energy conservation, relaxation, and stress management). Chronic bronchitis and emphysema are often associated with sleep disturbances. Obstructive sleep apnea is increasingly prevalent with disease severity. Thus activity and sleep patterns must be assessed to ensure that sleep is maximally restorative and not contributing to the patient's symptoms. Integral to an exercise prescription is the time of day it is to be performed. Exercise is prescribed when the patient is least fatigued, when he or she is most energetic, and when performing such a program is most convenient.

Aerobic exercise is a well-established essential component of the long-term management of the patient with chronic bronchitis to optimize the efficiency of oxygen transport overall including mobilization and removal of secretions.[42] The goal is to increase the exercise threshold intensity at which incapacitating dyspnea, perceived exertion, and desaturation occur.

Emphysema

Pathophysiology and Medical Management

Emphysema is associated with a prolonged history of smoking and chronic bronchitis and indicates significant irreversible lung damage. A less common type of emphysema not associated with smoking is alpha$_1$-antitrypsin deficiency. Antitrypsin is essential in balancing elastin production and degradation and in preserving optimal lung compliance. A deficiency of antitrypsin reduces lung elasticity and contributes to the characteristic increase in lung compliance that is the hallmark of emphysema. The pathophysiology of emphysema is detailed in Chapter 5. The principal pathophysiological deficits include irreversible alveolar damage resulting from loss of elastic recoil and the normal tethering of the alveoli, which renders the lung parenchyma excessively compliant and floppy. Excessive distension and dilatation of the terminal bronchioles and destruction of alveoli reduce the surface area for gas exchange. Hence diffusing capacity is correspondingly reduced. The dead space in the lungs and TLC increase significantly. Breathing at normal tidal volume, the patient's airways close beyond the degree normally occurring with aging, and this contributes to ventilation and perfusion mismatch and hypoxemia. Time constants are altered such that alveolar units are not evenly ventilated. In the nonacute, chronic stages the primary problems include inadequate and inefficient gas exchange resulting from the structural damage to the lungs and altered respiratory mechanics of the lungs and chest wall and their interaction. The lungs are hyperinflated, the chest wall becomes rigidly fixed in a hyperinflated position, the normal bucket handle and pump handle motions of the chest wall are impaired, the hemidiaphragms are flattened, the mediastinal structures are shifted, and the heart is displaced and rotated, making it mechanically inefficient.[40] The normal mucociliary transport system is ineffective because years of smoking destroy the cilia, reduce their number, and alter their configuration and orientation; thus their function is correspondingly obliterated or impaired. In addition, these patients are unable to generate high transpulmonary pressures and forced expiratory flow rates because of altered respiratory mechanics. Consequently, coughing is weak and ineffective. The administration of supplemental oxygen is limited because these patients rely on their hypoxic drive to breathe. This life-preserving drive can be attenuated with even moderate levels of oxygen. Thus oxygen administration is limited to low flows. The respiratory muscles are often weak, if not fatigued from being in a flattened position, and hence suboptimal on the length-tension curve.[43] The clinical consequences of hyperinflation include abnormal chest wall movement, impaired inspiratory muscle function, increased oxygen cost of breathing, impaired exercise capacity, hypoxemia and hypercapnia, and breathlessness. Overall, patients with emphysema, particularly severe emphysema, tend to be inactive and deconditioned, which further compromises the efficiency of the oxygen transport system and the capacity of other steps in the pathway to compensate.

Several physiological compensations occur in response to chronic hypoxemia. Stroke volume and cardiac output are increased. The red blood cell count increases (polycythemia); however, the blood becomes more viscous and requires more work to eject and distribute throughout the body. Thus the stroke work of the heart is further increased. This load on the heart occurs in addition to the increased afterload of the right ventricle because of an increase in pulmonary vascular resistance secondary to hypoxic vasoconstriction in the lungs. Over time the heart becomes enlarged and pumps even less efficiently. In the long-term management of the patient with emphysema, the primary pathophysiological problems are impaired alveolar ventilation, impaired gas exchange, reduced oxygen transport efficiency, and the work of breathing and of the heart. Unlike in chronic bronchitis, secretion accumulation may be less problematic in patients with emphysema during nonacute periods. Nonetheless, optimizing mucociliary transport is an ongoing goal of prevention in that the consequences of mucous retention and infection can be life-threatening.

Noninvasive positive pressure mechanical ventilation (NPPV) has been an important advance in the management of individuals with chronic lung disease.[44] Those with daytime hypercapnia with nocturnal hypoventilation may benefit most.[45] The efficacy of NPPV, however, is jeopardized by poor adherence to its use. Predictors of successful use include ability to protect the airway, acuteness of illness, and a good initial response within the first couple of hours. Barriers include discomfort of the nose piece or face mask, patient-ventilator asynchrony, excess sternocleidomastoid activity, unstable vital signs, prolonged hours of ventilator use, problems with adaptation, symptoms, and poor gas exchange. In addition to immediate clinical benefits, NPPV may help avoid or postpone respiratory failure and invasive mechanical ventilation and weaning in this population. Other benefits that may be associated with NPPV include improved sleep and quality of life and reduced hospitalization. The physical therapist needs to identify potential barriers and address these to maximize adaptation and adherence to NPPV. Patient subgroups of those who will benefit from NPPV must be identified. Technology research must improve comfort and adherence to NPPV.

Long-term outcome of lung volume reduction surgery for people with severe emphysema has been positive. Six months after surgery, right ventricular performance increases, particularly during exercise.[46]

Principles of Physical Therapy Management

The goals for long-term management of the patient with emphysema include the following:

- Maximize the patient's quality of life, general health, and well-being through maximizing his or her physiological reserve capacity
- Educate regarding emphysema, self-management, smoking reduction and cessation, medications, nutrition, weight control, stress management, infection control, and the role of a long-term rehabilitation program
- Optimize alveolar ventilation
- Optimize lung volumes and capacities and flow rates
- Optimize ventilation and perfusion matching
- Reduce the work of breathing
- Reduce the work of the heart
- Maximize aerobic capacity and efficiency of oxygen transport
- Optimize physical endurance and exercise capacity
- Optimize general muscle strength and thereby peripheral oxygen extraction
- Optimize respiratory muscle strength and endurance and overall respiratory muscle efficiency
- Ensure that sleep and rest are optimal
- Design comprehensive lifelong health and rehabilitation programs with the patient

Education focuses on teaching the patient about emphysema, self-management of the disease, the effect of smoking and smoking cessation, nutrition, weight control, hydration, relaxation, sleep and rest, stress management, activity pacing, energy conservation, and prevention (e.g., cold and flu prevention, flu shots, aerobic exercise, diet, sleep, and stress management).

Comparable to the patient with chronic bronchitis, sleep disturbances are common in the patient with emphysema. Activity and sleep patterns are assessed to ensure sleep is maximally restorative. If obstructive sleep apnea is disturbing the patient's sleep, recommendations can be made regarding optimal body positioning during sleep. Back elevation improves airway instability, and in some instances side-lying positions may reduce symptoms.[47] If noninvasive mechanical ventilation (e.g., nasal continuous positive airway pressure) is necessary, these body positions may help reduce the amount of ventilatory support required.

Patients are monitored for dyspnea, respiratory distress, inappropriate breathing pattern (depth and frequency), arterial desaturation, lightheadedness, discoordination; heart rate, blood pressure, and rate-pressure product also are monitored. Patients with cardiac dysfunction or low arterial oxygen tension require ECG monitoring, particularly during exercise. Subjectively, breathlessness is assessed using a modified version of the Borg scale of perceived exertion.

Medication that is necessary to maximize treatment response (e.g., bronchodilator) is administered before treatment. Knowledge of the type of medication, its administration route, and time to and duration of peak efficacy is essential if treatment is to be maximally efficacious. When patients are on multiple medications, the interactions and implications for treatment response must be identified.

The primary interventions for maximizing cardiovascular and pulmonary function and oxygen transport in patients with emphysema include some combination of education, aerobic exercise, strengthening exercise, ventilatory muscle training (strength and endurance) or ventilatory muscle rest, low flow oxygen, mechanical ventilatory support for home use, chest wall mobility exercises, range-of-motion exercises, body positioning, breathing control and coughing maneuvers, airway-clearance techniques, relaxation, activity pacing, and energy conservation. An ergonomic assessment of work and home environments may be indicated to minimize oxygen demands in these settings.

The benefits of aerobic and strengthening exercise in the long-term management of airflow limitation to optimize oxygen transport in patients with compromised oxygen delivery are well established.[48–50] Patients with severe limitations are often unable to exercise at a sufficient intensity to effect aerobic adaptations to the exercise stimulus. Benefits of exercise in these patients may be explained by desensitization of dyspnea, improved movement efficiency and hence movement economy, improved anaerobic capacity, improved ventilatory muscle strength and endurance, and increased motivation.[51,52] Exercise intensity is prescribed based on rating of breathlessness (modified Borg scale) (Chapters 18 and 19), in conjunction with objective and other subjective responses from the exercise test. Objective and subjective responses to exercise in patient populations, however, reflect many factors in addition to pathophysiology (see Chapter 19 for guidelines to maximize test validity).

Patients with chronic airflow limitation alter their breathing patterns so that they breathe on the most metabolically efficient portion of the pressure relaxation curve (see Chapters 5 and 31). These patients tend to breathe with prolonged expiratory phases to maximize gas transfer and mixing in the lungs in order to minimize the effects of altered ventilatory time constants. To facilitate such a breathing pattern, the patient tends to breathe through pursed lips, which may create back pressure to maintain the patency of the airways. The metabolic efficiency of the patient's breathing pattern may be improved further by altering breathing mechanics rather than imposing a different breathing pattern that may be suboptimal.[53] Altering breathing mechanics involves manipulating the patient's body position to promote alveolar ventilation, perfusion, and ventilation and perfusion matching, thereby reducing the work of the heart.

The increased intrathoracic pressures generated during chronic coughing limit venous return, cardiac output, and coronary perfusion. Blood pressure is also increased. These effects exert additional myocardial strain, lead to arterial desaturation, and increase the potential for cardiac dysrhythmias. Breathing control and coughing maneuvers coupled with body positioning and exercise are taught such that the work of breathing is minimized (i.e., alveolar ventilation and gas transfer are as efficient as possible) and coughing is as efficient as possible (i.e., maximally productive with the least energy expenditure).

Physical therapy is one component of a comprehensive rehabilitation program in the long-term management of people with emphysema. Such a program also needs to include information on health promotion and maintenance, ongoing review and a log of medications, respiratory support (e.g., oxygen aerosol therapy and mechanical ventilatory support), occupational therapy, sexual rehabilitation, psychosocial rehabilitation, and vocational rehabilitation.

Breathing control maneuvers (breathing exercises) warrant special mention. Breathing control has been thought to reduce the work of breathing. Inadvertent use of breathing exercises, however, can increase the work of breathing. Diaphragmatic breathing can reduce ventilatory efficiency in people with COPD.[54] Furthermore, these exercises are associated with greater oxygen cost than spontaneous breathing in stable patients with COPD.[53] The fact that patients do not breathe with the most energetically economic breathing pattern is of considerable clinical interest and suggests that biomechanical efficiency overrides economic efficiency. These findings support that an altered breathing pattern is the consequence of the underlying problem rather than the problem itself. Thus management should be focused on the factors that determine biomechanical efficiency and breathing pattern. Other than pursed-lip breathing, evidence for retraining breathing patterns in people with stable COPD is not well supported.[55]

Body positioning is a primary determinant of pulmonary function. Thus patients should be encouraged to perform coughing and other forced expiratory maneuvers in upright positions.[56] Leaning forward can increase intraabdominal and intrathoracic pressures, elevate the diaphragm, and increase expiratory flow rate.

Obstructive sleep apnea is often associated with COPD. This is complicated further by obesity in some patients. Upright positioning and weight loss can improve respiratory mechanics and oxygenation.[57] A more upright sleeping posture could improve nighttime oxygenation in this patient group.

Asthma

Pathophysiology and Medical Management

Asthma is a common respiratory condition that is characterized by hypersensitivity of the airways to various triggers resulting in reversible airway obstruction (i.e., bronchospasm and bronchial edema) (see Chapter 5).[39] In mild cases, no treatment other than prophylaxis may be needed. In severe cases, asthma can be life-threatening. Once affected by the trigger, the airways narrow, increasing the resistance to airflow and reducing oxygen delivery. Breathing through narrowed airways contributes to wheezing, reduced alveolar ventilation, rapid shallow breathing, shortness of breath, increased work of breathing, desaturation, and cyanosis. Increased inhomogeneity of the distribution of ventilation is present in some patients with nonacute asthma.[58] Expiratory flow-volume loops remain the cornerstone of monitoring asthma.[59] Although some triggers may produce mucous hypersecretion, even normal amounts of pulmonary secretions can obstruct narrowed airways and lead to atelectasis. Asthma that has well-defined triggers is easier to manage than cases in which the triggers are less specific.

Principles of Physical Therapy Management

The goals of long-term management of the patient with asthma include the following:

- Maximize the patient's quality of life, general health, and well-being through maximizing his or her physiological reserve capacity
- Educate regarding asthma, self-management, nutrition, weight control, air quality including smoking reduction and cessation, stress management, medications and their uses, prevention of asthmatic attacks, and infection control
- Reduce the work of breathing
- Maximize aerobic capacity and efficiency of oxygen transport
- Optimize physical endurance and exercise capacity
- Optimize general muscle strength and thereby peripheral oxygen extraction
- Design comprehensive lifelong health and rehabilitation programs with the patient

Patients are monitored for dyspnea, respiratory distress, inappropriate breathing pattern (depth and frequency), arterial desaturation, and cyanosis (delayed sign of desaturation); heart rate, blood pressure, and rate-pressure product are monitored. Patients with cardiac dysfunction or low arterial oxygen tension require ECG monitoring, particularly during exercise. Subjectively, breathlessness is assessed using a modified version of the Borg scale of perceived exertion.

Medication that is needed to maximize treatment response (e.g., bronchodilators and antiinflammatories) is administered before treatment. Knowledge of the type of medication, its administration route, and time to and duration of peak efficacy is essential if treatment is to be maximally efficacious. When patients are taking multiple medications, their interactions and the implications for management must be known.

The primary interventions for maximizing cardiovascular and pulmonary function and oxygen transport in patients with asthma include education, aerobic exercise, strengthening exercise, chest wall mobility exercises, range-of-motion exercises, relaxation, activity pacing, and stress management.

Education is central to self-management of asthma. The patient is taught the basic pathophysiology of the disease and its triggers. Other central topics, including preventive health practices, are also taught (e.g., cold and flu prevention; flu shots; medication types, administration, and effects; aerobic exercise; nutrition; weight control; hydration; air quality control including smoking reduction and cessation; relaxation and stress management; and the benefits of an integrative, lifelong, self-management rehabilitation program).

Special mention must be made regarding the use of medications and inhalers. These are frequently used unknowledgeably (i.e., the patient is unfamiliar with the basic pharmacokinetics of the medications being used and thus is not deriving optimal effects). Inhalers are often used improperly; therefore the patient does not derive the full benefit of the medication. The instructions provided by the supplier of the inhalers should be strictly followed. There are numerous types of inhalers, all with different applications. In not adhering to the instructions, the patient's time and effort are wasted by using the inhaler ineffectively, the patient does not derive the full benefit of the medication, an excessive amount of inhaler may be used to compensate for ineffective application, there may be increased exposure of the patient to the side effects of the medication, and there is considerable economic waste.

Knowledge of the triggers of increased airway sensitivity enables the patient to exert control over bronchospastic attacks. The patient is taught to record the frequency of bronchospastic attacks and identify what triggers and relieves them. In this way the patient learns to avoid or minimize their frequency, severity, and duration and minimizes the amount of medication required. In turn, doctor and hospital visits may be minimized. These are significant benefits.

The exercise prescription parameters are set below the bronchospasm threshold, which is established based on an exercise test (see Chapters 19 and 24). Specialized challenge tests are performed in a pulmonary function laboratory. Exercise training enables the patient to determine the balance between optimal aerobic capacity and medication and the optimal physical environment for exercise. Temperature and humidity can have significant effects on work output in patients with asthma.

Bronchiectasis

Pathophysiology and Medical Management

Bronchiectasis is characterized by dilatation and anatomical distortion of the airways and obliteration of the peripheral bronchial tree.[41] Bronchiectasis is often the sequela of prolonged chronic lung infection. The associated inflammation leads to occlusion of the airways, which results in atelectasis of the parenchyma and consequent dilatation of central airways by increased traction on the peribronchial sheath. In addition, chronic inflammation weakens the walls of the airways, leading to further dilatation. Fibrotic connective tissue changes in the wall contribute further to dilatation and airway distortion. These anatomical changes adversely affect normal respiratory mechanics and hence pressure volume characteristics of the lung. The chest wall becomes hyperinflated and assumes the barrel shape associated with chronic airflow limitation. The overall severity of bronchiectasis depends on the number of lung segments involved. There is often some reversible airflow limitation associated with bronchiectasis.

The patient with bronchiectasis has copious tenacious secretions, lung hyperinflation and impaired respiratory mechanics, an inefficient breathing pattern, reduced ability to clear secretions, and reduced aerobic capacity and is generally debilitated.

The increased intrathoracic pressures generated during bouts of chronic coughing limit venous return, cardiac output, and coronary perfusion. Blood pressure is also increased. These effects exert additional myocardial strain, lead to arterial desaturation, and increase the potential for cardiac dysrhythmias and dysfunction.

Principles of Physical Therapy Management

The goals of long-term management of the patient with bronchiectasis include the following:

- Maximize the patient's quality of life, general health, and well-being through maximizing his or her physiological reserve capacity and function
- Educate regarding bronchiectasis, self-management, nutrition, weight control, smoking reduction and cessation, stress management, medications and their use, and infection control
- Facilitate mucociliary transport
- Optimize secretion clearance
- Optimize alveolar ventilation
- Optimize lung volumes and capacities and flow rates
- Optimize ventilation and perfusion matching
- Reduce the work of breathing
- Maximize aerobic capacity and efficiency of oxygen transport
- Optimize physical endurance and exercise capacity
- Optimize general muscle strength and thus peripheral oxygen extraction
- Design comprehensive lifelong health and rehabilitation programs with the patient

Patients are monitored for dyspnea, respiratory distress, inappropriate breathing pattern (depth and frequency), arterial desaturation, and cyanosis (a delayed sign of desaturation); heart rate, blood pressure, and rate-pressure product are monitored. Patients with cardiac dysfunction or low arterial oxygen tension require ECG monitoring, particularly during exercise. Subjectively, breathlessness is assessed using a modified version of the Borg scale of perceived exertion.

Medication that is needed to maximize treatment response is administered before treatment. Knowledge of the type of medication, its administration route, and time to and duration of peak efficacy is essential if treatment is to be maximally efficacious.

The primary interventions for maximizing cardiovascular and pulmonary function and oxygen transport in patients with bronchiectasis include some combination of education, aerobic exercises, strengthening exercises, chest wall mobility exercises, range-of-motion exercises, body positioning, breathing control and coughing maneuvers, airway clearance interventions, optimizing rest and sleep, relaxation, pacing, and energy conservation. Factors that trigger symptoms are identified and avoided. An ergonomic assessment of the patient's work and home environments may be indicated to maximize function in these settings.

Education is a central component of the patient's long-term, self-management rehabilitation program. Preventative health practices are taught (e.g., cold and flu prevention, flu shots, smoking cessation, sleep, aerobic exercise, nutrition, weight control, hydration, relaxation, stress management, and the long-term benefits of an integrative rehabilitation program).

Cystic Fibrosis

Pathophysiology and Medical Management

Cystic fibrosis is a complex exocrine disease that has significant systemic effects.[39] The disease is congenital and is hallmarked by nutritional deficits contributing to impaired growth and development. Pulmonary function shows progressive decline with commensurate reductions in homogeneity of ventilation and inspiratory pressures.[58] Cardiovascular and pulmonary involvement can be classified into three groups: no physical signs in the chest; occasional cough and sputum; and constant cough, sputum, and other signs. Patients in each classification can benefit from physical therapy with respect to enhancing oxygen transport. Moderate and severe disease is characterized by significant airflow obstruction secondary to copious, tenacious secretions. In addition, pulmonary hypertension and right heart insufficiency may be manifested and eventual failure may ensue. Left ventricular diastolic failure may also be a feature of advanced disease.[60]

Between exacerbations, the medical priorities are to reduce the risk of infection and morbidity and promote optimal health, growth, and development.

Principles of Physical Therapy Management

The goals of long-term management of the patient with cystic fibrosis include the following:

- Maximize the patient's quality of life, general health, well-being, and growth and development through maximizing his or her physiological reserve capacity
- Educate the patient and family regarding cystic fibrosis, self-management, nutrition, avoidance of smokers, stress management and relaxation, prevention of acute exacerbations of the disease, infection control, and medication uses, modes of administration, pharmacokinetics, and times to peak efficacies
- Facilitate mucociliary transport
- Optimize secretion clearance
- Optimize alveolar ventilation
- Optimize lung volumes and capacities and flow rates
- Optimize ventilation and perfusion matching
- Reduce the work of breathing
- Reduce the work of and strain on the heart
- Maximize aerobic capacity and efficiency of oxygen transport
- Optimize physical endurance and exercise capacity
- Optimize general muscle strength and thereby peripheral oxygen extraction
- Design comprehensive lifelong health and rehabilitation programs with the individual (and the family if the patient is a child)

Patients are monitored for dyspnea, respiratory distress, inappropriate breathing pattern (depth and frequency), arterial desaturation, and cyanosis (a delayed sign of desaturation); heart rate, blood pressure, and rate-pressure product are monitored. Patients with cardiac dysfunction or low arterial oxygen tension require ECG monitoring, particularly during exercise. Subjectively, breathlessness is assessed using a modified version of the Borg scale of perceived exertion.

Medication that is needed to maximize treatment response is administered before treatment. Knowledge of the type of medication, its administration route, and time to and duration of peak efficacy is essential if treatment is to be maximally efficacious.

The primary interventions for maximizing cardiovascular and pulmonary function and oxygen transport in patients with cystic fibrosis include some combination of education, aerobic exercises, strengthening exercises, ventilatory muscle training (strength and endurance), ventilatory muscle rest, supplemental oxygen, mechanical ventilation for home use, chest wall mobility exercises, range-of-motion exercises, body positioning, breathing control and coughing maneuvers, airway clearance interventions, relaxation, pacing, and energy conservation.

Education focuses on teaching preventative health practices and infection control (e.g., avoidance of cold and flu, flu shots, aerobic exercise, nutrition, hydration, relaxation, stress management, activity pacing, and energy conservation).

Physical activity and aerobic exercise must be integrated early into the lifestyle of the child with cystic fibrosis.[61] As much as possible, the child is integrated into activities of his or her peer group. A prescribed aerobic exercise program is designed to optimize the efficiency of oxygen transport at all steps in the pathway and thereby enhance functional capacity overall. Physical activity and aerobic exercise enhance mucociliary transport and mucociliary clearance, maximize alveolar ventilation and ventilation and perfusion matching, increase ventilatory muscle strength and endurance and airway diameter, and stimulate a productive effective cough. Furthermore, physical activity and exercise have been associated with improved immunity and reduced risks of infection.[62,63] These are significant outcomes for patients with cystic fibrosis, who have thick, copious secretions.

In addition, breathing control and coughing maneuvers are included as a component of a long-term, self-management rehabilitation program. Postural drainage and manual techniques have been the mainstay of airway clearance in the past. Exercise, however, has a primary role in secretion mobilization and as an airway clearance intervention. Breathing control and coughing strategies are coupled with exercise to facilitate secretion clearance. The principles of autogenic drainage can be integrated into breathing control. This procedure focuses on eliciting coughing when it will be most productive, thereby minimizing less productive, exhaustive coughing. Patients with cystic fibrosis often cough so violently and uncontrollably that it leads to significant arterial desaturation, vomiting, and exhaustion and impedes venous return and cardiac output.

Ventilatory devices such as the positive expiratory pressure (PEP) mask and the flutter valve have shown benefit in some patients with cystic fibrosis with respect to reducing airway closure, clearing secretions, and enhancing gas exchange.[64,65] Such aids may be useful adjuncts in some patients; however, they do not replace the multiple benefits (including mobilizing and removing secretions) of physical activity and exercise on optimizing oxygen transport.

Individuals with Primary Pulmonary Disease: Restrictive Patterns

Interstitial Lung Disease

Pathophysiology and Medical Management

The pathophysiology of restrictive lung disorders and interstitial lung disease (ILD) in particular is described in Chapter 5. This classification of lung disease is associated with various occupations and the inhalation of inorganic and organic dust. As the disease progresses, TLC and vital capacity are reduced. Residual volume often remains the same. Maximal flow rates tend to be increased as compliance is reduced. The drive to breathe, breathing frequency, and the ratio of tidal volume to TLC are increased. Glandular hyperplasia may be present, leading to mucous hypersecretion in some patients. Diffusing capacity may be reduced, but this may be apparent only during exercise (i.e., arterial desaturation and dyspnea). Exercise-induced desaturation and reduction in partial pressure of arterial oxygen may also reflect shunt and ventilation and perfusion mismatch.

Hemodynamic changes may be present (e.g., increased pulmonary artery pressure). Chronically increased pulmonary artery pressures, and hence increased pulmonary vascular resistance, lead to increased right ventricular stroke work, hypertrophy, and right ventricular insufficiency. Partial pressure of oxygen in mixed venous blood may fall significantly during exercise, contributing to arterial hypoxemia.

Principles of Physical Therapy Management

The goals of long-term management of the patient with ILD include the following:

- Maximize the patient's quality of life, general health, and well-being through maximizing his or her physiological reserve capacity
- Educate regarding ILD, self-management, nutrition, weight control, smoking reduction and cessation, relaxation and stress management, medications and their uses, prevention, health promotion, and infection control
- Optimize alveolar ventilation
- Optimize lung volumes and capacities
- Optimize ventilation and perfusion matching
- Optimize mucociliary transport
- Reduce the work of breathing
- Reduce the work of the heart
- Maximize aerobic capacity and efficiency of oxygen transport
- Optimize physical endurance and exercise capacity
- Optimize general muscle strength and thereby peripheral oxygen extraction
- Design comprehensive lifelong health and rehabilitation programs with the patient

Patients are monitored for dyspnea, respiratory distress, and inappropriate breathing pattern (depth and frequency); arterial desaturation; in addition heart rate, blood pressure, and rate-pressure product are monitored. Patients with cardiac dysfunction or low arterial oxygen tension require ECG monitoring, particularly during exercise. Subjectively, breathlessness is assessed using a modified version of the Borg scale of perceived exertion.

Medication that is needed to maximize treatment response is administered before treatment. Knowledge of the type of medication, its administration route, and time to and duration of peak efficacy is essential if treatment is to be maximally effective.

The primary interventions for maximizing cardiovascular and pulmonary function and oxygen transport in patients with ILD include some combination of education, aerobic exercises, strengthening exercises, chest wall mobility exercises, range-of-motion exercises, body positioning, breathing control and coughing maneuvers, relaxation, pacing, and energy conservation. An ergonomic assessment of the patient's work and home environments may be indicated to maximize function in these settings.

Education is a central component of a comprehensive rehabilitation program for the management of ILD. Education includes information on preventative health practices (e.g., removal from the causative environment, cold and influenza prevention shots, triggers of disease exacerbations and their prevention, smoking reduction and cessation, nutrition, weight control, hydration, relaxation, activity pacing, and energy conservation).

During aerobic exercise, patients with ILD are prone to arterial desaturation.[66] Patients who desaturate during sleep require supplemental oxygen during exercise. The intensity of the exercise prescribed is based on arterial saturation, breathlessness, and work of the heart, in conjunction with other objective responses.

Lung Cancer

Pathophysiology and Medical Management

Lung cancer is a leading cause of death for men and the incidence is increasing for women. Once diagnosed, 80% of patients survive 1 year. Lung cancer is highly correlated with a history of smoking and exposure to coal tars, asbestos, and radioactive dusts. The majority of primary malignant tumors are bronchogenic carcinomas. They are centrally located and thus contribute to bronchial obstruction, atelectasis, and pneumonia. Pathophysiologically, lung cancer has features of both obstructive and restrictive lung disease. Presenting signs include airway obstruction, dyspnea, cough, and hemoptysis.[39] Treatment is limited to surgery, if metastasis has been ruled out, or conservative management with radiation and chemotherapy.

Bronchogenic carcinomas metastasize readily through the circulation and lymphatic channels to other organs including the brain, bone, liver, kidneys, and adrenal glands.

If detected early, thoracic surgery may be performed to excise the cancerous tumor (see Chapter 29). If inoperable, or in the case of metastases, a patient may be managed at home or in a hospice. Patients are debilitated, often undernourished, fatigued, short of breath, lethargic, depressed, and in pain. Although these patients are often extremely ill, there is a growing trend to manage these patients in the community whenever possible. As the disease progresses, maintaining function and reducing the rate of deterioration become primary goals.

End-of-life issues and palliative care must be discussed. If the patient is managed at home, these principles of care can be practiced in this setting, and they are common to other conditions as well.

Principles of Physical Therapy Management

The goals of long-term management of the medical patient with lung cancer include the following:

- Maximize the patient's quality of life, general health, and well-being through maximizing his or her physiological reserve capacity
- Educate the patient and family about the benefits of a palliative program
- Promote self-determination and pay particular attention to being an active listener
- Provide supportive care
- Optimize pain control
- Facilitate mucociliary transport
- Optimize secretion clearance and protect the airways
- Optimize alveolar ventilation
- Optimize lung volumes and capacities and flow rates
- Optimize ventilation and perfusion matching
- Reduce the work of breathing

- Maximize aerobic capacity and efficiency of oxygen transport
- Optimize physical endurance and exercise capacity
- Optimize general muscle strength and thereby peripheral oxygen extraction
- Optimize the benefits of sleep and rest
- Minimize the effects of restricted mobility and recumbency
- Design a rehabilitation program with the patient that is suited to his or her fluctuating needs

Patients are monitored for dyspnea, respiratory distress, inappropriate breathing pattern (depth and frequency), arterial desaturation, and cyanosis (a delayed sign of desaturation); heart rate, blood pressure, and rate-pressure product also are monitored. Patients who can be mobilized but have cardiac dysfunction or low arterial oxygen tensions require ECG monitoring. Subjectively, breathlessness is assessed using a modified version of the Borg scale of perceived exertion.

Medication that is necessary to maximize treatment response (e.g., analgesics or bronchodilators) is administered before treatment. Knowledge of the type of medication, its administration route, and time to and duration of peak efficacy is essential if treatment is to be maximally effective.

The primary interventions for maximizing cardiovascular and pulmonary function and oxygen transport in patients with lung cancer include some combination of education, mobilization, strengthening exercises, chest wall mobility exercises, body positioning, supplemental oxygen, mechanical respiratory support, breathing control and coughing maneuvers, airway clearance interventions, sleep and rest, relaxation, activity pacing, and energy conservation. Treatments are timed whenever possible to coincide with patients' peak energy level during the day.

Patients with lung cancer may benefit from the immunological effects, as well as oxygen transport effects, of mobilization and physical activity. The prescriptive parameters are adjusted each session, given the rapid changes in these patients' conditions.

Patients with lung cancer often cough up and expectorate blood in their sputum. The airways must be as clear as possible to avoid obstruction, atelectasis, infection, and pneumonia. Although airway clearance is an important goal, treatments should avoid contributing to bleeding and blood loss, if possible. This blood loss may contribute to anemia and fatigue.

Manual airway clearance interventions may be indicated in some patients. Postural drainage may be coupled with percussion and manual vibration. The impact of manual interventions, however, may contribute to bleeding; thus the patient requires stringent monitoring. Despite lack of evidence, metastases to the thoracic cavity and the ribs in particular may preclude percussion in favor of manual vibration being performed over unaffected areas. Treatment duration may be limited by the patient's tolerance. Tolerance may be improved by modifying body position or by shortening treatments but increasing their frequency.

Summary

This chapter reviews the pathophysiology, medical management, and comprehensive physical therapy management of individuals with chronic primary cardiovascular and pulmonary pathology. Exercise testing and training are major components of the comprehensive management of these conditions, and this topic is presented separately in Chapter 24. Given that the heart and lungs are interdependent and function as a single unit, primary lung or heart disease is considered with respect to the other organ and in the context of oxygen transport overall.

The principles of long-term management of people with chronic primary lung disease are presented first. Although there is no clear line between obstructive and restrictive patterns of lung disease as they often coexist, pathology can be generally defined based on the primary underlying pathophysiological problems. Thus the primary conditions presented included obstructive lung disease (i.e., chronic airflow limitation, asthma, bronchiectasis, and cystic fibrosis) and restrictive lung disease (i.e., interstitial pulmonary fibrosis). Lung cancer, which has the characteristics of both obstructive and restrictive patterns of pathology, is also presented.

The long-term cardiovascular and pulmonary management of people with chronic primary heart disease is then presented, with special attention to angina, myocardial infarction, and heart valve disease. Chronic vascular diseases including PVD, hypertension, and type 2 diabetes mellitus are also presented.

The principles of management of people with various chronic primary cardiovascular and pulmonary conditions are presented rather than treatment prescriptions, which cannot be discussed without consideration of a specific patient. These principles also are applied when one or more chronic primary cardiovascular and pulmonary conditions are secondary diagnoses for a patient, as such dysfunction may necessitate modifying the treatment prescription for some other condition or, minimally, indicate special monitoring.

Review Questions

1. Describe the chronic primary cardiovascular and pulmonary pathophysiology associated with airflow limitation (i.e., COPD), asthma, bronchiectasis, cystic fibrosis, interstitial pulmonary fibrosis, lung cancer, angina, myocardial infarction, valvular heart disease, PVD, hypertension, and type 2 diabetes mellitus, and how such pathology may affect an individual's participation in life or be a threat to it.
2. Relate cardiovascular and pulmonary physical therapy treatment interventions for individuals with each of the chronic conditions listed in question 1, and provide the rationale for your choice.

References

1. Ross J, Dean E: Integrating physiological principles into the comprehensive management of cardiopulmonary dysfunction. *Phy Ther* 69:255–259, 1989.
2. Wasserman K, Hansen JE, Sue DY, et al: *Principles of exercise testing and interpretation including pathophysiology and clinical applications.* Philadelphia, 2005, Lippincott Williams & Wilkins.
3. Pierson DJ: Translating new understanding into better care for the patient with chronic obstructive pulmonary disease. *Respir Care* 49:99–109, 2004.
4. Ferguson GT: Recommendations for the management of COPD. *Chest* 117:23S–28S, 2000
5. Langou RA, Wolfson S, Olson EG, et al: Effects of orthostatic postural changes on myocardial oxygen demands. *Am J Cardiol* 39:418–421, 1977.

6. Levine SA, Lown B: "Armchair" treatment of acute coronary thrombosis. *JAMA* 148:1365–1369, 1952.
7. Jackson HA, Jr: Sexual activity and the cardiovascular patient: guidelines. *Am J Cardiol* 84:6N–10N, 1999.
8. Aronow WS: Management of the older person with atrial fibrillation. *J Gerontol A Biol Sci Med Sci* 57:M352–M363, 2002.
9. Lanfranchi PA, Some VK, Braghiroli A, et al: Central sleep apnea in left ventricular dysfunction: prevalence and implications for arrhythmic risk. *Circulation* 107:727–732, 2003.
10. Mitani H, Hashimoto H, Isshiki T, et al: Health-related quality of life of Japanese patients with chronic heart failure: assessment using the Medical Outcome Study Short Form 36. *Circulation J* 67:215–220, 2003.
11. Gibbs CR, Jackson G, Lip GYH: ABC of heart failure. Non-drug management. *BMJ* 320:366–368, 2000.
12. Blake GJ, Ridker PM: Inflammatory bio-markers and cardiovascular risk prediction. *J Intern Med* 252:283–294, 2002.
13. Jiang W, Babyak MA, Rozanski A, et al: Depression and increased myocardial ischemic activity in patients with ischemic heart disease. *Am Heart J* 146:55–61, 2003.
14. Donker FJ: Cardiac rehabilitation: a review of current developments. *Clin Psychol Rev* 20:923–943, 2000.
15. Prakash R, Parmley WW, Dikshit K, et al: Hemodynamic effects of postural changes in patients with acute myocardial infarction. *Chest* 64:7–9, 1973.
16. Scordo KA: Effects of aerobic exercise training on symptomatic women with mitral valve prolapse. *Am J Cardiol* 67:863–868, 1991.
17. Spittell JA: *Peripheral vascular disease for cardiologists*. New York, 2004, Blackwell.
18. Dawson DL, Hiatt WR, Creager MA, et al: Peripheral arterial disease: medical care and prevention of complications. *Prev Cardiol* 5:119–130, 2002.
19. Lemaster JW, Reiber GE, Smith DG, et al: Daily weight-bearing activity does not increase the risk of diabetic foot ulcers. *Med Sci Sports Exerc* 35:1093–1099, 2003.
20. Doyle J, Creager MA: Pharmacotherapy and behavioral intervention for peripheral artery disease. *Rev Cardiovasc Med* 4:18–24, 2003.
21. Brevetti G, Annecchini R, Bucur R: Intermittent claudication: pharmacoeconomic and quality of life aspects of treatment. *Pharmacoeconomics* 20:169–181, 2002.
22. McDermott MM, Mandapat AL, Moates A, et al: Knowledge and attitudes regarding cardiovascular disease risk and prevention in patients with coronary or peripheral arterial disease. *Arch Intern Med* 163:2157–2162, 2003.
23. Gress TW, Nieto J, Shahar E, et al: Hypertension and antihypertensive therapy as risk factors for type 2 diabetes mellitus. *NEJM* 342:905–912, 2000.
24. Sun XG, Hansen JE, Oudiz RJ, et al: Pulmonary function in primary pulmonary hypertension. *J Am Coll Cardiol* 41:1028–1035, 2003.
25. Zarnke KB, McAlister FA, Campbell NR, et al: The 2001 Canadian recommendations for the management of hypertension: Part one—Assessment for diagnosis, cardiovascular risk, causes and lifestyle modification. *Can J Cardiol* 18:604–624, 2002.
26. Georgiades A, Sherwood A, Gullette EC, et al: Effects of exercise and weight loss on mental stress–induced cardiovascular responses in individuals with high blood pressure. *Hypertension* 36:171–176, 2000.
27. Brandao Rondon MU, Alves MJ, Braga AM, et al: Postexercise blood pressure reduction in elderly hypertensive patients. *J Am Coll Cardiol* 39:676–682, 2002.
28. Dean E, Ross J: Mobilization and exercise conditioning. In Zadai C, editor: *Pulmonary management in physical therapy*, New York, 1992, Churchill Livingstone.
29. Hall JE: *Guyton and Hall textbook of medical physiology*, ed 12, Philadelphia, 2010, Elsevier.
30. Bannister R, Mathais CJ: *Autonomic failure*, ed 4, New York, 2002, Oxford University Press.
31. Trujillo-Santos AJ: Diabetic muscle infarction. An undiagnosed complication of long-standing diabetes. *Diabetes Care* 26:211–215, 2003.
32. Lipman RL: Glucose tolerance during decreased physical activity in man. *Diabetes* 21:101–105, 1972.
33. Stannard SR, Johnson NA: Insulin resistance and elevated triglyceride in muscle: more important for survival than "thrifty" genes? *J Physiol* 554:595–607, 2004.
34. Malloy MJ, Kane JP: A risk factor for atherosclerosis: triglyceride-rich lipoproteins. *Adv Intern Med* 47:111–136, 2001.
35. American College of Sports Medicine (ACSM): *ACSM's guidelines for exercise testing and prescription*, ed 10, Philadelphia, 2009, Lippincott Williams & Wilkins.
36. Leon AS: Diabetes. In Skinner JS, editor: *(2005). Exercise testing and exercise prescription for special cases. Theoretical basis and clinical application*, ed 3, Philadelphia, 2003, Lippincott Williams & Wilkins.
37. Bates DV: *Respiratory function in diseases*, ed 3, Philadelphia, 1989, WB Saunders.
38. Gibbons RJ, Balady GJ, Bricker JT, et al: ACC/AHA 2002 guideline update for exercise testing: summary article. A report of the American College of Cardiology/American Heart Association Task Force on Practice Guidelines (Committee to Update the 1997 Exercise Testing Guidelines): (2002). American College of Cardiology/American Heart Association Task Force on Practice Guidelines. Available at: http://circ.ahajournals.org/cgi/content/full/106/14/1883. Retrieved September 2010.
39. Barrett KE, Barman SM, Boitano S, et al: *Ganong's review of medical physiology*, ed 23, New York, 2009, McGraw-Hill.
40. Mason RJ, Broaddus VC, Martin T, et al: *Murray and Nadel's Textbook of Respiratory Medicine*, ed 5, Philadelphia, 2010, Elsevier.
41. West JB: *Pulmonary pathophysiology: the essentials*, ed 7, Philadelphia, 2008, Lippincott Williams & Wilkins.
42. Oldenburg FA, Dolovich MB, Montgomery JM, et al: Effects of postural drainage, exercise, and cough on mucus clearance in chronic bronchitis. *Am Rev Respir Dis* 120:739–745, 1979.
43. Rochester DF, Arora NS: Respiratory muscle failure. *Med Clin North Am* 67:573–597, 1983.
44. Hill NS: Noninvasive ventilation in chronic obstructive pulmonary disease. *Clin Chest Med* 21:783–797, 2000.
45. Hill NS: Noninvasive ventilation for chronic obstructive pulmonary disease. *Respir Care* 49:72–87, 2004.
46. Mineo TC, Pompeo E., Rogliani P, et al: Effect of lung volume reduction surgery for severe emphysema on right ventricular function. *Am J Crit Care Med* 165:489–494, 2002.
47. Neill AM, Angus SM, Sajkov D, et al: Effects of sleep posture on upper airway stability in patients with obstructive sleep apnea. *Am J Respir Crit Care Med* 155:199–204, 1997.
48. Niederman MS, Clemente PH, Fein AM, et al: Benefits of a multidisciplinary pulmonary rehabilitation program: improvements are independent of lung function. *Chest* 99:798–804, 1991.
49. Ries AL, Ellis B, Hawkins RW: Upper extremity exercise training in chronic obstructive pulmonary disease. *Chest* 93:688–692, 1988.
50. ZuWallack RL, Patel K, Reardon JZ, et al: Predictors of improvement in the 12-minute walking distance following a six-week outpatient pulmonary rehabilitation program. *Chest* 99:805–808, 1991.
51. Belman MJ, Kendregan BA: Exercise training fails to increase skeletal muscle enzymes in patients with chronic obstructive pulmonary disease. *Am Rev Respir Dis* 123:256–261, 1981.
52. Belman MJ, Wasserman K: Exercise training and testing in patients with chronic obstructive pulmonary disease. *Basics Respir Dis* 10:1–6, 1981.
53. Jones AYM, Dean E, Chow CCS: Comparison of the oxygen cost of breathing exercises and spontaneous breathing in patients with stable chronic obstructive pulmonary disease. *Phys Ther* 83:424–431, 2003.
54. Gosselink RA, Wagenaar RC, Rijswijk H., et al. Diaphragmatic breathing reduces efficiency of breathing in patients with chronic obstructive pulmonary disease. *Am J Respir Crit Care Med* 151:1136–1142, 1995.
55. Dechman G, Wilson CR: Evidence underlying breathing retraining in people with stable chronic obstructive pulmonary disease. *Phys Ther* 84:1189–1197, 2004.
56. Badr C, Elkins MR, Ellis ER: The effect of body position on maximal expiratory pressure and flow. *Aust J Physiother* 48:95–102, 2002
57. Hakala K, Maasilta P, Sovijarvi AR: Upright body position and weight loss improve respiratory mechanics and daytime oxygenation in obese patients with obstructive sleep apnea. *Clin Physiol* 20:50–55, 2000.
58. Ross J, Bates DV, Dean E, et al: Discordance of airflow limitation and ventilation inhomogeneity in asthma and cystic fibrosis. *Clin Invest Med* 15:97–102, 1992.
59. Brand PL, Roorda, RJ: Usefulness of monitoring lung function in asthma. *Arch Dis Child* 88:1021–1025, 2003.
60. Koelling TM, Dec GW, Ginns LC, et al: Left ventricular diastolic function in patients with advanced cystic fibrosis. *Chest* 123:1488–1494, 2003.
61. Zach M, Oberwaldner B, Hausler F: Cystic fibrosis: physical exercise versus chest physiotherapy. *Arch Dis Child* 57:587–589, 1982.
62. Pyne DB: Regulation of neutrophil function during exercise. *Sports Med* 17:245–258, 1994.
63. Shephard RJ, Verde TJ, Thomas SG, et al: Physical activity and the immune system. Can *J Sports Sci* 16:163–185, 1991.
64. Pryor JA: *Respiratory care*. Edinburgh, 1993, Churchill Livingstone.
65. Pryor JA, Ammani Prasad S, editors: *Physiotherapy for respiratory and cardiac problems: adults and paediatrics*, ed 4, Edinburgh, 2008, Churchill Livingstone/Elsevier.
66. Arita KI, Nishida O, Hiramoto T: Physical exercise in "pulmonary fibrosis." *Hiroshima J Med Sci* 30:149–159, 1981.

V

Chapter 32

Individuals with Chronic Secondary Cardiovascular and Pulmonary Dysfunction

Elizabeth Dean and Donna Frownfelter

KEY TERMS

Ankylosing spondylitis
Cerebral palsy
Chronic renal insufficiency
Kyphoscoliosis
Multiple sclerosis
Muscular dystrophy
Obesity
Osteoporosis
Parkinson syndrome
Postpolio syndrome
Rheumatoid arthritis
Scleroderma
Spinal cord injury
Stroke
Systemic lupus erythematosus

CHAPTER OUTLINE

This chapter reviews the pathophysiology and medical management in relation to the comprehensive physical therapy management of individuals with chronic secondary cardiovascular and pulmonary pathology. Exercise testing and training are major components of the comprehensive physical therapy management of individuals with chronic secondary cardiovascular and pulmonary conditions, and this topic is presented separately in Chapter 25.

This chapter specifically addresses the comprehensive physical therapy management of chronic cardiovascular and pulmonary dysfunction secondary to neuromuscular, musculoskeletal, collagen vascular and connective tissue, and renal dysfunction. Considerations in the management of people who are overweight or obese are also addressed. The neuromuscular conditions that are presented include stroke, Parkinson syndrome, multiple sclerosis, cerebral palsy, spinal cord injury, chronic effects of poliomyelitis, and muscular dystrophy. The musculoskeletal conditions that are presented include thoracic deformity (kyphoscoliosis) and osteoporosis. The collagen vascular and connective tissue conditions that are presented include systemic lupus erythematosus (SLE), scleroderma, ankylosing spondylitis, and rheumatoid arthritis (RA). Finally, management of the patient with chronic renal insufficiency and management of the person who is obese are presented. The principles of physical therapy management are presented rather than treatment prescriptions, which cannot be given without consideration of a specific patient (see online Case Study Guide). In this context the goals of long-term management of each condition are presented, followed by the essential monitoring required and the primary interventions for maximizing cardiovascular and pulmonary function and oxygen transport. The selection of interventions for any given patient is based on the physiological hierarchy. The most physiological interventions are exploited, followed by less physiological interventions and those whose effectiveness is less well documented (see Chapter 17). With respect to physical therapy treatment prescription and monitoring, these principles must be considered when chronic secondary cardiopulmonary dysfunction is the diagnosis.

Principles of Physical Therapy Management in Chronic Secondary Dysfunction

Long-Term Physical Therapy Management Goals

Although short-term goals for patients with chronic cardiovascular and pulmonary secondary dysfunction are the immediate priority, long-term goals need to be considered from the outset. In addition to considering the patient's activity and participation needs, identifying the long-term goals early may help identify short-term component goals.

Physiological Management Goals

- Optimize lung volumes and capacities and flow rates
- Optimize ventilation and perfusion matching and gas exchange
- Facilitate mucociliary transport as needed
- Maximize aerobic capacity and efficiency of oxygen transport
- Optimize physical endurance and exercise capacity
- Optimize general muscle strength and thereby peripheral oxygen extraction

Psychosocial Management Goals

- Maximize the patient's quality of life, general health, and well-being through maximizing physiological reserve capacity
- Educate patient and/or family or caregiver regarding:
  - Cardiovascular and pulmonary manifestations of the condition
  - Self-management
  - Medication
  - Nutrition
  - Weight control
  - Smoking reduction and cessation
  - Stress management
  - Infection control
  - The role of a rehabilitation program
- As indicated, address multisystem conditions that affect presenting signs and symptoms (regarding comorbidities, see Chapters 6, 24, 25, and 31 and related parts of this chapter)
- Design lifelong health and rehabilitation programs with the patient

Among the primary goals in managing the needs of people with chronic conditions are teaching self-management skills and promoting lifestyle self-efficacy. Without attention to these components of management, short- and particularly long-term outcomes will be suboptimal.

Patient Monitoring

Patients with chronic secondary cardiovascular and pulmonary dysfunction should be monitored in a number of ways to ensure success in a rehabilitation program. These data points are necessary with most conditions discussed in this chapter, but not all. Dyspnea, for example, is not monitored for as part of an examination for osteoporosis because dyspnea is generally not part of the disease process. Exceptions to the data points mentioned are discussed in the individual monitoring discussions.

In general, patients with chronic secondary cardiovascular and pulmonary dysfunction should be monitored for the following:

- Dyspnea
- Respiratory distress
- Inappropriate breathing pattern (depth, symmetry, and frequency)
- Arterial saturation
- Cyanosis (delayed sign of desaturation)

The following values should be monitored:

- Heart rate
- Blood pressure
- Rate pressure product

The Borg scale for measuring perceived exertion is well established as a reliable tool for assessing and evaluating patients at rest and during and after exercise. Reduced exertion for a given level of work after training is an important indicator of improved oxygen transport capacity and fitness.

Medication Use

Medication(s), if necessary to maximize response, should be administered before treatment. Knowledge of the type of medication, its administration route, and time to and duration of peak efficacy is essential if treatment is to be maximally effective.

Primary Interventions

The primary interventions for maximizing cardiovascular and pulmonary function and oxygen transport in individuals with chronic secondary dysfunction are a combination of the following:

- Education
- Aerobic exercise
- Strengthening exercises
- Postural correction exercises
- Chest wall mobility exercises
- Range-of-motion exercises
- Airway clearance interventions
- Activity pacing
- Energy conservation

An ergonomic assessment of the patient's work and home environments may be indicated to minimize oxygen demand and energy expenditure in these settings for all patients with chronic secondary dysfunction.

Specific conditions require specific interventions; interventions particular to each condition are discussed in further detail in this chapter.

Patient Education

Education is a principal focus of the long-term management of all patients (see general principles and guidelines in Chapter 28), but it is especially important for those with secondary dysfunction. Patients should receive instruction in and information on the following health promotion and preventative practices:

- Infection control
- Smoking reduction and cessation
- Cold and flu prevention (including flu shots)
- Aerobic exercise
- Strengthening exercises
- Nutrition
- Weight control
- Hydration
- Pacing of activities
- Energy conservation

Information or instruction particular to each secondary condition is discussed in further detail in this chapter.

Individuals with Neuromuscular Conditions

Stroke

Pathophysiology and Medical Management

Stroke or hemiplegia affects cardiovascular and pulmonary function of the survivors either directly or indirectly. A cerebral infarct involving the vital centers of the brain can affect cardiovascular and pulmonary function. Such infarctions, however, are likely to be lethal or leave a person in a refractory vegetative state. More commonly, after a stroke, chest wall movement on the affected side is reduced, and myoelectrical activity can be reduced (flaccidity) or increased (spasticity). Facial and pharyngeal weakness contributes to an inability to control oral secretions, swallow effectively, and protect the upper airway. Altered respiratory mechanics and efficiency reflect impaired chest wall movement, asymmetry, and the degree of muscle paresis and spasm.

Individuals with stroke have associated problems that contribute to cardiovascular and pulmonary dysfunction. These patients tend to be older and hypertensive and have a high incidence of cardiac dysfunction. Muscle disuse and restricted mobility secondary to stroke lead to reduced cardiovascular and pulmonary conditioning and inefficient oxygen transport. Spasticity increases metabolic and oxygen demand. Hemiparesis results in gait deviations, which reduce movement efficiency and movement economy. Reduced movement economy results in an increased energy cost associated with ambulation, which may reduce exercise tolerance because of fatigue.[1] In addition, ambulating with a walking aid is associated with increased energy cost compared with normal walking. This increased energy cost reduces the patient's exercise tolerance further and increases fatigue.

The notion of a motor recovery plateau in the management of individuals with stroke has been challenged.[2,3] It has been argued that individuals adapt to the training stimulus and plateau when that stimulus no longer changes. Thus individuals are deprived of therapy unless they are responding. Capacity to improve can be augmented with changes in type of activity and the introduction of new exercises, as well as changes in the intensity, duration, and frequency of the exercises. Computer-assisted motivating rehabilitation employs the use of games and unconscious limb activation and movement, rather than engaging the patient in specific limb exercises.[2]

Individuals with stroke are at increased risk of having intercurrent ischemic heart disease, which compromises long-term survival and increases the risk of illness and inactivity.[4] Furthermore, concurrent congestive heart failure will adversely affect outcomes after stroke rehabilitation. Clinical assessment, even if patients are asymptomatic, must include a cardiac work-up to establish the degree to which cardiac insufficiency limits mobility, endurance, recovery, balance, and fatigue. An integrated multisystem approach will ensure improved rehabilitation outcomes and prevent complications.

Principles of Physical Therapy Management

GOALS OF LONG-TERM MANAGEMENT

The management of people with stroke is shifting from a primary sensorimotor focus to an integrated management approach of which aerobic conditioning is an integral component. Long-term management goals particular to patients with stroke include the following, in addition to the long-term management goals of all patients with secondary dysfunction:

- Optimizing aids and devices to reduce unnecessary energy demands by optimizing postural alignment
- Maximizing balance to also reduce unnecessary energy demands to maintain alignment
- Optimizing chest wall excursion and ventilation
- Optimizing secretion clearance as needed
- Reducing the work of breathing
- Reducing the work of the heart
- Protecting the airways from aspiration

Structured, progressive rehabilitation programs for people with stroke augment therapeutic gains with respect to endurance, mobility, and balance, compared with spontaneous recovery.[5]

Body weight support has been examined to support an individual with stroke in the upright position to facilitate treadmill walking as a means of conditioning and gait reeducation.[6]

Treadmill training with support appears to have a somewhat greater effect in ambulatory individuals with respect to improved walking speed than other interventions.

PATIENT MONITORING

Stroke is often associated with sleep disturbances (e.g., obstructive sleep apnea). Thus activity and sleep patterns must be assessed to ensure sleep is maximally restorative and not contributing to the patient's symptoms.

Traditional management approaches to stroke incorporate little exercise testing and monitoring; however, given stroke results from dysfunction of the cerebral vessels secondary to the same common pathway as ischemic heart disease and intermittent claudication, comparable monitoring and precautions must be instituted during treatment.

In addition to the monitoring necessary for all patients, patients with stroke and cardiac dysfunction require clearance from a cardiologist before participating in a rehabilitation program and may require electrocardiogram (ECG) monitoring, particularly during exercise.

MEDICATION

Medication that is needed to maximize treatment response (e.g., antihypertensive and cardiac medications) is administered before treatment. Knowledge of the type of medication, its administration route, and time to and duration of peak efficacy is essential if treatment is to be maximally effective.

PRIMARY INTERVENTIONS

Primary interventions for patients with stroke include the combination of global interventions previously discussed, and in addition they require the following:

- Body positioning instruction
- Breathing control and coughing maneuvers
- Spasticity control
- Gait reeducation

An ergonomic assessment of the patient's work and home, if applicable, may also help ensure the safety of the patient in those environments.

PATIENT EDUCATION

Patients with stroke will require the same instruction common to all patients with chronic secondary dysfunction.

Engagement of the social support network can have an important role in maximizing a patient's outcomes. Social support is recognized clinically as an important component of the comprehensive management of people with chronic conditions; however the literature in this area is scant. Family participation has been reported to improve the strength and mobility of an individual with stroke.[7]

EXERCISE

Aerobic exercise is an essential component of long-term management of the individual with stroke to optimize the efficiency of oxygen transport overall. Maximizing ventilation with mobilization is limited if the patient has severe generalized muscular weakness and increased fatigue. Although aggressive mobilization can be supported in these patients,[8] appropriate selection of patients for such a regimen, judicious exercise prescription, and monitoring must be instituted to ensure the treatment is optimally therapeutic and poses no risk to a patient in this high-risk group. Chest wall exercises include movement in all planes combined with rotation. Body positioning to optimize lung volumes and airflow rates is a priority. Breathing control and coughing maneuvers are essential and should be coupled with body movement and positioning. Exercise is conducted with the patient in upright positions to minimize the work of the heart and of breathing during physical exertion. Recumbent positions reduce lung volumes and expiratory flow rates, impair respiratory mechanics, increase closing volumes, increase thoracic blood volume, and increase compressive forces on both the lungs and the heart.[9] Thus, aerobic exercise for significant periods and intensities should be performed standing or sitting. Lower-extremity work is preferable to upper-extremity work in that the latter is associated with increased hemodynamic stress. Rhythmic exercise of large muscle groups is preferable to static exercise and exercise of small muscle groups, such as the arms, which produces smaller hemodynamic effects. Yoga-based exercise programs may be of some benefit for people with chronic stroke.[10] Resistance muscle training for the limbs increases their muscle power in a dose-dependent relationship without increasing spasticity.[11] Muscle training should be combined with aerobic training for optimal benefit and functional benefit.[12]

Ambulation or wheelchair locomotion should be as efficient as possible so that the metabolic demand of these functional activities is reduced. Performing these activities inefficiently on a frequent basis contributes to an excessive oxygen demand. The patient expends considerable energy in performing these activities uneconomically, which impairs the patient's tolerance and contributes to excessive fatigue. Conserving energy by performing these activities more economically from an energetic perspective will provide more energy to perform more of these or other activities.

PROPHYLACTIC MANAGEMENT

Patients with generalized neuromuscular weakness require prophylactic management because of their high risk of developing life-threatening respiratory infections and complications. Prophylaxis should include flu shots; avoidance of polluted, smoky environments; smoking reduction and cessation; control of the types of food eaten and chewing well to avoid choking; and regular deep breathing, frequent movement, and change in body positions (even just shifting and taking some deeper breaths while seated in a wheelchair) to promote mucociliary transport. An optimal time to take deep breaths and to cough is during transfers, which usually are physically exerting and stimulate hyperpnea.

Parkinson Syndrome

Pathophysiology and Medical Management

Parkinson syndrome is associated with reduced dopamine in the basal ganglia, resulting in the loss of normal reciprocal inhibitory and facilitatory neuronal input in the execution of smooth coordinated movement. The clinical manifestations of the disease include stooped posture; stiffness and slowed motion; a fixed, mask-like expression; and tremor of the limbs. Patients with Parkinson syndrome are hypertonic, rigid, and inflexible. Movement initiation is impaired, and once initiated, movement is not fluid. The patient walks with a quick, shuffling gait. These factors contribute to an increased energy cost of movement. Physical activity is restricted and function is compromised, contributing to impaired aerobic capacity, reduced movement efficiency, and hence reduced movement economy.

Although chest wall rigidity and respiratory muscle weakness are associated with a restrictive pattern of lung disease in the patient with Parkinson syndrome, the obstructive type of respiratory dysfunction has been reported (e.g., reduced midtidal flow rates, increase airway resistance, impaired distribution of ventilation, and an increase in functional residual capacity).[13] This obstructive defect may reflect parasympathetic hyperactivity, which has been associated with the disease. The degree to which these cardiovascular and pulmonary manifestations of the disease are offset with anticholinergic drugs (used to treat rest tremor and reverse dystonia) has not been reported.

The upper extremities are rigid and held slightly abducted from the chest wall during locomotion. The rigidity and dyskinesia associated with Parkinson syndrome lead to restricted movement and body positioning. The patient becomes deconditioned from disuse. Although the rigid, immobile chest coupled with reduced body position changes can contribute to restrictive cardiovascular and pulmonary pathology in this syndrome, chemoreceptor dysfunction has been documented.[14]

Principles of Physical Therapy Management

GOALS OF LONG-TERM MANAGEMENT

The goals of long-term management for the patient with Parkinson syndrome include all of the elements common to all other conditions, but also include the following:

- Optimize secretion clearance as needed
- Reduce the work of breathing
- Reduce the work of the heart
- Protect the airways from aspiration

PATIENT MONITORING

Patients with Parkinson syndrome require the same monitoring parameters common to all of the secondary conditions discussed in this chapter. Patients with additional cardiac dysfunction require ECG monitoring, particularly during exercise.

MEDICATION

Medication that is needed to maximize treatment response (e.g., L-dopa) is administered before treatment. Knowledge of the type of medication, its administration route, and time to and duration of peak efficacy is essential if treatment is to be maximally efficacious. In addition, patients with Parkinson syndrome may be taking a beta blocker to suppress action tremor. Because such medication reduces the heart rate and blood pressure, these patients are prone to orthostatic intolerance. In addition, heart rate and blood pressure responses to treatment and exercises will be less valid.

PRIMARY INTERVENTIONS

Primary interventions for patients with Parkinson syndrome include the combination of global interventions previously discussed, and in addition they require the following:

- Body positioning instruction
- Breathing control and coughing maneuvers
- Gait reeducation
- Flexibility exercise to facilitate participation in regular physical activity and exercise

For optimal functional outcomes, prescriptive parameters focus on cross training rather than a single aerobic type of exercise, and frequent, longer, less intense physical activity rather than less frequent, short, intense exercise.

PATIENT EDUCATION

Patients with Parkinson syndrome will require the same instruction common to all patients with chronic secondary dysfunction and in addition will likely also need instruction on airway protection.

EXERCISE

Aerobic exercise is an essential component of the long-term management of the patient with Parkinson syndrome to optimize the efficiency of oxygen transport overall, including maximizing alveolar ventilation and mobilizing secretions, as well as for its musculoskeletal benefits. Maximizing ventilation with mobilization is limited by the degree of hypertonicity and rigidity. Chest wall exercises include all planes of movement with a rotational component. Breathing control and coughing maneuvers are essential and should be coupled with body movement and positioning.

Multiple Sclerosis

Pathophysiology and Medical Management

Multiple sclerosis is a demyelinating disease of the central nervous system. The focal or patchy destruction of myelin sheaths is accompanied by an inflammatory response. The course of the disease consists of a variable number of exacerbations and remissions over the years from early adulthood. Exacerbations are also variable with respect to severity. The neurological deficits include visual disturbance; paresis of one or more limbs; spasticity; discoordination; ataxia; dysarthria; weak, ineffective cough; reduced perception of vibration and position sense; bowel and bladder dysfunction; and sexual dysfunction.[15] Breathing disturbances, including diaphragmatic paresis, may occur. Autonomic disturbance in the form of impaired cardiovascular reflex function at rest and attenuated heart rate and blood pressure responses during exercise are relatively common in patients with multiple sclerosis.[16]

Principles of Physical Therapy Management

GOALS OF LONG-TERM MANAGEMENT

In addition to all of the long-term management goals common to all other conditions, there are several more goals associated with this population:

- Protect the airways from aspiration
- Optimize secretion clearance as needed
- Reduce the work of breathing
- Reduce the work of the heart

Patients with multiple sclerosis may need prescriptive aids and devices to optimize function and activity.

PATIENT MONITORING

Patients with multiple sclerosis require the same monitoring parameters common to all of the secondary conditions discussed in this chapter. Patients with additional cardiac dysfunction require ECG monitoring, particularly during exercise.

Multiple sclerosis is associated with significant fatigue; thus activity and sleep patterns need to be assessed to ensure sleep is maximally restorative and not contributing to the patient's symptoms. Fatigue can be assessed subjectively using a modified version of the Borg scale or assessed objectively using a log of activity and rest. The log will help the patient identify the optimal time to rest.

MEDICATION

Medication that is needed to maximize treatment response (e.g., antispasticity medications) is administered before treatment. Knowledge of the type of medication, its administration route, and time to and duration of peak efficacy is essential if treatment is to be maximally effective. In addition, knowledge of the cardiovascular and pulmonary side effects of other medications is needed.

PRIMARY INTERVENTIONS

Primary interventions for patients with multiple sclerosis include the combination of global interventions previously discussed, and in addition these patients require the following:

- Body positioning instruction
- Breathing control and coughing maneuvers
- Gait reeducation
- Fatigue management

Prescriptive parameters are comparable to those for individuals with increased muscle tone—that is, frequent, less intense exercise, rather than the less frequent, intense exercise that might be appropriate for someone without such a condition.

PATIENT EDUCATION

Patients with multiple sclerosis require the same instruction common to all patients with chronic secondary dysfunction and in addition they will likely need instruction on fatigue management, as multiple sclerosis is associated with significant fatigue.

EXERCISE

Aerobic exercise is an essential component of the long-term management of the patient with multiple sclerosis to optimize the efficiency of oxygen transport overall. In mild-to-moderate cases the goals of aerobic exercise are to optimize cardiovascular and pulmonary conditioning and enhance movement economy. Optimizing cadence of walking or cycling is important to minimize discoordination, energy expenditure, and fatigue and to maximize safety. In more severe cases the goal is to maximize ventilation and gas exchange in the patient who has severe generalized muscular weakness, spasm, and excessive fatigue. Subjective parameters (i.e., fatigue and exertion) provide the basis for the intensity of the exercise program in conjunction with objective measures. Parameters such as intensity and duration may vary from session to session depending on the patient's general status, which tends to be variable. Aquatic exercise may be an alternative for patients whose discoordination precludes ambulation and cycling or who are troubled by heat. The use of a fan may also enhance the patient's work output.

Chest wall exercises include all planes of movement with a rotational component. Body positioning to optimize lung volumes and airflow rates is a priority. Breathing control and coughing maneuvers are coupled with body movement and positioning. If mucociliary clearance is impaired, leading to secretion retention, postural drainage may need to be instituted coupled with deep breathing and coughing maneuvers.

VENTILATORY STRATEGIES

Methods of facilitating effective coughing in patients with neuromuscular diseases are extremely important because they constitute life-preserving measures. Supported and unsupported coughing methods are described in detail in Chapters 22 and 23. Whenever possible, deep breathing and coughing are coordinated with chest wall movement to facilitate maximal inflation of the lungs before coughing and maximal exhalation of the lungs during coughing. Body positions are varied and changed frequently to simulate as much as possible the shifts in alveolar volume and ventilation and perfusion that occur with normal movement and body position changes.[17] In addition, body positioning is used to maximize the patient's coughing efforts.

PROPHYLACTIC MANAGEMENT

Patients with generalized neuromuscular weakness require prophylactic management, given their high risk of developing life-threatening respiratory infections and complications. Prophylaxis should include flu shots; avoiding polluted, smoky environments; smoking reduction and cessation; controlling the types of food eaten and chewing well to avoid choking; and regular deep breathing, frequent movement, and change in body positions (even just shifting and taking some deeper breaths while seated in a wheelchair) to promote mucociliary transport. An optimal time to take deep breaths and to cough is during transfers, which usually are physically exerting and stimulate hyperpnea.

Patients with multiple sclerosis often have remissions and exacerbations of their symptoms. Physical therapy focuses on all phases, with more intense treatment during stable periods. In this way it is hoped that periods between remissions are increased and exacerbations are less severe and shorter.

Cerebral Palsy

Pathophysiology and Medical Management

Cerebral palsy results from insult to the central nervous system that usually occurs before birth (e.g., from substance abuse and perinatal underoxygenation).[15] The clinical presentation includes spasticity and residual deformity from severe muscle imbalance, hyperreflexia, and mental retardation. Although there are varying degrees of cerebral palsy severity, patients most frequently seen by the physical therapist have significant functional deficits and require long-term care. The loss of motor control and hypertonicity of peripheral muscles often restrict the mobility of patients such that they are wheelchair dependent. Loss of motor function limits physical activity and the exercise stimulus needed to maintain an aerobic stimulus and optimal aerobic capacity. Often coupled with motor deficits are cognitive deficits and mental retardation. These afflictions limit the degree to which the patient can follow instructions, perform treatments, and participate actively in a long-term rehabilitation program. Patients with cerebral palsy who are able to ambulate do so at exceptional energy expenditure both with and without walking aids.[18] Central neurological deficits, generalized hypertonicity, and musculoskeletal deformity contribute to increased metabolic demand for oxygen and oxygen transport.

Principles of Physical Therapy Management

GOALS OF LONG-TERM MANAGEMENT

In addition to all of the long-term management goals common to all other conditions, patients with cerebral palsy should have several additional goals:

- Reduce spasticity to minimize undue energy cost
- Optimize secretion clearance as needed
- Reduce the work of breathing
- Reduce the work of the heart
- Protect the airways from aspiration

Maximizing aerobic capacity and efficiency of oxygen transport and optimizing general muscle strength pertain to the patient with cerebral palsy that is mild in severity. Many patients seen by physical therapists have poorly controlled spasticity and marked intellectual limitations, which preclude full participation in aerobic and strengthening exercise programs. These patients are at risk for the sequelae of restricted mobility and recumbency.

PATIENT MONITORING

Patients with cerebral palsy require the same monitoring parameters common to all of the secondary conditions discussed in this chapter. Physical therapists must keep in mind that unless the patient is only mildly affected, and not mentally incapacitated, patients with cerebral palsy are less able to provide subjective ratings of treatment response. The therapist must then rely particularly on clinical judgment in conjunction with the patient's objective responses to treatment.

MEDICATION

Medication that is needed to maximize treatment response (e.g., antispasticity medications) is administered before treatment. Knowledge of the type of medication, its administration route, and time to and duration of peak efficacy is essential if treatment is to be maximally effective.

PRIMARY INTERVENTIONS

Primary interventions for patients with cerebral palsy include the combination of global interventions previously discussed; in addition, they require the following:

- Body positioning instruction
- Breathing control and coughing maneuvers
- Mobilization and coordinated activity (aerobic stimulation)
- Strengthening exercises

Note that strength is often difficult to assess and treat because of overwhelming spasticity in patients with cerebral palsy.

PATIENT EDUCATION

In the case of patients with cerebral palsy, education should be directed at the patient whenever possible, but it more likely will be directed at the parents and/or care providers. Patients with cerebral palsy will require the same instruction common to all patients with chronic secondary dysfunction, and in addition will likely also need instruction on mobilization and coordinated activity.

Education on the importance of sleep and rest will also be important for patients in this population; individuals with cerebral palsy can be expected to have abnormal sleep patterns. Sleep patterns are often disrupted for the following reasons:

- Central cerebral involvement may affect the periodicity of breathing. During sleep, the effects of such dysfunction are accentuated. Loss of normal periodic breathing and interspersed sighs impairs mucociliary transport. Secretions may accumulate and contribute to airway obstruction and areas of atelectasis.
- Individuals with cerebral palsy are unable to reposition themselves during the night in response to cardiovascular-pulmonary and musculoskeletal stimuli.
- Patients often have poor swallowing and saliva control and thus are prone to aspiration and microatelectasis, particularly when recumbent at night. Inability to reposition themselves at night further increases the risk of aspiration and its sequelae.

MOBILIZATION

Mobilization is an essential component of the long-term management of the patient with cerebral palsy in order to stimulate aerobic metabolism and optimize the efficiency of oxygen transport overall, including maximizing alveolar ventilation and mobilizing and removing secretions.[19] Maximizing ventilation with mobilization is limited if the patient has generalized spasticity. Furthermore, mobilization stimuli are selected specifically to minimize eliciting further muscle spasm. Prescriptive hydrotherapy and equinotherapy (horseback riding) can provide effective stimulation to the cardiovascular and pulmonary system in the individual with multiple handicaps and can minimize the effects of spasticity. With training, coordination of ambulatory patients can be improved and aerobic energy expenditure reduced. In addition, energy is conserved for performing more activity. Chest wall exercises include all planes of movement with rotation. Body positioning to optimize lung volumes and airflow rates is a priority. Breathing control and coughing maneuvers are essential and should be coupled with body movement and positioning. If mucociliary transport is impaired and this leads to secretion retention, postural drainage and manual techniques may need to be instituted with appropriate monitoring to ensure they do not have a detrimental effect.[20]

VENTILATORY STRATEGIES

In this patient population, clearing oral secretions and coughing maneuvers require special attention. Ventilatory strategies for facilitating effective coughing in patients with neuromuscular diseases are extremely important because they constitute life-preserving measures. Supported and unsupported coughing methods are described in detail in Chapters 22 and 23. Whenever possible, deep breathing and coughing are coupled with chest wall movement to facilitate maximal inflation of the lungs before coughing and maximal exhalation of the lungs during coughing. Body positions are varied and changed frequently to simulate as much as possible shifts in alveolar volume and ventilation and perfusion that occur with normal movement and body position changes. Microaspirations are likely a common occurrence in this patient population, particularly at night. Nighttime positioning must be prescribed for a given patient to minimize aspiration.

PROPHYLACTIC MANAGEMENT

Individuals with generalized neuromuscular weakness require prophylactic management, given their high risk of developing life-threatening respiratory infections and complications. Prophylaxis should include flu shots; avoidance of polluted, smoky environments; control of the types of food eaten and chewing well to avoid choking; and stimulation of deep breathing, airway clearance, and frequent movement and change in body positions (even just shifting and eliciting deeper breaths while seated in a wheelchair) to promote mucociliary transport. Wheelchair design and seating are also important areas of concern in which the physical therapist is actively involved.

Spinal Cord Injury

Pathophysiology and Medical Management

The cardiovascular and pulmonary manifestations and complications of spinal cord injury are directly related to the level of the lesion.[21] Cardiovascular and pulmonary impairment results from the loss of supraspinal control of the respiratory muscles and the heart below the spinal cord lesion. Loss of diaphragmatic innervation results in ventilator dependency. Loss of abdominal and intercostal innervation reduces the ability to cough, mucociliary transport, and the ability to clear the airways. Denervation of the heart and orthostatism are less problematic in that the heart's autonomous function and increased responsiveness of the heart and blood vessels to circulating catecholamines adequately compensate. The cough mechanism of people with quadriplegia is ineffective in clearing the airways.[22]

Patients with quadriplegia are particularly prone to the effects of restricted mobility, given the extent of their functional motor loss and sensory deficits, particularly on cardiovascular and pulmonary function. Mobilization and physical activity are essential for the patient with a spinal cord injury to maintain optimal cardiovascular and pulmonary function and oxygen transport efficiency and the optimal strength and endurance of the respiratory muscles. Patients with partial cord lesions will have a greater probability of ambulation with or without aids. Walking with aids is enormously costly in terms of energy cost,[23] however, and may not be practical in daily life.

Because of the complexity and multisystem involvement of spinal cord lesions, the team works closely together. Even though the nurse may be primarily responsible for teaching and monitoring bowel and bladder routines, the physical therapist keeps informed of these because genitourinary and gastrointestinal problems can jeopardize physical therapy goals.

Principles of Physical Therapy Management

GOALS OF LONG-TERM MANAGEMENT

In addition to all of the long-term management goals common to all other neuromuscular conditions, patients with spinal cord injury have the following additional goals:

- Ensure that walking aids or wheelchairs used by the patient are optimal for the patient's needs for minimized energy cost, for optimal posture, and for safety.
- Optimize secretion clearance as needed
- Reduce the work of breathing
- Reduce the work of the heart
- Protect the airways from aspiration

PATIENT MONITORING

Patients with spinal cord injury require the same monitoring parameters common to all of the secondary conditions discussed in this chapter.

Patients with high spinal cord injuries are somewhat more hemodynamically unstable and have more ECG irregularities than age-matched control individuals; thus their cardiovascular and pulmonary status should be monitored during treatment.

MEDICATION

Medication that is needed to maximize treatment response (e.g., antispasticity agents) is administered before treatment. Knowledge of the type of medication, its administration route, and time to and duration of peak efficacy is essential if treatment is to be maximally efficacious.

PRIMARY INTERVENTIONS

Patients with spinal cord injury require a combination of the global primary interventions common to the secondary conditions discussed in this chapter. In addition, these patients will also need body positioning instruction and breathing control and coughing maneuvers.

PATIENT EDUCATION

Patients with spinal cord injury will require the same instruction common to all patients with chronic secondary dysfunction.

EXERCISE

Aerobic exercise is an essential component of the long-term management of the patient with spinal cord injury in order to optimize the efficiency of oxygen transport overall, including maximizing alveolar ventilation and mobilizing and removing secretions. With higher lesions, exercise is usually confined to upper-extremity work in the form of wheelchair ambulation. Preservation of upper-extremity muscle function and minimization of overuse are primary goals from the outset. Patients can maintain adequate cardiovascular and pulmonary conditioning with wheelchair exercise; however, exercise prescription should be conservative to maximize the benefit-to-risk ratio of cardiovascular and pulmonary conditioning that relies on upper-extremity work. Patients who are able to walk with leg braces and crutches expend considerable energy doing so. A decision must be made regarding the benefits of walking at high energy demand versus conserving energy for other activities. Chest wall exercises can be used and should include all planes of movement with a rotational component. Body positioning to optimize lung volumes and airflow rates is a priority. Breathing control and coughing maneuvers are essential and should be coupled with body movement and positioning. Coordination of respiration with aerobic activity and wheeling is taught to maximize work output.

VENTILATORY STRATEGIES

Ventilatory muscle training has a role in the long-term rehabilitation of some patients with high spinal cord lesions. Such muscle training has long been known to increase the strength and endurance of the respiratory muscles[24] and may improve the functional capacity of some patients. A stronger, endurance-trained diaphragm will not fatigue as readily as an untrained diaphragm. Standardizing the resistance of the training stimulus alone, however, is not sufficient to produce a training effect. It is essential that flow rate be controlled using a gauge.

Methods of facilitating effective coughing in patients with neuromuscular diseases are extremely important because they constitute life-preserving measures. Supported and unsupported coughing methods are described in detail in Chapters 22 and 23. Whenever possible, deep breathing and coughing are coupled with chest wall movement to facilitate maximal inflation of the lungs before coughing and maximal exhalation of the lungs during coughing. Body positions are varied and changed frequently to simulate as much as possible shifts in alveolar volume and ventilation and perfusion that occur with normal movement and body position changes.

A comprehensive program includes stretching of the chest wall and passive range-of-motion exercises of the shoulder girdle. Maximal insufflations are encouraged in optimal body positions. Glossopharyngeal breathing can enable high quadriplegic patients to be freed from mechanical ventilation for hours at a time. Assisted or unassisted coughing is coordinated with deep breathing and rhythmic rocking motion. Manual assisted coughing and mechanical coughing aids, including functional electrical stimulation and insufflation-exsufflation devices, can be useful.[25] The pneumobelt is a device that can facilitate ventilation without a tracheostomy. This device counters loss of abdominal tone and helps preserve normal thoracoabdominal interaction during respiration, which is lost because of reduced rib cage compliance and increased abdominal compliance.

PROPHYLACTIC MANAGEMENT

Patients with spinal cord injuries, particularly those with high lesions, require prophylactic management, given their risk of developing life-threatening respiratory infections and complications. Prophylaxis should include flu shots; avoiding polluted, smoky environments; smoking reduction and cessation; controlling the types of food eaten and chewing well to avoid choking; and regular deep breathing, airway clearance, and frequent movement and change in body positions (even just shifting and taking some deeper breaths while seated in a wheelchair are beneficial). An optimal time to take deep breaths and cough is during transfers, which usually are physically exerting and stimulate hyperpnea.

Chronic Effects of Poliomyelitis

Pathophysiology and Medical Management

The chronic effects of poliomyelitis affect a high proportion of survivors of poliomyelitis who contracted the disease during the epidemic of the 1950s. Three types of poliomyelitis were prevalent during the epidemic in the middle of the 20th century, namely, spinal (the majority of cases), bulbar, and encephalitic. Half of survivors report new symptoms consistent with postpolio syndrome (PPS) (see Chapter 6). New delayed symptoms include disproportionate fatigue, increased weakness, deformity, pain, reduced endurance, breathing and swallowing problems, and respiratory insufficiency. Although cardiovascular and pulmonary complications were not associated with the spinal form of poliomyelitis at onset, late-onset breathing and swallowing complications can appear as a late effect of the disease.[26] In addition, these patients may be deconditioned and have poor movement economy (i.e., expend excessive energy because of postural deformities).[1] Therefore, delayed-onset cardiovascular and pulmonary complications, coupled with the effects of overuse and general deconditioning, increase the risk of cardiovascular and pulmonary compromise, reduce the ability to recover from these, and increase surgical and anesthetic risk.

Because of the nonspecific symptoms associated with PPS, it is a diagnosis of exclusion based on a detailed history.

Principles of Physical Therapy Management

GOALS OF LONG-TERM MANAGEMENT

In addition to all of the long-term management goals common to other neuromuscular conditions, there are additional goals for patients with chronic effects of poliomyelitis:

- Ensure that the aids and devices used by the patient provide an optimal level of support for a specific muscle or extremity, or whole body as necessary
- Optimize movement economy
- Optimize secretion clearance as needed
- Reduce the work of breathing
- Reduce the work of the heart
- Protect the airways from aspiration

Although there are commonalities between the management of individuals with a history of poliomyelitis with and without PPS, injudicious management of the individual with PPS can lead to further deterioration. Special attention is therefore given to balancing rest with physical activity and developing modified exercise programs if they are indicated. Such programs are not indicated if an individual is exploiting maximal physiologic reserve capacity to meet the needs of each day. This individual has little reserve capacity and thus can lose functional capacity by increasing metabolic demands. With appropriate self-management and adherence to judicious recommendations, the prognosis for an individual with PPS can be favorable.

PATIENT MONITORING

Patients with chronic effects of poliomyelitis require the same monitoring parameters common to all of the secondary conditions discussed in this chapter, though additional monitoring of pain and fatigue is necessary as well.

Activity and sleep patterns must be monitored to ensure sleep is maximally restorative and not contributing to the patient's symptoms. Functional work capacity and activity tolerance may be increased by balancing activity with rest and maintaining fatigue below the patient's critical fatigue threshold (i.e., threshold requiring prolonged recovery time).

Subjective assessments of fatigue, breathlessness, and pain can all be made using analog scales, including modified versions of the Borg scale.

MEDICATION

Medication that is needed to maximize treatment response (e.g., analgesia) is administered before treatment. Knowledge of the type of medication, its administration route, and time to and duration of peak efficacy is essential if treatment is to be maximally effective.

PRIMARY INTERVENTIONS

Primary interventions for patients with PPS include the combination of global interventions previously discussed, and in addition these patients require the following:

- Body positioning instruction
- Breathing control and coughing maneuvers

Aids and devices should be reviewed to optimize energy expenditure (e.g., electric wheelchair or scooter versus manual wheelchair) and to reduce cardiovascular and pulmonary distress (e.g., home mechanical ventilation).

PATIENT EDUCATION

Patients with PPS will require the same instruction common to all patients with chronic secondary dysfunction; they will also need information on the importance of rest and monitoring sleep. Patients require varying schedules of activity to rest over the course of a day.

EXERCISE

Aerobic exercise is an essential component of the long-term management of the patient with the late sequelae of poliomyelitis to optimize the efficiency of oxygen transport overall. The two principal goals of exercise are to optimize cardiovascular and pulmonary conditioning and movement economy. Maximizing ventilation with exercise is limited if the patient has severe generalized muscular weakness and increased fatigue. Disproportionate fatigue and other symptoms experienced by patients with the late sequelae of poliomyelitis have been attributed to overwork of affected and unaffected muscles, terminal axon degeneration, and impaired impulse transmission. Exercise is therefore prescribed judiciously to provide an optimal aerobic training effect without contributing to further other use abuse (i.e., prescriptive parameters based on subjective responses using semiquantitative scales in conjunction with objective responses). Walking is the most functional type of aerobic exercise; however, aquatic exercise provides a useful medium for individuals with lower-extremity paresis who require crutches to walk or are confined to a wheelchair. Reducing physical activity and exercise is indicated in some patients to optimize aerobic and muscle power. The effect of resting affected and unaffected muscles enhances functional capacity.

Individuals with PPS are likely to experience greater functional decline over time compared with survivors of poliomyelitis without the syndrome. The need for aids, devices, manual wheelchairs, and electric wheelchairs and scooters should be anticipated for some people. These, however, can be introduced with their intermittent use to provide rest to overused muscles and joints, minimize local and general fatigue, and preserve remaining muscle function to the greatest degree. Excessive use as well as underuse of such aids can contribute to rapid deterioration and decline. Thus the rehabilitation program includes recommendations about the appropriate use of aids and devices to optimize function, and these recommendations require periodic review.

VENTILATORY STRATEGIES

Ventilatory strategies for facilitating effective coughing in patients with neuromuscular diseases are extremely important because they constitute a life-preserving measure. Supported and unsupported coughing methods are described in detail in Chapters 22 and 23. Whenever possible, deep breathing and coughing are coupled with chest wall movement to facilitate maximal inflation of the lungs before coughing and maximal exhalation of the lungs during coughing. Body positions are varied and changed frequently to simulate as much as possible shifts in alveolar volume and ventilation and perfusion that occur with normal movement and body position changes.

Progressive loss of pulmonary function in patients with ventilatory compromise at onset can lead to respiratory insufficiency. Comparable with other neuromuscular conditions, invasive mechanical ventilation is avoided. Alternatives include nasal and oral methods of noninvasive assisted mechanical ventilation. In addition, airway clearance can be further assisted with manual assisted coughing, glossopharyngeal breathing, mechanical exsufflation, and mechanical insufflation-exsufflation.[27]

Survivors of poliomyelitis with ventilatory compromise are comparable with other patients with generalized muscle weakness. Of particular concern in this population is the necessity to establish the role of mobilization and exercise as a first line of defense in the management and prevention of cardiovascular and pulmonary dysfunction. For patients with PPS and overuse abuse, however, additional exercise may be detrimental, though modified mobilization and exercise may be prescribed on an interval schedule (see Chapters 19 and 25).[28] The patient exercises for a period of time and then rests or reduces to a lower intensity of exercise to allow the muscles to rest. In addition to the multitude of benefits of mobilization and exercise on oxygen transport overall, these interventions also optimize respiratory muscle strength and endurance. If the patient does not recover within a few hours, the mobilization or exercise stimuli are excessive and should be modified. Chest wall mobility exercises to facilitate breathing and coughing may have a role.

PROPHYLACTIC MANAGEMENT

Patients with generalized neuromuscular weakness require respiratory prophylactic management, given their high risk of developing life-threatening respiratory infections and complications. Prophylaxis should include flu shots; avoiding polluted, smoky environments; controlling the types of food eaten and chewing well to avoid choking; and regular deep breathing, airway clearance, and frequent movement and change in body positions (even just shifting and taking some deeper breaths while seated in a wheelchair are beneficial). An optimal time to take deep breaths and cough is during transfers, which usually are physically exerting and stimulate hyperpnea.

Muscular Dystrophy

Pathophysiology and Medical Management

Individuals with muscular dystrophy and other types of degenerative neurological and muscular diseases have increased life expectancy and thus can expect prolonged morbidity. Prevention of complications as an individual becomes weaker and more limited in terms of participation in life is a priority. In addition to peripheral weakness, these conditions can lead to respiratory muscle weakness and alveolar hypoventilation. Vital capacity, forced expiratory volume, airflow rates, and maximum inspiratory and expiratory pressures are reduced. These patients are at risk for the development of atelectasis, impaired mucociliary transport, and pneumonia. In addition, long-term generalized muscular weakness, particularly of the thoracic cavity and abdomen, as well as restricted mobility and confinement to a wheelchair predispose the patient to thoracic deformities (e.g., scoliosis and dropping of the ribs and further muscle disuse). Patients with Duchenne muscular dystrophy are susceptible to dysphagia and upper airway obstruction secondary to gag reflex depression and hypotonia of the pharyngeal structures.[21] These factors further compromise or threaten cardiovascular and pulmonary function and oxygen transport.

Cardiac dysfunction has also long been reported in progressive muscular dystrophy.[29] Although the majority of patients have no clinical evidence of cardiac dysfunction, a high proportion have abnormal ECGs at rest or during exercise and abnormal echocardiograms and radionuclide ventriculograms showing reduced left ventricular ejection fraction and abnormal ventricular wall motion. Fatty and fibrous tissue infiltrate the myocardium and conduction system, and electrical conduction is slowed. Thus subclinical cardiac involvement is prevalent in patients with muscular dystrophy and may explain sudden death in this patient population.

Chronic respiratory muscle weakness is characteristic of muscular dystrophy and other neuromuscular disorders. Because the cardiovascular and pulmonary systems are seldom stressed owing to musculoskeletal dysfunction in these patients, respiratory muscle weakness is seldom detected. Such weakness is significant, however, in that it contributes to several other serious problems, including thoracic mechanical abnormalities, diffuse microatelectasis, reduced lung compliance, a weak cough with impaired mucociliary transport and secretion accumulation, ventilation and perfusion imbalance, and nocturnal hypoxemia. Progressive respiratory muscle weakness has long been known to increase the risk of respiratory muscle fatigue and failure.[30,31]

The severity of disease is not consistently correlated with compromised pulmonary function; thus cardiovascular and pulmonary function must be assessed individually in each patient. Patients with mild-to-moderate involvement of peripheral muscles may exhibit disproportionate respiratory compromise. This may be explained by differential changes in the degree of involvement of the diaphragm and the abdominal and intercostal muscles. Over time, musculoskeletal changes of the chest wall lead to spinal deformity and stiffness with loss of its elastic recoil. Chronic alveolar hypoventilation leads to respiratory insufficiency and the need for ventilatory assistance. With progressive respiratory insufficiency, nocturnal hypoventilation with hypercapnia and hypoxemia develop. Nocturnal respiratory support should be considered early to postpone the need for intubation and mechanical ventilation, which is associated with a poor prognostic outcome in patients who have chronically reduced vital capacities and weak cough.

Clinically, patients with muscular dystrophy demonstrate low functional capacity commensurate with the extent of muscle weakness and impaired cardiovascular and pulmonary function, including alveolar hypoventilation, orthopnea (shortness of breath on reclining), impaired mucociliary transport, difficulty clearing secretions, and increased work of breathing. Abdominal muscle strength provides an index of pulmonary function in that it is correlated with vital capacity and expiratory flow rates. The significant progressive functional loss associated with Duchenne muscular dystrophy increases the patient's susceptibility to the sequelae of restricted mobility, including cardiovascular and pulmonary deconditioning and reduced efficiency of oxygen transport, circulatory stasis, muscular weakness, and bone loss.

Improved medical management of the complications of myopathies has significantly increased the life expectancy of patients such as those with Duchenne muscular dystrophy over the past 20 years. With advancing age, further complications will arise from age-related changes in cardiovascular and pulmonary function.[32,33] Thus in the years ahead an increasing number of patients with myopathies will be requiring cardiovascular and pulmonary management and prophylaxis.

Principles of Physical Therapy Management

GOALS OF LONG-TERM MANAGEMENT

The goals of long-term management for the patient with muscular dystrophy are to reduce the impact of progressive debility and prolonged morbidity throughout their longer life spans. Respiratory complications may advance from mild respiratory distress to the need for nocturnal noninvasive mechanical ventilation. Respiratory failure is the primary cause of death.

In addition to all of the long-term management goals common to other neuromuscular conditions, the following are additional goals for patients with muscular dystrophy:

- Optimize capacity with judiciously prescribed and appropriately introduced aids and devices consistent with the patient's changing needs (e.g., walking aids, wheelchair, and dressing and activities of daily living aids)

- Optimize aerobic capacity with a balance of judicious exercise, energy conservation, and rest
- Optimize secretion clearance as needed
- Reduce the work of breathing
- Reduce the work of the heart
- Protect the airways from aspiration

PATIENT MONITORING

Patients with muscular dystrophy require the same monitoring parameters common to all of the secondary conditions discussed in this chapter; however, those with additional cardiac dysfunction need to be cleared by a cardiologist before starting a rehabilitation program, particularly when it involves a mobilization or exercise program, to refine the prescriptive parameters of the program.

If supplemental oxygen is used, the fraction of inspired oxygen (FiO_2) administered is recorded.

Assessment of nighttime and daytime cardiovascular and pulmonary function is needed because respiratory insufficiency often begins with nocturnal hypoxemia in patients with Duchenne muscular dystrophy.

Activity and sleep patterns must be assessed to ensure sleep is maximally restorative and not contributing to the patient's symptoms; obstructive sleep apnea is related to hypotonia of the upper airway musculature and obesity.

MEDICATION

Medication that is needed to maximize treatment response is administered before treatment. Knowledge of the type of medication, its administration route, and time to and duration of peak efficacy is essential if treatment is to be maximally effective.

PRIMARY INTERVENTIONS

Primary interventions for patients with muscular dystrophy include the combination of global interventions previously discussed; in addition, they require the following:

- Body positioning instruction
- Breathing control and coughing maneuvers
- Mobilization, primarily in the form of functional activities
- Strengthening exercises, primarily in the form of functional activities (to maintain strength or reduce rate of decline)
- Ventilatory muscle training
- Deformity prevention

An assessment of the patient's living and working environments should include a review of aids and devices (e.g., wheelchair type, weight, and size and noninvasive mechanical ventilation). Aids and devices are selected to minimize energy demand such that energy is conserved for other activities and undue fatigue is reduced.

The use of supplemental oxygen depends on the severity of the disease. Some patients have no need for supplemental oxygen, some need it only during exercise, and some patients require continuous oxygen with proportionately more delivered during activity and exercise compared with rest.

PATIENT EDUCATION

Patients with muscular dystrophy will require the same instruction common to all patients with chronic secondary dysfunction and would additionally benefit from information on weight control.

Weight control is an important goal in patients with chronic neuromuscular diseases because they have the least capacity to compensate for the cardiovascular and pulmonary sequelae of obesity. Obesity is also related to obstructive sleep apnea.

MOBILIZATION

Mobilization is an essential component of long-term management of the patient with muscular dystrophy. It is prescribed to optimize the efficiency of oxygen transport overall and minimize the sequelae of restricted mobility. Maximizing ventilation with mobilization is limited if the patient has severe generalized muscular weakness and increased fatigue. Functional activities provide the basis for the mobilization prescription. Although heavy resistive strengthening exercise has been advocated for these patients,[34,35] a conservative approach including an exercise program based on functional goals and energy conservation is more justifiable physiologically.[36] Chest wall mobility exercises include all planes of movement combined with a rotational component. Body positioning to optimize lung volumes and airflow rates is a priority. Breathing control and coughing maneuvers are coupled with body movement and positioning. If mucociliary transport is impaired and leads to secretion accumulation, which is refractory to mobilization and body positioning, it may be necessary to institute postural drainage coupled with deep breathing and coughing maneuvers.

VENTILATORY STRATEGIES

Although the primary factor contributing to respiratory compromise is respiratory muscle weakness, ventilatory muscle training may have a role in selected patients (Chapter 26). Improved respiratory muscle endurance and strength may have a generalized effect on functional capacity. The effect of walking alone, however, may be superior to the effect of ventilatory muscle training on ventilatory muscle strength and endurance. Ventilatory muscle training should therefore be used selectively to elicit effects over and above those resulting from functional activities such as walking, given the multisystem and functional benefits of walking.

Patients with signs of ventilatory muscle fatigue, as opposed to weakness, benefit from ventilatory support at night. Rest of the respiratory muscles at night with continuous positive airway pressure or bi-level positive airway pressure optimizes their function during the daytime.

EXERCISE

Methods of facilitating effective coughing in individuals with neuromuscular diseases are extremely important because they constitute life-preserving measures. Supported and unsupported coughing methods are described in detail in Chapters 22 and 23. Patients on noninvasive ventilatory support who are unable to generate adequate peak cough expiratory flow rates can benefit from manual assisted coughing and mechanical insufflation-exsufflation, thereby minimizing the need for endotracheal suctioning.[37] Tracheostomy is delayed as long as possible. Significantly reduced maximal insufflation capacity, however, is an indication for tracheostomy.

Whenever possible, deep breathing and coughing are coupled with chest wall movement. This facilitates maximal inflation of the lungs before coughing by increasing pulmonary compliance[38] and maximal exhalation of the lungs during coughing. Body positions are varied and changed frequently to simulate shifts in alveolar volume and ventilation and perfusion that occur with normal movement and body position changes. Glossopharyngeal breathing is a nonmechanical method of assisting ventilation. The patient is taught to use the tongue and pharyngeal muscles to swallow boluses of air past the vocal cords and into the trachea. The efficiency of training is monitored with spirometry to ensure the patient is able to achieve acceptable vital capacities. Some patients are able to support their ventilation, ventilator-free, for several hours in a day.

One intervention that is prolonging the life of patients with muscular dystrophy, as well as of patients with other progressive neuromuscular diseases, is the use of mechanical ventilatory support.[39] Home mechanical ventilation provides a noninvasive method of providing positive airway pressure through an oral or nasal mask. This provides considerable advantage over invasive, full body or tracheostomy ventilatory support. If used in conjunction with an insufflation-exsufflation device, pulmonary complications can be minimized and life expectancy increased. Other forms of noninvasive mechanical ventilation include intermittent abdominal pressure ventilation, rocking bed, negative pressure tank ventilator, and chest shell ventilator. The type of ventilation is determined individually based on the indications for ventilation and the patient's status. The use of ventilatory aids as a component of a comprehensive rehabilitation program maintains pulmonary compliance and cough efficacy. Introduction of these devices early will facilitate increased use as the respiratory muscles progressively weaken. These aids are introduced to meet the individual's needs and are changed over time. Excessive use or dependence can contribute to deterioration.

PROPHYLACTIC MANAGEMENT

Patients with generalized neuromuscular weakness require prophylactic management because of their high risk of developing life-threatening respiratory infections and complications. Prophylaxis should include flu shots; avoidance of polluted, smoky environments; smoking reduction and cessation; controlling the types of food eaten and chewing well to avoid choking; and regular deep breathing, frequent movement, and change in body positions (even just shifting and taking some deep breaths while seated in a wheelchair) to promote mucociliary transport. An optimal time to take deep breaths and to cough is during transfers, which usually are physically exerting and stimulate hyperpnea. Wheelchair design is important for comfort, biomechanical and metabolic efficiency, and reduction of unnecessary energy expenditure.

Individuals with Musculoskeletal Conditions

Thoracic Deformities

Pathophysiology and Medical Management

Respiratory insufficiency can result from abnormalities of the chest wall secondary to congenital deformity, acquired neuromuscular disease, and trauma.[21] Congenital deformity of the chest wall reduces the mobility of the bony thorax, thereby increasing the work of breathing. Shallow, rapid breathing often results. Minute ventilation is increased at the expense of alveolar ventilation. Severe deformity leads to compression of the mediastinal structures. The heart can be displaced and rotated, impeding its mechanical function. Examples of chronic deformities that impinge on pulmonary function are kyphoscoliosis secondary to poliomyelitis, tuberculous osteomyelitis, and other causes and ankylosing spondylitis. Other examples of deformity include traumatic injury of the vertebral column, ribs, and sternum. Routine cardiovascular and pulmonary assessment should include a musculoskeletal examination of the spinal column and thoracic cavity.

Normal pulmonary function and gas exchange depend on symmetry of cardiovascular and pulmonary anatomy and physiological function. Asymmetry of the chest wall interferes with normal lung mechanics, regional gradients of ventilation and perfusion in the lungs, and the distribution of inspired gas. Significant decrease in lung compliance and increase in work performed against the elastic resistance of the lung are characteristic of kyphoscoliosis. Altered pressure gradients and uneven lung movement during the respiratory cycle may contribute to altered lung water balance and impaired lymphatic drainage. The effects of physiological dead space and shunt may be magnified, producing hypoxemia and hypercapnia. With severe chest deformity, a cycle of respiratory acidosis, pulmonary hypertension, and right-sided heart failure can result in a life-threatening situation.

Principles of Physical Therapy Management

GOALS OF LONG-TERM MANAGEMENT

In addition to all of the long-term management goals common to all other musculoskeletal conditions, there are five additional goals for patients with thoracic deformity:

- Optimize secretion clearance
- Optimize movement economy
- Reduce the work of breathing
- Reduce the work of the heart
- Protect the airways from aspiration

Treatment is directed at the underlying problem contributing to threatened or impaired oxygen transport. In addition, the underlying problems that limit the individual's activities and participation are addressed primarily, with the exception of life-threatening impairments.

PATIENT MONITORING

Patients with thoracic deformities require the same monitoring parameters common to all of the secondary conditions discussed in this chapter. Patients with additional cardiac dysfunction require ECG monitoring, particularly during exercise.

PRIMARY INTERVENTIONS

Primary interventions for patients with thoracic deformity include the combination of global interventions previously discussed, and in addition they require the following:

- Body positioning instruction
- Breathing control and coughing maneuvers
- Gait reeducation
- Postural correction exercises

PATIENT EDUCATION

Patients with thoracic deformity will require the same instruction common to all patients with chronic secondary dysfunction.

EXERCISE

Aerobic exercise is an essential component of the long-term management of the patient with thoracic deformity in order to optimize the efficiency of oxygen transport overall. Abnormal postural alignment may contribute to excessive energy cost and reduced movement economy. Improving alignment will help offset this effect. In severe cases, surgical correction is indicated.

Maximizing ventilation with exercise in patients with severe deformity may be limited. Optimizing alignment to minimize the cardiovascular and pulmonary limitations of the deformity during physical activity, exercise, and rest is a priority. Chest wall exercises include all planes of movement with a rotational component. Body positioning to optimize lung volumes and airflow rates is a priority. Breathing control and coughing maneuvers are essential and should be coupled with body movement and positioning. If mucociliary transport is impaired leading to secretion retention, postural drainage may need to be instituted, coupled with deep breathing and coughing maneuvers.

Ventilatory muscle training may have a role in the management of patients with reduced inspiratory pressures and associated decreases in total lung capacity and hypoxemia.

Methods of facilitating effective coughing in patients with musculoskeletal deformity are extremely important because they constitute life-preserving measures. Supported and unsupported coughing methods are described in detail in Chapters 22 and 23. Whenever possible, deep breathing and coughing are coupled with chest wall movement to facilitate maximal inflation of the lungs before and maximal exhalation during coughing. Body positions are varied and changed frequently to simulate as much as possible shifts in alveolar volume and ventilation and perfusion that occur with normal movement and body position changes.

PROPHYLACTIC MANAGEMENT

Patients with chest wall deformities secondary to neuromuscular conditions require prophylactic management because of their high risk of developing life-threatening respiratory infections and complications. Prophylaxis should include flu shots; avoidance of polluted, smoky environments; smoking reduction and cessation; control of the types of food eaten and chewing well to avoid choking; and regular deep breathing, airway clearance, and frequent movement and change in body positions (even just shifting and taking some deep breaths while seated in a wheelchair are beneficial). An optimal time to take deep breaths and cough is during transfers, which usually are physically exerting and stimulate hyperpnea.

Osteoporosis

Pathophysiology and Medical Management

Osteoporosis is a condition associated with reduced bone mass per unit volume and appears to be on the increase (see Chapter 1). Age-related bone loss begins earlier and accelerates faster in women, particularly after menopause, than in men. Lifestyle factors, such as diet, exercise, and smoking, have a significant role in reducing bone mass. Caffeine has also been implicated as a contributing factor to bone loss secondary to increasing urinary calcium loss.

Osteoporosis is classified as idiopathic osteoporosis unassociated with other conditions, osteoporosis associated with other conditions (e.g., malabsorption, calcium deficiency, immobilization, or metabolic bone disease), osteoporosis as a feature of an inherited condition (e.g., osteogenesis imperfecta and Marfan syndrome), osteoporosis associated with paralytic conditions prohibiting weight bearing and activity, and osteoporosis associated with other conditions but with a pathogenesis that is not understood (e.g., RA, alcoholism, diabetes mellitus, or chronic airflow limitation).[15]

The most common clinical features are vertebral pain and spinal deformity resulting from vertebral compression and collapse. Vertebral bodies tend to collapse anteriorly, contributing to cervical lordosis, thoracic kyphosis, postural slumping, and loss of height. Acute episodes may be relieved by restricted mobility. Straining and sudden changes in position can exacerbate an acute episode. Cardiovascular and pulmonary complications of osteoporosis are secondary to spinal deformity, chest wall rigidity, and cardiovascular and pulmonary deconditioning resulting from restricted mobility. Vertebral compression fractures are also a feature of advanced osteoporosis. Collapse of the anterior surfaces of the vertebrae leads to kyphosis.

Osteoporosis is a condition associated with aging and older age groups. The pain of acute episodes leads to periods of restricted mobility and significant cardiovascular and pulmonary dysfunction in older persons.[32,40] Exercise that is weight bearing and loads the muscles around bone maintains bone density and decelerates bone loss and thus has a central role in preserving bone health. Generally, the growth and remodeling of bone depends highly on the exercise prescription parameters (e.g., type of exercise, intensity, duration, and frequency). Bone mineral content is more closely related to cardiovascular and pulmonary conditioning than physical activity level. Furthermore, any detrimental effect of exercise on osteoporosis appears to relate more to malalignment and injury rather than activity itself.

The primary physiological mechanism underlying osteopenia and osteoporosis is negative calcium balance. Loss of calcium is associated with lack of exercise, smoking, alcohol consumption, consumption of caffeine, and meat consumption. Calcium supplementation is only part of the remedy, as calcium loss may be the greater concern.

Principles of Physical Therapy Management

GOALS OF LONG-TERM MANAGEMENT

The etiology of osteoporosis is diverse; thus management must consider the underlying pathophysiology and that several factors may be contributing to the presentation of osteoporosis in the same patient.

In addition to all of the long-term management goals common to all other musculoskeletal conditions, patients with osteoporosis should have as an additional goal the reduction of the risk of falls and instruction on fall prevention strategies.

PATIENT MONITORING

Patients with osteoporosis require most of the monitoring parameters common to other secondary cardiovascular and pulmonary conditions discussed in this chapter; monitoring for dyspnea, respiratory distress, inappropriate breathing pattern or arterial desaturation, and cyanosis may be less indicated.

These patients also require serial bone density assessments conducted over time. It is essential to obtain a bone density assessment early for reference over time.

MEDICATION

Medication that is needed to maximize treatment response (e.g., analgesics) is administered before treatment. Knowledge of the type of medication, its administration route, and time to and duration of peak efficacy is essential if treatment is to be maximally effective.

PRIMARY INTERVENTIONS

Patients with osteoporosis require the same global interventions common to all of the secondary conditions discussed in this chapter.

PATIENT EDUCATION

Patients with osteoporosis will require the same instruction common to other patients with chronic secondary cardiovascular and pulmonary dysfunction.

EXERCISE

Aerobic and strength training are essential components of the long-term management of the individual with osteoporosis to optimize the efficiency of oxygen transport overall. Upright, weight-bearing aerobic exercise is essential to maintain bone density or reduce the rate of bone loss. Maximizing ventilation with exercise is limited if the patient has severe generalized muscular weakness and increased fatigue. Balance problems have also been identified in patients with osteoporosis, and these need to be addressed to minimize the risk of falling and its severe complications.

Chest wall exercises may have a role and include all planes of movement with a rotational component. Breathing control and coughing maneuvers are essential and should be coupled with body movement and positioning. Straining, Valsalva maneuvers, and jarring activity and exercise are contraindicated.

Methods of facilitating effective coughing in patients with osteoporosis are extremely important because they constitute life-preserving measures. Some patients fracture ribs and vertebrae during coughing. Patients at risk should rely on huffing maneuvers that do not require closing the glottis and do not generate high intrathoracic pressures.

Individuals with Collagen Vascular, Connective Tissue, and Rheumatoid Conditions

Systemic Lupus Erythematosus

Pathophysiology and Medical Management

SLE is a condition characterized by the presence of multiple antibodies that contribute to immunologically mediated tissue inflammation and damage.[41] The condition affects the major organ systems, including the central nervous, musculoskeletal, pulmonary, vascular, and renal systems. Symptoms include arthralgic and myalgic stiffness, pain, and fatigue.

The cardiovascular and pulmonary manifestations of SLE include atelectasis, which results from inflammation of the alveolar walls and perivascular and peribronchial connective tissue, effusions secondary to lung infarction, reduced surface tension, and splinting secondary to pleuritic pain. Other manifestations include pleuritis with or without effusion, pneumonitis, interstitial fibrosis, pulmonary hypertension, diaphragmatic dysfunction, pulmonary hemorrhage, systemic hypertension, myocarditis, constrictive pericarditis, dysrhythmias, tamponade, pericardial pain, arteritis, and defects of the mitral and aortic valves.[42] Other manifestations that affect cardiovascular and pulmonary function include anemia, leukopenia, thrombocytopenia, thrombosis, splenomegaly, ascites, gastrointestinal bleeding, nephritis, and renal insufficiency.[15]

Principles of Physical Therapy Management

GOALS OF LONG-TERM MANAGEMENT

In addition to all of the long-term management goals common to all other collagen vascular and connective tissue diseases, there are four additional goals for patients with SLE:

- Reduce the work of breathing
- Reduce the work of the heart
- Protect the airways from aspiration
- Optimize secretion clearance

PATIENT MONITORING

Patients with SLE require all of the monitoring parameters common to all of the secondary conditions discussed in this chapter. Patients with additional cardiac dysfunction should be cleared by a cardiologist before being prescribed an exercise program.

Subjectively, discomfort, pain, and fatigue can be assessed using analog scales.

MEDICATION

Medication that is needed to maximize treatment response (e.g., analgesic and antiinflammatory agents) is administered before treatment. Knowledge of the type of medication, its administration route, and time to and duration of peak efficacy is essential if treatment is to be maximally effective.

PRIMARY INTERVENTIONS

Primary interventions for patients with SLE include the combination of global interventions previously discussed, and in addition these patients require instruction in body positioning and breathing control and coughing maneuvers.

PATIENT EDUCATION

Patients with SLE will require the same instruction common to all patients with chronic secondary dysfunction.

EXERCISE

Aerobic exercise is an essential component of the long-term management of the patient with SLE in order to optimize the efficiency of oxygen transport overall, including maximizing alveolar ventilation and mobilizing and removing secretions. Parameters of the exercise prescription are based on subjective responses (e.g., discomfort, pain, breathlessness, and perceived exertion in conjunction with objective responses). Optimal types of aerobic exercise include walking and cycling. Aquatic exercise may be preferable for patients with musculoskeletal involvement that precludes walking and cycling. Chest wall exercises can be used and should include all planes of movement with a rotational component. Body positioning to optimize lung volumes and airflow rates is a priority. Breathing control and coughing maneuvers are essential and should be coupled with body movement and positioning. If mucociliary transport is impaired, leading to secretion retention, it may be necessary to institute postural drainage coupled with deep breathing and coughing maneuvers.

Scleroderma

Pathophysiology and Medical Management

Scleroderma is characterized by the overproduction of collagen and progressive fibrosis of cutaneous and subcutaneous tissues.[43] The cardiovascular and pulmonary manifestations of this condition result in interstitial pulmonary fibrosis with significantly reduced vital capacity, diffusing capacity, and arterial oxygen tension.[15] Reduced static compliance is the primary mechanical deficit. Pulmonary hypertension may be a complicating factor. Bronchoalveolar lavage is consistent with an acute inflammatory process. Cardiomyopathy is associated with ischemia, areas of infarction, and myocardial fibrosis.[43] Fibrosis of the conduction system predisposes the patient to conduction defects and dysrhythmias. Other cardiovascular and pulmonary manifestations include pericarditis with or without effusion and pulmonary and systemic hypertension from renal involvement. Half of patients with scleroderma have renal involvement including intimal hyperplasia, fibrinous necrosis of the afferent arterioles, and thickening of the glomerular basement membrane. Fibrotic changes and stenoses occur in the small arteries and arterioles systemically. Similar changes in the lymphatic vessels may obliterate lymph flow.

Esophageal involvement contributes to regurgitation of gastric contents, which is exacerbated when the patient is recumbent or bends over. Bloating and abdominal discomfort may reflect paralytic ileus and intestinal obstruction. Ascites and fluid accumulation in the gut increase abdominal pressure and encroach on diaphragmatic motion.

Principles of Physical Therapy Management

GOALS OF LONG-TERM MANAGEMENT

In addition to all of the long-term management goals common to all other collagen vascular and connective tissue diseases, there are four additional goals for patients with scleroderma:

- Reduce the work of breathing
- Reduce the work of the heart
- Protect the airways from aspiration
- Optimize secretion clearance

PATIENT MONITORING

Patients with scleroderma require all of the monitoring parameters common to all of the secondary conditions discussed in this chapter. Patients with additional cardiac dysfunction require ECG monitoring, particularly during exercise. If supplemental oxygen is used, the FiO_2 administered is recorded.

MEDICATION

Medication that is needed to maximize treatment response (e.g., immunosuppressive agents and antiplatelet therapy) is administered before treatment. Knowledge of the type of medication, its administration route, and time to and duration of peak efficacy is essential if treatment is to be maximally effective.

PRIMARY INTERVENTIONS

Primary interventions for patients with scleroderma include the combination of global interventions previously discussed; in addition, these patients require instruction in body positioning and breathing control and coughing maneuvers.

Patients with esophageal involvement are not treated or exercised immediately after a meal. These patients have frequent, small meals, take antacids between meals, and do not lie down for a few hours after eating. When recumbent, these patients have the head of bed elevated to minimize the risk of aspiration of gastric contents.

PATIENT EDUCATION

Patients with scleroderma will require the same instruction common to all patients with chronic secondary dysfunction.

EXERCISE

Aerobic exercise is an essential component of the long-term management of the patient with scleroderma to optimize the efficiency of oxygen transport overall. The exercise program is modified according to the signs and symptoms (see Chapter 25). Chest wall exercises can be used and should include all planes of movement with a rotational component. Body positioning to optimize lung volumes and airflow rates is a priority. Breathing control and coughing maneuvers are essential and should be coupled with body movement and positioning. If mucociliary transport is impaired and this leads to secretion retention, it may be necessary to institute postural drainage coupled with deep breathing and coughing maneuvers.

Ankylosing Spondylitis

Pathophysiology and Medical Management

Ankylosing spondylitis results in reduced total lung capacity, vital capacity, and inspiratory muscle function. Ventilatory capacity is preserved, given that the respiratory muscles are not involved. The condition can result in spinal and chest wall rigidity; thus there is greater reliance on diaphragmatic contribution to ventilation (84%) compared with healthy persons (68%). The patient with ankylosing spondylitis has an increased dependence on diaphragmatic function and therefore is at risk if administered respiratory depressant medications or if he or she undergoes thoracic or upper abdominal surgery. These changes can lead to an increased respiratory rate during exercise to meet ventilatory demands. In combination with impaired respiratory mechanics, the work of breathing can increase.

During exercise, patients with ankylosing spondylitis show minimal chest wall expansion compared with otherwise healthy people. Although peak workload is reduced, diaphragmatic fatigue is more likely to be the limiting factor than ventilatory capacity, ventilation-perfusion mismatch, or abnormal blood gases.

Principles of Physical Therapy Management

GOALS OF LONG-TERM MANAGEMENT

In addition to all of the long-term management goals common to all other collagen vascular and connective tissue diseases, there are two additional goals for patients with ankylosing spondylitis:

- Optimize alveolar ventilation
- Optimize spinal mobility

PATIENT MONITORING

Patients with ankylosing spondylitis require all of the monitoring parameters common to all of the secondary conditions discussed in this chapter.

PRIMARY INTERVENTIONS

Primary interventions for patients with ankylosing spondylitis include the combination of global interventions previously discussed; in addition, these patients require the following:

- Body positioning instruction
- Breathing control and coughing maneuvers
- Gait reeducation
- Ventilatory muscle training

PATIENT EDUCATION

Patients with ankylosing spondylitis will require the same instruction common to all patients with chronic secondary dysfunction.

EXERCISE

Aerobic exercise is an essential component of the long-term management of the patient with ankylosing spondylitis in order to optimize the efficiency of oxygen transport overall. Maximizing ventilation with mobilization is limited if the patient has extreme spinal rigidity. Chest wall exercises can be used and should include all planes of movement with a rotational component. Body positioning to optimize lung volumes and airflow rates is a priority. Breathing control and coughing maneuvers are essential and should be coupled with body movement and positioning. Ventilatory muscle training in conjunction with exercise may have some additional benefit in maximizing aerobic capacity.

Consistent with the physical activity and exercise pyramid recommendations of daily exercise, individuals with ankylosing spondylitis can benefit from frequent, prolonged, low-intensity cross training to offset the potential for loss of flexibility and range.

Rheumatoid Arthritis

Pathophysiology and Medical Management

RA is a multisystemic condition that is associated with well-documented cardiovascular-pulmonary effects, including pleuritis with or without effusions, interstitial fibrosis, pulmonary vasculitis, an increased incidence of bronchitis and pneumonia myocarditis, epicarditis, endocarditis, dysrhythmias, neuritis, and vasculitis.[44]

Individuals with RA have significant cardiovascular risk factors. Compared with individuals without RA, diastolic blood pressure and levels of thrombotic variables are elevated.[45] Risk factor modification has an important role in the comprehensive management of individuals with RA.

Functional capacity is limited by pain and stiffness in the affected muscles and joints, weakness, the number of joints affected, fatigue, and whether the patient is having an acute episode. Self-limited physical activity and exercise contributes to cardiovascular and pulmonary deconditioning. Movement such as walking is often inefficient because of limping. Peak exercise tests are limited by musculoskeletal complaints; thus submaximal tests are more functional in this population. Tests of cardiovascular status must be non–weight bearing to enable the patient to reach an acceptable stress level without confounding joint pain.

Prolonged use of steroids contributes to bone fragility. Thus physical activity and exercise prescriptions are modified accordingly.

RA is hallmarked by exacerbations and remissions. A lifelong health program helps to reduce the frequency and severity of exacerbations and enhance recovery from these.

Furthermore, such a program may help reduce the need for potent medication.

Principles of Physical Therapy Management

GOALS OF LONG-TERM MANAGEMENT

Traditionally the approach to the physical therapy management of RA has been largely from the orthopedic perspective. Exercise and stress of the oxygen transport system, however, are major components of overall management. Thus the secondary cardiovascular and pulmonary manifestations must be assessed to ensure that exercise prescription is safe as well as maximally therapeutic.

In addition to all of the long-term management goals common to all other collagen vascular and connective tissue diseases, there are five additional goals for patients with RA:

- Reduce the work of breathing
- Reduce the work of the heart
- Protect the airways from aspiration
- Optimize secretion clearance
- Optimize alveolar ventilation

PATIENT MONITORING

Patients with RA require all of the monitoring parameters common to all of the secondary conditions discussed in this chapter.

MEDICATION

Medication that is needed to maximize treatment response (e.g., steroids, nonsteroidal antiinflammatory drugs, and analgesics) is administered before treatment. Knowledge of the type of medication, its administration route, and time to and duration of peak efficacy is essential if treatment is to be maximally efficacious. Gentle, rhythmic, nonjarring exercise is prescribed, particularly for patients at risk of loss of bone mass secondary to long-term steroid use.

PRIMARY INTERVENTIONS

Primary interventions for patients with RA include the combination of global interventions previously discussed; in addition, these patients require instruction in body positioning and breathing control and coughing maneuvers. A review of mobility aids and devices is carried out to maximize the patient's function and exercise tolerance.

PATIENT EDUCATION

Patients with RA will require the same instruction common to all patients with chronic secondary dysfunction.

EXERCISE

Aerobic exercise is an essential component of the long-term management of the patient with RA in order to optimize the efficiency of oxygen transport overall with respect to both cardiovascular and pulmonary conditioning and improving movement economy. Mild-to-moderate exercise during subacute periods can be beneficial. Cycling efficiency of patients with RA is comparable to that of healthy persons. The efficiency of walking, however, is less in patients with RA because of limping and associated deformity and pain. Non–weight-bearing exercise is beneficial in patients with severe deformity and pain (e.g., aquatic exercise or water walking). Given the fluctuations in the patient's condition from day to day, exercise prescription is modified frequently in consideration of the patient's changing condition. Chest wall exercises include all planes of movement with a rotational component. Body positioning to optimize lung volumes and airflow rates is a priority. Breathing control and coughing maneuvers are essential and should be coupled with body movement and positioning.

For patients with RA, 15 to 35 minutes of graded, low-intensity aerobic exercise performed three times a week can be sufficient to enhance aerobic capacity. In addition to improving aerobic capacity, such an exercise prescription results in increased exercise time, reduced affected joint count, improved activities of daily living, and reduced joint pain and general fatigue. Should a joint flare-up occur while the patient is participating in an exercise program, a few days or weeks of restricted mobility and abstinence from exercise frequently ameliorate the symptoms. Gentle mobilization (preferably weight bearing) coupled with range-of-motion exercises during this period will minimize the negative effects of reduced activity.

Individuals with Chronic Renal Insufficiency

Pathophysiology and Medical Management

Patients with chronic renal disease have significant systemic complications. Cardiovascular and pulmonary manifestations include left ventricular hypertrophy and congestive heart failure secondary to chronic volume and pressure overload. Patients have a high incidence of atherosclerosis, coronary artery disease, glucose intolerance, and diabetes. Also, generalized muscle weakness and fatigue compromise functional work capacity.

Chronically increased fluid volume, although regulated with dialysis, contributes to increased stroke work of the heart and cardiomegaly and hypertension. With respect to pulmonary function, increased fluid volume increases peribronchial fluid and airway closure. After dialysis, the reduction in body weight is related to a reduction in closing volume, increased vital capacity, and forced expiratory flow rates.

The pulmonary-renal syndromes reflect the close relationship between the lungs and kidneys. These syndromes are characterized by altered immunological status, alveolar hemorrhage, interstitial and alveolar inflammation, and pulmonary vascular involvement.

The kidneys have a primary role in the production and regulation of certain humoral regulators of metabolism, hemodynamics, fluid balance, and oxygen transport. Thus pathology of the kidneys affects those life-sustaining processes. Patients may be taking potent medications that are associated with severe side effects that can further compromise function.

Principles of Physical Therapy Management

Goals of Long-Term Management

In addition to all of the long-term management goals common to all other collagen vascular and connective tissue diseases, there are five additional goals for patients with chronic renal insufficiency:

- Reduce the work of breathing
- Reduce the work of the heart
- Protect the airways from aspiration
- Optimize secretion clearance
- Optimize alveolar ventilation

Patient Monitoring

Patients with chronic renal insufficiency require all of the monitoring parameters common to all of the secondary conditions discussed in this chapter.

Medication

Medication that is needed to maximize treatment response is administered before treatment. Knowledge of the type of medication, its administration route, and time to and duration of peak efficacy is essential if treatment is to be maximally effective. A lifelong health program has the potential to reduce the need for potent medications for renal dysfunction.

Primary Interventions

Postural correction exercises, chest wall mobility exercises, range-of-motion exercises, airway clearance interventions, activity pacing, and energy conservation techniques, which were all mentioned as global primary interventions, are not strictly necessary for patients with chronic renal insufficiency. These patients do require a combination of the other global interventions previously discussed; they will in addition need instruction on body positioning and breathing control and coughing maneuvers.

Patient Education

Patients with chronic renal insufficiency will require the same instruction common to all patients with chronic secondary dysfunction.

Exercise

Aerobic exercise is an essential component of the long-term management of the patient with chronic renal insufficiency in order to optimize the efficiency of oxygen transport overall. Maximizing ventilation with exercise is limited if the patient has severe generalized muscular weakness and increased fatigue. Maximal oxygen uptake increases in hemodialysis patients along with improvement in other indices of cardiovascular and pulmonary conditioning. Patients may decrease or eliminate the need for antihypertension medications. Exercise carried out during hemodialysis treatment sessions is feasible and safe for appropriate patients. Because hemodialysis treatments require sessions of several hours multiple times weekly, aerobic training (e.g., cycle ergometry) can be effectively incorporated into treatment time. The exercise prescription of patients with blood glucose abnormalities and coronary artery disease is modified accordingly.

Chest wall exercises can be used and should include all planes of movement with a rotational component. Body positioning to optimize lung volumes and airflow rates is a priority. Breathing control and coughing maneuvers are essential and should be coupled with body movement and positioning.

Individuals Who Are Obese

Pathophysiology and Medical Management

Obesity and its multisystem sequelae are epidemic in industrialized countries; thus obesity must be managed by the physical therapist as a primary condition as well as secondary to other diagnoses. Any other pathology or problem is accentuated when compounded with obesity, and morbidity and mortality are increased for all health concerns.[46,47]

A detailed assessment is conducted to identify organ systems that are affected and may limit exercise. Central abdominal obesity (apple obesity) constitutes a greater cardiovascular risk than hip obesity (pear obesity).[48,49] In younger people, low aerobic fitness in people who are obese appears to reflect deconditioning rather than a primary cardiac problem.[50] Individuals who are morbidly obese, however, may develop heart failure. Noninvasive approaches to weight control are superior to invasive approaches in terms of promoting lifelong change and multisystem benefit, health and well-being, and cost-effectiveness.

Pharmacological approaches and surgery are extreme measures whose use is generally not restricted to those with morbid obesity. Vertical banded gastroplasty is increasingly being performed on patients with morbid obesity. One study that compared exercise responses before and 6 months after weight loss with surgery showed that cardiac diastolic function is improved, along with V_{O_2} and anaerobic threshold.[51] The extent to which these and additional benefits would have occurred with conservative weight loss, however, and the long-term changes effected by both, were not studied.

Health risks associated with obesity are multisystemic (see Chapters 1 and 6). The cardiovascular and pulmonary risks are life-threatening. In particular, the work of breathing, owing to alveolar hypoventilation, and the work of the heart are increased with increasing body mass. The heart may enlarge to accommodate increased workload, even at rest. Body mass over the chest wall can lead to alveolar hypoventilation and airway closure and reduced oxygenation. Individuals who are obese have problems when recumbent, particularly during sleep (e.g., obstructive sleep apnea, dysrhythmias, and shortness of breath). These problems are identified in the comprehensive assessment.

Principles of Physical Therapy Management

Goals of Long-Term Management

Obesity can be a primary referred problem or a secondary condition. Physical therapists are uniquely suited to counsel and coach patients with weight problems and promote physically active lifestyles, recommend exercise programs, and provide basic knowledge on nutrition and diet commensurate with supporting these activities. Lessons learnt from tobacco control and smoking cessation have been extrapolated for use in the management of the obesity epidemic.[52]

Physical activity through the course of the day must be increased, and patients who are obese need to participate in a regular program of exercise. The goals of long-term management for the obese patient include all of the elements common to all other conditions.

Patient Monitoring

Patients with obesity require all of the monitoring parameters common to all of the secondary conditions discussed in this chapter.

Maintaining a healthy weight is a function of optimal nutrition and exercise (see recommendations in Chapter 1). The individual's readiness to change dietary and activity patterns must be assessed to determine the optimal time to introduce a structured program to maximize and sustain long-term outcomes (see Chapters 1 and 28).

A weight loss program is introduced concurrently with an increasing volume of regular physical activity and a structured exercise program. The parameters of the prescription, however, may require modification because of biomechanical stress and discomfort. As weight is lost, the prescriptive parameters are modified to increase the intensity and volume of exercise that is performed. Also, the individual's movement economy and efficiency will improve as the body's biomechanics normalize. Initially the hemodynamic responses to even low levels of exercise are likely to be excessive because of the weight that the individual carries during the performance of the activity. Before significant loss of weight, cycling may initially be preferable to walking if the person's biomechanics limit endurance. Physical activity must be comfortable both for sustainability and injury avoidance.

The role of the physical therapist as health coach is critically important in providing both support to the individual who is obese and long-term follow-up. The probability of success is increased with the involvement of a health care provider and follow-up. Facilitating weight loss and adopting long-term healthy lifestyle behaviors can be lifesaving for a patient. Given the current epidemic of obesity, assisting an individual to attain a healthy lifestyle through optimal nutrition, exercise, and weight loss is a singularly important health outcome.

Summary

This chapter reviews pathophysiology and medical management as they relate to the comprehensive physical therapy management of individuals with chronic secondary cardiovascular and pulmonary pathology. Exercise testing and training are major components of the comprehensive management of these conditions and are presented separately in Chapter 25.

This chapter specifically presents the comprehensive physical therapy management of chronic cardiovascular and pulmonary dysfunction secondary to neuromuscular, musculoskeletal, collagen vascular and connective tissue, and renal dysfunction. The neuromuscular conditions that are presented include stroke, Parkinson syndrome, multiple sclerosis, cerebral palsy, spinal cord injury, chronic effects of poliomyelitis, and muscular dystrophy. The musculoskeletal conditions that are presented include thoracic deformity (kyphoscoliosis) and osteoporosis. The collagen vascular and connective tissue conditions that are presented include SLE, scleroderma, ankylosing spondylitis, and RA. Finally, management of the patient with chronic renal insufficiency and the person who is obese is presented.

The principles of patient management are presented rather than treatment prescriptions, which cannot be given without specific consideration of an individual patient. In this context, the goals of long-term management of patients with each condition are presented, followed by the essential monitoring required, and the primary interventions for maximizing cardiovascular and pulmonary function and oxygen transport. The selection of interventions for any given patient is based on the physiological hierarchy. The most physiological interventions are exploited, followed by less physiological interventions and those whose effectiveness is less well documented.

These principles must be considered if a patient has a chronic secondary cardiovascular and pulmonary condition as a secondary diagnosis for which the patient is being treated by the physical therapist. These principles have implications for treatment prescription and monitoring in the management of the condition for which the patient is being primarily treated.

Review Questions

1. Analyze the limitations in participation and related activities that are associated with chronic cardiovascular and pulmonary pathophysiology that occurs secondary to stroke, Parkinson syndrome, multiple sclerosis, cerebral palsy, spinal cord injury, late sequelae of poliomyelitis, muscular dystrophy, kyphoscoliosis, osteoporosis, SLE, scleroderma, ankylosing spondylitis, RA, chronic renal insufficiency, and obesity.
2. Relate cardiovascular and pulmonary physical therapy treatment interventions to the underlying pathophysiology of each of the chronic conditions listed in question 1 that a person may have, and provide the rationale for your choice.

References

1. Dean E, Ross J: Movement energetics of individuals with a history of poliomyelitis. *Arch Phys Med Rehabil* 74:478–483, 1993.
2. Bach-y-Rita P, Wood S, Leder R, et al: Computer-assisted motivating rehabilitation for institutional, home, and educational late stroke programs. *Top Stroke Rehabil* 8:1–10, 2002.
3. Page SJ, Gater DR, Back-Y-Rita P: Reconsidering the motor recovery plateau in stroke rehabilitation. *Arch Phys Med Rehabil* 85:1377–1381, 2004.
4. Roth EJ: Heart disease in patients with stroke. Part II. Impact and implications for rehabilitation. *Arch Phys Med Rehabil* 75:94–101, 1994.

5. Duncan P, Studenski S, Richards L, et al: Randomized clinical trial of therapeutic exercise in subacute stroke. *Stroke* 34:73–80, 2003.
6. Moseley AM, Stark A, Cameron ID, et al: Treadmill training and body weight support for walking after stroke. *Cochrane Database and Systematic Review* CD002840, 2003.
7. Maeshima S, Ueyoshi A, Osawa A, et al: Mobility and muscle strength contralateral to hemiplegia from stroke: benefit from self-training with family support. *Am J Phys Med Rehabil* 82:456–462, 2003.
8. Malouin F, Potvin M, Prevost J: Use of an intensive task-oriented gait training program in a series of patients with acute cerebrovascular accidents. *Phys Ther* 72:781–793, 1992.
9. Ross J, Dean E: Body positioning. In Zadai C, editor: *Pulmonary management in physical therapy*, New York, 1992, Churchill Livingstone.
10. Bastille JV, Gill-Body KM: A yoga-based exercise program for people with chronic poststroke hemiparesis. *Phys Ther* 84:33–48, 2004.
11. Badics E, Wittmann A, Rupp M, et al: Systematic muscle building exercises in the rehabilitation of stroke patients. *Neuro Rehabilitation* 17:211–214, 2002.
12. National clinical guidelines for stroke: a concise update. *Clin Med* 2:231–233, 2002.
13. Neu HC, Connolly JJ, Schwertley FW, et al: Obstructive respiratory dysfunction in Parkinsonian patients. *Am Rev Respir Dis* 95:33–47, 1966.
14. Serebrovskaya T, Karaban I, Mankovskaya I, et al: Hypoxic ventilatory responses and gas exchange in patients with Parkinson's disease. *Respiration* 65:28–33, 1998.
15. Kasper DL, Braunwald E, Fauci A, et al, editors: Harrison's principles of internal medicine, ed 16, New York, NY, 2004, McGraw-Hill Professional.
16. Merkelbach S, Dillmann U, Kölmel C, et al: Cardiovascular autonomic dysregulation and fatigue in multiple sclerosis. *Mult Scler* 7:320, 2001.
17. Ray JF, 3rd, Yost L, Moallem S, et al: Immobility, hypoxemia, and pulmonary arteriovenous shunting. *Arch Surg* 109:537–541, 1974.
18. Mossberg KA, Linton KA, Friske K: Ankle-foot orthoses: effect of energy expenditure of gait in spastic diplegic children. *Arch Phys Med Rehabil* 71:490–494, 1990.
19. Braverman JM: Airway clearance dysfunction associated with cerebral palsy: An overview. Advanced Respiratory. 2001, www.lagunahealth.de/vest_1/Zerebr.pdf. Retrieved September 2011.
20. Kirilloff LH, Owens GR, Rogers RM, et al: Does chest physical therapy work? *Chest* 88:436–444, 1985.
21. Mason RJ, Broaddus VC, Martin T, et al: *Murray and Nadel's textbook of respiratory medicine*, ed 5, Philadelphia, 2010, Elsevier.
22. Estenne M, Gorino M: Action of the diaphragm during cough in tetrapelgic subjects. *J Appl Physiol* 72:1074–1080, 1992.
23. Smith WE, Clark PF, MacArthur D, et al: Oxygen costs using a reciprocating gait orthosis in a paraplegic (T9) patient with a bilateral below-knee amputation: case report. *Spinal Cord* 35:121–123, 1997.
24. McCool FD, Tzelepis GE: Inspiratory muscle training in the patient with neuromuscular Disease. *Phys Ther* 75:1006–1114, 1995.
25. Linder SH: Functional electrical stimulation to enhance cough in quadriplegia. *Chest* 103:166–169, 1993.
26. Dean E, Ross J, Road JD, et al: Pulmonary function in individuals with a history of poliomyelitis. *Chest* 100:118–123, 1991.
27. Bach JR, Smith WH, Michaels J, et al: Airway secretion clearance by mechanical exsufflation for post-poliomyelitis ventilator-assisted individuals. *Arch Phys Med Rehabil* 74:170–174, 1993.
28. McArdle WD, Katch FI, Katch VL: *Exercise physiology, North American Edition: Nutrition, Energy, and Human Performance*, ed 7, Philadelphia, 2009, Lippincott Williams & Wilkins.
29. Moorman JR, Coleman E., Packer DL, et al: Cardiac involvement in myotonic muscular dystrophy. *Medicine* 64:371–387, 1985.
30. Macklem PT, Roussos CS: Respiratory muscle fatigue: A cause of respiratory failure? *Clin Sci Mol Med* 53:419–422, 1977.
31. Laghi F, Tobin MJ: Disorders of the respiratory muscles. *Am J Respir Crit Care Med* 168: 10–48, 2003.
32. Dean E: Advances in rehabilitation for older persons with cardiopulmonary dysfunction. In Katz PR, Mezey MD, Kane RL, editors: *Emerging systems in long-term care: Advances in long-term care*, ed 4, New York, 1999, Springer.
33. Janssens JP, Pache JC, Nicod LP: Physiological changes in respiratory function associated with ageing. *Eur Respir J* 13: 197–205, 1999.
34. Aitkens SG, McCrory MA, Kilmer DD, et al: Moderate resistance exercise program: Its effect in slowly progressive neuromuscular disease. *Arch Phys Med Rehabil* 74:711–715, 1993.
35. Kilmer DD, McCrory MA, Wright NC, et al: The effect of a high resistance exercise program in slowly progressive neuromuscular disease. *Arch Phys Med Rehabil* 75:560–563, 1994.
36. Kilmer DD: Response to resistive strengthening exercise training in humans with neuromuscular disease. *Am J Phys Med Rehabil* 81(Suppl):S121–S126, 2002.
37. Bach JR: Mechanical insufflation-exsufflation. Comparison of peak expiratory flows with manually assisted and unassisted coughing techniques. *Chest* 104:1553–1562, 1993.
38. Lechtzin N, Shade D, Clawson L, et al: Supramaximal inflation improves lung compliance in subjects with amyotrophic lateral sclerosis. *Chest* 129:1322–1329, 2006.
39. Gomez-Merino E, Bach JR: Duchenne muscular dystrophy: prolongation of life by noninvasive ventilation and mechanically assisted coughing. *Am J Phys Med Rehabil* 81:411–415, 2002.
40. Dean E: Cardiopulmonary development. In Bonder BR, Wagner MB, editors: *Functional performance in older adults*, ed 2, Philadelphia, 2001; F.A. Davis.
41. Segal AM, Calabrese LH, Ahmad M, et al: The pulmonary manifestations of systemic lupus erythematosus. *Semin Arthritis Rheum* 14:202–224, 1985.
42. Dickey BF, Myers AR: Pulmonary manifestations of collagen-vascular diseases. In Fishman AP, Elias JA, Fishman JA, et al, editors: *Fishman's pulmonary diseases and disorders*, ed 4, New York, 2008, McGraw Hill.
43. Gray IR: Cardiovascular manifestations of collagen vascular diseases. In Julian DG, Camm AJ, Fox KM, et al, editors: *Diseases of the heart*, ed 2, Philadelphia, 1996, W.B. Saunders.
44. Ekblom B, Nordemar R: Rheumatoid arthritis. In Skinner J, editor: *Exercise testing and training for special cases*, ed 3, Philadelphia, 2003, Lippincott Williams & Wilkins.
45. McEntegart A, Capell HA, Creran D, et al: Cardiovascular risk factors, including thrombotic variables, in a population with rheumatoid arthritis. *Rheumatology* 40:640–644, 2001.
46. Desapriya E: Obesity epidemic. *Lancet* 364:1488, 2004.
47. Orzano AJ, Scott JG: Diagnosis and treatment of obesity in adults: an applied evidence-based review. *J Am Board Fam Pract* 17:359–369, 2004.
48. Kahn HS, Williamson DF: Abdominal obesity and mortality risk among men in nineteenth-century North America. *Int J Obes* 18:686–691, 1994.
49. Flodmark CE, Sveger T, Nilssonehle P. Waist measurement correlates to a potentially atherogenic lipoprotein profile in obese 12–14-year-old children. *Acta Paediatr* 83:941–945, 1994.
50. Rowland T, Bhargava R, Parslow D, et al: Cardiac response to progressive cycle exercise in moderately obese adolescent females. *J Adolesc Health* 32:422–427, 2003.
51. Kanoupakis E, Michaloudis D, Fraidakis O, et al: Left ventricular function and cardiopulmonary performance following surgical treatment of morbid obesity. *Obes Surg* 11:552–558, 2001.
52. Mercer SL, Green LW, Rosenthal AC, et al: Possible lessons from the tobacco experience for obesity control. *Am J Clin Nutr* 77(Suppl 4):1073S–1082S, 2003.

Part VI

Cardiovascular and Pulmonary Physical Therapy: Intensive Care

PART VI OUTLINE

VI

Chapter 33

Comprehensive Management of Individuals in the Intensive Care Unit

Elizabeth Dean and Christiane Perme

KEY TERMS

Early mobilization
End-of-life issues
Evidence-based practice
Function optimization
Goals
High-quality care
Humanity
Outcomes and measures
Prevention
Scientific evidence
Team
Treatment prescription

CHAPTER OUTLINE

Cardiovascular and pulmonary physical therapy in the intensive care unit (ICU) is a subspecialty within cardiovascular and pulmonary physical therapy. This chapter presents the principles of clinical and nonclinical aspects of patient management in this setting. An overview of the general goals of management and the rationale for prioritizing treatments according to a physiological hierarchy is described. End-of-life issues are also addressed.

The thrust toward evidence-based practice in health care and the development of conceptual bases for practice have had major implications for cardiovascular and pulmonary physical therapy in the ICU.[1-4] Superior knowledge of cardiovascular and pulmonary physiology, pathophysiology, pharmacology, multisystem dysfunction and its medical management, and ICU equipment and changing technology is essential. Clinical decision making in the ICU and rational management of patients is based on a tripod approach: knowledge of the underlying pathophysiology and basis for general care; knowledge of the physiological and scientific evidence for treatment interventions; and clinical reasoning and decision making in prioritizing treatments, prescribing their parameters, and performing serial evaluation to assess outcomes and further modify treatment (Figure 33-1). High-quality care is a function of these three areas of knowledge and expertise. Evidence-based practice and excellent problem-solving ability

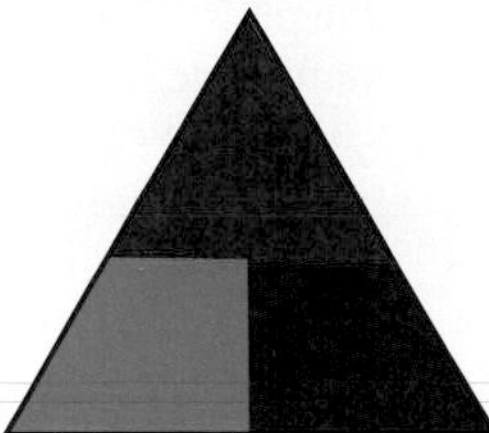

Fig. 33-1 Tripod approach to patient management.

will optimize outcomes[5] and maximize the benefit-to-risk ratio of cardiovascular and pulmonary physical therapy interventions.

Specialized Expertise of the Intensive Care Unit Physical Therapist

Effective clinical decision making and practice in the ICU demand specialized expertise and skill, including advanced, state-of-the-art knowledge in cardiovascular and pulmonary and multisystem physiology and pathophysiology and in medical, surgical, nursing, and pharmacological management (Box 33-1). Physical therapists in the ICU need to be first-rate diagnosticians and observers. Given the multitude of factors that contribute to impaired oxygen transport,[6] the physical therapist needs to analyze these to define the patient's specific oxygen transport deficits and problems. Optimizing oxygen delivery in the patient who is critically ill[7] by exploiting noninvasive interventions is the priority.

The role of the ICU physical therapist is to promote healing and recovery and to return the patient to the highest possible level of life participation and satisfaction. Therefore the physical therapist must be capable of processing considerable amounts of objective information quickly, interpreting this information, and integrating it to provide the basis for a treatment prescription (i.e., the specific selection, prioritization, and implementation of treatment interventions). The ability to integrate and interpret the vast amount of multiorgan system data is perhaps the single most important skill in ICU practice and treatment prescription. With these data the physical therapist identifies the indications for treatment, contraindications, and optimal timing of interventions. The condition of the patient in the ICU can change rapidly. The physical therapist works within narrow windows of opportunity to effect an optimal treatment response. Treatments are variable with respect to their intensity, duration, and frequency. The maximally beneficial outcome with the least risk to the patient is the objective of every treatment. Although principles of management may be the same, specific knowledge requirements will differ depending on the type of critical care setting (e.g., burn, coronary care, neurosurgery, spinal cord injury, and trauma). Alternatively, a community hospital with a small general ICU will have a cross section of patients that the physical therapist will need to manage.

Box 33-1 Specialized Expertise and Skill of the Intensive Care Unit Physical Therapist

- Detailed, comprehensive knowledge of cardiopulmonary physiology and pathophysiology and pharmacology.
- Thorough working knowledge of the monitoring systems routinely used in the intensive care unit (ICU) and an understanding of the interpretation of the output of these monitoring systems (e.g., electrocardiogram [ECG], arterial blood gases, fluid and electrolyte balance, hemodynamic monitoring, chest-tube drainage systems, intracranial pressure monitoring). This information is an integral component for assessing the underlying problems and selecting, prioritizing, and progressing or modifying treatment.
- Extensive expertise in cardiopulmonary assessment and treatment prescription; general experience in medicine and surgery is recommended.
- Detailed understanding of multisystem physiology and pathophysiology and the cardiopulmonary manifestations of systemic disease.
- Ability to practice effectively under pressure and in congested, suboptimal working conditions.
- Knowledge regarding all emergency procedures, including those for respiratory and cardiac arrest, equipment problems, and power failure.
- Knowledge regarding the paging system used in the unit for being contacted as well as for contacting other team members when they are out of the unit or out of the hospital.
- On-call service, 24 hours a day, 7 days a week, is a common practice and should be considered in units without this service.
- Knowledge regarding the roles of all team members.
- Sensitivity toward each patient's psychosocial situation, culture, and values and promotion of active involvement of the patient and family in clinical decision making, whenever feasible.
- Superior communication skills (e.g., ability to work cooperatively with other members of the ICU team [Figure 33-3] and give verbal presentations and discuss patients at rounds).

Goals and General Basis of Management

The ultimate goals of cardiovascular and pulmonary physical therapy in the ICU include the following:

1. Return the patient to his or her premorbid functional level or a higher level if possible
2. Reduce complications, morbidity, premature mortality, and length of ICU and overall hospital stay

As precursors to achieving these goals, the immediate goals relate initially to maximizing oxygen transport, hence, cardiovascular and pulmonary function; and second to maximizing musculoskeletal and neurological function. In the ICU the physical therapist needs to recognize the implications of cardiovascular and pulmonary insufficiency on neuromuscular status and that apparent impairment of neuromuscular status is not necessarily indicative of neurological dysfunction.

Rather, reduced cardiac output and blood pressure, hypoxemia, hypercapnia, and increased intracranial pressure (ICP) may be responsible for these changes indirectly. Musculoskeletal and neurological complications can become life-threatening and therefore need to be detected early and managed.

Key elements of the assessment of the patient in the ICU include risk factors for a suboptimal clinical outcome. In addition to age and comorbidity, risk factors include poor indices of PaO_2 with a high FIO_2, platelet count, cardiac index, blood urea nitrogen, creatinine, and renal function. Other risk factors include peritoneal dialysis or hemodialysis, continuous infusion of antidysrhythmic agents, base deficit, reduced consciousness, pain, and cardiac arrest. Thus patients with one or more of these risk factors, conditions and interventions, require close monitoring and management.

Many elements of the assessment of patients in the ICU are comparable to those for patients with acute conditions who are not critically ill but require respiratory support and mechanical ventilation (see Chapter 44). The primary difference is that for patients in the ICU the adequacy of the steps in the oxygen transport pathway are monitored closely, and the status and function of multiple organ systems are monitored in a serial (repeated at regular or judicious intervals) manner to observe trends over time so that treatment modifications can be titrated to the patient's responses. Serial vital signs including pain and distress are recorded along with arousal and cognitive status, neuromuscular status, musculoskeletal status, and functional mobility. Assessment of functional mobility ranges from the smallest movement to walking (see Figure 33-2 and Box 33-4). Often it includes bed mobility, transfers to chair, and walking, which may require assistive devices. Related laboratory investigations are noted, including the electrocardiogram (ECG), radiographs, scans, blood work, blood sugar level, and fluid and electrolyte balance, and are followed closely to quickly detect improvement or deterioration so that treatment can be correspondingly modified.

Mechanical ventilation and its modes and parameters are described in Chapter 44. The ventilator settings including the fraction of inspired oxygen (FIO_2) are important indicators of changes in the patient's status and therefore must be included in the assessment and recorded at each treatment. Similarly, changes in FIO_2 are important outcomes and indicators of treatment response. This information is used collectively in clinical decision making before, during, and after weaning from mechanical ventilation.

In patients who are medically stable, invasive mechanical ventilation is titrated judiciously to ensure that the patient is initiating breaths as much as possible, which facilitates weaning. Depending on the patient's response to ventilation, however, sedation and neuromuscular blockade may be indicated. These interventions limit the patient's capacity to cooperate fully with treatment. Breathing patterns imposed by the mode of mechanical ventilation influence venous return and aortic pressures[8]; thus mobilization needs to be prescribed accordingly. Furthermore, weaning patients with chronic obstructive pulmonary disease (COPD) and neuromuscular conditions is complicated by respiratory muscle weakness and fatigue (see Chapter 26), which may indicate respiratory muscle training or rest. Because of these challenges, weaning necessitates close cooperation and coordination within the team to maximize weaning success.

As for patients who are not critically ill, the assessment data are evaluated, problems and diagnoses made, and interventions prescribed based on the patient's needs and goals. Physical therapy has a prominent role in the management of patients who are on mechanical ventilation.[9,10] With each treatment, the responses are reviewed and prescription parameters of the interventions are refined to progress the patient

Restricted Mobility and Recumbency

Hospitalization, particularly in the ICU, is associated with a considerable reduction in mobility (i.e., loss of exercise stimulus) and recumbency (i.e., loss of gravitational stimulus) (see Chapters 18 and 20).[11-13] These two factors are essential for normal oxygen transport; thus their removal has dire consequences for the patient with or without cardiovascular and pulmonary dysfunction.

In terms of a physiological hierarchy of treatment interventions (see Chapter 17), exploiting the physiological effects of acute mobilization, upright positioning, and their combination is the most physiologically justifiable primary intervention to maximize oxygen transport and prevent its impairment in patients who are critically ill.

Recumbency is nonphysiological; it is a position in which, all too often, most patients are injudiciously confined. Changing the position of the body from erect to supine positions results in significant physiological changes that may jeopardize the patient's already compromised or threatened oxygen transport system (Box 33-2) (see Chapter 20).

The culmination of these deleterious effects offsets the increased homogeneity of ventilation and perfusion and their

Box 33-2 Physiological Changes When Changing from the Upright to the Supine Position

- Cephalad displacement of the visceral contents and diaphragm
- Compression of the dependent lung fields
- Cephalad fluid shift to the central circulation
- Increased stroke volume and cardiac output and over days a reduction caused by renal compensation
- Decreased total lung capacity
- Decreased vital capacity
- Decreased functional residual capacity
- Decreased residual volume
- Decreased forced expiratory volumes
- Increased airway resistance
- Increased closing volumes of small airways
- Increased restriction of chest wall and decreased diaphragmatic excursion
- Decreased pulmonary and chest wall compliance
- Decreased arterial oxygen levels
- Decreased cough effectiveness
- Increased preload, afterload, and myocardial work
- Decreased myocardial efficiency
- Decreased sympathetic stimulation and decreased peripheral vascular resistance

matching in the supine position. These effects compound the superimposed factors of restricted mobility, recumbency-induced central fluid shifts, prolonged lying without the normal stimulation or will to turn the body, and underlying pathophysiology or trauma that may contribute to impaired cardiovascular and pulmonary function and oxygen transport. Theoretically, the more compromised the patient, the greater the priority to maximize time spent in the upright position in conjunction with exploiting the benefits of acute mobilization.

Specificity of Cardiovascular and Pulmonary Physical Therapy

Physical therapy interventions in the ICU (see Chapter 17 and Part III) are more specifically geared toward the status of each organ system, taking into consideration the pathophysiological basis for the patient's signs and symptoms, the rationale for each intervention, and the physiological and scientific evidence supporting the effectiveness of the intervention.[14] Physical therapy provides both prophylactic and therapeutic interventions for the patient in the ICU. Conservative, noninvasive measures constitute initial treatments of choice to avert or delay the need for additional invasive monitoring and treatment including supplemental oxygen, pharmacological agents, and the need for intubation and mechanical ventilation. The physical therapist aims to avoid, reduce, or postpone for as long as possible the need for respiratory support. Even if the patient is mechanically ventilated, maintaining some level of spontaneous breathing, no matter how minimal, is associated with improved oxygenation and outcomes.[15] In addition, the physical therapist helps to prevent the multitude of side effects of restricted mobility and recumbency during bed rest. A summary of general information required before treatment of the patient in the ICU is presented in Box 33-3. This provides the basis for establishing a patient's readiness to be mobilized and the progressive steps for doing so (Box 33-4 and Figure 33-2).

Maximizing Function

Maximizing function refers to maximizing the capacity to participate in one's life roles and associated activities. This necessitates promotion of optimal physiological functioning at an organ system level, as well as promoting maximal functioning of the patient as a whole. In critical care, primary goals related to function optimization are initially focused on cardiovascular and pulmonary function. With improvement in oxygen transport, increased attention is given to optimal functioning of the patient with respect to self-care, self-positioning, sitting up, and walking. General physical therapy goals related to function optimization are shown in Box 33-5. Outcomes can be tracked objectively by recording the length of time a patient sits over the edge of the bed, sits in a chair at bedside, stands, and walks. Also, the weight a patient lifts as well as the number of repetitions and sets he or she performs can be readily quantified.

Consistent with being primarily a noninvasive practitioner, the physical therapist exploits noninvasive interventions to achieve therapeutic goals. Outcomes related to reduced reliance on invasive interventions are important physical therapy outcomes. These include reducing FIO_2; avoiding mechanical ventilation; minimizing mechanical ventilator support; increasing the amount of spontaneous breathing, even minimally, if the patient is mechanically ventilated; and reducing medication (e.g., bronchodilators, inotropes, chronotropes, sedation, narcotics, and analgesics).

Box 33-3 General Information Required before Treatment of the Patient in the Intensive Care Unit

- Sex and age
- Premorbid status (e.g., lifestyle, ethnicity, culture, work situation, stress, cardiopulmonary conditioning, and oxygen transport reserve capacity)
- Knowledge of patient's life roles and related activities for optimal return to daily life
- Medical and surgical histories
- General multisystem assessment findings
- Pharmacological support
- Smoking history
- Hydration and nutritional status: deficiencies, obesity, or asthenia
- Time of onset and course of present condition
- Existing or potential medical instability
- Indications or necessity for intubation and mechanical ventilation
- Mode and parameters of mechanical ventilation
- FIO_2
- Invasive monitoring, lines, leads, and catheters
- Existence of or potential for complications and multiorgan system failure
- Cognition or coma scale score
- Presence of elevated intracranial pressure (ICP) and the need for ICP monitoring
- Risk or presence and site(s) of infection
- Quality of sleep and rest periods
- Nutritional support during intensive care unit stay
- Pain control regimen

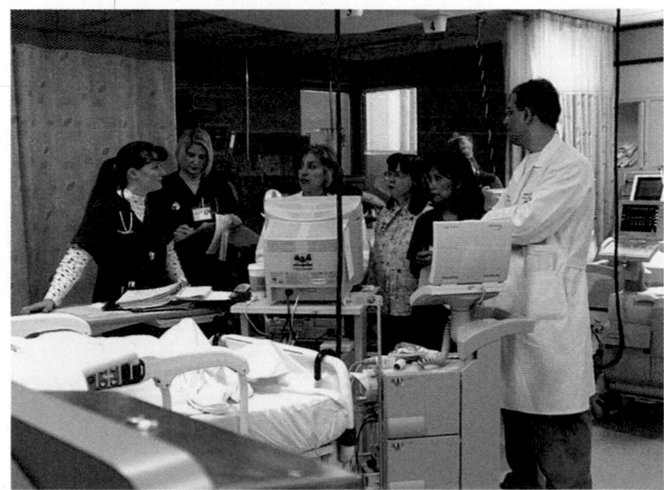

Fig. 33-2 Progressive sequence for mobilizing patients (i.e., being upright and moving).

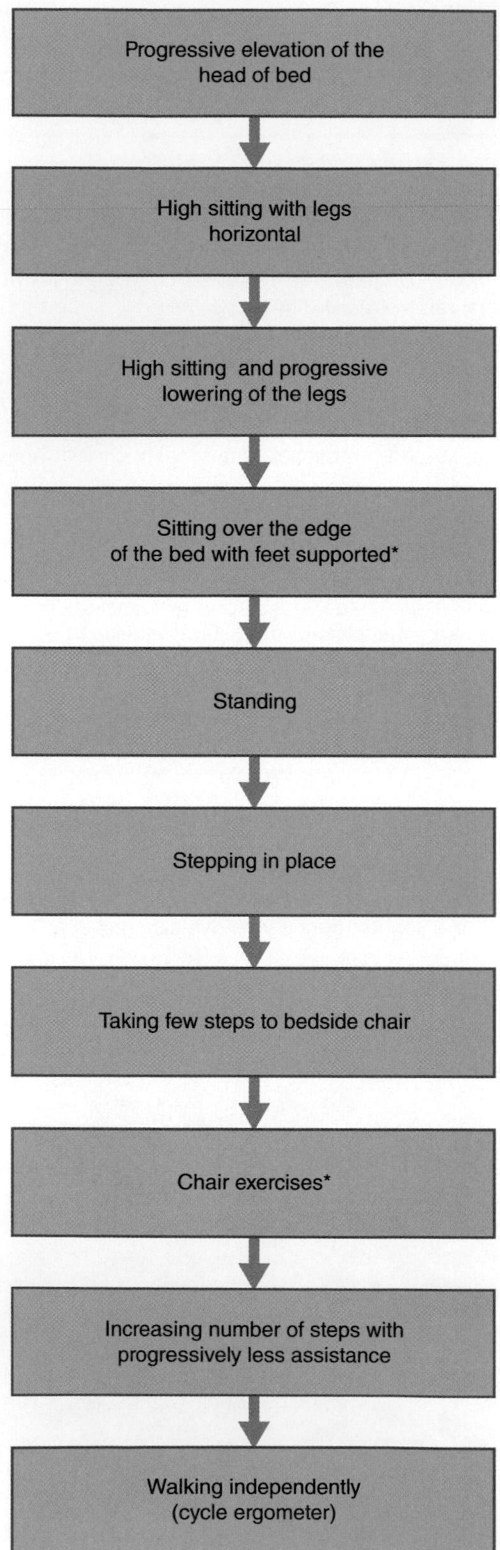

Fig. 33-3 Multidisciplinary rounds in the intensive care unit (ICU). Team work in the ICU is essential to facilitate communication and patient outcome. Note the presence of the nurse, respiratory therapist, pharmacist, social worker, physical therapist, and physician. *When indicated, add resistance muscle exercise with aids and devices such as weights, belts, leg press, and ergometer pedals; progression is based on safety considerations and anticipated therapeutic responses.

Box 33-4 Guiding Principles for Mobilizing Patients in the Intensive Care Unit

Based on a multisystem assessment and discussion with the team:

- Determine the patient's readiness for mobilization—that is, perform multisystem assessment including arousal, medications, lines and leads, mechanical ventilation and respiratory support; responses to gravitational and mobilization challenge tests; contraindications and precautions and clearance by team.
- Establish therapeutic and safe parameters for a given patient based on objective and subjective measures.
- Prescribe the parameters of the gravitational and mobilization stimuli (types of mobilization and exercise, their intensities, duration, and frequencies) by titrating them to the patient's immediate and longer term responses (see Fig 33-2 for progression of mobilization). Principles for progressing the mobilization stimulus:
  - Progression to successive steps is based on the patient's responses.
  - If the patient's physiological responses change appropriately and commensurately with the increment in mobilization load and the patient's condition remains stable, then the next step may be attempted.
  - If untoward responses occur, then the patient can return to the previous level or potentially to sitting or supine to regain resting status.
  - The patient is reassessed before each bout of mobilization and evaluated throughout and afterward.
- Monitor the patient during and after each of the levels shown in the following schema, and record the responses and outcomes.
- Progress patient:
  - Increased intensity. Increase is commensurate with reduction of support and assistance, and increased duration to increase volume of exercise overall, and with improvement—that is, the patient tolerates greater gravitational stress and exercise stress with reduced physiologic demands within therapeutic and safe limits)
  - With increased intensity and increased duration, frequency of the mobilization sessions may be reduced.
  - Some patients quickly progress through these steps, and others progress more slowly based on their individual responses.
- Monitor response to recovery and rest and qualitative and quantitative evaluation of return to resting baseline.

Prophylaxis

General aspects of patient care related to physical therapy practice include the role of prophylaxis or prevention. The complications of restricted mobility and recumbency are described in Chapter 18 and relate primarily to the status of the cardiovascular and pulmonary, neuromuscular, and musculoskeletal systems and overall functional capacity. In the ICU the negative physiological effects of restricted mobility are amplified in patients who are severely ill and older. A primary objective of the physical therapist therefore is to avoid or reduce these untoward effects on the patient's recovery and

Box 33-5 General Physical Therapy Goals toward Function Optimization in the Patient in the Intensive Care Unit

- Establish a detailed baseline of outcome measures and measures to be recorded serially to assess change.
- Maintain or restore adequate alveolar ventilation and perfusion and their matching in unaffected and affected lung fields and thereby optimize oxygen transport overall.
- Prolong spontaneous breathing (to the extent that is therapeutically indicated) and thereby avoid, postpone, or minimize need for mechanical ventilation.
- Minimize the work of breathing.
- Minimize the work of the heart.
- Design a positioning schedule to maintain comfort and postural alignment (distinct from therapeutic body positioning to optimize oxygen transport).
- Maintain or restore general mobility, strength, endurance, and coordination within the limitations of the patient's condition and consistent with the patient's anticipated rehabilitation prognosis (distinct from therapeutic mobilization to optimize oxygen transport).
- Maximally involve the patient in a daily routine including self-care, changing body position, standing, transferring, sitting in a chair, and ambulating in patients for whom these activities are indicated.
- Optimize treatment outcome by interfacing physical therapy with the goals and patient-related activities of other team members; coordinating treatments with medication schedules; and treating the patient specifically, on the basis of both results of objective monitoring available in the intensive care unit and subjective findings.

the patient's length of stay in the ICU. Ventilator-associated pneumonia (VAP) is the most common nosocomial infection in the ICU and is associated with poor outcomes and high cost of ICU care.

Preventive physical therapy goals include reducing the deleterious effects of restricted mobility and pathology on cardiovascular and pulmonary and neuromuscular function and reducing the risk of musculoskeletal deformity, neurological dysfunction, and decubitus ulcers over pressure areas (back of the head, shoulders, elbows, sacrum, and heels). Special mattresses or a special bed may be indicated. The negative sequelae of recumbency and restricted mobility, which can be life-threatening in people who are critically ill, are largely preventable. Particular care must be taken to avoid pressure sores because these increase the risk of infection and deterioration and can be life-threatening. Physical therapists as well as nurses need to pay particular attention to individuals at risk and to examine routinely for sites of redness, pressure, and potential skin lesions in every patient, regardless of expected length of stay in the ICU.[16] The texture of bed covers, their smoothness, bunching of the bed gown, and irritation from lines and catheters to the patient must be routinely monitored. Prevention is key, given the potentially reduced immunity and capacity to heal of patients in the ICU.[17] Although pressure sores are largely preventable, the need to be vigilant remains, given the deleterious consequences they may have on recovery. Unrelieved pressure and equipment failure have been identified as key causes of pressure sores in the patient after trauma.[18] These causes of pressure sores are 100% avoidable with vigilance and monitoring. Physical therapists have a role for making recommendations about patient positioning between treatments in the interest of preventing deleterious sequelae of recumbency and restricted mobility.

Preparation for Treating the Patient in the Intensive Care Unit

Patients in the ICU are generally characterized by some degree of life-threatening medical instability or its risk. Before treating a given patient in the ICU, the physical therapist should be thoroughly familiar with the specific information shown in Box 33-6. Depending on the level of care in the ICU, nursing care is usually 1:1 or 1:2. Coordinating treatment with nursing interventions is efficient. It is helpful to have the nurse at hand to assist as required, particularly if the patient is beginning physical therapy. Alternatively, if the nursing care proved strenuous for the patient, physical therapy may be more beneficial if delayed.

General Clinical Aspects of the Management of the Intensive Care Unit Patient

Assessment and Evaluation

The fundamental assessment procedures for the cardiovascular and pulmonary systems are described in detail in Part II. Laboratory reports, procedures, sputum culture, and radiographs supplement the findings of inspection, palpation, and auscultation of the chest. Of particular importance are the blood work, arterial blood gases (including SaO_2), ECG, fluid and electrolyte balance, hemodynamic monitoring, and ICP monitoring. These are the most commonly monitored parameters in the ICU in addition to vital signs, temperature, respiration rate, heart rate, blood pressure, respiratory distress, and pain.

Although the priority in the ICU is survival, greater attention is now being placed on thriving after the episodes of care in the ICU and hospital (see Chapters 16 and 17). Therefore assessment and evaluation in the ICU focus on activity, participation, and quality of life as well as factors related to conventional oxygen transport deficits and multisystem function, in anticipation of the patient's return to community living.

Monitoring

Maximizing the effects of physical therapy treatment depends on exploiting information from the ICU monitoring systems. Monitoring systems can be used to establish the indications and contraindications for treatment as well as parameters of the treatment prescription and progression, and to assess the patient. Physical therapy uses of monitoring systems in the ICU are summarized in Box 33-7. Physical therapists need to exploit the considerable amount of objective data available to them in patient management. A thorough knowledge and routine use of monitoring systems for each patient in the ICU cannot be overemphasized in terms of contributing to

Box 33-6 Specific Patient Information Required before Treatment of the Patient in the Intensive Care Unit

- Detailed knowledge of the patient's history, including the differential diagnosis on admission to the intensive care unit (ICU) and relevant medical, surgical, and social histories.
- Knowledge of premorbid status related to the International Classification of Functioning, Disability and Health (see Chapters 1 and 17) (i.e., limitations of structure and function [impairment], activities, and social participation [health-related quality of life]—these will provide a baseline of outcome measures on which clinical decisions about ICU discharge and hospital discharge will be made).
- Detailed understanding and knowledge of the medications administered to the patient, their indications, and side effects (especially those affecting response to physical therapy).
- Knowledge regarding the stability of vital signs since admission, including heart rate and rhythm, respiration rate and rhythm, blood pressure, skin color, core temperature, and hemodynamic stability.
- Detailed knowledge of relevant findings of laboratory tests, procedures, and biopsies, including arterial blood gases, blood analysis, fluid and electrolyte balance, electrocardiogram (ECG), radiographs, thoracentesis, central venous pressure (CVP), left atrial pressure (LAP), pulmonary artery wedge pressure (PAWP), microbiology and biochemistry reports, and urinalysis.
- Detailed understanding of the rationale for the ventilatory mode and parameters used if the patient is ventilated.
- With respect to establishing a patient database:
  - Conduct a thorough, detailed clinical assessment specific to the patient's condition(s), including inspection, palpation, percussion, and auscultation of the chest, as well as a neuromusculoskeletal assessment to rule out any secondary effects of cardiopulmonary dysfunction and to establish rehabilitation prognosis.
  - Establish a physical diagnosis and problem list and prioritize the treatment goals and overall treatment plan.
  - Determine the optimal assessment and treatment outcome measures and be knowledgeable about their interpretation.
  - Conduct serial measurements to predict the patient's oxygen transport reserve capacity before treatment and stressing the oxygen transport system.
- As treatment progresses, record objective and relevant subjective treatment outcome measures and revise treatment goals as indicated by the patient's progress.

improved quality of care with less risk to the patient. Subjective responses of the patient are particularly important in the ICU, where the patient's power and self-responsibility are compromised. Eliciting subjective responses can be achieved through a sign system, use of analog scales, and communication devices. The patient needs to be able to communicate basic needs if possible (e.g., discomfort or /pain, anxiety, fear, and general distress). Patients have been reported to experience significant levels of stress when being managed in the ICU—in turn, worsening outcomes.[19]

Box 33-7 Physical Therapy Uses of Monitoring Systems in the Intensive Care Unit

- Establish the indications for and contraindications to cardiopulmonary physical therapy
- Define treatment intensity, duration, and frequency for optimal treatment outcome
- Determine the appropriateness of response to a specific intervention
- Assess the need for supplemental oxygen before, during, and after treatment
- Determine appropriate patient positioning between, during, and after treatments
- Establish whether the patient is responding positively or negatively to treatment or there is no change and whether treatment should be modified or discontinued

The monitoring systems described in Chapter 16 provide essential information with respect to the management of the patient in the ICU. Information regarding arousal, acid-base imbalance, and fluid and electrolyte balance helps to establish specific treatment goals. The Swan-Ganz catheter in situ permits measurement of pulmonary artery pressure and wedge pressure, which provide an index of myocardial sufficiency and specifically left-sided heart function. Central venous pressure gives an indication of fluid loading and the ability of the right side of the heart to cope with changes in circulating body fluids. Pressures related to heart function give the physical therapist an indication of pulmonary status and help to determine whether heart dysfunction is affecting lung function or lung dysfunction is affecting heart function, or both. Cardiovascular and pulmonary stress alerts the physical therapist to modify workloads or the physical demands of treatment to keep the patient medically stable and avoid undue fatigue and deterioration. The physical therapist conducts ongoing monitoring of the patient's responses to invasive care in the ICU (e.g., responses to medication and fluid resuscitation, indications for intervention and refinement of its prescription) to ensure patient safety.

Changes in ECG may reflect heart disease, lung disease, altered acid-base, and electrolyte and fluid balance. The physical therapist is responsible for identifying the patient's heart rhythm and ECG changes, which can be expected with improvement or deterioration in oxygen transport and secondary to medical management, drug intervention, changes in the course of the disease, and response to treatment generally.

Pharmacological Agents

The physical therapist needs a thorough knowledge of the common pharmacological agents used in intensive care (see Chapter 45). With this knowledge, the physical therapist can augment the effects of these agents and optimize physical therapy treatment response when treatments are coordinated with medication schedules. Most medications have optimal dosages for any given patient, optimal sensitivity, and peak response time. Most medications have side effects. Side effects may cause deterioration in the patient's condition, create apparent signs and symptoms suggestive of other disorders, or alter response to treatment. The physical therapist therefore needs to identify the medications each patient is taking and their side effects. Medication that contributes to suboptimal therapeutic outcomes warrants discussion with the team in terms of finding an alternative. One physical therapy outcome is the minimization of medication with effective physical therapy.

Certain medications, such as anxiolytics, bronchodilators, sedatives, mucolytic agents, antianginal medications, and analgesics, help the patient to cooperate and tolerate treatment. Special consideration must always be given to the different peak response times of different medications. The patient can cooperate more actively in the treatment if pain and anxiety are reduced and breathing is easy. An enhanced treatment effect is therefore more likely. These advantages can result in shorter, more cost-effective treatment and more effective use of the physical therapist's time.

Some medication can attenuate a patient's response to mobilization and exercise and activity. Patients on beta-blocking agents, for example, may not show the normal changes in heart rate and blood pressure in response to exercise. In addition, beta-blockers contribute to fatigue. Therefore, caution needs to be observed when prescribing exercise for patients taking beta-blockers. Another classification of drugs called *vasopressor agents* regulates blood pressure and heart rate. Patients taking these agents may also exhibit abnormal mobilization and exercise responses. Monitoring is essential; however, vital signs to assess treatment response may be rather limited for patients taking drugs that act on the cardiovascular system.

Narcotics are a commonly used classification of drug in the ICU and are often administered for their analgesic effects jointly with sedatives and tranquilizers. Despite pain relief, narcotics, particularly in combination with other sedative-type drugs, interfere with physical therapy treatments because of the patient's reduced arousal, monotonous ventilation, and inability to cooperate with treatment. Furthermore, narcotics tend to have multisystem effects rather than localized effects. Because physical therapy is the most physiological and noninvasive intervention available to the patient in the ICU, it behooves the physical therapist to ensure that pharmacological agents that are effective and more selective than narcotics in achieving the desired effect have been considered. Thus as a team member the physical therapist has a major role during rounds to ensure an integrative management program for each patient.

Treatment Prescription in the Intensive Care Unit

Physical therapy treatments in the ICU are judiciously selected in a goal-specific manner. As a general guideline, treatments descend in a physiological hierarchy (Chapter 17). Mobilization, exercise, and body positioning are exploited first with respect to their direct and potent effects on oxygen transport overall.[20] Early mobilization and walking are priorities regardless of whether the patient is mechanically ventilated.[21-23] At the other end of the treatment intervention hierarchy (i.e., least physiological interventions that have a more limited effect on the steps in the oxygen transport pathway overall) are conventional interventions such as airway clearance techniques and suctioning. Assessment of the oxygen uptake and delivery relationship is essential given the high metabolic demands of patients in the ICU[24] and the documented associated exercise and stress responses associated with physical therapy.[25]

Supplemental Oxygen

Supplemental oxygen is usually administered continuously, whether the patient is ventilated or not, to maintain PaO_2 level within an optimal range.[26] Oxygen concentrations can be increased before treatment to help compensate for associated stress. Oxygen, however, should always be increased to 100% and inspired for at least 3 minutes before and after suctioning. Should arterial desaturation be apparent during treatment, oxygen may need to be increased. If the patient is spontaneously breathing without oxygen, supplemental oxygen may also be indicated during treatment to avoid desaturation. Oxygen administration is regulated by the ICU team based on arterial blood gas levels including arterial saturation and subjective distress. Severe hypoxemia is known to result in irreversible tissue damage within minutes, but hyperoxia can also produce harmful effects within hours. By maximizing alveolar ventilation, gas exchange, and ventilation and perfusion matching, supplemental oxygen can be optimally used and the effects of acidemia minimized.

Treatment for respiratory acidosis in individuals with chronic pulmonary disease is aimed at increasing alveolar ventilation to improve the exchange of carbon dioxide and oxygen. Because the respiratory center is depressed by increased amounts of carbon dioxide (carbon dioxide narcosis), the lowered oxygen tension of the blood becomes the stimulus for respiration. If the patient inhales high concentrations of oxygen, the stimulation for respiration may be removed. For this reason, oxygen is never given to patients with carbon dioxide narcosis.

Low-flow oxygen (1 to 3 L/min) is given to a patient with chronic pulmonary disease who maintains a chronically elevated arterial PCO_2 in the presence of arterial hypoxemia. If intermittent positive pressure breathing is indicated, compressed or room air is used instead of oxygen.

Severe hypoxemia usually suppresses cardiac output to some degree. Cardiac output may be further compromised immediately after a patient has been placed on a mechanical ventilator because of impaired venous return resulting from the elevated transpulmonary pressure.[27] An attempt is made to carefully balance ventilation with an optimal or adequate cardiac output by shortening inspiratory time and minimizing transpulmonary pressures by using lower tidal volumes.

Breathing and Coughing Maneuvers

If the patient is nonventilated or was recently extubated, breathing and coughing maneuvers in conjunction with moving and body positioning are emphasized to promote ventilation, flow rates, and secretion clearance; decrease minute ventilation and respiratory rate; increase tidal volume; and improve arterial blood gases. Breathing exercises for individuals who breathe with long-time constants (e.g., patients with chronic pulmonary disease) are believed to be most effective if pursed-lip breathing is performed in conjunction with mechanical pressure applied over the abdomen. To derive the maximum benefits, breathing and coughing maneuvers should be performed in body positions that are most mechanically and physiologically optimal. In addition, they can be performed in the postural drainage positions to augment mucociliary clearance. To avoid airway closure, patients should not breathe below the end of normal tidal ventilation.

Mucociliary Transport and Secretion Clearance

The patient in the ICU needs special attention regarding fluid balance to carefully regulate hydration and fluid volume. Inhaled humidified air is a significant additional source of body fluid. Normally the alveolar gas is saturated with water vapor. The lining of the tracheobronchial tree is therefore protected from erosion and potential infection. This is particularly important in the patient who requires frequent suctioning. The effect of humidification can be assessed by the consistency of the patient's secretions. Thick secretions suggest humidification may be inadequate, and the patient may be dehydrated.

If the effects of mobilization on mucociliary transport and secretion accumulation have been exploited and further secretion clearance is warranted, postural drainage may be indicated. Postural drainage may be contraindicated in patients with unstable vital signs and is usually contraindicated immediately after feedings and meals. In some institutions, however, patients on continuous 24-hour tube feedings are tipped after feeding has been discontinued for 15 minutes. The cuff in the artificial airway is inflated to avoid aspiration. The specific postural drainage positions to be used are determined on the basis of the pathology, radiographs, and clinical examination. The recommended positions for the bronchopulmonary segments involved should be approximated as closely as possible (see Chapter 21) and modified as needed. Frequently, specific positioning in the ICU is compromised as a result of the patient's status, intolerance to lying flat or being tipped, or limitations imposed by the monitoring apparatus or ventilator.

The role of manual techniques has long been questioned because they have been associated with desaturation, atelectasis, musculoskeletal trauma, discomfort, cardiac dysrhythmias, and cardiac arrest.[28] Thus these techniques must be applied rationally, with appropriate monitoring, and modified accordingly. The precise sequence, duration, intensity, and frequency of treatment are based on treatment outcome rather than time. Oxygen demand has been shown to increase with manual airway techniques, and the hemodynamic and metabolic responses have been reported to resemble the response to exercise.[24] The increases in cardiac output and blood pressure are thought to reflect increased sympathetic activity from stress as well as the exercise-like response.[25] The stressful responses to ICU procedures as well as conventional airway clearance procedures have been reported to be effectively modulated with medication.[29] A recent study reported no significant changes in $\dot{V}O_2$ and mean arterial pressure with conventional airway clearance interventions compared with undisturbed side-lying positions.[30] These discrepant findings may reflect differences in the intervention and subjects studied (stable patients who are ventilated). The application of manual techniques in the head-down position is contraindicated in patients with acute myocardial infarction and increased ICP. Relative contraindications include hemorrhage, bronchopulmonary fistula, acute chest trauma, lung abscess, and gastric reflux.[31] Given the adverse effects of manual airway clearance interventions that have been reported, the physical therapist needs to ensure that more physiological alternatives associated with fewer risks have been exploited.

Bagging or Manual Hyperinflation

Although not universally accepted, bagging is practiced to varying degrees in ICUs. The purpose of manually hyperinflating the lungs with a resuscitation bag is to provide extra-large breaths during treatment, to maintain some degree of positive end-expiratory pressure, to assess lung compliance, and to facilitate the effect of instillation of a small volume of saline solution into the tracheobronchial tree to loosen secretions. A self-inflating breathing bag is temporarily connected to the airway. Bagging must be performed cautiously. Aggressive bagging can produce bronchospasm. The lungs are manually inflated for a few breaths. The use of bagging in conjunction with suctioning is controversial. Some clinicians prefer to bag after suctioning to avoid the possibility of the positive pressure pushing the mucus distally. Others maintain that because the mucus adheres to the walls of the airways and because the airways dilate in response to positive pressure, bagging does not propel the mucus distally. Rather, it is believed that bagging before suctioning promotes air entry distal to the mucous plugs and movement of plugs centrally on expiration.

Certain body positions present a particular problem when a pressure-cycled ventilator is being used. The efficiency of the ventilator is greatly reduced when the patient's head is positioned below the hips because of an increase in total pulmonary resistance caused by the pressure of the abdominal contents. Therefore the use of a self-inflating breathing bag may be required to maintain pressure when changing from one position to another and during some postural drainage positions. Adequate tidal volume can be maintained by an assistant while the physical therapist assists the patient with bronchial drainage. With the use of the self-inflating bag, the physical therapist needs to ensure the patient is adequately ventilated and takes a larger than tidal breath every minute or so.

As soon as possible, spontaneous breathing is encouraged in conjunction with postural drainage. The small airways dilate slightly on inspiration and cause mucus to peel away from the walls; thus during expiration, mucus plugs are moved centrally toward the trachea. The degree to which chest wall percussion, shaking, and vibration facilitate this movement has remained equivocal in the literature.[14,28] Thus these less substantiated, less physiological conventional procedures (i.e., manual techniques) should be considered carefully and only after other more supported and physiological treatments have been exploited. Furthermore, because of their documented hemodynamic and adverse effects,[32] it is essential that the patient be continuously monitored for safety reasons and to establish a favorable treatment outcome. For the patient who is unconscious or paralyzed, the ventilator or self-inflating bag can be used to increase inflation volumes. Research is needed to examine the role of bagging in removal of mucus.

Instillation

Instillation is another procedure that should be used selectively in patients. A mucolytic effect of saline has not been well established. Beneficial effects may be more apparent in neonates.

Weaning from the Mechanical Ventilator

Depending on the institution and country, the physical therapist, the respiratory therapist, or both are often responsible for assisting physicians in weaning the patient from mechanical ventilation. Coordinating goals and working with the ICU team to ensure that the weaning process is carried out expediently and with the least risk of weaning complications (e.g., postextubation atelectasis, aspiration, and hypoxemia) are priorities. Expediting weaning is an important ICU goal, as patient outcomes improve with shorter periods of mechanical ventilation.[33] Evidence-based guidelines have been documented.

Weaning can increase cardiovascular and psychological stress, and in turn $\dot{V}O_2$. Patients at particular risk of weaning failure must be identified and monitored by the physical therapist during this process. One study reported that cardiovascular responses to weaning in patients after heart surgery depended on the type of surgery.[34] Cardiac index, for example, was greater after abdominal aortic surgery than after bypass or transplantation surgery. Although the oxygen extraction ratio remained stable after aortic surgery, it increased somewhat after bypass surgery and markedly after transplantation surgery. Weaning patients with cardiac dysfunction from mechanical ventilation can lead to pulmonary edema because of increased venous return and release of catecholamines, reduced left ventricular compliance, compression of the heart by the lungs, and increased left ventricular afterload.

Because of its profound effect on pulmonary function and gas exchange, body position must be optimized for weaning to maximize weaning success and avoid the need for reintubation because of weaning failure. Patients who are overweight warrant particular attention. Low tidal volume and high respiratory rates can jeopardize weaning success. In patients who are obese, a semirecumbent position may favor weaning, compared with a 90-degree upright position, which may cause the abdomen to encroach on the underside of the diaphragm and limit its excursion.[35]

Blood gas analysis and pulmonary function provide the indications for weaning. Ideally the patient's spontaneous tidal volume should approximate that delivered by the ventilator. Forced vital capacity should be two to three times the patient's required tidal volume. Weaning is not usually indicated if the patient requires positive end-expiratory pressure greater than 5 cm H_2O or if FIO_2 is greater than 0.4. In addition, patients who are unable to generate a negative inspiratory pressure of −20 mm Hg or greater are unlikely to be able to generate sufficient intrathoracic pressures for deep breathing and airway clearance and thus are poor candidates for weaning. Minute ventilation and maximum voluntary ventilation can be measured at bedside and contribute to the decision regarding whether to wean. Although weaning protocols differ depending on the patient and the ventilatory mode used, general guidelines for this common ICU procedure are outlined in Box 33-8.

Box 33-8 General Steps in Weaning a Patient from the Mechanical Ventilator

1. An individualized weaning schedule is designed for each patient in which periods of time are spent off the ventilator and on a T tube that delivers appropriate oxygen and humidity.
2. The initial time period off the ventilator is carefully selected; mornings are often good times.
3. (a) Physical activity should be at a minimum during this period (e.g., not during or after physical therapy, not after meals, tests, or procedures, and not during family visits). (b) Supplemental oxygen and humidity are given.
4. The physical therapist offers support and reassurance.
5. Monitoring of vital signs and for signs and symptoms of respiratory distress is performed continuously during weaning.
6. The patient is not left unattended in the initial weaning sessions until periods off the ventilator are reliably tolerated well for several successive minutes.
7. (a) Deterioration of vital signs or blood gases and evidence of distress indicate that the patient will have to return to ventilatory assistance imminently. (b) Rest periods of at least an hour are strategically interspersed in the weaning schedule.
8. Blood gas evaluations are performed at regular intervals (e.g., 15, 30, 60, 90, and 120 minutes, or more or less frequently as indicated).
9. If blood gas levels stabilize to within acceptable limits during the weaning period and the patient is generally tolerating the procedure well, the time off the ventilator is increased.
10. Patients with underlying cardiopulmonary disease who are older, malnourished, or obese or who smoke can be expected to take longer to be completely weaned from the ventilator.
11. Weaning is generally faster in patients who have required a shorter period of mechanical ventilation.
12. To hasten the weaning process, synchronized intermittent mandatory ventilation (SIMV) has been reported to be useful in some patients. Others, however, have observed that the use of SIMV tends to fatigue the patient and delay the patient's progress in weaning. Thus SIMV is used cautiously, and individual variability is considered in terms of its effectiveness. Assist-control ventilation is a well-tolerated alternative.

Special Noninvasive Intensive Care Unit Priorities and Considerations

Intubation and mechanical ventilation are usually delayed as long as possible, particularly in individuals with COPD. These individuals have poor blood gas levels in combination with poor CO_2 ventilatory drive. Once mechanically ventilated, the patient tends to deteriorate rapidly, and the risk of failure to wean is increased. Noninvasive mechanical ventilation (see Chapter 44) has been a more recent advance to provide low-risk ventilatory support as a means of avoiding associated risks of invasive ventilation. It is used for patients in whom short-term mechanical ventilation is anticipated.

Discharge from the Intensive Care Unit

Every ICU should have and use admission and discharge criteria. The criteria may differ from ICU to ICU and hospital to hospital. The discharge criteria are likely to be met in situations in which there is no need for mechanical ventilation, airway protection, or invasive hemodynamic monitoring and there is resolution of the medical problems that necessitated the admission.

The physical therapist is responsible for documenting the physical therapy treatment priorities and frequent progress notes during the ICU stay so that the team responsible for the patient after discharge can continue management with reduced risk of disruption of care or regression of the patient's condition. The patient should be informed continually of his or her progress and the plans made by the team and family.[36] The patient should be given as many choices as possible about his or her care and should be actively involved in long-term management planning.

Nonclinical Aspects of the Management of the Patient in the Intensive Care Unit

Teamwork

Comprehensive patient care in the ICU must include a multidisciplinary team. The ICU team usually includes non–health care professionals and health care professionals. The non–health care professionals include the patient, family or immediate support network, case manager, and possibly a spiritual or religious leader. The health care professionals typically include dieticians, nurses and nursing assistants, occupational therapists, physical therapists, physicians, respiratory therapists, social workers, and speech therapists. Teamwork is the essence of maximal patient care and must include the patient and family as much as possible, particularly in the ICU. The physical therapist interacts frequently with other team members, particularly the medical staff, nurses, and respiratory therapists if in the ICU, regarding observations and changes in the patient's condition, medications, mechanical ventilation requirements, treatment goals, and treatment response (see Figure 33-2). In addition to providing therapy for patients and planning for discharge, the physical therapist is often consulted regarding early mobility, ambulation, body positioning, transferring, chair sitting, and self-care.

Nutrition

Patients who are critically ill are hypermetabolic. Metabolic demand and oxygen consumption are increased after surgery and secondary to healing and repair, increased temperature, and altered thermoregulation. Patients with chronic cardiovascular and pulmonary limitation who are admitted to the ICU are often undernourished because of the effort required to purchase, prepare, and consume food. Furthermore, these patients have increased $\dot{V}O_2$ and energy expenditure secondary to the increased work of breathing. Without adequate nutrition, patients incur the effects of deconditioning faster and are debilitated, less capable of responding optimally to therapy, and more susceptible to infection. Intravenous or external hyperalimentation is typically instituted early to maintain optimal nutritional status and avoid excessive physical wasting and deterioration. If a tracheostomy has been performed, the patient is able to eat normally, provided risk of aspiration is minimal.

Regardless of the means by which nutritional support is provided, carbohydrate may be limited because of the increased CO_2 production resulting from its metabolism.

Infection Control

Infection control has become an even greater concern in hospitals and particularly ICUs now that "superbugs" have become prevalent. Superbugs are microorganisms that are resistant to broad-spectrum antibiotics. The prevalence of these microorganisms has been attributed to the fact that many people today, over the course of their lives, have taken antibiotics, which has made them more susceptible to certain microorganisms and less sensitive to antibiotics. In addition, more patients with critical illness are surviving owing to advances in management. Personal hygiene and good hygienic practice on the part of the physical therapist are mandatory because of the inherently high rate of infection in the ICU and compromised immunity of the patients. Patients in the ICU are prone to infection. Meticulous hand washing with an antiseptic detergent between patients is essential. Soaping for 30 seconds or more with a thorough scrubbing motion followed by thorough rinsing should be carried out. After contact with infected wounds, saliva, blood, pus, vomit, urine, or stool, the physical therapist must be particularly conscientious about washing immediately. Physical protection, including gowning, gloving, capping, and masking, is often required, given the concerns regarding infection, and has in fact become routine practice in many ICUs.

There are several levels of infection control, and there may be differences across ICUs in different hospitals. Some patients need to be protected from infection transmitted across patients in the ICU by health care staff—hence the need for meticulous hand washing. Some patients have types of infections from which the health care staff need protection. Often a combination of both types of precautions is indicated. The physical therapist needs to know the different level of infection control and precautions for each patient. In respiratory isolation, the patient remains in an isolated room for treatment. Masking and gloving will be required, and possibly gowning. Depending on the patient's diagnoses, eye protection may also be required. Contact isolation requires maximal infection control by those who come into contact with the patient; however, the patient can leave the room or restricted area according to the hospital's policies.

The Patient as a Person

Although constraints do exist in the high technology environment of the ICU, the patient's dignity is observed as much as possible regardless of the reason for admission, the level of consciousness, or combative behavior directed toward the ICU staff. Gestures such as using the patient's preferred name, explaining aspects of the patient's care, continually orienting the patient regarding person, place, time, and day, and having an interpreter available if necessary are widely practiced. A supportive caring atmosphere is created in which the patient is free to make choices and ask questions as much as possible. With endotracheal intubation, patients are unable to talk. Communication strategies are assessed to ensure the patient is maximally able to communicate his or her needs and maintain a sense of perceived control. Some strategies include mouthing (silent speech), use of a spelling board, writing, pointing to pictures, and responding with yes and no signs.

Other considerations that must be observed are related to disrobing, modesty, and privacy. These may reflect sex, age, physical image, culture, and individual differences. The patient needs to be asked about his or her comfort level with these and also whether he or she is more comfortable with family present during treatment. Accommodating these individual differences is extremely important if the patient is to be maximally motivated to participate in treatment and adhere to recommendations between treatment sessions.

Patients may be in varying stages of cognitive awareness, from completely comatose to semicomatose to a reduced state of arousal. Patients who are comatose have been reported to have some awareness of their environment and later can recall having been talked about or wanting to communicate and having been unable to do so. In addition, mechanical ventilation is a barrier to communication; thus methods of communicating need to be identified.

The Intensive Care Unit as a Healing Environment

The physical environment of the ICU has a profound effect on the patient's recovery independent of the level of care received. Outside windows with daylight orient the patient to day and night. Other benefits include reduced number and types of complications and reduced length of stay in the ICU and in the hospital overall.[37,38] Also, exposure to daylight may reduce the need for analgesia.[39] Minimizing the sense of social isolation is important, so family is encouraged to be present as much as permitted by the ICU visiting policy. Pet therapy may have some role in the ICU, as it has been shown to have benefits in other care settings.[40] Circadian rhythms are associated with fluctuations in physiological and hormonal functions important to the patient's healing, recovery, and well-being, and these are compromised with bed rest deconditioning. Normalizing circadian rhythms can be achieved by optimizing a sleep schedule with more wakeful periods during the day and reduction of noise at night.[41]

End-of-Life Issues

Palliative care is provided to patients in the ICU with the goal of improving the quality of life of patients and their families facing life-threatening illness. Palliative care treatment focuses on the prevention, assessment, and treatment of pain and other symptoms, as well as the provision of psychological, spiritual, and emotional support. Anticipation of dying and death are traumatic for the patient, family and friends, and the health care team. The phases of dying[42] that can be anticipated when caring for the patient who is at the end of life are presented in Box 33-9.

The psychosocial issues in conjunction with support of the patient's physical status and comfort are priorities.[43] Communicating effectively and being responsive to an individual's dignity and needs are important. Each individual differs with respect to his or her needs, and time must be taken to identify these in an open and honest environment. Touching has a particularly important role in providing support and comfort as the end of life nears.

Box 33-9 Characteristics of the Patient Who Is at the End of Life

- Failure of the peripheral circulation and profuse sweating, causing body cooling
- Loss of strength, motion, and reflexes in the legs and then in the arms
- Decreased sensitivity to touch, deep pressure, and pain tends to remain
- May experience pain, acute loneliness, and fear
- May have increased spiritual needs, particularly at night
- An interval of quiescence just before death
- Can be conscious until death

From Kinney MR, Packa DR: Andreoli's comprehensive cardiac care, *ed 8, St. Louis, Mosby, 1996.*

As the goal shifts from the provision of active treatment to supportive palliative care, the physical therapist needs to adjust treatment accordingly. Comfort and symptom management are the primary goals toward the end of an individual's life. If the patient is able to participate, modified active treatment in conjunction with a high level of support and attention to comfort can be of benefit. As the goals are revised, and if appropriate for the patient, he or she may remain actively engaged in planning and scheduling treatments.

If the patient is unable to cooperate actively with treatment, physical and psychological comfort and symptom management are maximized from a noninvasive perspective to support pharmacological support. Treatments may include relaxation, provision of comfort and human contact, noninvasive pain control strategies, breathing control and coughing maneuvers, and family education.

Principles of Physical Therapy Management

The family and friends of the patient who is dying have special needs that must be considered, and in fact constitute an integral part of the patient's overall care. In general the physical comfort and personal hygiene of the patient, as well as the quality of the immediate psychosocial environment, are paramount concerns. Optimal functional capacity is maintained as much as possible[44] and has been shown to improve even in patients whose course is unstable.[45] Nonetheless, the individual's priorities and needs may change quickly. The physical therapist needs to be flexible to accommodate these fluctuations and sensitive to indications for no intervention. This may be a time for providing support and touching, if the patient wishes. Compassion, understanding, and respect for the patient and the family must be forthcoming from the ICU team as a whole. The ability to be attentive, comforting, and compassionate is an invaluable personal quality that needs to be developed to a high degree in the critical care area. The team members need to attend to how the patient, if sufficiently alert, is dealing with the possibility of dying and must take their cues from the patient with respect to the role they need to play. If requested by the patient or family, spiritual care leaders are summoned.

If life support systems are being continued, the physical therapist may provide treatment to keep the patient as comfortable as possible. Conservative prophylactic cardiovascular and pulmonary physical therapy may be provided to reduce the work of breathing (body positioning and stress reduction, both of which can minimize oxygen cost). Treatments are kept to a minimum in terms of number and duration if death is inevitable. Range-of-motion exercises and skin care may help to reduce the discomfort of restricted mobility, facilitate nursing management and the basic care of the patient, and prevent complications. Analgesics may be continued along with other medications to reduce pain and suffering and maximize comfort. If so, these are prudently coordinated with treatments, if appropriate. In the presence of life supports the patient's needs may have to be anticipated somewhat more than without life supports because they severely limit communication. The dignity and modesty of the patient continue to be observed even after death.

The patient who has had life supports removed receives the same level of palliative care as the patient with supports. Weakness and wasting may contribute to the fatigue induced by treatment and coughing. Facilitated and supported coughing may help reduce the effort required to cough productively.

One's humanity is one of the most important attributes a health care provider can bring to the care of patients, and this is particularly true in palliative care. The use of human touch and talking (or being silent) may be the most important means of communicating with and providing support to the patient who is dying and may be unable to communicate or disinterested in doing so. Supportive touching and handholding may be even more important to the patient on life support systems, as the supports may be experienced as a physical barrier between the patient and those around him or her.

Summary

Cardiovascular and pulmonary physical therapy in the ICU is a unique subspecialty. Despite the high-tech environment and severity of illness, most people are discharged after their ICU stays, which are highly variable in duration. Management focuses on returning the patient to a premorbid level of function or higher and in the process minimizing morbidity, premature mortality, and length of hospital stay. The general goals of critical care are maximizing function (consistent with the International Classification of Functioning, Disability and Health) and prophylaxis. Specific primary goals are defined by the underlying cardiovascular and pulmonary pathophysiology and multisystem dysfunction and their sequelae. Specific secondary goals are defined by the presence of or the potential for complications including musculoskeletal and neuromuscular dysfunction. Early mobilization that is safe, feasible, and effectively prescribed is essential both for its direct and potent effects of oxygen transport and minimization of complications and as a precursor for transitioning the patient effectively to community living. Strong interprofessional teamwork and an ICU culture that promotes early mobilization can maximize the effectiveness of this intervention. This chapter elaborated on general aspects of managing the physical therapy priorities of patients in the ICU. The knowledge base and experience of physical therapists practicing in the ICU were presented. A broad overview of the objectives of treatment and the rationale for prioritizing treatments according to a physiological hierarchy were described. General clinical and nonclinical aspects of patient management were discussed. Finally, end-of-life issues of relevance to the physical therapist in the ICU were presented.

Review Questions

1. Describe the elements of evidence-based practice in cardiovascular and pulmonary physical therapy.
2. Describe the general goals and principles of cardiovascular and pulmonary physical therapy in the ICU.
3. How do these goals reflect the International Classification of Functioning, Disability and Health (i.e., limitations in participation and activity as well as structure and function)?
4. Explain the role of monitoring in cardiovascular and pulmonary physical therapy of the patient who is critically ill.
5. Describe what is meant by "bringing one's humanity" to the management of people who are critically ill.
6. End-of-life issues are not a concern in only the ICU. What attributes of the physical therapist are especially important in managing an individual at the end of life, irrespective of setting?

References

1. Barlow DH, Hayes SC, Nelson RO: *The scientist practitioner: research and accountability in the age of managed care.* Boston, 1999, Allyn & Bacon.
2. Cook DJ, Sibbald WJ, Vincent J-L, et al: Evidence based critical care medicine: what is it and what can it do for us? *Crit Care Med* 24:334–337, 1996.
3. Dean E: Oxygen transport: a physiologically-based conceptual framework for the practice of cardiopulmonary physiotherapy. *Physiotherapy* 80:347–355, 1994.
4. Ross J, Dean E: Integrating physiological principles into the comprehensive management of cardiopulmonary dysfunction. *Phys Ther* 69:255–259, 1989.
5. Thomas DC, Kreizman IJ, Melchiorre P, et al: Rehabilitation of the patient with chronic critical illness. *Crit Care Clin* 18:695–715, 2002.
6. Dean E: Invited commentary to "Are incentive spirometry, intermittent positive pressure breathing, and deep breathing exercises effective in the prevention of postoperative pulmonary complications after upper abdominal surgery? A systematic overview and meta-analysis." *Phys Ther* 74:10–15, 1994.
7. Kelly KM: Does increasing oxygen delivery improve outcome? Yes. *Crit Care Clin* 12:635–644, 1996.
8. Frédéric M: Changes in arterial pressure during mechanical ventilation. *Anesthesiology* 103:419–428, 2005.
9. Pohlman MC, Schweickert WD, Pohlman AS, et al: Feasibility of physical and occupational therapy beginning from initiation of mechanical ventilation. *Crit Care Med* 38:2089–2094, 2010.
10. Schweickert, WD, Pohlman, MC, Pohlman, AS, et al: Early physical and occupational therapy in mechanically ventilated, critically ill patients: a randomised controlled trial. *Lancet* 373:1874–1882, 2009.
11. Dean E: Physiotherapy skills: positioning and mobilization of the patient. In Pryor JA, Ammani Prasad S, Webber BA, editors: *Physiotherapy for respiratory and cardiac problems: adults and paediatrics*, ed 3, St. Louis, 2002, Harcourt Health Sciences Group.
12. Timmerman RA: A mobility protocol for critically ill adults. *Dimens Crit Care Nurs* 26:175–178, 2007.

13. Vollman KM: Progressive mobility in the critically ill. *Crit Care Nurs* 30:S3–S16, 2010.
14. Dean E, Ross J: Discordance between cardiopulmonary physiology and physical therapy. *Chest* 101:1694–1698, 1992.
15. Hedenstierna G, Lattuada M: Gas exchange in ventilated patients. *Curr Opin Crit Care* 8:39–44, 2002.
16. Stillwell S: *Mosby's critical care nursing reference*. St Louis, 1992, Mosby.
17. Williams DT, Harding K: Healing responses of skin and muscle in critical illness. *Crit Care Med* 31:S547–S557, 2003.
18. O'Sullivan KL, Engrav LH, Maier RV, et al: Pressure sores in the acute trauma patient: incidence and causes. *J Trauma* 42:276–278, 1997.
19. Schelling G, Richter M, Roozendaal B, et al: Exposure to high stress in the intensive care unit may have negative effects on health-related quality-of-life outcomes after cardiac surgery. *Crit Care Med* 31:1971–1980, 2003.
20. Hopkins RO, Spuhler VJ, Thomsen GE: Transforming ICU culture to facilitate early mobility. *Crit Care Clin* 23:81–86, 2007.
21. Bell L: Achieving early mobility in mechanically ventilated patients. *Am J Crit Care* 18:222, 2009.
22. Needham DM: Mobilizing patients in the intensive care unit. Improving neuromuscular weakness and physical function. *J Am Med Assoc* 305:437–522, 2011.
23. Perme C, Chandrashekar R: Early mobility and walking program for patients in intensive care units: creating a standard of care. *Am J Crit Care* 18:212–221, 2009.
24. Weissman C, Kemper M: Stressing the critically ill patient: the cardiopulmonary and metabolic responses to an acute increase in oxygen consumption. *J Crit Care* 8:100–108, 1993.
25. Horiuchi K, Jordan D, Cohen D, et al: Insights into the increased oxygen demand during chest physiotherapy. *Crit Care Med* 25:1347–1351, 1997.
26. Dantzker DR, Schay SM, Fletcher J: *Cardiopulmonary critical care*, ed 3, Philadelphia, 1997, Elsevier.
27. Jardin F, Farcot JC, Boisante L, et al: Influence of positive end-expiratory pressure on left ventricular performance. *N Engl J Med* 304:387–392, 1981.
28. Kirilloff LH, Owens GR, Rogers RM, et al: Does chest physical therapy work? *Chest* 88:436–444, 1985.
29. Cohen D, Horiuchi K, Kemper M, et al: Modulating effects of propofol on metabolic and cardiovascular and pulmonary responses to stressful intensive care unit procedures. *Crit Care Med* 24:612–617, 1996.
30. Berney S, Denehy L: The effect of physiotherapy treatment on oxygen consumption and hacmodynamics in patients who are critically ill. *Aust J Physiother* 49:99–105, 2003.
31. Lynn-McHale DJ, Carlson, KK: *AACN procedure manual for critical care*, ed 4, Philadelphia, 2000, Elsevier.
32. Patman S, Jenkins S, Bostock S, et al: Cardiovascular responses to manual hyperinflation in post-operative coronary artery surgery patients. *Physiother Theory Pract* 14:5–12, 1998.
33. MacIntyre NR: Evidence-based guidelines for weaning and discontinuing ventilatory support. A Collective Task Force Facilitated by the American College of Chest Physicians; the American Association for Respiratory Care; and the American College of Critical Care Medicine. *Chest* 120(6 Suppl):375S–396S, 2001.
34. De Backer D, El Haddad P, Preiser JC, et al: Hemodynamic responses to successful weaning from mechanical ventilation after cardiovascular surgery. *Intensive Care Med* 26:1201–1206, 2000.
35. Burns SM, Egloff MB, Ryan B, et al: Effect of body position on spontaneous respiratory rate and tidal volume in patients with obesity, abdominal distension and ascites. *Am J Crit Care* 3:102–106, 1994.
36. Curtis JR, White DB: Practical guidance for evidence-based ICU family conferences. *Chest* 134:835–843, 2008.
37. Gelling L: Causes of ICU psychosis: the environmental factors. *Nurs Crit Care* 4:22–26, 1999.
38. Keep P, James J, Inman M: Windows in the intensive therapy unit. *Anaesthesia* 35:257–262, 1980.
39. Walch J, Rabin B, Day R, et al: The effect of sunlight on postoperative analgesic medication use: a prospective study of patients undergoing spinal surgery. *Psychosom Med* 67:156–163, 2005.
40. Cullen L, Titler M, Drahozai R: Family and pet visitation in the critical care unit. *Crit Care Nurse* 23:62–67, 2003.
41. Shiraishi M, Kamo T, Nemoto S, et al: Blood pressure variability during 120-day head-down bed rest in humans. *Biomed Pharmacother* 57(Suppl 1):35S–38S, 2003.
42. Kinney MR, Packa DR: *Andreoli's comprehensive cardiac care*, ed 8, St. Louis, MI, 1996, Mosby.
43. Kuhl D: *What dying patients want: practical wisdom for the end of life*. Toronto, 2002, Random House of Canada Ltd.
44. Santiago-Palma J, Payne R: Palliative care and rehabilitation. *Cancer* 92:1049–1052, 2001.
45. Sliwa JA, Marciniak C: Physical rehabilitation of the cancer patient. *Cancer Treat Res* 100:75–89, 1999.

VI

Chapter 34

Intensive Care Management of Individuals with Primary Cardiovascular and Pulmonary Dysfunction

Elizabeth Dean and Christiane Perme

KEY TERMS

Cardiovascular and pulmonary failure
Coronary artery disease
Obstructive lung disease
Primary cardiovascular and pulmonary dysfunction
Restrictive lung disease
Status asthmaticus

CHAPTER OUTLINE

This chapter presents the principles of cardiovascular and pulmonary physical therapy in the management of patients who are critically ill with primary cardiovascular and pulmonary dysfunction that can lead to cardiovascular and pulmonary failure. Common conditions seen by physical therapists in the intensive care unit (ICU) that are presented include obstructive lung disease, status asthmaticus, restrictive lung disease, and coronary artery disease (medical and surgical conditions). Each condition is presented in two parts. The related pathophysiology and pertinent aspects of the medical management of each condition are presented as a basis for and in relation to the principles of physical therapy management. These are not mutually exclusive for each category because considerable overlap may exist when conditions coexist. Invasive care and noninvasive care have common goals and thus are complementary. Special considerations for the physical therapy management of patients in the ICU, predominantly for mobilization and body positioning, are highlighted for the conditions described.

The principles of physical therapy management that are described are not treatment prescriptions. Rather, each patient must be assessed and treated individually, taking into consideration all factors that contribute to impaired oxygen transport (i.e., recumbency, restricted mobility, extrinsic factors related to the patient's care, intrinsic factors related to the patient, and the underlying pathophysiology) (see Chapter 2).

Cardiovascular and Pulmonary Failure

Pathophysiology and Medical Management

The heart and lungs work interdependently; thus failure of one organ has implications for the function of the other organ. Insufficiency or failure of the cardiovascular and pulmonary systems refers to the inability of these systems to maintain adequate oxygen and carbon dioxide homeostasis.

Pulmonary failure reflects a gas exchange defect or defect of the ventilatory pump. Table 34-1 shows the classification of pulmonary failure by specific causes and the mechanisms involved. Some common predisposing conditions include primary cardiovascular and pulmonary conditions (e.g., chronic lung disease, overwhelming pneumonia, and myocardial infarction [MI]) and cardiovascular and pulmonary conditions that are secondary to other conditions (e.g., motor neuron diseases, spinal cord injury, stroke, and muscular dystrophy) (see Chapter 35). The oxygen and carbon dioxide tensions that have been used to define failure are variable because they depend on factors such as premorbid status, general health, age, prior blood gas profile, and the time frame for the development of failure. Arterial blood gases and pH are essential in the assessment of cardiovascular and pulmonary failure, which is usually diagnosed when the PaO_2 falls below 50 to 60 mm Hg and the $PaCO_2$ rises above 50 mm Hg.[1]

Primary cardiac failure reflects failure of the myocardium to pump blood to the pulmonary and systemic circulations and maintain adequate tissue perfusion. Significant dysfunction of the left ventricle can lead to pulmonary vascular congestion and cardiogenic pulmonary edema (i.e., congestive heart failure). Conditions affecting the heart that can lead to failure include significant myocardial damage as a result of infarction or myopathy, valvular heart disease, and congenital defects.

Both primary pulmonary and cardiac failure can be classified into acute and chronic stages. The compensation mechanisms that occur in the two stages are distinct. With adequate physiological compensation, patients can tolerate some degree of chronic failure. Patients with a mild degree of failure can live reasonably independent lives. Moderate failure is significantly more limiting; these patients may require home ventilatory support (e.g., supplemental oxygen and nighttime ventilation). Severe failure necessitates hospitalization, mechanical ventilatory support, and supplemental oxygen support.

Obstructive Lung Disease

Pathophysiology and Medical Management

Obstructive lung disease can result in ventilatory failure and admission of the patient to the ICU, or it can complicate management if the patient is admitted for other reasons.[2] If conservative management fails or is unlikely to improve critically impaired oxygen transport and gas exchange and to adequately remove copious and tenacious secretions, intubation and mechanical ventilation are indicated (see Chapter 43). Complicating factors include impaired oxygen delivery, polycythemia, impaired respiratory mechanics secondary to lung damage and increased time constants impairing optimal inhalation and exhalation, flattened hemidiaphragms, rigid barrel-shaped chest wall, increased accessory muscle use and work of breathing, reduced diffusing capacity, impaired mucociliary transport, secretion accumulation, ineffective cough mechanism, increased oxygen consumption, increased work of the heart, and general debility and weakness.

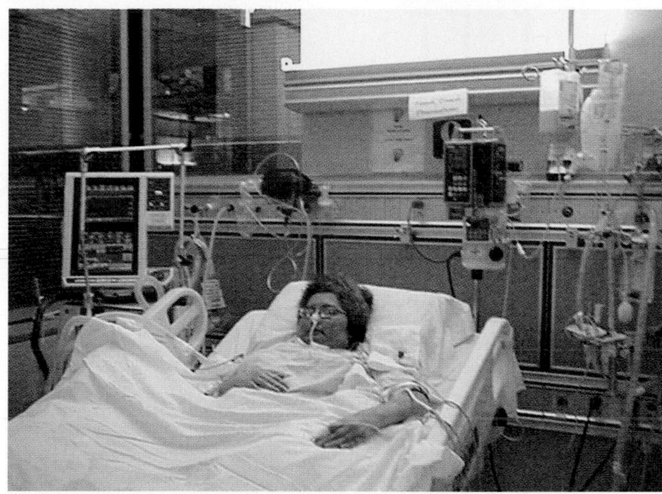

Fig. 34-1 Patient receiving mechanical ventilation.

The goal of intubation and mechanical ventilation is to support breathing by providing an airway and adequate alveolar ventilation and is based on arterial blood gas analysis. A tidal volume and a respiratory rate that provide satisfactory blood gas and pH values are established and maintained unless the clinical condition changes. The precise regulation of mechanical ventilation helps to restore adequate blood gases and cardiovascular and pulmonary function, reduce the work of breathing, rest fatigued ventilatory muscles, and provide an optimal fraction of inspired oxygen (FIO_2) and humidification (Figure 34-1).

Minute ventilation can be seriously impaired with a leak in the mechanical ventilator circuitry. The tubes connecting sites are often the sites of air leakage. Complete disconnection at the endotracheal or tracheostomy connection may inadvertently occur in patients with high pulmonary resistance. Close monitoring of the exhaled tidal volume and end-tidal carbon dioxide will ensure that the patient is receiving sufficient ventilation.

Positive end-expiratory pressure (PEEP) is useful in promoting greater opportunity for gas exchange at end-expiration in mechanically ventilated patients. Venous return, myocardial perfusion, and cardiac output, however, may be impaired during positive-pressure ventilation with PEEP administration.[3] Excessive stimulation to cough in these ventilated patients should be avoided because this accentuates the cardiovascular side effects of PEEP. Continuous positive airway pressure (CPAP) can maintain airway patency during spontaneous ventilation. This mode of ventilation, however, seems to be preferred in children, whereas PEEP is used more commonly in adults.

Interference with the gag reflex in the patient with an endotracheal tube increases the risk of aspiration of the oropharyngeal and gastric contents and can result in pneumonitis and pneumonia. Risk of aspiration from the oropharyngeal cavity can be reduced by suctioning through the airway with the cuff of the airway inflated, in addition to suctioning the oropharynx after suctioning via the airway.

Suctioning can be performed frequently in a patient with an artificial airway and is less traumatic. Patients should be suctioned only as indicated because this procedure can

Table 34-1 Classification of Respiratory Failure by Cause and Mechanism

Origin	Drugs	Metabolic	Neoplasms	Infections	Trauma	Other
Brain	Narcotics Barbiturates Sedatives Poisons Anesthetics	Hyponatremia Hypocalcemia Hypercapnia Alkalosis Hyperglycemia Myxedema	Primary Metastatic	Meningitis Encephalitis Abscess Bulbar polio	Direct injury Increased pressure	Central alveolar hypoventilation Obstructive sleep apnea
Nerves and muscles	Curariform drugs Arsenic Aminoglycosides	Hypophosphatemia Hypomagnesemia	Primary Metastatic	Polio Tetanus	Direct injury	Motor neuron disease Myasthenia gravis Multiple sclerosis Muscular dystrophy Guillain-Barré syndrome
Upper airway			Tonsillar adenoid hyperplasia Goiter Polyps Malignant tumors	Epiglottitis Laryngotracheitis	Vocal cord paralysis Tracheomalacia Cricoarytenoid arthritis Laryngeal edema	
Chest bellows					Flail chest Burn with keloids	Scleroderma Pleural interposition (fibrosis, fluid, tumor, air) Spondylitis Scoliosis Kyphosis
Contributing factors						Massive obesity Ascites Ileus Pain Recumbency
Lower airway and parenchyma				Viral (bronchiolitis, bronchopneumonia) Bacterial (bronchitis, pneumonia, abscess, bronchiectasis) Fungal Mycoplasma	Contused lung	Bronchospasm Heart failure: congestive, restrictive, obstructive COPD Respiratory distress syndrome Interstitial lung disease Atelectasis Cystic fibrosis Pulmonary emboli

From Civettia, J.M. Taylor, R.W. & Kirby, R.R (1988). *Critical care*, Philadelphia: JB Lippincott.

produce significant desaturation (up to 60%), particularly in the ventilated patient.[4] Administration of 100% oxygen for 3 minutes before and after suctioning (i.e., hyperoxygenation) minimizes this desaturation effect. This can be accomplished by manual bagging before treatment (i.e., manual hyperventilation) or by presetting of the mechanical ventilator. Risk of aspiration of gastric contents is reduced by the use of a nasogastric tube.

A common cause of acute respiratory failure is advanced chronic airflow limitation.[5] The pathophysiological deficits include significant loss of alveolar tissue, increased compliance of alveolar tissue, hyperinflated chest wall, impaired respiratory mechanics, flattened hemidiaphragms, impaired breathing efficiency, and reduced diffusing capacity. Proportional changes in lung volumes and capacities in patients with chronic airway limitation compared with healthy persons are presented in Figure 9-5. The primary abnormalities are significantly increased residual volume and inspiratory reserve volume and hence total lung capacity. Failure of oxygen transport ensues secondary to ventilation and perfusion mismatch, ventilatory muscle fatigue, reactive pulmonary hypertension, and right ventricular failure. Correcting the complications of respiratory failure, however, is often more problematic than treating the specific cause. Hypoxemia and hypercapnia are often present. Hypoxemia is usually improved with supplemental oxygen in the absence of significant diffusion defect or shunt.

Cardiovascular complications are among the most prevalent observed in ventilatory failure. Marked hypercapnia (increased arterial P_{CO_2}) with acidemia (reduced pH) can produce extreme vasodilatation and hypotension resulting from the local action on blood vessels.[2] Mild hypercapnia can produce reflex vasoconstriction and hypertension. Occasionally, systemic hypertension is observed during weaning from the ventilator with the presence of a moderate degree of hypercapnia.

Right-sided heart failure (formerly called cor pulmonale) is a well-known complication of chronic lung disease and congestive heart failure. Both hypoxia and reduced pH cause pulmonary vasoconstriction and an increase in pulmonary artery pressure. Consequently, reversing bronchospasm, hypoxemia, hypercapnia, and acidemia can often reduce pulmonary vasoconstriction, lower pulmonary artery pressure, and thereby improve hemodynamics.

End-stage respiratory failure results in a progressive increase in airway resistance, work of breathing, oxygen consumption, and carbon dioxide production. In areas of bronchial obstruction, marked alveolar hypoventilation results and ventilation and perfusion are severely mismatched. Hypoxemia and respiratory acidosis produce reactive pulmonary hypertension and further ventilatory failure. Profound carbon dioxide retention, refractory hypoxemia, and respiratory acidemia may terminate in a fatal dysrhythmia.[6]

Acidemia from respiratory causes with a pH of less than 7.25 is often harmful with respect to dysrhythmia production. Conversely, hypoventilation is equally harmful, and pH elevations greater than 7.5 may cause neurological and cardiovascular complications. In acute respiratory failure with profound acidemia, intravenous bicarbonate is used to buffer the hydrogen ion concentration until the underlying disorder has been corrected. Bicarbonate infusion is guided by frequent pH measurements.

Transport of oxygen and carbon dioxide to and from the tissues depends on adequate pulmonary and systemic circulation. Frequently, blood volume has to be restored by fluids or blood replacement or both. Inotropic agents are used to maintain adequate circulation by augmenting myocardial contractility.

Of increasing interest in recent years has been the experience of illness and its contribution to disability. After their first episode of respiratory failure, patients with chronic obstructive pulmonary disease (COPD) report worse cognitive function and overall health status. After several months, however, these conditions may return to levels reported by individuals with similar disease severity who are being conservatively managed and have had no ICU admission.[7] The Nottingham Health Profile and Mini-Mental State Examination can be useful tools for ongoing assessment of perceived health and cognition.

Principles of Physical Therapy Management

The principles of management of acute respiratory failure secondary to an exacerbation of COPD are based on interventions that will enhance oxygen transport (i.e., oxygen delivery, oxygen consumption, and oxygen extraction) and facilitate carbon dioxide removal. Thus the steps of the oxygen transport pathway that have been identified as impaired or threatened by the patient's condition (i.e., restricted mobility, recumbency, and extrinsic and intrinsic factors in addition to the underlying pathophysiology) (see Chapter 2) are the focus of treatment.[8] On the basis of a detailed analysis of these factors, treatments are selected, prioritized, and applied to optimize the steps in the pathway that are affected. These may include treatments to maximize the patency of the airways, increase alveolar ventilation, facilitate mucociliary transport, facilitate airway clearance, optimize the mechanical position of the diaphragm, optimize ventilation and perfusion matching, optimize pH, eliminate carbon dioxide, optimize peripheral circulation and tissue perfusion, and reduce the work of breathing and of the heart. To optimize oxygen transport, the primary goals of physical therapy management include the following:

1. Improve or maintain arterial oxygen tension (Pa_{O_2}) or prevent its deterioration
2. Improve or maintain arterial oxygen saturation (Sa_{O_2}) or prevent its deterioration
3. Improve or maintain arterial carbon dioxide levels (Pa_{CO_2}) and pH or prevent their deterioration
4. Optimize oxygen delivery and oxygen consumption relationship

The means by which these goals are fulfilled depends on each patient's clinical presentation and the specific factors that contribute to cardiovascular and pulmonary dysfunction.

Mobilization: Special Considerations

Mobilization and ambulation are required for normal physiological functioning of the human body (i.e., to stimulate exercise stress and gravitational stress and thereby optimize oxygen transport).[9,10] Although patients in the ICU are encouraged to move, exercise, sit up, stand, sit in chairs, take a few steps, and in some circumstances ambulate across the unit even if they are ventilated, therapeutic mobilization is prescribed to exploit its acute effects, long-term cumulative effects, and preventive effects (see Chapter 18). These effects are physiologically distinct and need to be prescribed specifically to address each patient's problems. With the monitoring capability in the ICU to ensure safety, patients who are critically ill can move and be moved within safe as well as therapeutic limits.

Given that cardiovascular and pulmonary physical therapy is among those activities that are the most metabolically demanding for patients in the ICU,[11-14] the patient's capacity to meet a given increase in oxygen demand must be determined before treatment. Even though cardiovascular and pulmonary physical therapy stresses the oxygen transport system as a means of improving the function and efficiency of this system, unnecessary or excessive energy expenditure is undesirable and thus should be minimized. Interventions that can minimize oxygen demand include relaxation, judicious body positioning to facilitate oxygen transport, coordination of treatments with other interventions, scheduling of treatments at appropriate times, timing of treatments with medications so the maximal effect is achieved, pain control, and coordination of treatments with peak energy periods and around rest periods.

Mobilization and exercise are at the top of the hierarchy of physiological treatments in the management of patients in the ICU[15-17]; therefore the potent and direct effects of these interventions are exploited first (see Chapter 17). Being moved to (passive) or moving into (active) the upright position promotes improved cardiovascular and pulmonary function and gas exchange. A supported chair should be available beside every ICU bed to provide greater opportunity for the patient to be upright when out of bed. The benefits of the upright sitting position are different from those of sitting propped up in bed. Stretcher chairs are particularly useful for patients who are unable to bear weight (Figure 34-2). There are also beds that are designed to position patients sitting. Even minimal ability of the patient to assist with his or her bed mobility and transferring must be exploited, even if the maneuver takes several minutes and multiple assistants. These minimal efforts must be exploited, or the patient's oxygen transport system will decondition further, which also will reduce the patient's tolerance for being mobilized. What justifies this time and personnel cost is the greater therapeutic outcome that can be expected compared with passive interventions. The ultimate goal is enhanced recovery, reduced discomfort, reduced morbidity and mortality, and reduced ICU and hospital stay.

Significant benefit can be gained from standing the ventilated patient, provided there are no absolute contraindications to being upright in terms of cardiovascular and pulmonary function, neuromuscular and musculoskeletal status, and skin integrity. Ambulating the patient who is ventilated is the priority whenever possible.[18-20] The potential risks, however, must be recognized. In a prospective study, Bailey and colleagues (2007)[21] documented a total of 1449 "activity events" in 103 patients with respiratory failure. These activity events included 233 (16%) instances of sitting on the bed, 454 (31%) instances of sitting in a chair, and 762 (53%) instances of ambulating. In patients with an endotracheal tube, there were 593 activity events reported, of which 249 (42%) were ambulation. Fewer than 1% adverse activity-related events were reported (including fall to the knees without injury, feeding tube removal, systolic blood pressure greater than 200 mm Hg, systolic blood pressure less than 90 mm Hg, and desaturation less than 80%). No patient was extubated during an activity event. Thus activity and mobilization are feasible and safe in patients with respiratory failure. Of note, the majority of survivors (69%) were able to ambulate over 100 feet at discharge from the ICU. These findings have been corroborated by others.[22,23] Mobilization and exercise must be prescribed specifically, however, to ensure that the exercise stimulus is therapeutic (i.e., provides an adequate stressor to the oxygen transport pathway yet is not hazardous).

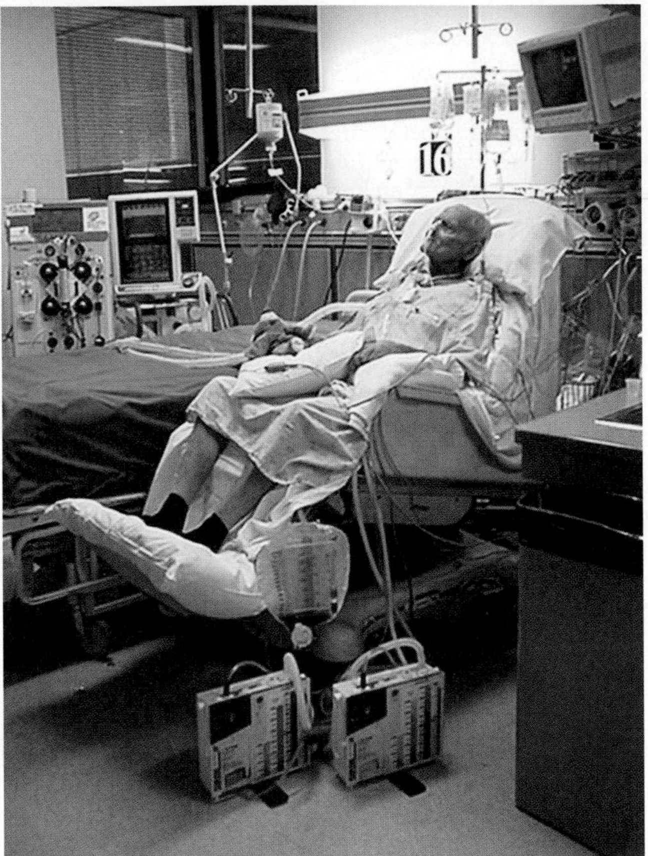

Fig. 34-2 Intensive care unit patient sitting in a stretcher chair.

Standing and walking even a few steps can be extremely strenuous with respect to oxygen demand for the patient in the ICU. Such activities need to be introduced gradually and with continuous monitoring to ensure that the patient does not exceed the prescribed therapeutic intensity needed to maximize oxygen transport. Standing and walking are coordinated with other aspects of the patient's care and should be carried out in several stages (Figure 34-3). Monitoring of the electrocardiogram (ECG) and arterial saturation of the critically ill patient while he or she performs activities such as standing or walking cannot be overemphasized. In anticipation of an increased workload, ventilatory parameters for ventilated patients may require adjusting. A greater concentration of oxygen should be delivered for at least 3 to 5 minutes before the activity and continued afterward for 10 minutes or so until the patient has recovered from the increased exertion and the heart rate and blood pressure have returned to within 5% to 10% of baseline values.

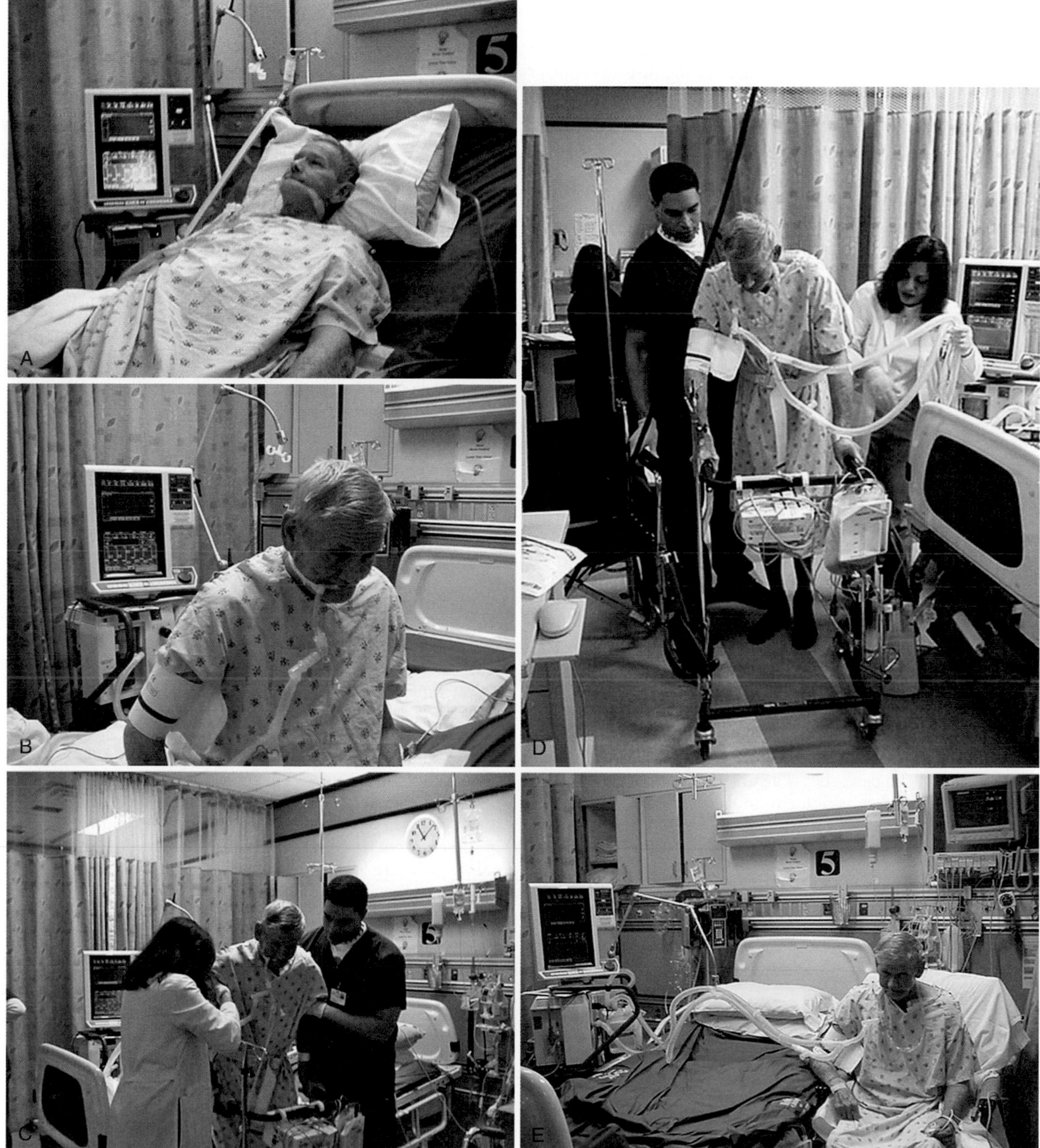

Fig. 34-3 Intensive care unit patient receiving physical therapy. **A,** Patient is on mechanical ventilation with an oral endotracheal tube. **B,** Patient sitting on the edge of the bed. **C,** Standing at the edge of bed with walker and assistance of two people. **D,** Walking around the bed. **E,** Patient sitting on a bedside chair after physical therapy treatment. Specific safety precautions must be followed at all times to safely mobilize the patient and to prevent accidental extubation.

Active movements have greater therapeutic effect on oxygen transport than assisted or passive movements; thus the benefits of active movements are exploited first. Movement recruiting large muscle groups minimizes the disproportionate hemodynamic stress associated with movement of small muscle groups or movements requiring excessive dynamic stabilization. If active movements cannot be performed or excessively stress the oxygen transport system, then active assisted movements are indicated. A recent randomized controlled clinical trial reported evidence supporting that early exercise training (including use of a bedside ergometer for 20 minutes daily either passively or actively) enhanced the recovery of functional exercise capacity in patients in the ICU, their self-perceived functional status, and their muscle force at hospital discharge.[24]

Passive movements have a role primarily when the patient is paralyzed or so hemodynamically unstable that his or her condition deteriorates with active movement. With respect to cardiovascular and pulmonary benefits, passive movement stimulates changes in ventilatory and circulatory patterns.[25] These can be particularly beneficial in patients who have significant mobility restriction; however, they should not substitute for active and active-assisted movements, which are associated with even greater benefit because they are higher-order activities on the physiologically based treatment hierarchy (see Chapter 17).

A study reported on the use of electrical stimulation in combination with active exercise of the limbs in patients with severe COPD who were mechanically ventilated.[26] Muscle strength was improved, and the number of days to transfer from bed to chair was reduced. The study's design precludes electrical stimulation as being superior to extended active exercise and progressive mobilization to the chair and ambulation. Another recent study demonstrated that electrical stimulation is well tolerated and seems to preserve the muscle mass of critically ill patients.[27] The use of electrical stimulation as a preventive and rehabilitative tool in patients in the ICU with polyneuromyopathies, however, needs to be further investigated and should not replace mobilization. Deep sedation and bed rest are common in the routine medical care for many mechanically ventilated patients[20] and need to be reconsidered in light of rehabilitation initiatives to prevent iatrogenic effects of care and to maximize short- and long-term functional outcomes.

Body Positioning: Special Considerations

Body positioning is a potent therapeutic intervention that promotes optimal oxygen transport and gas exchange in two ways: one, from the physiological benefits accrued from the specific positions themselves, and two, from the physiological benefits accrued from physically changing from one position to another (see Chapter 20). Body position can be used preferentially to augment alveolar volume, alveolar ventilation, ventilation and perfusion matching, respiratory mechanics, cough effectiveness, central and peripheral hemodynamics and fluid shifts, mucociliary transport, and secretion clearance (see Chapter 20). Both ventilation and perfusion are enhanced in the inferior lung fields. Therefore in postural drainage positions the superior lung being treated is neither preferentially ventilated nor perfused. The less-affected lung fields therefore may be contributing more substantially to improving arterial gases. Hence the physical therapist must consider the goals of treatment with respect to pulmonary function in both the involved and less-involved lung fields. During postural drainage, the length of time in a given position needs to be monitored to avoid drainage of secretions into the less-involved, functional, inferior lung fields and to avoid the possibility of compression atelectasis in the inferior lung.

Although positions can be predicted that will optimize ventilation and perfusion matching, each patient will respond differently, depending on such factors as pathology, age, weight, depth of breathing, and mechanical ventilation.[28,29] Therefore the patient's response to specific positioning must be observed, documented, and objectively monitored with respect to the effect on oxygen transport variables.

Another important goal of body positioning is to potentiate position-dependent fluid shifts to optimize cardiovascular function. For this reason the patient should be positioned upright as often as possible commensurate with tolerance and hemodynamic stability. There are other beneficial effects of the upright position on pulmonary function (e.g., maximize lung volumes and capacities, minimize alveolar collapse, decrease airway resistance, increase lung compliance and thereby reduce ventilator system pressure). To maximize the effect of gravity on promoting fluid shifts, the legs should be positioned dependently at frequent intervals. In a patient who is not self-supporting with or without assistance, fluid shifts can be stimulated with a high Fowler position coupled with the use of the bed knee-break. Between sessions of therapeutic body positioning, a schedule of four-point turning (supine, left side, prone, right side) is ideal and should be attempted even in the ventilated patient if not strictly contraindicated.[30]

Extreme 360-degree body position changes (e.g., randomized positioning in supine, prone, right and left side-lying) have been reported to have beneficial effects on oxygen transport in patients with acute respiratory failure.[31] The head-down position has been shown to reduce respiratory distress in some patients with obstructive lung disease.[32] The abdominal viscera are displaced cephalad, thereby elevating the typically flattened hemidiaphragms and placing them in a mechanically advantageous position. This effect may be mimicked in other body positions by manual abdominal compression and abdominal binders. In some patients, however, the additional load imposed by the increased intraabdominal pressure on the underside of the diaphragm may inadvertently increase the work of breathing and increase respiratory distress. The prone position has been reported to be beneficial in patients with hypoxemia and acute respiratory failure.[33-35] A variant of the prone position, semiprone, may be more beneficial in some patients by reducing intraabdominal pressure. In addition, the semiprone position may be safer and more comfortable for the mechanically ventilated patient. The prescription of any body positioning must be based on its anticipated benefits on oxygen transport. The more extreme positions should be introduced in progressive stages and the patient's response monitored to ensure the response is favorable.

Time alone is an inadequate parameter for prescribing the duration a patient should remain in one position. Adverse responses including discomfort should serve as guides in addition to the therapeutic goals. Although patients tend to be turned every 2 hours or less across ICUs, there is considerable variability with respect to this practice.[36] Positioning is a clinically important evidence-based intervention for maximizing oxygen transport and minimizing multisystemic complications when a patient is unable to be mobilized or between mobilization episodes.

Status Asthmaticus

Pathophysiology and Medical Management

Status asthmaticus is a potentially life-threatening situation. The pathophysiological features include marked airway resistance secondary to bronchospasm, edema, and mucous secretion and retention. The work of breathing is markedly increased, resulting in respiratory distress. A cycle results in which the patient becomes more hypoxemic and hypercapnic secondary to alveolar hypoventilation, bronchospasm increases, and reactive pulmonary hypertension may ensue, along with a further increase in the work of breathing and anxiety.

The classic signs and symptoms of a severe asthmatic attack that may progress to status asthmaticus include tachypnea, dyspnea, labored breathing, audible wheezing, tachycardia, cyanosis, anxiety, and panic. If the patient is able to cooperate with spirometric testing, the degree of reduced vital capacity, peak flow, and forced expiratory volume provide indices of the severity of airway obstruction.

Medical management is aimed at administering drugs and fluids to reduce hypoxemia with oxygen, decrease airway inflammation and resistance, and hence reduce the work of breathing and anxiety. Intravenous sodium bicarbonate helps to reverse respiratory acidosis and possibly metabolic acidosis.[5]

Principles of Physical Therapy Management

The prime objective of physical therapy is to optimize oxygen transport and avoid or delay the need for mechanical ventilation. Physical therapy can augment the medical management of the patient with status asthmaticus. In an attempt to avert intubation and mechanical ventilation the physical therapist coordinates treatment with the patient's medications (i.e., bronchodilators, muscle relaxants, steroids, and supplemental oxygen). The physical therapist promotes breathing control, enhances ventilation and perfusion matching, promotes mucociliary transport and secretion clearance, reduces hypoxemia, and teaches the patient to coordinate relaxed breathing with general body movement. Caution needs to be observed to avoid stimuli that potentiate bronchospasm and deterioration of the patient's condition (e.g., body positions that increase respiratory distress rather than relieve it, chest wall percussion, forced expiration maneuvers, aggressive bagging, and possibly instillation). Attention to relaxation and reduction of excessive oxygen demands is a priority, as was described for the patient with chronic airflow limitation. Certain body positions may have to be avoided (e.g., because of the patient's intolerance and exacerbation of symptoms in those positions). Because of the altered pulmonary function in different positions, positioning (especially in patients in respiratory distress) must be applied cautiously within the patient's tolerance. Body positions that reduce respiratory distress and the work of breathing and maximize alveolar ventilation, oxygen saturation, and blood gases are the positions of choice.

Major problems in status asthmaticus are alveolar hypoventilation, airway obstruction secondary to bronchospasm, mucosal edema, and secretions. Therefore maximizing alveolar ventilation and facilitating mucociliary transport are priorities. Other problems include significantly increased work of breathing because of an inefficient breathing pattern and an ineffective cough. Obtaining a productive cough without augmenting bronchospasm is a challenge. Deep breathing with pursed-lip expiration helps to prolong expiration and maintain the patency of the small airways. Deep, slow, and relaxed breathing is emphasized, along with periodic effective, controlled huffing, and avoidance of forced expiratory maneuvers.[37]

Despite aggressive noninvasive management, blood gases may deteriorate and mechanical ventilation may be inevitable. Relaxation, maximizing alveolar ventilation, and reducing airway collapse and obstruction continue to be the primary goals; however, the means of achieving these goals differ when the patient is mechanically ventilated. Optimal prescriptive body positioning is the intervention of choice. Secretion clearance is achieved by judicious suctioning. Suctioning is performed as required because it can contribute to reduced oxygenation, airway collapse, atelectasis, increased arousal, increased work of breathing, and generally increased respiratory distress. Once the patient is medically stable, a progressive mobilization program is initiated to prevent the side effects of bed rest as well as augment oxygen transport.

Restrictive Lung Disease

Pathophysiology and Medical Management

Acute respiratory failure can be associated with primary restrictive lung disease (i.e., interstitial pulmonary fibrosis). This is distinct from restrictive defects secondary to neuromuscular and musculoskeletal diseases (e.g., Guillain-Barré syndrome, myasthenia gravis, and neuromuscular poisonings are common neuromuscular disorders that can precipitate respiratory failure in the absence of underlying primary lung disease) (see Chapter 35).

Restrictive lung dysfunction may complicate the management of patients admitted to the ICU for reasons other than cardiovascular and pulmonary disease. The lung parenchyma, the chest wall, or both may be involved. The underlying cause of respiratory failure may therefore reflect ventilatory pump failure, gas exchange failure, or both. The specific restrictions to cardiovascular and pulmonary function need to be identified and treated individually to optimize treatment. Obstructive and restrictive patterns of cardiovascular and pulmonary function frequently coexist; thus the contribution of both types of defects to a patient's oxygen transport must be determined. Typically in restrictive lung disease, all lung volumes and capacities are reduced, although tidal volume can be relatively normal (see Figure 9-5). Patients with severe interstitial pulmonary fibrosis have increased pulmonary artery pressures with an associated increase in right ventricular work. These patients are at high risk of desaturating with minimal activity.

Principles of Physical Therapy Management

Restrictive ventilatory dysfunction is commonly associated with both medical and surgical conditions. The principles of management of acute respiratory failure associated with these differ in that medical conditions are associated with underlying irreversible lung damage, whereas in the surgical patient the pulmonary restriction is reversible. The natural course of disease in the medical patient will be determined in part by the patient's premorbid status. The majority of surgical patients, however, will have had normal lung function before surgery and the development of cardiovascular and pulmonary complications (see Chapter 30). Regardless of whether mechanical ventilation is indicated, tissue oxygenation, carbon dioxide removal, regulation of blood pH, and an effective cardiac output are priorities. Supplemental oxygen is often effective in improving tissue oxygenation in conditions associated with restrictive lung disease in the absence of a right-to-left shunt. In the presence of shunt, supplemental oxygen does not reverse hypoxemia.

A judicious turning regimen can also be designed to optimize cardiovascular and pulmonary function (even if the patient is mechanically ventilated), reduce risks of cardiovascular and pulmonary complications, reduce musculoskeletal deformities and skin breakdown, and promote comfort. It is essential with body positioning for any purpose that the patient not be confined unnecessarily and not assume any position for too long. Although lines, leads, monitoring devices, and catheters may be required, these are anchored as securely as possible with sufficient length to allow the patient to move spontaneously, be mobilized as much as possible, undergo as many positioning changes as possible, and facilitate routine patient care.

Mobilization and general body movement, particularly in upright positions, are always priorities in the ICU, as much and as often as possible given the patient's condition and safety considerations. Owing to the possibility of activity-induced desaturation, an appropriate plan of care for oxygen titration during physical therapy interventions should be established in coordination with the ICU team. Movements may be totally assisted but more often are likely to be active-assisted and active. No matter how weak the patient may be, active-assisted and active movements are the mainstay of the movement interventions performed by the physical therapist, particularly if these can be performed in near-upright positions. Assisted or passive movements should not be performed unless specifically indicated (i.e., the patient is unable to execute these movements completely alone). Even modest attempts at active-assisted movements, with perhaps only a minimal number of repetitions, benefit the patient considerably more, in terms of treatment goals related to both cardiovascular and pulmonary and musculoskeletal function, than assisted movements that do not contribute to muscle strength, endurance, and coordination. Injudicious application of totally assisted movements will contribute to the patient's deconditioning and physical deterioration. Regardless of the type of mobilization, the patient is observed closely for arterial desaturation, discomfort, respiratory distress, cyanosis, fatigue, and extent of cooperation if assisted-active and active movements are being performed.

Assisted movements are indicated to promote oxygen transport via their effects on ventilatory and circulatory patterns.[25] In addition the goal is to maintain joint range of motion and prevent adaptive shortening of periarticular soft tissue in particular. Care must therefore be taken to perform these movements through the complete range of movement for each joint, with special attention to rotary components of joint movement. Lax joints can maintain range with one complete range of motion daily. Lax joints are unprotected and vulnerable to excessive strain. Protection may best be effected in these joints by moving the joint more slowly through the extremes of joint range and just short of complete range. In the presence of spasticity or limb splinting because of discomfort, the involved joints will benefit from two or more excursions through full range daily.

One approach that may be particularly beneficial in altering the distribution of ventilation and blood flow is use of general body and range-of-motion exercises, particularly of the upper limbs. If the patient is able to assist, however, greater cardiovascular and pulmonary stress occurs with upper limb exercise; thus heart rate, ECG, and blood pressure must be monitored. Lower-extremity movements, such as hip and knee flexion, may help to position the diaphragm for improved excursion. Lower-extremity movements will also increase venous return, which may or may not be desirable, depending on the patient. The goals of upper- or lower-extremity work must therefore be clearly defined. Possible benefits and untoward effects must be identified to ensure that the patient benefits optimally from the prescribed exercise.

The treatment of choice in all patients is to simulate conditions that maintain optimal oxygen transport in health or approximate those conditions as closely as possible. That is, the most physiological interventions are exploited first and the least physiological interventions are exploited last or when more physiological interventions are not possible. Physiological interventions such as mobilization may be contraindicated in patients whose oxygen delivery is too low. Without some reserve capacity in oxygen transport, the patient cannot sustain the additional metabolic load that mobilization imposes. Patients whose condition is this critical are often put on neuromuscular blocking agents to reduce muscle tone and thereby reduce oxygen demand. Because these patients are in induced paralytic states, mobilization is not possible. In such cases, optimizing oxygen transport using body positioning and then nonphysiological interventions may be considered. Extreme caution must be observed when positioning these patients and moving their limbs because they are at risk of joint subluxation, strains, bruising, and pressure sores.

Interventions to promote mucociliary transport and secretion clearance are applicable to all situations in which secretions, mucosal edema, bronchospasm, or a combination of these factors is present. If postural drainage is indicated to further facilitate mucociliary transport and secretion clearance, caution needs to be exercised to avoid inducing bronchospasm and hypoxemia; thus the use of percussion should be considered carefully.

Myocardial Infarction

Pathophysiology and Medical Management

The initial priority of management in the acute phase of MI is the correction of the immediate problems including dysrhythmias, myocardial insufficiency, reduced cardiac output, hypoxemia, chest pain, and anxiety, followed by implementation of a progressive rehabilitation program ranging from the acute medically stable phase to the postdischarge rehabilitation phase.[38,39] On admission to the coronary care unit or medical ICU, continuous monitoring of the heart rate and rhythm is established. An intravenous line is routinely started for the administration of medications and fluids. An arterial line may be started for serial blood sampling for blood gases and enzyme measures. Initially pain medications, coronary vasodilators, and diuretics are frequently used to minimize the work of the heart, anginal pain, and discomfort. Drugs such as morphine serve to depress the respiratory drive; thus the physical therapist must be aware of corresponding changes in vital signs. Less-potent sedatives and tranquilizers are more routinely prescribed. Increased pain and anxiety potentially worsen the patient's cardiac status by increasing myocardial oxygen demand and altering normal breathing pattern and gas exchange.

The primary purpose of oxygen administration to the cardiac patient is to reduce hypoxemia, myocardial work, and angina. Dyspnea, however, is commonly observed in the initial phases of MI and can be effectively controlled by supplemental oxygen administered by nasal cannula or mask. Oxygen may also correct potential ventilation-perfusion mismatching and hypoxemia. Oxygen is always administered with humidity to avoid drying the airways.

Blood gas analysis is performed within an hour of initiating oxygen therapy to establish a baseline of arterial saturation. In this way the oxygen dose can be altered to regulate blood gases and acid-base balance.

Myocardial Infarction Conservatively Managed

Principles of Physical Therapy Management

A primary principle of the management of the patient after MI is to reduce myocardial oxygen demand and workload. The myocardium needs rest for optimal healing. Judicious rest of the myocardium is a priority that can often be balanced with gentle rhythmic, nonstatic movements. Box 34-1 illustrates several ways of reducing myocardial workload in patients with cardiovascular and pulmonary conditions.

Physical therapists need to work closely with the interprofessional team members in the ICU to provide safe and effective therapeutic interventions. The physical therapist should also be watchful at all times for signs of impending or silent infarction, including generalized or localized pain anywhere over the thorax, upper limbs, and neck, palpitations, dyspnea, lightheadedness, syncope, sensation of indigestion, hiccups, and nausea.

Box 34-1 Means of Reducing Myocardial Workload in Patients with Cardiopulmonary Dysfunction

- Provide a quiet environment without excessive noise and stimulation.
- Prescribe low-intensity activity until medical stability has been maintained and patient shows signs of physical improvement.
- Begin progressive mobilization in conjunction with patient's medical status, electrocardiographic stability, and unchanging or resolving enzyme levels.
- Reduce patient's anxiety about his or her condition, self-care activities, and family and work responsibilities.
- In general, begin gentle mobilization exercises, deep breathing, and coughing immediately as prophylactic measures unless, as frequently is the case in coronary patients, crepitations are audible in the bases of the lungs; treatments need to minimize pulmonary congestion and cardiac stress.
- Promote relaxation with low-intensity activity.
- All levels of activity, including breathing exercises, are to be performed in a coordinated, rhythmic manner.
- Breath holding, Valsalva maneuvers, and intense isometric muscle contractions (i.e., isometric exercise and exercise involving significant muscle or postural stabilization) are contraindicated during all activities in patients with coronary artery disease and should not be performed.

Depending on the degree of MI and damage, varying lengths of modified mobility may be recommended.[38] Shorter initial periods of restricted mobility are safe and promote faster functional recovery.[40] During this period the physical therapist concentrates on rhythmic breathing exercises, gentle coughing exercises or huffing, and modified positioning with the bed head elevated at least 30 degrees to facilitate the gravity-dependent mechanical action of the heart and thereby reduce myocardial oxygen demand. Intermittent exposure to orthostatic stress by imposing the upright position is recommended for patients after acute MI.[41] The patient is encouraged to perform deep breathing and coughing every hour during the day. Bed exercises including rhythmic, unresisted hip, knee, foot, and ankle exercises are usually performed as frequently as possible by the patient or when the patient turns in bed. The patient is cautioned to exercise one leg at a time, sliding one heel up and down the bed and guarding against lifting the leg off the bed. These exercises, when performed correctly and coordinated with inspiration and expiration, require relatively little effort from and induce little additional physical stress on the individual with MI. Comparable with the management of the postoperative patient, these exercises are performed prophylactically to reduce the risk of venous stasis and formation of thromboemboli. In addition, they may help to regulate more coordinated breathing, encourage deep breaths and mucociliary transport, and reduce atelectasis. The patient is cautioned against performing the Valsalva maneuver and straining because these activities increase intrathoracic pressure and reduce cardiac output.

Electrocardiographic monitoring of the patient with cardiac disease is the responsibility of all members of the health care team involved in the patient's care. The physical therapist has a special responsibility to be proficient in ECG interpretation in the coronary care unit because physical therapy is one of the most metabolically demanding interventions for patients.[11,14] The physical therapist often has the responsibility of initiating new activities with the cardiac patient, which might include sitting over the edge of the bed, engaging in self-care (particularly involving the arms being maintained in a raised position), getting in and out of bed, sitting in a chair, going to the bathroom, walking around the room or in the hallways, and eventually exercising on the treadmill or ergometer. Changes in the ECG must be watched for, particularly in introducing new activities and increasing the intensity of workload in activities. Careful attention to ECG changes and serum enzyme levels will contribute to enhanced physical therapy care of the acute MI patient by optimizing the treatments prescribed and the margin of safety with which activities are performed.

Congestive heart failure may be unavoidable in cases of severe infarction or even milder infarction coupled with lung disease. Fluid intake and output and daily weight measurements promote early detection of congestive heart failure. Signs of imminent and established congestive heart failure are listed in Box 34-2. The work of the heart can be significantly reduced in the upright position.[42]

Patients with cardiac conditions are prone to anxiety about their conditions and prognoses. The patient is given realistic guidelines at each stage of recovery with respect to the level of activity that can be safely performed, which can potentially avert deterioration and promote recovery. Involving the patient in rehabilitation planning from the outset facilitates the patient's planning realistically for the future and may help to reduce the depression often experienced by the acute MI patient.

The initial rehabilitation program is planned with the long-range rehabilitation goals in mind. The program designed for the cardiac patient is progressive in terms of types of activities, usually beginning with activities of daily living, and with respect to the intensity, duration, and frequency of these activities.[39] The patient's tolerance and changes in ECG and vital signs are used as indicators for establishing and modifying the treatment program. These physiological parameters must be observed carefully as the patient progresses to optimize the potential benefits of the therapeutic regimens as early as possible without endangering the patient.

Patient education and prevention of infarction are particularly important for the cardiac patient. As soon as the patient is alert and able to cooperate, information about his or her condition with guidelines about activity, diet, and stress management is reinforced. The more involved and informed the patient is in self-management, the greater the likelihood of receptivity and adherence to a rehabilitation regimen after discharge.

Box 34-2 **Signs of Imminent Congestive Heart Failure**

- Development of tachydysrhythmias
- Development of a ventricular gallop
- Pulmonary crackles and other persistent adventitiae
- Development of dyspnea
- Development of increased jugular venous pressure and distension

Open Heart Surgery

Principles of Physical Therapy Management

Patients scheduled for open heart surgery are considered moderately risky surgical candidates because of the nature and invasiveness of this type of surgery (Figure 34-4), regardless of their general level of health before surgery. Whenever possible, patients prepare for surgery in advance by decreasing or stopping smoking, by avoiding exposure to respiratory tract infections, by avoiding stress, by eating a balanced diet, and by getting adequate sleep. Patients can benefit from a modified, prescriptive exercise program before surgery to maximize their aerobic capacity and thereby improve their perioperative course.

Preoperative teaching coupled with a conditioning program before hospitalization has a role in reducing hospital stay and complications (see Chapters 18, 29, and 30). During the preoperative period the physical therapist may spend additional time with patients scheduled for open heart surgery to provide teaching of the basic anatomy and physiology related to the surgery to be performed; the effect of anesthesia; the role of intubation and mechanical ventilation; the incision lines to be expected over the chest, and the legs if veins are to be removed for bypass surgery; the lines, leads, chest tubes, and catheters that will be in place after surgery; interventions beginning during the postanesthesia and recovery period (breathing control and coughing maneuvers, body positioning, foot and ankle exercises, and early mobilization); and the course of recovery the patient might expect, barring complications (see Chapter 17). The emphasis on patient education in most open heart surgery units may contribute to the generally low incidence of complications and mortality.

Some special considerations in physical therapy management of the patient after open heart surgery appear in

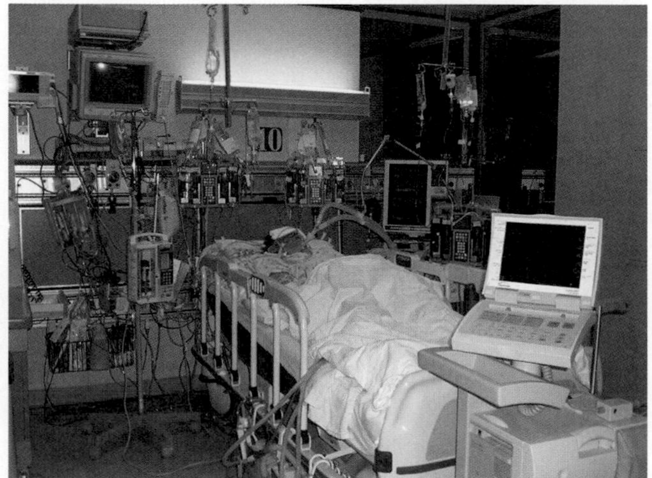

Fig. 34-4 Patient after open heart surgery. Note mechanical ventilator, mediastinal drains and chest tubes, intraaortic balloon pump, and multiple intravenous drips.

Table 34-2 and these expand on the concurrent medical course of patients in phase I cardiac rehabilitation (see Chapter 31). Patients are extubated early, and rehabilitation is commenced as soon as possible.[43] These guidelines are to be applied thoughtfully and cautiously with regard to each specific patient's condition and observed recovery. Intermittent orthostatic stress and exercise stress are encouraged.[41] These guidelines suggest the upper limit of intensity of physical therapy, which should be applied if all is progressing well initially and reduced if warranted by the patient's condition. Progression from one stage to the next is based on an optimal and reliable treatment response at each level before

Table 34-2 Stages of and Guidelines for Physical Therapy for the Patient after Open Heart Surgery

Stage	Guidelines
Stage 1	Postanesthesia and recovery is where the patient is hemodynamically stabilized. The patient may be seen in the postanesthesia and recovery room for a physical therapy assessment; the patient is usually extubated within 24 hours after surgery. Although the patient must be permitted to rest as much as possible in the initial 24-hour period, judicious body positioning is instituted to stimulate physiological "stir-up." Usually, once extubated, the patient is positioned side to side for deep breathing and coughing at least four times in the first 24 hours, is progressively positioned in the upright position, and low-intensity mobilization is initiated. Medications are administered before treatment to ensure optimal effect during treatment. Depending on the findings of radiography, physical examination, and arterial blood gases, the patient may require vibrations and possibly percussion. If postural drainage is indicated, positions are modified to avoid tipping the patient head-down and causing increased myocardial strain. A sputum sample for culture and sensitivity testing may be taken at this time. The patient can usually tolerate being dangled over the edge of the bed for a few minutes. Special care is taken for all heart patients to avoid the Valsalva maneuver, forced coughing, and huffing and to maintain a semirecumbent or upright position for treatment. Blood pressure is checked before, during, and after treatment. Mobilization is progressed.
Stage 2	Deep breathing and coughing maneuvers coupled with mobilization are continued. Positioning for enhanced alveolar ventilation and ventilation and perfusion matching may be indicated. If secretion accumulation is a problem and the patient is too unstable to be optimally mobilized or positioned, postural drainage and possibly percussion and/or vibration may be indicated. Upper limb and neck exercises are introduced. Neck exercises are withheld if central venous pressure lines are still in place in the neck veins. The patient can sit in a chair at bedside as tolerated. The patient is encouraged to stand erect for a minute or so on transferring back and forth to the chair.
Stage 3	The patient takes short walks as tolerated. Ambulation is usually commenced after the arterial lines and the Swan-Ganz catheter have been capped or removed, respectively (policies may differ across ICUs). Vital signs are monitored before and after standing and walking. Deep breathing and coughing maneuvers are continued even if the chest is clear, until the patient is up and about within reasonable limits as tolerated. The patient is encouraged in grooming and self-care.
Stage 4	Deep breathing and coughing should be done by the patient without supervision. The presence of atelectasis on radiograph or from assessment findings, however, would indicate the need for continuation of mobilization and body positioning with breathing exercises. Ambulation is increased as tolerated.*
Stage 5	The patient can participate in individual or class activities, concentrating on trunk mobility, range of motion, coordinated breathing activities, posture, biomechanics, and gradually increasing endurance.
Stage 6	The patient can attempt six to eight stairs if progress has been satisfactory and as indicated. Aortic repairs in the first week or so are prone to rupture. Elevation of the blood pressure is therefore avoided to reduce the risk of breakdown of the aortic suture line. Vital signs are always monitored.
Stage 7	The patient depends primarily on ambulation for maintaining optimal alveolar ventilation and mucociliary transport rather than breathing and coughing exercises. The patient is cautioned to balance a period of exertion with a period of rest. The patient may be discharged. The physical therapist ensures that the patient fully understands the specific details of the home exercise program. The emphasis of exercise for cardiac patients continues to be on rhythmic, coordinated dynamic movements on discharge, avoiding isometric, static exercise, in conjunction with breathing control. Precautions are reinforced with respect to avoiding stress to the incision, and this includes postponing driving for several weeks. If possible, the patient is invited to participate in a reconditioning and health promotion program as an outpatient in a physical therapy department. Follow-up medical and physical therapy visits are arranged before discharge for 4 to 6 weeks after surgery.

*The physical therapist must guard against excessively intense treatment of post–open heart surgery patients as well as other patients receiving prophylactic anticoagulants.

proceeding. Different institutions may advocate different practices, depending on their facilities, the experience of the surgical and ICU team, and the incidence of postoperative complications and survival for that institution.

The physical therapist must guard against excessively intense treatment of both patients after open heart surgery and patients for whom periods of relatively restricted mobility are anticipated. In addition to the fact that these patients may be hemodynamically unstable initially, they may be susceptible to soft tissue bruising from being on a prophylactic course of anticoagulants.

Patients are monitored for complications (see Chapters 16 and 36) and to guide treatment progression and detect untoward responses to treatment. After cardiac surgery, $\dot{V}O_2$ tends to increase owing to increased cardiac output and oxygen delivery.[44] The oxygen extraction ratio may increase and $S\bar{v}O_2$ decrease if cardiac function deteriorates.

Depression has been reported in patients in the ICU, particularly in those admitted for coronary care who are experiencing a physiological loss.[45] Signs and symptoms of depression warrant monitoring and reporting to the team to maximize clinical and psychosocial outcomes.

Complications do occur in high-risk ICU settings. Risk assessment is a fundamental component of the assessment (see Chapter 17). Common complications often related to premorbid status include restricted mobility, inability to wean from mechanical ventilation, deep vein thrombosis, pulmonary emboli, and stroke. Other complications are related to surgery (e.g., internal bleeding, overwhelming pneumonia, and lung collapse) or medication reaction. Complications are better managed if anticipated and detected early. Depending on the nature of the complication, physical therapy interventions may be stepped up in terms of intensity, duration, and frequency; modified; or discontinued until the patient is cleared with respect to stability.

Physical therapy follow-up should continue for several months beyond discharge, at which point the patient should be well integrated into a cardiac rehabilitation program. Continuity and continuation of physical therapy throughout the entire rehabilitation period, from the acute period to long term, cannot be overemphasized, given that achieving maximal recovery from surgery is the priority.

Summary

This chapter described the principles of cardiovascular and pulmonary physical therapy in the management of critically ill patients with primary cardiovascular and pulmonary dysfunction. Cardiovascular and pulmonary failure secondary to chronic lung disease and heart disease were described. Cardiovascular and pulmonary physical therapy management is based on the specific underlying pathophysiological mechanisms of these various disorders. These principles, however, cannot be interpreted to be guidelines for specific treatment because each patient is an individual whose condition reflects multiple factors contributing to impaired cardiovascular and pulmonary function or threatening to cause it (i.e., the effects of recumbency, restricted mobility, extrinsic factors related to the patient's care, and intrinsic factors related to the patient in addition to the underlying pathophysiology). Special considerations with respect to body positioning and mobilizing patients with primary cardiovascular and pulmonary dysfunction are described.

Review Questions

1. With respect to the management of patients in the ICU with conditions associated with primary cardiovascular and pulmonary dysfunction (e.g., cardiovascular and pulmonary failure, obstructive lung disease, status asthmaticus, restrictive lung disease, and coronary artery disease), describe the pathophysiology of primary cardiovascular and pulmonary dysfunction or threats associated with each condition and how these threaten life.
2. Relate cardiovascular and pulmonary physical therapy treatment interventions to the underlying pathophysiology of each of the conditions listed in question 1 in the individual who is critically ill, and provide the rationale for your choice.
3. Identify special considerations with respect to positioning and mobilizing a patient with each condition.

References

1. Shoemaker WC, editor: *Textbook of critical care*, ed 4, Philadelphia, 1999, Elsevier.
2. Lynn-McHale DJ, Carlson KK: *AACN procedure manual for critical care*, ed 4, Philadelphia, 2000, Elsevier.
3. Jardin F, Farcot JC, Boisante L, et al: Influence of positive end-expiratory pressure on left ventricular performance. *N Engl J Med* 304:387–392, 1981.
4. Walsh JM, Vanderwarf C, Hoscheit D, et al: Unsuspected hemodynamic alterations during endotracheal suctioning. *Chest* 95:162–165, 1989.
5. Kirby RR, Taylor RW, Civetta JM: *Critical care*, ed 2, Philadelphia, 1996, Lippincott Williams & Wilkins.
6. Weissman C, Kemper M, Elwyn DH, et al: The energy expenditure of the mechanically ventilated critically ill patient. *Chest* 2:254–259, 1989.
7. Ambrosino N, Bruletti G, Scala V, et al: Cognitive and perceived health status in patients with chronic obstructive pulmonary disease surviving acute chronic respiratory failure: a controlled study. *Intensive Care Med* 28: 170–177, 2002.
8. Wong WP: Physical therapy for a patient in acute respiratory failure. *Phys Ther* 80:662–670, 2000.
9. Dean E: Mobilizing patients in the ICU: Evidence and principles of practice. *Acute Care Perspect* 17:2–9, 2008.
10. Dean E, Ross J: Mobilization and body conditioning. In Zadai C, editor: *Pulmonary management in physical therapy*, New York, 1992, Churchill Livingstone.
11. Dean E, Murphy S, Parrent L, et al: *Metabolic consequences of physical therapy in critically ill patients*. Washington, DC, 1995, Proceedings of the World Confederation of Physical Therapy Congress.
12. Horiuchi K, Desmond J, Cohen D, et al: Insights into the increased oxygen demand during chest physiotherapy. *Clin Invest* 25:1347–1351, 1997.
13. Weissman C, Kemper M: Stressing the critically ill patient: the cardiopulmonary and metabolic responses to an acute increase in oxygen consumption. *J Crit Care* 8:100–108, 1993.
14. Weissman C, Kemper M, Damask MC, et al: Effect of routine intensive care interactions on metabolic rate. *Chest* 86:815–818, 1984.
15. Dean E: Getting the ICU patient "upright and moving": evidence-based clinical decision making. *Physiother News Bull* 13(5):2–4, 2009.
16. Morris PE, Goad A, Thompson C, et al: Early intensive care unit mobility therapy in the treatment of acute respiratory failure. *Crit Care Med* 36:2238–2243, 2008.
17. Needham DM, Korupolu R, Zanni JM, et al: Early physical medicine and rehabilitation for patients with acute respiratory failure: a quality improvement project. *Arch Phys Med Rehabil* 91: 536–542, 2010.
18. Bell L: Achieving early mobility in mechanically ventilated patients. *Am J Crit Care* 18:222, 2009.

19. Burns RJ, Jones FL Letter: early ambulation of patients requiring ventilatory assistance. *Chest* 68:608, 1975.
20. Needham DM: Mobilizing patients in the intensive care unit. Improving neuromuscular weakness and physical function. *JAMA* 305:437–522, 2011.
21. Bailey P, Thomsen G, Spuhler V, et al: Early activity is feasible and safe in respiratory failure patients. *Crit Care Med* 35:139–145, 2007.
22. Perme C, Chandrashekar R: Early mobility and walking program for patients intensive care units: creating a standard of care. *Am J Crit Care* 18:212–221, 2009.
23. Hanekom S, Gosselink R, Dean E. et al: The development of a clinical management algorithm for early physical activity and mobilization of critically ill patients: synthesis of evidence and expert opinion and its translation into practice. *Clin Rehabil* 25:771–787, 2011.
24. Burtin C, Clerckx B, Robbeets C, et al: Early exercise in critically ill patients enhances short-term functional recovery. *Crit Care Med* 37:2499–2505, 2009.
25. West JB: *Respiratory physiology: The essentials*, ed 8, Baltimore, 2008, Williams & Wilkins.
26. Zanotti E, Felicetti G, Maini M, Fracchia C: Peripheral muscle strength training in bed-bound patients with COPD receiving mechanical ventilation: effect of electrical stimulation. *Chest* 124:292–296, 2003.
27. Gerovasili V, Stefanidis K, Vitzilaios K, et al: Electrical muscle stimulation preserves the muscle mass of critically ill patients: a randomized study. *Crit Care* 13(R161):1–8, 2009.
28. Clauss RH, Scalabrini BY, Ray JF, III, et al: Effects of changing body position upon improved ventilation-perfusion relationships. *Circulation* 37 (Suppl 4):214–217, 1968.
29. Ray JF, III, Yost L, Moallem S, Sanoudos GS, et al: Immobility, hypoxemia, and pulmonary arteriovenous shunting. *Arch Surg* 109:537–541, 1974.
30. Dean E: Physiotherapy skills: positioning and mobilization of the patient. In Pryor JA, Prasad SA, Webber BA, editors: *Physiotherapy for respiratory and cardiac problems: adults and paediatrics*, St. Louis, 2002, Harcourt.
31. Kim MJ, Hwang HJ, Song HH: A randomized trial on the effects of body positions on lung function with acute respiratory failure patients. *Int J Nurs Stud* 39:549–555, 2002.
32. Barach AL, Beck GJ: Ventilatory effects of head-down position in pulmonary emphysema. *Am J Med* 16:55–60, 1954.
33. Blanch L, Mancebo J, Perez M, et al: Short-term effects of prone position in critically ill patients with acute respiratory distress syndrome. *Int Care Med* 23:1033–1039, 1997.
34. Douglas WW, Rehder K, Beynen FM, et al: Improved oxygenation in patients with acute respiratory failure: the prone position. *Am Rev Respir Dis* 115:559–566, 1977.
35. Piehl MA, Brown RS: Use of extreme position changes in acute respiratory failure. *Crit Care Med* 4:13–14, 1976.
36. Goldhill DR, Badacsonyi A, Goldhill AA, Waldmann C: A prospective observational study of ICU patient position and frequency of turning. *Anaethesia* 63:509–515, 2008.
37. Nunn JF, Coleman AJ, Sachithanandan T, et al: Hypoxemia and atelectasis produced by forced expiration. *Br JAnaesth* 37:3–12, 1965.
38. Kinney MR, Packa DR: *Andreoli's comprehensive cardiac care*, ed 8, St. Louis, MI, 1996, Mosby.
39. Froelicher VF, Myers JN: *Exercise and the heart, clinical concepts*, ed 4, Philadelphia, 2000, WB Saunders.
40. Herkner H, Thoennissen J, Nikfardjam M, et al: Short versus prolonged bed rest after uncomplicated acute myocardial infarction: a systematic review and meta-analysis. *J Clin Epidemiol* 56:775–781, 2003.
41. Convertino VA: Value of orthostatic stress in maintaining functional status soon after myocardial infarction or cardiac artery bypass grafting. *J Cardiovasc Nurs* 26:105–116, 2003.
42. Levine SA, Lown B: "Armchair" treatment of acute coronary thrombosis. *J Am Med Assoc* 148:1365–1368, 1952.
43. Cheng DC, Karski J, Peniston C, et al: Morbidity outcome in early versus conventional tracheal extubation after coronary artery bypass grafting: a prospective randomized controlled trial. *J Thorac Cardiovasc Surg* 112:755–764, 1996.
44. Routsi C, Vincent JL, Bakker J, et al: Relation between oxygen consumption and oxygen delivery in patients after cardiac surgery. *Anesth Analg* 77:1104–1110, 1993.
45. Johnson LH, Roberts SL: A cognitive model for assessing depression and providing nursing intervention in cardiac intensive care. *Intensive Crit Care Nurs* 12:138–146, 1996.

Chapter 35

Intensive Care Management of Individuals with Secondary Cardiovascular and Pulmonary Dysfunction

Elizabeth Dean and Christiane Perme

KEY TERMS

Burns	**Morbid obesity**	**Neuromuscular dysfunction**
Head injury	**Musculoskeletal trauma**	**Spinal cord injury**

CHAPTER OUTLINE

This chapter describes the principles and practice of cardiovascular and pulmonary physical therapy in the management of cardiovascular and pulmonary dysfunction secondary to other conditions that can lead to cardiovascular and pulmonary failure. Some common categories of conditions described include neuromuscular disease, morbid obesity, musculoskeletal trauma, head injury, spinal cord injury, and burns. Each category of condition is presented in two parts. The related pathophysiology and pertinent aspects of the medical management of the condition are presented in relation to the principles of physical therapy management. Invasive care and noninvasive care have common goals and thus are complementary. The principles presented are not treatment prescriptions. Each patient must be assessed and treated individually, taking into consideration the contribution of recumbency, restricted mobility, extrinsic factors related to the patient's care, and intrinsic factors related to the individual patient (see Chapter 17) in addition to the underlying pathophysiology. Special considerations related to physical therapy intervention such as body positioning and mobilization for cardiovascular and pulmonary failure secondary to other conditions are emphasized.

Neuromuscular Conditions

Pathophysiology and Medical Management

Amyolateral sclerosis, Guillain-Barré syndrome, myasthenia gravis, muscular dystrophy, multiple sclerosis, stroke, poliomyelitis, and neuromuscular poisonings are common neuromuscular disorders that can precipitate respiratory failure in the absence of underlying primary heart and lung disease. If paralyzed, the patient will likely be dependent on ventilatory assistance. Noninvasive mechanical ventilation has been an important advance in prolonging the lives of individuals with these serious progressive conditions. As respiratory failure becomes imminent, however, invasive mechanical ventilation is warranted.

Cardiovascular and pulmonary physical therapy has a central role in minimizing the need for mechanical ventilation in these patients because their prognosis for weaning is poor. Progressive respiratory insufficiency is best addressed early with the institution of nighttime ventilation at home before the development of failure and necessity for hospitalization. Patients with progressive neuromuscular conditions (e.g., muscular dystrophy) are living longer; thus cardiovascular and pulmonary insufficiency will be compounded by age-related changes of the cardiovascular and pulmonary system.[1,2]

Neuromuscular conditions contribute to cardiovascular and pulmonary dysfunction in numerous ways (see Chapters 6, 22, and 23).[3] With progressive deterioration of inspiratory and expiratory muscle strength and endurance, respiratory insufficiency and failure can ensue. Depending on the specific pathology, such deficits include reduced lung volumes and flow rates, reduced alveolar ventilation, increased airway resistance, ventilation and perfusion mismatch, impaired mucociliary transport, accumulation of mucus, reduced cough and gag reflexes, relatively unprotected airway secondary to impaired glottic closure and weakness of the pharyngeal and laryngeal structures, and increased work of breathing.

Iatrogenic effects of medications can confound muscle weakness. Muscle relaxants and corticosteroids are used commonly in the intensive care unit (ICU) and can lead to muscle weakness. The clinical diagnosis of ICU-acquired weakness is achieved by clinical assessment, electrophysiological studies, and morphologic analysis of muscle and nerve tissue.[4]

Principles of Physical Therapy Management

A patient with restrictive pulmonary disease secondary to neuromuscular conditions is at considerable risk of succumbing to the negative cardiovascular and pulmonary sequelae of reduced mobility and recumbency, in addition to the pathophysiological consequences of respiratory failure. Provided the patient has some residual muscle power, the balance between oxygen demand and supply will determine the degree to which mobilization can be exploited to maximize oxygen transport.[5] The treatment goals for these patients are to maximize oxygen delivery, enhance the efficiency of oxygen uptake and usage, and thereby reduce the work of breathing. In these patients, minimizing oxygen demand overall (i.e., during mobilization as well as at rest) is a priority. Mobilization needs to be prescribed in body positions that enhance oxygen transport and its efficiency so that the benefits of mobilization can be exploited more fully without worsening arterial oxygenation. The patient requires continuous monitoring of oxygen transport and hemodynamic monitoring to ensure the exercise stimulus is optimally therapeutic and not excessive.

Although the mechanisms are different, patients with neuromuscular dysfunction, much like patients with chronic airflow limitation, can benefit from body positioning to reduce respiratory distress. Upright and lean-forward positions will reduce distress to the greatest extent.

The patient's body position and length of time in any one position must be carefully monitored and recorded to minimize the risks of positions that are deleterious to oxygenation and ensure that a beneficial position is not assumed for too long because of the diminishing benefits over time. This is particularly important for the patient who is incapable of positioning himself or herself, who is incapable of communicating a need to turn, and in whom muscle wasting, bony prominences, and thinning of the skin may predispose the patient to skin breakdown. Educating the family and caregiver to work with the patient is an essential component of the physical therapy management of patients with neuromuscular conditions.

Patients who are hypotonic and generally weak and debilitated fail to adapt normally to position-dependent fluid shifts and thus are more prone to orthostatic intolerance.[6] Gravitational stimulation is essential to maintain the volume-regulating mechanisms. Tilt tables should be used judiciously given the potential risks in these patients, which are compounded by the loss of the lower-extremity muscle pump mechanism. Stretcher chairs may be preferable. Because of potential adverse reactions to fluid shifts and the potential for desaturation, falling PaO_2 levels, and dysrhythmias, the patient's hemodynamic status must be monitored closely during gravitational challenges.

The importance of chest wall mobility to optimize three-dimensional chest wall excursion in individuals with chronic neurological conditions is emphasized in Chapters 22 and 23. This goal is particularly challenging if complicated by acute respiratory insufficiency. The goal is to promote alveolar ventilation, reduce areas of atelectasis, and optimize ventilation and perfusion matching and breathing efficiency to augment and minimize reliance on respiratory support (i.e., supplemental oxygen and mechanical ventilation) while minimizing respiratory distress. This is especially important because patients with neuromuscular conditions are poor candidates for being weaned off mechanical ventilation. In addition, these patients are prone to microaspiration. Promotion of mucociliary transport is therefore essential to facilitate clearing of aspirate and minimize bacterial colonization and risk of infection.

Another major problem for patients with restrictive lung disease secondary to generalized weakness and neuromuscular disease is an ineffective cough. Cough facilitation techniques (e.g., body positioning, abdominal counter pressure, and tracheal tickle; see Chapters 22 and 23) can be used to increase intraabdominal and intrathoracic pressures and cough effectiveness. A natural cough, even when facilitated, is preferable and more effective in dislodging mucus from the sixth or seventh generation of bronchi than repeated suctioning. Even a weak, facilitated cough may be effective in dislodging secretions to the central airways for removal by suctioning or for redistribution of peripheral secretions.[7] Huffing, a modified cough performed with the glottis open and with abdominal support, may help mobilize secretions in patients with generalized weakness. In some cases suctioning may be the only means of eliciting a cough and clearing secretions simultaneously. Coughing attempts are usually exhausting for these patients. Thus ample rest periods must be interspersed during treatment, particularly for the ventilated patient. Coughing maneuvers must be strategically planned. Even though the patient may be able to effect only a series of a few weak coughs, it is essential that these attempts be maximized (i.e., the patient, optimally rested and medicated [e.g., bronchodilators, analgesia, reduced sedation and narcotics], is physically positioned to optimize length-tension relationship of the diaphragm and abdominal muscles; is positioned vertically to optimize inspiratory lung volumes and expiratory flows and avoid aspiration; and is provided thoracic and abdominal support during expiration to maximize intrathoracic and intraabdominal pressures) (see Chapter 22). These supportive measures will ensure that the benefits of the normal physiological cough mechanism, which is the single best secretion clearance technique, are maximized (i.e., the most productive cough with the least energy expenditure).[8] Forced chest wall compression or forced expiratory maneuvers are contraindicated because of airway closure and impairment of gas exchange.[9]

Impaired mobility, inability to cough effectively, decreased airway diameter, and bronchospasm contribute to impaired mucociliary transport and secretion accumulation. In addition, impaired glottic closure and increased risk of reflux in this patient population expose the airway to risk of aspiration. Prophylactically, multiple body positions and frequent position changes will minimize the risk of secretion accumulation and stasis. If mechanically ventilated, these patients are suctioned as indicated. If pulmonary secretions become a significant problem despite these preventative measures, postural drainage positions are selected to achieve the optimal effect (i.e., secretion mobilization and optimal gas exchange). Given the treatment response, manual techniques, of which manual vibration would have the greatest physiological justification, may yield some benefit.

Patients with chronic neuromuscular dysfunction and residual musculoskeletal deformity pose an additional challenge to the cardiovascular and pulmonary physical therapist in that cardiovascular and pulmonary function is less predictable because of altered lung mechanics and possibly cardiac dynamics. Thus, clinical decision making is more experiential in these patients, and they require close monitoring.

Obesity

Pathophysiology and Medical Management

Restriction of cardiovascular and pulmonary function secondary to morbid obesity is called the *alveolar hypoventilation syndrome.* In this syndrome the weight of excess adipose tissue over the thoracic cage and abdominal cavity restricts chest wall movement and movement of the diaphragm and abdominal contents, respectively, during respiration. In very heavy individuals, cardiovascular and pulmonary function can be significantly impaired, resulting in hypoxemia and cardiovascular and pulmonary failure. The major pathophysiological mechanisms include significant alveolar hypoventilation, reactive hypoxic pulmonary vasoconstriction, increased pulmonary vascular resistance, myocardial hypertrophy, increased right ventricular work, altered position of the thoracic structures, abnormal compression of the heart, lungs, and mediastinal structures, abnormal position of the heart, cardiomegaly, increased intraabdominal pressure, elevated hemidiaphragms with resulting pressure on the underside of the diaphragm, impaired cough effectiveness, impaired mucociliary transport, mucous obstruction of airways, airway narrowing, bronchospasm, impaired mechanical efficiency of diaphragmatic excursion, and impaired respiratory mechanics and breathing efficiency. In addition, such patients are likely to have poor cardiovascular and pulmonary reserve capacity secondary to increased metabolic rate and minute ventilation at submaximal work rates, increased metabolic cost of breathing, and increased work of breathing. Moderately heavy patients whose pulmonary function is normally not compromised may exhibit cardiovascular and pulmonary dysfunction when their oxygen transport systems are stressed because of illness.

Mechanical ventilation can be a challenge in that the system pressure required to inflate the lungs may predispose the patient to barotrauma. Furthermore, high system pressures contribute to reduced stroke volume and cardiac output. Adequate circulation is essential to fulfill the goals of medical management (i.e., to optimize tissue oxygenation and carbon dioxide removal). Thus a delicate balance among adequate alveolar ventilation, cardiac output, and peripheral circulation is maintained.

Principles of Physical Therapy Management

The patient who is obese can be treated aggressively provided there are no contraindications and he or she is being fully monitored. Treatments must be intense, to the limits of the patient's tolerance, provided this is not contraindicated. An aggressive approach is essential given that the obese patient is at greater risk of deteriorating between treatments than a nonobese patient. Recumbency is tolerated poorly by an individual who is obese. Positional decrements in PaO_2 and SaO_2 can induce dysrhythmias. The weight of the abdominal viscera limits diaphragmatic descent and elevates the resting position of the diaphragm, impeding its mechanical efficiency. Furthermore, these patients are likely to become distressed if positioned prone because of restriction of chest wall mobility. Half-prone positions in which the abdominal contents are displaced forward, however, may be well tolerated.

These patients need to be aggressively mobilized; both whole-body exercise stress and range-of-motion exercises between mobilization sessions are required. Active and active-assisted upper-extremity range-of-motion exercises are associated with increased hemodynamic stress; thus the patient must be monitored closely. Lower-extremity exercise, such as pedaling and hip and knee flexion and extension exercises may help position and improve the excursion of the diaphragm. Lower-extremity movement will augment venous return. Depending on the patient and the work of the heart, the effect of lower-extremity movement will require monitoring to ensure that myocardial work is not increased excessively.

The patient should be encouraged to sit out of bed as much as possible when tolerated. The erect upright position is optimal to augment ventilation and reduce the work of the mechanical ventilator and the risk of barotrauma. The upright position coupled with leaning forward displaces the abdominal contents forward, thereby reducing intraabdominal pressure and facilitating diaphragmatic descent. The posterior lung fields, particularly of the bases, are at risk for dynamic airway closure and atelectasis. Numerous positions and position changes ensure that the dependent alveoli remain open. The time spent in the supine position should be minimized. In fact, greater emphasis should be placed on nursing these patients in the upright position (i.e., the position of least risk and its variants). In addition to its pulmonary benefits, the upright position can reduce compression of the heart and mediastinal structures, and there is a potential decrease in stroke volume and cardiac output. The weight of the chest wall, in addition to the weight of internal fat deposits in and around the cardiovascular and pulmonary unit, can compromise cardiac output and contribute to dysrhythmias. Thus during all body position changes the patient should be monitored hemodynamically to ensure the position is being tolerated well. People who are obese often slump after being positioned in the upright position. It is crucial that the position of these patients be checked frequently and corrected. The slumped position can be counterproductive in that the benefits of the upright position are significantly reduced and can lead to deterioration.

Although patients who are obese do not tolerate the prone position well, the semiprone position can be beneficial by simulating the benefits of the upright lean-forward position on the displacement of the abdominal viscera.[10] This position also simulates the prone abdomen-free position, which is associated with even greater benefit than the prone abdomen-restricted position. The benefits of the prone position for the obese individual include increased lung compliance and enhanced gas exchange and oxygenation. The full prone abdomen-restricted position is contraindicated in the obese individual with cardiovascular and pulmonary failure, however, because this position can compromise diaphragmatic descent and contribute to further cardiovascular and pulmonary distress and failure and possibly cardiac arrest.

Mucociliary transport is slowed and ineffective in individuals who are obese with cardiovascular and pulmonary failure. Frequent body positioning will facilitate mucociliary transport and lymphatic drainage. The postural drainage positions can be effective in mobilizing secretions should accumulation become a problem. Manual techniques are not likely to add much benefit, particularly in the person who is morbidly obese. Suctioning is essential to clear pulmonary secretions from the central airways.

A person who is obese is at risk for postextubation atelectasis. Thus, aggressive mobilization, numerous positions, and frequent position changes must be continued.

The spontaneously breathing patient who is obese may have a weak ineffective cough, which will be even less effective after a period of intubation and mechanical ventilation. These patients are taught deep breathing and coughing maneuvers comparable with those described for the patient with neuromuscular disease. Body positioning to facilitate coughing and supported coughing must be instituted to maximize cough effectiveness. These maneuvers should be carried out in conjunction with hourly extreme position shifts.

People who are morbidly obese have a high incidence of upper airway obstruction and sleep apnea secondary to floppy compliant pharyngeal tissue. Thus the quality of their sleep and rest is suboptimal, and they are apt to desaturate while sleeping. These patients are also at high risk for esophageal reflux and aspiration. The optimal resting position is with the head of the bed up.

Individuals who are obese must be positioned upright and mobilized particularly aggressively because of their cardiovascular and pulmonary risks. Positioning and mobilizing can be facilitated with hinged beds, heavy-duty lifts, and reinforced stretcher chairs and walking frames. These items are essential to ensure that the patients are physiologically perturbed as much as possible and to minimize biomechanical injury to staff. The physical therapist has to ensure that the optimal devices are selected such that the individual is actively involved as much as possible and optimal but not excessive support is provided. The care of the individual who is morbidity obese is a particular challenge in the ICU and places increased demand on coordinated teamwork in the unit.

Musculoskeletal Trauma

Pathophysiology and Medical Management

Crush and penetrating injuries of the chest are commonly seen in the ICU. Damage to the chest wall, lung parenchyma, and heart contributes to the risk of cardiovascular and pulmonary failure (Table 35-1). Associated injuries of the head, spinal cord, and abdomen may also contribute. Fractures of long bones and the pelvis are associated with fat emboli, which pose the threat of pulmonary embolism. In addition, fluid loss in multiple trauma contributes to loss of blood volume, hypovolemia, and hemodynamic instability. The more extensive the injuries, the greater the pain and requirement for analgesia. Pain contributes significantly to reduced alveolar ventilation, airway closure, and inefficient breathing patterns.

Paradoxical motion of the chest wall associated with flail chest and rib fractures results from instability of portions of the rib cage after trauma to the chest. If severe, patients may require surgical stabilization of the ribs or stabilization by continuous ventilatory management. Chest wall injuries and rib fractures are particularly painful.

The presence of blood or air in the chest cavity and in the potential spaces of the pericardial sac and intrapleural cavity impairs cardiac distension and contraction, impairs

Table 35-1 Factors Contributing to Cardiovascular and Pulmonary Failure after Trauma and Their Diagnostic Signs

Airway obstruction	Respiratory insufficiency Respiratory distress Impaired blood gases
Inadequate ventilation	Reduced thoracic movement Paradoxical thoracoabdominal movement
Tension pneumothorax	Cyanosis Unilaterally absent breath sounds Distended neck veins Subcutaneous emphysema
Cardiac tamponade	Distended neck veins Muffled heart sounds Narrowed pulse pressure Paradoxical pulse
Open pneumothorax	Decreased breath sounds Penetration of thoracic wall
Myocardial contusion	Dysrhythmia
Flail chest	Loose segment Multiple palpable fractured ribs Decreased or moist breath sounds Hemoptysis

ventilation, promotes retention of secretions, interferes with effective clearance, and impairs lymphatic drainage.

The presence of a pneumothorax or hemothorax can severely compromise lung expansion. A tension pneumothorax results when air collects under tension in the pleural cavity. The tension pneumothorax promotes lung collapse on both the ipsilateral and contralateral sides, which further threatens respiratory failure. Phrenic nerve injuries inhibit diaphragmatic function. The affected hemidiaphragm rests higher in the thoracic cavity, a position that may restrict ventilation to the lung base and contribute to airway closure and basal atelectasis. Diaphragmatic injuries directly affect ventilation in two ways. First, the bellows action of the lungs is compromised. Second, the lung is displaced by herniation of the abdominal contents into the thoracic cavity.

Analysis of blood gases in the patient who has sustained traumatic injuries to the chest often shows severe hypoxemia and moderate elevations of arterial PCO_2. The presence of acidemia is common, which may have both respiratory and metabolic components. Patients with severe injuries have improved outcomes if hemodynamic status can be optimized.[11] Being less than 40 years of age is the best predictor of achieving optimal levels. Increasing DO_2 and maintaining normal SVO_2 are particularly relevant goals.[12]

Principles of Physical Therapy Management

Severe restlessness and dyspnea in a patient with chest injury are classic indications of respiratory failure. Auscultation and percussion can usually reveal an underlying pneumothorax or hemothorax. Tension pneumothorax is confirmed by chest radiograph or aspiration of the chest with a needle and syringe.

Flail chest refers to the asynchronous movement of the chest wall with two or more fractured ribs at two or more sites. This results in instability of the chest wall. The so-called "flail segment" is usually apparent on physical examination. Paradoxical movement of the flail segment can often be observed. The chest is depressed rather than elevated over the site during inspiration. Rib fractures are indicated by tenderness and crepitations on physical examination and from x-ray examination findings. Nonventilatory management of chest injuries in the absence of severe hypoxemia is preferred in these patients.

Analgesia is timed such that peak effect is achieved at the time of treatment to maximize comfort, minimize distress, and maximize cooperation, motivation, and tolerance for as well as duration of treatment.

Rib Fractures

Simple uncomplicated rib fractures often receive no specific treatment. Pain from complicated fractures may be treated with intercostal nerve blocks and transcutaneous electrical nerve stimulation and analgesia. Optimizing alveolar ventilation and mucociliary transport and avoiding pulmonary complications are primary goals. Strapping the chest is avoided because this further restricts and compromises chest wall expansion.

The current method of therapy for flail chest is internal stabilization of the chest and use of a mechanical ventilator. Slight hyperventilation will usually reduce the respiratory drive of most patients to allow the ventilator to take over the full work of breathing. The flail segment is then stabilized by internal expansion of the lungs. The treatment ensures adequate ventilation with the least pain possible. After 2 weeks the flail segment is usually stable.

When the patient can maintain a reasonable tidal volume and normal blood gases, weaning is begun. As soon as tidal volume and forced vital capacity are within acceptable limits, oxygen can be administered through an endotracheal tube with a T-tube assembly. Arterial blood gases are monitored closely during T-tube trials. Once the blood gases are in acceptable ranges over a reasonable period of time (i.e., 12 to 24 hours), the endotracheal tube is removed.

Pneumothorax and Hemothorax

Air or blood in the pleural cavity after chest trauma must be removed through a chest tube. For a pneumothorax the chest tube is positioned in the second or third intercostal space in the midclavicular line. For a hemothorax the chest tube is positioned in the sixth intercostal space in the posterior axillary line. Usually the chest tubes are sutured and taped into position and therefore are not easily dislodged. If the tubes are pulled out, subcutaneous emphysema or a pneumothorax results. A pneumothorax will also result if the tube is disconnected from the underwater seal. This is the reason for securing the collecting reservoirs of a chest tube drainage system to the floor with tape. Mobilizing and frequently repositioning the patient facilitates chest tube drainage and reexpansion of collapsed alveoli. Care must be taken to avoid kinking or straining chest tubes during patient treatment.

A bronchopulmonary fistula can be responsible for a major loss of the tidal volume delivered by the ventilator. Small leaks can be tolerated and are usually compensated for by an increase in tidal or minute ventilation.

Multiple Trauma

The management of multiple trauma is a major challenge for the ICU team. Multisystem involvement and complications often present a precarious situation in which priorities have to be defined for each individual situation. Multiple trauma can include head injury, chest wall injuries, fractures, lung contusions, diaphragm injury, pleural space disorders, internal injuries, thromboemboli, fat emboli, and cardiac contusions. Deep vein thrombosis occurs in 20% to 40% of patients in the absence of prophylaxis.[13] Shock and acute respiratory distress syndrome (ARDS) may ensue (see Chapter 36). Early intervention with body positioning significantly lowers the incidence of ARDS compared with later intervention in patients with multiple trauma.[14] The clinical picture of the patient with multiple trauma is compounded by the mobilization and positioning restrictions imposed.[15] Positive end-expiratory pressure (PEEP) is frequently used to reduce the effects of lung congestion secondary to shock or ARDS. Arterial blood gases are assessed to evaluate the effectiveness of PEEP in effecting improved oxygen transfer.

Multiple Fractures

Multiple trauma patients are assumed to have spinal involvement, particularly of the cervical spine, until ruled out with appropriate scans and radiographs. Meanwhile the physical therapist performs repeated assessments to establish a baseline position for the patient and recommend positions that will maximize oxygen transport. Treatment to enhance oxygen transport and mucociliary transport is primarily restricted to body positioning using log-rolling maneuvers and selected range-of-motion exercises (i.e., not of the head or neck, nor possibly the shoulders).

Fixation, traction, and casting of fractures and dislocations of the limbs complicate the management of the trauma patient. Restrictions to mobilization and body positioning are primary concerns of the physical therapist. Mobilization in the upright position provides both a gravitational stimulus and an exercise stimulus, both of which are essential to optimize oxygen transport. This is preferable to mobilization exercises in the recumbent position. In some cases, traction can be transferred from over the end of the bed to over a chair. A strict routine of body positioning is maintained, although severe limitations often exist with respect to the specific positions and the degree of turning permitted. Lower limb traction can be maintained when the patient is positioned in a modified side-lying position. Coordinating treatments with analgesia schedules reduces the patient's pain and fatigue, thereby improving tolerance to treatment and prolonging the treatment. These patients usually tolerate the head-down position well, provided head injury does not complicate the clinical picture.

The acute effects of mobilization that will benefit the patient with musculoskeletal trauma include augmentation of ventilation, perfusion, and ventilation and perfusion matching and promotion of mucociliary transport and cough effectiveness. General mobilization exercises and proprioceptive neuromuscular facilitation can be used to promote a mobilization stimulus. Cycle pedals can be attached to a chair or the end of the bed to provide a low-intensity exercise challenge for some patients. Maximal work output can be achieved within the patient's capacity using an interval training type schedule (i.e., schedule of work to rest periods). A mobilization program that promotes the long-term effects of exercise can be prescribed that involves as many large muscle groups as possible in rhythmic, dynamic exercise.

Frequent deep breathing and coughing are continued during and between treatments, depending on whether the patient requires mechanical ventilation. Body positioning is carried out within the limits of the patient's traction and casts. Impaired mucociliary transport is treated with body positioning and frequent position changes. Secretion accumulation may necessitate postural drainage. Modified positions may be indicated because of the positioning restrictions imposed by the fractures, traction, and fixation devices. If indicated, manual techniques may be coupled with postural drainage. Care must be taken to ensure that the addition of manual techniques is beneficial and is tolerated by the patient.

Relaxation interventions, both active and passive, should be integrated into the treatment regimen for the trauma patient to reduce excessive oxygen consumption and promote comfort.[16] *Active relaxation* refers to relaxing the patient through participation of the patient in relaxation procedures. *Passive relaxation* refers to relaxing the patient using passive procedures (e.g., body positioning, physical supports, talking slowly and calmly, and taking adequate time for conducting treatments). Taking time to implement mobilization is essential. First, mechanically moving and having patients who have multiple injuries move, requires a prolonged period of time. In addition, the cardiovascular and pulmonary systems of patients who are critically ill need time to adapt to new positions physiologically and to control discomfort. Prolonged periods of time may be required to turn a patient, dangle him or her over the bed, or transfer him or her to a chair with continuous monitoring. Every effort is made to maintain the patient's spirits, reduce stress, and encourage a positive attitude toward active participation early in the rehabilitation program that begins in the ICU.

Care must be taken to avoid undertreating or overtreating individuals with traumatic injury. A clear chest can rapidly regress because of general immobility and limitations to body positioning imposed by traction and pain. Treatments should always be coordinated with the patient's analgesics to optimize treatment response and for the patient's comfort. Whenever possible, the patient should be equipped with slings and pulleys and weights at bedside and a trapeze bar overhead for bed mobility and upper-extremity exercise. In addition to their cardiovascular and pulmonary benefits, all activities are taught in conjunction with breathing control exercises and coordination with the respiratory cycle.

Head Injury

Pathophysiology and Medical Management

Hypoxemia is observed in many patients with injury to the central nervous system. This may reflect primary damage to the cardiovascular and pulmonary centers of the brain or secondary effects of associated trauma. Arterial blood gases are therefore closely monitored in these patients.

Acute cerebral edema with sudden increase in intracranial pressure (ICP) and reduction in cerebral perfusion pressure rapidly affects central control of respiration. Advancing cerebral edema is evidenced by deterioration in level of consciousness, pupillary reflexes, ocular reflexes, and pattern of respiration and exaggerated muscle tone and posture. The sequence of these clinical signs corresponds to progressively increasing ICP from the cortex toward the medullopontine region. With involvement of the brainstem, respiration becomes variable and uncoordinated. With loss of central control and imminent cessation of breathing, respiration is shallow and ataxic. The appearance of the jaw and laryngeal jerk with each inspiratory effort suggests a poor prognosis.

Physical therapy and the patient's normal routine may have a dramatic effect on the ICP. ICP can be elevated indirectly by an increase in intrathoracic pressure as a result of physical therapy or suctioning. Turning and positioning may produce obstruction to cerebral venous outflow. Noxious stimuli, such as arterial and venous punctures or cleansing wounds, and relatively innocuous stimuli, such as noise or pupil checks, can elevate ICP. Whether these factors elevate ICP depend on cerebral blood volume and intracranial compliance. On cerebral stimulation, a chain reaction is initiated. Cerebral activity is increased, which in turn elevates metabolic rate, blood flow, and hence volume and ICP. Alternatively, increased cerebral blood volume secondary to gravitational effects increases ICP and reduces cerebral perfusion pressure.

The head of the bed is usually maintained at 30 to 40 degrees to promote venous drainage and thereby reduce ICP.

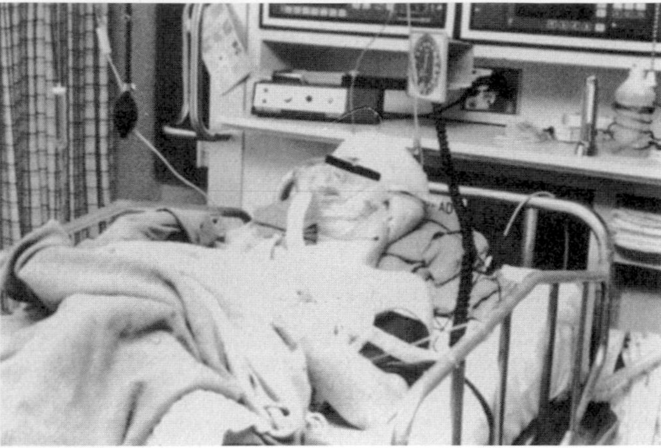

Fig. 35-1 Patient after neurosurgery procedure; head of bed elevated 20 degrees to help reduce intracranial pressure.

The patient's head and neck can be fixed in a neutral position by halo traction or by sandbags positioned on either side (Figure 35-1). Mechanical hyperventilation is used to maintain PCO_2 below normal limits but above 20 mm Hg. Arterial blood gases are checked during or immediately after hyperventilation. Prolonged hyperventilation is avoided.

Barbiturate coma may be induced to decrease the cerebral metabolic rate for oxygen and hence cerebral blood flow. The reduction in cerebral metabolic rate exceeds the reduction in blood flow, and thus oxygen supply exceeds demand, which is a desirable treatment outcome. Invasive hemodynamic monitoring is instituted in conjunction with barbiturate coma because barbiturates contribute to hemodynamic instability.

A complication of head injuries is acute lung injury, specifically neurogenic pulmonary edema (see Chapter 36). Autonomical nervous system dysfunction contributes to hypertension and neurogenic pulmonary edema. The endothelial tight junctions in the pulmonary capillaries leak protein into the interstitium along with fluid. Constriction of the lymphatic vessels may also contribute to fluid accumulation by impeding the removal of lung water. Increased fluid accumulation in the interstitium may progress to the alveoli, contributing further to impaired gas exchange and reduced lung compliance.

Box 35-1 Physical Therapy Priorities in the Management of the Patient with Cardiovascular and Pulmonary Dysfunction Secondary to Head Injury

1. Prevent cerebral hypoxia by maintaining a patent airway
2. Reduce intracranial pressure and optimal cerebral perfusion pressure
3. Position the patient within the limits of fracture stabilization and elevated intracranial pressure to promote alveolar ventilation and ventilation and perfusion matching
4. Position the patient to reduce pathological patterns of muscle synergy and thereby promote ventilation and reduce oxygen consumption
5. Position the patient to reduce myocardial stress
6. Avoid activities and stimuli that increase intracranial pressure
7. Reduce atelectasis and its risk
8. Shift lung fluid accumulations and areas of atelectasis
9. Promote lymphatic drainage
10. Promote mucociliary transport and reduce pooling of secretions and risk of chest infection
11. Reduce the work of breathing and improve the efficiency of the muscles of respiration, particularly if long-term disability is a risk
12. Perform active, active-assisted, or passive movements as soon as possible to enhance cardiovascular and pulmonary function and secondarily to preserve musculoskeletal and neuromuscular function and reduce the risk of thromboemboli

Principles of Physical Therapy Management

Physical therapy priorities in the management of the patient with cardiovascular and pulmonary dysfunction secondary to head injury are shown in Box 35-1. Body positioning, a mainstay of treatment for the patient with reduced consciousness, is based on a detailed assessment, consideration of multisystem status, and serial monitoring of the patient's response.[17]

ICP may increase with treatment and in particular with turning or suctioning. An ICP of up to 30 mm Hg may be acceptable provided the pressure returns to normal immediately after the removal of the pressure-potentiating stimulus. Specific guidelines with respect to the maximum ICP for a given patient need to be obtained in consultation with the medical team. Prolonged elevation of ICP suggests low cerebral compliance and the possibility of potential brain damage unless pressure is reduced. Thus all interventions must be performed guardedly with due consideration given to corresponding changes in ICP. Typically, management of patients with central nervous system trauma includes judicious tracheal suctioning, a stringent turning regimen, lung hyperinflation with the manual breathing bag in the nonventilated patient, or deep breathing with occasionally increased tidal volumes or sighs in the ventilated patient.

If the ICP is unstable and a risk of brain damage exists, physical therapy should follow sedation. Ideally treatments should be performed when the ICP is low and intracranial compliance is satisfactory. Patients whose cerebral compliance is compromised need monitoring during position changes.[18] The head-down position is contraindicated. Noise and noxious stimulation that increases ICP should be kept to a minimum.

If the ICP is elevated, all noxious stimuli should be removed. In severe conditions a decision may have to be made by the team to limit or withdraw interventions that lead to an excessive ICP increase that does not remit instantly (e.g., physical therapy, positioning, suctioning, or neurological assessment).

Movement of the limbs is performed gently and in a relaxed manner. Patients in a comatose state may experience passive limb movement noxiously. ICP may be elevated as a result. Passive movements, however, may have the added benefit of promoting improved tidal ventilation in the nonventilated patient by providing afferent stimulation to the respiratory center via peripheral muscle and joint receptors.

Severe head injury may produce flexor or extensor posturing. These synergies may be inhibited by appropriately positioning the patient. Judicious body positioning, in turn, reduces oxygen consumption and the patient's overall energy requirements.

Although arousing the patient and increasing oxygen consumption occur with cardiovascular and pulmonary physical therapy, arousal and oxygen consumption are generally minimized to reduce hemodynamic and metabolic demands in the patient with a head injury.

Spinal Cord Injury

Pathophysiology and Medical Management

The principal cause of death in the early stages of acute spinal cord injury, particularly for the high lesions, is cardiovascular and pulmonary complications. Lung volumes are reduced with the exception of residual volume, which increases. Vital capacity increases in the supine compared with the sitting position in quadriplegic patients. This does not, however, counter the negative effects of reduced functional residual capacity (FRC) and increased airway closure in this position and reduced flow rates.

Spinal cord injuries above C3 result in loss of phrenic nerve innervation, necessitating a tracheostomy and mechanical ventilation. The lower the level of the spinal cord lesion, the lower the cardiovascular and pulmonary risk. All patients with spinal cord injuries are at risk for developing atelectasis and pneumonia. The coughing mechanics of patients with quadriplegia are abnormal and contribute to ineffective airway clearance.[19] In addition, the quadriplegic patient is at risk for developing pulmonary emboli. Prophylactic low-dose heparin is used routinely unless the presence of pulmonary emboli is suspected and higher doses are indicated.

Patients with suspected spinal cord injuries usually undergo immediate spinal fixation on admission. Depending on the level of injury determined by clinical signs and radiographs, traction and fixation may be localized to the head and neck, or spinal support and casting may be required in the thoracic or lumbar regions.

Principles of Physical Therapy Management

Because of the need to maintain relative immobility in the acute stabilization period of suspected spinal cord injury, therapeutic body positioning rather than mobilization is a primary intervention for optimizing oxygen transport. Although modified body positioning can be achieved, the provision of optimal care under these restricted conditions is a singularly important challenge to the physical therapist, particularly with respect to the management of adequate oxygen transport while the patient is in the ICU. Patients with high spinal cord lesions can be positioned in all positions within the limits of the cervical traction device being used, barring head injury. Both head- and foot-tipped positions, however, are introduced cautiously and with hemodynamic monitoring because both positions can have significant cardiovascular and pulmonary and hemodynamic consequences secondary to spinal nerve loss and hence sympathetic nerve loss to the peripheral blood vessels. Turning frames such as the Stryker frame facilitate turning and tipping of these hemodynamically labile patients in the supine and prone positions.[20]

Effective body positioning, despite the need in some cases for extensive modification, may be sufficient to optimize oxygen transport secondary to improved regional ventilation and perfusion to all lung fields. In the spontaneously breathing patient, deep breathing and coughing maneuvers need to be coupled with position changes to optimize mucociliary transport. Some patients may not tolerate numerous positions and position changes and thus have impaired mucociliary transport. If secretion accumulation and stasis develop, postural drainage can be instituted; however, tipping must be attempted very cautiously. Patients should be monitored closely during and after treatment. Because of the hemodynamic lability of acute quadriplegic patients and the well-documented side effects of percussion and vibration,[8] these procedures must be applied cautiously, should they be indicated, depending on the severity of any complicating fracture-dislocation(s), the stability of fixation, the condition of the lungs, the presence of chest wall injuries, and hemodynamic lability.

The high-frequency oscillating ventilator may have some benefit in the management of multiple trauma patients with spinal injuries who require ventilation. The advantages of the high-frequency oscillating ventilator include improved spontaneous mucociliary clearance and reduced incidence of atelectasis. Weaning patients with high spinal cord lesions off the ventilator requires special skill because of the impaired function of the respiratory muscles. For these patients, weaning can be particularly fatiguing, frightening, and frustrating. Patients are weaned lying supine when they are alert and able to cooperate. Short periods off the ventilator on the T-piece are used initially. Use of the accessory muscles of respiration and any other muscular reserves is encouraged to compensate for the loss of function of the respiratory muscles. In some centers, patients are started in the weaning period on respiratory muscle training. The physical therapist must be well versed and practiced in this procedure before using it in conjunction with weaning the quadriplegic patient off the ventilator. Because of the potential risk of inappropriate application and of danger to the patient, respiratory muscle training must be effected knowledgeably to optimize its benefits for each individual patient.

Respiratory muscle weakness and fatigue, two physiologically distinct entities, are probably much more common in patients in the ICU than appreciated. These states need to be recognized and detected early because both are well known to cause respiratory muscle failure.[21] The distinction between the two conditions is that weakened muscles respond to resistive muscle training, whereas fatigued muscles do not. Exposing fatigued respiratory muscles to resistive loads can accentuate respiratory failure. The indication for respiratory muscle training, therefore, is weak rather than fatigued respiratory muscles. Rest is indicated for fatigued respiratory muscles. Whether the respiratory muscles are weak or fatigued must be established before respiratory muscle training is prescribed. Patients with quadriplegia with weak respiratory muscles, even if ventilated for a prolonged period, potentially may be weaned (low-level injury) or minimally may breathe independently for brief periods after a course of inspiratory muscle training.[22] For further detail on respiratory muscle training refer to Chapter 26.

The combination of immobilization and cardiovascular and pulmonary involvement secondary to multiple trauma may result in disuse atrophy and weakness of the diaphragm similar to that observed in other skeletal muscles. Respiratory muscle weakness and fatigue can be components of both obstructive and restrictive patterns of lung disease. Patients with spinal cord injuries do not have the same advantage of performing coordinated general body activity and relaxation maneuvers to help reduce the work of breathing. This contributes to a marked decrease in respiratory muscle strength and endurance, resulting in reduced vital capacity, rib cage mobility, and ability to cough. For these reasons, patients with paralysis and demonstrated respiratory muscle weakness are particularly well suited for respiratory muscle training. The quadriplegic patient has lost the function of the intercostal muscles, which are important muscles of inspiration and responsible for thoracic cage expansion. In addition, the absence of the abdominal muscles, which are the primary expiratory muscles, drastically reduces the ability to cough effectively and perform a forced expiration. The diaphragm and the accessory muscles of inspiration, namely the scalene and sternocleidomastoid muscles, then become the quadriplegic patient's respiratory muscles. These factors as well as the effects of heat, humidity, and the vertical position, all predispose the individual with quadriplegia to the development of respiratory muscle weakness and failure.

Maximum inspiratory mouth pressure and vital capacity can be measured routinely to monitor change in diaphragmatic function. The level of inspiratory resistance and the duration for which the patient can use each resistor are indications of the endurance of the inspiratory muscles. Measurement of vital capacity and maximum inspiratory and expiratory mouth pressures provide an index of the strength of the inspiratory muscles.

Certain precautions must be observed with respiratory muscle training. Each time a new resistance is tried, the physical therapist should be with the patient. The patient selects his or her own rate and pattern of breathing. The inspiratory rate is usually constant. Breathing that is too shallow is inefficient, and breathing that is too slow and deep may result in accumulation of carbon dioxide. The patient is cautioned about avoiding hyperventilation. The physical therapist, or the patient when he or she is capable, should check the valving system on the respiratory muscle trainer before each training session to ensure it is functioning properly.

Burns

Pathophysiology and Medical Management

Cardiovascular and pulmonary complications are common in patients with smoke inhalation with or without severe burns and are a major cause of death. Smoke and chemical inhalation produce edema, bronchospasm, cough, mucosal sloughing, hemorrhage, hoarseness, stridor, and profuse carbonaceous secretions. Irritation of the alveoli and acute pulmonary edema can result in a condition resembling ARDS (see Chapter 36).

On admission of the patient with burns to the hospital, the patency of the airway is assessed immediately. Inhalation injuries are common in burn patients, resulting from smoke inhalation, heat trauma, and chemical and gas inhalation. Oxygen and humidification are usually administered immediately. Heat may cause laryngeal and bronchial edema. If airway occlusion from impending edema threatens, intubation is performed. If indicated early, intubation may prevent respiratory distress within the critical 24-hour period after admission. Particular care is given to children and older adults with inhalation injury because these patients have a higher risk of developing secondary cardiovascular and pulmonary complications.

Carbon monoxide poisoning may complicate the clinical picture further and seriously threaten tissue oxygenation. Hemoglobin has a higher affinity for binding with carbon monoxide than oxygen. A carboxyhemoglobin level greater than 20% denotes carbon monoxide poisoning. Levels in excess of 50% may produce irreversible neurological damage. The principal danger of carbon monoxide poisoning is that arterial PaO_2 can be adequate and tissue oxygen tension inadequate. Administration of high levels of oxygen is an initial priority to reduce the half-life of carbon monoxide from several hours to 1 hour.

Depending on the severity and extent of the burns, treatment ranges from conservative medical interventions to multiple surgeries related to progressive debridement and skin grafting. Both second- and third-degree burns can result in severe disfigurement and disability. Second-degree burns are partial thickness burns and tend to be painful. Third-degree burns are full thickness burns; these tend to be anesthetic in that the nerves themselves have been destroyed.

Treatment is directed at improving arterial saturation, maintaining fluid balance, and preventing infection. Hypoxemia is effectively treated with the administration of oxygen and maintenance of clear airways. If the patient is breathing spontaneously, oxygen is given via nasal cannulas or mask at flows of 1 to 5 L/min, depending on the arterial oxygen saturation. Moisture can be administered through a face tent with a heated nebulizer. Fluid balance is particularly challenging in the patient with burns because of the loss of skin, which is essential to the retention and compartmentalization of body fluids and in the regulation of fluid and electrolyte loss from the body. In addition, these patients may lose blood because of injury at the time of the accident. There is also a period without fluid replacement from before the injury to the time medical attention is available and intravenous fluid resuscitation commenced. Because of the nature of burns, even when fluid resuscitation has begun, fluid and electrolyte balance remains a challenge until considerable healing and repair have occurred. Fluid and electrolyte imbalances have considerable implications for hemodynamics and cardiovascular and pulmonary function (see Chapter 16) and contribute to hemodynamic instability, which necessitates modification of the physical therapy management.

An airway may be inserted initially with burns to the face, airway, and lungs in anticipation of progressive edema, which would make the insertion of the airway considerably more difficult hours or days later. Ventilatory assistance is indicated with evidence of respiratory insufficiency secondary to smoke inhalation and with burns of the nose, face, throat, airway, lungs, and chest wall. A nasotracheal tube is preferred to a tracheostomy tube because complications with a tracheostomy tube are greater in patients with burns.

Cardiovascular and pulmonary complications are generally related to sepsis or fluid overload in the initial stage. Acute pulmonary edema and congestion are largely preventable with careful fluid therapy. Central venous pressure can be misleading in the burn patient because of severe fluid loss and may remain at low values despite pulmonary edema. Pulmonary artery pressure more accurately reflects the status of the pulmonary circulation in these patients. Treatment of pulmonary edema consists typically of digitalis, diuretics, and mechanical ventilation. PEEP is usually indicated in the ventilated burn patient. Mist or aerosol inhalation is also used to reduce the thickness of pulmonary secretions.

Complications must be anticipated and prevented in the burn patient. These include impaired thermoregulation, hypermetabolism and increased energy expenditure, ileus and gastric distension, pain, and infection. Eschar formation associated with circumferential burns of the chest wall mechanically restricts chest wall movement and can lead to respiratory failure. Tissue edema that can continue for a few days after the burn contributes to increased tissue pressure and impaired tissue perfusion, potentiating tissue ischemia and necrosis. Late complications include gastrointestinal bleeding secondary to stress ulceration and the continued high risk of infection.

Principles of Physical Therapy Management

Cardiovascular and pulmonary physical therapy is often required immediately for the patient with inhalation damage to maintain the patency of the airways, prevent atelectasis and retention of secretions, and improve or maintain gas exchange. Pulmonary function may be severely impaired as the net result of inhalation damage, burns and trauma to the chest wall, pain, and fluid imbalance.

Cardiovascular and pulmonary physical therapy often has to be modified in the patient with burns. Mobilization to enhance oxygen transport is exploited as much as possible; however, because of blood volume and hemodynamic problems, orthostatic intolerance may limit mobilization and positioning alternatives. With more severe burns and more extensive burn distribution, body positioning is the primary intervention. Positioning for an optimal therapeutic effect on oxygen transport is challenging because of the significant physical limitations that may exist. Given that body positioning profoundly influences ventilation and perfusion matching,[23] the reduced number of positioning alternatives will contribute to shunt, ventilation and perfusion mismatch, and hypoxemia. This effect will be accentuated if the patient is mechanically ventilated (see Chapter 33).

Body positioning to optimize oxygen transport is life-preserving; however, positioning and limb splinting must also be considered from the outset to minimize deformity and restore optimal neuromuscular and musculoskeletal status. Positioning priorities in burn patients must address both these aspects of management.

Patients who have skin grafts require particular care during moving or positioning because of the danger of shearing forces on the graft, which can disrupt the circulation, nutrition, and healing of the new skin. Sterile procedures must be observed at all times. The physical therapist is usually required to cap, gown, mask, and glove before treating the patient with extensive exposed areas and to cover the chest with a sterile drape. Facilitating mucociliary transport is a priority if the patient has significant mobility and positioning restrictions because of the burn severity. Wherever possible, mobilization in conjunction with multiple body positions and position changes is attempted to maximize mucociliary clearance.[24] If secretions have accumulated, positioning for postural drainage requires the same consideration as positioning for improved alveolar ventilation and ventilation and perfusion matching. In the spontaneously breathing patient, postural drainage positions can be used selectively to increase alveolar volume in the superior lung fields and alveolar ventilation to inferior lung fields, in addition to facilitating drainage of the superior bronchopulmonary segments. If the patient is mechanically ventilated, however, the superior lung fields are preferentially ventilated (see Chapter 33). Should the addition of manual techniques be indicated, percussion may not be comfortably tolerated in the presence of first- and second-degree burns. Manual vibration may be substituted. Manual techniques are contraindicated over freshly grafted skin; however, manual vibration may be transmitted from a more distal site to a lung field that cannot be vibrated directly.

Risk of aspiration is increased if tube feedings are not discontinued for at least 1 hour before treatment. A nasogastric tube is often used and should be correctly positioned, particularly during treatment.

Stimulating exercise and gravitational stress may initially consist of being in the upright position, preferably with the legs dependent, performing selected limb movements and dangling over the edge of the bed for a few minutes if this can be tolerated. In patients with severe burns and fluid imbalance, however, active and active-assisted moments in an upright position that can be tolerated may be substituted. As the patient's tolerance increases, free, unsupported sitting can progress to standing and walking. Ambulation during ventilator-assisted breathing should always be considered for any patient for whom this activity is not contraindicated. The upright position and physical activity in the upright position are likely to markedly enhance the patient's cardiovascular and pulmonary and neuromuscular function and improve the patient's strength and endurance in preparation for long-term rehabilitation. If sitting up and ambulation are not imminent, appropriate limb movements, preferably active, can help provide an exercise stimulus that can enhance oxygen transport. Aggressive passive full range-of-motion exercises and positioning, in addition, are required to maximize joint range (a distinct goal from that of enhancing oxygen transport) wherever possible.

Positioning to minimize deformity is a priority given the potential consequences for cardiovascular and pulmonary function and oxygen transport, as well as musculoskeletal and biomechanical reasons. Positioning a burn patient, regardless of the goal, should take into consideration alignment, pressure points, muscle balance, and effect on healing and grafted skin.

Certain precautions have to be observed in the management of the burn patient. First, skin loss contributes to substantial fluid loss, often resulting in labile fluid and electrolyte imbalance. This situation enhances myocardial irritability and the risk of dysrhythmia. Hemodynamic and electrocardiogram monitoring is performed routinely during physical therapy treatment. Second, large areas of skin loss increase the risk of infection; therefore the physical therapist must be familiar with sterile technique.

Organ Transplantation

An increasing number of patients have received organ transplantation with excellent results in terms of survival because of improved surgical techniques and new immunosuppressive drugs. Organ transplantation is a surgical procedure that can save and prolong the lives of patients with end-stage heart, lung, liver, kidney, pancreas, and small bowel diseases.

Optimal nutrition and exercise have been advocated as means of improving outcomes before and after transplantation.[25] The benefits of regular physical exercise have been well documented for patients who have had transplants. The benefits, however, begin in the ICU, where mobilization is prescribed to reap similar benefits including improved oxygen transport and physical conditioning and to potentially reduce or attenuate the side effects of immunosuppression.[26,27] In addition, the progression from mobilization in the ICU and hospital to the community can also help to address conditions that are often seen in these patients, including hypertension, type 2 diabetes mellitus, hyperlipidemia, and other cardiovascular risks. Once discharged, patients may attain a similar or even higher level of health and conditioning than their peers who have not undergone transplantation surgery.

As with other highly invasive surgeries, the degree to which a patient thrives long term versus merely survives has become a focus of interest. The quality of life is usually measured in terms of a patient's ability to function, from both physical and psychosocial standpoints, and his or her perceived sense of well-being. Physical therapists play a pivotal role in helping patients regain their highest levels of function after organ transplantation and minimizing postoperative complications.

Summary

This chapter has described the principles and practice of physical therapy in the management of people with cardiovascular and pulmonary dysfunction secondary to neuromuscular and musculoskeletal conditions that can lead to cardiovascular and pulmonary failure. Conditions included were neuromuscular conditions, musculoskeletal conditions, morbid obesity, head injury, spinal cord injury, burns, and organ transplantation. A detailed understanding of the underlying pathophysiology of these conditions and their medical management provides a basis for defining the physical therapy goals and prescribing treatments and their parameters. The principles of management described in this chapter cannot be interpreted as complete treatment prescriptions because each patient is an individual whose condition reflects multiple factors contributing to impaired oxygen transport or threat to it (i.e., the effects of recumbency, restricted mobility, extrinsic factors related to the patient's care, and intrinsic factors related to the patient in addition to the underlying pathophysiology). Special considerations with respect to physical therapy management with attention to body positioning and mobilization have been emphasized.

Review Questions

1. With respect to patients who are critically ill, describe the pathophysiology of cardiovascular and pulmonary dysfunction secondary to the following conditions: neuromuscular dysfunction, morbid obesity, musculoskeletal trauma, head injury, spinal cord injury, burns, and organ transplantation.
2. Relate cardiovascular and pulmonary physical therapy treatment interventions to the underlying pathophysiology of each of the conditions listed in question 1 in the patient who is critically ill, and provide the rationale for your choice.

References

1. Dean E: Oxygen transport: a physiologically-based conceptual framework for the practice of cardiopulmonary physiotherapy. *Physiother* 80:347–359, 1994.
2. Leblanc P, Ruff F, Milic-Emili J: Effects of age and body position on "airway closure" in man. *J Appl Physiol* 28:448–451, 1970.
3. Dean E: Oxygen transport deficits in systemic disease and implications for physical therapy. *Phys Ther* 79:476–487, 1997.
4. Stevens R, Marshall SA, Cornblath DR, et al: A framework for diagnosing and classifying intensive care unit-acquired weakness. *Crit Care Med* 37S:299–308, 2009.
5. Needham DM, Korupolu R: Rehabilitation quality improvement in an intensive care unit setting: implementation of a quality improvement model. *Top Stroke Rehabil* 17:271–281, 2010.
6. Marini JJ, Wheeler AP: *Critical care medicine—The essentials*, ed 2, Baltimore, 1997, Lippincott Williams & Wilkins.
7. Hasani A, Pavia D, Agnew JE, et al:The effect of unproductive coughing /FET on regional mucus movement in the human lungs. *Resp Med* 85(Suppl A): 23–26, 1991.
8. Kirilloff LH, Owens GR, Rogers RM, et al: Does chest physical therapy work? *Chest* 88:436–444, 1985.
9. Nunn JF, Coleman AJ, Sachithanandan T, et al: Hypoxaemia and atelectasis produced by forced expiration. *Br J Anesth* 37:3–12, 1965.
10. Ross J, Dean E: Body positioning. In Zadai C, editor: *Clinics in physical therapy, pulmonary management in physical therapy*, New York, 1992, Churchill Livingstone.
11. Velmahos GC, Demetriades D, Shoemaker WC, et al: Endpoints of resuscitation of critically injured patients: normal or supranormal? A prospective randomized trial. *Ann Surg* 232:409–418, 2000.
12. Kremzar B, Spec-Marn A, Kompan L, et al: Normal values of SvO_2 as therapeutic goal in patients with multiple injuries. *Intensive Care Med* 23:65–70, 1997.
13. Piotrowski JJ, Alexander JJ, Brandt CP, et al: Is deep vein thrombosis surveillance warranted in high-risk trauma patients? *Am J Surg* 172:210–213, 1996.
14. Pape HC, Remmers D, Weinberg A, et al: Is early kinetic positioning beneficial for pulmonary function in multiple trauma patients? *Injury* 29:219–225, 1998.
15. Ray JF, III, Yost L, Moallem S, et al: Immobility, hypoxemia, and pulmonary arteriovenous shunting. *Arch Surg* 109:537–541, 1974.
16. Malamed SF: *Sedation: A guide to patient management*, ed 4, Philadelphia, 2002, Elsevier.
17. Sullivan J: Positioning of patients with severe traumatic brain injury: research-based practice. *J Neurosci Nurs* 32:204–209, 2000.
18. Mavrocordatos P, Bissonnette B, Ravussin P: Effects of neck position and head elevation on intracranial pressure in anaesthetized neurosurgical patients: preliminary results. *J Neurosurg Anesthesiol* 12:10–14, 2000.
19. Estenne M, Gorino M: Action of the diaphragm during cough in tetrapelgic subjects. *J Appl Physiol* 72:1074–1080, 1992.
20. Douglas WW, Rehder K, Beynen FM, et al: Improved oxygenation in patients with acute respiratory failure: The prone position. *Am Rev Respir Dis* 115:559–566, 1977.
21. Macklem PT, Roussos CS: Respiratory muscle fatigue: A cause of respiratory failure? *Clin Sci Mol Med* 53:419–422, 1977.
22. Gutierrez C, Harrow J, Haines F: Using an evidence-based protocol to guide rehabilitation and weaning of ventilator-dependent cervical spinal cord injury patients. *J Rehabil Res Dev* 40 2; 99–110, 2003.

23. Clauss RH, Scalabrini BY, Ray JF, III, et al: Effects of changing body position upon improved ventilation-perfusion relationships. *Circulation* 37(Suppl 4): 214–217, 1968.
24. Wolff RK, Dolovich MB, Obminski G, et al: Effects of exercise and eucapnic hyperventilation on bronchial clearance in man. *J Appl Physiol* 43:46–50, 1977.
25. Vintro AQ, Krasnoff JB, Painter P: Roles of nutrition and physical activity in musculoskeletal complications before and after liver transplantation. *AACN Clin Issues* 13:333–347, 2002.
26. Kjær M, Beyer N, Secher NH: Exercise and organ transplant. *Scand J Med Sci Sports* 9:1–14, 1999.
27. Painter P: Exercise following organ transplantation: A critical part of the routine post transplant care. *Ann Transplant* 10:28–30, 2005.

VI

Chapter 36

Intensive Care Management of Medical and Surgical Complications

Elizabeth Dean and Christiane Perme

KEY TERMS

Acute lung injury
Acute respiratory distress syndrome
Extracorporeal life support
Multiorgan system failure
Perioperative complications
Respiratory failure
Sepsis
Shock
Systemic inflammatory response syndrome

CHAPTER OUTLINE

The purpose of this chapter is to describe some common complications seen in patients who are critically ill that have implications for physical therapists practicing in the intensive care unit (ICU). Complications arising from the following conditions are included: respiratory failure, surgery, acute lung injury and ARDS, shock, sepsis, and multiorgan system failure (MOSF). Furthermore, the implications for cardiovascular and pulmonary physical therapy are presented. Complications add further complexity to the diagnosis of the multiple factors contributing to impaired oxygen transport and to the challenge of prescribing treatment parameters effectively. Understanding the pathophysiological deficits in these complex conditions is the basis for delivering effective management, reducing the risk of an untoward treatment response, and preventing worsening of the patient's condition. In addition, risks such as age, comorbidity, severity of trauma, extent of surgery, obesity, deconditioning, smoking, and FiO_2 greater than 0.5 have been reported.[1] Compared with nonsurvivors, survivors of these conditions have increased right ventricular ejection fraction, PaO_2, FiO_2, and oxygen consumption ($\dot{V}O_2$).[2] With respect to vasoactive substances, atrial natriuretic peptide, catecholamines, renin, and vasopressin are lower in survivors. Cardiac index is not different between survivors and nonsurvivors, and there is no correlation between hemodynamics and circulating vasoactive substances. Impending life threat is associated with global energetic failure secondary to cellular oxygen deficits. Despite the severity of illness of patients in the ICU, physical therapy has a well defined role in this setting.[3] More recently, the integration of physical therapy has been included in a quality control model of ICU care.[4] Although treatment options may be more restricted in patients with complications and greater severity of illness, judiciously prescribed physical therapy can have an important role in reducing further complications, enhancing weaning from mechanical ventilation, and reducing ICU stay.[5]

Common Complications of Medical and Surgical Etiologies

Complications that arise in the ICU either directly or indirectly relate to threat or dysfunction of oxygen transport. Medical and surgical complications often coexist. Medical complications include metabolic dysfunction, pulmonary dysfunction related largely to mechanical ventilation, acid-base abnormalities, fluid and electrolyte disturbance, cardiac dysrhythmias, thromboembolism, myocardial dysfunction, gastrointestinal dysfunction, neurological dysfunction, and renal dysfunction. Surgical complications include hypoxemia, pain, deep vein thrombosis, and pulmonary embolism. The implications of these complications for physical therapy assessment and management are presented.

In severe cases of heart and lung failure, extracorporeal life support with artificial heart and lung, commonly called extracorporeal membrane oxygenation (ECMO), may be indicated. Rather than being a treatment, ECMO is a temporary means of providing partial or total life support. ECMO stabilizes the patient by regulating gas exchange and perfusion and facilitates recovery from the primary problem.[6] The major limitations to widespread applications are the need for anticoagulation and bleeding complications. Advances in ECMO have minimized the risk of bleeding and need for anticoagulants. They hold promise for prolonged extracorporeal circulation in patients with severe respiratory and cardiac failure.

Metabolic Dysfunction

Complications associated with respiratory failure that can further impair tissue oxygenation are described in Box 36-1. The metabolic consequences of these complications and impairment of oxygen transport are life-threatening for the patient. Thus prevention of their development is a priority. Should complications develop, however, early detection and definitive management become the priorities if the patient is to survive.

A hallmark of these complications is the impairment of multiple steps in the oxygen transport pathway, which adds to the complexity of management.[7] The three major components of oxygen transport (i.e., oxygen delivery, consumption, and extraction) can be affected individually or in combination.[8,9]

In healthy individuals, the ratio of oxygen consumption to delivery is low (i.e., 23%, which ensures an oversupply of oxygen as a safety margin) (see Chapter 2). This safety margin also ensures that most patients are able to recover from insults to the oxygen transport system. If the insult is extreme, however, such as that resulting from complications of respiratory failure, surgery, acute lung injury and acute respiratory distress syndrome, shock, sepsis, and MOSF, metabolic dysfunction secondary to tissue hypoxia can result.

The relationship between oxygen consumption and delivery has elucidated our understanding of hemodynamic and metabolic changes observed in critical illness.[10] The phenomenon of oxygen-delivery dependence of oxygen consumption occurs when a patient's oxygen transport system is unable to supply sufficient oxygen to meet basal oxygen demand.[11] Oxygen delivery below 300 mL/min/m^2 limits the oxygen diffusion gradient and reduces oxygen extraction and usage at the cellular level. This is termed the *critical level of oxygen delivery.* When oxygen delivery exceeds 300 mL/min/m^2, $\dot{V}O_2$ does not depend on delivery. Thus the greater the delivery in relation to $\dot{V}O_2$, the greater the safety margin. When oxygen transport is so severely compromised that oxygen delivery falls below the critical level, anaerobic metabolism is triggered. Anaerobic metabolism, however, may also be triggered at levels of oxygen delivery that exceed the normal critical threshold for anaerobic metabolism.[12] This so-called "pathological dependence" of oxygen consumption on oxygen delivery occurs when the cells are inadequately extracting and using oxygen even in the presence of supranormal oxygen delivery levels. This phenomenon is observed in patients with ARDS and shock (discussed later this chapter).

Given that physical therapy is one of the most metabolically demanding ICU interventions,[13,14] the physical therapist needs to be able to calculate this safety margin to prescribe the type of treatment and its parameters (i.e., intensity, duration, and frequency) such that treatment is maximally beneficial and associated with the least risk to the patient.

The ultimate treatment outcome measures are markers of oxygen tissue metabolism.[8,15,16] In addition, continuous assessment of oxygen delivery, consumption, and extraction provide the basis for directing management of oxygen transport deficits.

Box 36-1 Complications of Respiratory Failure

- Life-threatening impairment of oxygen transport and tissue oxygenation
- Fluid and electrolyte imbalances
- Cardiac dysrhythmias and hemodynamic instability
- Myocardial dysfunction
- Metabolic dysfunction
- Thromboembolism
- Neurological dysfunction
- Gastrointestinal dysfunction
- Renal dysfunction
- Metabolic and blood sugar irregularities
- Infection
- Nutritional deficits
- Complications of intubation and mechanical ventilation, including increased risk of infection
- Complications of oxygen therapy

Pulmonary Dysfunction

Complications of the cardiovascular and pulmonary systems can lead to respiratory failure (see Box 36-1).[17,18] Some of these, such as ventilator-associated pneumonia, relate to being mechanically ventilated. Certain technical problems related to the cuffs used in conjunction with artificial airways may occur (e.g., overinflation, distortion, and herniation of the orifice of the tube). Mucus plugs can occlude the endotracheal tube or tracheostomy and impede ventilation. The common complications can be reduced if the tube is changed frequently and if minimal amounts of air are used for cuff inflation.

Prolonged endotracheal intubation can result in laryngeal edema, ulceration, and fibrosis. Mechanical ventilation may also rupture a bleb on the surface of the lung and produce a pneumothorax with rapid tension development. Chest tubes are inserted immediately to relieve the tension. Blebs occur when alveoli rupture, causing air to track to subpleural sites.

Mechanical ventilators can be a source of infection. The physical therapist can help minimize this risk by not directly handling the ventilator attachments that communicate with the airflow channels. Condensation from the hose should not be drained toward the ventilator or toward the patient. The physical therapist should be masked and gloved when connecting and disconnecting the patient to and from the ventilator.

Oxygen toxicity is a significant clinical complication of mechanical ventilation. Mechanical ventilators have precise oxygen controls to deliver the lowest possible inspired oxygen concentration needed to maintain arterial oxygen tensions. Because of the iatrogenic complications of high FiO_2 levels (i.e., denitrogen atelectasis and oxygen toxicity), oxygen above the patient's needs is never indicated other than for short periods of hyperoxygenation before suctioning or in preparation for, during, and immediately after mobilization.

Acid-Base Abnormalities

Any combination of acid-base imbalance may occur either acutely or chronically during respiratory failure. Severe alkalemia associated with potassium and chloride losses may occur after mechanical ventilation and can precipitate serious cardiovascular and neurological complications (see Chapter 16). Significantly impaired oxygen delivery to peripheral tissue may contribute to increased anaerobic metabolism and metabolic acidosis.[12]

Fluid and Electrolyte Abnormalities

Fluid retention can occur with prolonged mechanical ventilation in a patient with no evidence of cardiac failure. Pulmonary edema, weight gain, decreased pulmonary compliance, and reduced oxygen transport are common signs. Fluid overload is a common cause of this fluid retention. Individuals who are mechanically ventilated are therefore usually maintained underhydrated. Because of a tendency for sodium retention and hence fluid retention, intravenous saline solution is kept to a minimum. Humidifiers attached to mechanical ventilators are responsible for adding a considerable amount of water by absorption through the lungs.

Cardiac Dysfunction

When the heart fails to the point of cardiac output being compromised, intracardiac volumes and pressures can be monitored. Flow-directed pulmonary artery catheters (i.e., Swan-Ganz catheters) are commonly used in the ICU for monitoring patients who develop such hemodynamic complications. Although inserted through the venous side of the circulation through the right atrium and ventricle to lodge in a branch of the pulmonary artery, they provide useful measures and indices of right-sided and left-sided heart function and the adequacy of fluid resuscitation and pharmacological support. These catheters are also associated with some complications (see Chapter 16). Infection may lead to bacteremia and septicemia. Judicious selection and application of any invasive procedure is warranted to minimize undue hazard. The presence of these catheters limits head and neck positions and requires mobilization be carried out cautiously within the patient's hemodynamic tolerance.

Cardiac dysrhythmias are a common complication of respiratory failure. In addition, patients in respiratory failure tend to be older adults who as a group have a greater incidence of dysrhythmias secondary to cardiac disease. Electrocardiographic monitoring is therefore essential for all patients requiring ventilatory assistance in addition to patients with overt or suspected heart disease. Both atrial and ventricular tachydysrhythmias are seen in acute respiratory failure. Sinus tachycardia and premature ventricular contractions, however, are particularly common. Ventricular fibrillation or death may occur with rapid lowering of arterial PCO_2.

In the presence of respiratory failure and absence of cardiac disease, the management of cardiac dysrhythmias lies predominantly in the correction of blood-gas abnormalities. Effective supportive management can usually be achieved with pharmaceutical agents. Electrolyte replacement may also be required.

A thorough understanding of the clinical presentation, diagnosis, and correct management of cardiac dysrhythmias is fundamental to the optimization of physical therapy treatments in the ICU and minimization of any risk to the patient. Cardiac dysrhythmias resulting from any cause necessarily require ongoing evaluation and therapy.

The physical therapist must be able to treat the patient with any dysrhythmia optimally and safely when associated with other medical or surgical conditions. The implications of the dysrhythmia for the patient's clinical presentation as well as treatment selection and response must be recognized by the physical therapist and considered in designing the treatment plan.

Thromboembolism

A high incidence of pulmonary thrombosis or embolism exists in patients in acute respiratory failure. Early diagnosis and management of pulmonary thromboembolism have been greatly facilitated by the use of serial ultrasound procedures and scans. Physical therapy has a key role in preventing the development of thromboemboli by promoting frequent changes in position; specific bed exercises, particularly of the lower limbs; and passive range-of-motion exercises if indicated. It is essential that movement and repositioning be performed regularly to maximize their cardiovascular and pulmonary protective benefits. Pneumatic extremity cuffs apply pressure intermittently over the lower legs to minimize venous pooling and assist venous return (see Chapter 33). Compression stockings also may be applied over the feet and legs to increase circulatory transit time in the dependent areas and reduce circulatory stasis.

Myocardial Dysfunction

As in any clinical situation, acute myocardial infarction can occur during the management of acute respiratory failure. The risks are increased because patients in respiratory failure tend to be older and more susceptible to positional hypoxemia. The probability of heart failure and associated dysrhythmias is increased and compounds the problems of the patient in respiratory failure.

Gastrointestinal Dysfunction

Stress ulceration leading to peptic ulcers is commonly associated with chronic airway obstruction. The stress of respiratory failure predisposes the patient to peptic ulceration. Profound hemorrhage may occur and blood replacement is necessitated.

Gastric dilation may occur in patients who are receiving mechanical ventilation. Gastric dilation is best managed by a nasogastric tube and intermittent suction. Care must be exercised to avoid hypokalemia and hypochloremia caused by excessive gastric suctioning. Special care is also taken to avoid fecal impaction, particularly in the patient who is paralyzed. This risk can be reduced with suitable fluid balance, mobilization, and frequent turning in conjunction with appropriate trunk and lower-limb movements.

Muscular and Neurological Dysfunction

A close correlation exists between state of consciousness and arterial PO_2 and PCO_2. In addition, alteration in blood gases causes changes in alertness, personality, memory, and orientation. Motor changes include generalized or localized weakness, tremors, twitching, myoclonic jerks, gross clonic movements, convulsions, and flaccidity. Neurological complications of respiratory failure must be differentiated from those of nonpulmonary origin. The physical therapist must be aware of the spectrum of neurological complications that can result from respiratory failure and recognize that apparent improvement of neurological signs may reflect improved cardiovascular and pulmonary status.

Critical illness neuropathy and critical illness myopathy are serious complications of critical illness and are associated with metabolic disturbance during illness, paralysis, neuromuscular blockade, recumbency, and restricted mobility.[19,20] Prevention is a primary goal and includes early detection. Detection of risk factors is an important component of the physical therapy assessment. Additional risk factors include ICU stays over 7 days, sepsis and systemic inflammatory response syndrome (SIRS), multiorgan system dysfunction, a high Acute Physiology and Chronic Health Evaluation III (APACHE III) score, the use of high-dose steroids, and patients who have had organ transplantation, patients with severe neurological or muscle disease, and those with hyperglycemia.[21]

Periodic nerve electrical stimulation has been one means of establishing nerve conduction integrity during an assault of critical illness requiring neuromuscular blockade and sedation. Medical management is focused on addressing its causes and reversing them. Because rehabilitation potential is threatened in the presence of critical illness neuropathy and critical illness myopathy, physical therapy goals focus not only on reducing the possibility of neuropathy and myopathy and their functional sequelae but also on facilitating weaning and improving clinical outcomes overall including functional independence.[21]

Renal Dysfunction

Lung and kidney dysfunction are closely related.[22] The development of renal failure greatly compromises the chances of the patient's survival. Renal failure can result from gastrointestinal bleeding, sepsis associated with shock, drug-induced nephrotoxicity, and hypotension. Urinary outputs are maintained with adequate fluid and diuretics, with care not to induce pulmonary edema. Dialysis may need to be instituted if more conservative management fails.[23] If dialysis is anticipated, the physical therapist should review existing treatment goals to modify treatment accordingly.

Systemic Inflammatory Response Syndrome

Localized inflammation is a physiological protective response. Typically this response is controlled by the body at the site of injury.[24] Loss of local control or an overly active response results in an exaggerated systemic response that is known as *systemic inflammatory response syndrome* (SIRS). Compensatory mechanisms and outcome (such as resolution, or potentially multiple organ dysfunction syndrome or death) depend on the balance of SIRS and the effectiveness of the compensatory mechanisms. The effectiveness of therapies to date remains equivocal.

Common Complications of Surgical Etiology

Respiratory failure in a patient postoperatively is usually associated with a low PaO_2 and a high $PaCO_2$. This situation is likely to be more common than generally appreciated. If the patient is in good general health and is free from underlying cardiovascular and pulmonary conditions, recovery is usually rapid. Otherwise, more severe complications and cardiovascular and pulmonary failure may result and progress to a life-threatening situation. The effects of surgery on oxygen transport and on the various organ systems are described in Chapter 23. Common perioperative complications and their causes are listed in Boxes 36-2 and 36-3. With severely reduced arterial oxygen content, hence oxygen delivery, oxygen extraction increases.[25]

Hypoxemia

The most common postoperative complication is hypoxemia secondary to alveolar hypoventilation, reduced functional residual capacity (FRC), airway closure, and postsurgical atelectasis.[26,27] Adequate oxygenation, however, can be present despite hypoventilation when oxygen is being administered. The presence or absence of cyanosis may be an unreliable sign because peripheral cyanosis can occur despite adequate arterial PO_2. Morbidity and mortality have been reported to be reduced in patients with severe respiratory failure and system involvement when supranormal levels of oxygen delivery are achieved.[21,28]

Box 36-2 Common Postoperative Complications

- Hypoxemia
- Hypercapnia
- Increased work of breathing
- Increased work of the heart
- Fluid shifts and third spacing
- Fluid and electrolyte imbalances
- Metabolic and blood sugar abnormalities
- Reduced blood volume
- Cardiac dysrhythmias
- Reduced cardiac output
- Reduced tissue perfusion and oxygenation
- Anemia
- Pain
- Alveolar hypoventilation
- Airway collapse
- Atelectasis
- Physiological shunting
- Ventilation and perfusion mismatching
- Impaired mucociliary transport
- Accumulation of mucus and stasis
- Pneumonia
- Thromboemboli
- Pulmonary embolus
- Coagulopathies
- Sepsis
- Shock
- Multiorgan system failure

Pain

Pain, in addition to the effects of anesthesia, frequently contributes to alveolar hypoventilation and atelectasis after abdominal or thoracic surgery. Rapid, shallow, and monotonous breathing may be spontaneously adopted by the patient to avoid pain and coughing. Although minute ventilation is favored, alveolar ventilation is compromised by the increased ratio of dead space to tidal volume. Furthermore, in the absence of deep breaths, coughs, and sighs, atelectasis may develop in the underventilated portions of the lungs. The ventilation-perfusion ratio is disturbed because blood flow to underventilated lung segments is ineffective, physiological shunting occurs, and arterial P_{O_2} tends to drop although P_{CO_2} may be unchanged. An abnormally high transpulmonary pressure is then needed to reinflate these atelectatic alveoli. The physical therapist ensures good pain control before intervention, including mobilization. Patient-controlled analgesia is used if the patient is able to cooperate sufficiently, as well as conventionally administered analgesia, as required.

Pulmonary Embolism and Deep Vein Thrombosis

Pulmonary embolism is a life-threatening complication. Pulmonary embolism usually results from a thrombus forming in the veins of the lower limbs, in the pelvis, in the right atrium, or in the right ventricle. Patients may be at risk if they have varicose veins, chronic heart failure, or cancer or if they are obese, pregnant, or taking oral contraceptives.

Box 36-3 Factors Contributing to Perioperative Complications that Affect Oxygen Transport

- Premorbid cardiovascular and pulmonary status
- Premorbid oxygen transport (aerobic) capacity
- Premorbid systemic disease
- Premorbid general health and immune status
- Smoking history
- Age and sex
- Lifestyle factors: nutritional status, stress, work situation, family situation, psychosocial support system, and substance abuse
- Obesity
- Pregnancy
- Pain and anxiety
- Reduced arousal
- Reduced mobility
- Recumbency
- Medications (e.g., narcotics)
- Nutritional deprivation
- Reduction in normal sleep quality and quantity
- Type of surgery
- Extent of physical manipulation and compression of lung parenchyma, phrenic nerves, diaphragm, and the heart
- Fever and increased oxygen consumption
- Duration of surgery
- Position assumed during surgery
- Duration of static positioning during surgery
- Type, depth, and duration of anesthesia and sedation
- Use of an airway
- Use of mechanical ventilation
- Oxygen therapy
- Neuromuscular blockade
- Fluid loss and chest tube drainage
- Fluid accumulation and third spacing
- Infusion of blood products
- Site, number, and extent of incisions
- Dressings and binders
- Traction and splinting devices
- Placement of lines, leads, catheters, and monitoring devices
- Invasive monitoring equipment (e.g., Swan-Ganz catheter, Foley catheter, intracranial pressure monitor, central venous line, arterial lines, intravenous lines, and intraaortic balloon counter pulsation pump)
- Need for cardiopulmonary bypass machine
- Duration of cardiopulmonary bypass machine use
- Infection

The patient with a pulmonary thromboembolism usually has a sudden onset of tachypnea, radiating chest pain, and apparent anxiety. Occasionally, right-sided heart failure follows. Enzymes are often elevated. Right-sided heart strain may be evidenced on an echocardiogram or electrocardiogram (ECG). Right bundle branch block, peaked P waves, and inverted T waves may be seen. There may be no abnormality noted on chest radiographs.

Treatment consists of primary ventilatory and circulatory support, with adequate oxygenation of peripheral tissues. Anticoagulants, such as heparin, are infused intravenously to minimize further formation of thromboembolic substrates.

Principles of Physical Therapy Management

Impairments in lung volume, mechanics, and gas exchange uniformly occur after anesthesia and tissue dissection. The extent and duration of these changes increase with the magnitude of the operative procedure, the degree of anesthesia required, and the patient's premorbid risk factors. These abnormalities observed in the postoperative period are characterized by gradual and progressive alveolar collapse. Total lung capacity, FRC, and residual volume are decreased in patients who develop complications. Because of the decrease in FRC (30% or more), lung compliance is decreased, and therefore the work of breathing is increased. Hypoxemia secondary to transpulmonary shunting usually becomes maximal within 72 hours after surgery and often is completely resolved with conservative management within 7 days. The FiO_2 will depend on the mode of supplemental oxygen administration. Low oxygen flows and low amounts of FiO_2 tend to be delivered via nasal cannulas. Higher flows can deliver higher amounts of FiO_2 via oxygen masks and masks with reservoir bags. The FiO_2 must always be taken into account in interpreting arterial blood gases. The FiO_2 is selected to provide adequate oxygenation with the lowest oxygen concentration possible.

On the basis of patient assessment, arterial blood gases, fluid and electrolyte balance, hemodynamic status, and radiographs, a decision is made as to which treatments on the physiological hierarchy will optimize oxygen transport and what parameters will be used for each treatment. Positioning these patients upright and mobilizing them whenever possible will maximize FRC and reduce closing volumes and hence enhance gas exchange and oxygenation. What precludes mobilizing these patients even minimally is their lack of alertness, which must be explained. If the patient is unable to respond to treatment because of narcotics, for example, this can be discussed at rounds, and other medications should be considered so that the patient is able to cooperate more. Thus even extreme body positioning will achieve more favorable results.[29-31]

Endotracheal intubation and mechanical ventilation may be indicated if blood gases fail to improve with conservative management. The treatment priorities for the ventilated patient before and during weaning are presented in Chapter 33. Special attention in the postoperative patient is given to the pulmonary complications associated with diminished ability to move spontaneously, surgical pain, restrictions imposed by dressings and binders, and diminished ability to cooperate and to periodically hyperventilate the lungs.

Facilitating mucociliary transport is a primary goal in these patients. Impaired mucociliary transport can be precipitated by alveolar hypoventilation, perhaps the most common cause of postoperative complications. Sufficient impairment can lead to mucus stasis, airway obstruction, atelectasis, and infection. Multiple positions, including upright positions and 360-degree axial turns, and multiple position changes facilitate mucociliary transport. In the event of accumulation of mucus and difficulty in removing pulmonary secretions, specific body positions are selected to optimize postural drainage of the affected bronchopulmonary segments and to maximize alveolar volume and ventilation. The addition of manual techniques can be detrimental in severely ill patients; thus their use needs to be considered carefully.

Suctioning may be most effective immediately before and after position changes. The appropriate oxygen transport variables are monitored to assess treatment outcome and minimally to ensure that the condition of the patient, which may be unstable, is not deteriorating. If the patient's condition begins to deteriorate, treatment is discontinued until the condition stabilizes. Why the patient's condition deteriorated is determined so that a decision can be made as to whether treatment can be reintroduced and, if so, what modifications are indicated.

Pain management is integral to the management of the surgical patient. Noninvasive and nonpharmacological pain control strategies need to be exploited for all surgical patients to augment or reduce the need for potent analgesics, especially narcotics. Chapter 30 describes some physical therapy pain-control strategies for surgical patients that can be applied with modification to the patient with surgical complications. Of these, use of electrotherapy modalities, such as transcutaneous electrical nerve stimulation, may be limited in the ICU because of electrical interference with monitoring devices.

Rest is prescribed as judiciously as treatment interventions to enable the patient to physiologically restore between and within treatments. This is particularly important for ICU patients who are hypermetabolic and have increased oxygen demands. Particular care must be observed in prescribing treatment threshold parameters for these patients. Suprathreshold states can be associated with an inappropriate balance between oxygen delivery and oxygen consumption such that the patient becomes compromised (e.g., patient becomes hemodynamically unstable, cardiovascular and pulmonary distress is precipitated, or both). A greater volume of a mobilization stimulus, however, may be delivered to these patients with an intermittent mobilization regimen than with a single prolonged course of mobilization. Thus the benefits that would be accrued would be correspondingly increased.

Prevention of thromboemboli is a major treatment objective and is best achieved with mobilization, body positioning, passive movements, and physical devices, such as pneumatic cuff devices and stockings, to augment low-dose anticoagulants in patients at risk. Patients who develop pulmonary emboli are treated medically, and physical therapy must be correspondingly modified to minimize oxygen consumption until the patient is in no imminent danger.

Complications Resulting in Secondary Cardiovascular and Pulmonary Dysfunction

Acute Lung Injury and Acute Respiratory Distress Syndrome

Acute lung injury results from damage to the alveolar epithelium.[32] The extent of the damage reflects damage to the type I and type II alveolar cells. Damage to the type I cells results in alveolar edema, atelectasis, and loss of lung compliance secondary to loss of structural integrity of the alveoli provided by the type I alveolar cells. Damage to the type II cells also contributes to atelectasis and loss of lung compliance, but the mechanism relates to impairment of the production of surfactant and pulmonary fluid that covers the alveolar epithelium.

Pulmonary edema refers to the accumulation of vascular fluid in the interstitial spaces and alveoli. In acute lung injury the mechanism of pulmonary edema involves increased water movement across the pulmonary endothelial cells and increased permeability of the endothelium to protein. This type of pulmonary edema is referred to as *noncardiogenic pulmonary edema.* Pulmonary edema that is cardiogenic in origin results from left ventricular failure. An increase in hydrostatic pressure damages the interstitial tight spaces, which normally provide an effective barrier between the pulmonary circulation and alveoli. The critical distinction between the two types of pulmonary edema is that cardiogenic pulmonary edema primarily involves the movement of water across the alveolar capillary membrane, whereas noncardiogenic pulmonary edema involves the movement of protein and water into the interstitial and alveolar spaces. The clinical consequences reflect the location of the edema (i.e., interstitial, alveolar, or both) and the amount of fluid accumulation.

Acute lung injury is characterized as a clinical spectrum of parenchymal cell dysfunction. Mild injury reflects predominantly endothelial cell dysfunction and noncardiogenic edema. Severe injury reflects a progression to both endothelial and epithelial cell dysfunction and ARDS. The clinical spectrum of acute lung injury and the clinical manifestations of mild and severe injury are shown in Figure 36-1. The clinical presentation of moderate injury falls between these two extremes.

ARDS results from major insult to the lung and injury to the alveolar-capillary membrane. Some of the causes of ARDS include shock, severe trauma or infection, overwhelming pneumonia, and inhaled toxins. Increased vascular permeability resembling that of the inflammatory response is a common feature. Fluid seeps into the interstitial spaces and overwhelms the alveoli, leading to pulmonary edema. Lung compliance and gas exchange are severely compromised. Thus the patient manifests severe dyspnea and hypoxemia. Diffuse pulmonary infiltrates appear on radiographs. Arterial hypoxemia results primarily from underventilated but perfused lung units and right-to-left shunt. In this situation, hypoxemia is relatively refractory to increases in FIO_2.

Fibrinogen in the fluids leaking into the alveoli contributes to fibrosis and reduction of lung compliance associated with ARDS. Increased lung surface tension and alveolar collapse tend to result from an inactivation of surfactant with the accumulation of fluid in the alveolar spaces. Thus, reduced lung compliance produces a decrease in FRC in the patient with ARDS.

The signs and symptoms of ARDS may take up to 48 hours to fully manifest. Survival rate has increased over the past decade from 50% to 80%.[33] The explanation for this improvement is unclear; however, the shift to an integrated management approach may be responsible.[34,35] Hypoxemia is a principal feature of the syndrome, resulting from ventilation-perfusion mismatch and from a right-to-left shunt, whereby fluid-filled alveoli are ineffectively ventilated.[36] Hyperventilation and labored respiration can be expected in conjunction with hypoxemia. Oxygen therapy has little effect in the

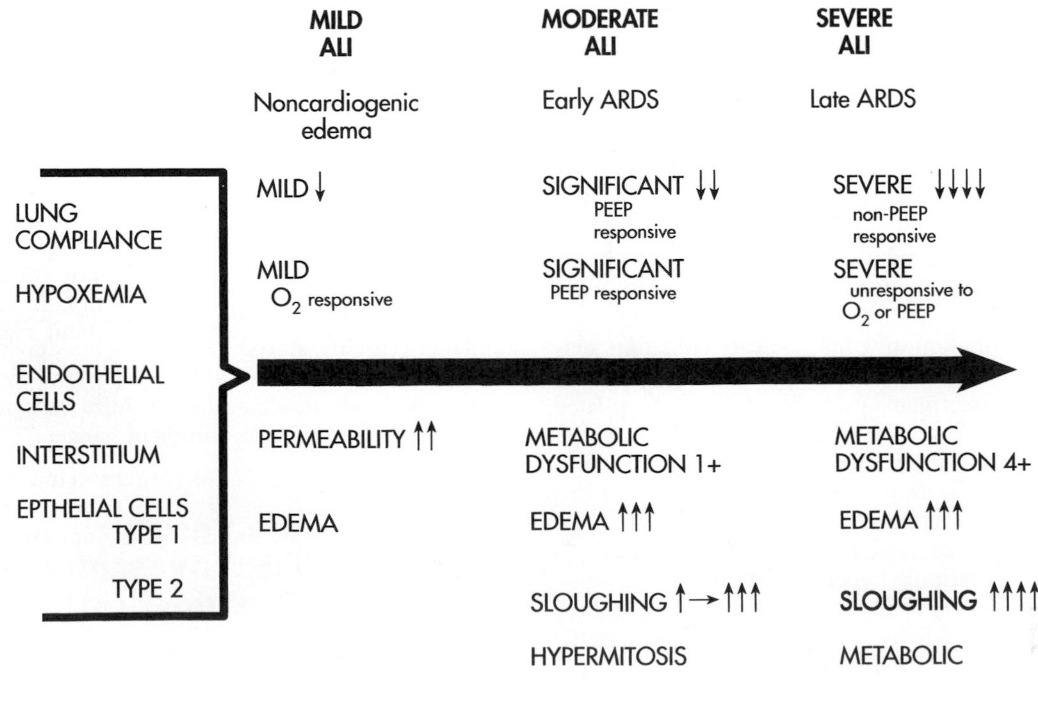

Fig. 36-1 Major pathophysiological manifestations composing the spectrum of acute lung injury from mild to severe disease. *(From Shapiro BA, Peruzzi WT: Changing practices in ventilator management: a review of the literature and suggest clinical correlates,* Surgery *117:121–133, 1991.)*

presence of shunting. Hypercapnia is not usually a major problem in the patient with ARDS.

The metabolic perturbations that can result include problems with oxygen delivery, consumption, and extraction, as discussed previously. When oxygen delivery falls below the critical level, anaerobic metabolism is triggered, resulting in increased lactate production. Elevated serum lactates are associated with a poor prognosis. Changes in oxygenation may not be reflected in $S\bar{v}O_2$ because of the abnormal dependence of oxygen consumption and delivery. Positive end-expiratory pressure (PEEP) can worsen DO_2 in patients with ARDS who are mechanically ventilated and sedated. In turn, $\dot{V}O_2$ may become oxygen supply dependent; thus peripheral extraction may be increased.

Recent advances in the medical management of ARDS include the use of partial liquid ventilation. Although not widely adopted, this form of ventilation may be more effective in recruiting dependent alveoli than conventional mechanical ventilation and may augment the benefits of exogenous surfactant replacement, inhaled nitric oxide, and prone positioning.[37] In addition to improving oxygenation and respiratory mechanics, partial liquid ventilation may reduce ventilator-induced lung damage.[38]

Over the past decade there has been greater interest in long-term outcomes of patients after a course of ICU care, with evidence to support poor long-term functional outcomes. Herridge and colleagues,[39] for example, followed 109 survivors of ARDS at 3, 6, and 12 months after hospital discharge. The patient characteristics were mean age 45 (36 to 58 years); mean APACHE II score 23 (17 to 27); mean ventilator days, 21 (12 to 40); and mean ICU stay, 25 days (15 to 45). All patients reported poor function and attributed this to the loss of muscle bulk, proximal weakness, and fatigue. Only 49% reported working at 12 months. Thus survivors of ARDS may have persistent functional disability 1 year after discharge from the ICU. Furthermore, extrapulmonary conditions such as muscle wasting and weakness were common.

Principles of Physical Therapy Management

As in the management of other conditions, physical therapists need to address the immediate short-term needs of the patient related to maximizing oxygen transport as well as long-term functional outcomes, including aerobic capacity and general physical conditioning, that meet the needs of daily living.

With respect to the short-term goals of maximizing oxygen transport in patients with ARDS (comparable to others with severe respiratory distress), patients will be intubated and mechanically ventilated. Intubation and ventilatory support are implemented if arterial blood gases are severely affected and respiratory distress worsened. An endotracheal tube can be placed through the nose or mouth or a tracheostomy can be performed in cases in which prolonged ventilatory support is anticipated. A high level of PEEP maintains the alveoli open and thereby optimizes gas transfer at end expiration. Arterial oxygenation is usually improved with PEEP because the effect of shunting is reduced and a given FiO_2 tends to be more effective. Although the FiO_2 may be reduced, which reduces the possibility of oxygen toxicity, supranormal oxygen delivery can be beneficial in these patients. Survival may be improved and frequency of MOSF reduced.

Further monitoring of respiratory status in conjunction with arterial blood gases is essential for following the progress of the syndrome. In addition to the oxygen transport variables, the principal parameters monitored in ARDS are reduced lung compliance, tachypnea, and the concentration of inspired oxygen needed to maintain acceptable levels of the arterial blood gases.

ARDS is characterized by a major pathophysiological restrictive component; hence the principles of management of restrictive lung disease are applied. Changes in lung compliance and FiO_2 requirements provide guidelines to treatment required, treatment response, and course of the syndrome. Patients with ARDS require close monitoring and often treatments aimed at promoting optimal gas exchange because of the severity of the syndrome and high incidence of mortality associated with it.

Initially, if the patient is sedated, body positioning is exploited to maintain blood gases, and optimal range of motion and skin care are the focus of management. In severe ARDS the patient usually requires a high degree of ventilatory support with high FiO_2, and sedation. Severely affected patients may require neuromuscular blockade to reduce their oxygen demand and enable them to respond to ventilatory assistance more effectively. Handling and positioning patients on neuromuscular blockade requires particular care because these patients lack muscle tone to protect their muscles and joints. Rotating beds can be extremely beneficial for patients who are either too hemodynamically unstable or difficult to turn manually. These mechanical beds slowly rotate side to side through an arc, thus changing the patient's body position continuously.[40,41] When the effects of continuous axial rotation on a kinetic bed are compared with the effects in prone position, they have been shown to be comparable.[42]

The prone position can have immediate benefit in remediating hypoxemia in patients with ARDS,[43,44] and oxygenation can be significantly improved over supine.[45] This position and semirecumbent positions can augment the effects of mechanical ventilation.[46] The prescriptive parameters of the prone position in patients with ARDS, however, need to be based on a careful analysis of the pros and cons for each patient, and no single position will be maximally beneficial all the time. There are other physiological benefits to shifting the patient's position rather than maintaining a single position (see Chapter 20), provided that oxygenation is not compromised. With improvement of ARDS (e.g., less ventilator support, reduced FiO_2, and satisfactory gases), the patient may be able to be mobilized with careful monitoring of vital signs, ECG, saturation, and subjective tolerance. Body positioning is initiated as soon as patients can tolerate it without significant desaturation. Special attention is given to body positioning to promote ventilation and perfusion matching and mucociliary transport and to minimize the effect of restriction of diaphragmatic and chest wall excursion. Some patients, for example, benefit from side-lying positions in which excursion of the inferior hemidiaphragm is favored. Other patients, however, seem to deteriorate from apparent restriction of the inferior lung in side-lying positions.

The underlying pathophysiology associated with ARDS is primarily related to respiratory mechanics, which could explain why improvements in oxygenation have not been associated with secretion clearance.[47] Each patient's condition and specific areas of lung involvement must be taken into consideration when a turning regimen is prescribed. The effect of the patient's body position on blood gases helps to establish a suitable regimen on a rational basis. Optimal positioning can result in reduced supplemental oxygen needs.[48] The sitting position optimizes lung capacity even when a patient is intubated and mechanically ventilated. The airway can dislodge, however, so caution must be observed and the artificial airway properly secured before any mobility activity. The use of a reclining chair at the bedside should be considered in the management of patients with acute lung injury. Theoretically, the potential function of all lung fields will be benefited with the lungs in a more upright position. Patients who are too unstable to tolerate upright positions and whose oxygenation is compromised in this position[49] may respond favorably to extreme body positions and the prone position.[50,51] The clinical benefits of the prone position in the management of the majority of patients with ARDS have been well documented over the past 20 years; thus physical therapists need to consider positioning these patients prone as a common practice barring contraindications.

Improvements in oxygenation in patients with acute lung injury and ARDS with the prone position, including prone abdomen free, have been well documented in adult and pediatric populations.[33,52-55] The benefits can persist when the patient is returned to the supine position, and furthermore, the prone position does not adversely affect hemodynamics.[56] The use of the prone position in the management of ARDS has been reported to be independently associated with survival.[57] The literature is inconsistent, however, regarding whether patients respond differently depending on the underlying ARDS pathophysiology (pulmonary or nonpulmonary). Some investigators report no differences,[58] whereas others have reported marked differences with respect to radiographic changes, respiratory mechanics, and time course of oxygenation.[54] These differences may be explained by pathophysiological differences in the primary disease insult responsible for ARDS, stage and severity, and comorbidity.

The mechanisms for improved gas exchange in prone positions in these severely ill patients have been the subject of much interest. Hypotheses have included improved alveolar recruitment and lung volumes; homogeneous distributions of ventilation and perfusion[59]; increased static lung compliance[60]; and reduced compressive forces compared with the supine position.[61,62] In the posterior lung fields in the prone position, in the areas where atelectasis, shunt, and ventilation-perfusion mismatch are most prevalent, transpulmonary pressure exceeds airway opening pressure without apparently compromising anterior lung fields.[63] A decrease in $PaCO_2$ with prone positioning predicts survival.[64]

Problems with positioning patients in prone have been reported to be rare. Studies have been focusing on the differences between patients who respond favorably and those who do not (i.e., responders versus nonresponders). Patients may respond better in the early stages in which pulmonary edema is present versus the later stages in the presence of pulmonary fibrosis.[65] Alveolar recruitment procedures are more effective in improving PaO_2 in the prone position, and lower PEEP levels are needed to sustain improved PaO_2 compared with the supine position.[66] In addition, positive inspiratory pressure, hence barotrauma, and FiO_2 can be reduced.[59] The effects of mechanical ventilation including PEEP,[67] airway pressure release ventilation,[68] and certain pharmacological agents (inhaled nitric oxide) may be augmented in the prone position.[69] Other studies have reported a particular beneficial effect of the prone position. One study reported that the prone position rather than PEEP improved oxygenation.[70] Another study reported that prone positioning improves oxygenation more than inhaled nitric oxide in patients with severe ARDS.[71]

Although considerable evidence supports the clinical effectiveness of the prone position to improve oxygenation, this position should be considered for the management of hypoxemia associated with other conditions as a means of simulating the normal effects of gravity on cardiovascular and pulmonary function. Favorable results have been reported in the management of hypoxemia associated with acute respiratory failure in acute myeloid leukemia,[72] pulmonary hemorrhage,[73] and subarachnoid hemorrhage.[74]

Few complications have been reported with the use of body positioning, and in particular the prone position. Normal precautions are taken to ensure that ventilator tubing and lines and leads are not compromised. Despite beneficial effects of oxygenation in patients with ARDS related to trauma,[75] complications associated with prone positioning have been reported for such patients, including facial and chest wall skin necrosis, wound dehiscence, and cardiac arrest.[76] Special precautions are necessary in this subgroup. Brachial plexopathy has also been reported when positioning patients prone in the ICU.[19] In addition to frequent body position changes, the semiprone position may help to avoid the adverse effects of prone positioning in some patients.[77]

Shock

Common causes of shock include hypovolemia, septicemia, heart failure, and direct insult to the central nervous system. Some of the classical features of shock are hypotension, reduced cardiac output, tachycardia, hyperventilation, diaphoresis, pallor, confusion, nausea, and incontinence. Inadequate tissue perfusion results in extracellular acidemia and loss of potassium ions from the cells. The pulmonary blood vessels constrict in response to hypoxemia, which tends to increase pulmonary artery pressures.

Failure of cellular function secondary to shock can result from a deficiency of substrate for energy production, a reduced ability to use the nutrients for energy production, or both. The pathophysiological mechanisms responsible include hypoperfusion of the tissues, hormonal and metabolic cellular changes, and the toxic effects of the metabolic changes. Collectively, these produce cellular damage. With hypoperfusion and decreased oxygen delivery and other nutrients, the production of adenosine triphosphate is reduced. The maintenance and repair of cell membranes is disrupted, resulting in swelling of the endoplasmic reticulum and eventually the mitochondria. Persisting cellular hypoxia contributes to rupture of the lysosomes, which releases enzymes that contribute to intracellular digestion and calcium deposition. Once the lysosomes have ruptured and intracellular digestion has been triggered, irreversible cell damage ensues, impairing oxygen extraction and uptake.[9]

The dependence between oxygen consumption and delivery is a marker for septic shock and thus provides justification for increasing oxygen delivery (see Chapter 2).[78] The relationship of oxygen consumption and delivery has been used to evaluate patients who are critically ill with SIRS and predict metabolic stress on this basis.[79]

The pathology of shock and the effect on the respiratory membranes of the mitochondria follow a similar course regardless of cause. Swelling of the interstitial tissue disrupts the perfusion of the pulmonary capillaries. Congestive atelectasis and pulmonary edema ensue. In the advanced stages, hyaline membrane changes and pneumonitis may occur.

When shock is associated with heart failure, ventricular assist devices or an intraaortic balloon pump may be indicated. These devices reduce the degree to which the patient can be positioned and moved; therefore consultation with the team is essential in progressing such a patient.

Septic shock is a serious condition; patients manifest hypotension despite intensive medical treatment. Persistent hypotension leads to decreased blood flow to vital organs and can result in acute MOSF. Poulsen and colleagues (2009)[80] followed 174 patients in the ICU to evaluate the physical outcomes of survivors 1 year after septic shock. Survivors were interviewed about their physical function and socioeconomic status. Seventy-eight patients were invited to participate, and 70 replied. After 12 months, two thirds of the patients reported that they had not regained their preadmission physical status, and 81% attributed this to loss of muscle mass. Physical function is substantially reduced in survivors of septic shock 1 year after discharge; thus recovery of physical function warrants being identified as a long-term goal.

Principles of Physical Therapy Management

Foremost, the physical therapist must be knowledgeable about the relationship of oxygen delivery and consumption in patients with shock, as well as the implications of the pathophysiological processes on oxygen extraction. The type of treatments and their parameters are based on a careful analysis of oxygen transport variables. Treatments are prescribed within the patient's safety margin. Physical therapists in the ICU must also be knowledgeable about the signs and symptoms associated with impending and frank shock. By recognizing and understanding the components of the different types of shock and the effect on the cardiovascular and pulmonary systems, the physical therapist can better prescribe a rational treatment plan for the short- and long-term management of the patient.

Although physical therapy may be limited in reversing the signs and symptoms of shock, physical therapy can help to restore and maintain optimal cardiovascular and pulmonary function, reduce the risk of complications associated with restricted mobility and recumbency, and maintain physical status at an optimal level during the episode and in anticipation of the patient's recovery. The primary objective, however, is to minimize oxygen demand. A minimal objective is not to worsen the patient's condition by imposing excessive metabolic demand. This is the case in patients whose oxygen delivery is approaching the critical level with respect to oxygen consumption dependence. Excessive demands in these patients can be life-threatening.

Patients in shock are usually unresponsive. The course of the shock episode is often complicated by the sequelae of restricted mobility and recumbency. The specific goals related to optimization of cardiovascular, pulmonary, and musculoskeletal function and prevention of further complications associated with cardiovascular and pulmonary function in particular are priorities.

Treatment goals are therefore critically appraised and prioritized throughout each day to target physical therapy treatment only to the very immediate and essential needs of the patient, avoiding unnecessary fatigue. Prudent patient positioning is a priority because of the relative immobility and reduced spontaneous movement observed in these patients, and recumbency. Approximations to the upright position (i.e., head of bed up and foot of bed down) can augment sympathetic stimulation and improve hemodynamic status and reduce sympathomimetic medications. In addition, this position simulates the upright sitting position (although not perfectly) with respect to its beneficial effects on pulmonary and cardiac function.

Late stages of refractory shock leading to renal failure may necessitate dialysis. If hemodialysis is indicated, the patient is connected to a unit that dialyzes the blood externally. This process takes several hours and is usually repeated every few days.

Comparable to the management of other patients who are unstable and severely ill, physical therapy may consist of primarily supportive care and comprehensive monitoring in the patient with severe effects of shock regardless of whether he or she is in an acute or chronic stage.

Sepsis and Multiorgan System Failure

Sepsis is the response to bacteremia or other byproducts of bacteria in the blood. The clinical features of sepsis include fever, tachycardia, tachypnea, and respiratory alkalemia. Metabolic abnormalities are also a common feature of sepsis. Sepsis is the most common predisposing factor contributing to MOSF, which typically involves failure of more than two organ systems.[81,82] Table 36-1 shows the major organs affected and their clinical manifestations (i.e., pulmonary, gastrointestinal, hepatic, renal, cardiovascular, hematological, and central nervous systems). The cascade of pathophysiological features of MOSF is precipitated by multiple mediator systems. The release of these mediators impairs oxygen delivery and usage of oxygen by the cells. Inadequate tissue oxygenation may be a mechanism underlying MOSF. Thus, the supply of the major energy source to the cell, adenosine triphosphate, is reduced, which leads to structural and functional damage of the various organ systems. The mortality rate ranges from 60% to 80%.

Conditions that predispose a patient to MOSF include sepsis, overwhelming infection, multiple trauma and tissue injury, inflammation, and tissue perfusion deficits. Patients who are older, have chronic conditions, are immunosuppressed, or have a severe initial presentation have an increased risk of failure and mortality.

Sepsis causes damage to peripheral nerves and muscles as well as organs and is termed critical illness polyneuropathy (CIP).[83] Although the pathogenesis is not understood, these effects must be detected early and addressed to avoid clinical manifestations including muscle weakness, prolonged recovery, and delayed weaning. The systemic inflammatory response and MOSF have been implicated, and neuromuscular blockers and steroids can exacerbate these manifestations. The use of steroids and muscle relaxants should be minimized. Stabilizing the underlying critical condition and avoiding sepsis are of major importance in preventing CIP.

Table 36-1 Presentation of Multiorgan System Failure

Organ	Clinical Presentation	Syndrome
Lungs	Hypoxemia, lung compliance, diffuse infiltrates	Acute lung injury, ARDS
Kidneys	Creatine >2 mg/dL	
	Urine output <500 mL/24 h	Oliguric ARF
	Urine output >500 mL/24 h	Nonoliguric ARF
Liver	Bilirubin 2 mg/dL, SGOT and LDH	Jaundice
	Intractable hyperglycemia or hypoglycemia	Hepatocyte failure
	Cholecystitis	Acalculous cholecystitis
Gut	Upper gastrointestinal bleed	Stress ulceration
Coagulation	Thrombocytopenia, prolonged PT and PTT	Hypofibrinogenemia, DIC
Heart	Hypotension, CI	Heart failure
CNS	Response only to painful stimuli	Obtundation

Modified from Kirby RR, Taylor RW, Civetta JM: Critical care, *ed 2, Philadelphia, 1996, Lippincott Williams & Wilkins.*

ARDS, Acute respiratory distress syndrome; ARF, acute renal failure; CNS, central nervous system; CI, cardiac index; DIC, disseminating intravascular coagulation; LDH, lactate, dehydrogenase; PT, prothrombin time; PTT, partial thromboplastin time; SGOT, serum glutamic-oxaloacetic transaminase.

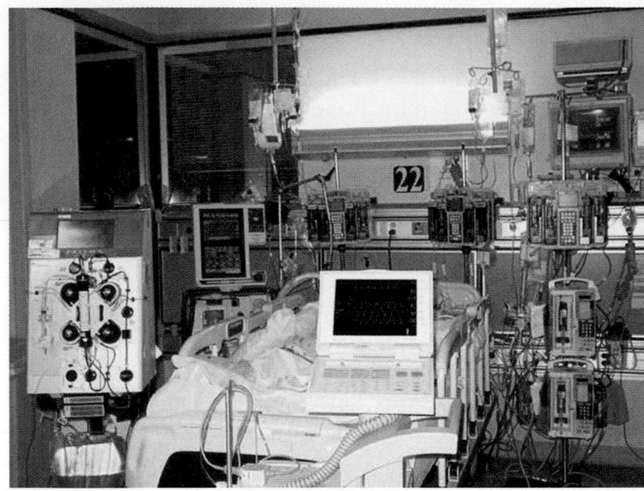

Fig. 36-2 Patient in the intensive care unit with multiorgan system failure. Note the ventilator, continuous dialysis, intraaortic balloon pump, and multiple intravenous drips.

General guidelines for current medical strategies for sepsis and septic shock have been documented.[84] These include life support measures including fluid resuscitation, blood product administration, vasopressor and inotropic support, bicarbonate therapy, and hemodynamic stabilization. To control the sepsis process requires identification and management of the source of sepsis, as well as antibiotic and steroid administration. Sedation, analgesia, neuromuscular blockade, and glucose control are instituted to reduce excess metabolic demand. In the event of renal dysfunction, hemofiltration may be required, along with intermittent hemodialysis. The management of acute renal failure in patients who are hemodynamically unstable with fluid overloaded may include continuous renal replacement therapy (CRRT). CRRT is a dialysis treatment provided as a continuous 24-hour-per-day therapy. Intermittent dialysis treatments are treatments that are provided for brief intervals, usually every day or every 2 or 3 days as needed.

Preventive strategies are implemented to avoid the sequelae of recumbency and restricted mobility, which include risk of deep vein thrombosis and embolism. Like other patients who are critically ill, they are at risk of stress ulceration, thus, stress ulceration prophylaxis is a component of routine medical management.

Principles of Physical Therapy Management

The patient with sepsis and MOSF, like the patient in shock, is gravely ill and unlikely to be able to cooperate with treatment (Figure 36-2). The principles of management are comparable to those for managing the patient in shock; however, oxygen delivery is likely to be consistently compromised in these patients. If oxygen delivery is critically low, $\dot{V}O_2$ depends on oxygen delivery and the patient is in a state of metabolic acidosis (see Chapter 2). In this situation—when oxygen delivery is compromised to the point of not meeting tissue oxygen demands—the goal of treatment is to maximize oxygen delivery[85] and minimize oxygen demand so that oxygenation of vital organs is threatened to the least extent. Thus the physical therapist must estimate the oxygen reserve capacity (i.e., the balance between oxygen demand and oxygen supply) in every assessment to select optimal treatment that is associated with the least risk. Treatments are selected to improve the efficiency of oxygen transport and usage and thereby reduce the work of the heart and of breathing. Above all, treatment should not worsen the patient's oxygen transport status. Selective body positioning, including the prone position, can augment oxygen transport and maximize the effective FiO_2.[86] Even though the patient will likely benefit more from some positions than others, frequent body position changes, preferably a 360-degree turning regimen, are still necessary to avoid the sequelae of static body positioning. Semiprone positions can substitute well for full prone positions if the patient is too hemodynamically unstable. Semiprone positions may be tolerated better by the patient and may be safer. Even though hourly position changes may not be feasible in these severely ill patients, prolonged periods in a static position (more than 2 hours) are deleterious. Thus a balance between these two concerns must be achieved.

Promoting optimal mucociliary transport remains a priority even in the absence of secretion accumulation. Frequent position changes and numerous positions ensure that pulmonary secretions are continually being redistributed to prevent accumulation and enhance removal. Should postural drainage be indicated, these positions may need to be modified.

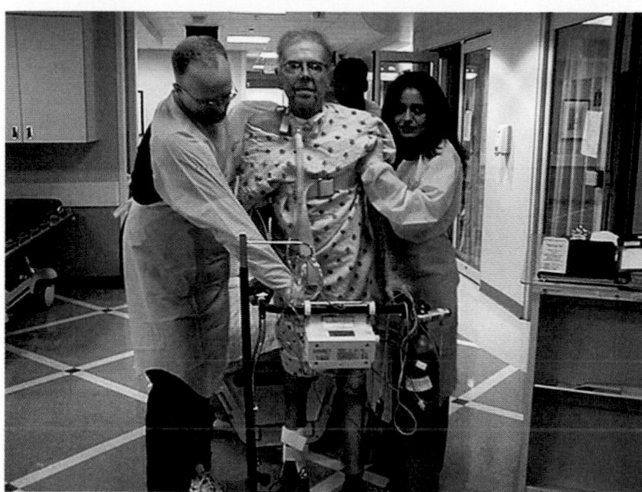

Fig. 36-3 Mobilizing a patient with critical illness polyneuropathy in the intensive care unit. Note the presence of marked muscle atrophy on both lower extremities.

Head-down positions in particular may not be tolerated well. The relative benefits of superimposing manual techniques must be established on the basis of careful assessment because these procedures are associated with an increased metabolic demand to which the patient is not readily able to adapt. Increasing the oxygen demand of these patients may worsen their condition.

The assessment of neuromuscular function is challenging and inaccurate in patients who are severely ill. Patients may have marked weakness related to CIP and myopathy[87,88] and from interventions themselves (e.g., resting of the respiratory muscles with mechanical ventilation; pharmacological agents including glucocorticoids, some antibiotics, and neuromuscular blockers) (Figure 36-3). Thus these interventions may be risk factors, and their use needs to be assessed.

Summary

This chapter presents several major complications that can develop in a patient secondary to various conditions in the ICU. These have implications for physical therapy management. Complications add to the complexity of the physical therapy diagnoses of the patient's underlying problems with respect to oxygen transport and cardiovascular and pulmonary management. The complications highlighted in this chapter include those that impair multiple steps in the oxygen transport pathway and hence jeopardize metabolism at the cellular level. This sequence of events is most frequently associated with the complications of respiratory failure, surgery, ARDS, shock, sepsis, and MOSF.

Physical therapy treatments in critical care areas are typically short and frequent and should always be effective. Patients with complications however, are usually severely compromised and often less able to cooperate with treatment, which necessitates particularly short and frequent sessions. Because of the severity of illness, patients with the complications described may require treatments that are more passive (i.e., stress to the oxygen transport system must be minimal, thus the treatments are lower on the physiological treatment hierarchy). These patients require frequent and comprehensive monitoring (often several times daily) of their oxygen transport capacity (i.e., the relationship between oxygen delivery and consumption, and oxygen extraction, to establish if and when treatment is indicated and the specific parameters of treatment). If a patient is thought to be too unstable for treatment at a given time, continued monitoring of her or his status is essential so that small windows of opportunity can be exploited during stable periods. During periods of monitoring (as opposed to periods of active treatment intervention), the physical therapist continues to have an important role in recommending body positions and frequency of body position changes so that these can yield the greatest benefit to oxygen transport. Treatment continues to progress in preparation for discharge to the ward. Physical therapy assessment and evaluation are ongoing to determine the precise moment when intervention can commence or needs to be modified or withdrawn until the patient has stabilized again. Physical therapy care is imperative throughout a patient's stay in the ICU because patients remain at risk of turns for the worse, which may occur suddenly. Prevention remains the overriding goal until the patient is discharged from the unit.

Review Questions

1. Describe the complications associated with respiratory failure.
2. Describe the implications for cardiovascular and pulmonary physical therapy (assessment and management) of respiratory failure, surgical complications, acute lung injury, ARDS, shock, sepsis, and MOSF.
3. Few longitudinal studies have examined the long-term prognosis for survivors of complications in the ICU. Identify some research questions related to long-term physical therapy outcomes (consistent with the International Classification of Functioning, Disability and Health), and design some studies to address these.
4. Describe some methodological challenges related to physical therapy research in the ICU and how these might be addressed.

References

1. Marx G, Vangerow B, Hecker H, et al: Predictors of respiratory function deterioration after transfer of critically ill patients. *Intensive Care Med* 24:1157–1162, 1998.
2. Boldt J, Menges T, Kuhn D, et al: Alterations in circulating vasoactive substances in the critically-ill: a comparison between survivors and non-survivors. *Intensive Care Med* 21:1836–1849, 1995.
3. Denehy L, Berney S: Physiotherapy in the intensive care unit. *Phys Ther Rev* 11:49–56, 2006.
4. Needham DM, Korupolu R: Rehabilitation quality improvement in an intensive care unit setting: implementation of a quality improvement model. *Top Stroke Rehabil* 17:271–281, 2010.
5. Malkoc M, Karadibak D, Yıldırım Y: The effect of physiotherapy on ventilatory dependency and the length of stay in an intensive care unit. *Int J Rehabil Res* 32:85–88, 2009.
6. Bartlett RH, Gattinoni L: Current status of extracorporeal life support (ECMO) for cardiopulmonary failure. *Minerva Anestesiol* 76:534–540, 2010.
7. Dantzker DR, Schay SM, Fletcher J: *Cardiopulmonary critical care*, ed 3, Philadelphia, 1997, Elsevier.
8. Pallares LCM, Evans TW: Oxygen transport in the critically ill. *Respir Med* 86:289–295, 1992.

9. Wysocki M, Besbes M, Roupie E, et al: Modification of oxygen extraction ratio by change in oxygen transport in septic shock. *Chest* 102:221–226, 1992.
10. Vincent JL: Advances in the concepts of intensive care. *Am Heart J* 121:1859–1865, 1991.
11. Phang PT, Russell JA: When does VO_2 depend on DO_2? *Respir Care* 38:618–630, 1993.
12. Fenwick JC, Dodek PM, Ronco JJ, et al: Increased concentrations of plasma lactate predict pathologic dependence of oxygen consumption on oxygen delivery in patients with adult respiratory distress syndrome. *J Crit Care* 5:81–86, 1990.
13. Dean E, Murphy S, Parrent L, et al: *Metabolic consequences of physical therapy in critically ill patients.* Washington, DC, 1995, Proceedings of the World Confederation of Physical Therapy Congress.
14. Weissman C, Kemper M: Stressing the critically ill patient: the cardiopulmonary and metabolic responses to an acute increase in oxygen consumption. *J Crit Care* 8:100–108, 1993.
15. Dantzker DR: Adequacy of tissue oxygenation. *Crit Care Med* 21:S40-S43, 1993.
16. Nightingale P: Optimization of oxygen transport to the tissues. *Acta Anaesthesiol Scand* 98:32–36, 1993.
17. Lynn-McHale DJ, Carlson KK: *AACN procedure manual for critical care*, ed 4, Philadelphia, 2000, Elsevier.
18. Kirby RR, Taylor RW, Civetta JM: *Critical care*, ed 2, Philadelphia, 1996, Lippincott Williams & Wilkins.
19. Goettler CE, Pryor JP, Reilly PM: Brachial plexopathy after prone positioning. *Critical Care* 6:540–542, 2002.
20. Puthucheary Z, Hart N: Intensive care unit acquired muscle weakness: when should we consider rehabilitation? *Critical Care* 13:167, 2009.
21. Yu DTW: 2010. Early rehabilitation in intensive care unit. Hong Kong Respiratory Medicine. www.hkresp.com/index.php/administrator/128-critical-care/666-2010-may-early-rehabilitation-in-intensive-care-unit. Retrieved February 2011.
22. Pierson DJ: Respiratory considerations in the patient with renal failure. *Respiratory Care* 51:413–422, 2006.
23. Phipps WJ, Monahan FD, Sands J, editors: Medical-surgical nursing: concepts and clinical practice, ed 7, Philadelphia, 2002, Elsevier.
24. Davies MG, Hagen PO: Systemic inflammatory response syndrome. *Br J Surg* 84:920–935, 1997.
25. Polonen P, Hippelainen M, Takala R, et al: Relationship between intra- and postoperative oxygen transport and prolonged intensive care after cardiac surgery: a prospective study. *Acta Anaesthesiol Scand* 41:810–817, 1997.
26. Leblanc P, Ruff F, Milic-Emili J: Effects of age and body position on "airway closure" in man. *J Appl Physiol* 28:448–451, 1970.
27. Ray JF, III, Yost L, Moallem S, et al: Immobility, hypoxemia, and pulmonary arteriovenous shunting. *Arch Surg* 109:537–541, 1974.
28. Hayes MA, Yau EHS, Timmins AC, et al: Response of critically ill patients to treatment aimed at achieving supranormal oxygen delivery and consumption. *Chest* 103:886–895, 1993.
29. Clauss RH, Scalabrini BY, Ray JF, III, et al: Effects of changing body position upon improved ventilation-perfusion relationships. *Circulation* 37 (Suppl 4):214–217, 1968.
30. Douglas WW, Rehder K, Beynen FM, et al: Improved oxygenation in patients with acute respiratory failure: the prone position, *Am Rev Respir Dis* 115:559–566, 1977.
31. Piehl MA, Brown RS: Use of extreme position changes in acute respiratory failure. *Crit Care Med* 4:13–14, 1976.
32. Gattinoni L, Bombino M, Pelosi P, et al: Lung structure and function in different stages of severe adult respiratory distress syndrome. *JAMA* 271:1772–1779, 1994.
33. Ullrich R, Lorber C, Roder G, et al: Controlled airway pressure therapy, nitric oxide inhalation, prone position, and extracorporeal membrane oxygenation (ECMO) as components of an integrated approach to ARDS. *Anesthesiology* 91:1577–1586, 1999.
34. Houston P: An approach to ventilation in acute respiratory distress syndrome. *Can J Surg* 43:263–268, 2000.
35. Stocker R, Neff T, Stein S, et al: Prone positioning and low-volume pressure-limited ventilation improves survival in patients with severe ARDS. *Chest* 111:1008–1017, 1997.
36. Sinclair SE, Albert RK: Altering ventilation-perfusion relationships in ventilated patients with acute lung injury. *Intensive Care Med* 23:942–950, 1997.
37. Wiedemann P: Partial liquid ventilation for acute respiratory distress syndrome. *Clin Chest Med* 21:543–554, 2000.
38. Suh GY, Chung MP, Park SJ, et al: Partial liquid ventilation shows dose-dependent increase in oxygenation with PEEP and decreases lung injury associated with mechanical ventilation. *J Crit Care* 15:103–112, 2000.
39. Herridge MS, Cheung AM, Tansey CM, et al: One-year outcomes in survivors of the acute respiratory distress syndrome. *N Engl J Med* 348:683–693, 2003.
40. Gentilello L, Thompson DA, Tonnesen AS, et al: Effect of a rotating bed on the incidence of pulmonary complications in critically ill patients. *Crit Care Med* 16:783–786, 1988.
41. Pape HC, Regel G, Borgman W, et al: The effect of kinetic positioning on lung function and pulmonary haemodynamics in posttraumatic ARDS: a clinical study. *Int J Care Injured* 25:51–57, 1994.
42. Staudinger T, Kofler J, Mullner M, et al: Comparison of prone positioning and continuous rotation of patients with adult respiratory distress syndrome: results of a pilot study. *Crit Care Med* 29:51–56, 2001.
43. Blanch L, Mancebo J, Perez M, et al: Short-term effects of prone position in critically ill patients with acute respiratory distress syndrome. *Intensive Care Med* 23:1033–1039, 1997.
44. Lan MJ, He XD: Prone positioning ventilation for treatment of acute lung injury and acute respiratory distress syndrome. *Clin J Traumatol* 12:238–242, 2009.
45. Vollman KM, Bander JJ: Improved oxygenation utilizing a prone positioner in patients with acute respiratory distress syndrome. *Intensive Care Med* 22:1105–1111, 1996.
46. Rouby JJ, Puybasset L, Nieszkowska A, et al: Acute respiratory distress syndrome: lessons from computed tomography of the whole lung. *Crit Care Med* 31(4 Suppl):S285–295, 2003.
47. Gillart T, Bazin JE, Guelon D, et al: Effect of bronchial drainage on the improvement in gas exchange observed in vertical decubitus in ARDS [English abstract]. *Ann Fr Anesth Reanim* 19:156–163, 2000.
48. Swanlund SL: Body positioning and the elderly with adult respiratory distress syndrome: implications for nursing care. *J Gerontol Nurs* 22:46–50, 1996.
49. Bittner E, Chendrasekhar A, Pillai S, et al: Changes in oxygenation and compliance as related to body position in acute lung injury. *Am Surg* 62:1038–1041, 1996.
50. Albert RK, Leasa D, Sanderson M, et al: The prone position improves arterial oxygenation and reduces shunt in oleic-acid-induced acute lung injury. *Am Rev Respir Dis* 135:626–633, 1987.
51. Langer M, Mascheroni D, Marcolin R, et al: The prone position in ARDS patients. A clinical study. *Chest* 94:103–107, 1988.
52. Curley MA: Prone positioning of patients with acute respiratory distress syndrome: a systematic review. *Am J Crit Care* 8:397–405, 1999.
53. Curley MA, Thompson JE, Arnold JH: The effects of early and repeated prone positioning in pediatric patients with acute lung injury. *Chest* 118:156–163, 2000.
54. Lim CM, Kim EK, Lee JS, et al: Comparison of the response to the prone position between pulmonary and extrapulmonary acute respiratory distress syndrome. *Intensive Care Med* 27:477–485, 2001.
55. Tobin A, Kelly W: Prone ventilation—it's time. *Anaesth Intensive Care* 27:194–201, 1999.
56. Jolliet P, Bulpa P, Chevrolet JC: Effects of the prone position on gas exchange and hemodynamics in severe acute respiratory distress syndrome. *Crit Care Med* 26:1934–1935, 1998.
57. Venet C, Guyomarc'h S, Pingat J, et al: Prognostic factors in acute respiratory distress syndrome: a retrospective multivariate analysis including prone positioning in management strategy. *Intensive Care Med* 29:1435–1441, 2003.
58. Rialp G, Betbese AJ, Perez-Marquez M, et al: Short-term effects of inhaled nitric oxide and prone position in pulmonary and extrapulmonary acute respiratory distress syndrome. *Am J Crit Care Med* 164:243–249, 2001.
59. Breilburg AN, Aitken L, Reaby L, et al: Efficacy and safety of prone positioning for patients with acute respiratory distress syndrome. *J Adv Nurs* 32:922–929, 2000.
60. Servillo G, Roupie E, De Robertis E, et al: Effects of ventilation in ventral decubitus position on respiratory mechanics in adult respiratory distress syndrome. *Intensive Care Med* 23:1219–1224, 1997.
61. Albert RK: Prone ventilation. *Clin Chest Med* 21:511–517, 2000.
62. Albert RK, Hubmayr RD: The prone position eliminates compression of the lungs by the heart. *Am J Respir Crit Care Med* 161:1660–1665, 2000.
63. Lamm WJ, Graham MM, Albert RK: Mechanism by which the prone position improves oxygenation in acute lung injury. *Am J Respir Crit Care Med* 150:184–193, 1994.
64. Gattinoni L, Vagginelli F, Cariesso E, et al: Decrease in $PaCO_2$ with prone position is predictive of improved outcome in acute respiratory distress syndrome. *Crit Care Med* 31:2727–2733, 2003.

65. Nakos G, Tsangaris I, Kostanti E, et al: Effect of the prone position on patients with hydrostatic pulmonary edema compared with patients with acute respiratory distress syndrome and pulmonary fibrosis. *Am J Respir Critical Care Med* 161:360–368, 2000.
66. Kacmarek RM: Strategies to optimize alveolar recruitment. *Curr Opin Crit Care* 7:15–20, 2001.
67. Lim CM, Koh Y, Chin JY, et al: Respiratory and haemodynamic effects of the prone position at two different levels of PEEP in a canine lung injury model. *Eur Respir J* 13:163–168, 1999.
68. Varpula T, Pettila V, Nieminen H, et al: Airway pressure release ventilation and prone positioning in severe acute respiratory distress syndrome. *Acta Anaesthesiol Scand* 45:340–344, 2001.
69. Johannigman JA, Davis K, Jr, Miller SL, et al: Prone positioning and inhaled nitric oxide: synergistic therapies for acute respiratory distress syndrome. *J Trauma* 50:589–595, 2001.
70. Gainnier M, Michelet P, Thirion X, et al: Prone position and positive-end expiratory pressure in acute respiratory distress syndrome. *Crit Care Med* 31:2719–2726, 2003.
71. Dupont H, Mentec H, Cheval C, et al: Short-term effect of inhaled nitric oxide and prone positioning on gas exchange in patients with severe acute respiratory distress syndrome. *Crit Care Med* 28:304–308, 2000.
72. Schmidt JE, Tamburro RF, Sillos EM, et al: Pathophysiology-directed therapy for acute hypoxemic respiratory failure in acute myeloid leukemia with hyperleukocytosis. *J Pediatr Hematol Oncol* 25:569–571, 2003.
73. Hayes-Bradley C: Hypoxia from vasculitis pulmonary haemorrhage improved by prone position ventilation. *Br J Anaesth* 92:754–757, 2004.
74. Reinprecht A, Greher M, Wolfsberger S, et al: Prone position in subarachnoid hemorrhage patients with acute respiratory distress syndrome: effects on cerebral tissue oxygenation and intracranial pressure. *Crit Care Med* 31:1831–1838, 2003.
75. Fridrich P, Krafft P, Hochleuthner H, et al: The effects of long-term prone positioning in patients with trauma-induced adult respiratory distress syndrome. *Anesth Analg* 83:1139–1140, 1996.
76. Offner PJ, Haenel JB, Moore EE, et al: Complications of prone ventilation in patients with multisystem trauma with fulminant acute respiratory distress syndrome. *J Trauma* 48:224–228, 2000.
77. Schmitz TM: The semi-prone position in ARDS: five case studies. *Crit Care Nurs* 11:22–30, 1991.
78. Friedman G, de Backer D, Shahla M, et al: Oxygen supply dependency can characterize septic shock. *Intensive Care Med* 14:118–123, 1998.
79. Moriyama S, Okamoto K, Tabira Y, et al: Evaluation of oxygen consumption and resting energy expenditure in critically ill patients with systemic inflammatory response syndrome. *Crit Care Med* 27:2133–2136, 1999.
80. Poulsen JB, Moller K, Kelet H, et al: Long-term physical outcome in patients with septic shock. *Acta Anaesthsiol Scand* 53:724–730, 2009.
81. Carrico CJ, Meakins JL, Marshall JC: Multiple organ failure syndrome. The gastrointestinal tract: the motor of MOF. *Arch Surg* 121:197–208, 1993.
82. Vincent JL: Oxygen transport in severe sepsis. *Acta Anaesthesiol Scand* 37(Suppl 98):29–31, 1993.
83. Hund EF, Fogel W, Krieger D, et al: Critical illness polyneuropathy: clinical findings and outcomes of a frequent cause of neuromuscular weaning failure. *Crit Care Med* 24:1328–1333, 1996.
84. Dellinger RP, Carlet JM, Masur H, et al: Surviving Sepsis Campaign guidelines for management of severe sepsis and septic shock. *Crit Care Med* 32:858–873, 2004.
85. Yu M, Levy MM, Smith P, et al: Effect of maximizing oxygen delivery on morbidity and mortality rates in critically ill patients: A prospective, randomized, controlled study. *Crit Care Med* 21:830–838, 1993.
86. Chiumello D, Cressoni M: Respirator management of sepsis-related respiratory failure. *Curr Infect Dis Rep* 11:365–371, 2009.
87. Latronico N, Recupero D, Candiani A, et al: Critical illness myopathy and neuropathy. *Lancet* 347:1579–1582, 1996.
88. Fan E, Zanni JM, Dennison CR, et al: Critical illness neuromyopathy and muscle weakness in patients in the intensive care unit. *AACN Adv Crit Care* 20:243–253, 2009.

Part VII

Cardiovascular and Pulmonary Physical Therapy: Special Cases

PART VII OUTLINE

VII

Chapter 37

Infants and Children with Cardiovascular and Pulmonary Dysfunction

Mary Rahlin and Victoria A. Moerchen

KEY TERMS

Atrioventricular septal defect
Bronchopulmonary dysplasia
Cardiac defect
Cardiovascular development
Cerebral palsy
Chest physical therapy with infants/children
Childhood asthma
Cystic fibrosis
Down syndrome
Endocardial cushion defect
Exercise
Handling for ventilation
Muscular dystrophy
Obesity
Patent ductus arteriosus
Pediatric cardiac rehabilitation
Pediatric pulmonary rehabilitation
Pulmonary development
Respiratory distress syndrome
Transitional circulation
Trunk-ventilation interaction

CHAPTER OUTLINE

Pediatrics entails a special application of cardiovascular and pulmonary physical therapy. This chapter stresses that cardiovascular and pulmonary development and its related vulnerabilities form the basis for neonatal and pediatric practice in this area.

The objectives of this chapter are to review cardiovascular and pulmonary development and related vulnerabilities; relate developmental pathologies to issues of adequate ventilation and oxygen transport; identify cardiovascular and pulmonary co-morbidities associated with reduced physical activity and obesity; present principles and precautions of direct respiratory care; and incorporate these principles into suggestions for practice.

This chapter begins with a brief description of critical events and important characteristics of cardiac and pulmonary development. Relevant pediatric conditions are then presented to build on to this developmental perspective and stress that cardiovascular and pulmonary pathology and ventilatory compromise are often related to developmental vulnerabilities. Obesity is presented as a complicating factor in the cardiovascular and pulmonary health of children with and without clinical diagnoses. Finally, treatment approaches are described, including pediatric cardiac rehabilitation, pulmonary care for neonates, infants and children, pediatric pulmonary rehabilitation, and developmental therapeutic handling used to improve trunk alignment and ventilatory muscle function.

Knowledge of cardiovascular and pulmonary development, congenital and developmental cardiovascular and pulmonary pathology, and appropriate pediatric interventions is essential for any pediatric therapist. Most children require ongoing attention to respiratory function, whether as a primary focus of physical therapy or as an inherent aspect of motor development. This chapter is relevant to therapists who perform direct cardiovascular and pulmonary care and to those who incorporate a cardiovascular and pulmonary awareness into developmental motor therapy and the promotion of wellness in children.

Cardiovascular and Pulmonary Development

The application of cardiovascular and pulmonary physical therapy to infants and children requires a special understanding of developmental anatomy and physiology. Knowledge of normal development and its inherent points of vulnerability will help the reader understand some of what is known about cardiovascular and pulmonary pathology in pediatric populations.

Cardiac Development

Differences in fetal and neonatal gas exchange account for differences in the anatomy and physiology of fetal and neonatal circulation. A basic review of developmental circulation is essential for the discussion of congenital heart defects and the role of pediatric cardiovascular and pulmonary physical therapy.

Fetal Circulation

Placental oxygenation is a major characteristic of fetal circulation. Additionally, in fetal circulation, blood flow through the right and left sides of the heart occurs in parallel, and therefore cardiac output is actually combined ventricular output (CVO).[1] This is possible as a result of shunts present in fetal circulation.[2]

Three points of shunting during fetal circulation are at the ductus venosus, foramen ovale, and ductus arteriosus. The oxygenated blood from the umbilical vein passes through the ductus venosus to the foramen ovale.[1] The foramen ovale allows right-to-left blood flow through the atria, bypassing the lungs.[1,2,3] Left ventricular output (LVO) enters the ascending aorta and flows to the brain and upper body. The ductus arteriosus similarly allows the lungs to be bypassed, as most of the right ventricular output (RVO) flows to the descending aorta and from there to the lower body.[1,4]

RVO is larger than LVO (59% and 41%, respectively).[5] Fetal blood flow to the lungs from the right ventricle is low because of high pulmonary vascular resistance during fetal circulation. Only 10% to 12% of CVO goes to the lungs,[5-7] and its function is to nourish the developing lung tissue rather than to provide gas exchange.

Neonatal Circulation

Adult-like circulation occurs at or shortly after birth, with separation from the placenta and ventilation of the lungs resulting in closure of the ductus venosus, foramen ovale, and ductus arteriosus.[1,8] This process, referred to as transitional circulation, occurs early in neonatal life and increases the efficiency of oxygen uptake and transport.[2,4,9]

The initiation of breathing and removal of lung fluid increase pulmonary blood flow. Whereas fetal circulation is characterized by high pulmonary vascular resistance and low systemic resistance, separation from the placenta causes a rise in systemic resistance and a decrease in pulmonary vascular resistance. As this shift in relative pulmonary and systemic resistances occurs, the shunts close and the ventricles shift from working in parallel to working in series.[9,10]

CLOSURE OF FORAMEN OVALE

The increase in left atrial pressure that occurs during transitional circulation results in apposition of the valve of foramen ovale against the interatrial septum, functionally closing this site of fetal circulatory shunting.[10,11] The anatomical closure occurs several weeks to several months later.[11]

CLOSURE OF DUCTUS ARTERIOSUS

Functional closure or constriction of the ductus arteriosus occurs within the first 24 to 48 hours after birth in response to increased arterial oxygen saturation. Anatomical closure of ductus arteriosus occurs by 2 to 3 weeks in most term neonates.[4] The responsiveness of the ductal smooth muscle to arterial oxygen tension and to endogenous prostaglandins is affected by gestational age at birth.[4,12]

Pulmonary Development

Structural and functional characteristics of pulmonary development in infants and children are significant because they may contribute to specific aspects of respiratory vulnerability.[10]

Newborn Respiration

The pulmonary anatomy of the term infant is markedly different from the adult but also different from the child. An infant's airways are narrower from the nares to the terminal bronchioles. This presents a point of pulmonary vulnerability because a smaller-diameter airway is more easily obstructed by mucus, edema, foreign objects, and enlarged lymphatic tissue. The infant also has a higher larynx.[10] Although this position of the larynx enables the newborn to breathe and swallow simultaneously, it may also contribute to predominant patterns of infant nasal breathing, which may result in increased work to breathe during any compromise of the nasal airway.

Even without airway compromise, the work of breathing is increased during the neonatal period. The initial low compliance of the newborn's lungs requires increased effort for ventilation, which results in a high respiratory rate and increased oxygen consumption.

Although the process of transitional circulation allows more efficient oxygen transport in the neonate than in the fetus, gas exchange in the newborn is still somewhat inefficient because of immature alveolar structure and function, with significantly lower number of alveoli present in the lungs of a newborn as compared to an adult.[3] The surface area for gas exchange in a newborn is one-twentieth that of an adult,[13] and the diffusion distance across the alveoli-capillary membrane is increased because of thick alveolar walls.[14] Functional characteristics of infant pulmonary development are also significant in terms of understanding possible contributions to pulmonary distress in infants. The diaphragm of a newborn has fewer type I (fatigue-resistant) muscle fibers (20% compared with 50% in an adult).[10] This difference predisposes an infant to earlier diaphragmatic fatigue when stressed.

A biomechanical difference between the infant and child is the circular and horizontal alignment of the ribs and the concomitant horizontal angle at which the diaphragm inserts on the ribs during newborn and early infant chest development.[8,10,15] This, along with the more cartilaginous nature of the ribcage, results in less efficient chest wall mechanics, leading to increased work of breathing (see Chapter 39 for a more complete discussion of chest development).

Respiration in the Child

Two residual structural differences exist beyond the newborn period and have potential implications for pulmonary vulnerability in the child. First, the somewhat horizontal angulation of the ribs persists until approximately 10 years of age and results in less efficient chest wall mechanics.[16] Second, although lymphatic tissues, including tonsils and adenoids, grow in proportion to skeletal growth from 1 to 11 years of age,[17] they may be a potential source of upper airway obstruction in some children.

As infants and children grow and develop, however, most structural and functional disadvantages disappear. An aspect of growth and development that can be protective for infants and younger children is alveolar multiplication. This begins in the first year of life and continues until approximately 8 years of age.[3,8]

Cardiovascular and Pulmonary Considerations in the Preterm Infant

All of the cardiovascular and pulmonary structural and functional characteristics of neonates that have been previously discussed apply to the premature infant. Additionally, there are significant gestational aspects of cardiovascular and pulmonary vulnerability that are more pronounced and create more problems in premature infants (Table 37-1).

Table 37-1 Factors Contributing to Cardiovascular and Pulmonary Dysfunction in the Premature Infant

Anatomical	Physiological
Capillary beds not well developed before 26 weeks of gestation	Increased pulmonary vascular resistance leading to right-to-left shunting
Type II alveolar cells and surfactant production not mature until 35 weeks of gestation; elastic properties of lung not well developed; lung space decreased by relative size of the heart and abdominal distention	Decreased lung compliance
Decreased responsiveness of ductus arteriosus to oxygen tensions; delayed ductal closure	Left-to-right shunting
Type I, high-oxidative fibers compose only 10% to 20% of diaphragm muscle	Diaphragmatic fatigue: respiratory failure
Highly vascular subependymal germinal matrix not resorbed until 35 weeks of gestation, increasing the vulnerability of the infant to hemorrhage	Decreased or absent cough and gag reflexes; apnea
Lack of fatty insulation and high surface area to body/weight ratio	Hypothermia and increased oxygen consumption

Modified from Crane LD: Physical therapy for the neonate with respiratory disease. In Irwin S, Tecklin JS, editors: *Cardiopulmonary physical therapy,* St Louis, 1995, Mosby.

Recall that the transitional circulation of a term newborn includes a decrease in pulmonary vascular resistance over the first day. In preterm infants, however, lung immaturity and abnormal surfactant function[18] may result in retained high pulmonary resistance (poor lung compliance), hypoperfusion, and respiratory distress syndrome.[3,19,20] Persistent pulmonary hypertension will reinforce persistent right-to-left shunting through the ductus arteriosus.[21] Respiratory distress syndrome (RDS) has been identified as the best predictor of prolonged patency of ductus arteriosus.[22]

As the respiratory distress of the premature infant improves with neonatal intensive care, cardiovascular and pulmonary vulnerabilities can then occur in the opposite circulatory direction. Given the gestationally related responsiveness of ductus arteriosus to oxygen, some preterm infants retain patency of the ductus even when pulmonary vascular resistance falls.[23] The result is left-to-right shunting that leads to excessive pulmonary blood flow and the need for supplemental oxygen and mechanical ventilation,[24] which increases the risk for bronchopulmonary dysplasia.[25,26] Therefore the immature status of cardiovascular and pulmonary anatomy in preterm infants predisposes them to hypoxia under any conditions that require increased oxygen.[14,18] Cardiovascular and pulmonary pathophysiology and the stressors inherent to medical care often present challenges beyond the adaptive capacities of these fragile little systems.

Common Pediatric Diagnoses

The sections that follow present and discuss specific cardiac and pulmonary conditions. Common neuromuscular or developmental diagnoses that carry an inherent risk for compromised respiration or associated cardiovascular and pulmonary disease are also discussed. This list is not all-inclusive but merely represents an attempt to provide a preliminary knowledge of underlying pathologies and medical management of children with conditions commonly encountered in the practice of pediatric cardiovascular and pulmonary physical therapy.

Cardiac Diagnoses

Patent ductus arteriosus, endocardial cushion defects, and tetralogy of Fallot are the cardiac defects discussed within the limits of this chapter. Additionally, Table 37-2 provides a

Table 37-2 Common Pediatric Diagnoses and Associated Heart Defects and Conditions

Diagnosis	Heart Defect/Condition
Duchenne's muscular dystrophy[27]	Cardiomyopathy (adolescence)
Fetal alcohol syndrome[28]	Atrial septal defect Ventricular septal defect Tetralogy of Fallot Pulmonary valve stenosis Patent ductus arteriosus
Friedreich's ataxia[29,30]	Cardiomyopathy Ventricular hypertrophy Congestive heart failure
HIV-1 infection[31,32]	Myocarditis Ventricular dysfunction
Juvenile rheumatoid arthritis[33]	Pericarditis Myocarditis Endocarditis
Marfan syndrome[34]	Aortic aneurysm Aortic/mitral insufficiency
Noonan's syndrome[35]	Pulmonary stenosis
Prematurity[24,36]	Patent ductus arteriosus
Trisomy 13 (Patau syndrome)[37,38]	Ventricular septal defect Atrial septal defect Patent ductus arteriosus
Trisomy 18 (Edward's syndrome)[39]	Ventricular septal defect Patent ductus arteriosus (large)
Trisomy 21 (Down syndrome)[40]	Endocardial cushion defect Ventricular septal defect Atrial septal defect Tetralogy of Fallot
Turner syndrome[41]	Aortic abnormalities
Williams syndrome[42]	Supravalvular aortic stenosis Supravalvular pulmonary stenosis

summary of common developmental diagnoses and their associated cardiac defects and conditions.

Patent Ductus Arteriosus

Patent ductus arteriosus (PDA), already introduced as a cardiopulmonary complication in preterm infants, is the most common heart defect during the neonatal period.[24,36] In term newborns, however, PDA incidence is 1 in 2000 births (5% to 10% of infants with congenital heart disease).[4]

Gestational age, the presence of lung disease, the size of the ductus, and the direction of the shunt mediate the clinical features of PDA.[24,36,43] The preterm infant with very low birth weight will have the most extreme clinical picture. An infant or child with a large ductus will also have an obvious clinical presentation. Tachycardia, an ejection systolic murmur, bounding peripheral pulses, increased respiratory distress, and poor feeding or poor weight gain are the classical signs of PDA.[4,23,36] In the term infant, PDA may be more clinically subtle, especially when the ductus is small.[4]

Depending on the extent of the PDA, medical management includes nonsurgical (intravenous) use of indomethacin or direct, minimally invasive surgical closure.[24,36,44-46]

Endocardial Cushion Defects and Atrioventricular Septal Defects

Endocardial cushion defects (ECD) or atrioventricular septal defects (AVSD) represent a spectrum of defects characterized by malformation of the atrial septum, the mitral and tricuspid valves, and/or the ventricular septum.[47] Combinations of these defects are categorized as complete, transitional/intermediate, and partial, depending on degree of ventricular septal deficiency.[48-50] In the complete form, all of the structures are deficient. In the partial form of ECD, only an atrial septal defect with a cleft mitral valve is present.[47-49]

There is marked variation in the underlying anatomy of this class of cardiac defects, such that clinical features are equally varied and difficult to summarize inclusively. In neonates with a complete defect, heart failure may manifest in infancy. Children with milder forms of this defect, however, may not be symptomatic until much later in life, and sometimes, not until adulthood.[49] Additionally, it is common for ECD to be associated with other cardiac defects.[47]

Although the total incidence of endocardial cushion defects in infancy is 1% to 4%, the incidence in infants and children with Down syndrome is 40% to 50%.[51,52] A complete AVSD is associated with this genetic disorder.[50] Operative management of infants and children with ECD depends on the morphology of the defect, the degree of pulmonary hypertension, and the extent of mitral valve regurgitation.[48] For infants with complete AVSD, early surgical repairs are indicated.[52,53,50]

Tetralogy of Fallot

Tetralogy of Fallot (TOF) is named for its tetrad of defects: ventricular septal defect, right ventricular outflow obstruction, right ventricular hypertrophy, and aortic override.[54,55] A neonate with TOF will have symptoms dependent on the extent of right ventricular tract obstruction, which results in decreased pulmonary blood flow and the presence of right-to-left shunting.[54] The classical picture is one of cyanosis, especially with crying or agitation.[47,55] Although most infants have sufficient pulmonary blood flow at birth, the cyanosis usually increases within a few weeks or months after that.[54]

In neonates, initial medical management may include treatment of hypoxemia by pharmacologically maintaining patency or reopening the ductus arteriosus for additional pulmonary blood flow.[55,56] The elimination of conditions that produce hypoxemia may also include pharmacological agents to increase systemic vascular resistance and decrease myocardial contractility.[54] Surgical repairs are generally performed between 3 and 6 months of age.[54,55]

Pulmonary Diagnoses

The section that follows provides a brief discussion of common pulmonary disorders for which chest physical therapy is indicated. Additional physical therapy intervention and interactions of select diagnoses with obesity are described later in this chapter.

Respiratory Distress Syndrome

The most common respiratory disorder in infants born prematurely is respiratory distress syndrome (RDS), or hyaline membrane disease. The higher incidence of RDS has been linked to lower birth weights, and this condition has been described as the primary cause of mortality and morbidity in this population.[3,18,20] A correlation between RDS and increased morbidity, including apnea, bradycardia, and pneumonia, has been reported.[57]

RDS results from lung immaturity, insufficient number of alveoli, and an inadequate amount of surfactant.[3,7,20] Surfactant decreases alveolar surface tension and prevents alveoli collapse during expiration. The surfactant deficiency results in alveolar collapse and increased work of breathing.[20] Antenatal corticosteroids[20,58] and surfactant replacement are standard care for prematurely born neonates to reduce symptoms and sequelae of RDS.[3,59,60] Respiratory failure is common in these infants and necessitates oxygen therapy and assisted ventilation, which, in turn, may lead to further respiratory problems, lung injury, and bronchopulmonary dysplasia.[3,61,62]

Chest physical therapy (CPT) has been commonly advocated for airway clearance and to decrease postintubation atelectasis in infants with RDS.[63-66] However, concerns have been raised about possible brain damage associated with CPT in infants with extreme prematurity and very low birth weight.[65,67] Evidence supporting the application of this intervention with preterm infants has been insufficient and, at times, contradictory.[66,67,68] The results of a Cochrane review of effects of percussion and vibration on the pulmonary system in mechanically ventilated infants were also inconclusive but showed no increase in risk for intraventricular hemorrhage associated with these CPT techniques.[66]

Bronchopulmonary Dysplasia

As more preterm newborns survive neonatal respiratory distress, the prevalence of chronic lung disease, or bronchopulmonary dysplasia (BPD), has increased.[62,69] Although in the past the etiology of BPD was strongly linked to high-pressure positive pressure ventilation and oxygen therapy in the treatment of respiratory distress during the neonatal period,[18,70] this condition is now also seen in infants who initially may need only low-pressure ventilation and minimal oxygen supplementation but whose respiratory function deteriorates over time, with an increased demand for oxygen and ventilatory support seen later, after prolonged mechanical ventilation.[62] Oxygen toxicity, combined with damage to the alveoli caused by mechanical ventilation, leads to inflammation, pulmonary edema, and fibrosis.[61,62,71]

The risk for BPD is highest in infants born at 32 weeks of gestation or earlier, with a birth weight ≤1200 grams, and in those who have more severe RDS.[3,62,71] Table 37-3 displays the definition and diagnostic criteria for BPD.[71]

Medical management of BPD is primarily supportive. Long-term oxygen therapy is often necessary for infants who exhibit persistent severe hypoxemia. The target oxygen saturation levels administered via several different strategies is 90% to 95%.[72] The most promising reported ventilatory strategies include avoiding intubation whenever possible, administering surfactant early if the infant has to be intubated, and using noninvasive ventilation, such as nasal continuous positive airway pressure (CPAP) or synchronized nasal intermittent positive pressure ventilation (SNIPPV).[72,73] Such sequelae of BPD as congestive heart failure, cor pulmonale, and pulmonary edema warrant diuretic therapy for these infants.[18]

Many infants with BPD require rehospitalization before 1 year of age, with respiratory symptoms persisting beyond infancy and into childhood, adolescence, and even adulthood. Decreased lung function in these children[3] has been linked to the duration of oxygen supplementation.[72] Because BPD survivors demonstrate decreased growth and increased incidence of neurodevelopmental sequelae, including cerebral palsy, impairments in gross and fine motor skills, cognition and language development, many of them require developmental interventions, such as physical, occupational, and speech therapies.[18,72,74] Evidence related to CPT application for airway clearance with infants born preterm has been discussed earlier in this chapter.

Table 37-3 Definition of Bronchopulmonary Dysplasia: Diagnostic Criteria

Gestational Age	<32 wk	≥32 wk
Time point of assessment	36 wk PMA or discharge to home, whichever comes first	>28 d but <56 d postnatal age or discharge to home, whichever comes first
Treatment with oxygen >21% for at least 28 d **plus:**		
Mild BPD	Breathing room air at 36 wk PMA or discharge, whichever comes first	Breathing room air by 56 d postnatal age or discharge, whichever comes first
Moderate BPD	Need* for <30% oxygen at 36 wk PMA or discharge, whichever comes first	Need for <30% oxygen at 56 d postnatal age or discharge, whichever comes first
Severe BPD	Need* for ≥30% oxygen and/or positive pressure (PPV or NCPAP) at 36 wk PMA or discharge, whichever comes first	Need for ≥30% oxygen and/or positive pressure (PPV or NCPAP) at 56 d postnatal age or discharge, whichever comes first

BPD, Bronchopulmonary dysplasia; *NCPAP*, nasal continuous positive airway pressure; *PMA*, postmenstrual age; *PPV*, positive-pressure ventilation.

*A physiologic test confirming that the oxygen requirement at the assessment time point remains to be defined. This assessment may include a pulse oximetry saturation range. BPD usually develops in neonates being treated with oxygen and positive pressure ventilation for respiratory failure, most commonly respiratory distress syndrome. Persistence of clinical features of respiratory disease (tachypnea, retractions, rales) are considered common to the broad description of BPD and have not been included in the diagnostic criteria describing the severity of BPD. Infants treated with oxygen >21% and/or positive pressure for nonrespiratory disease (e.g., central apnea or diaphragmatic paralysis) do not have BPD unless they also develop parenchymal lung disease and exhibit clinical features of respiratory distress. A day of treatment with oxygen >21% means that the infant received oxygen >21% for more than 12 h on that day. Treatment with oxygen >21% and/or positive pressure at 36 wk PMA, or at 56 d postnatal age or discharge, should not reflect an "acute" event, but should rather reflect the infant's usual daily therapy for several days preceding and following 36 wk PMA, 56 d postnatal age, or discharge.Reproduced with permission from Jobe AH, Banclari E: Bronchopulmonary dysplasia, *Am J Respir Crit Care Med* 163:1723-1729, 2001.

Transient Tachypnea of the Newborn

Transient tachypnea of the newborn (TTNB) is another neonatal problem considered in the differential diagnosis of RDS. It is associated with delayed clearance of amniotic fluid from the lungs, and is the most common cause of respiratory distress in neonates.[47,75] It is a self-limiting condition that usually resolves spontaneously, with symptoms lasting from 2 hours to 2 days. Risk factors for TTNB include cesarean section delivery, macrosomia (birth weight of greater than 4000 grams), male sex, and maternal asthma or diabetes.[75]

Meconium Aspiration Syndrome

Meconium is the content of fetal and newborn bowels. Meconium aspiration syndrome (MAS) is respiratory distress in a full-term or post-term neonate born through meconium-stained amniotic fluid (MSAF). This diagnosis is made in absence of any other explanation.[76,77] Meconium aspiration may occur with the first postnatal breaths or with gasping in utero just before delivery.[76,78,79] Although in the past, it was suggested that MAS could be prevented if the upper and lower airways were suctioned immediately after birth,[80] more recent research showed no benefit from routine intrapartum oronasopharyngeal suctioning and yielded varied recommendations regarding endotracheal intubation and lower airway suctioning performed immediately after delivery.[77,81,82] Generally, intubation is recommended for "depressed" but not "vigorous" infants born through MSAF. A systems approach to prevention of MAS has been proposed, including careful monitoring of the delivery by a well-trained interdisciplinary rapid response team and an evidence-based decision-making process regarding the need for endotracheal intubation and suctioning.[81]

Aspiration of meconium may result in serious and devastating pathophysiology. Most commonly, the meconium will partially or completely block the peripheral airways.[76-79] Atelectasis is the classical finding, but with partial obstruction, hyperexpanded areas will also be observed as the result of air trapping in distal, small airways after inspiration. Common complications of MAS include tension pneumothorax, persistent pulmonary hypertension, bronchiolitis, and meconium-induced chemical pneumonitis.[76-79] Additionally, long-term pulmonary sequelae, such as BPD, and neurological and neurodevelopmental disorders, such as seizures, cerebral palsy and global delays, have been reported in these infants.[76,83,84]

Medical management of MAS includes respiratory support via supplemental oxygen and, if necessary, mechanical ventilation; extracorporeal membrane oxygenation (ECMO); and surfactant administration.[82] CPT has been advocated for infants with MAS,[85,86] but more research is needed to confirm its benefits for this patient population.

Pneumonia

NEONATAL PNEUMONIA

The most common organisms producing neonatal septicemia associated with pneumonia in neonates are group B streptococcus and *Haemophilus influenzae.*[47] Neonatal pneumonia mimics RDS in clinical presentation and chest radiographs.

ASPIRATION PNEUMONIA

Aspiration is an unfortunate result of small children's "indiscreet curiosity"[87] in exploring their environment and relying on their mouths for sensory learning. Aspiration can also result from gastroesophageal reflux[88] and decreased upper airway neuromuscular control.[89]

Bronchial drainage techniques are often indicated as part of the medical management of infants and children after aspiration to aid with airway clearance and reduce the possibility of bacterial superinfection.

PNEUMOCYSTIS JIROVECI PNEUMONIA IN CHILDREN INFECTED WITH HIV

In infants with perinatally acquired HIV, *Pneumocystis jiroveci* pneumonia (PCP) frequently occurs within the first 12 months of life, with the peak incidence reported at 3-6 months of age. Although in the United States there has been a decline in the rate of PCP infection, it remains the leading cause of death in children with HIV/AIDS in Africa.[90]

The clinical presentation of PCP includes failure to thrive, cough, dyspnea, tachypnea, fever, hypoxemia, and chest radiograph evidence of diffuse parenchymal infiltrates of reticulogranular quality.[90,91] PCP is most definitively diagnosed after bronchoalveolar lavage studies. Chemoprophylaxis is recommended to prevent the first episode of this disease. Treatment includes antibiotic therapy, antiretroviral therapy, nutritional support, short courses of corticosteroids, and surfactant administration in severe cases.[90]

Asthma

Although asthma is described in detail in Chapter 5, a discussion of pediatric pulmonary problems would not be complete without mentioning this common cause of childhood lung disease. Currently, approximately 22% of school children in the United States have asthma, with this disease prevalence ranging from 15.5% to 28.3% among different states.[92]

Childhood asthma can begin at any age, and its clinical etiology and clinical course are variable. Children with early medical histories that include very low birth weight, bronchopulmonary dysplasia, and respiratory syncytial virus (RSV) infection may be at increased risk for developing asthma.[93-95] Common triggers for asthma symptoms and exacerbations are allergens, respiratory viral infections, tobacco smoke, air pollutants and irritants, extreme temperatures and high humidity, excessive weight gain and low physical fitness, stress, and exercise leading to bronchospasm.[96]

Medical management usually includes avoidance of known precipitants, bronchodilator drugs, and corticosteroids (in chronic, severe cases). Other measures include immunotherapy and child, parent, and health-care provider education, as well as monitored exercise to maintain healthy weight and fitness.[96,97]

Asthma is underdiagnosed and undertracked among minority groups and children from families with low socioeconomic status (SES).[98] Some studies suggest that detection and treatment in schools may be part of the solution.[98,99] Similarly, education regarding asthma management of children from minority or low SES families may be effectively implemented in schools by positioning the school nurse as the case manager.[98-101] In a school district that does not have a full-time nurse in each school, the physical therapist may need to track and be aware of asthma in the child before he or she engages in physical exertion.

Cystic Fibrosis

Cystic fibrosis (CF) is a complex, autosomal-recessive disorder that occurs at a frequency of one in 3500 live births.[102] A defect in a single gene, the CF transmembrane conductance regulator (CFTR), leads to pathological changes in exocrine glands, including airways, sweat glands, pancreas, biliary tract, and gut.[103,104]

The Cystic Fibrosis Foundation Consensus Statement on the Diagnosis of CF[102] includes recommendations for newborn screening (NBS) to identify infants at risk for CF and for the sweat chloride test as the primary method used to confirm the diagnosis. The diagnostic pathway for screened newborn babies differs from that used for patients who present with clinical symptoms of CF. Positive results of NBS warrant a sweat chloride test, which, if also positive, is followed by genetic testing. In patients with signs and symptoms of CF and a family history of the disease, a sweat chloride test is performed, followed by a clinical evaluation, genetic testing, pancreatic function tests, and tests for specific pathogens, such as *Staphylococcus aureus* or *Pseudomonas aeruginosa,* present in the respiratory tract. Clinical symptoms of CF are chronic productive cough, respiratory infections with CF pathogens, abnormal chest radiographs, airway obstruction, nasal polyps, and clubbing of the digits. Other symptoms include gastrointestinal and nutritional problems, systemic loss of salt, and male genital abnormality.[102] The disease progression is one of chronic lung infection that results in fibrosis and bronchiectasis that lead to respiratory insufficiency, the primary factor in morbidity by the second or third decade of life.[103,104] Chronic nocturnal hypoxia becomes a stimulus for the development of pulmonary hypertension and right ventricular failure and is associated with poor prognosis.[105]

The chronic pulmonary disease in CF is related to increased secretion of abnormally viscous mucus, impaired mucociliary transport, airway obstruction, bronchiectasis, overinflation, and infection.[102] Early detection and early treatment are key to the management of CF. The major marker of pulmonary disease in this population is forced expiratory volume in 1 second (FEV_1).[106] However, one study that used high resolution computed tomography (HRCT) to examine the lungs of children 6 through 10 years of age who had no abnormality of FEV_1 revealed air trapping and bronchiectasis.[107] Similarly, when $FEV_{0.5}$ was used as a marker, airway function was noted to be diminished soon after diagnosis in infants with CF.[108] These results support the importance of early intervention in children for whom detection occurs during infancy.[106] Further development of genetic diagnostics and gene therapy may enhance early identification and address effective, if not preventive, early treatment.[109,110]

Medical management includes early nutritional support, treatment of pancreatic dysfunction, judicious use of antibiotics, and preventive infection control measures.[111] The early institution of prophylactic pulmonary physical therapy, such as airway clearance techniques, helps to control or decrease the effects of bronchiolar and bronchial obstruction. Involvement of the child and family in pulmonary care is particularly important. Family understanding of the nature of the disease and the purpose of each therapeutic measure promotes successful intervention. An individualized home program of CPT should be established, taking into consideration the child's ongoing pulmonary needs and the family's unique contributions and constraints.

Bronchial drainage is an aspect of conventional treatment for CF with several options that allow both efficacy and patient independence.[112] Airway clearance techniques (ACT) are described in detail in Chapter 21, but alternatives to traditional percussion and postural drainage warrant mention within the context of CPT for children with CF. Specifically, the forced-expiration technique (FET) as part of the active cycle of breathing (ACB) technique, the use of a positive expiratory pressure (PEP) mask, autogenic drainage (AD), the use of the flutter device, and the application of high-frequency chest compression (HFCC) through an inflatable vibrating vest have been shown to be effective in assisting sputum expectoration, often in greater amounts and in less time per treatment compared with other interventions.[113-119] The efficacy of PEP in this population remains equivocal.[120,121]

Although postural drainage, percussion, and vibration are the treatment of choice for infants and children who are unable to be instructed in techniques that use specific patterns of voluntary breathing, other techniques are available for children who can follow breathing instructions and who can perform a reliable pulmonary function test. Children as young as 2 to 3 years of age can be taught to "huff" as part of FET;[113] the PEP mask has been used with children as young as three years;[115] and AD can reportedly be taught to children at 4 to 6 years of age.[116] The Cystic Fibrosis Foundation CF Pulmonary Guidelines[119] recommend ACT for patients with CF to maintain lung function, clear sputum, and improve their quality of life. Because none of these techniques have been shown to be superior to others, it is recommended to base their prescription on the child's age, specific technique preference, and incidence of adverse events associated with the use of ACT.[119] In patients diagnosed with CF, an airway clearance program should be initiated in early infancy.[111] The benefits of each technique should be carefully considered relative to each child's cognitive, respiratory, and motor planning abilities when choosing or modifying the airway clearance program, and the child's response to any technique must be carefully monitored. The head-down position should not be used for infants and toddlers younger than 2 years of age because it may exacerbate gastroesophageal reflux and affect oxygen saturation in infants with CF who have gastroesophageal reflux disease.[111,119,122]

Ventilatory muscle training is an important aspect of pulmonary treatment in older children with CF. Studies have demonstrated that training to improve the endurance of ventilatory muscles decreases dyspnea and increases general exercise tolerance in patients with CF.[123,124] The role of general exercise in the cardiovascular and pulmonary management of children with CF is discussed within the context of pulmonary rehabilitation later in this chapter. It is important to mention that the use of aerobic exercise for patients with CF is recommended for general health and fitness benefits, as well as a component of the airway clearance program.[104,119]

Special Respiratory Problems Associated with Intubation and Tracheostomy

Once an infant or child develops respiratory failure, intubation and mechanical ventilation are usually required.[3,125] The goals of medical management are then to treat the cause of the respiratory failure as aggressively as possible and to wean the child from mechanical ventilation as quickly as possible. If a child's condition necessitates long-term mechanical ventilation, if an artificial airway is needed to bypass an upper airway obstruction, or if there is a risk for aspiration, a tracheostomy is usually performed.[126]

Infants and children who have a tracheostomy and are intubated for long periods of time require vigorous prophylactic airway management, such as bronchial drainage and airway suctioning. Several studies showed that CPT, including postural drainage and vibration emphasizing right upper lobe segments, significantly decreased the incidence of postextubation atelectasis in infants intubated for more than 24 hours.[64,127] However, as discussed in the RDS section of this chapter, there is insufficient current research evidence to support or refute the use of CPT with infants with extreme prematurity and low birth weight.[66]

Pulmonary Considerations in Children with Movement Disorders

Although cardiovascular and pulmonary symptoms may not be the primary reason for referral to physical therapy in children with neurological, neuromuscular, and other developmental movement disorders, these children do have motor involvement that can result in respiratory and postural muscle weakness, chest immobility, and hypoventilation. Furthermore, many of these children have medical histories remarkable for cardiovascular and pulmonary complications or have progressive disorders that will result in cardiovascular and pulmonary compromise.

Table 37-4 provides an extensive summary of the interactions between trunk musculature and ventilation in children with atypical development. Although the biomechanical deviations noted are frequently seen in children with abnormal muscle tone, they are also common in children with scoliosis, sternal deformity, or general immobility of the thorax. These deviations and other aspects of ventilatory compromise are discussed with regard to motor diagnoses common to pediatric practice.

Cerebral Palsy

Children with cerebral palsy (CP) generally have weak trunk and postural muscles, related to muscle tone abnormalities. A combination of atypical neural mechanisms and muscle weakness produces atypical movement patterns and deviations in functional alignment, leading to decreased chest expansion and lung function.[128] The trunk control and respiration relationships described in Table 37-4 are consistent with the clinical picture of external pulmonary development in children with CP.

Although the extent of mobility impairment is variable among children with CP, hypoventilation, increased work of breathing, inefficient cough, increased risk for aspiration, and poor breath support for vocalization can occur.[129] These children demonstrate decreased movement variability,[130] which contributes to thoracic stiffness. A high chest, flattened anteriorly, with excessive rib flaring is common in these children (Figure 37-1).

Table 37-4 Functional Relationship of Trunk Control and Respiration

Biomechanical Component	Postural/Trunk Control Consequences	Respiratory Consequences
Weak abdominal obliques	Passive lumbar lordosis Protruding tummy Lower rib flaring Decreased trunk rotation Unable to weight shift Dependence on rectus abdominis	Ineffective cough High chest Retained horizontal rib alignment Tight rectus abdominis may lead to pectus excavatum Child may use diaphragm for trunk control, limiting its function as a primary muscle of respiration Decreased support of abdominal contents under diaphragm
Tight pectoralis minor	Forward shoulders Scapula pulled laterally and anteriorly, away from the thoracic wall Upper thoracic flexion	Anterior upper chest cannot adequately expand
Weak serratus anterior	Weak upper fibers—medial edge of scapula leaves the thoracic wall	Decreased structural reinforcement of the posterior chest wall Interdigitation of the lower fibers of serratus anterior with the external abdominal oblique will interact to affect the dynamic stability of the ribcage
Decreased active upper thoracic extension	Kyphotic upper trunk Passive overlengthening of the scapular retractors	Approximation of upper ribs → decreased upper chest mobility → decreased oxygenation of the upper lobe → abdominal breathing
Decreased ribcage stability	Serratus anterior will elevate the ribs rather than stabilize the scapula against the thoracic wall	Decreased structural support for the respiratory muscles to work from

Modified from Moerchen VA: Respiration and motor development: a system perspective. *Neurology Report* 18:8-10, 1994. Reprinted from the *Neurology Report* with the permission of the Neurology Section, APTA.

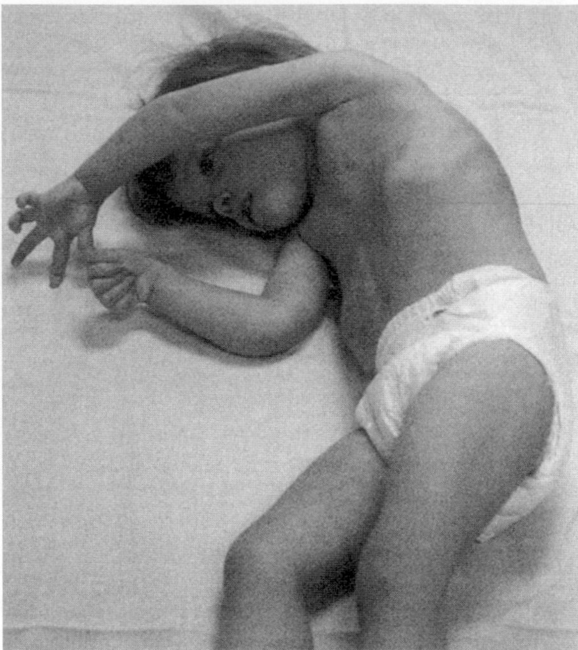

Fig. 37-1 Flattened anterior chest with marked rib flaring in a child with cerebral palsy.

Therapeutic attention to respiration should first identify possible aspiration[131] and suggest modifications for positioning during feeding. Additionally, certain postures for sleep and play may be less restrictive for chest excursion and should be incorporated into a home program.[131,132]

CPT, including postural drainage, percussion and vibration techniques, may be indicated if the child develops a primary pulmonary complication. Because gastroesophageal reflux is a common comorbidity observed in children with CP, head-down positioning should not be used for postural drainage.[131,133] Prophylactic postural drainage can also be integrated into many sensory stimulation programs for more severely involved children. Additional "handling" to address ventilatory function will be discussed in a subsequent section on motor approaches to respiratory treatment.

Myelomeningocele

Myelomeningocele, or spina bifida, is a diagnosis that physical therapists generally equate with issues of ambulation and mobility; however, central ventilatory dysfunction is prevalent in infants, children, and adolescents who also have an associated Arnold-Chiari type II malformation.[134-137]

The Arnold-Chiari type II malformation, which occurs in 57% to 76% of infants with myelomeningocele, is a hindbrain malformation consisting of a caudal herniation of the cerebellum and brainstem into the cervical canal.[138] Ventilatory problems associated with a symptomatic Arnold-Chiari type II malformation include inspiratory stridor (vocal cord paralysis), central apnea, and respiratory distress.[134,137,139] Abnormal ventilatory patterns, however, have also been observed in asymptomatic infants[136] and adolescents.[135] Ventriculoperitoneal shunting for management of hydrocephalus and, if necessary, cervical decompression are the surgical approaches to treatment of life-threatening ventilatory complications in this population.[137,138,140]

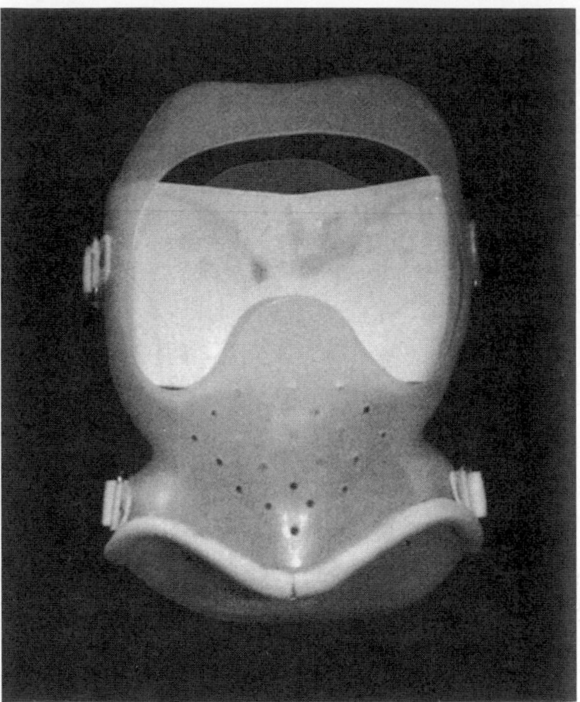

Fig. 37-2 An anterior cut-out and elastic support in a body jacket/spinal orthosis aids diaphragm function.

Other pulmonary issues in children with myelomeningocele warrant discussion. Trunk weakness and hypotonia are observed early in the motor development of infants and toddlers with this condition.[140] In children with thoracic and high lumbar level lesions, abdominal muscle support for diaphragm function may be insufficient. The use of abdominal binders and spinal orthoses/body jackets with anterior (diaphragm) cut-outs and an elastic insert are indicated to aid in diaphragm function (Figure 37-2).

Spinal deformities, such as congenital or acquired scoliosis, kyphosis, lordosis, or their combinations limit chest expansion and decrease ventilatory function in these children. In addition, sudden progression of scoliosis may be indicative of unstable neurology (tethered cord).[140] Therefore close attention to ventilatory ability is necessary both for general monitoring and for possible preoperative evaluation.

Down Syndrome

Respiratory complications are the most common cause of hospitalization in children with Down syndrome.[141-143] These complications are related to structural airway abnormalities and pulmonary hypoplasia, such as tracheomalacia, subglottic stenosis, decreased number of alveoli, increased alveoli size, and widened alveoli ducts. Frequent respiratory infections, pneumonia, sleep-disordered breathing, and interstitial lung disease have been reported in these children.[143]

Impaired pulmonary function in children with Down syndrome is also related to generalized weakness of trunk musculature.[144] The postural deviations common in these children (Figure 37-3) reflect inefficient muscle function for both ventilation and movement.[145] The trunk control-ventilation relationships delineated in Table 37-4 summarize the clinical presentation of external pulmonary development in these

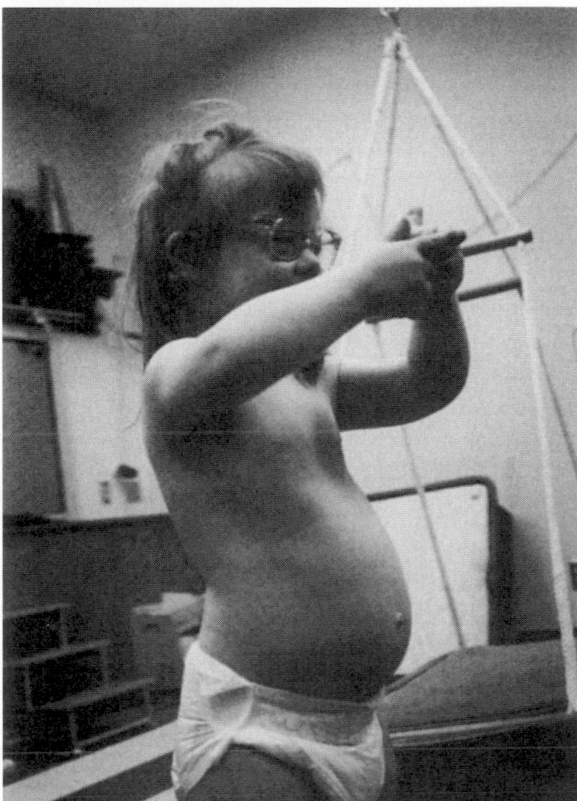

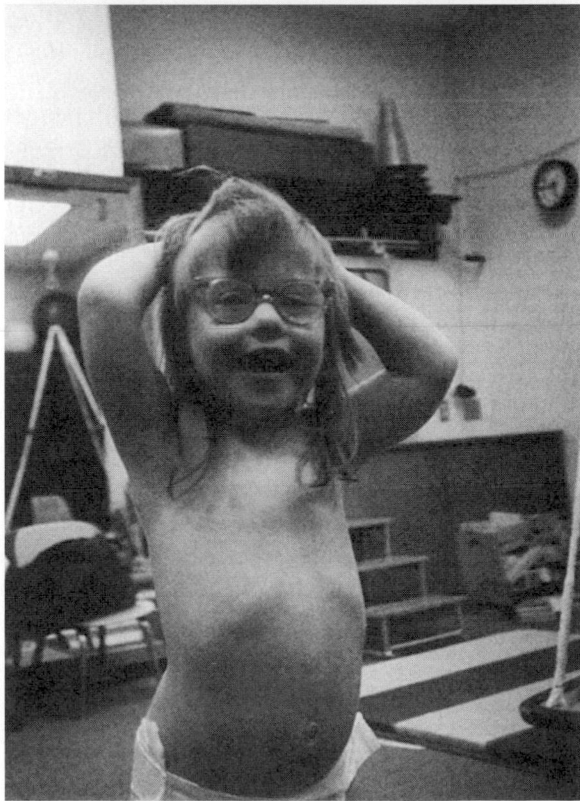

Fig. 37-3 A, Characteristic posture of a child with Down syndrome/hypotonia. Note the abdominal protrusion and sternal retraction. **B,** Rib flaring with upper extremity movement; the abdominal obliques are not stabilizing the lower ribs. *(Photos from Moerchen VA: Respiration and motor development: a systems perspective,* Neurology Report *18:8-10, 1994. Reprinted with the permission of the Neurology Section, APTA.)*

children. Too often, physical therapists who are treating children with Down syndrome address only motor development. Respiration needs to be considered if therapy goals include increased vocalization or improved exercise tolerance.

Duchenne Muscular Dystrophy

Duchenne muscular dystrophy (DMD) is an example of a diagnosis in which the neuromotor and chest wall impairments together lead to ventilatory failure. End-stage respiratory failure in this disease results from progressive respiratory muscle weakness, thoracic deformity, reduced lung compliance, retained secretions, ventilation-perfusion imbalance, and hypoxemia.[146-148] In 70% to 90% of these patients, death is directly related to restrictive respiratory complications. In addition to ventilatory failure, cardiac function also deteriorates in DMD. Dilated cardiomyopathy or congestive heart failure develops during or after puberty.[27,149]

Physical therapists are typically involved in treatment of these patients for preservation of motor function. Early attention to ventilation, however, is warranted. Spinal fusion to prevent scoliosis-related compromise of ventilation in these patients considers both the progression of the spinal curvature and vital capacity (VC).[148,150]

CPT should be a component of the overall physical therapy management of children with muscular dystrophy. Deep breathing, coughing, and activities to address endurance are recommended but will require ongoing modification as the disease progresses.[148] Research has demonstrated positive effects of inspiratory muscle training on ventilatory muscle strength and endurance in these children[151-153] and suggested that these effects are dose dependent.[151,153] Significant correlation between these variables was found in children with VC decline of less than 10% per year before training, but not in children with a greater rate of the disease progression.[151]

Respiratory dependence does occur as the disease progresses. Close monitoring of VC and nocturnal hypoventilation can allow respiratory support to be implemented before the onset of acute respiratory failure.[146,148,154,155] The speed of progression of the disease is significant to the timing of noninvasive positive pressure ventilation (NPPV). Symptoms of nocturnal hypoventilation may be treated initially with continuous positive airway pressure (CPAP), especially if obstructive sleep apnea is noted.[156,157] Transitioning to NPPV is typically required when diurnal hypercapnia is noted,[158] unless severe bulbar weakness is present.[159] Furthermore, when NPPV in combination with insufflation/exsufflation is used to treat adolescents with end-stage DMD, pulmonary complications requiring hospitalization have been reduced.[154] Peak cough flow is greater with in/exsufflation than with manual cough techniques.[160] Progressing to tracheostomy (invasive) ventilation is elective and may be avoidable with combined noninvasive methods initiated earlier in the disease process.

Miscellaneous Conditions

Children with many other diagnoses and musculoskeletal conditions may present with clinical signs (decreased strength, atypical alignment, and limited mobility) that should cue the therapist's attention to pulmonary function. Genetic disorders that involve chest wall deformity, such as Marfan syndrome, Poland syndrome, or osteogenesis imperfecta,[161] may entail ventilatory compromise. Children with juvenile rheumatoid arthritis (JRA) may have inflammation of thoracic joints or may splint through their trunks when they try to move painful extremities. Decreased respiratory muscle strength and lung function have been reported in children with polyarticular and systemic JRA.[162] With these children, breathing exercises will have a role both in pulmonary care and in pain management.

Pain, weakness, or chest wall deformity may lead to the development of compensatory movement patterns that limit the mechanics of the child's thorax. Conversely, inadequate oxygenation may lead to the development of compensatory movement patterns that support ventilation. Therefore attention to ventilation should be an inherent aspect of observing motor development and quality of movement in all children.

Obesity as a Cardiovascular and Pulmonary Comorbidity

The childhood obesity epidemic that is occurring worldwide, across cultures and socioeconomic groups, cannot go unmentioned as a comorbity associated with cardiovascular and pulmonary disorders.[163,164] In addition, overeating and immobility (either elective or secondary to motor impairments) create an additional set of risk factors for the development of cardiovascular and pulmonary disease.[164-166] A brief review of these comorbidities is provided.

Obesity and Asthma

Asthma and obesity present an interaction of factors that are somewhat cyclical in their effects. Children with asthma may be less active, especially if their asthma is exercise induced and they have not been instructed in how to prepare for physical activity. Inactivity superimposed on excessive energy intake (overeating) leads to an overweight status. Among children with asthma, children with obesity wheeze more, use their inhalers more frequently, and have higher bronchial hyperreactivity than do children with normal body mass index (BMI).[167] It has been debated whether high BMI is a risk factor for asthma or whether chest symptoms related to obesity mimic asthma.[166,168,169] A systematic review of the literature has pointed to a strong association between childhood obesity and the development of asthma in adolescents.[170]

Obesity and Obstructive Sleep Apnea

The incidence of obstructive sleep apnea (OSA) related to obesity in clinical as well as nonclinical populations of children is alarming. In typically developing children, the severity of OSA is positively related to degree of obesity.[171-173] Additionally, obesity and obstructive sleep apnea in children are associated with elevated blood pressures and other cardiovascular comorbidities.[172-174]

In clinical populations with known low neuromotor tone of the upper airways, such as children with Down syndrome and Prader Willi syndrome, obesity is associated with higher incidence of obstructive sleep apnea.[175-178]

Physical Therapy Intervention Approaches

Postoperative Pediatric Cardiac Rehabilitation

Postoperative physical therapy consists largely of techniques to increase respiration, mobilize secretions, and progress physical mobility.[179] Positional rotation for pulmonary care is possible if the child has a stabilized sternum. Breathing exercises and coughing will need to be modified based on the patient's age and cognitive level. Huckabay and Daderian (1990)[180] reported improved postoperative cooperation in children 3 to 10 years of age when choice making was incorporated into a breathing program. Another study showed significant reduction in risk for postsurgical pulmonary complications in children who underwent preoperative and postoperative cardiovascular and pulmonary physical therapy as compared with postoperative physical therapy alone.[179]

Immobilization after cardiac surgery is to be avoided as much as medically possible.[179,181] Passive range of motion may be initiated immediately, taking care to avoid compromising arterial lines. Ambulation is generally initiated once the child is extubated and has had atrial and groin lines removed.[181]

Child and family education as part of pediatric cardiac rehabilitation has been observed to reduce parent and child anxiety related to safe levels of physical activity.[182-184] Although studies of pediatric cardiac rehabilitation have focused on children older than 6 years, monitored exercise has been shown to produce such effects as a safe increase in peak oxygen consumption and a decrease in resting heart rate.[182-184]

Exercise prescription for cardiovascular and pulmonary rehabilitation of older children who have undergone cardiac repairs at an early age will require careful monitoring. Lower exercise $\dot{V}O_2$ values, lower cardiac output, and lower values of diffusion capacity of the lung for carbon monoxide have been observed in response to exercise in children who have undergone cardiac surgery compared to healthy peers.[185-187] In addition, lower functional health status has been reported in these children.[188] Exercise recommendations for this clinical population include submaximal performance[186,189] and technique training to increase the biomechanical efficiency of movement while decreasing the associated metabolic costs.[185]

CPT for Neonates and Infants

The primary goal of CPT for neonates and infants is to improve airway clearance. If techniques of bronchial drainage can increase the diameter of the airways through secretion mobilization, then ventilation may also be improved and the work of breathing reduced. These techniques should be judiciously applied for prophylaxis and treatment in infants who have or are at risk for developing airway clearance problems. Applying bronchial drainage techniques to infants requires a thorough understanding of each infant's condition and the precautions and considerations inherent to any technique or combination of techniques.

Positional Rotation

Frequent changing of position will prevent prolonged dependency of any one portion of the lung so that pooling of secretions can be limited or avoided and improved ventilation can

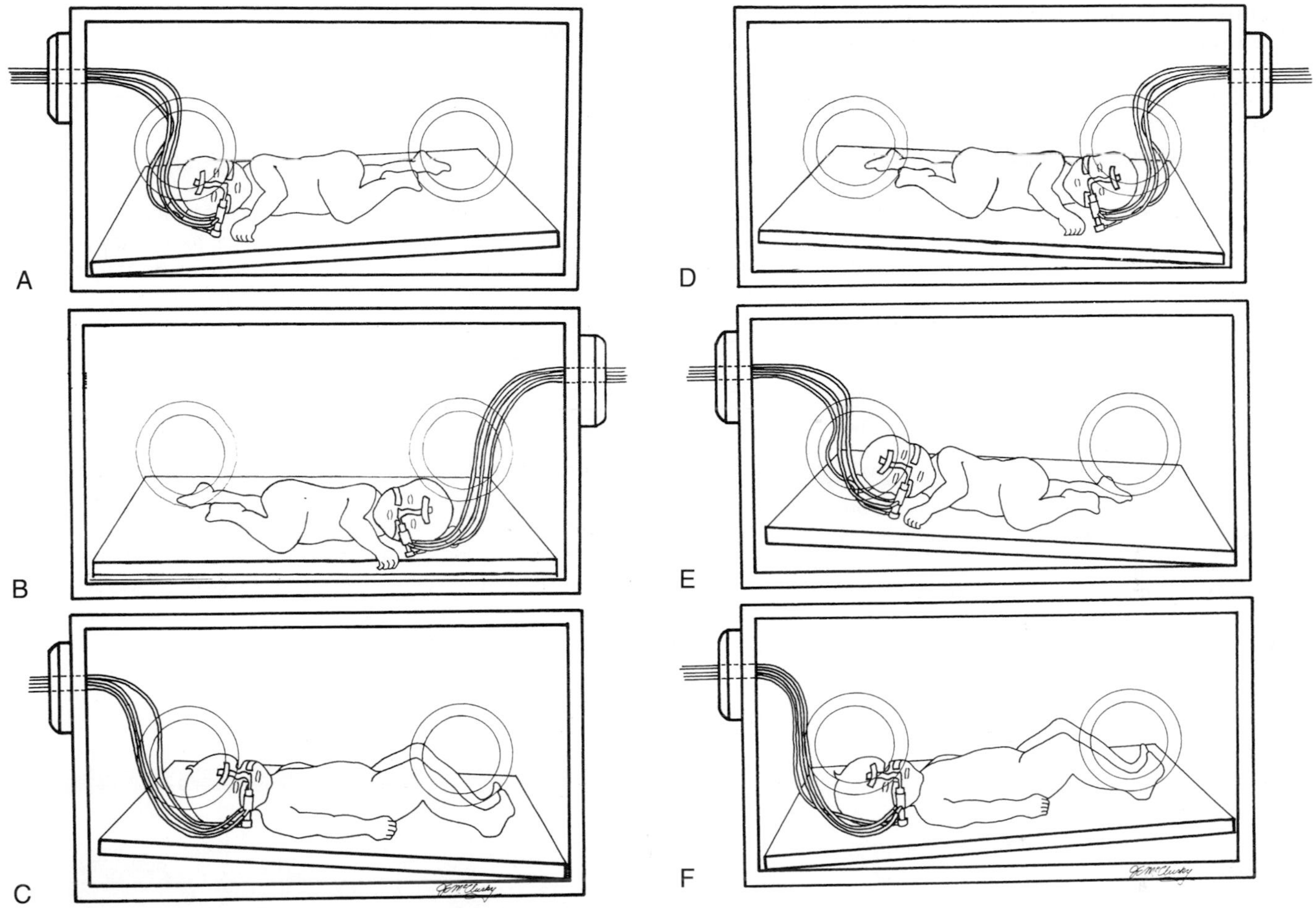

Fig. 37-4 Sequence for positional rotation. *Position 1:* Segments that come off the left lower bronchus posteriorly are drained by positioning the infant on his or her right side, three-fourths prone with a head-down angle. *Position 2:* The posterior segment of the right upper lobe is drained by positioning on the left side, three-fourths prone with the bed flat. *Position 3:* The anterior segments of the upper lobes are drained by positioning supine with the head of the bed elevated or flat. *Position 4:* Segments that come off the right lower lobe bronchus posteriorly are drained by positioning on the left side, three-fourths prone with a head-down angle. *Position 5:* The posterior segment of the left upper lobe is drained by positioning on the right side, three-fourths prone with the head of the bed elevated. *Position 6:* Segments that come off the tracheobronchial tree anteriorly are drained by positioning supine with a head-down angle. *Positions 7 and 8:* Segments such as the right middle lobe or lingula that come off the tracheobronchial tree anterolaterally will be drained in a three-fourths supine position, slightly head down (see Figure 37-5). Babies on ventilators may also be positioned prone. This is usually done by the therapist rather than in a routine positional rotation (see Figure 37-6).

be achieved.[190] Whereas positional rotation programs for adults emphasize the lower lobes, positional programs for infants must emphasize all lung areas (Figure 37-4). The upper lobes and right middle lobe (Figure 37-5) are common sites of airway collapse and atelectasis in infants, and the right middle lobe bronchus is surrounded by a collar of lymph nodes, making it vulnerable to extrinsic compression. Important considerations and essentials of a positional rotation program for infants are outlined in Box 37-1.

Infants born preterm do tolerate and benefit from prone positioning (Figure 37-6). Studies have demonstrated improved oxygenation, tidal volume, dynamic lung compliance, and synchrony of chest wall movement when preterm neonates are placed in prone positions.[191-194] Additionally, nested prone and side-lying positioning, with boundaries provided for comfort, has been shown to decrease stress behaviors in these infants.[3,195] However, when healthy infants born

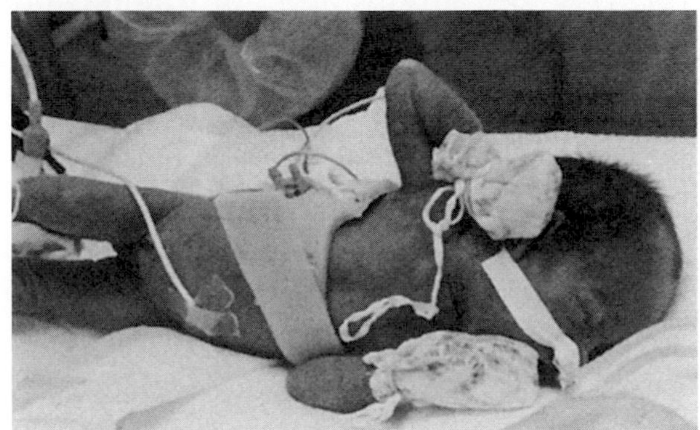

Fig. 37-5 Three-fourths supine position for right middle lobe. Lingula is the same three-fourths supine position with the patient lying on his or her right side.

prematurely approach their discharge to home, the benefits of prone over supine positioning in decreasing their work of breathing are no longer observed.[194]

Positional rotation is generally performed manually every 2 hours, and although this provides pulmonary benefit, it may also contribute to the disruption of homeostasis that has been documented to occur in the course of neonatal intensive care.[3,195,196] Murai and Grant (1994)[197] demonstrated that the use of continuous positional oscillation nursery beds as compared with manual repositioning decreased the duration of oxygen supplementation without adversely affecting the cardiovascular and pulmonary status of the neonates.

Box 37-1 Essentials of a Positional Rotation Program

1. Care should be taken to coordinate any change in the infant's position with other nursing procedures to avoid unnecessary stimulation.
2. Infants should never be left unattended when in a head-down position.
3. Vital signs should be monitored closely by respiration and heart rate monitors. The alarms should be turned on.
4. The infant's chest should be auscultated for adventitious breath sounds after positioning.
5. While the infant is in a drainage position, secretions will be more easily mobilized. The infant's trachea or endotracheal tube should be suctioned as needed.
6. Avoid placing the infant in a head-down position for approximately one hour after eating to avoid aspiration of regurgitated food.
7. Any change in the infant's position should be done slowly to minimize stress on the cardiovascular system.
8. Infants with umbilical arterial lines can be placed on their abdomens; however, one should always check that the line has not been kinked.
9. Some infants might require modified drainage positions. Infants with CF, as well as infants with severe cardiovascular instability and infants with or at risk for intracranial bleeding should not be placed in a head-down position.

Postural Drainage

Postural drainage positions to promote gravity-assisted drainage of specific segmental airways can be safely applied to infants and children. In the acute care setting, however, many of the head-down positions are modified according to tolerance and precautions or contraindications (Table 37-5). The rule for modification of any position for postural drainage is that the position used should be as close to the classical (anatomically correct) position for that segment as safely possible. Examples of the classical postural drainage positions for each bronchopulmonary segment are pictured in Figure 37-7.

Tiny infants (especially those weighing less than 800 grams) usually require and benefit from modification of the head-down position. Horizontal to slightly elevated positioning of the head may be best.[198] This modification is primarily due to changes in oxygenation[198] and the high incidence of intraventricular hemorrhage in infants born preterm.[199-201] In addition, Trendelenburg positioning is contraindicated for infants with cystic fibrosis and cerebral palsy because of high incidence of gastroesophageal reflux disease observed in this patient population.[111,119,122,131,133]

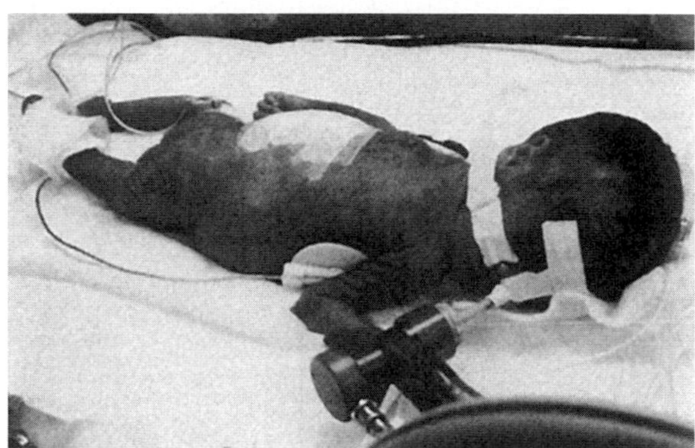

Fig. 37-6 Infants born prematurely (even those on ventilators with numerous catheters) may be placed prone when care is taken.

Table 37-5 Precautions and Contraindications for Postural Drainage in a Neonate

Position	Precaution	Contraindication
Prone	Umbilical arterial catheter Continuous positive airway pressure in nose Excessive abdominal distention Abdominal incision Anterior chest tube	Untreated tension pneumothorax
Trendelenburg position (head down)	Distended abdomen SEH/IVH* (grades I and II) Chronic congestive heart failure or cor pulmonale Persistent fetal circulation Cardiac dysrhythmias Apnea and bradycardia Infant exhibiting signs of acute respiratory distress Hydrocephalus Less than 28 weeks' gestational age	Untreated tension pneumothorax Recent tracheoesophageal fistula repair Recent eye or intracranial surgery Intraventricular hemorrhage (grades III and IV) Acute congestive heart failure or cor pulmonale

**SEH/IVH*, Subependymal hemorrhage/intraventricular hemorrhage.
From Crane LD: Physical therapy for the neonate with respiratory disease. In Irwon S, Tecklin JS, editors: *Cardiopulmonary physical therapy*, St Louis, 1995, Mosby.

Chest Percussion and Vibration

Percussion and vibration are used in conjunction with postural drainage to augment the effect of gravity in the removal of secretions.[63,66] There are several ways to perform percussion on infants. For a larger infant, it is possible to use a cupped hand in a manner similar to percussing an adult's chest. For a smaller infant, some modification of this technique is needed. Chest percussion for a smaller infant is accomplished by tenting three or four fingers or using any of the commercially available percussion devices made for neonates (Figure 37-8). A small anesthesia mask or "palm cup" can also be used effectively.[63,66]

Precautions for chest percussion in the infant include, but are not limited to, unstable cardiovascular or oxygenation status (although percussion may be provided safely if continuous transcutaneous monitoring is available), coagulopathy, subcutaneous emphysema, or intraventricular hemorrhage.

A

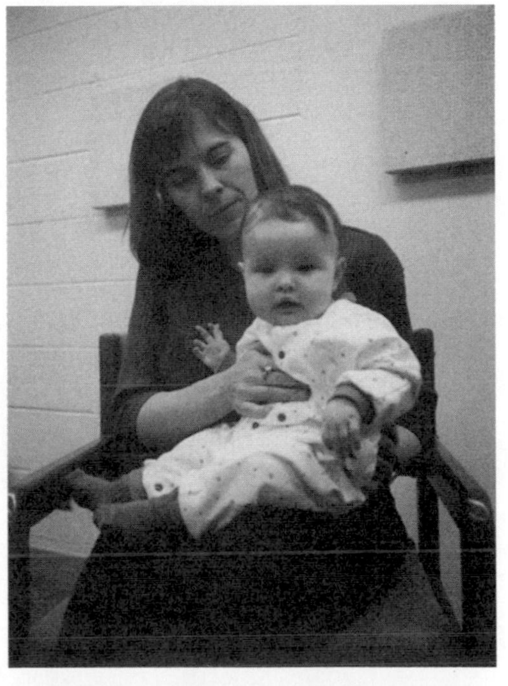

B

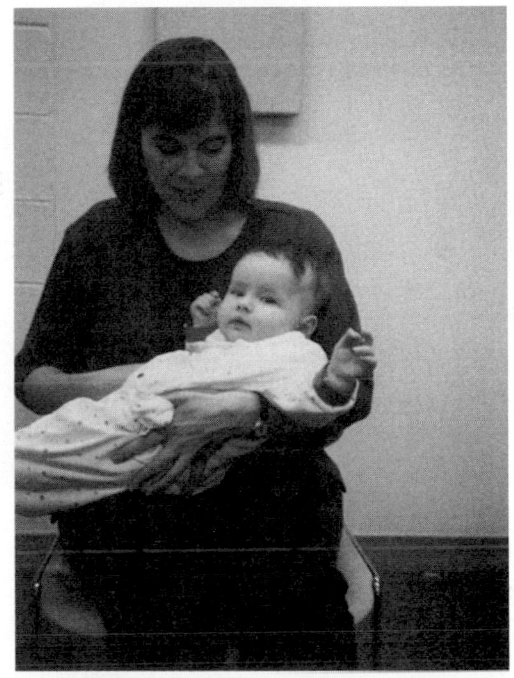

C

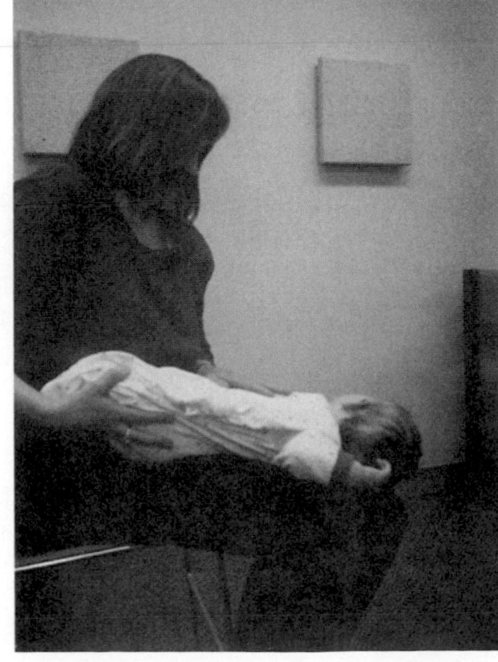

D

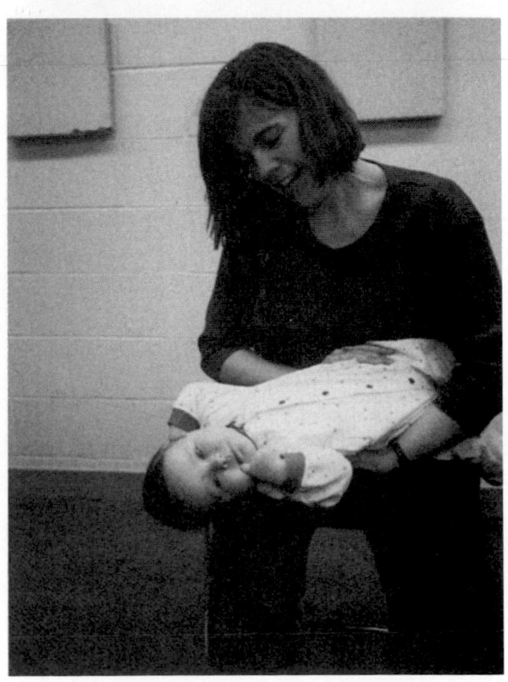

Fig. 37-7 Postural drainage with an infant. **A,** Both upper lobes—apical segments. **B,** Left upper lobe—anterior segment. **C,** Right upper lobe—anterior segment. **D,** Lingula.

Continued

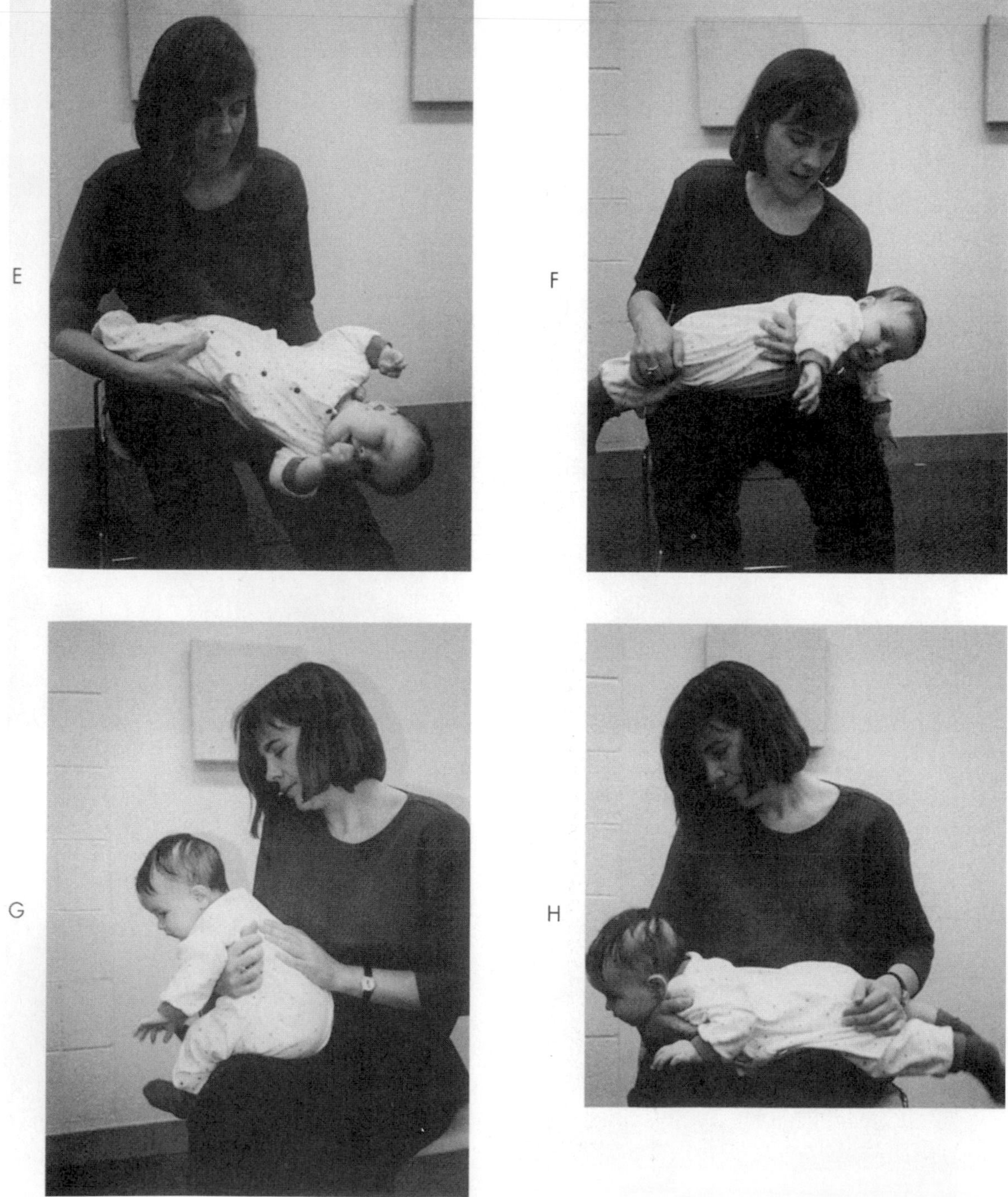

Fig. 37-7, cont'd E, Right middle lobe. **F,** Right upper lobe—posterior segment. **G,** Left upper lobe—posterior segment. **H,** Both lower lobes—apical (superior) segments.

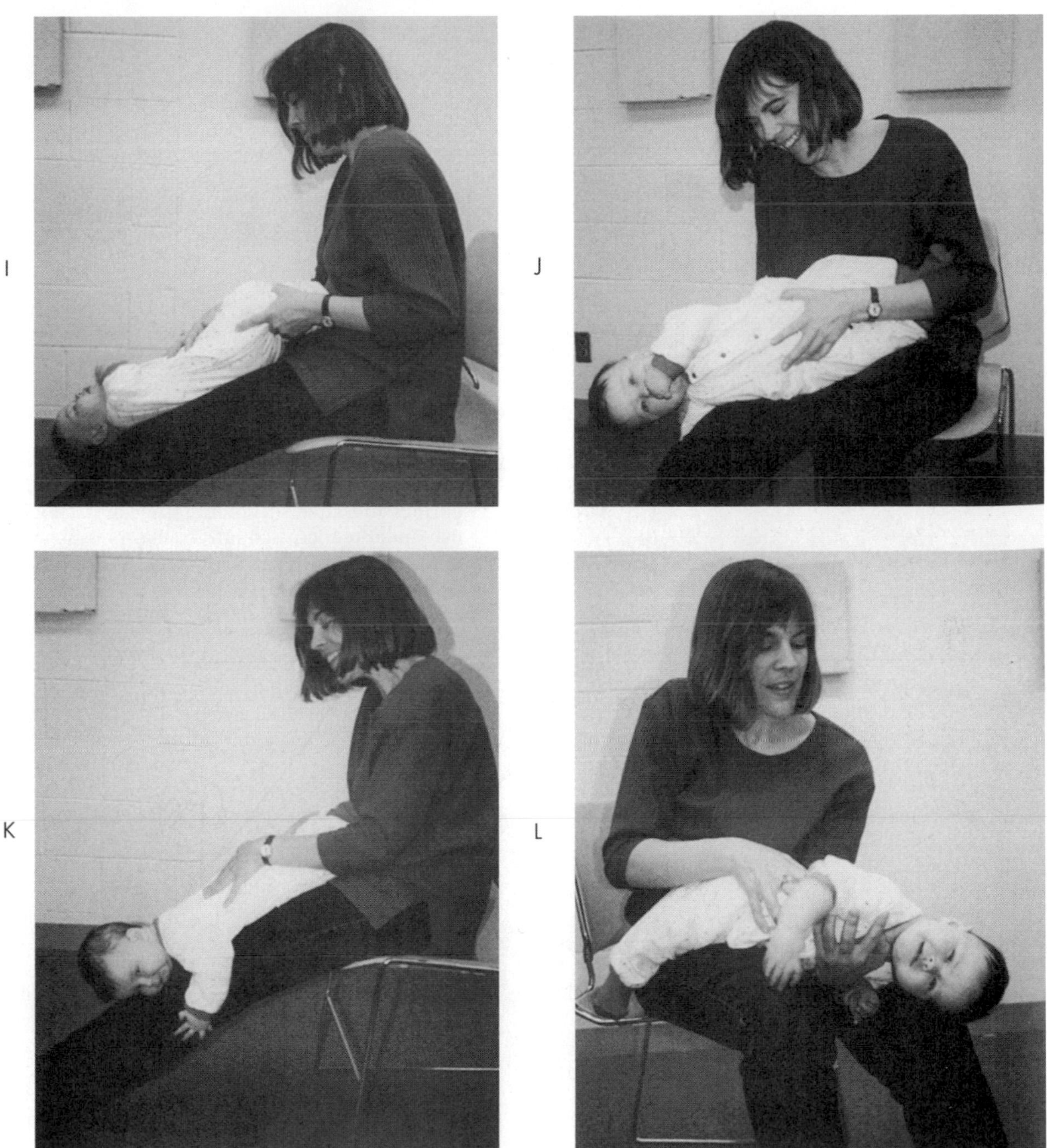

Fig. 37-7, cont'd I, Both lower lobes—anterior basal segments. **J,** Left lower lobe—lateral basal segment; right lower lobe—medial segment. **K,** Both lower lobes—posterior basal segments. **L,** Right lower lobe—lateral basal segment.

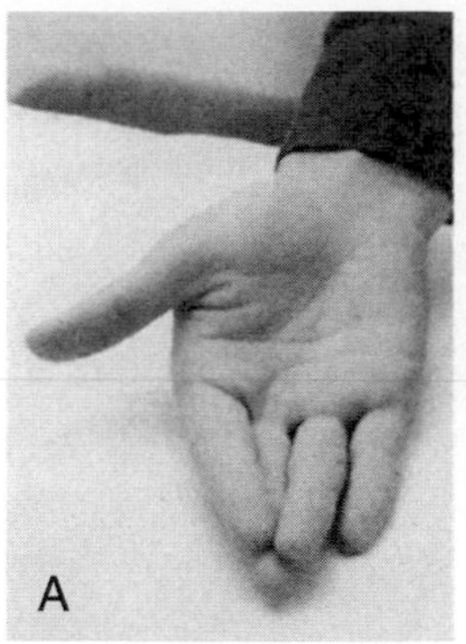

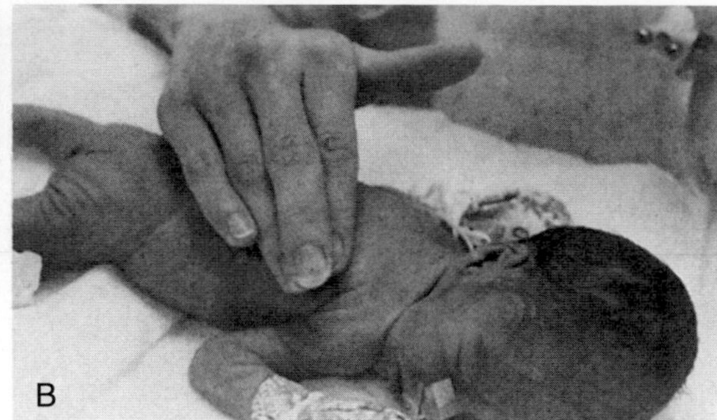

Fig. 37-8 "Tenting" of the fingers for percussion of premature infants or small children.

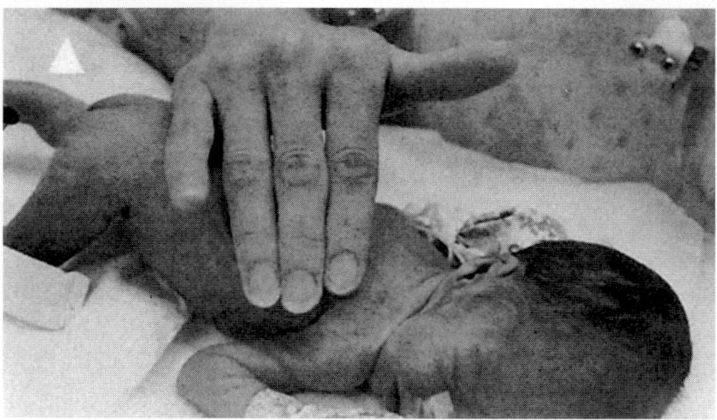

Fig. 37-9 Manual chest wall vibration of an infant born preterm.

Additionally, percussion is generally contraindicated over a healing thoracotomy incision or if the child displays irritability and signs of respiratory distress with the treatment.

Vibration is accomplished either through manual vibratory motion of the therapist's fingers on the infant's chest wall (Figure 37-9) or through the use of a mechanical vibrator. An electric toothbrush can be adapted by padding the bristle portion with foam.[63,66] Vibration has been observed to occasionally increase irritability and may be less well tolerated than percussion. The most common precaution for vibration is increased irritability with the development of bradycardia and respiratory distress.

The decision to use chest percussion and vibration will depend on the reviewed principles and precautions, the medical condition of the infant, and the infant's tolerance to handling. Continuation of percussion and vibration will depend on the day-to-day medical status of the infant and his or her response to treatment.

Airway Suctioning

Sterile airway suctioning is discussed in detail in Chapter 44; however, some special considerations for suctioning the airway of an infant must be highlighted.[202-205]

1. If possible, suction with a transcutaneous oxygen monitor in place. These monitors give continuous feedback regarding the infant's oxygenation status.
2. Bagging should be done only with a bag attached to a pressure manometer to ensure that sufficient pressures are being used without exceeding the maximum safe levels (these limits should be similar to the ventilator settings).
3. Suction for no more than 5 seconds with each catheter withdrawal.
4. Infants should be carefully hyperoxygenated when hyperventilated so as to minimize hyperoxia and hypoxia. Bagging usually does not need to continue for more than 5 to 10 seconds to maintain adequate oxygen levels.
5. Monitor the blood pressure of preterm infants before, during, and after suctioning. Change in blood pressure may indicate increased intracranial pressure and risk for intracranial hemorrhage.

In intubated infants, the need for endotracheal tube (ETT) suctioning should be carefully assessed. Clinical indications for ETT suctioning include respiratory pattern and rate changes, presence of secretions in the ETT (observed visually or heard during respiration), abnormal breath sounds audible upon chest auscultation, decrease in oxygen saturation and Pa_{O_2}, increase in Pa_{CO_2}, bradycardia, ventilator waveform changes related to proximal airway pressure, and agitated behavior.[205]

CPT for Children

The goals for CPT in children (2 years of age and older) include more than improving airway clearance. Children are capable of following directions and imitating a therapist's demonstration of deep breathing, coughing, and active exercise. CPT in children is focused on improving ventilation and efficiency of breathing;[179] increasing general strength and endurance with an emphasis on muscles of respiration; improving posture; and addressing relaxation, breathing control, and pacing.[206]

The application of CPT with children often requires patience and creative adaptation. The challenge is to make it seem less like a treatment and more like a game. It is important, however, to be honest in your explanations and to speak to children with respect and at a level appropriate for their age and development.

Involving the family in CPT treatment of a child can be invaluable.[179,207,208] In some cases, the parent may do most of the "hands-on" and repeat instructions to the child under the direct guidance of the therapist. This arrangement will also help reinforce parent and family education for carry-over of home therapy.

Positional Rotation

The goal of positional rotation and postural drainage is to prevent the accumulation of secretions and to aid in their removal. Any child who is immobile, receiving artificial ventilation, or not expanding his or her chest adequately should have his or her position changed at least every 2 hours. Recall that positional changes will enhance oxygen transport and promote pulmonary drainage.[190] If the child is reluctant to have his or her position changed, changing the location of the television may be helpful. Be creative!

YOUNG CHILDREN

In younger children (18 months to 3 years of age), deep breathing is usually encouraged by blowing bubbles, tissue paper, mobiles, or simple horns. To achieve maximal chest expansion, the child should be positioned on each side while playing blowing games or singing. The theory behind the side-lying position is that the downside lung ventilates more effectively (see Chapter 19). Additionally, if the poorly ventilated lung is uppermost, stretch techniques can facilitate deeper breathing (see Chapter 23).

Spontaneous coughing in younger children often occurs with a change in position or with crying. For the child who does not cough spontaneously or whose cough is inadequate to clear secretions, nasopharyngeal suctioning may be necessary.

OLDER CHILDREN

School-age children can be more specifically instructed in various breathing exercises, such as diaphragmatic breathing, pursed-lips breathing, and segmental lateral costal breathing. They may also be candidates for using relaxed deep breathing for control and pacing of activity. Cooperation with this age group, however, still remains higher if some aspect of therapy is fun. Elaborate whistles are available that encourage deep breathing; they make therapy fun by challenging the patient to make the whistle components move. Additionally, pediatric incentive spirometers are available with cheerful, "cool" pictures to make respiratory exercises seem more like a game.

Older children (not infants) can be stimulated to cough by applying a firm pressure over the trachea in the suprasternal notch. Be aware that coughing, whether spontaneous or stimulated, may elicit gagging and vomiting, especially if airway clearance is scheduled too soon after a child has eaten.

Preoperative and Postoperative Care

The efficacy of postoperative CPT is highly related to preoperative care.[179] The appropriate application of preoperative assessment, instruction, and direct therapeutic intervention helps to decrease the incidence of postoperative complications.

Preoperative teaching is extremely important for both the child and the family. Parents may often be more anxious than the child, so patient and family education is important. The level of preoperative training with the child will depend on his or her age.

If the child is very young (under two years of age), the therapist needs to meet with the parents and explain the purpose of bronchial drainage treatments, potential airway clearance problems, and possible complications. The preventive nature of these interventions should be stressed, and procedures that can be done with the child after surgery should be demonstrated and discussed. These may include positioning, chest percussion, vibration, and airway suctioning. In addition, the physical therapist should always allow time for the parents to ask questions.

If the child is able to understand simple concepts, the therapist can, in addition to parent education, instruct the child in various breathing games, use of an incentive spirometer, coughing, and general upper and lower extremity exercises.

Postoperative procedures can be effectively explained and demonstrated to children starting at approximately 8 years of age and older. The importance of bronchial hygiene should be stressed during demonstration of deep breathing and coughing. The child can be shown how to splint the incision using a pillow or a stuffed animal to assist with comfort while coughing. Do not tell the child that coughing will not hurt; be honest but reinforce that splinting will help. Teach the child diaphragmatic and pursed-lips breathing with an inspiratory-hold maneuver, and, if appropriate, teach the child how to use an incentive spirometer.

Postoperative pulmonary complications may not be as prevalent in the pediatric age group as in adults, but they still occur. The most common complications are atelectasis, infection secondary to pooling of secretions, and airway obstruction. Infants and children with the following characteristics will be at risk for developing postoperative pulmonary complications: preexisting lung disease, thoracic or upper abdominal location of incision, prolonged postoperative bed rest or restricted mobility, and neuromuscular involvement that affects the ability to move, cough, and breathe deeply.

Postoperative interventions generally focus on increasing ventilation, coughing, and active mobility.[179,181] Specific bronchial drainage is used only if the child is unable to clear his or her airway or is at risk because of chronic lung disease.

After high abdominal or thoracic surgery, there may be a tendency for the child to splint on the side of the incision. Arm, shoulder, and trunk movement should be encouraged to prevent any postoperative complications. For the younger child, chest mobility can be encouraged by clapping the hands overhead or by dramatizing songs such as "The Itsy Bitsy Spider." More conventional exercises may be taught to the older child.

Children tend to mobilize very quickly (unless their movement is limited by motor involvement or a specific surgical procedure). In general, once the child is out of bed and moving about, with clear lungs and an effective cough, postoperative CPT can be discontinued.

Pediatric Pulmonary Rehabilitation

Rehabilitation programs for children with chronic lung disease include the same components and have essentially the same goals as adult pulmonary rehabilitation. However, the specific diagnoses most prevalent in children differ from those in adults. Asthma and CF are the most common conditions among children who may benefit from pulmonary rehabilitation.

Exercise and Asthma

Exercise and conditioning are very important interventions for children with asthma. Improved chest and trunk mobility, control of breathing, strength, posture, increased exercise capacity, and improved quality of life are all goals that can be addressed in the design of exercise programs for these children.[209-211]

The transient airflow obstruction associated with physical exertion may render children (and their parents) wary of exercise. Several approaches may be beneficial at promoting and maintaining exercise in this population. First, aerobic conditioning will reduce the ventilation requirement for activity, thus reducing the increased rate of ventilation with exertion. Second, wearing a face mask and inhaling through the nose will warm up and humidify the inhaled air before it moves to the intrathoracic region, thus raising the threshold for exercise-induced bronchospasm.[212-214] Third, because many younger children perform bursts of activity at unpredictable times of day and may not be allowed to carry their inhalers with them in school or during sports events, the physical therapist may be influential in communicating with the child's physician to identify longer-acting medications that might be given at home.[213] Finally, exercise-induced symptoms may be reduced in some children with the use of 10- to 15-minute warm-up and warm-down exercise periods.[212,214] Recommendations for warm-up exercise include submaximal activity performed at up to 60% maximal heart rate[214] and repeated activity that varies in intensity and includes high burst periods.[212]

Part of a pulmonary rehabilitation program may involve providing recommendations for the child's participation in physical education (PE).[209] Certain aspects of exercise relative to pulmonary function in children with asthma need to be communicated to the PE teacher. Running is the form of exercise most likely to aggravate exercise-induced asthma, especially if performed in a cool, dry environment. Swimming, by contrast, is an excellent activity.[104,209,211] Strenuous or continuous exercise may induce bronchospasm, whereas short periods of exercise (less than 5 continuous minutes) may be beneficial for conditioning without bronchial aggravation.[209,214] PE teachers should also be aware that the child may need to use a pre-exercise inhaler to participate in PE without pulmonary consequence.[209,214]

Exercise and CF

Physical activity designed to improve exercise tolerance helps children with CF to mobilize secretions and improve body image. In terms of preventing opportunistic infections in these children, exercise is also associated with an increased immune responsiveness.[215] Furthermore, quality-of-life measures and subjective reports also indicate improvement when exercise is part of the overall management program of children with CF.[216-218]

An individualized exercise program should be developed for each child with CF. A pre-exercise examination and evaluation should include the following components:

1. Evaluation of the range of motion, strength, and posture
2. Complete chest evaluation
3. Evaluation of neuromuscular control, including muscle recruitment patterns during breathing and arm and trunk movements
4. Evaluation of ADL tolerance and limitations
5. Inspiratory muscle strength (maximal inspiratory negative pressure at the mouth) and endurance testing (The inspiratory endurance testing can be done with an inspiratory muscle training device by having the child breathe for a predetermined length of time at progressively increased resistances until tolerance is reached.)
6. Cardiovascular and pulmonary exercise testing performed with electrocardiogram, blood pressure, and oxygen monitoring, to assess exercise capacity by determining the peak oxygen uptake or VO_{2peak}

A basic exercise program for children with CF should include activities to elongate tight musculature; retrain and strengthen weak musculature; transfer postural, range of motion, and strength gains to preferred functional physical activities; and address overall endurance.[216-218] Vigorous exercise and fitness training in these children requires careful monitoring of pulmonary response. Considerable research exists to support aerobic and anaerobic training in children with CF.[104,216,217] Physical therapists should pay special attention to promotion of enjoyment of exercise by offering a variety of different activities and supporting the child's self-esteem, with a goal of improving the overall exercise compliance.[219]

Among hospitalized children with CF, those who followed either aerobic or resistance training protocols had better aerobic and strength outcomes, respectively, than children in a standard CPT program, with no significant differences between the exercise and nonexercise groups in disease severity or length of hospital stay.[217] Attention to nutritional status in these children is paramount to prevent decreased activity and promote exercise tolerance and quality of life.[220-222] The evidence base suggests that the benefits of exercise will likely outweigh the risks in this population when other aspects of health are optimized.[104]

Therapeutic Handling to Maximize Trunk and Ventilatory Function

Attention to pulmonary function is easily accomplished within any "handling" approach to motor therapy for children with trunk weakness, tightness, alterations in tone, or general immobility. Most handling consistent with a neurodevelopmental treatment (NDT) approach lends itself readily to a dual focus on movement quality and ventilation. Extrinsic pulmonary development is clearly interrelated with musculoskeletal and motor development of the trunk.[223]

After an observational assessment of chest mobility, trunk posture and muscle recruitment strategies during breathing and functional activities, intervention should begin with initial handling for functional range of motion through the trunk. This will typically require elongation of the pectoral, sternocleidomastoid, upper trapezius, and rectus abdominis muscles. Manual lowering of the rib cage will also be necessary to work toward maximizing chest mobility (Figure 37-10).

Passive elongation of muscles must always be followed by active elongation. Controlled prone extension on a large inflated ball is both fun for the child and effective for the therapist (Figure 37-11). Manual guidance for upper extremity abduction and external rotation will facilitate active elongation of the pectoral muscles via active firing of the scapular

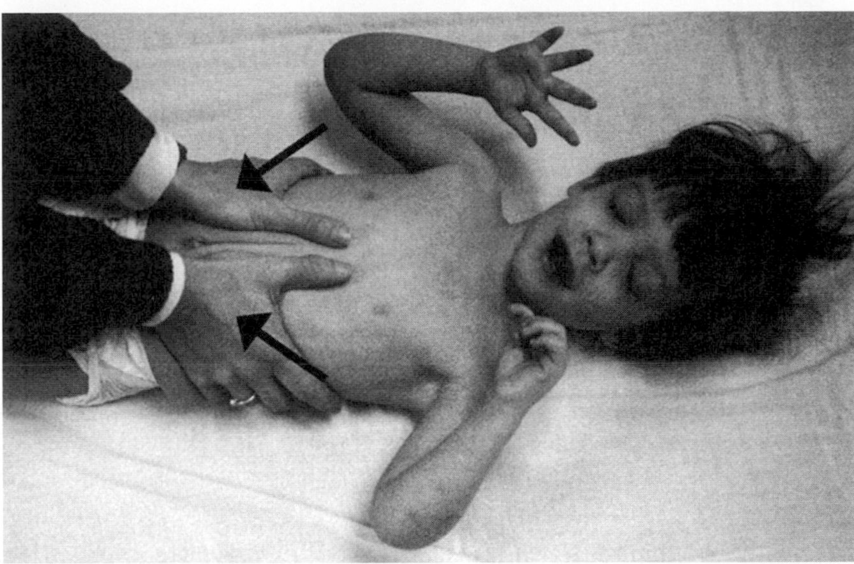

Fig. 37-10 Manual lowering of the rib cage. *Arrows* indicate direction of therapist's hand movement (caudal and medial).

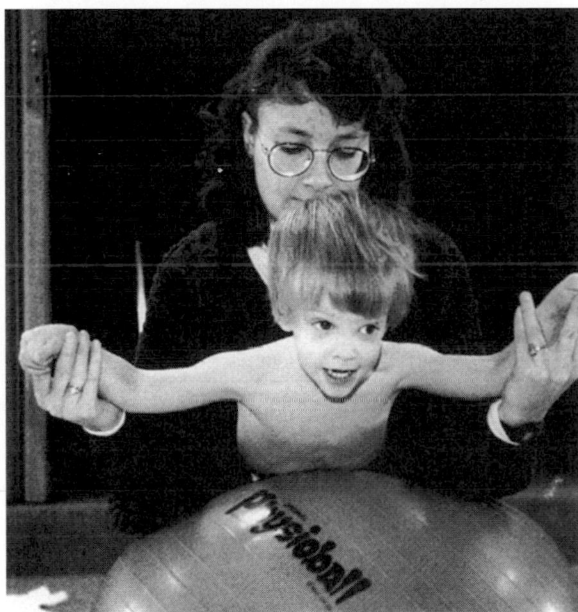

Fig. 37-11 Handling to facilitate active upper thoracic extension as a means of opening the anterior chest and lengthening the rectus abdominis muscle while supporting the lower ribcage on the ball.

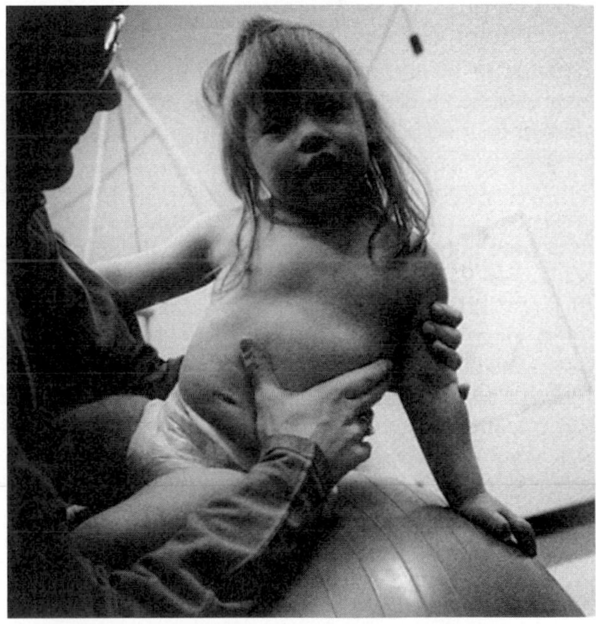

Fig. 37-12 Handling to reinforce upper chest expansion and abdominal oblique stabilization of the lower ribs.

retractors.[224] The ball can be used to impart movement and support the lower rib cage. This elongates the anterior trunk (rectus abdominis), lengthens intercostal muscles, and facilitates increased upper chest expansion.

Handling to achieve proprioceptive input of the scapulae on the posterior thorax will help to reinforce active thoracic extension and anterior chest expansion.[223,224] The therapist's hands can stabilize the rib cage to reinforce the abdominal oblique muscle function during movement (Figure 37-12). Activities requiring alternating extension-rotation and flexion-rotation will recruit control of the abdominal obliques and maintain active upper trunk extension. Bubble blowing, using whistle toys, and singing are excellent means of monitoring the ventilatory changes that occur with active use of increased upper chest expansion. As tidal volume increases, vocalizations should increase in frequency, sound higher, and become louder.

The concept of functional carryover is central to the treatment approach presented here. Addressing ventilation and trunk control simultaneously has intuitive appeal based not only on shared musculoskeletal relationships but also on the necessity of pulmonary tolerance for motor activity.

Summary

Cardiovascular and pulmonary physical therapy with infants and children begins with an understanding of the issues related to development and developmental vulnerabilities. In this chapter, specific cardiovascular and pulmonary conditions in pediatrics are described and treatment recommendations provided. Cardiovascular and pulmonary development and function are the basis for indications and precautions for treatment of neonates, infants, children, and adolescents.

The link between pulmonary and motor functions is also important. Many children with motor involvement are at risk for or have medical histories remarkable for cardiovascular and pulmonary dysfunction. Motor approaches that maximize ventilatory function are critical, because efficient oxygenation is a priority not only for children with primary cardiovascular and pulmonary diagnoses but also for children with motor disorders.

Acknowledgement

Dedicated to Linda D. Crane, the first author of the first two editions of this chapter.

Review Questions

1. Discuss the importance of changes in pulmonary blood flow during transitional circulation, and relate these changes to closure of foramen ovale and ductus arteriosus.
2. Describe six characteristics of an infant's pulmonary anatomy that contribute to the increased work of breathing and potential for pulmonary distress in this age group.
3. Identify and discuss two aspects of cardiovascular and pulmonary vulnerability in the preterm infant.
4. Compare pulmonary disorders commonly seen in preterm neonates with those seen in full-term neonates.
5. Compare the goals of chest physical therapy for infants and older children. What are the similarities and differences?
6. When the therapist treats infants to improve airway clearance, what are the precautions for and/or considerations of each of the following?
   - Positional rotation
   - Postural drainage
   - Percussion
   - Vibration
   - Airway suctioning
7. How might neuromotor (neuromuscular) dysfunction affect pulmonary development?
8. Identify two cardiovascular and pulmonary comorbidities of obesity in typically developing children.
9. Describe goals, precautions, and suggested monitoring for exercise in children who have the following:
   - A history of cardiac surgery
   - Asthma
   - Cystic fibrosis

References

1. Kiserud T: Physiology of fetal circulation. *Seminars in Fetal and Neonatal Medicine* 10:493–503, 2005.
2. Sadler TW: Cardiovascular system. In Sadler TW, editor: *Langman's medical embryology*, ed 8, Philadelphia, 2000, Lippincott Williams & Wilkins.
3. Rahlin M: Impaired ventilation, respiration/gas exchange and aerobic capacity/endurance associated with respiratory failure in the neonate. In Frownfelter D, editor: *Cardiopulmonary essentials: preferred physical therapist practice patterns*, Thorofare, 2007, SLACK, Inc.
4. Schneider DJ, Moore, JW: Patent ductus arteriosus. *Circulation* 114:1873–1882, 2006.
5. Mielke G, Benda, N: Cardiac output and central distribution of blood flow in the human fetus. *Circulation* 103:1662–1668, 2001.
6. Koff PB: Development of the cardiopulmonary system. In Koff PB, Eitzman D, Neu J, editors: *Neonatal and pediatric respiratory care*, St Louis, 1993, Mosby.
7. Phelan PD, Olinsky A, Robertson CF, editors: *Respiratory illness in children.* Boston, 1994, Blackwell-Scientific Publications.
8. Cech DJ, Martin S: Cardiovascular and pulmonary system changes. In Cech DJ, Martin S, editors: *Functional movement development across the life span*, ed 2, Philadelphia, 2002, WB. Saunders.
9. Lapointe A, Barrington KJ: Pulmonary hypertension and the asphyxiated newborn. *The Journal of Pediatrics* 158:e19–24, 2011.
10. Starr JA, Tucker CA: The cardiopulmonary system. In Effgen SK, editor: *Meeting the physical therapy needs of children*, Philadelphia, 2005, FA. Davis.
11. Hughes EA, Sperle CK: Fetal and newborn cardiopulmonary physiology. In Beachey W, editor: *Respiratory care anatomy and physiology: foundations for clinical practice*, ed 2, St Louis, 2007, Mosby.
12. Hermes-DeSantis ER, Clyman RI: Patent ductus arteriosus: pathophysiology and management. *Journal of Perinatology* 26:S14–S18, 2006.
13. Johnson TR, Moore WM, Jeffries JE: *Children are different: developmental physiology*, ed 2, Columbus, Ohio, 1978, Ross Laboratories.
14. Blackburn S: Alterations of the respiratory system in the neonate: implications for clinical practice. *Journal of Perinatal Nursing* 6:46–58, 1992.
15. Massery M: Chest development as a component of motor development: implications for pediatric physical therapists. *Pediatric Physical Therapy* 3:3–8, 1991.
16. Hicks GH: The respiratory system. In Wilkins RL, Stoller JK, Kacmarek RM, editors: *Egan's fundamentals of respiratory care*, ed 9, St Louis, 2009, Mosby.
17. Arens R, McDonough JM, Corbin AM, et al: Linear dimensions of the upper airway structure during development. *American Journal of Respiratory and Critical Care Medicine* 165:117–122, 2002.
18. Kahn-D'Angelo L, Unanue Rose RA: The special care nursery. In Campbell SK, Vander Linden DW, Palisano RJ, editors: *Physical therapy for children*, ed 3, St Louis, 2006, Saunders.
19. Walther FJ, Benders MJ, Leighton JO: Persistent pulmonary hypertension in premature neonates with severe respiratory distress syndrome. *Pediatrics* 90:899–903, 1992.
20. Crowley P, Roberts D, Dalziel S, et al: *Antenatal corticosteroids to accelerate fetal lung maturation for women at risk of preterm birth: protocol for a Cochrane review. The Cochrane Library 1.* Chichester, 2004, John Wiley & Sons, Ltd.
21. Deming DS, Specht NL: Neonatal and pediatric respiratory disorders. In Wilkins RL, Stoller JK, Kacmarek RM, editors: *Egan's fundamentals of respiratory care*, ed 9, St Louis, 2009, Mosby.
22. Milne MJ, Sung RYT, Fok TF, et al: Doppler echocardiographic assessment of shunting via the ductus arteriosus in newborn infants. *American Journal of Cardiology* 64:102–105, 1989.
23. Archer N: Patent ductus arteriosus in the newborn. *Arch Dis Child* 69(5 Spec No): 529–532, 1993.
24. Eichenwald EC, Stark AR: Management and outcomes of very low birth weight. *The New England Journal of Medicine* 358:1700–1711, 2008.
25. Bancalari E, Claure N, Gonzales A: Patent ductus arteriosus and respiratory outcome in premature infants. *Biology of Neonate* 88:192–201, 2005.
26. Rocha G, Ribeiro O, Guimarães H: Fluid and electrolyte balance during the first week of life and risk of bronchopulmonary dysplasia in the preterm neonate. *Clinics* 65:663–674, 2010.
27. Birnkrant DJ, Ashwath ML, Noritz GH, et al: Cardiac and pulmonary function variability in Duchenne/Becker muscular dystrophy: and initial report. *Journal of Child Neurology* 25:1110–1115, 2010.
28. Burd L, Deal E, Rios R, et al: Congenital heart defects and fetal alcohol spectrum disorders. *Congenital Heart Disease* 2:250–255, 2007.
29. Koeppen AH: Friedreich's ataxia: pathology, pathogenesis, and molecular genetics. *Journal of the Neurological Sciences* 303:1–12, 2011.
30. Tsou AY, Paulsen EK, Lagedrost SJ, et al: Mortality in Friedreich Ataxia. *Journal of the neurological Sciences.* Advance online publication, 2011.
31. Barbaro G: HIV-associated cardiomyopathy etiopathogenesis and clinical aspects. *Herz* 30:486–492, 2005.
32. Lai H, Redheuil A, Tong W, et al: HIV infection and abnormal regional ventricular function. *International Journal of Cardiovascular Imaging* 25:809–817, 2005.

33. Oguz D, Ocal B, Ertan U, et al: Left ventricular diastolic functions in juvenile rheumatoid arthritis. *Pediatric Cardiology* 21:374–377, 2000.
34. Yetman AT, Graham T: The dilated aorta in patients with congenital cardiac defects. *Journal of the American College of Cardiology* 53:461–467, 2009.
35. Hatemi AC, Gursoy M, Tongut A, et al: Pulmonary stenosis as a predisposing factor for infective endocarditis in a patient with Noonan syndrome. *Texas Heart Institute Journal* 37:99–101, 2010.
36. Musewe NN, Olley PM: Patent ductus arteriosus. In Freedom RM, Benson LN, Smallhorn JF, editors: *Neonatal heart disease*, London, 1994, Springer-Verlag.
37. Capobianco G, Cherchi PL, Ambrosini G, et al: Alobar holoprosencephaly, mobile proboscis and trisomy 13 in a fetus with maternal gestational diabetes mellitus: a 2D ultrasound diagnosis and review of the literature. *Archives of Gynecology and Obstetrics* 275:385–387, 2007.
38. Hsu HF, Hou JW: Variable expressivity in Patau syndrome is not all related to trisomy 18 mosaicism. *American Journal of Medical Genetics Part A* 143A:1739–1748, 2007.
39. Kaneko Y, Kobayashi J, Achiwa I, et al: Cardiac surgery in patients with trisomy 18. *Pediatric Cardiology* 30:729–734, 2009.
40. Pandit C, Fitzgerald DA: Respiratory problems in children with Down syndrome. *Journal of Paediatrics and Child Health*. Advance online publication. doi: 10.1111/j.1440-1754.2011.02077X, 2011.
41. Kim HK, Gottliebson W, Hor K, et al: Cardiovascular anomalies in Turner syndrome: spectrum, prevalence, and cardiac MRI findings in a pediatric and young adult population. *American Journal of Roentgenology* 196:454–460, 2011.
42. Bajracharya P, Bhatnagar S, Pauliks LB: Mitral valve diseases in Williams syndrome: case report and review of the literature. *Echocardiography*. Advance online publication. doi: 10.1111/j.1540-8175.2011.01423X, 2011.
43. Madan JC, Kendrick D, Hagadorn JI, et al: Patent ductus arteriosus therapy: impact on neonatal and 18-month outcome. *Pediatrics* 123:674–681, 2009.
44. Georgeson KE, Robertson DJ: Minimally invasive surgery in the neonate: review of current evidence. *Seminars in Perinatology* 28:212–220, 2004.
45. Moore JW, Levi DS, Moore SD, et al: Interventional treatment of patent ductus arteriosus in 2004. *Catheter Cardiovascular Intervention* 64:91–101, 2005.
46. Smyth JM, Collier PS, Darwish M, et al: Intravenous indomethacin in preterm infants with symptomatic patent ductus arteriosus. A population pharmacokinetic study. *British Journal of Clinical Pharmacology* 58:249–258, 2004.
47. Emmanouilides GC, Baylen BG: *Neonatal cardiopulmonary distress*. Chicago, 1988, Year Book Medical Publishers.
48. Merrill WH, Hoff SJ, Bender HW: Surgical treatment of atrioventricular septal defects. In Mavroudis C, Backer CL, editors: *Pediatric cardiac surgery*, St Louis, 1994, Mosby.
49. Amin A, Davis M, Auseon A: Isolated cleft posterior mitral valve leaflet: an uncommon cause of mitral regurgitation. *European Journal of Endocardiography* 10:173–174, 2009.
50. Calabrò R, Limongelli G: Complete atrioventricular canal. *Orphanet Journal of Rare Diseases* 1:8, 2006.
51. Freedom RM, Smallhorn JF: Atrioventricular septal defect. In Freedom RM, Benson LN, Smallhorn JF, editors: *Neonatal heart disease*, London, 1992, Springer-Verlag.
52. Tanamati C, Suguimoto RL, Atik E, et al: Complete repair in total atrioventricular canal defect with cyanosis. *Arquivos Brazileiros de Cardiologia* 87:e1–e3, 2006.
53. Ono M, Goerier H, Boethig D, et al: Improved results after repair of complete atrioventricular septal defect. *Journal of Cardiac Surgery* 24:732–737, 2009.
54. Apitz C, Webb GD, Redington AN: Tetralogy of Fallot. *Lancet* 374:1462–1471, 2009.
55. Bailliard F, Anderson RH: Tetralogy of Fallot. *Orphanet Journal of rare Diseases* 4:2, 2009.
56. Freedom RM, Benson LN: Tetralogy of Fallot. In Freedom RM, Benson LN, Smallhorn JF, editors: *Neonatal heart disease*, London, 1992, Springer-Verlag.
57. As-Sanie S, Mercer B, Moore J: The association between respiratory distress and nonpulmonary morbidity at 34 to 36 weeks' gestation. *American Journal of Obstetrics and Gynecology* 189:1053–1057, 2003.
58. Crowther CA, Harding J: *Repeat doses of prenatal corticosteroids for women at risk of preterm birth for preventing neonatal respiratory disease "Cochrane Review". The Cochrane Library 1*. Chichester, 2004, John Wiley & Sons, Ltd.
59. Ainsworth S, Milligan D: Surfactant therapy for respiratory distress syndrome in premature neonates. A comparative review. *American Journal of Respiratory Medicine* 1:417–433, 2002.
60. Bevilacqua G, Parmigiani S: An observational study of surfactant treatment in infants of 23–30 weeks' gestation: comparison of prophylaxis and early rescue. *Journal of Maternal-Fetal and Neonatal Medicine* 14:197–204, 2003.
61. Attar M, Donn S: Mechanisms of ventilator-induced lung injury in premature infants. *Seminars in Neonatology* 7:353–360, 2002.
62. Bancalari E, Claure N, Sosenko IRS: Bronchopulmonary dysplasia: changes in pathogenesis, epidemiology and definition. *Seminars in Neonatology* 8:63–71, 2003.
63. Crane L: Physical therapy for neonates with respiratory dysfunction. *Physical Therapy* 61:1764–1773, 1981.
64. Finer NN, Boyd J: Chest physiotherapy in the neonate: a controlled study. *Pediatrics* 61:282–285, 1978.
65. Giannantonio C, Papacci P, Ciarniello R, et al: Chest physiotherapy in preterm infants with lung diseases. *Italian Journal of Pediatrics* 36:65, 2010.
66. Hough JL, Flenady V, Johnston L, et al: *Chest physiotherapy for reducing respiratory morbidity in infants requiring ventilatory support. "Cochrane Review". The Cochrane Library 3*. Chichester, 2008, John Wiley & Sons, Ltd.
67. Harding JE, Miles FKI, Becroft DMO, et al: Chest physiotherapy may be associated with brain damage in extremely premature infants. *Journal of Pediatrics* 132:440–444, 1998.
68. Knight DB, Bevan CJ, Harding JE, et al: Chest physiotherapy and porencephalic brain lesions in very preterm infants. *Journal of Paediatrics and Child Health* 37:554–558, 2001.
69. D'Angelo CT, Maniscalco WM: Bronchopulmonary dysplasia in preterm infants: pathophysiology and management strategies. *Paediatric Drugs* 6:303–330, 2004.
70. Northway WH, Rosan RC, Porter DY: Pulmonary disease following respirator therapy of hyaline membrane disease: bronchopulmonary dysplasia. *New England Journal of Medicine* 276:357–368, 1967.
71. Jobe AH, Bancalari E: Bronchopulmonary dysplasia. *American Journal of Respiratory and Critical Care Medicine* 163:1723–1729, 2001.
72. Bhandari A, Bhandari V: Pitfalls, problems, and progress in bronchopulmonary dysplasia. *Pediatrics* 123:1562–1573, 2009.
73. Bhandari V, Gavino RG, Nedrelow JH, et al: Meconium aspiration syndrome: current concepts. *Indian Journal of Maternal and Child Health* 7:1–7, 1996.
74. Luu TM, Lefevre F, Riley P, et al: Continuing utilisation of specialised health services in extremely preterm infants. Archives of Disease in Childhood. *Fetal and Neonatal Edition* 95:F320–F325, 2011.
75 Hermansen CL, Lorah KN: Respiratory distress in the newborn. *American Family Physician* 76:987–994, 2007.
76. Klingner MC, Kruse J: Meconium aspiration syndrome: pathophysiology and prevention. *The Journal of the American Board of Family Practice* 12:450–466, 1999.
77. Fanaroff AA: Meconium aspiration syndrome: historical aspects. *Journal of Perinatology* 28:S3–S7, 2008.
78. Wiswell TE, Bent RC: Meconium staining and the meconium aspiration syndrome. *Pediatric Clinics of North America* 40:955–981, 1993.
79. Wiswell TE: Advances in the treatment of the meconium aspiration syndrome. *Acta Paediatrica Supplement* 90:28–30, 2001.
80. Wiswell TE, Tuggle JM, Turner BS: Meconium aspiration syndrome: have we made a difference? *Pediatrics* 85:715–721, 1990.
81. Bhutani VK: Developing a systems approach to prevent meconium aspiration syndrome: lessons learned from multinational studies. *Journal of Perinatology* 28:S30–S35, 2008.
82. Vain NE, Szyld EG, Prudent LM, et al: What (not) to do at and after delivery? Prevention and management of meconium aspiration syndrome. *Early Human Development* 85:621–626, 2009.
83. Ellwanger DL, Weber-Hardy LA: Neonatal pulmonary disorders. In Czervinske MP, editor: *Perinatal and pediatric respiratory care*, ed 2, St Lois, 2008, Saunders.
84. Beligere N, Rao R: Neurodevelopmental outcome of infants with meconium aspiration syndrome: report of a study and literature review. *Journal of Perinatology* 28:S93–S101, 2008.
85. Reference deleted in proofs.
86. Gadzinowski J: Contemporary treatment options for meconium aspiration syndrome. *Croatian Medical Journal* 39:158–164, 1998.
87. Waring WW: Respiratory diseases in children: an overview. *Respiratory Care* 20:1138–1145, 1975.
88. Kumar M, Biswal N, Bhuvaneswari V, et al: Persistent pneumonia: underlying cause and outcome. *Indian Journal of Pediatrics* 76:1223–1226, 2009.
89. Sullivan PB, Morrice JS, Vernon-Roberts A, et al: Does gastrostomy tube feeding in children with cerebral palsy increase the risk of respiratory morbidity? *Archives of Disease in Childhood* 91:478–482, 2006.

90. Mofenson LM, Brady MT, Danner SP, et al: 2009). Guidelines for the prevention and treatment of opportunistic infections among HIV-exposed and HIV-infected children; recommendations from CDC, the National Institutes of Health, the HIV Medicine Association of the Infectious Diseases Society of America, the Pediatric Infectious Disease Society, and the American Academy of Pediatrics. *Morbidity and Mortality Weekly Report Recommendations and Reports* 58(RR-11):1–166, 2009.
91. Berdon WE, Mellins RB, Abramson SJ, et al: Pediatric HIV infection in its second decade: the changing pattern of lung involvement. Clinical, plain film, and computed tomographic findings. *Radiol Clin North Am.* 31(3):453–463, 1993 May.
92. Eaton DK, Kann L, Kinchen S, et al: Youth risk behavior surveillance—United States, 2009. *Morbidity and Mortality Weekly Report Surveillance Summaries* 59(SS05):1–142, 2010.
93. Crump C, Winkleby MA, Sundquist J, et al: Risk of asthma in young adults who were born preterm: a Swedish national cohort study. *Pediatrics* 127:e913–e920, 2011.
94. Baraldi E, Carraro S, Filippone M: Bronchopulmonary dysplasia: definitions and long-term respiratory outcome. *Early Human Development* 85:S1–S3, 2009.
95. Jackson DJ, Lemanske RF: The role of respiratory virus infections in childhood asthma inception. *Immunology and Allergy Clinics of North America* 30:513–522, 2010.
96. Bacharier LB, Boner A, Carlsen K-H, et al: Diagnosis and treatment of asthma in childhood: a PRACTALL consensus report. *Allergy* 63:5–34, 2008.
97. Towns SJ, van Asperen PP: Diagnosis and management of asthma in adolescents. *The Clinical Respiratory Journal* 3:69–76, 2009.
98. Galant SP, Crawford LJ, Morphew T, et al: Predictive value of a cross-cultural asthma case-detection tool in an elementary school population. *Pediatrics* 114:307–316, 2004.
99. Knorr RS, Condon SK, Dwyer FM, et al: Tracking pediatric asthma: the Massachusetts experience using school health records. *Environmental Health Perspectives* 112:1424–1427, 2004.
100. Homer SD: Effect of education on school-age children's and parent's asthma management. *Journal for Specialists in Pediatric Nursing* 9:95–102, 2004.
101. Taras H, Wright S, Brennan J, et al: Impact of school nurse case management on students with asthma. *Journal of School Health* 74:213–219, 2004.
102. Farrell PM, Rosenstein BJ, White TB, et al: Guidelines for diagnosis of cystic fibrosis in newborns through older adults: Cystic Fibrosis Foundation consensus report. *Journal of Pediatrics* 153:S4–S14, 2008.
103. Staab D: Cystic fibrosis: therapeutic challenge in cystic fibrosis children. *European Journal of Endocrinology* 151(Suppl 1):S77–S80, 2004.
104. Philpott J, Houghton K, Luke A; Canadian Paediatric Society, Healthy Living and Sports Medicine Committee, Canadian Academy of Sport Medicine, Paediatric Sport and Exercise Medicine Committee: Physical activity recommendations for children with specific chronic health conditions: juvenile idiopathic arthritis, hemophilia, asthma and cystic fibrosis. *Paediatric and Child Health* 15:213–225, 2010.
105. Milross MA, Piper AJ, Dobbin CJ, et al: Sleep disordered breathing in cystic fibrosis. *Sleep Medicine Reviews* 8:253–255, 2004.
106. McColley SA: Cystic fibrosis lung disease: when does it start, and how can it be prevented? *The Journal of Pediatrics* 145:6–7, 2004.
107. Brody AS, Klein JS, Molina PL, et al: High-resolution computed tomography in young patients with cystic fibrosis: distribution of abnormalities and correlation with pulmonary function tests. *The Journal of Pediatrics* 145:32–38, 2004.
108. Ranganathan SC, Stocks J, Dezateux C, et al: The evolution of airway function in early childhood following clinical diagnosis of cystic fibrosis. *American Journal of Respiratory and Critical Care Medicine* 169:928–933, 2004.
109. Griesenbach U, Geddes DM, Alton EW: Gene therapy for cystic fibrosis: an example for lung gene therapy. *Gene Therapy* 11(Suppl 1):S43–S50, 2004.
110. Griesenbach U, Alton EW: Current status and future directions of gene and cell therapy for cystic fibrosis. *BioDrugs* 25:77–88, 2011.
111. Borowitz D, Robinson KA, Rosenfeld M, et al: Cystic fibrosis foundation evidence-based guidelines for management of infants with cystic fibrosis. *The Journal of Pediatrics* 155:S73–S93, 2009.
112. Davis PB: Evolution of therapy for cystic fibrosis. *New England Journal of Medicine* 331:672–673, 1994.
113. Pryor JA: The forced expiration technique. In Pryor JA, editor: *Respiratory care*, London, 1991, Churchill-Livingstone.
114. Pryor JA, Webber BA: An evaluation of the forced expiration technique as an adjunct to postural drainage. *Physiotherapy* 65:304–307, 1979.
115. Mahlmeister MJ, Fink JB, Hoffman GL, et al: Positive-expiratory-pressure mask therapy: theoretical and practical considerations and a review of the literature. *Respiratory Care* 36:1218–1229, 1991.
116. Shoni MH: Autogenic drainage: a modern approach to physiotherapy in cystic fibrosis. *Journal of the Royal Society of Medicine* 82(Suppl 16):32–37, 1989.
117. Konstan MW, Stern RC, Doershuk CF: Efficacy of the Flutter device for airway mucus clearance in patients with cystic fibrosis. *Journal of Pediatrics* 124:689–693, 1994.
118. Hansen LG, Warwick WJ: High-frequency chest compression system to aid in clearance of mucus from the lung. *Biomedical Instrumentation and Technology* 24:289–294, 1990.
119. Flume PA, Robinson KA, O'Sullivan BP, et al: Cystic fibrosis pulmonary guidelines: airway clearance therapies. *Respiratory Care* 54:522–537, 2009.
120. Elkins MR, Jones A, van der Schans C: Positive expiratory pressure physiotherapy for airway clearance in people with cystic fibrosis [review]. *The Cochrane Database of Systematic Reviews* 4, 2004.
121. Darbee JC, Ohtake PJ, Grant BJ, et al: Physiologic evidence for the efficacy of positive expiratory pressure as an airway clearance technique in patients with cystic fibrosis. *Physical Therapy* 84:524–537, 2004.
122. Button BM, Heine RM, Catto-Smith AG, et al: Chest physiotherapy, gastroesophageal reflux, and arousal in infants with cystic fibrosis. *Archives of Disease in Childhood* 89:435–439, 2004.
123. Keens TG, Krastins IRS, Wannamaker EM, et al: Ventilatory muscle training in normal subjects and patients with cystic fibrosis. *American Review of Respiratory Disease* 116:853–860, 1977.
124. Reid WD, Loveridge BM: Ventilatory muscle endurance training in patients with chronic obstructive airway disease. *Physiotherapy Canada* 35:197–205, 1983.
125. Santillanes G, Gausche-Hill M: Pediatric airway management. *Emergency Medicine Clinics of North America* 26:961–975, 2008.
126. Davis GM: Tracheostomy in children. *Pediatric Respiratory Reviews* 75:S206–S209, 2006.
127. Finer NN, Moriartey RR, Boyd J, et al: Postextubation atelectasis: a retrospective review and a prospective controlled study. *Journal of Pediatrics* 94:110–113, 1979.
128. Ersöz M, Selçuk B, Gündüz R, et al: Decreased chest mobility in children with spastic cerebral palsy. *The Turkish Journal of Pediatrics* 48:344–350, 2006.
129. Alexander R: Respiratory and oral-motor functioning. In Connolly BH, Montgomery PC, editors: *Therapeutic exercise in developmental disabilities*, ed 2, Hixson, Tenn, 1993, Chattanooga Group.
130. Hadders-Algra M: Variation and variability: key words in human motor development. *Physical Therapy* 90:1823–1837, 2010.
131. Fitzgerald DA, Follett J, Van Asperen PP: Assessing and managing lung disease and sleep disordered breathing in children with cerebral palsy. *Paediatric Respiratory Reviews* 10:18–24, 2009.
132. Littleton SR, Heriza CB, Mullens PA, et al: Effects of positioning on respiratory measures in individuals with cerebral palsy and severe scoliosis. *Pediatric Physical Therapy* 23:159–169, 2011.
133. Campanozzi A, Capano G, Miele E, et al: Impact of malnutrition on gastrointestinal disorders and gross motor abilities in children with cerebral palsy. *Brain Development* 29:25–29, 2007.
134. Hays RM, Jordan RA, McLaughlin JF, et al: Central ventilatory dysfunction in myelodysplasia: an independent determinant of survival. *Developmental Medicine and Child Neurology* 31:366–370, 1989.
135. Swaminathan S, Paton JY, Ward SLD, et al: Abnormal control of ventilation in adolescents with myelodysplasia. *Journal of Pediatrics* 115:898–903, 1989.
136. Ward SLD, Jacobs RA, Gates EP, et al: Abnormal ventilatory patterns during sleep in infants with myelomeningocele. *Journal of Pediatrics* 4:631–634, 1986.
137. Juranek J, Salmon MS: Anomalous development of brain structure and function in spina bifida myelomeningocele. *Developmental Disabilities Research Reviews* 16:23–30, 2010.
138. Mayer S, Weisser M, Till H, et al: Congenital myelomeningocele: do we have to change our management? *Cerebrospinal Fluid Research* 7:17, 2010.
139. Dauvilliers Y, Stal V, Abril B, et al: Chiari malformation and sleep related breathing disorders. *Journal of Neurology, Neurosurgery & Psychiatry* 78:1344–1348, 2007.
140. Hinderer KA, Hinderer SR, Shurtleff DB: Myelodysplasia. In Campbell SK, Vander Linden DW, Palisano RJ, editors: *Physical therapy for children*, ed 3, Philadelphia, 2006, WB. Saunders Company.

141. Yang Q, Rasmussen SA, Friedman JM: Mortality associated with Down's syndrome in the USA from 1983 to 1997: a population-based study. *Lancet* 359:1019–1025, 2002.
142. Bruijn M, van der Aa LB, van Rijn RR, et al: High incidence of acute lung injury in children with Down syndrome. *Intensive Care Medicine* 33:2179–2182, 2007.
143. Reference deleted in proofs.
144. Dichter CG, Darbee JC, Effgen SK, et al: Assessment of pulmonary function and physical fitness in children with Down syndrome. *Pediatric Physical Therapy* 5:3–8, 1993.
145. Moerchen VA: Respiration and motor development: a systems perspective. *Neurology Report* 18:8–10, 1994.
146. Bach JR, O'Brien J, Krotenberg R, et al: Management of end stage respiratory failure in Duchene muscular dystrophy. *Muscle and Nerve* 10:177–182, 1987.
147. Smith PEM, Calverley PMA, Edwards RHT, et al: Practical problems in the respiratory care of patients with muscular dystrophy. *New England Journal of Medicine* 316:1197–1205, 1987.
148. Stuberg W: Muscular dystrophy and spinal muscular atrophy. In Campbell SK, Vander Linden DW, Palisano RJ, editors: *Physical therapy for children*, ed 3, Philadelphia, 2006, WB. Saunders Company.
149. Cox GF, Kunkel LM: Dystrophies and heart disease. *Current Opinion in Cardiology* 12:329–343, 1997.
150. Takaso M, Nakazawa T, Imura T, et al: Surgical management of severe scoliosis with high risk pulmonary dysfunction in Duchenne muscular dystrophy: patient function, quality of life and satisfaction. *International Orthopaedics* 34:695–702, 2010.
151. Winkler G, Zifko U, Nader A, et al: Dose-dependent effects of inspiratory muscle training in neuromuscular disorders. *Muscle and Nerve* 23:1257–1260, 2000.
152. Koessler W, Wanke T, Winkler G, et al: 2 years' experience with inspiratory muscle training in patients with neuromuscular disorders. *Chest* 120:765–769, 2001.
153. Topin N, Matecki S, Le Bris S, et al: Dose-dependent effect of individualized respiratory muscle training in children with Duchenne muscular dystrophy. *Neuromuscular Disorders* 12:576–583, 2002.
154. Bach JR, Isikawa Y, Kim H: Prevention of pulmonary morbidity for patients with Duchene muscular dystrophy. *Chest* 112:1024–1028, 1998.
155. Bach JR, Chaudhry SS: Standards of care in MDA clinics. *American Journal of Physical Medicine and Rehabilitation* 79:193–196, 2000.
156. Hukins CA, Hillman DR: Daytime predictors of sleep hypoventilation in Duchene muscular dystrophy. *American Journal of Respiratory Critical Care Medicine* 161:166–170, 2000.
157. Vianello A, Bevilacqua M, Salvador V, et al: Long-term nasal intermittent positive pressure ventilation in advanced Duchenne's muscular dystrophy. *Chest* 105:445–448, 1994.
158. Raphael JC, Chevret S, Chastang C, et al: Randomised trial of preventive nasal ventilation in Duchenne muscular dystrophy. French multicentre cooperative group on home mechanical ventilation assistance in Duchenne de Boulogne muscular dystrophy. *Lancet* 343:1600–1604, 1994.
159. Shneerson JM, Simonds, AK: Noninvasive ventilation for chest wall and neuromuscular disorders. *European Respiratory Journal* 20:480–487, 2002.
160. Bach JR: Mechanical insufflation/exsufflation: has it come of age? [commentary]. *European Respiratory Journal* 21:385–386, 2003.
161. Kotzot D, Schwabegger AH: Etiology of chest wall deformities: a genetic review for the treating physician. *Journal of Pediatric Surgery* 44:2004–2011, 2009.
162. Reference deleted in proofs.
163. Vos MB, Welsh J: Childhood obesity: update on predisposing factors and prevention strategies. *Current Gastroenterology Reports* 12:280–287, 2010.
164. Raj M, Kumar RK: Obesity in children and adolescents. *The Indian Journal of Medical Research* 132:598–607, 2010.
165. Daniels SR: Complications of obesity in children and adolescents. *International Journal of Obesity* 33:S60–S65, 2009.
166. Yamaki K, Rimmer JH, Lowry BD, et al: Prevalence of obesity-related chronic health conditions in overweight adolescents with disabilities. *Research in Developmental Disabilities* 32:280–288, 2011.
167. Bibi H, Shoseyov D, Feigenbaum D, et al: The relationship between asthma and obesity in children: is it real or a cause of overdiagnosis? *Journal of Asthma* 41:403–410, 2004.
168. Chinn S: Obesity and asthma: evidence for and against a causal relation. *Journal of Asthma* 40:1–16, 2003.
169. Chinn S, Rona RJ: Obesity and asthma in children (comment). *American Journal of Respiratory and Critical Care Medicine* 170:95, 2004.
170. Noal RB, Menezes AMB, Macedo EC, et al: Childhood body mass index and risk of asthma in adolescence: a systematic review. *Obesity Reviews* 12:93–104, 2010.
171. Arens R, Marcus CL: Pathophysiology of upper airway obstruction: a developmental perspective [review]. *Sleep* 27:997–1019, 2004.
172. Ng DK, Lam YY, Kwok KL, et al: Obstructive sleep apnea in children. *Hong Kong Medical Journal* 10:44–48, 2004.
173. Arens R, Muzumdar H: Childhood obesity and obstructive sleep apnea syndrome. *Journal of Applied Physiology* 108:436–444, 2010.
174. Bhattacharjee R, Kim J, Kheirandish-Gozal L, et al: Obesity and obstructive sleep apnea syndrome in children: a tale of inflammatory cascades. *Pediatric Pulmonology* 46:313–323, 2011.
175. Dyken ME, Lin-Dyken DC, Poulton S, et al: Prospective polysomnographic analysis of obstructive sleep apnea in Down syndrome. *Archives of Pediatrics and Adolescent Medicine* 157:655–660, 2003.
176. de Miguel-Díez J, Villa-Asensi JR, Alvarez-Sala JL. Prevalence of sleep-disordered breathing in children with Down syndrome: polygraphic findings in 108 children. *Sleep* 26(8):1006–1009, 2003 Dec 15.
177. Schrander-Stumpel CT, Curfs LM, Sastrowijoto P, et al: Prader-Willi syndrome: causes of death in an international series of 27 cases. *American Journal of Medical Genetics* 124:333–338, 2004.
178. Cassidy SB, Driscoll DJ: Prader-Willi syndrome. *European Journal of Human Genetics* 17:3–13, 2009.
179. Felcar JM, Guitti JC, Marson AC, et al: Preoperative physiotherapy in prevention of pulmonary complications in pediatric cardiac surgery. *Revista Brasileira de Cirurgia Cardiovascular* 23:383–388, 2008.
180. Huckabay L, Daderian AD: Effect of choices on breathing exercises post-open heart surgery. *Dimensions of Critical Care Nursing* 9:190–201, 1990.
181. Johnson B: Postoperative physical therapy in the pediatric cardiac surgery patient. *Pediatric Physical Therapy* 3:14–22, 1991.
182. Balfour IC, Drimmer AM, Nouri S, et al: Pediatric cardiac rehabilitation. *American Journal of Disease in Childhood* 145:627–630, 1991.
183. Calzolari A, Turchetta A, Biondi G, et al: Rehabilitation of children after total correction of tetralogy of Fallot. *International Journal of Cardiology* 28:151–158, 1990.
184. Mathews RA, Nixon PA, Stephenson RJ, et al: An exercise program for pediatric patients with congenital heart disease: organizational and physiologic aspects. *Journal of Cardiac Rehabilitation* 3:467–475, 1983.
185. Gildein P, Mocellin R, Kaufmehl K: Oxygen uptake transient kinetics during constant-load exercise in children after operations of ventricular septal defect, tetralogy of Fallot transposition of the great arteries, or tricuspid valve atresia. *American Journal Cardiology* 74:166–169, 1994.
186. Tomassoni TL, Galioto FM, Vaccaro P: Cardiopulmonary exercise testing in children following surgery for tetralogy of Fallot. *American Journal of Disease in Childhood* 145:1290–1293, 1991.
187. Müller J, Christov F, Schreiber C, et al: Exercise capacity, quality of life, and daily activity in the long-term follow-up of patients with univentricular heart and total cavopulmonary connection. *European Heart Journal* 30:2915–2920, 2009.
188. Manlhiot C, Knezevich S, Radojewski E, et al: Functional health status of adolescents after the Fontan procedure: comparison with their siblings. *The Canadian Journal of Cardiology* 25:e294–e300, 2009.
189. Moalla W, Maingourd Y, Gauthier R, et al: Effect of exercise training on respiratory muscle oxygenation in children with congenital heart disease. *European Journal of Cardiovascular Prevention and Rehabilitation* 13:604–611, 2006.
190. Ross J, Dean E: Integrating physiological principles into the comprehensive management of cardiopulmonary dysfunction. *Physical Therapy* 69:255–259, 1989.
191. Hutchinson AA, Ross KR, Russell G: The effects of posture on ventilation and lung mechanics in preterm and light-for-date infants. *Pediatrics* 64:429–432, 1979.
192. Lioy J, Manginello FP: A comparison of prone and supine positioning in the immediate postextubation period of neonates. *Journal of Pediatrics* 112:982–984, 1988.
193. Martin RJ, Herrell N, Rubin D, et al: Effects of supine and prone positions on arterial oxygen tension in the preterm infant. *Pediatrics* 63:528–531, 1979.
194. Levy J, Habib RH, Lipsten E, et al: Prone versus supine positioning in the well preterm infant: effects on work of breathing and breathing patterns. *Pediatric Pulmonology* 41:754–758, 2006.
195. Grenier I, Bigsby R, Vergara E, et al: Comparison of motor self-regulatory and stress behaviors of preterm infants across body positions. *American Journal of Occupational Therapy* 57:289–297, 2003.

196. Long JG, Phillip AGS, Lucey JF: Excessive handling as a cause of hypoxemia. *Pediatrics* 65:203–207, 1980.
197. Murai DT, Grant JW: Continuous oscillation therapy improves pulmonary outcome of incubated newborns: results of a prospective, randomized, controlled trial. *Critical Care Medicine* 22:1147–1154, 1994.
198. Thoresen M, Cowan F, Whitelaw A: Effect of tilting on oxygenation in newborn infants. *Archives of Disease in Childhood* 63:315–317, 1988.
199. Crane LD, Zombek M, Krauss AN, et al: Comparison of chest physiotherapy in infants with HMD. *Pediatric Research* 12:559, 1978.
200. Emery JR, Peabody JL: Head position affects intracranial pressure in newborn infants. *Journal of Pediatrics* 103:950–953, 1983.
201. Stoll BJ, Hansen NI, Bell EF, et al: Neonatal outcomes of extremely preterm infants from the NICHD Neonatal Research Network. *Pediatrics* 126:443–456, 2010.
202. Durand M, Sangha B, Cabal LA, et al: Cardiopulmonary and intracranial pressure changes related to endotracheal suctioning in preterm infants. *Critical Care Medicine* 17:506–510, 1989.
203. McFadden R: Decreasing respiratory compromise during infant suctioning. *American Journal of Nursing* 81:2158–2161, 1981.
204. Perlman JM, Volpe JJ: Suctioning in the preterm infant: effects on cerebral blood flow velocity, intracranial pressure, and arterial blood pressure. *Pediatrics* 72:329–334, 1983.
205. Gardner DL, Shirland L: Evidence-based guideline for suctioning the intubated neonate and infant. *Neonatal Network* 28:281–302, 2009.
206. Edelschick J, Seal D: Pediatric cardiopulmonary physical therapy. In Hillegass E, editor: *Essentials of cardiopulmonary physical therapy*, ed 3, St Louis, 2011, Saunders.
207. Tibbals J, Henning R, Robertson CF, et al: A home respiratory support programme for children by parents and layperson carers. *Journal of Paediatrics and Child Health* 46:57–62, 2010.
208. Clark NM, Brown R, Joseph CLM, et al: Effects of a comprehensive school-based asthma program on symptoms, parent management, grades, and absenteeism. *Chest* 125:1674–1679, 2004.
209. Magee CL: Physical therapy for the child with asthma. *Pediatric Physical Therapy* 3:23–28, 1991.
210. Nixon PA: Role of exercise in the evaluation and management of pulmonary disease in children and youth [review]. *Medicine and Science in Sports and Exercise* 28:414–420. 1996.
211. Basaran S, Guler-Uysal F, Ergen N, et al: Effects of physical exercise on quality of life, exercise capacity and pulmonary function in children with asthma. *Journal of Rehabilitation Medicine* 38:130–135, 2006.
212. de Bisschop C, Guenard H, Desnot P, et al: Reduction of exercise-induced asthma in children by short, repeated warm ups. *British Journal of Sports Medicine* 33:100–104, 1999.
213. Milgrom H, Taussig LM: Keeping children with exercise-induced asthma active. *Pediatrics* 104:38–42, 1999.
214. Randolph C: Exercise-induced bronchospasm in children. *Clinical Reviews in Allergy and Immunology* 34:205–216, 2008.
215. Boas SR, Danduran MJ, McBride AL, et al. Postexercise immune correlates in children with and without cystic fibrosis. *Med Sci Sports Exerc* 32(12):1997–2004, 2000 Dec.
216. Klign PH, Oudshoorn A, van der Ent CK, et al: Effects of anaerobic training in children with cystic fibrosis: a randomized controlled study. *Chest* 125:1299–1305, 2004.
217. Selvadurai HC, Blimkie CJ, Meyers N, et al: Randomized controlled study of in-hospital exercise training programs in children with cystic fibrosis. *Pediatric Pulmonology* 33:194–200, 2002.
218. Massery M: Musculoskeletal and neuromuscular interventions: a physical approach to cystic fibrosis. *Journal of the Royal Society of Medicine* 98(Supplement 45):55–66, 2005.
219. van Brussel M, van der Net J, Hulzebos E, et al: The Utrecht approach to exercise in chronic childhood conditions: the decade in review. *Pediatric Physical Therapy* 23:2–14, 2011.
220. Boucher GP, Lands LC, Hay JA, et al: Activity levels and the relationship to lung function in children with cystic fibrosis. *American Journal of Physical Medicine and Rehabilitation* 76:311–315, 1997.
221. Marin VB, Velandia S, Hunter B, et al: Energy expenditure, nutrition status, and body composition in children with cystic fibrosis. *Nutrition* 20:181–186, 2004.
222. Moorcroft AJ, Dodd ME, Webb AK: Long-term change in exercise capacity, body mass, and pulmonary function in adults with cystic fibrosis. *Chest* 111:338–343, 1997.
223. Boehme R: Assessment and treatment of the respiratory system for breathing, sound production, and trunk control. *Team Talk* 2:2-8, 1992.
224. Boehme R: How do I get scapular stability in my patients? *Team Talk* 1:1-3, 1991.

The Aging Patient

Elizabeth J. Protas

KEY TERMS

Aging
Autonomic
Cardiovascular changes
Exercise changes
Pulmonary changes

CHAPTER OUTLINE

Cardiovascular, pulmonary, and autonomic nervous system functions are dynamic and undergo changes as people age. It is important for physical therapists to be aware of changes that occur with normal aging to better understand the impact of pathological conditions and impairment on these systems' functions. In addition, a clear understanding of how these systems respond to exercise training will assist the clinician in prescribing and evaluating exercise interventions in older adults.

Understanding aging is more complicated than simply taking into account chronological age. As people age, greater variability occurs among individuals, making predictions about any one individual challenging. The trends of some changes are probably not linear but curvilinear, with changes accelerating after the age of 65. Thus many of the physiological studies that have been done with 60-year-olds may not apply to individuals who are 80, 90, or 100 years of age. Many of the studies that are available on exercise in older individuals have been conducted with people who are less than 65 years of age. The vast majority of these studies used only men as subjects or had a small number of women in the sample. Sex may be an important variable in relation to exercise and aging, but the data available on this issue are limited.

Another consideration is the composition of study populations. With increasing age there is a greater incidence of pathology and co-morbidities. Latent cardiovascular disease and histories of chronic illnesses are common in older populations. Co-morbidities are frequently encountered in older adults. It may be more common for a person over 75 years of age to have health problems than to be healthy. The physical therapist may be more interested in the responses of a frail 85- or 90-year-old woman who has a history of hypertension, coronary artery disease, and diabetes than someone who is healthy at this age because this reflects the population most often referred to physical therapy. The occurrence of pathological states in study populations may affect the cardiovascular and pulmonary responses to exercise. Furthermore, the study of the physiological aspects of exercise and aging is still evolving. The literature can be confusing and contradictory, making conclusions and generalizations difficult. An attempt is made in this chapter to provide some direction in this confusing maze of information.

An additional issue is a model of aging that might sort out some of the determinants of aging (Figure 38-1). The model identifies biological factors, disuse, pathology, and psychosocial concerns as determinants of aging. Biological factors address genetics, sex, cellular mechanisms, and metabolic and physiological responses that influence aging. Disuse is implicated in the more sedentary lifestyle led by many older adults, which results in loss of exercise capacity.[1] With exercise training, it should be possible to reverse or attenuate capacities that decline as a result of disuse. This chapter focuses on the biological and disuse characteristics of aging. The impact of various pathological conditions is discussed in other chapters.

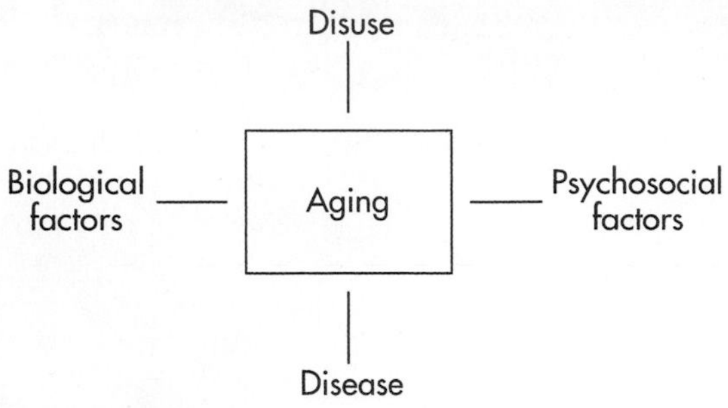

Fig. 38-1 A model of aging that identifies the major determinants underlying the aging process.

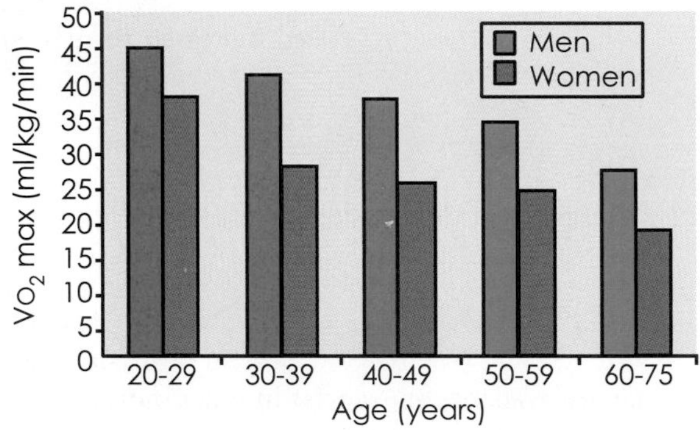

Fig. 38-2 Decline in $\dot{V}O_{2max}$ from 20 to 75 years of age in both men and women. *(From Hossack KF, Bruce RA: Maximal cardiac function in sedentary normal men and women: Comparison of age-related changes,* Journal of Applied Physiology *53:799-804, 1982.)*

Psychosocial issues related to exercise and aging are not addressed.

Cardiac Changes with Aging

Aerobic Capacity

Aerobic capacity is the maximum ability to perform exercise with large muscle groups. This ability is produced by interaction of the lungs, heart, and peripheral tissues. The most common indirect measure of aerobic capacity is maximum oxygen consumption ($\dot{V}O_{2max}$), or the maximum amount of oxygen used during exercise. $\dot{V}O_{2max}$ is directly related to cardiac output (the amount of blood pumped by the heart) and the arteriovenous oxygen content difference (the amount of oxygen extracted in the periphery). Cardiac output is the product of heart rate and stroke volume. Aerobic capacity reflects the central cardiac function and the efficiency of the peripheral tissues to extract and use oxygen.

$\dot{V}O_{2max}$ declines with age[2,3] at a rate of 0.40 to 0.50 mL/kg/min per year for men and between 0.20 to 0.35 mL/kg/min per year for women (Figure 38-2).[4] The reduction is approximately 10% per decade. The decline is faster and greater in men than women; however, men have a larger aerobic capacity overall than women.[5,6] $\dot{V}O_{2max}$ is related to body size, which is generally smaller in women than men. $\dot{V}O_{2max}$ is associated with peripheral vascular reserve in older men but not in women.[7] Increases in body weight along with aging result in reduced $\dot{V}O_{2max}$, even if aerobic capacity remains the same, because relative oxygen consumption is related to body weight. Reduced physical activity with aging also contributes to a loss of $\dot{V}O_{2max}$.

Considerable disagreement exists regarding the mechanisms that contribute to the decline in $\dot{V}O_{2max}$ with age. Both cardiac and peripheral changes contribute to this loss. Maximum cardiac output declines with age similarly in men and women.[7] A reduction in maximum cardiac output may account for 50% to 100% of the total reduction in $\dot{V}O_{2max}$.[8-10] McGuire and colleagues (2001)[2], however, suggested that reductions in peripheral oxygen extraction were the dominant mechanism responsible for reduced $\dot{V}O_{2max}$ with age. A major component to the decline in maximum cardiac output is decreased maximum heart rate.[3,9,11] The decline in heart rate is linearly related to age and occurs in both sedentary and active people.[5,12] Discrepancies in the age-related response of maximum stroke volume also exist; studies have reported reduced, preserved, and increased maximum stroke volume with age.[2,3,9,13] The decline in $\dot{V}O_{2max}$ associated with aging is most likely attributable to decreased maximum heart rate, stroke volume, and arteriovenous oxygen content difference, although each component's contribution varies.[8,14]

Cardiac Mechanics

Age-related changes in cardiac structure occur in the form of left ventricular wall thickness[13,15] and are attributed to an increase in size of cardiac myocytes[16] and increased collagen.[13] Additional cardiac structural changes include increases in vascular intimal thickness, vascular stiffness, and left arterial dimension.[13,17]

The diastolic properties (cardiac filling) of the heart alter with age. Diastole requires relaxation of the myocardial fibers, sufficient venous return to rapidly fill the heart, and timing of the atrial contraction to contribute to the end-diastolic volume. Relaxation may be hampered by increased ventricular stiffness, although there is limited evidence of this in humans.[14] The period of the isovolumetric myocardial relaxation (the time between aortic valve closing and mitral valve opening) is prolonged with aging.[15] Likewise, the peak rate of left ventricular filling during early diastole is progressively reduced so that between the ages of 20 and 80 years, the average rate can be reduced up to 50%.[13] Despite the changes in early diastole, the resting left ventricular end-diastolic volume remains the same because of an enhanced left atrial contribution to ventricular filling.[13] This is accompanied by an enlarged left atrium and an audible fourth heart sound in most older adults.[13,18]

Considerable disagreement exists regarding what happens to diastolic function during exercise. End-diastolic volume index (end-diastolic volume normalized for body surface) increases similarly in both young and older men during submaximal exercise; however, only older men remain at these elevated levels during exhaustive exercise.[13] Filling pressures during exercise in men increase with age.[19] In addition, peak left ventricular diastolic filling rate during submaximal and maximal exercise decreases with aging.[20,21] Decreased filling rate is associated with increased ventricular stiffness and prolonged relaxation time.[22]

Resting measures of systolic and cardiac pump function do not change with aging. The resting end-systolic volume and stroke volume do not change with age. Likewise, ejection fraction at rest (end-diastolic volume – [end-systolic volume/end-diastolic volume]) is similar in healthy older and younger individuals.[13]

Unlike resting systolic function, the pumping function of the heart changes considerably in response to exercise. Myocardial contractility as measured by the ratio of end-systolic volume to systolic arterial pressure declines during exercise as people age.[14] The end-systolic volume index increases, whereas the ejection fraction decreases during exercise.[13] Reduced contractile performance is related to decreased response to beta-adrenergic stimulation, changes in the myocardium, increased systolic blood pressure, and ventricular wall abnormalities.[8]

Exercise Training

For older people who remain active, the rate of decline in $\dot{V}O_{2max}$ is reduced to 5% per decade, compared with an anticipated decline of 10% per decade in sedentary adults.[11] A meta-analysis of 29 studies on endurance training, which included 1030 men and 466 women between the ages of 61 and 78 years, concluded that endurance training increases functional capacity in young older adults.[23] Less improvement was seen with increasing age, a shorter length of training, low $\dot{V}O_{2max}$ before training, and short duration of exercise sessions. The analysis suggests that a healthy 68-year-old individual who exercises for 30 minutes three times per week for 4 to 6 months can improve $\dot{V}O_{2max}$ by 14%.[23] Similar improvements occur in both men and women.[24,25]

The mechanisms underlying improvements in $\dot{V}O_{2max}$ in older adults who engage in endurance training are not clear. One consistent finding, however, is greater extraction of oxygen in the exercising skeletal muscle, which produces a wider arteriovenous oxygen content difference in both older men and women.[9,22,26] This implies that adaptations in the peripheral skeletal muscles account for some of the increase in $\dot{V}O_{2max}$ in older adults. The impact of exercise training on maximum cardiac output is uncertain.[22] Maximum cardiac output can either remain the same or increase after exercise training, depending on the effect of training on maximum stroke volume and maximum heart rate. Maximum heart rate remains the same in older men regardless of activity level, suggesting that the decline in maximal heart rate depends on factors other than exercise and physical fitness.[27] A decrease in response to circulating catecholamines is most often cited as the reason for changes in maximum heart rate with aging.[28] Relatively intense endurance training for a year or more can increase peak stroke volume in men.[29-31] Adaptations to exercise training in older women have been attributed predominantly to peripheral changes in arteriovenous oxygen content difference rather than central changes in cardiac function.[32,33] This apparently occurs despite intensive endurance training over a year-long period. In contrast, a relatively recent study that compared men and women who were masters athletes with healthy sedentary older adults, healthy young persons, and sedentary controls reported that stroke volume for any given filling pressure was greater for masters athletes compared with age-matched sedentary older adults.[34]

A recent study followed a small group of competitive distance-running men for 10 years with measures of the cardiovascular, pulmonary, and metabolic systems.[35] The 5-kilometer race time slowed over the 10 years, along with decreased training mileage, intensity, and frequency. Consistent with this, the peak exercise heart rate and oxygen consumption declined. Another intriguing study indicates that telomere length, a measure of the ability of cells to replicate, is preserved in healthy, older adults who engage in vigorous aerobic exercise.[36] The preservation of telomere length is positively related to maximum oxygen consumption, suggesting that exercise reduces cell senescence with aging. Further studies examining the outcomes of prolonged, sustained endurance training in older men and women are needed to characterize the adaptations that occur in women.

The diastolic changes that occur with aging can be reversed with exercise training.[20] Levy and colleagues intensively endurance trained 13 rigorously screened older men aged 60 to 82 years (mean age 68 years) and 11 younger men in their 20s, for 6 months. The training produced increased resting, submaximal, and peak filling rates for the older group comparable to the changes observed in the younger group.[20] End-diastolic peak volume at rest and exercise also increase after lengthy endurance training.[30] Thus training may reduce the age-associated diastolic changes. In contrast, endurance athletes who were followed for 10 years after age 65 showed deterioration in diastolic left ventricular function indices consistent with decreased cardiovascular diastolic function.[35] Another study demonstrated that 1 year of vigorous exercise training in sedentary seniors did not improve cardiac stiffening, but improved left ventricular mass and reduced arterial elastance.[37] The mechanisms of these responses are uncertain in humans. Studies in rats have shown that exercise training increases calcium uptake in cardiac sarcoplasmic reticulum, decreases relaxation time, reduces the decline of left ventricular pressure, enhances fatty acid oxidation, and increases cytochrome c oxidase levels.[20,38,39] All these changes have been associated with reduced diastolic function with aging.

Exercise training can also improve systolic performance in older men as reflected by the increase in exercise stroke volume. Increased peak stroke volume occurs with an increased exercise ejection fraction, a decrease in end-systolic volume, and greater left ventricular wall mass.[3,30,31] These changes apparently do not occur in older, estrogen-deficient women.[33] Table 38-1 summarizes these changes.

Vascular and Autonomic Changes with Aging

Aging increases arterial stiffness because of a loss of elastin, elastin fractures, and an increase in collagen and calcification.[17,40] Sex may influence some of these changes. Some evidence suggests that aortic stiffness may be greater in women after menopause than men.[41] Arterial wall thickness and diameter and resting systolic pressure also increase (Figure 38-3).[14,17] It is unclear whether peripheral vascular resistance increases in normotensive older adults. Changes in the structure, size, and reactivity of the arteries increase the work of the left ventricle and have been directly implicated in the increase in cardiac myocyte size.

Complaints of dizziness when an older patient moves from supine to standing are frequently encountered by the physical therapist. Postural hypotension, or orthostatic intolerance, generally does not occur in healthy community-dwelling older adults but is common in individuals over 70 years of age who

Table 38-1 Cardiac Changes with Aging

	Because of Aging	After Exercise Training
MAXIMUM EXERCISE		
Oxygen consumption	↓	↑
Heart rate	↓	↔
Stroke volume	↓	↑, ↔
Arteriovenous oxygen difference	↓	↑
Cardiac output	↓	↑, ↔
CARDIAC FUNCTION		
Diastolic		
Left ventricular wall thickness	↑, ↓ after 80	↑
Left ventricular filling rate	↓	↑
End-diastolic volume	↔	↑
Systolic		
Myocardial contractility	↓	↑, ↔*
End-systolic volume	↑	↓, ↔*
Ejection fraction	↓	↑, ↔*

↑, Increase; ↓, decrease; ↔, no change.
*In women.

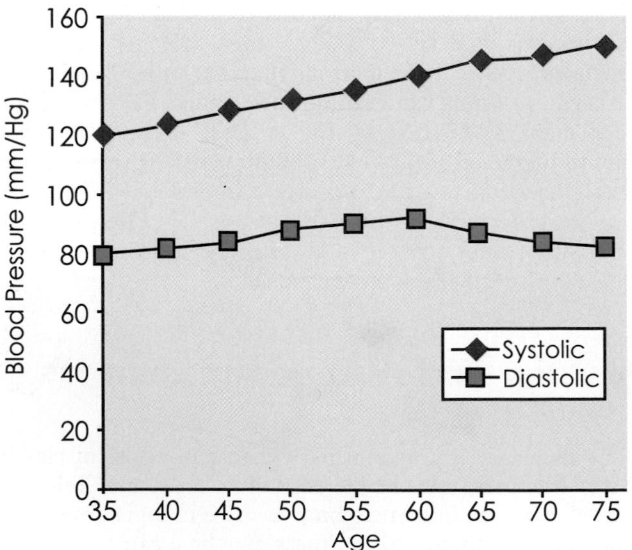

Fig. 38-3 Changes in systolic and diastolic blood pressures as people age. *(From Timiras PS: Cardiovascular alterations with age: Atherosclerosis, coronary heart disease and hypertension. In PS Timiras, editor:* Physiological basis of aging and geriatrics. *Boca Raton, Fla, 1988, CRC.)*

are debilitated and in hospitals or nursing homes.[42,43] Orthostatic intolerance is associated with decreased resting diastolic function, possibly decreased stroke volume, extreme inactivity, and, in individuals with hypertension, high systolic blood pressure.[44]

There are decreases in baroreceptor and cardiopulmonary reflexes with aging.[14,45] Arterial and venous dilation are reduced, but vasoconstriction is relatively spared. The heart demonstrates an overall decrease in responsiveness to autonomic stimulation. Older individuals experience higher central venous and mean arterial pressures, but lower forearm blood flow and forearm vascular resistance in response to passive leg raising.[45]

Response to Exercise

During submaximal and maximal exercise, arterial blood pressure is either unchanged or increased when younger subjects are compared with older subjects.[46] There also appears to be impaired peripheral vasodilation in skeletal muscle in response to exercise.[9] Redistribution of blood flow during exercise normally involves the shunting of blood from inactive limbs and viscera. There seems to be an enhanced vasoconstriction in inactive muscles during dynamic exercise in healthy older men.[47]

Exercise Training

Exercise training improves peripheral blood flow in skeletal muscle in 60-year-old men and women.[3,48] Exercise training, specifically aerobic training, has been reported to decrease blood pressure.[49] Meta-analysis revealed that 4 or more weeks of aerobic training can decrease systolic and diastolic blood pressure[50] and mean arterial blood pressure responses in older individuals when compared with sedentary individuals.[48] Adults who regularly exercise compared with sedentary individuals have smaller or no age-associated stiffness of the large arteries and have improved vascular endothelial function.[51] Aerobic training also reduces the age-related decline in cardiovagal baroreflex sensitivity and partially restores diminished cardiovagal baroreflex sensitivity in older men.[52] Aerobic training alters the autonomic nervous system and its control over resting heart rate by enhancing parasympathetic activity and attenuating sympathetic activity.[53] During vigorous exercise, the predominant activity of the autonomic nervous system is to increase sympathetic nerve activity, producing an increase in norepinephrine concentrations and increasing blood flow via dilation of the large arteries and constriction of the veins (Table 38-2).[13,54] Long-term aerobic training, however, reduces sympathetic nerve activity for a given work rate, thereby lowering exercise heart rate at a given work rate.[53] In summary, habitual exercise can improve characteristics of arterial aging, preserve vascular function, and possibly reduce the risk for cardiovascular disease.[51]

Pulmonary Changes with Aging

Structure and Function

Two major changes to the pulmonary system associated with aging are decreased elastic recoil and stiffening of the chest wall.[8,55] Elastic recoil of the lungs depends on the composition of the connective tissue, the structure of the connective tissue, and alveolar surface tension produced by surfactant.[8] Limited evidence suggests that the structure of the connective tissue may be the primary mechanism for age-associated change in

Table 38-2 Vascular and Autonomic Changes with Aging

	Because of Aging	After Exercise Training
Arterial wall thickness	↑	?
Systolic blood pressure	↑	↓
Diastolic blood pressure	↑ and ↔	↓
Orthostatic tolerance	↔	?
Arterial and venous dilation	↓	?
Vasoconstriction	↔	↔
Central venous pressure	↑	?

↑, Increases; ↓, decreases; ↔, unchanged; ?, insufficient data on older adult subjects.

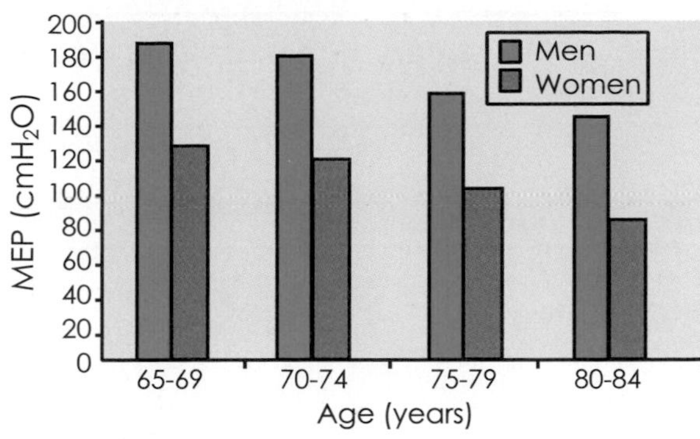

Fig. 38-4 Decrease in maximum expiratory pressures between 65 and 84 years of age for both men and women. This is a measure of respiratory muscle strength. *(From Enright PL, Kronmal RA, Monlio TA, et al: Respiratory muscle strength in the elderly,* American Journal of Respiratory Critical Care Medicine *149:430-438, 1994.)*

elastic recoil. Chest wall stiffness is accompanied by an increase in chest anterioposterior diameter, costal cartilage calcification, narrowing of the intervertebral disks, and changes in the rib to vertebrae articulations.[55-57] Postural changes such as kyphosis from osteoporosis limit expansion of the thoracic cage during inspiration and place the diaphragm at a mechanical disadvantage.[56]

Decreases occur with the alveolar-capillary surface area, the alveolar septal surface area, and the total surface area of lung parenchyma.[58] This reduces the alveolar surface area available for gas exchange and increases the amount of physiological dead space.[55]

Loss of elastic recoil with aging is directly associated with reduced forced expiratory flow.[59] Limitations in exhalation are caused by airway narrowing and closure at all lung volumes, thus reducing forced expiratory volume in 1 second (FEV_1).[8] Additionally, early airway closure also produces an early closing volume and a relative increase in the total residual volume. The combination of reduced elastic recoil and increased chest wall stiffness further increases residual volume and leads to a decrease in forced vital capacity in older individuals.[60,61] Flow rates are also lower in women and African-Americans than in white men at any age.[8]

Respiratory muscle strength, as reflected by the ability to create pressure over a range of lung volumes and flow rates, is similar when comparing healthy 30- and 70-year-olds.[62] This suggests that respiratory muscle strength does not change with aging; however, transdiaphragmatic pressure is reduced in older compared with younger individuals, suggesting reduced diaphragmatic strength.[56] Decline in diaphragmatic strength can contribute to diaphragmatic fatigue and ventilator weaning failure in older individuals.[56] Maximal inspiratory and expiratory pressures have been reported to decrease 15% between the sixth and eighth decades (Figure 38-4).[63] Perhaps these observed differences are similar to the differences observed with submaximal and maximal cardiac responses with the dynamic pressure measures over a range of volumes and flows considered submaximal.

Changes in the surface area result in a decrease in the diffusion capacity of the lung.[60,64] Both the loss of surface area and a decrease in pulmonary capillary blood volume contribute to reduced and uneven ventilation-to-perfusion matching in older adults. The resting partial arterial pressure of oxygen declines 5 to 10 mm Hg between the ages of 25 and 75 years.[8] These changes do not affect the arterial oxymyoglobin saturation or oxygen content. Parallel changes in the peripheral vasculature, pulmonary vascular resistance, and pulmonary arterial pressure at rest increase (Table 38-3).

Responses to Exercise

In addition to the structural and functional changes at rest, several changes occur in breathing during acute exercise. Expiratory flow limitations occur at lower exercise intensities as people age. A normal, healthy 69-year-old will begin to experience flow limitations even in response to moderate exercise.[8] Practically, the individual may experience this by having greater difficulty catching his or her breath during exercise.

Normally as people exercise, the tidal volume increases directly with increasing exercise intensity up to about 50% to 60% of the vital capacity. This remains unchanged as people age, although the vital capacity for older adults is reduced.[65] Likewise, as exercise and the tidal volume increase, there is a slight drop in the ratio of dead space to tidal volume. This drop is not affected by aging, although the older person will breathe more (have a higher minute ventilation) in response to submaximal exercise.[66] Of interest, the short-term modulation of the exercise ventilatory response does not change in healthy older men compared with healthy younger men, despite changes in ventilatory capacity with aging.[67]

The work of breathing is increased during exercise as people age as a result of several factors. Older adults require an increased ventilatory response to exercise to attain the same alveolar ventilation and $PaCO_2$.[66] Combined with the loss of elastic recoil, which causes airway closure at higher lung volumes, expiratory flow limitation occurs at moderate exercise intensities (an expiratory volume of 70 to 100 $L \cdot min^{-1}$), producing a hyperinflation, a noticeable increase in elastic and flow-resistive work of breathing, and shortness of breath.[66] In addition, an increase in the end-expiratory lung volume with increasing exercise results in breathing that occurs at a stiffer point in the lung-volume relationship. The increased stiffness imposes a higher elastic recoil on the ventilatory muscles, requiring greater pressure generated by the inspiratory muscles. The increase in expiratory flow resistance likewise requires greater pressure development by the expiratory

Table 38-3 Pulmonary Function Changes with Aging

	Because of Aging	After Exercise Training
STRUCTURE AND FUNCTION		
Elastic recoil	↓	
Chest wall stiffness	↑	
Alveolar-capillary surface area	↓	
Forced expiratory flow	↓	
Total residual volume	↑	
Forced vital capacity	↓	
Maximum inspiratory and expiratory pressure	↓	
Ventilation-perfusion matching	↓	
Partial arterial pressure oxygen	↓	
Oxygen saturation	↔	
Pulmonary vascular resistance	↑	
EXERCISE RESPONSE		
Expiratory flow limitation	↑	↔
Minute ventilation	↑	↓*, ↑†
Work of breathing	↑	↓
Respiratory muscle oxygen consumption	↑	↓
Arterial hypoxemia	↔, ↑	↑
Pulmonary artery pressure	↑	↔
Pulmonary wedge pressure	↑	↔

↑, Increases; ↓, decreases; ↔, unchanged.
*Submaximal.
†Maximal.

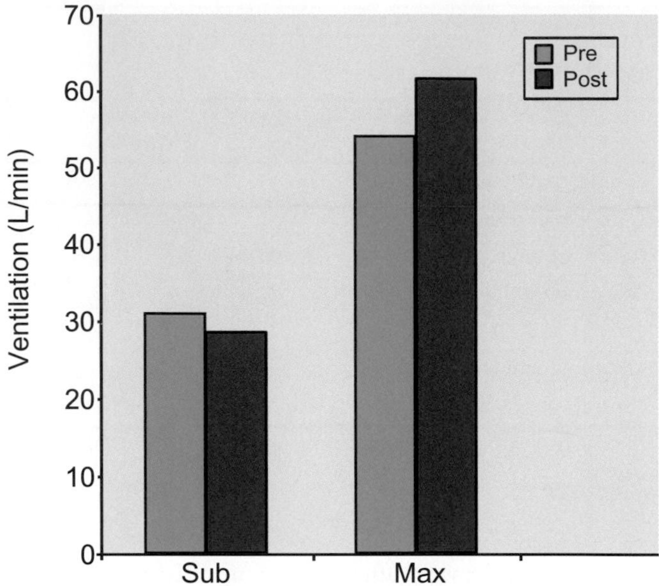

Fig. 38-5 Submaximum and maximum minute ventilation preexercise and postexercise training with a 12-week walking program in women whose mean age was 72.5 years. *(From Warren BJ, Nieman DC, Dotson RG, et al: Cardiorespiratory responses to exercise training in septuagenarian women,* International Journal of Sports Medicine *14:60-65, 1993.)*

muscles. Both the inspiratory and expiratory changes increase the work of breathing. The increase in the work of breathing increases the respiratory muscle oxygen consumption so that the respiratory muscles alone may require 10% to 12% of the total body oxygen consumption during maximal exercise in a sedentary 70-year-old man.[8]

What is also apparent is that the reserves used to respond to exercise represent a greater percentage of the available capacity. An older individual can exceed 50% of inspiratory muscle capacity even during moderate exercise. This is in contrast to the younger individual who rarely exceeds 50% of the inspiratory muscle capacity with exercise.[8] Thus the reserve capacity to generate pleural pressure is reduced in older adults because greater capacity is needed for even moderate exercise.

The variability characteristic of exercise responses in older individuals is particularly evident when considering gas exchange and pulmonary-vascular hemodynamics. In general, most individuals demonstrate only slight changes in arterial blood-gas homeostasis, but some individuals demonstrate arterial hypoxemia with exercise.[8] This response may be a factor of fitness. More fit older individuals appear to exhibit progressive arterial hypoxemia and carbon dioxide retention during mild-to-moderate exercise.[68,69]

Pulmonary artery pressure increases with age at any oxygen consumption or cardiac output during exercise.[70] In addition, the maximum pulmonary artery pressure at maximal exercise is reached at substantially lower oxygen consumption and cardiac output levels in older individuals compared with younger people. Pulmonary wedge pressure also increases with age and can exceed 25 mm Hg during peak supine exercise.[8] Limited data suggest that these high pressures may in turn induce pulmonary edema during intense exercise in older adults. Pulmonary edema would limit diffusion and may contribute to ventilation-perfusion maldistribution.[8]

Exercise Training

Aerobic training in older adults may offset some of the changes that have been described. Studies that address some of these changes, such as chest wall compliance or pulmonary artery pressure, are limited or nonexistent. The studies that are available deal with relatively young subjects who are 60 to 70 years of age, which does not provide insight into what exercise might do for individuals in their 70s and 80s, or beyond.

Aerobic training can decrease submaximal minute ventilation.[25,71] One study used a walking program with 70-year-old women over a 12-week period and demonstrated a 7.7% drop in submaximal minute ventilation (Figure 38-5).[25] Decreased minute ventilation is accompanied by a decrease in carbon dioxide production, respiratory exchange ratio (carbon dioxide production/oxygen consumption), and blood lactate level for any given level of submaximal exercise.[25,71] Thus the improved ventilatory efficiency after training may have more to do with improved efficiency in the periphery rather than an impact on the pulmonary system directly. Improved peripheral metabolic efficiency results in the production of less carbon dioxide; therefore the lungs do not have to work as hard to eliminate carbon dioxide. The important functional results of these changes are that the older adults who engage in exercise training will feel less breathlessness, experience a lower perceived exertion, and use a lower proportion of their maximal ventilatory capacity during exercise.[72]

Exercise training also increases maximum ventilatory responses during maximal exercise.[25,72] The 12-week walking program referred to above increased maximum minute ventilation by 14% in 70-year-old women (see Figure 38-5).[72] These women walked five days per week at an intensity of 78% of the maximal treadmill heart rate, or 118 beats per minute on average, so even though the program was not very strenuous, it produced substantial changes in maximum ventilation. Exercise training can improve submaximal ventilatory efficiency and increase maximum ventilation in older adults. Table 38-3 summarizes the pulmonary changes seen with aging and exercise.

Summary

As people age, profound changes occur at rest and in response to submaximal and maximal exercise. Many of these changes can be reduced or reversed as a result of exercise training. The implication is that many of these changes may have more to do with disuse than aging per se. Sedentary individuals tend to show these changes to a greater extent than more active seniors. Prevailing evidence suggests that older adults at any age can derive benefits from exercise training. Even very modest, short-term interventions can be effective. Older individuals should be encouraged to engage in regular physical activity to improve their exercise capacity and health overall.

Review Questions

1. What are the major changes that occur with aging in the cardiovascular system?
2. What outcomes will exercise training produce in an older adult's cardiovascular system?
3. What are the major changes that occur with aging in the autonomic nervous system in response to exercise, and which of these changes can be influenced by exercise training?
4. What are the major changes that occur in the pulmonary system with aging and in response to exercise?
5. Describe the possible impact of exercise training on the aging pulmonary system.

References

1. Bortz WM: The physics of frailty. *Journal American Geriatric Society* 41:1004–1008, 1993.
2. McGuire DK, Levine BD, Williamson JW, et al: A 30–year follow–up of the Dallas bed rest and training study. *Circulation* 104:1350–1357, 2001.
3. Beere PA, Russell SD, Morey MC, et al: Aerobic exercise training can reserve age–related peripheral circulatory changes in healthy older men. *Circulation* 100:1085–1094, 1999.
4. Buskirk ER, Hodgson JL: Age and aerobic power: the rate of changes in men and women. *Federation Proceedings* 46:1824–1829, 1987.
5. Cunningham DA, Paterson DH, Koval JJ, et al: A model of oxygen transport capacity changes for independently living older men and women. *Canadian Journal of Applied Physiology* 22:439–453, 1999.
6. Hossack KF, Bruce, RA: Maximal cardiac function in sedentary normal men and women: comparison of age–related changes. *Journal of Applied Physiology* 53:799–804, 1982.
7. Ridout SJ, Parker BA, Smithmeyer SL, et al: Age and sex influence the balance between maximal cardiac output and peripheral vascular reserve. *Journal of Applied Physiology* 108:483–489, 2010.
8. Dempsey JA, Seals DR: Aging, exercise, and cardiopulmonary function. In Holloszy J, editor: *Perspectives in exercise science*, New York, 1995, Williams & Wilkins.
9. Ogawa T, Spina RJ, Martin WH 3rd, et al: Effects of aging, sex, and physical training on cardiovascular responses to exercise. *Circulation* 86:494–503, 1992.
10. Saltin B: The aging endurance athlete. In Sutton, JR, Brock RM, editors: *Sports medicine for the mature athlete*, Indianapolis, 1986, Benchmark Press.
11. Hagberg JM: Effect of training on the decline of $\dot{V}O_{2max}$ with aging. *Federation Proceedings* 46:1830–1833, 1987.
12. Sidney KH, Shephard RJ: Maximum and submaximum exercise tests and men and women in the seventh, eighth, and ninth decades of life. *Journal of Applied Physiology* 43:280–287, 1977.
13. Lakatta EG: Age–associated cardiovascular changes in health: impact on cardiovascular disease in older persons. *Heart Failure Review* 7:29–49, 2002.
14. Lakatta EG: Cardiovascular regulatory mechanisms in advanced age. *Physiology Review* 73:413–467, 1993.
15. Gates PE, Tanaka H, Graves J, et al: Left ventricular structure and diastolic function with human aging. *European Heart Journal* 24:2213–2220, 2003.
16. Olivetti G, Melissari M, Capasso JM, Anversa P: Cardiomyopathy of the aging human heart. Myocyte loss and reactive cellular hypertrophy. *Circulation Research* 68:1560–1568, 1991.
17. Lakatta EG: Arterial and cardiac aging: major shareholders in cardiovascular disease enterprises. Part 1: Aging arteries: a "set up" for vascular disease. *Circulation* 107:139–146, 2003.
18. Fleg JL, Gerstenbleth G, Lakatta EG: Pathophysiology of the aging heart and circulation. In Messerli FH, editor: *Cardiovascular disease in the elderly*, ed 2, Boston, 1988, Martinus Nihoff.
19. Ehrsam RE, Perruchoud A, Oberholzer M, et al: Influence of age on pulmonary hemodynamics at rest and during supine exercise. *Clinical Science* 65:653–660, 1983.
20. Levy WC, Cerqueira MD, Abrass IB, et al: Endurance exercise training augments diastolic filling at rest and during exercise in healthy young and older men. *Circulation* 88:116–126, 1993.
21. Schulman DD, Lakatta EG, et al: Age–related decline in left ventricular filling at rest and exercise. *American Journal of Physiology* 263:H1932–H1938, 1992.
22. Ehsani AA: Cardiovascular adaptations to exercise training in the elderly. *Federation Proceedings* 46:1840–1843, 1989.
23. Green JS, Crouse SF: The effects of endurance training on functional capacity in the elderly: a meta–analysis. *Medical Science of Sport Exercise* 27:920–926, 1995.
24. Kohrt WM, Malley MT, Coggan AR, et al: Effects of gender, age, and fitness level on response of $\dot{V}O_{2max}$ to training in 60–71 year olds. *Journal of Applied Physiology* 71:2004–2011, 1991.
25. Warren BJ, Nieman DC, Dotson RG, et al: Cardiorespiratory responses to exercise training in septuagenarian women. *International Journal of Sports Medicine* 14:60–65, 1993.
26. Wilmore JH, Stanforth PR, Gagnon J, et al: Cardiac output and stroke volume changes with endurance training: the heritage family study. *Medicine and Science in Sports and Exercise* 33:99–106, 2001.
27. Seals DR, Hagberg JM, Hurley BF, et al: Endurance training in older men and women. I. Cardiovascular response to exercise. *Journal of Applied Physiology* 57:1024–1029, 1985.
28. Rodeheffer RJ, Gerstenblith G, Becker JL, et al: Exercise cardiac output is maintained with advancing ages in healthy human subjects: cardiac dilatation and increased stroke volume compensate for diminished heart rate. *Circulation* 69:203–213, 1984.
29. Coudert J, Praagh EV: Endurance exercise training in the elderly: effects on cardiovascular function. *Current Opinion in Clinical Nutrition and Metabolic Care* 3:479–483, 2000.
30. Ehsani AA, Ogawa T, Miller TR, et al: Exercise training improves left ventricular systolic function in older men. *Circulation* 83:96–103, 1991.
31. Seals DR, Hagberg JM, Spina RJ, et al: Enhanced left ventricular performance in endurance trained older men. *Circulation* 89:198–205, 1994.
32. Spina RJ: Cardiovascular adaptations to endurance exercise training in older men and women. *Exercise and Sports Science Review* 27:317–332, 1999.

33. Spina RJ, Ogawa T, Kohrt WM, et al: Differences in cardiovascular adaptations to endurance exercise training between older men and women. *Journal of Applied Physiology* 75:849–855, 1993.
34. Arbab–Zadeh A, Dijk E, Prasad A, et al: Effect of aging and physical activity on left ventricular compliance. *Circulation* 110:1799–1805, 2004.
35. Muster AJ, Kim H, Kane B, et al: Ten–year echo/Doppler determination of the benefits of aerobic exercise after the age of 65 years. *Echocardiography* 27:5–10, 2010.
36. LaRocca TJ, Seals DR, Pierce GL: Leukocyte telomere length is preserved with aging in endurance exercise-trained adults and related to maximal aerobic capacity. *Mech Ageing Dev* 131:165–167, 2010.
37. Fujimoto N, Prasad A, Hastings JL, et al: Cardiovascular effects of 1 year of progressive and vigorous exercise training in previously sedentary individuals older than 65 years of age. *Circulation* 122:1797–1805, 2010.
38. Tate CA, Taffet GE, Hudson EK, et al: Enhanced calcium uptake of cardiac sarcoplasmic reticulum in exercise–trained old rats. *American Journal of Physiology* 27:H431–H435, 1990.
39. Starnes JW, Beyer RE, Edington DW: Myocardial adaptations to endurance exercise in aged rats. *American Journal of Physiology* 245:H560–H566, 1983.
40. Roach MR, Burton AC: The effect of aging on the elasticity of human iliac arteries. *Canadian Journal Biochemistry Physiology* 37:557–570, 1959.
41. Lee H–Y, Oh B–H: Aging and arterial stiffness. Circulation *Journal* 74:2257–2262, 2010.
42. Tsutsui Y, Sagawa S, Yamauchi K, et al: Cardiovascular responses to lower negative pressure in the elderly: role of reduced leg compliance. *Gerontology* 48:133–139, 2002.
43. Lipsitz LA: Orthostatic hypotension in the elderly. *New England Journal Medicine* 321:952–957, 1989.
44. Harris T, Lipsitz LA, Kleinman JC, et al: Postural change in blood pressure associated with age and systolic blood pressure. Journal Gerontology Medicine *Science* 46:M159–M163, 1991.
45. Cleroux J, Giannattasio C, Bolla G, et al: Decreased cardiorespiratory reflexes with aging in normotensive humans. *American Journal of Physiology* 257:H961–H968, 1989.
46. Seals DR: Influence of aging on autonomic–circulatory control in humans at rest and during exercise. In Gisolfi CV, Lamb DR, Nadel ER, editors: *Perspectives in exercise science and sports medicine, ed 6. Exercise, heat, and thermoregulation*, Dubuque, 1993, Brown & Benchmark.
47. Taylor JA, Hand GA, Johnson DG, et al: Augmented forearm vasoconstriction during dynamic exercise in healthy older men. *Circulation* 86:1789–1799, 1992.
48. Martin WH, 3rd, Ogawa T, Kohrt WM, et al: Effects of aging, gender, and physical training on peripheral vascular function. *Circulation* 84:654–664, 1991.
49. American College of Sports Medicine: Position stand on exercise and hypertension. *Medicine and Science in Sports and Exercise* 36:533–553, 2004.
50. Halbert JA, Silagy CA, Finucane P, et al: The effectiveness of exercise training in lowering blood pressure a meta–analysis of randomised controlled trials of 4 weeks or longer. *Journal of Hypertension* 11:641–649, 1997.
51. Seals DR, DeSouza CA, Donato AJ, et al: Habitual exercise and arterial aging. *Journal of Applied Physiology* 105:1323–1332, 2008.
52. Monahand KD, Dinenno FA, Tanaka H, et al: Regular aerobic exercise modulates age–associated declines in cardiovagal baroreflex sensitivity in healthy men. *Journal of Physiology* 529:263–271, 2000.
53. Carter JB, Banister EW Blaber AP: Effect of endurance exercise on autonomic control of the heart. *Sports Medicine* 33:33–46, 2003.
54. Ng AV, Callister R, Johnson DG, et al: Endurance exercise training is associated with elevated basal sympathetic nerve activity in healthy older humans. *Journal of Applied Physiology* 77:1366–1374, 1994.
55. Zaugg M, Lucchinetti E: Respiratory function in the elderly. *Anesthesiology Clinics of North America* 18:47–58, 2000.
56. Sharma G, Goodwin J: Effect of aging on respiratory system physiology and immunology. *Clinical Interventions in Aging* 1:253–260, 2006.
57. Crapo RO: The aging lung. In Mahler DA, editor: *Pulmonary disease in the elderly*, New York, 1993, Marcel Dekker.
58. Brody JS, Thurlbeck WM: Development, growth, and aging of the lung. In Fishman AP, editor: *Handbook of physiology*, ed 3, 1985.
59. Babb TG, Rodarte JR: Mechanism of reduced maximal expiratory flow with aging. *Journal of Applied Physiology* 89:505–511, 2000.
60. Mahler DA, Fierro–Carrion G, Baird JC: Evaluation of dyspnea in the elderly. *Clinic in Geriatric Medicine* 19:19–33, 2003.
61. Janssens JP, Pache JC, Nicod LP: Physiological changes in respiratory function associated with aging. *European Respiratory Journal* 13:197–205, 1999.
62. Johnson BD, Dempsey JA: Demand vs. capacity in the aging pulmonary system. In Holloszy J, editor: *Exercise and sport sciences review*, ed 19, Baltimore, 1991, Williams & Wilkins.
63. Enright PL, Kronmal RA, Manolio TA, et al: Respiratory muscle strength in the elderly. *American Journal Respiratory Critical Care Medicine* 149:430–438, 1994.
64. Murray JF: *Aging in the normal lung*, ed 2, Philadelphia, 1986, WB Saunders.
65. McClaran SR, Babcock MA, Pegelow DF, et al: Longitudinal effects of aging on lung function at rest and exercise in healthy active fit elderly adults. *Journal of Applied Physiology* 78:1957–1968, 1995.
66. Dempsey JA, Sheel AW, Haverkamp HC, et al: The John Sutton lecture CSEP, 2002: pulmonary system limitations to exercise in health. *Canadian Journal of Applied Physiology* 28(Suppl):S3–S24, 2003.
67. Wood HE, Mitchell SM, Babb TG: Short–term modulation of the exercise ventilatory response in older men. *Respiratory Physiology & Neurobiology* 173:37–46, 2010.
68. Prefaut C, Anselme F, Caillaud C, et al: Exercise–induced hypoxemia in older athletes. *Journal of Applied Physiology* 76:120–126, 1994.
69. Anselme F, Caillaud C, Couret I, et al: Histamine and exercise–induced hypoxemia in highly trained athletes. *Journal of Applied Physiology* 76:127–132, 1994.
70. Reeves JT, Dempsey JA, Grover RF: Pulmonary circulation during exercise. In Weir EK, Reeves JT, editors: *Pulmonary vascular physiology and pathophysiology*, New York, 1989, Marcel Dekker.
71. Makrides L, Heigenhauser GJ, Jones NL: Physical training in young and older healthy subjects. In Sutton JR, Brock RM, editors: *Sports medicine for the mature athlete*, Indianapolis, 1986, Benchmark Press.
72. Jones NL: The lung of the Master's athlete. In Sutton JR, Beck RM, editors: *Sports medicine for the mature athlete*, Indianapolis, 1986, Benchmark Press.

Multisystem Clinical Implications of Impaired Breathing Mechanics and Postural Control

Mary Massery

KEY TERMS

Abnormal or compensatory breathing patterns
Abdominal binder
Breathing mechanics
Cardiac mechanics
Gastrointestinal impairments
Gravitational influence on physical development
Integumentary impairments
Internal organs
Multisystem interactions
Musculoskeletal impairments
Neuromuscular impairments
Normal and abnormal chest wall development
Paradoxical breathing
Pelvic floor
Postural control
Reflux
Sandifer's syndrome
Scoliosis
Soda Can Model of respiratory and postural control
Spinal cord injury
Vocal folds/glottis

CHAPTER OUTLINE

The cardiovascular and pulmonary systems provide both physiological support (oxygen delivery) (see Chapters 2 and 4) as well as a mechanical support (respiratory and trunk muscle control) for movement. This chapter focuses on breathing mechanics and their interactions with other organ systems in both health and dysfunction. Its three main premises are:

1. Breathing is a three-dimensional motor task that is influenced by gravity in the three planes of motion.
2. Breathing is influenced by multisystem interactions that simultaneously support respiratory and postural control during motor tasks.
3. The mechanics of breathing influence both health and motor performance outcomes related to participation.

The four motor impairment categories identified in the *Guide to Physical Therapist Practice,* second edition, are incorporated into this chapter.[1] A fifth category, the internal organs, has been added (Box 39-1). In addition to addressing the impact of these impairment categories on health and motor performance from a ventilatory perspective, we present a method to cross-reference impairment-based findings with functional limitations. Six common functional tasks that require the integration of breathing and movement are shown in Box 39-2. Children and adults with multiple physical challenges are patients in whom the interaction between respiratory control and postural control is particularly relevant.

Box 39-1 Motor Impairment Categories

Neuromuscular system
Musculoskeletal system
Integumentary system
Cardiovascular and pulmonary systems
Internal organs, especially the gastrointestinal system

Modified from American Physical Therapy Association: Guide to physical therapist practice, ed 2, *Physical Therapy* 81:29,133, 2001.

Box 39-2 Daily Tasks That Require the Integration of Respiratory and Postural Demands of the Trunk for Function

Breathing
Coughing
Sleeping
Eating
Talking
Moving

The role of multisystem interaction in effective breathing and postural control is an emerging field; hence it lacks rigorous evidence from experimental evaluation. Nonetheless, the physiologic evidence supporting the interactions among systems and their impact on breathing and posture (see Chapter 6) is compelling and sufficient to inform contemporary approaches to patient care in physical therapy practice. As an area of research, multisystem interaction represents a relatively new frontier that could have far-reaching implications for research in other physical therapy areas with respect to assessment, intervention, and evaluation.

Breathing: A Three-Dimensional Gravity-Dependent Activity

Planes of Ventilation and Gravitational Influence

Ventilation is a three-dimensional activity. With each breath, the chest wall expands in the anterior-posterior plane, the inferior-superior plane, and the medial-lateral plane (Figure 39-1). The muscles that support breathing are resisted by gravity in one direction, assisted by gravity in another direction, and relatively unaffected in other directions. When a person is upright, superior expansion of the chest wall is resisted by gravity while inferior expansion is assisted, and other movements of the chest wall (anterior, posterior, and lateral expansion) are relatively unaffected by gravity. The adverse effects of gravity are counteracted by muscles that can function effectively in the presence of gravitational force. If the respiratory muscles become dysfunctional due to weakness, paralysis, or fatigue; or pathological conditions, the patient may no longer breathe effectively within gravity's influence.[2,3] Further, the impact of posture on breathing mechanics, as well as on cardiovascular function, has been well documented (see Chapter 20).[4] Therefore, when physical therapists are positioning patients with impaired breathing mechanics or posture, they need to consider how gravity can affect the muscles that support breathing and posture in each body position, as well as how it affects oxygen transport overall.

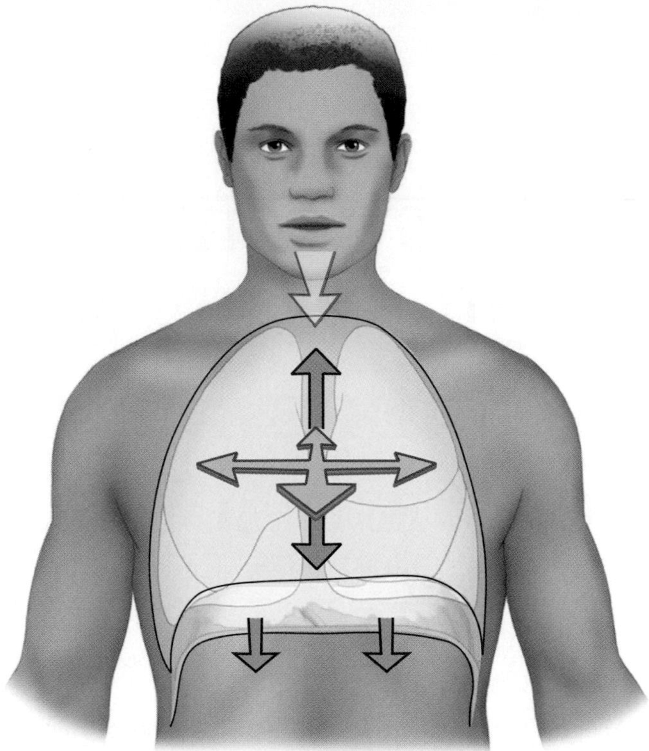

Fig. 39-1 Planes of respiration: anterior-posterior, inferior-superior, and lateral.

Effects of Gravity on Normal and Abnormal Chest Wall Development

Gravitational force is crucial in the normal development of the skeleton. Typically developing infants move freely in and out of a range of body positions (prone, hands and knees, and standing), allowing gravity to alternately assist or resist their movements. Moving through these positions, the infant strengthens muscle groups and learns to interact with the gravitational force in his or her physical environment and compensate as needed.[5] The development of the bones, muscles, and joints that constitute the trunk is influenced by genetic factors and movements performed in a gravitational field. Infants with limited ability to move and counteract gravity develop malaligned joints and impaired muscle support that, in turn, impair breathing mechanics, or vice versa.[6-8] Cerebral palsy, spinal muscle atrophy, stroke, head trauma, and spinal cord injury are conditions that can cause such muscle imbalance in children.[3] Weakness or fatigue of the trunk muscles can result from conditions outside the neuromuscular system[9] (for example, oxygen transport deficits from bronchopulmonary dysplasia and congenital heart defects and nutrition-related deficits such as gastroesophageal reflux and malabsorption; see Chapters 6 and 32). Such symptoms can impair breathing mechanics, as well as muscle tone

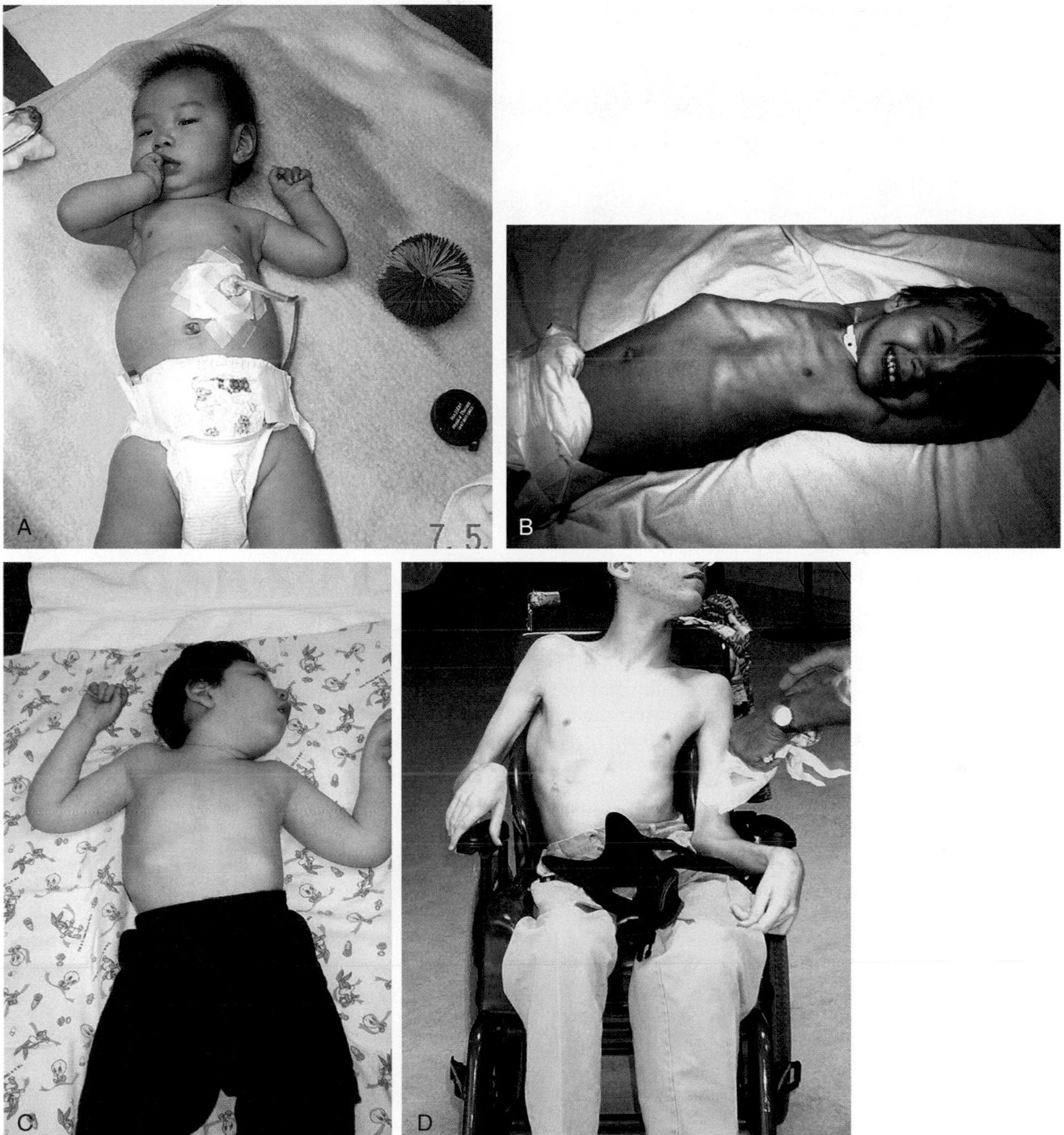

Fig. 39-2 A, Caitlin, six months of age. Caitlin has spinal muscle atrophy, type I. Note persistent immature triangular shaping of chest wall secondary to pronounced muscle weakness and an inability to counteract gravity effectively. **B,** Melissa, three-and-a-half years of age. Melissa has a C5 complete spinal cord injury due to birth trauma. Melissa's chest wall has become more deformed than Caitlin's chest wall due to the prolonged exposure to the severe muscle imbalance of the respiratory muscles within gravity's constant influence. Note the marked pectus excavatum and anteriorly flared ribs in supine. **C,** Carlos, 5 years of age and **D,** Kevin, 17 years of age. Both have spastic cerebral palsy. Note the lateral flaring of the lower ribcage, the asymmetry of the trunk, and the flattening of the entire anterior ribcage, all of which are more noticeable in the older child.

(as in hypertonicity or hypotonicity), and can contribute to deficits in motor planning and learning.[10]

Children who have impaired breathing mechanics and are recumbent for prolonged periods are exposed to abnormal gravitational stress. Over time, this leads to pathological changes and deformities such as retention of the primitive triangular shape of the newborn chest wall (Figure 39-2, *A*). In some cases, the child's diaphragm remains functional in the presence of weak or paralyzed abdominal and intercostal muscles. In turn, this can affect skeletal development (Figure 39-2, *B*). Pronounced imbalance of the thoracic muscles can result in chest wall deformity, compromising the child's ability to meet his or her ventilatory needs. Musculoskeletal abnormalities include anteriorly flared lower ribs, dynamic pectus deformity (most often, pectus excavatum; less often, pectus carinatum), laterally flared ribs, and chest wall asymmetry

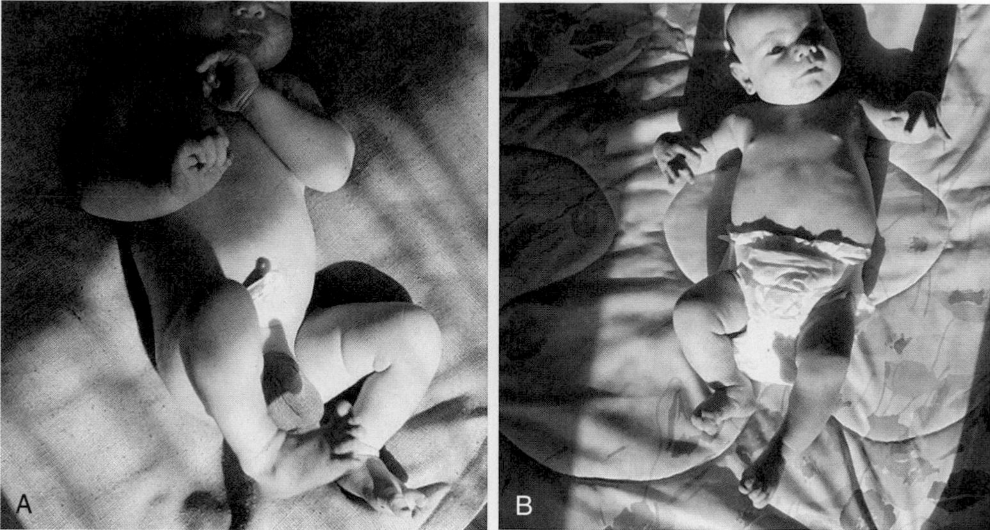

Fig. 39-3 A and **B,** Chest wall of a newborn. Note triangular shape, short neck, narrow and flat upper thorax, round barreled lower thorax. Muscle tone is primarily flexion and breathing is primarily diaphragmatic and in one plane: inferior.

(Figure 39-2, *B, C, D*).[6,8,11] These deformities have varying impact on ventilation depending on the gravitational consequences of each position.

Understanding chest wall development in typically healthy children is essential for the physical therapist to assess chest wall deformities and their impact on oxygen transport.[11] Chapter 37 describes normal growth and development of the cardiovascular and pulmonary systems during infancy and childhood. The present chapter takes this information a step further, and considers the impact of musculoskeletal and neuromuscular impairments on typical childhood development. Initially the newborn's chest wall is triangular: narrow and flat in the upper portion and wider and rounded in the lower portion (Figure 39-3). The infant's short neck reduces the effectiveness of the upper accessory muscles as ventilatory muscles. The infant's arms tend to be flexed and adducted across the chest wall, hampering lateral or anterior movement of the chest wall. The infant, largely a diaphragmatic breather, shows disproportionate development of the lower chest wall, which promotes a triangular shape of the ribcage. Newborns breathe primarily in a single plane (inferior), rather than in three planes apparent in adults.

From 3 to 6 months of age, the infant develops more trunk extension tone and spends more time on his or her elbows in prone. The baby begins to reach with the arms into the environment. This facilitates development of the anterior upper chest wall. Continuous stretching and upper extremity weight bearing helps to expand the anterior upper chest wall both anteriorly and laterally, while increasing posterior stabilization.[5] An increase in the strength of the intercostal muscles and pectoralis muscles improves the infant's ability to counteract gravity exerted on the anterior upper chest wall in the supine position, leading to the development of a slight convex configuration of the area and a rectangular shaping of the thorax from the frontal plane (Figure 39-4). The baby begins to breathe more effectively in multiple planes as the muscles' length-tension relationships become more efficient.

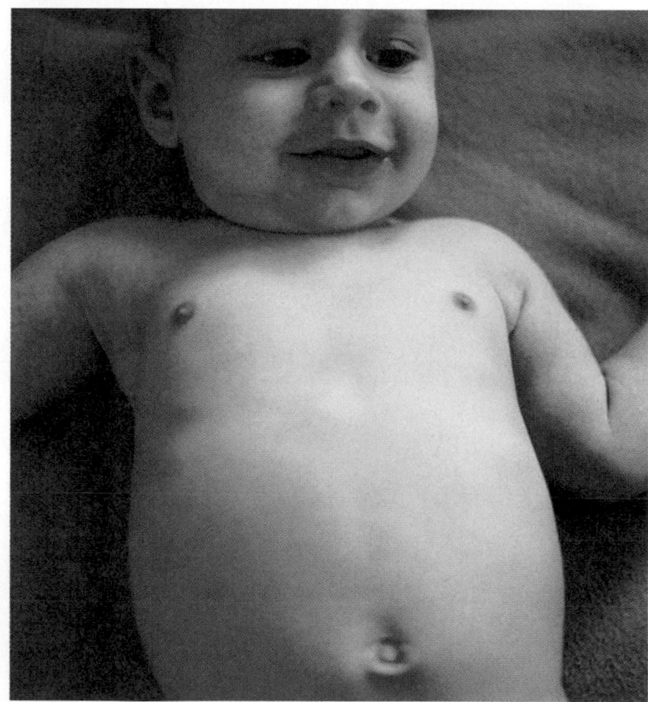

Fig. 39-4 Infant chest wall at 3 to 6 months of age. Increased upper thorax width. More convex shaping of entire chest wall occurs as antigravity movements are becoming possible. Note the short neck and two functionally separate chambers: thorax and abdomen.

The next step in development occurs when the child assumes erect body positions independently (i.e., sitting, kneeling, and standing). Until this time, the ribs are aligned relatively horizontally, with narrow intercostal spacing (Figure 39-3). The newborn's chest wall accounts for about one-third of the trunk cavity. As the child progressively moves against gravity, the ribs, with the aid of the abdominal muscles, rotate downward (more so in the longer lower ribs), creating the sharp angle of the ribs (Figure 39-5). This elongates the ribcage until it eventually occupies over half of the trunk cavity (Figure 39-6). Chest x-rays of newborns and adults, as

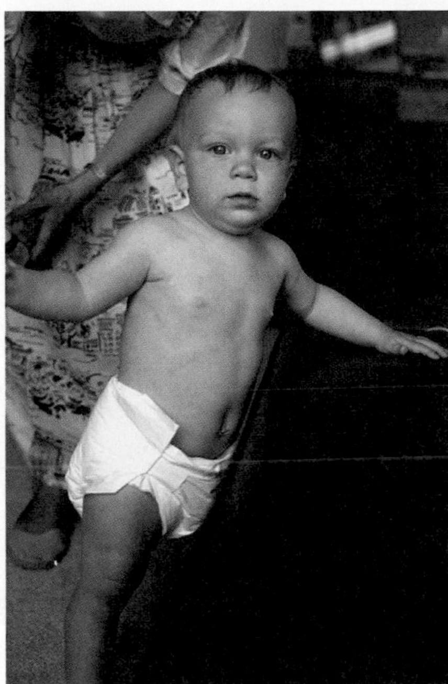

Fig. 39-5 Infant chest wall at 6 to 12 months of age. The infant spends more time upright. The activation of abdominal muscles, gravity's influence, and increased postural demands result in a more elongated chest wall, wider rib spacing, and increased intercostal muscle activation, as well as a functional interface of the ribcage onto the abdomen with the abdominal and intercostal muscles. This improves both the respiratory dynamics by giving more external support to the diaphragm at the mid-trunk level and the postural stabilization potential needed for more complex motor tasks. Note that the base of the ribcage is no longer barrel-shaped as it is in the newborn.

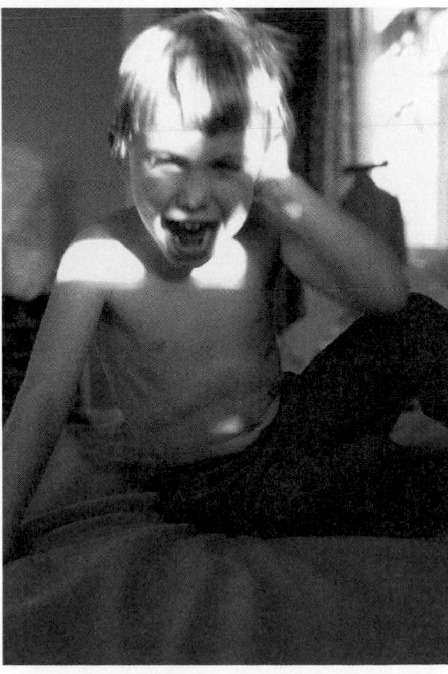

Fig. 39-6 A 4-year-old boy. Note the elongated chest wall, which occupies more than half of the trunk space, the wide intercostal spacing, the effective muscle stabilization of the lower ribcage with the abdominal muscles, the rectangular shaping of the chest wall from a frontal view, and the elliptical shaping of the chest wall from a transverse view.

Table 39-1 Typical Chest Wall Development from Infant to Adulthood

Chest Wall Components	Infant	Adult
Size	Thorax occupies one third thoracic cavity	Thorax occupies more than half thoracic cavity
Shape	Triangular frontal plane, circular anterior-posterior plane	Rectangular frontal plane, elliptical anterior-posterior plane
Upper thoracic	Narrow, flat apex	Wide, convex apex
Lower thoracic	Circular, flared lower ribs	Elliptical, lower ribs integrated with abdominals
Ribs	Evenly horizontal	Rotated downward, especially inferiorly
Intercostal spacing	Narrow, limits movement of thoracic spine and cavity	Wide, allows for individual movement of ribs and spine
Diaphragm	Adequate, minimal dome shape	Adequate, large dome shape
Accessory muscles	Nonfunctional	Functional

well as pictures of infants, illustrate these developmental trends (Figure 39-7, *A, B*); details are further summarized in Table 39-1.

Optimum respiratory function cannot be expected in a person with an underdeveloped or deformed chest wall, spine, or both.[3] As long as the condition that caused the trunk muscle imbalance persists, regardless of whether that deficit was a neuromuscular disorder or an impairment in another motor impairment category (see Box 39-1), the chest wall and spine will likely develop atypically.

Strategies to optimize trunk development include:

- Frequent body position changes
- Management of adverse neuromuscular tone
- Facilitation of weakened chest wall muscles
- Promotion of optimal breathing patterns
- Incorporation of ventilatory strategies with movement
- The alignment of physical therapy goals with the child's development and medical program

Influence of Multisystem Interactions on Motor Performance: Relationship Between Respiratory and Postural Control

Normal human movement reflects the interactions of multiple organ systems. If these interactions are atypical or inadequately compensated when impaired, motor impairments can result. Thus it is recommended that every physical therapy examination and evaluation include multisystem screening of the five impairment categories (Box 39-1) in order to determine the impact of each organ system on total motor performance. The following Soda Can Model of respiratory and

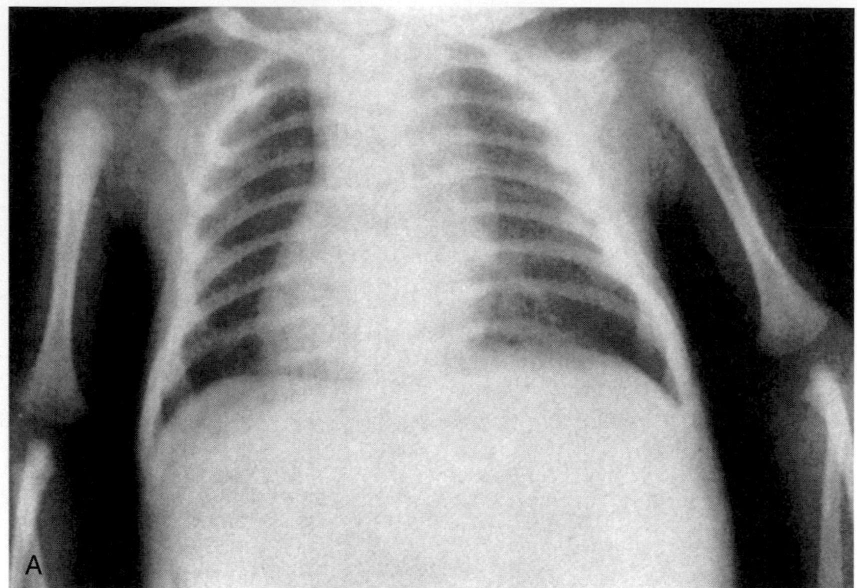

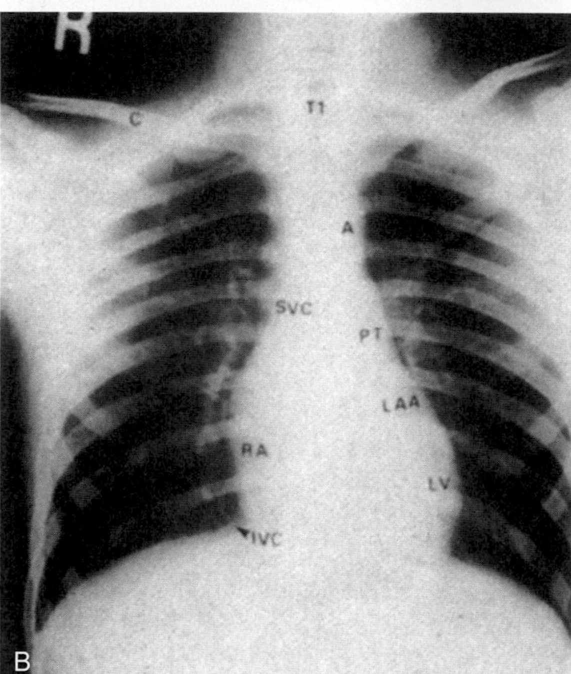

Fig. 39-7 A, Chest x-ray of a newborn. Note triangular shaping of ribcage and narrow intercostal spacing. **B,** Typical adult chest x-ray. Chest wall shape is rectangular, ribs angled downward, upper and lower thorax equally developed.

postural control was developed to facilitate the clinician's understanding of the multisystem interactions between the mechanics of breathing and the simultaneous needs of postural control

Soda Can Model of Respiratory and Postural Control

The muscles of respiration are muscles of postural support and vice versa.[14] Each muscle that originates from or inserts onto the trunk is both a respiratory muscle and a postural muscle. This duality of function means that respiratory and postural control should not be evaluated separately. External and internal forces that affect the function of the respiratory muscles also affect postural responses. The Soda Can Model illustrates this dual function.

Structurally Weak, Yet Functionally Strong

The shell of a soda or soft drink can is made of thin aluminum that is easily compressed when the can is open and empty. This same can, however, unopened and full, is almost impossible to compress or deform without puncturing the exterior shell. The strength of the can is derived from the positive pressure it exerts against atmospheric pressure and gravity through its closed (unopened) system (Figure 39-8, *A*). As soon as the closed system is compromised by either opening or puncturing the can, it loses its functional strength. It is no longer capable of counteracting the positive pressure forces acting on it. Once the can is opened, it is possible to compress it completely (Figure 39-8, *B*).

The structural integrity of the trunk of the body is similar to that of the soda can described in the Soda Can Model. The

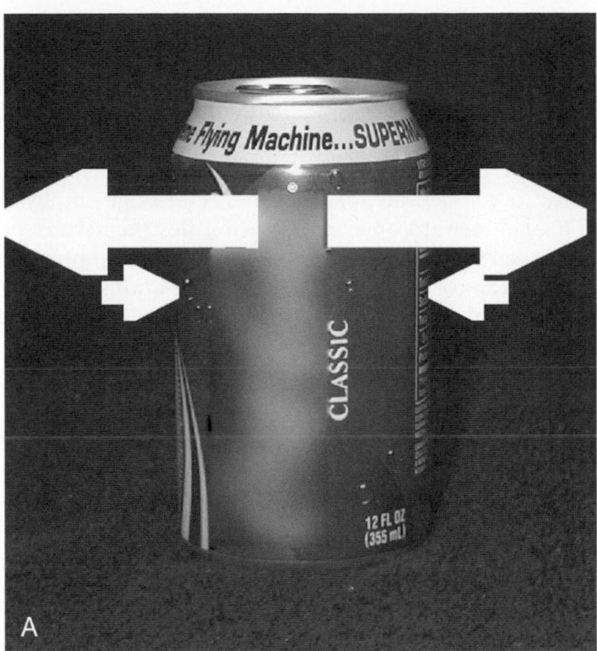

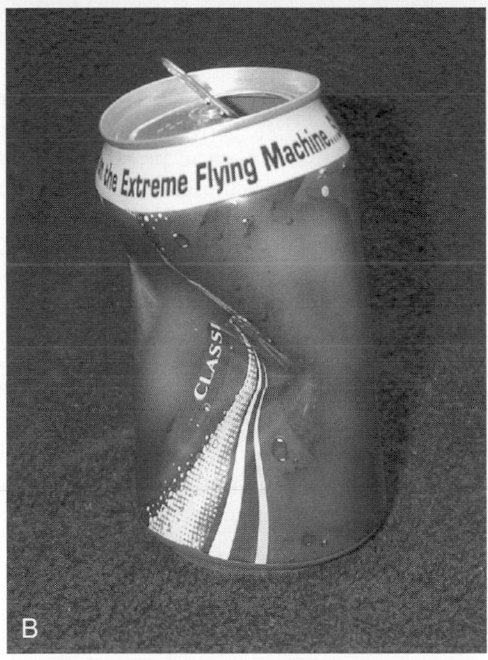

Fig. 39-8 Soda Can Model of respiratory and postural control. **A,** A soda can derives its functional strength because the internal pressure of the carbonated drink is higher than the atmospheric pressure acting on it, not because of its thin aluminum shell. **B,** Without the internal pressure support, the aluminum can is easily deformed and compressed.

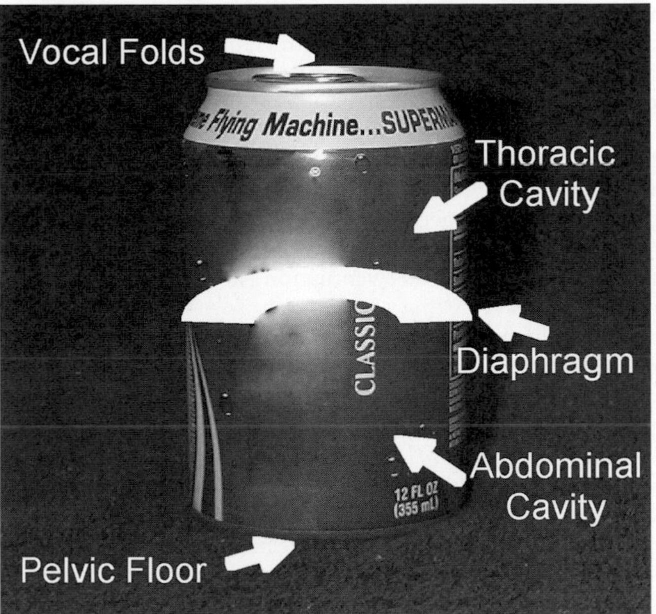

Fig. 39-9 A soda can as a three-dimensional model for trunk muscle support for breathing and postural control. Note that the control of pressure begins at the level of the vocal folds and extends down to the pelvic floor. A breach in pressure anywhere along the cylinder impairs the total function of the can (or, in the human analogy, the function of the patient's trunk).

skeletal support of the trunk is not inherently strong. The spine and ribcage alone cannot maintain their alignment against gravity without muscular support that enables them to generate pressure that is capable of countering gravitational pull. This is commonly observed in patients in intensive care. Weakened from prolonged illnesses and medical procedures, patients in the intensive care unit (ICU) typically slump into a forward, flexed posture when they sit up initially. This is associated with less ability to generate pressure through muscle activation to support alignment of the pelvis, spine, and ribcage in an upright position. In pediatric patients, the effects can be particularly alarming. Melissa provides such an example. She incurred a C5 spinal cord lesion from a vaginal birth injury and experienced marked collapse of the pelvis, ribcage, and spine when sitting upright. Melissa was incapable of making an effective inspiratory effort in this position, which explained her intolerance to upright activities. Figuratively, her "soda can" was compressed, and correspondingly, her breathing mechanics were severely compromised (Figure 39-8, *C*).

Positive Pressure Support Instead of More Skeletal Support

The aluminum can is a chamber. Once the chamber is filled with carbonated fluid and sealed, carbonated gases are released, leading to positive pressure pushing outward, which lends dynamic support to the metal. Likewise, the trunk of the body is composed of thoracic and abdominal chambers that are dynamically supported by muscle activity that generates the positive pressure in both chambers needed to support both respiration and posture.

The thoracic and abdominal chambers are separated by the diaphragm (Figure 39-9). The chambers are "sealed" at the top by the vocal folds, at the bottom by the pelvic floor, and circumferentially by the trunk muscles. Muscle support allows these chambers to match or exceed the positive pressure exerted on them by external forces to support the "flimsy" skeletal shell. The primary muscles involved in this support are the (1) intercostal muscles, which generate and maintain transthoracic pressure[15]; (2) the abdominal muscles, especially the transverse abdominus, which generate and maintain transabdominal pressure[16,17]; (3) the diaphragm, which regulates and uses the pressure in both chambers[18,19]; (4) the back muscles, which stabilize the spine to optimize its alignment and articulation with the ribcage[20]; (5) the pelvic floor muscles, which work synchronously with the diaphragm to support breathing and urinary control[21,22]; and (6) the vocal folds, which regulate intrathoracic pressure to stabilize the diaphragm and upper extremities.[23] These muscles work synergistically to adjust the pressure in both chambers so that the demands of ventilation and posture are met simultaneously.[24]

The following synopsis of the biomechanics of breathing describes the interactions among the diaphragm, intercostals muscles, and abdominal muscles within the construct of a positive pressure chamber.[24-27] The diaphragm is the primary muscle of respiration, but its function as a pressure regulating muscle may be less well recognized. The diaphragm separates the thoracic and abdominal cavities, thus creating and using the difference in pressure between the two chambers to support the simultaneous needs of respiration and trunk stabilization. The interactions among the diaphragm, intercostal muscles, and abdominal muscles, along with support from other trunk muscles, work synergistically to generate, regulate, and maintain thoracic and abdominal pressures necessary for the concurrent needs of breathing and motor control of the trunk.[28] In summary, the diaphragm depends on the intercostal and abdominal muscles for effective and efficient breathing, and likewise, the trunk depends on the diaphragm for muscular support and pressure support during activities, particularly those with high postural demands.[20,28-30]

When the diaphragm contracts to effect inhalation, its central tendon descends inferiorly, creating negative pressure in the thoracic cavity. This draws air into the lungs due to the pressure difference with atmospheric pressure. Simultaneously, the intercostal muscles are activated to counter the negative pressure that draws them inward.[7,31-34] Inadequate intercostal muscle support tends to collapse the chest wall, which in the long-term can cause musculoskeletal deformity (e.g., pectus excavatum) and secondary loss of chest wall compliance (see Figure 39-2, *B*).[6,7,35,36] With descent of the diaphragm, positive pressure is created within the abdominal cavity and augmented by counterpressure exerted by the abdominal muscles, particularly the deepest muscle, the transverse abdominus.[37] This pressure equals the negative pressure created in the thorax, based on Newton's Law—that is, for every action, there is an equal and opposite reaction.[38] Further, positive abdominal pressure provides a fulcrum for the diaphragm to stabilize its central tendon. This central stability mechanically supports the contractions of the lateral (peripheral) fibers up and over the abdominal viscera (lateral and superior chest wall expansion).[24] That is, the coupling among the intercostals, abdominals, and diaphragm is greater than the sum of their parts for maximal respiratory function.[26,39]

The abdominal cavity has relatively higher pressure at rest than the thoracic cavity, as reflected by the position of the diaphragm within the trunk. Its dome is convex superiorly because the higher pressure from the abdominal cavity pushes it upward. In lung disease, the relationship between the abdominal and thoracic pressures may reverse and compromise the mechanics of breathing. For example, patients who have obstructive lung disease such as emphysema, trap air distally in the diseased lung segments.[40] Air trapping and other manifestations of the condition cause the thoracic cavity to become the higher-pressure chamber at rest, pushing the diaphragm inferiorly and flattening its dome. The diaphragm's mechanical support becomes compromised to the extent that it no longer functions well as an inspiratory muscle. To compensate, patients with end-stage emphysema tend to lean forward on extended arms, flex their trunks, and activate their abdominal muscles to increase abdominal pressure as a means of restoring the pressure relationship with the thoracic chamber. If successful, these patients are able to displace the dome of the diaphragm upward to enable it to function more effectively as an inspiratory muscle, thereby relieving dyspnea.[41]

Top and Bottom of the "Soda Can": The Vocal Folds and Pelvic Floor

VOCAL FOLDS AND VOCAL APPARATUS

Positive thoracic pressure is needed for both postural support of the upper trunk and expiratory maneuvers such as talking, coughing, and bowel and bladder evacuation.[42-44] The vocal apparatus, including the vocal folds, provides the superior valve for pressure regulation of the thoracic chamber. If the vocal folds are compromised because of an impairment of the upper airway or because they are bypassed with a tracheostomy or endotracheal tube, the patient is incapable of generating and sustaining positive thoracic pressure support. After the patient has inhaled and achieved higher pressure inside than outside the lungs, the air is simply expired. There is no valve at the top to hold the pressure within the chest. Activities of the trunk that require positive thoracic pressure will be compromised. Without functioning vocal folds to regulate the controlled release of thoracic pressure during exhalation, the patient has no means of slowly, or eccentrically, releasing the air for speaking or performing eccentric trunk or extremity activities. The therapist may observe impairments such as dysfunctional speech and eccentric motor activity. The same is true for concentric contractions. Without the vocal folds being able to serve as the pressure valve, the patient is unable to generate intrathoracic pressure to elicit an effective cough.[45] Similarly, if the patient is unable to close the glottis and direct thoracic positive pressure toward the pelvic floor, bowel and bladder evacuation may be compromised.[46-49] Patients with tracheostomies often experience constipation. Bowel motility usually improves with decannulation when the vocal folds are restored as an active component of thoracic pressure regulation. The patient with compromised vocal folds can briefly generate positive expiratory pressure for activities such as coughing and yelling by concentrically contracting the trunk flexors, primarily the abdominal muscles, pelvic floor muscles, pectoralis muscles, latissimus dorsi muscles, or some combination, at peak inspiratory lung volume. This positive thoracic expiratory pressure, however, cannot be sustained because the expiratory pathway (e.g., tracheostomy tube or paralyzed vocal folds) is wider than the opening of the vocal folds, resulting in a larger volume of air to be expelled per second. Unlike patients with obstructive lung disease who have an abnormally prolonged expiration, patients with impaired pressure regulation at the top of the chamber have no mechanism to prolong exhalation for either eccentric or concentric motor tasks.

In addition to regulating airflow from the lungs, the vocal folds have a role in generating increased thoracic pressure needed for stabilization associated with balance or activities such as lifting, pushing, and upper extremity weight-bearing activity.[23,50-52] This response is called the glottal effort closure reflex.[43] The vocal folds adduct and prevent air leakage while the chest wall, back, abdominal, and pelvic floor muscles contract to increase abdominal and thoracic pressures. Increased trunk pressure stabilizes the shoulder complex to enhance force production of the muscles of the upper extremities. For example, a tennis player with a strong serve often takes advantage of the glottal effort closure reflex. The server throws the ball up while taking a deep breath, then he or she closes the glottis at the peak of inspiration to trap the inspired air and activate the chest wall and abdominal muscles to increase thoracic pressure. When the tennis racket contacts the ball, the server explosively expels the air (usually with a grunt) to maximize the force production for the serve. This concept is used in every day life to perform tasks such as pushing open a heavy door, lifting a heavy box, or leaning on a table with one arm and reaching across to lift an object with the other arm. This mechanism is also used by infants to bear weight on their arms during activities such as crawling. These types of activities require full or partial glottal closure to increase the functional strength of the arms. This concept is consistent with that of the Soda Can Model, that is, providing a means of regulating pressure to augment functional strength and control.

The importance of the vocal folds as the superior (i.e., uppermost) pressure regulator of the trunk may be observed in a child with a tracheostomy necessitated because of an airway impairment or a paralyzed vocal fold, or in a child with poor vocal control due to other reasons. The physical therapist may observe that the infant crawls with elbow flexion rather than on extended arms, even though there is no muscle weakness in the arms. It is possible that the inability of the vocal folds to maintain adequate positive pressure within the thoracic cavity during weight bearing (glottal effort closure reflex) causes the elbows to flex (rather than weak triceps). In this case, strengthening the vocal folds, or adding a Passy Muir® valve (speaking valve) to a tracheostomy tube may improve the child's potential to generate the positive thoracic pressure needed for energetically demanding postural activities. In other words, restoring the trunk's pressure support system (analogous to the soda can) may lead to greater functional gain than focusing on exercises for the upper extremities.

Other types of vocal fold interactions can influence speech, breathing, and postural control through their effects on this pressurized system. For example, the function of the vocal folds may be improved as a speech valve if the abdominal pressure is improved with an abdominal binder in patients with spinal cord injury.[53,54] For children with upper airway obstruction such as laryngeal malacia, excessive inspiratory flow rates, which create excessive negative pressure in the upper airway, may decrease vocalization or elicit exercise-induced asthma.[55]

PELVIC FLOOR

The pelvic floor muscles provide support at the inferior end of the cylinder, that is, at the base of the abdominal cavity. Dysfunction of these muscles can impair the potential of the abdominal cavity to generate positive pressure.[23] For example, when abdominal pressure is intended to be directed toward the vocal folds for coughing, sneezing, yelling, and laughing, insufficient pelvic floor muscle strength or motor control may reduce positive pressure through the pelvic opening. This is often expressed as urinary stress incontinence, rendering the intended respiratory or postural maneuver less effective.[56,57] Numerous conditions compromise the integrity of the pelvic floor, but most common is the overstretching of pelvic floor muscles during childbirth leading to pelvic floor muscle weakness and inadvertent incontinence, especially during activities such as sneezing, coughing, and running. Women with this condition may cross their legs or perform other pressure-supporting compensatory behaviors to reduce urinary incontinence until their pelvic floor muscles heal. In other conditions, such as cystic fibrosis, women have a high incidence of urinary stress incontinence secondary to repetitive stress on the pelvic floor from the positive pressure associated with chronic coughing.[58,59] Incontinence is not restricted to patients with primary pulmonary disease. Women with low back pain and impaired postural responses also have been reported to have a higher incidence of incontinence.[56]

INTERNAL ORGANS

The organs of the thoracic and abdominal cavities generate or use pressure changes in the thorax and abdomen to augment their functions. The neuromuscular system, for example, creates pressure changes in the thorax and abdomen. The lungs and esophagus use this pressure change to effect efficient breathing and augment upper gastrointestinal motility. The cardiovascular system contributes to small changes in thoracic pressure. Using these changes and the changes from the respiratory mechanics, the heart and vasculature can optimize circulation, blood pressure, and tissue perfusion. The abdomen also uses pressure changes to optimize internal organ function. Rhythmic abdominal pressure is transmitted through the intestines to stabilize the lumbar spine, augment lower gastrointestinal motility, and optimize movement of body fluids including lymphatic drainage (Figure 39-10).[60]

Without pressure support, which includes the rhythmic change in the thorax from negative to positive pressure and the rhythmic change in the abdomen from neutral to positive pressure (making the abdomen the relatively higher pressure system), the function of the internal organs may be compromised. Dysfunction may be expressed as a decrement in blood pressure (hypotension), inefficient breathing, gastroesophageal reflux with or without abnormal posturing such as in Sandifer's syndrome, inadequate bladder emptying (increasing risk for urinary tract infections), and constipation.[61-64] Although these dysfunctions may not result solely from reduced pressure support, it is a major contributor.

Soda Can Model Summary

The Soda Can Model of respiratory and postural control provides a three-dimensional, dynamic illustration of how the trunk meets its concurrent needs for breathing, postural control, and function of the internal organs. When the patient has reduced ability to generate, regulate, and maintain pressure within the thoracic and abdominal chambers, the mechanics of breathing and other body functions may be

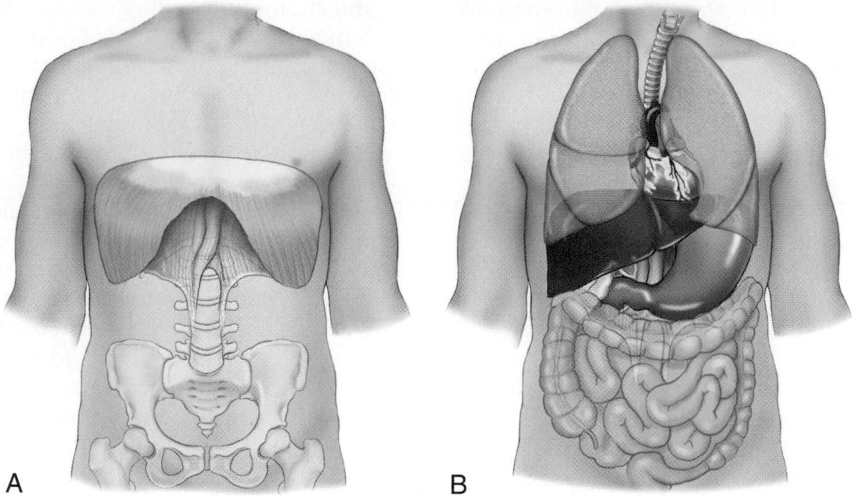

Fig. 39-10 A, Note the position of the diaphragm, which serves as the internal pressure regulator between the thoracic and abdominal cavities. The vocal folds and pelvic floor serve as the external pressure valves. **B,** Note the number and alignment of the internal organs within the thorax and abdomen that are affected by the changes in the diaphragm's position during respiration.

impaired. Inadequate pressure support may begin with an impairment of the mechanics of breathing, such as in a neuromuscular or musculoskeletal disorder. Alternatively, the problem may originate in conjunction with another impairment—for instance, an impairment of the cardiovascular, pulmonary, integumentary, or internal organ system—that nonetheless leads to impaired breathing mechanics. Breathing mechanics are best assessed from a multisystem perspective.

Compensatory Breathing Patterns Associated with Insufficient Muscular Support

As illustrated in the Soda Can Model, the trunk muscles provide the pressure changes necessary for breathing. What happens, however, if the muscles are weak, paralyzed, fatigued, or otherwise nonsupportive? What types of compensatory breathing patterns can be used? Six compensatory breathing patterns are described below and summarized in Table 39-2.

Paradoxical Breathing

Paradoxical breathing refers to opposite movements of the chest wall during normal breathing (occasionally termed belly breathing, see-saw breathing, or reverse breathing). The most common type of paradoxical breathing is caused by strong contraction of the diaphragm in the absence of adequate muscular support from the intercostal muscles and abdominal muscles. The diaphragm contracts, the abdomen rises excessively because weak or paralyzed abdominal muscles do not increase positive abdominal pressure, which limits the descent of the diaphragm. The upper chest wall collapses inward because of inadequate stabilization from the intercostal muscles (see Figure 39-2, *A*). Although not efficient, paradoxical breathing can be sufficient for breathing without mechanical ventilator support for patients with neuromuscular weakness.[7,11]

Table 39-2 Compensatory Breathing Patterns Associated with Insufficient Muscular Support

Paradoxical breathing	a. Functioning diaphragm with paralyzed or weak intercostals and abdominal muscles b. Paralyzed or weak diaphragm with functional accessory muscles; may or may not have functioning abdominal muscles
Diaphragm and upper accessory breathing	a. Paralyzed or weak intercostals
Upper accessory muscles breathing	a. Paralyzed or weak diaphragm and intercostals; abdominal muscles may or may not be functional
Asymmetrical breathing	a. Paralyzed or weak thoracic muscles on one side b. Often associated with hemiparesis or scoliosis
Lateral or "gravity-eliminated" breathing	a. Generalized weakness, no paralysis b. Breathing takes place in the plane with the least resistance to gravity c. Often associated with weakness due to prolonged illness
Shallow breathing	a. Small tidal volumes b. Often associated with high neuromuscular tone or painful conditions

Another type of paradoxical breathing is observed when the diaphragm is weak or paralyzed and the upper accessory

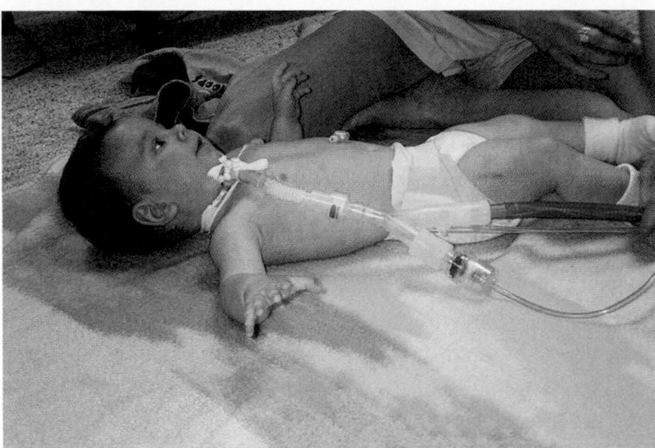

Fig. 39-11 Nicholas, 1 year of age. Nicholas was born with both hemidiaphragms paralyzed and requires full-time mechanical ventilation. When he is off the ventilator for brief periods of time to assess his independent breathing pattern, he demonstrates the second type of paradoxical breathing: a rising upper thorax and falling abdomen during inhalation.

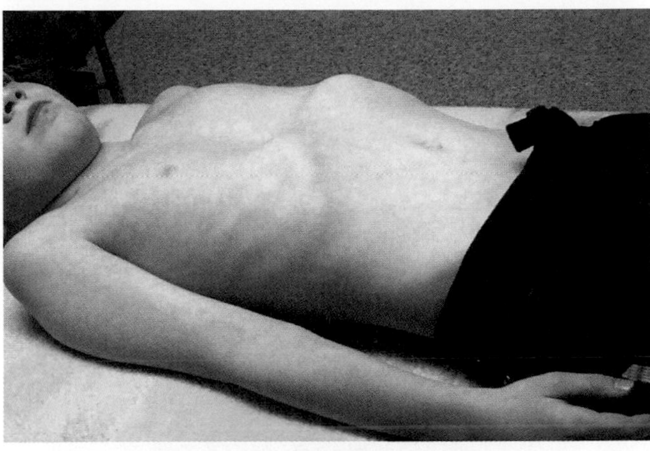

Fig. 39-12 Justin, 9 years of age. Justin has a congenital pectus excavatum. No neurological impairment. His breathing pattern is primarily diaphragm and upper accessory muscles. Note the persistent elevation of the ribcage and the inward collapse of the lower sternum (pectus excavatum). Justin's sternum moved paradoxically with every inspiratory effort, especially during high respiratory and postural demand.

muscles remain intact. The abdominal muscles may or may not be functional. The inspiratory action is opposite to the motion that was described for the most common type of paradoxical breathing (Figure 39-11). The abdomen is drawn inward by the negative pressure in the thorax created by the upper accessory muscle during inhalation. The chest wall rises and the abdomen falls. Generally, this type of paradoxical breathing requires at least partial mechanical ventilatory support because the accessory muscles cannot adequately meet the needs of long-term independent ventilation. In addition, they are more likely to fatigue and lead to respiratory distress. The loss of the diaphragm as the primary respiratory muscle results in greater inspiratory volume deficits than the loss of just the accessory-muscles support observed in the prior paradoxical breathing pattern. Loss of the diaphragm as the primary pressure regulator for the trunk also contributes to deficits in postural control.

Diaphragm and Upper Accessory Muscles Only (Paralyzed or Nonfunctional Intercostal Muscles)

Another type of compensatory breathing pattern can be observed when the intercostal and abdominal muscles are paralyzed or weak but the diaphragm and upper accessory muscles continue to function (i.e., patients with tetraplegia, high paraplegia, some congenital pectus excavatum deformities, upper airway obstruction, and asthma). These patients counterbalance the strength of the diaphragmatic inferior pull by using their sternocleidomastoid muscles and possibly their scalene, trapezius, and pectoralis muscles. Allowing for superior and possibly some anterior and lateral expansion of the chest wall, this compensatory breathing pattern minimizes the collapse of the upper chest wall that is observed in paradoxical breathing. This must be cognitively coordinated with inspiration. This pattern can be an effective breathing pattern for patients with neuromuscular weakness but may be less efficient for patients with asthma. On assessment, these patients can present with shortened neck muscles. Intercostal retractions (the collapsing of the intercostal spaces on inspiration) may be observed, especially at the level of the xiphoid. Paralyzed or weak intercostal muscles will be sucked in toward the lungs during negative pressure generated within the thoracic cavity, which can lead to intercostal retractions and can develop into a pectus excavatum in the long-term (Figure 39-12).[6,65]

Upper Accessory Muscles Only

If the patient cannot recruit the diaphragm, intercostal, and abdominal muscles, then independent breathing can be achieved only by using the upper accessory muscles in the superior plane and limited anterior expansion. These patients often require mechanical ventilation to augment their breathing independently because the lung volumes they are able to generate are insufficient to support the oxygen needs of the body.

Asymmetrical Breathing

Asymmetrical movement of the chest wall in patients with stroke, scoliosis, or other conditions is often associated with an asymmetric breathing pattern. This pattern is generally sufficient for breathing without mechanical ventilation because the strong side compensates for the weak side.[66] This compensation, however, may lead to asymmetric alignment of the trunk that adversely affects postural control in upright body positions. In addition, the adverse effects on posture can lead to adverse musculoskeletal changes over time, especially in the pediatric patient whose musculoskeletal system is still maturing.[67] Prevention of these secondary changes is a clinical priority[68] (Figure 39-13).

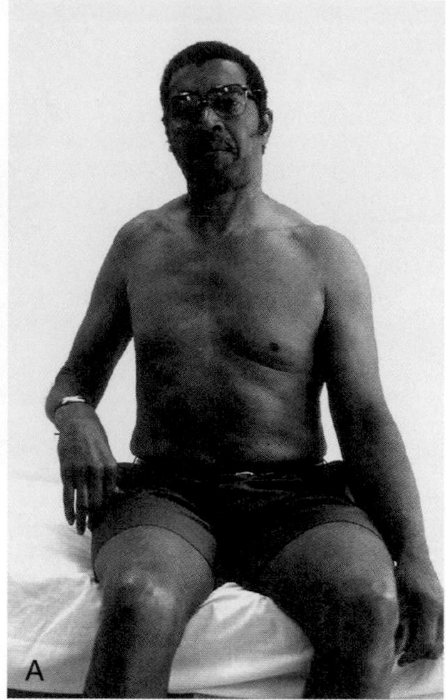

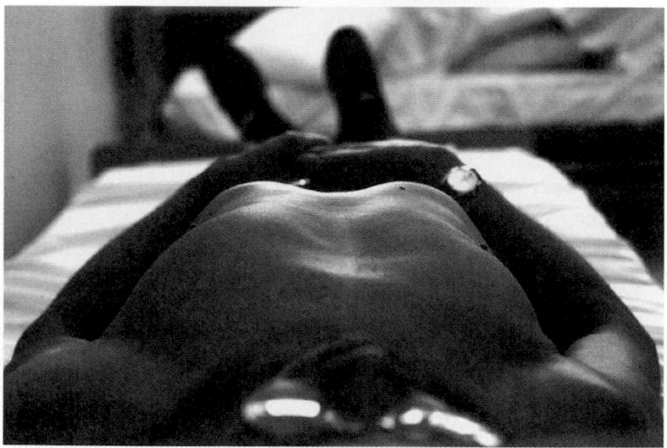

Fig. 39-13 Charles. Right hemiparesis from a stroke. **A,** Note asymmetry of the trunk in sitting during breathing and postural control. **B,** Note the weakness in the right upper thorax. Charles' right upper thorax moved less during inhalation than the left, which accentuated his asymmetrical trunk alignment and may have been a contributing factor to his impaired posture and upper extremity function in stance and during gait.

Lateral or Gravity-Eliminated Breathing

Patients with generalized weakness such as that associated with benign hypotonia, prolonged illness, or incomplete spinal cord injury, may breathe wherever gravity provides the least resistance. For example, in a supine position, patients with weakened chest wall muscles cannot effectively oppose the force of gravity in the anterior plane; thus they alter their breathing patterns to expand their chest walls primarily in the lateral plane in which gravity is eliminated. In sitting, these patients tend to breathe inferiorly where gravity assists the movement. Likewise, in a side-lying position, they tend to breathe in the anterior plane. Because their muscles are weak rather than paralyzed, these patients have a positive prognosis with respect to breathing retraining methods.

Shallow Breathing

Shallow breathing can result from injuries to the central nervous system. Such impairments include high tone associated with Parkinson syndrome, head injuries, and cerebral palsy. Shallow breathing occurs secondary to high neuromuscular tone (e.g., spasticity, rigidity, and tremors), which severely limits chest wall expansion in any plane; cerebellar discoordination; and/or improper neuromotor sequencing because of lesions in the brain, most commonly associated with medullary lesions. Shallow breathing may also occur secondary to pain, including low back pain. In such cases, breathing patterns are altered less from muscle weakness and more from the patient limiting his or her thoracic movement, thereby changing thoracic pressure. The breathing pattern is usually symmetrical, shallow, sometimes asynchronous, and frequently tachypneic (respiratory rates over 25 breaths/min for adults). Initiation and follow-through of a volitional maximal inspiration can be difficult or impossible for patients. This will markedly curtail the ability to produce an effective cough, maintain bronchial hygiene, or yell.[29]

Application of the Soda Can Model to a Clinical Example

Inherent in the Soda Can Model of respiratory and postural control is the concept that impaired pressure regulation of the trunk may result from an impairment in any organ system that generates or uses this pressure. Organ systems therefore need to be screened for their role in the motor dysfunction of breathing, postural control or both. Five impairment categories were identified at the beginning of this chapter (see Box 39-1) as well as six functional activities that require the effective coordination of the mechanics of breathing and the postural demands of motor tasks (see Box 39-2). A clinical case illustrating these points follows.

Multisystem Evaluation, Examination, and Intervention

Case History

Katie is a 9-year-old girl (Figure 39-14, *A*) diagnosed with congenital idiopathic scoliosis (infantile scoliosis) that required surgical stabilization of two upper thoracic vertebrae when she was 3 years old. After surgery, several ribs became fused on the concave side of the scoliosis and contributed to progressive kyphoscoliosis as Katie matured. Spinal fusion from T1 to S1 was planned when she was 9½ years old, when the scoliosis reached 98° despite conservative bracing from 3 years of age and close monitoring by the orthopedic surgeon.

The presurgical work-up revealed that Katie's lungs were severely restricted by her musculoskeletal impairment; the pulmonologist was unsure she would survive surgery. Figuratively speaking, Katie's soda can was crushed, resulting in dysfunction of multiple organ systems, even though the original impairment was in a single system, the musculoskeletal system. Katie was referred to physical therapy with the goal of improving her restrictive lung pathology so that she could become a viable surgical candidate. Katie had not been referred to physical therapy previously.

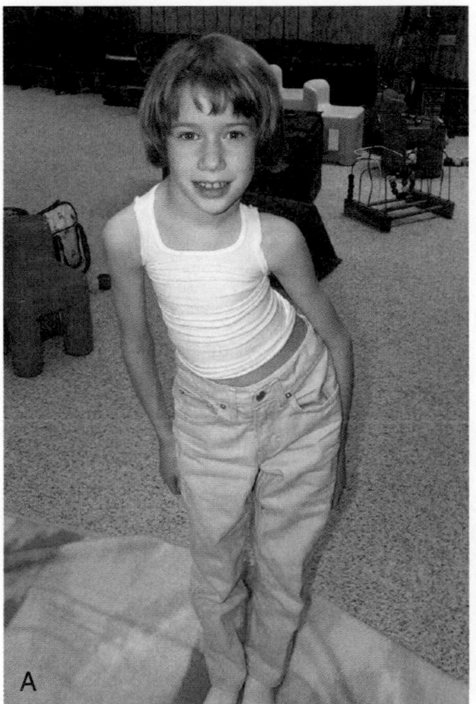

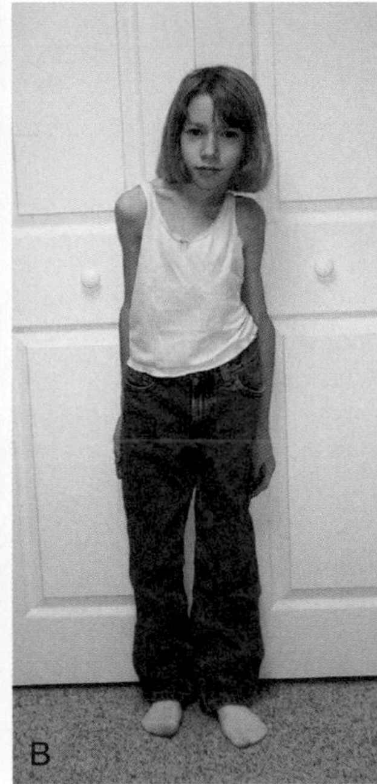

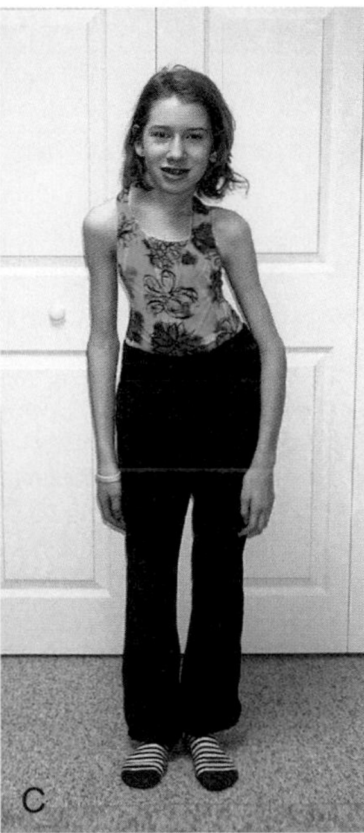

Fig. 39-14 A, Katie, 9 years of age; diagnosis of infantile scoliosis. Presurgical workup showed her FVC at 33% of predicted value. **B,** Katie, age 10 years old. 1 year later. Her surgeon believed that the improvements in lung volumes and a slight reduction in the scoliosis would allow him to postpone the surgery, giving Katie more time to grow before the surgery blunted her adult height. Katie's loose shirt partially occludes the severity of the spinal deformity. **C,** Katie, age 13 years old. 6 months after back surgery. Scoliosis was reduced as much as possible given her fused ribs (from surgery as a toddler) and other joint limitations.

IMPAIRMENT CATEGORIES

Based on a multisystem examination and evaluation based on the Soda Can Model, Katie's pathology was no longer regarded as motor dysfunction resulting from one system. The progression of her impairments, starting with the original insult to the musculoskeletal system, is described in Table 39-3.

1. Katie's pathology originated in the musculoskeletal system, specifically her spine. Her skeletal support, the "aluminum can," had collapsed over her growing years. Katie's muscle support matured around those deformities and did not develop optimal length tension relationships. Her weakness primarily involved the muscles of the trunk and proximal joints. Her distal extremity muscles showed less weakness. In particular, her intercostal muscles were so weak from disuse that the negative pressure of inhalation caused her chest wall to be drawn inward (paradoxical breathing). She was unable to generate sufficient muscle force to counteract the internal negative pressure associated with normal inspiratory lung volumes. Although the paradoxical movement had not led to a pectus excavatum, this possibility remained. Her hips and shoulders matured around her malaligned spine, which resulted in additional joint dysfunction. Katie's mother reported that her daughter had never been a physically active child, which was expected given her multiple joint limitations.
2. Katie's musculoskeletal weakness resulted in a secondary neuromuscular problem. Her muscle recruitment and balance strategies developed to compensate for atypical musculoskeletal alignment that neither supported the symmetrical development of her body nor effectively supported the concurrent demands of thoracic pressure support for the control of respiration and posture. As a result, Katie's breathing pattern was atypical (paradoxical) and this likely contributed to reduced lung volumes.
3. Reduced lung volumes and limited physical activity could explain Katie's marked endurance and mechanical impairments related to the cardiovascular and pulmonary systems. Her breathing mechanics and potential lung space were compressed to the extent that she developed severe restrictive lung pathology. No heart or vascular problems were reported by her physician based on her initial evaluation. Right heart failure, however, which can develop secondary to chronic pulmonary dysfunction, was a risk for Katie as she matured.
4. The shape of the scoliosis severely compressed Katie's stomach, causing internal organ impairment and, in turn, undernutrition and dehydration. Katie ate less than 200 calories at each meal due to premature satiety. Fluids made her feel full faster, which further compromised her hydration and capacity to consume sufficient calories. Fortunately, she did not develop gastroesophageal reflux from the abnormal thoracic and abdominal pressures and musculoskeletal malalignment.
5. Katie's integumentary system appeared to have adapted to her deformities. Her surgical scars had healed and had not adhered to underlying structures. Despite severe spinal deformity, the connective tissue around Katie's trunk and extremities was easily moved. This permitted maximum mobility of the underlying skeletal structures. Adhered integument and connective tissue were possibilities.

Table 39-3 Identifying Katie's Motor Impairments from a Multisystem Model and Planning a Targeted Intervention Strategy

Impairment Categories	Musculoskeletal	Neuromuscular	Cardiovascular/ Pulmonary	Integumentary	Internal Organs
Identify primary pathology	Scoliosis				
Identify the progression of impairments	Musculoskeletal→	Neuromuscular→	Cardiovascular/ Pulmonary→	Internal organs→	(Integumentary)
List current impairment problems	**Musculoskeletal**: Abnormal joint alignment, proximal worse than distal; abnormal length tension relationship of all muscles affected by joint malalignment resulting in weakness proximal > distal **Neuromuscular**: Trunk muscle weakness and malalignment resulting in the development of inadequate postural control strategies and a constant conflict between breathing and postural needs **Cardiovascular/pulmonary**: severe restrictive lung condition resulting in significant endurance impairments; impaired breathing mechanics, including paradoxical breathing (weak intercostal muscles); RR 32 breaths/min (tachypneic); forced exhalations even at rest; weak cough; chronic nocturnal hypoventilation; inadequate respiratory reserves for inhalation or exhalation demands; 3-5 syllables/breath (normal 8-10); sustained phonation 2-3 sec (normal 10 seconds); no cardiac symptoms (yet) **Integumentary**: No connective tissue limitations around scars from previous surgeries or around her shoulders or pelvis **Internal organs**: Malnutrition; dehydration; no reflux;				
Functional limitations and impact on participation	Functional limitations were noted in all activities that required greater oxygen or caloric fuel than Katie's restricted body could provide or that required effective coordination of breathing with movement. This resulted in limitations from the most basic motor activity of breathing to limitations in coughing, sleeping, talking, eating, and moving, thus causing severe limitations in Katie's ability to participate in normal childhood activities such as running, walking, biking, etc.				
Prioritize the current problems by categories	Internal organs→	Musculoskeletal→	Neuromuscular→	Cardiovascular/ Pulmonary→	(Integumentary)
Diagnosis	Nine-year-old girl with congenital idiopathic progressive kyphoscoliosis with severe secondary restrictions to her breathing mechanics and lung growth, nutritional health, strength and alignment of the entire musculoskeletal frame, resulting in pain, endurance impairments, significant health risks, and overall limitations in the child's physical capabilities and participation.				
Prognosis	Marked compromises of the musculoskeletal and neuromuscular support for breathing and movement, combined with Katie's poor nutritional status, limit the pulmonary status she needs immediately for surgical clearance. I believe that Katie can improve the alignment, mobility, strength, and control of her ribcage and respiratory mechanics necessary to meet the pulmonary demands of surgery if given enough time to achieve a true change in the muscle function (minimum of 4-6 weeks of training). After surgery, Katie will need an aggressive physical therapy program to develop new neuromuscular strategies that effectively utilize her new musculoskeletal alignment to maximize breath support and postural control in order to reduce her long-term cardiopulmonary, nutritional, and musculoskeletal health risks, as well as to increase her potential to participate in normal childhood activities.				
Pre- and postsurgical goals	**Presurgery**: Improve nutritional status, hydration, skeletal alignment of the trunk, and strength and control of the thoracic musculature in order to improve Katie's breathing mechanics and cough effectiveness so that she can survive the scoliotic reduction surgery and the recovery phase. **Postsurgery**: Use Katie's improved breathing mechanics to initiate an effective airway clearance program and to develop neuromuscular strategies to utilize and maintain her new spine alignment in order to reduce the risk for postsurgical pulmonary complications and to maximize breath support and postural control long term in order to reduce her ongoing cardiopulmonary, nutritional, and musculoskeletal health risks and to increase her potential to participate in normal childhood activities.				
Interventions specific to Katie's short-term goal of surgical readiness	**Musculoskeletal**: Rib mobilization to maximize inspiratory lung volumes; other ROM of joints as needed. **Neuromuscular**: Neuromuscular reeducation to increase intercostal activation for inspiratory lung volumes and chest wall stabilization; neuromuscular reeducation to reduce recruitment of abdominal muscles for forced exhalation strategies; incorporation of new breathing pattern into postural demanding tasks starting with low level activities such as walking. **Cardiovascular/pulmonary**: Endurance training—ventilator muscle training, including both resistive inspiratory and expiratory devices to increase respiratory endurance and low level power production; power training—using peak flow meter and incentive spirometers for visual feedback for maximal effort breathing; coughing strategies for improved airway clearance. **Integumentary**: No short-term interventions needed. **Internal organs**: Devised plan for increasing overall hydration and caloric intake through multiple small meals/snacks and constant sipping of water throughout the day, including school hours; school approval was critical to carryover.				

FUNCTIONAL LIMITATIONS

A functional assessment was conducted to cross-reference the evaluation from both perspectives: impairments and functional limitations. The functional findings were consistent with the impairment findings: Katie had marked functional limitations due to impaired breathing mechanics that were impacting her quality of life.

1. Katie's breathing pattern at rest showed excessive diaphragmatic excursion, underuse of the intercostal muscles (especially on the left, concave side of her chest wall), and paradoxical breathing. Her respiratory rate (RR) was 32 breaths per minute with forced exhalations (normal RR is 10 to 20 breaths/minute). With minor increased physical workload, such as walking fast, she responded by breathing faster rather than deeper. Consistently, Katie had limited physical endurance compared with her peers. Her forced vital capacity (FVC) was 33% of predicted for her sex, age, and height, indicating severe restrictive lung pathology.
2. Her cough neuromotor sequence was normal, but the small lung volume impaired her expiratory force. Her peak expiratory flow rate (PEFR) was 59% of predicted. Clinically, less than 60% of predicted PEFR has been associated with an ineffective cough and increased risk of secondary pulmonary complications.
3. Katie's teachers reported that she fell asleep most afternoons in school and often complained of headaches. Given her severe restrictive lung pathology and weak thoracic muscles, nocturnal hypoventilation was suspected. A sleep study 3 years earlier showed no abnormalities. Hypoventilation due to fatigue can contribute to poor lung function during the day and could account, in part, for her limited growth. Her pulmonologist concurred and ordered another sleep study. Chronic hypoventilation was confirmed.
4. According to her mother, Katie had always been a quiet child. The question was whether she was naturally quiet or whether she was conserving energy. Her speech consisted of three to five syllables per breath. Normal speech consists of 8 to 10 syllables per breath.[43] Katie's sustained phonation of a vowel was 2.4 to 3.1 seconds (normal is 10 seconds).[43] Katie yelled on demand, but her mother reported that she rarely did so spontaneously. Her lack of breath support could explain her quiet speech, short answers, and apparent reserved style. It was not possible to establish whether Katie was quiet by nature or had become quiet as a result of a lifetime of poor breath support.
5. Katie's stomach was compromised by kyphoscoliosis, which contributed to her feeling full after consuming fewer than 200 calories. Not only did Katie have poor weight gain as she grew, but as she aged and needed more calories for vertical growth, she lost weight. Furthermore, she failed to achieve even conservative vertical height goals that had been anticipated by her orthopedic surgeon prior to scheduling Katie for a spinal fusion.
6. Katie had marked endurance limitations for age-appropriate physical activities. She fatigued when walking more than 1½ lengths of the school gym or riding her bike more than 1½ blocks. Katie's weak muscles and impaired breathing mechanics, combined with malnutrition, dehydration, and impaired oxygen delivery, meant that she had less physiological reserve capacity for activities beyond those for basic survival. Katie's body was unable to meet the needs of both breathing and high postural demands of childhood activities.[28,30] Katie preferred to engage in low energy cost activities such as playing the violin, reading, and playing quietly.

PRIORITIES OF INTERVENTIONS

Understanding Katie's progression of impairments streamlined the screening process. The status of Katie's pulmonary system precluded her having surgery. Her primary pathology, however, had not originated in the pulmonary system. This presented several questions: How had all five motor impairment categories contributed to her current pulmonary status? How could treatment interventions be prioritized to meet Katie's short-term respiratory and surgical goals? In the short term, the evaluation led to the several interventions that are described below. Katie's long-term health and participation goals were developed after surgery.

1. Katie's poor nutritional status meant she had minimal energy reserve to participate effectively in a conditioning program to strengthen her respiratory muscles in preparation for surgery. Likewise, her dehydrated state could reduce the mobility of pulmonary secretions, thus increasing her postsurgical risk for atelectasis and pneumonia. Thus, addressing Katie's nutritional and hydration needs was the first priority. Katie was instructed to eat at least six meals daily rather than three. She was permitted to use a water bottle in class. In school, she was encouraged to drink at the start of every new subject. Her nutritional intake was managed by her pediatrician.
2. Surgery was the recommended intervention to improve the alignment of Katie's spine and ribcage. In the short term, however, manual mobilization of her ribcage was a priority to gain movement to augment lung volumes.
3. After Katie's ribcage mobility was increased and a body position identified that gave her the best support for chest wall movement, specifically, sitting, a neuromuscular rehabilitation program was initiated to improve her respiratory mechanics. The goals of the program were:
   a. To increase recruitment, strength, and function of the intercostal muscles as inspiratory muscles (to increase lung volume) and as chest wall stabilizers (to minimize paradoxical breathing), while decreasing the use of forced abdominal muscle exhalations, thus reducing the energy cost of breathing (by manipulating thoracic pressure more effectively).
   b. To increase the power generated by both the inspiratory and expiratory muscles needed to increase lung volumes and cough effectiveness. This was achieved with the use of peak flow meters and incentive spirometers that provided Katie with visual feedback of specific targeted performance (large effort, low repetitions).
   c. To increase endurance and overall fitness of the respiratory muscles through use of an aggressive daily ventilatory muscle training program involving both the inspiratory and expiratory muscles (low resistance, high repetitions) (see Chapter 26). Ventilatory resistance muscle training was used instead of a traditional fitness training program such as treadmill walking because Katie's weakness, malalignment, and painful joints likely would have prevented her from exercising

sufficiently to elicit a favorable response and may have contributed to additional joint problems.

d. To improve Katie's ability to meet the conflicting needs of respiration and postural control required for functional endurance and motor performance, low-level activities (e.g., walking) were prescribed initially, with distance being increased over time (with increased endurance). Katie was instructed how to use the new breathing pattern during functional tasks designed to challenge her balance and breathing simultaneously.

4. In anticipation of orthopedic surgery, ensuring effective pulmonary hygiene was the goal. The contributions of her various body systems to the efficiency and effectiveness of her breathing mechanics, lung volumes, cough effectiveness, endurance, and posture were targeted through multiple interventions.
5. Katie's integumentary system did not show any impairment and was not a major contributor to her limited pulmonary status. After surgery, however, dehydration predisposed her to skin breakdown and poor tissue healing. She was monitored for residual problems.

DIAGNOSIS AND PROGNOSIS

Katie's musculoskeletal pathology impaired the structural support of her trunk and respiratory mechanics. Musculoskeletal restrictions contributed to dysfunction in other systems due to their various interactions. She was referred to physical therapy for one reason, to improve breathing mechanics so that she could undergo surgery to correct the initial pathology, the scoliosis. Based on the physical therapy examination, the pulmonologist was informed that Katie's condition showed potential for improvement. A minimum of 4 to 6 weeks was needed to achieve a training effect that would sustain her through the long surgery. Surgery was postponed for 8 weeks to allow Katie the maximum benefit of the physical therapy intervention. With respect to the long-term goals of health and participation in typical childhood activities, improving her breathing mechanics was only one goal. Other goals were to be addressed after surgery.

OUTCOMES

Katie and her mother understood the risks of surgery and were motivated to participate in an aggressive physical therapy program that relied heavily on home participation. Katie and her mother were instructed regarding the necessity of a home exercise program five days a week for 5 to 6 weeks in order to increase muscle strength and endurance. Katie was enthusiastic: exercising every day. Pulmonary function improvements are shown below, along with their influence on her surgical status.

1. Katie's pulmonary function baseline for FVC was 0.45 L (33% of predicted, or 1.36 L), and her PEFR was 1.64 L/s (59% of predicted).
   a. Three weeks later, Katie's FVC improved to 0.57 L (42% of predicted).
   b. Five months later, FVC had increased to and stabilized at 0.63 L (45% of predicted).
   c. Three months after initiating her program, Katie's PEFR improved to 2.31 L/s (81% of predicted), which is within a normal range for effective coughing.
   d. Two years later, after a sleep study confirmed chronic hypoventilation and after successful initiation of noninvasive mechanical ventilatory support at night, that is, bi-level positive airway pressure (BiPAP), Katie's FVC had improved to 0.71 L, but this value was now only 40% of predicted for her sex, age, and height (1.78 L). Pulmonary function progressively increases with age until adulthood, but Katie's lungs did not keep pace with expectations for a typically developing child. A predicted FVC of 60% is often used as the clinical index of adequate lung volume necessary for normal pulmonary maneuvers such as coughing, sighing, and sneezing. With an FVC of 40% of predicted, she was still at long-term risk for secondary respiratory problems due to impaired lung volumes.
2. At 4 months, the orthopedic surgeon recommended postponing surgery because her scoliosis was reduced progressively from 98° to 91°. He believed that her improved pulmonary status had a positive effect on her skeletal frame and that as long as she remained stable, it was worth postponing surgery to give her every chance to grow and continue making respiratory gains before undergoing a spinal fusion (Figure 39-14, *B*).
   a. Katie's surgery was postponed for over 3 years, until she was 12 years old, allowing her to achieve more vertical growth before surgery. The orthopedic surgeon expressed surprise that surgery had not been indicated before Katie reached 10 years of age.
   b. Katie continued to do her exercises three to four days a week over the course of intervention. She had no postoperative respiratory complications. Her scoliosis was markedly reduced (Figure 39-14, *C*). Additional surgeries may eventually be required for her shoulders, hips, and fused ribs.

Katie's ongoing care included interventions such as gastric surgery for placement of a gastrostomy tube that was needed to improve her nutrition, growth hormone administration, BiPAP nocturnal support to reverse chronic hypoventilation and its effects on her physical endurance and growth, and a comprehensive physical therapy program focusing on her growth and postural maturation. This case history focused on the initial physical therapy intervention to illustrate how a multisystem assessment can be used to develop a differential diagnosis regarding her physical and pulmonary limitations. Katie's scoliosis and muscle development made her incapable of generating, maintaining, and regulating adequate pressures in her thoracic and abdominal cavities to support normal respiration, postural control, and internal organ function. The Soda Can Model helped explain why the impairment of her musculoskeletal system had major implications for her health and the function of other systems.

QUALITY OF LIFE

In addition to Katie's medical improvement, her mother reported that the respiratory and multisystem approach to her daughter's physical therapy program "absolutely saved her life." Katie appeared increasingly confident in her abilities, which was noted at the second physical therapy visit, during which she appreciated the positive results of her diligent adherence to the home program. Within 6 months of the initiation of the physical therapy program, Katie's paradoxical breathing was eliminated, she no longer used forced abdominal exhalations, her chest wall expansion improved, and her sustained phonation improved 50% (from 3.1 seconds to 4.7 seconds); all of which appeared to contribute to her increased physical activity. She began swimming lessons, joined recreational softball, and generally reported that she "likes this new feeling; it's easier to move and breathe." Her mother reported that Katie smiled more often.

CLINICAL RELEVANCE OF THIS CASE REGARDING IMPAIRED RESPIRATORY MECHANICS AND POSTURAL CONTROL

The cardiovascular and pulmonary systems are systems that create and use pressure support within the trunk's cavities to maximize performance; thus they should not be assessed or treated in isolation. Rather, they need to be assessed in conjunction with other organ systems. The body functions as a whole with individual systems interacting and supporting one another. In particular, postural control and mechanical support for breathing are interdependent; yet breathing necessarily takes precedence over postural requirements. Therefore mechanical support for breathing needs to be assessed and treated within the context of the mechanical support for postural control because both activities use the same muscles.

Although Katie's initial pathology originated in the musculoskeletal system, her more important problems, clinically, involved the neuromuscular system (motor planning and strength), the cardiovascular and pulmonary systems (severely impaired respiratory mechanics, inadequate respiratory endurance, and the risk for cardiac impairments), and the internal organs (persistent undernutrition and dehydration). If Katie had been treated based on an impairment of one system, she may not have achieved comparable clinical and functional outcomes that allowed her surgeon to delay her surgery for 3 years and allowed her to achieve other health and functional outcomes.

Application

Pathologies stemming from any motor impairment category may result in impaired breathing mechanics, a conflict in postural control and breathing that interferes with motor performance, or both. For example, a patient with a neuromuscular condition such as a spinal cord injury (SCI), cerebral palsy, stroke, or head injury will have impaired breathing mechanics and impaired postural control due to paralysis, weakness, or impaired motor planning or execution. The physical therapist needs to assess such a patient from a neuromotor perspective, as well as from that system's interaction with the musculoskeletal, cardiovascular, pulmonary, integumentary systems and the internal organs. This helps ensure that the major limitations affecting motor performance and health are identified and prioritized for intervention. Improvements in chest wall and thoracic alignment can be achieved in the long term from a multisystem approach. See Melissa's changes from 3 to 12 years of age after an SCI incurred at birth (compare Figures 39-15 and 39-16 with Figures 39-2, *B*, and 39-8, *C*). Melissa's chest wall and spinal deformities were almost completely reversed after years of interventions from a multiprofessional team approach to her multisystem impairments.[11] Melissa was

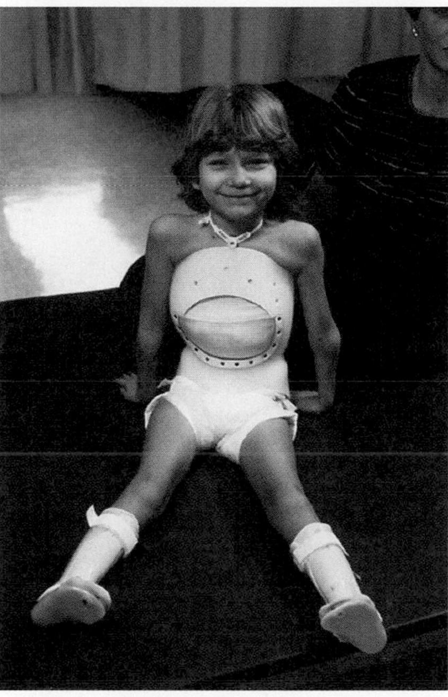

Fig. 39-15 Melissa, 6 years of age. Note the use of the thoracic-lumbar-sacral orthosis with an abdominal cutout supported by an abdominal binder. This provided support for her developing spine and trunk while still allowing for optimal support for breathing mechanics. Note that the TLSO provided ideal alignment of the proximal extremity joints (shoulders and hips), as well as ideal head alignment for normal functions such as talking and eating.

not assessed or treated by a physical therapist or other rehabilitation professional until she was 3½ years old. Key long-term interventions and outcomes follow.

1. Melissa used an abdominal binder whenever she was upright to provide the abdominal pressure needed for internal organ support, improved breathing mechanics, and lumbar stabilization. This is a lifelong intervention.
2. Melissa also needed a body jacket or thoracic-lumbar-sacral orthosis (TLSO) with an abdominal cutout and abdominal binder. An abdominal binder alone would not provide adequate support for her developing spine and proximal joints. She still developed a scoliosis, but she did not develop a kyphosis or axial rotation of the curve. The orthopedic surgeon stated that this made surgical correction easier, safer, and faster.
3. An aggressive neuromuscular reeducation program was implemented to teach Melissa how to engage her upper accessory muscles, especially her pectoralis muscles, as substitute chest wall stabilizers and how to use them as long-term inspiratory muscles to balance the excessive inward pressure generated by the isolated contractions of the diaphragm. She was also instructed on how to use her breath support (ventilatory strategies) to improve the efficiency of her mobility skills such as in rolling over and reaching.
4. An airway clearance program was developed to minimize the family's reliance on suctioning. Melissa and her family learned multiple manual assistive coughing techniques that effectively expectorated mucus. They reduced her suctioning from 24 to 36 times daily to one to three times

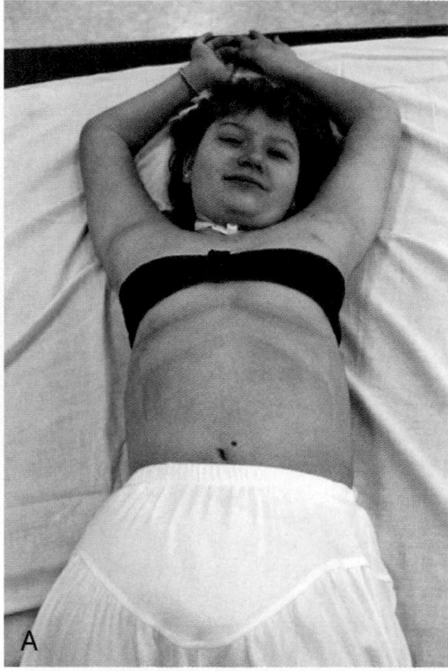

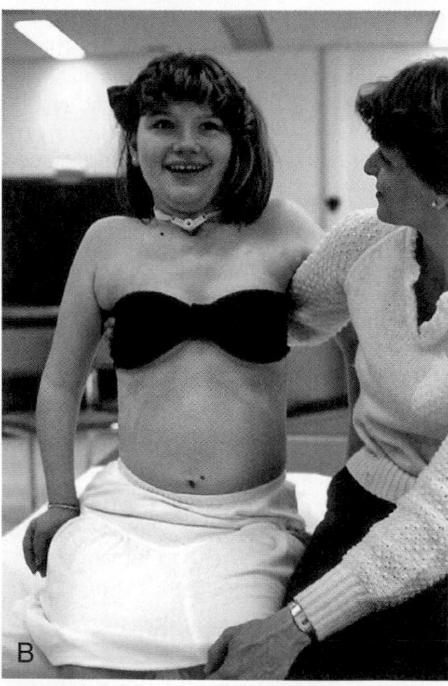

Fig. 39-16 Melissa, 12 years of age, after orthopedic surgery to reduce scoliosis. **A,** Note that the chest wall deformities that were prevalent at 3 years old are almost absent. The only apparent skeletal restriction is the slight reduction in mid-thoracic expansion around ribs 6 and 7, which looks like a high "waistline" just under her bra-strap line in supine position. The intercostal muscles, which were paralyzed, are the only muscles supporting the ribcage at that level. Melissa used her upper accessory muscles, especially her pectoralis muscles, to support breathing and chest wall alignment around ribs 1-5 and her diaphragm around ribs 8-10. **B,** Melissa continues to wear an abdominal binder in upright postures, but it was removed for this picture.

daily. She had multiple bouts of pneumonia in her first 3½ years of life, but none from age 3 to 12 years of age.

5. Melissa's nutrition and hydration needs were addressed by the health care team by increasing her caloric intake and improving her hydration. A picture taken when she was 12 years old shows that she had been consuming sufficient calories for growth. (A gastrostomy tube was not inserted because it had not yet been invented when Melissa was a young girl.)
6. Nocturnal positive pressure ventilatory support was initiated when Melissa was approximately 6 years of age because of nocturnal hypoventilation and the conflict between the use of calories for growth and breathing. The positive pressure support relieved her work of breathing and rested her muscles. In addition, it appeared to reverse forces that could contribute to pectus deformity of her anterior chest wall.

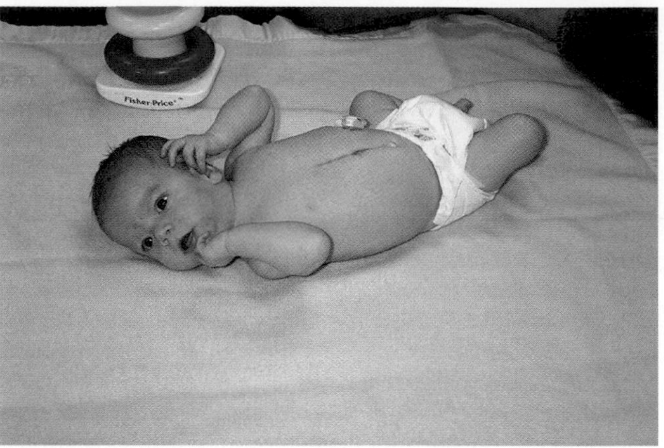

Fig. 39-17 Jonathan, 6 months of age. His severe gastroesophageal reflux required surgical support (gastrostomy tube and Nissen fundoplication procedures) at 5 months of age. His mother reports that his favorite posture when he is supine is extreme trunk extension and right head rotation. This is a typical compensatory strategy in response to the noxious stimulus of reflux and/or upper airway obstruction.

The same concept can be applied to other impairment categories. For example, in Katie's case, if her integumentary system showed connective tissue restrictions secondary to kyphoscoliosis, her integumentary system would be the primary limiting factor to improving pulmonary status rather than the neuromuscular system and internal organs. In other words, if Katie's ribcage could be mobilized but overlying taut skin disallowed movement, breathing strategies to increase her lung volumes would be ineffective. This is observed in patients who have connective tissue involvement such as in the case of scar formation, scleroderma, or severe burns. In these cases, the skin has insufficient mobility to allow the underlying muscles to move the chest wall. If the chest wall moves inadequately, lung volumes will not be sufficient to deliver sufficient oxygen to working muscle. The severity of the condition and damage to the integumentary and proximal underlying structures will determine the extent of impaired breathing mechanics.

Conditions related to the internal organs may have a subtle influence on postural control and breathing. Infants with severe gastroesophageal reflux, for example, may assume a posture of trunk hyperextension and right head rotation in supine (Sandifer's syndrome) (Figure 39-17).[63,69-72] Such posturing may be mistaken for a neuromuscular lesion. In fact, the infant may use this posturing to move away from the noxious stimulus of reflux experienced whenever he or she moves into a flexed trunk posture of head turning and lateral trunk bending to the left. If the child is not assessed from a multisystem perspective, the physical therapist may focus on treating the excessive extensor tone and asymmetry of the trunk rather than the underlying cause of the motor behavior, which stems from the internal organs. If untreated, these infants may develop further spinal extension and upper thoracic breathing strategies to avoid exacerbating the reflux and increasing intraabdominal pressure. Reflux can be exacerbated with descent of the diaphragm onto an irritable stomach and by increased intraabdominal pressure. Over time, the infant may develop impairments in all motor systems, potentially affecting overall health and participation. For example, children with cystic fibrosis were traditionally tipped downward for postural drainage to improve lung function; however, this treatment predisposed many of these children to gastroesophageal reflux and a worsening of their pulmonary status.[73,74] The outline below describes how the motor systems could be affected by a pathology originating in the internal organs.

1. Internal organs: The pathology originates within these organs.
2. Neuromuscular system: Inadequate motor control of trunk flexors, necessary for balance, forced expiratory maneuvers, and lumbar stabilization, may develop. Pathology of the internal organs may predispose the child at a later stage to low back dysfunction and pain because normal positive pressure stabilization motor strategies, especially from the diaphragm and abdominal muscles, are not developed in childhood.
3. Musculoskeletal system: Sequelae of associated pathology may include (a) excessive ligamentous shortening of lumbar vertebrae secondary to the chronic lordotic posture and/or (b) elevated ribcage alignment, which results when the trunk flexors do not actively engage in pulling the ribcage inferiorly and the over-recruitment of upper accessory muscles continues to promote this position, which can contribute to (c) increased risk for low back pain secondary to poor lumbar stabilization strategies, weak abdominal muscles, and atypical vertebral alignment.
4. Cardiovascular and pulmonary systems: Limited overall endurance may result if the child develops an upper thoracic breathing pattern as his or her primary breathing pattern in response to the noxious feedback received in response to using the diaphragm as the primary respiratory muscle. This could also predispose the child to neck and shoulder dysfunction because the conflict between the respiratory recruitment of the upper accessory muscles and the dual role these muscles play in upper quadrant movement may contribute to overuse and later complaints of symptoms such as pain, fatigue, and headaches.
5. Integumentary system: This system is less commonly a contributor to motor impairments, but can be in cases such as surgical scars, where tight connective tissue in the skin restricts flexion of the trunk, shoulder, or hip.

Impaired breathing mechanics do not occur strictly because of a direct impairment of the lungs, airways, or chest wall muscles. Impaired breathing mechanics can occur from insults to any organ or system that influences motor performance. The cardiovascular and pulmonary systems should be seen as integral parts of motor assessment in order to determine whether the mechanics of breathing are facilitating or impairing the patient's overall motor performance. That is, breathing mechanics may be the cause or the consequence of motor dysfunction. A thorough multisystem evaluation helps the clinician distinguish the two. Respiratory muscle testing has a role in determining the degree to which impairments are respiratory or postural in origin.[75] With an analysis based on a Soda Can Model, the physical therapist can identify the sources of the underlying impairments and target interventions accordingly.

Summary

In this chapter, the role of respiratory mechanics as they relate to a range of body systems has been explored. Gravity was described as a major influence on both the potential movement of the chest wall and development of the chest wall, trunk, and thoracic structures. The dual role of the trunk to support both respiratory and postural control was introduced in the context of the Soda Can Model. Clinical cases based on multiple motor impairment categories were described to illustrate how trunk control, breathing, and internal organ function depend on the ability of the body to generate, maintain, and regulate pressure in the thoracic and abdominal cavities, the control of which extends from the vocal folds down to the pelvic floor. In the clinical examples, the five motor impairment categories—musculoskeletal, neuromuscular, cardiovascular and pulmonary, and integumentary systems and the internal organs—were screened with respect to their roles in motor performance and breathing mechanics; each system influences the performance of the others. Such analysis provided the basis for designing treatment plans that targeted the primary impairments. Anticipated motor outcomes involving the trunk and breathing were achieved.

Review Questions

1. Explain the role of gravity in normal chest wall development of infants.
2. Explain how the pressures in the thorax and abdomen provide postural support for the trunk and the role of the diaphragm in that process.
3. Explain the role of the vocal folds and the pelvic floor in normal respiration and in high postural demanding activities.
4. Explain the relationship between the gastrointestinal system and respiration.
5. Using one of your patients as a case study, apply the concepts of multisystem evaluation, examination, and intervention planning as discussed in this chapter.

References

1. APTA: Guide to Physical Therapist Practice, ed 2. *Physical Therapy* 81, 2001.
2. Panitch HB: The pathophysiology of respiratory impairment in pediatric neuromuscular diseases. *Pediatrics* 123(Suppl 4):S215–S218, 2009.
3. Inal-Ince D, Savci S, Arikan H, et al: Effects of scoliosis on respiratory muscle strength in patients with neuromuscular disorders. *Spine J* 9(12):981–986, 2009.
4. Coonan TJ, Hope CF: Cardio-respiratory effects of change in body position. *Canadian Anaesthetists' Society Journal* 30:424–437, 1983.
5. Piper MC, Darrah J: *Motor assessment of the developing infant*, Philadelphia, 1994, Sanders.

6. Bach JR, Bianchi C: Prevention of pectus excavatum for children with spinal muscular atrophy type 1. *American Journal of Physical Medicine and Rehabilitation* 82:815–819, 2003.
7. Lissoni A, Aliverti A, Tzeng AC, et al: Kinematic analysis of patients with spinal muscular atrophy during spontaneous breathing and mechanical ventilation. *American Journal of Physical Medicine and Rehabilitation* 77:188–192, 1998.
8. Papastamelos C, Panitch HB, Allen JL: Chest wall compliance in infants and children with neuromuscular disease. *American Journal Respiratory Critical Care Medicine* 154:1045–1048, 1996.
9. West JB: *Pulmonary pathophysiology: the essentials*, ed 7, Philadelphia, 2008, Lippincott Williams and Wilkins.
10. Toder DS: Respiratory problems in the adolescent with developmental delay. *Adolescent Medicine* 11:617–631, 2000.
11. Massery MP: Chest development as a component of normal motor development: implications for pediatric physical therapists. *Pediatric Physical Therapy* 3:3–8, 1991.
12. Massery M: Theoretical model: The interaction and inter-dependence of breathing and postural control. Unpublished manuscript for doctoral classwork at Rocky Mountain University of Health Professions, Provo, UT:1–15, 2003.
13. Massery M: Musculoskeletal and neuromuscular interventions: a physical approach to cystic fibrosis. *Journal of the Royal Society of Medicine* 98(Supplement 45):55–66, 2005.
14. Hodges PW, Gandevia SC: Activation of the human diaphragm during a repetitive postural task. *Journal of Physiology* 522:165–175, 2000.
15. Hudson AL, Butler JE, Gandevia SC, et al: Interplay between the inspiratory and postural functions of the human parasternal intercostal muscles. *J Neurophysiol* 103(3):1622–1629, 2010.
16. Hodges PW, Cresswell AG, Thorstensson A: Intra-abdominal pressure response to multidirectional support-surface translation. *Gait Posture* 20(2):163–170, 2004.
17. Morris SL, Allison GT: Effects of abdominal muscle fatigue on anticipatory postural adjustments associated with arm raising. *Gait Posture* 24(3):342–348, 2006.
18. Rehan VK, McCool FD: Diaphragm dimensions of the healthy term infant. *Acta Paediatr* 92(9):1062–1067, 2003.
19. Dimitriou G, Greenough A, Kavvadia V, et al: Diaphragmatic function in infants with surgically corrected anomalies. *Pediatr Res* 54(4):502–508, 2003.
20. Hodges PW, Gurfinkel VS, Brumagne S, et al: Coexistence of stability and mobility in postural control: evidence from postural compensation for respiration. *Experimental Brain Research* 144:293–302, 2002.
21. Smith MD, Russell A, Hodges PW: Disorders of breathing and continence have a stronger association with back pain than obesity and physical activity. *Australian Journal of Physiotherapy* 52(1):11–16, 2006.
22. Hodges PW, Sapsford R, Pengel LHM: Postural and respiratory functions of the pelvic floor muscles. *Neurourology & Urodynamics* 26(3):362–371, 2007.
23. Orlikoff RF: Voice production during a weightlifting and support task. *Folia Phoniatrica et Logopedica* 60(4):188–194, 2008.
24. Flaminiano LE, Celli BR: Respiratory muscle testing. *Clinics in Chest Medicine* 22:661–677, 2001.
25. De Troyer A, Kirkwood PA, Wilson TA: Respiratory action of the intercostal muscles. *Physiol Rev* 85(2):717–756, 2005.
26. De Troyer A, Leduc D: Role of pleural pressure in the coupling between the intercostal muscles and the ribs. *J Appl Physiol* 102(6):2332–2337, 2007.
27. Butler JE, Gandevia SC: The output from human inspiratory motoneuron pools. *Journal of Physiology* 586(5):1257–1264, 2008.
28. Hodges PW, Heijnen I, Gandevia SC: Postural activity of the diaphragm is reduced in humans when respiratory demand increases. *Journal of Physiology* 537:999–1008, 2001.
29. Grimstone SK, Hodges PW: Impaired postural compensation for respiration in people with recurrent low back pain. *Experimental Brain Research* 151:218–224, 2003.
30. Gandevia SC, Butler JE, Hodges PW, et al: Balancing acts: respiratory sensations, motor control and human posture. *Clinical and Experimental Pharmacology and Physiology* 29:118–121, 2002.
31. Bach JR, Baird JS, Plosky D, et al: Spinal muscular atrophy type 1: management and outcomes. *Pediatric Pulmonology* 34:16–22, 2002.
32. Wilson TA, Legrand A, Gevenois PA, et al: Respiratory effects of the external and internal intercostal muscles in humans. *Journal of Physiology* 530:319–330, 2001.
33. De Troyer A, Gorman RB, Gandevia SC: Distribution of inspiratory drive to the external intercostal muscles in humans. *Journal of Physiology* 546:943–954, 2003.
34. Ratnovsky A, Elad D, Halpern P: Mechanics of respiratory muscles. *Respiratory Physiology & Neurobiology* 163:82–89, 2008.
35. Canavan PK, Cahalin L: Integrated physical therapy intervention for a person with pectus excavatum and bilateral shoulder pain: a single-case study. *Arch Phys Med Rehabil* 89(11):2195–2204, 2008.
36. Skjodt NM, Farran RP, Hawes HG, et al: Simulation of acute spinal cord injury: effects on respiration. *Respiratory Physiology* 127:3–11, 2001.
37. Hodges PW, Gandevia SC: Changes in intra-abdominal pressure during postural and respiratory activation of the human diaphragm. *Journal of Applied Physiology* 89:967–976, 2000.
38. Serway R, Faughn J: *College physics*, Orlando, Fla, 1992, Harcourt Brace Jovanovich.
39. Schilero, G. J., Spungen AM, Bauman WA, et al: Pulmonary function and spinal cord injury. *Respir Physiol Neurobiol* 166(3):129–141, 2009.
40. Mason RJ, Broaddus VC, Martin T, et al: *Murray and Nadel's Textbook of Respiratory Medicine*, ed 5, Philadelphia, 2010, Elsevier.
41. Spahija, J, de Marchie M, Grassino A: Effects of imposed pursed-lips breathing on respiratory mechanics and dyspnea at rest and during exercise in COPD. *Chest* 128(2):640–650, 2005.
42. Pierce RJ, Worsnop CJ: Upper airway function and dysfunction in respiration. *Clinical and Experimental Pharmacology and Physiology* 26:1–10, 1999.
43. Deem JF, Miller L: *Manual of voice therapy*, ed 2, Austin, Tex, 2000, PRO-ED, Inc.
44. Irwin RS, Boulet LP, Cloutier MM, et al: Managing cough as a defense mechanism and as a symptom. A consensus panel report of the American College of Chest Physicians. *Chest* 114:133–181, 1998.
45. Bach JR, Saporito LR: Criteria for extubation and tracheostomy tube removal for patients with ventilatory failure. A different approach to weaning. *Chest* 110:1566–1571, 1996.
46. Borowitz SM, Borowitz KC: Gastroesophageal reflux in babies: impact on growth and development. *Infants and Young Children* 10:14–26, 1997.
47. Borowitz SM, Sutphen JL: Recurrent vomiting and persistent gastroesophageal reflux caused by unrecognized constipation. *Clinical Pediatrics* 43:461–466, 2004.
48. Iannaccone ST: Modern management of spinal muscular atrophy. *Journal of Child Neurology* 22(8):974–978, 2007.
49. Corcia, P, Meininger V Management of amyotrophic lateral sclerosis. *Drugs* 68(8):1037–1048, 2008.
50. Hayama S, Honda K, et al: Air trapping and arboreal locomotor adaptation in primates: a review of experiments on humans. *Zeitschrift fur Morphologie und Anthropologie* 83:149–159, 2002.
51. Hagins M, Lamberg EM: Natural breath control during lifting tasks: effect of load. *European Journal of Applied Physiology* 96(4):453–458, 2006.
52. Massery M: *The effect of airway control on postural stability (doctoral dissertation)*. Provo, UT, Rocky Mountain University of HealthProfessions, 2011.
53. Hoit JD, Banzett RB, Brown R: Binding the abdomen can improve speech in men with phrenic nerve pacers. *American Journal of Speech-Language Pathology* 11(1):71–76, 2002.
54. Wadsworth B, Haines TP, Cornwell PL, et al: *The effect of an abdominal binder on respiratory function and voice in people with acute tetraplegia*. The Australian Physiotherapy Annual Conference. Sydney, Australia, 2009.
55. Mandell DL, Arjmand EM: Laryngomalacia induced by exercise in a pediatric patient. *International Journal of Pediatric Otorhinolaryngology* 67(9):999–1003, 2003.
56. Sapsford RR, Hodges PW, Richardson CA, et al: Co-activation of the abdominal and pelvic floor muscles during voluntary exercises. *Neurourology and Urodynamics* 20:31–42, 2001.
57. Button BM, Sherburn M: Cough and the pelvic floor: prevent, control and treat urinary incontinence. *Pediatric Pulmonology, Supplement* 31:114 –115, 2008.
58. Langman H, Orr A, et al: Urinary incontinence in CF: why does it happen? Eighteenth Annual North American Cystic Fibrosis Conference, St. Louis, Mo. *Pediatric Pulmonology* 27(Suppl):154–155, 2004.
59. Dodd ME, Langman H: Urinary incontinence in cystic fibrosis. *Journal of The Royal Society of Medicine* 98(Suppl 45):28–36, 2005.
60. De Looze D, Van Laere M, De Muynck M, et al: Constipation and other chronic gastrointestinal problems in spinal cord injury patients. *Spinal Cord* 36:63–66, 1998.
61. Noreau L, Proulx P, Gagnon L, et al: Secondary impairments after spinal cord injury: a population-based study. *American Journal of Physical Medicine and Rehabilitation* 79:526–535, 2000.
62. Zimmer MB, Nantwi K, Goshgarian HG: Effect of spinal cord injury on the respiratory system: basic research and current clinical treatment options. *Journal of Spinal Cord Medicine* 30:319–330, 2007.

63. Frankel EA, Shalaby TM, Orenstein SR: Sandifer syndrome posturing: relation to abdominal wall contractions, gastroesophageal reflux, and fundoplication *Digestive Diseases & Sciences* 51(4):635–640, 2006.
64. Bhatia J, Parish A: GERD or not GERD: the fussy infant. *J Perinatol* 29(Suppl 2):S7–11, 2009.
65. Massery M: Asthma: multisystem implications. In Campbell S, Palisano R, Vander Linden D, Editors: *Physical therapy for children*, Philadelphia, Pa: WB. Saunders, 2005.
66. Lanini B, Bianchi R, Romagnoli I, et al: Chest wall kinematics in patients with hemiplegia. *American Journal of Respiratory and Critical Care Medicine* 168:109–113, 2003.
67. McNamara D: *Diaphragmatic Hernia Survivors Do Well. Chest Physician*, Morristown, NJ, 2011, Elsevier, Inc. for The American College of Chest Physicians. 6: 1 & 5.
68. Sobus KML, Horan SM, et al: Respiratory management of neuromuscular diseases in children. *Physical Medicine and Rehabilitation: State of the Art Reviews* 14:285–299, 2000.
69. Lehwald N, Krausch M, Franke C, et al: Sandifer syndrome—a multidisciplinary diagnostic and therapeutic challenge. *European Journal of Pediatric Surgery* 17:203–206, 2007.
70. Demir E, Saka E, Aysun S: A case of Sandifer's syndrome with hand tremor. *Turkish Journal of Pediatrics* 43:348–350, 2001.
71. de Ybarrondo L, Mazur JL: Sandifer's syndrome in a child with asthma and cerebral palsy. *Southern Medical Journal* 93(10):1019–1021, 2000.
72. Kostakis A, Manjunatha NP, Kumar A: Abnormal head posture in a patient with normal ocular motility: Sandifer syndrome *Journal of Pediatric Ophthalmology & Strabismus* 45(1):57–58, 2008.
73. Button BM, Heine RG, Catto-Smith AG, et al: Chest physiotherapy in infants with cystic fibrosis: to tip or not? A five-year study. *Pediatric Pulmonology* 35:208–213, 2003.
74. Button BM, Heine RG, Catto-Smith AG, et al: Chest physiotherapy, gastro-esophageal reflux, and arousal in infants with cystic fibrosis. *Archive of Diseases in Childhood* 89:435–439, 2004.
75. Nicot F, Hart N, Forin V, et al: Respiratory muscle testing: a valuable tool for children with neuromuscular disorders. *American Journal of Respiratory and Critical Care Medicine* doi:10.1164/rccm.200512-1841OC, 2006.

VII

Chapter 40

The Transplant Patient

Susan A. Scherer

KEY TERMS

Heart transplant
Lung transplant
Rehabilitation
Aerobic capacity
Oxygen

CHAPTER OUTLINE

The ability to transplant an organ from one individual to another is a relatively new phenomenon. New advances in surgical techniques and immunosuppressive drugs, ability to detect and treat rejection, and improved outcomes have made transplantation of solid organs a viable treatment option for patients with end-stage cardiac and pulmonary conditions. The increased life expectancy of transplant patients means that physical therapists have many opportunities for patient intervention both before and after transplant in various settings. Trends in patient demographics indicate that a physical therapist may see a transplant patient not only in a regional medical center setting but also in outpatient and rural clinics. This chapter contains guidelines for managing patients with heart or lung transplants.

Background

Transplantation of tissues and organs has been of interest to physicians and surgeons since the 18th century. Advances in our understanding of the immune system, development of immunosuppressive medications, and techniques such as cardiopulmonary bypass have provided the opportunity for successful organ transplants. In 1954, the first kidney was successfully transplanted. Other successful organ transplants include the first heart transplant in 1968, combined heart-lung transplant in 1981, and single-lung transplant in 1983.[1]

Organ transplantation has become a viable alternative to medical treatment of many conditions. Because of the success rates, many types of transplants are no longer considered experimental but are considered appropriate treatment for organ failure. As a result of improved survival, long-term outcomes are as important as short-term outcomes as a measure of successful transplantation. The number of Medicare-approved medical centers that perform lung and heart-lung transplants has grown to 50 in the United States, and there are 110 certified heart transplant centers.[2] Over 2000 heart transplants and 1000 lung transplants have been performed annually since 2000. The 5-year survival rates for heart transplants of all status levels are reported as 70.9%; for lung transplants, 43.1%. Other national data on median waiting time and survival rates are presented in Table 40-1.

Organ Donation

The major cause of limitation in the number of organ transplants is the lack of organ supply with an increasing demand for organ transplantation. The number of patients who could benefit from transplant significantly exceeds the number of organs available. The Organ Procurement and Transplantation Network (OPTN) is an organization whose primary goal is to increase the availability of donated organs available and improve organ sharing. OPTN was established by the National

Table 40-1 **Heart/Lung Transplantation National Data**

	Heart	Lung
Number of transplants, 2005-2010	12,660	8744
Median waiting time (in days), 2003-2004	Status 1A, 50 Status 1B, 78 Status 2, 309	Cystic fibrosis, 587 COPD, 1349 Pulmonary fibrosis, 1115
1-year survival (all status)	87.3%	83.1%
5-year survival	70.9%	46.3%

Data from: http://optn.transplant.hrsa.gov/latestData/step2.asp?

Box 40-1 **General Criteria for Transplant Waiting Lists**

- Age (under 65)
- Terminal illness (expected life span less than 1 year)
- Nonsmoker
- Adequate social support system
- Disease free in other systems

Organ Transplant Act of the United States Congress in 1984 and is administered by the private, nonprofit organization United Network for Organ Sharing (UNOS), under contract with the U.S Department of Health and Human Services. An organ procurement organization (OPO) coordinates the management of the organ donor and family, the transplant center, and the recipient.[3]

The number of organs available for transplant remains well below the need for donor organs. Currently, there are over 110,000 individuals on the national waiting list for all organs, with over 3200 candidates waiting for heart transplant and approximately 1800 candidates waiting for lung transplant. A general list of criteria for patient selection for transplant is presented in Box 40-1. Names of patients on the waiting list are filed in the UNOS Organ Center, a centralized database that links transplant centers with OPOs. Once an organ donor has been identified, a computer-generated list of potential recipients is ranked, according to the criteria established for each organ. Criteria may include blood or tissue type, size of organ, medical status of the patient, and amount of time a patient has been on the waiting list. The organ procurement coordinator confers with the transplant surgeons until a potential recipient is identified. Surgical teams then travel to the donor hospital while the recipient is concurrently prepared for surgery. Heart, lung, and liver transplantation success is optimized when transplant occurs within 6 hours after removing the donated organ. Surgical methods that allow for longer travel times or changes in management of the donor organ have increased the number of available organs; however, the number of available organs still remains significantly below the need.

Policies were updated by the UNOS in 2006 to decrease the number of patients dying while waiting for transplant. These changes increased the number of transplants for the most severely ill patients awaiting heart transplant.[4]

Issues Associated with Transplantation

There are many ethical, psychological, and social concerns surrounding organ transplantation. Ethical issues relate to increasing potential donor sources and distributing available organs. Psychological issues include stress due to an unknown waiting time, the potential of moving from one's home to a location near a transplant center, and possible employment disruption. The transplant process affects not only the individual patient, but the patient's social support systems as well. This is highly significant because adequate social support is a factor in long-term transplant success and quality of life.[5]

Ethical Considerations

The ethical considerations of organ transplantation relate to increasing potential donor sources and distributing available organs. The bioethical issues involved in the selection of appropriate organ donors continue to generate considerable debate. For example, one important issue is whether the donor's family should be compensated monetarily for the organ donation. Currently, there can be no legally accepted monetary gain from organ donation in this country.

Other bioethical considerations include how to allocate the available organs to individuals waiting for transplant. All patients are screened for medical and psychological conditions that would adversely affect the outcome of transplantation. The specific acceptance criteria are different for each organ; lung transplant criteria differ from heart transplantation criteria. OPTN policies specify that each transplant center will create its own specific policies.[6] In general, waiting list time remains the primary factor that determines who is next in line to receive an available organ; however, other matching factors are considered for each available organ. Patients who are current smokers are not candidates for lung transplantation, although most centers allow former smokers to qualify for a lung transplant. Patients with documented alcohol abuse are not candidates for transplantation. Criteria are used so that individual preferences of team members are not given priority. In addition, ethnicity, gender, religion, and financial status are not part of the transplant criteria.

Psychological and Social Considerations

There are many psychological issues associated with organ transplantation, such as feelings of uncertainty, upheaval associated with moving, and issues of psychological adjustment. The time spent waiting for a transplant can vary considerably. During the waiting period, patients struggle with the need to carry on their lives, knowing that at any moment they may be called to the hospital for transplant. In addition, the patient is torn between wanting to remain hopeful that a transplant will provide new life and the reality of knowing they have a terminal condition. Anxiety and depression have been identified as prevalent psychological issues related to transplant.[7]

The number of transplant centers in the United States is limited. Because donor organs are viable for only hours after removal from the donor, patients waiting for transplant are frequently required to live within a several-hour radius of the transplant center. Patients need information and logistics assistance for relocation to a transplant center. They may also require emotional and financial support for this transition.[8] The demands of waiting and relocation to the transplant city put considerable stress on the patient and their significant others. Those patients who relocate to transplant centers may have the most difficult time psychologically, especially when they leave family and significant others behind. The psychological stresses are somewhat different for spouses. Spouses speak of the struggle to remain hopeful, yet plan for a future that may not include their loved one. If the patient and spouse move together to a new city to wait for transplant, they may find themselves with more time together than previously. In this "forced retirement" situation, new stresses are added to relationships. Transplant teams usually include a psychologist or social worker to whom patients may be referred for individual or family counseling if needed.

Other concerns include psychological adjustment and the effect of social supports on mediating coping skills. Feelings of being useless are common because patients waiting in a new city are outside of their own environment and must find some meaningful activities. Coping strategies appear to strengthen psychological outcomes. After transplant, patients are often emotionally overwhelmed with a feeling of gratefulness that they are alive and feelings of guilt that someone else's grief has given them a chance to rejoice. A strong support system is considered an essential component of a successful transplant and improves psychosocial outcomes after transplantation.[9] Therapists can assist patients by listening to feelings, being supportive, and encouraging participation in support groups. Support groups that include patients waiting for transplants as well as posttransplant patients can offer significant psychosocial support. Spouses and significant others also benefit from group support.

Physical Therapy Considerations

As important members of the transplant team, physical therapists need an understanding of the physiological components of both the pretransplant disease and posttransplant state, as well as knowledge of the influence of surgery, medications, or rejection on musculoskeletal structure and function. In addition, physical function may be decreased due to the primary cardiopulmonary condition and overall deconditioning. Knowledge of medical management, including medications, ventilatory support, and hemodynamic monitoring, assists the therapist in determining whether modifications are needed during rehabilitation.

Physical therapists have a role in the management of the transplant patient in all stages of transplant: before transplant, during the acute postoperative phase, and throughout the rehabilitation phase. The purpose of physical therapy before transplant is to identify baseline function and to screen for impairments that may limit rehabilitation goals. The pretransplantation period offers an opportunity to address limitations in strength and range of motion or endurance and to improve physical function. Because of the surgical intervention, bed mobility, ventilation, secretion management, range of motion, and pain control are important areas to address in the immediate postoperative phase. In the posttransplantation rehabilitation phase, physical therapy goals are to return the patient to the highest functional level. Upper and lower extremity muscle strength and range of motion are addressed, as well as posture, shoulder and trunk mobility, breathing pattern, breath sounds, and functional mobility.

Oxygen Transport

Cardiac and pulmonary conditions leading to transplant produce limitations in the oxygen transport pathway. An understanding of the limitations in the oxygen transport pathway assists the therapist in designing a plan of care specific for each individual. Oxygen transport may be affected by the primary disease process, the surgical or medical intervention, or the medications used posttransplant. Cardiac conditions lead to impairments in myocardial function, leading to decreased oxygen availability for daily activities. Peripheral muscle dysfunction often occurs concurrently with the myocardial condition.

Pulmonary conditions lead to impairments in the mechanics of the lungs and chest wall, as well as diffusion abnormalities, producing a low blood oxygen content that is inadequate for daily activities. Myocardial function may be decreased secondary to increased vascular resistance in the lung. Likewise, peripheral utilization of oxygen may be decreased as a result of the pulmonary condition or inactivity.

Surgical and Medical Considerations

Physical therapists need to consider the effect of surgery, medication, or rejection on oxygen transport and functional ability. In patients who have undergone a surgical procedure, physical therapists must identify and manage problems related to anesthesia, pain control, hemodynamic instability, and alterations in muscle function, depending on the site of surgical incisions. The medication regimen for patients following organ transplant is complex and, in many cases, more cumbersome than the medical management of the underlying condition. Patients must take immunosuppressant medications for the rest of their lives. These medications, along with others used to manage the symptoms related to the immunosuppressants, have consequences for peripheral muscle function and energy production. Limitations in physical function may be due to the primary condition, the lack of physical activity, and the side effects of medications. Specifics will be covered later in this chapter.

The principal limitation to survival is graft rejection. Although advances in immune suppression have been successful, graft rejection remains a difficult medical problem. During the first year after transplant, the primary causes of morbidity and mortality relate to acute cellular rejection and infection. In the long term, chronic rejection is problematic. In heart transplant patients, cardiac allograft vasculopathy, an accelerated form of atherosclerosis, remains a primary limitation to long-term survival.

Rehabilitation of the Transplant Patient

To assist in management of the patient with transplant, rehabilitation is categorized into the following four phases: (1) pretransplant, (2) surgery and the postoperative acute phase, (3) postoperative outpatient phase, and (4) community- or home-based phase. Although the ultimate goal of transplant rehabilitation is to improve the patient's function and quality of life, each phase of rehabilitation has its own emphasis.

Pretransplant Rehabilitation

Heart Transplant and End-Stage Cardiac Disease

Patients are referred for heart transplantation for end-stage cardiac conditions. The primary diagnoses for adults requiring a heart transplant are severe coronary artery disease (38%) and end-stage cardiomyopathy/heart failure (53%). In children under 1 year, the primary diagnosis requiring transplant is congenital cardiac abnormalities; for ages 1-10, cardiomyopathy.[10]

Patients with heart failure report symptoms of fatigue, dyspnea, and orthopnea. Physical signs include the presence of a third heart sound, pulmonary rales that do not reverse with coughing, jugular venous distension, peripheral edema, and hepatomegaly. Compensatory mechanisms include increased sympathetic nervous system activity, increasing resting heart rate, and activation of the rennin-angiotensin system, increasing blood pressure.

Patients with heart failure generally meet the heart transplant selection criteria if they have New York Heart Association (NYHA) class III or IV heart failure that is unresponsive to medical management. Specific criteria for recipient status vary somewhat from center to center, although International Society for Heart and Lung Transplantation (ISHLT) criteria for listing are generally followed.[11] Exercise testing criteria can be used to guide transplantation. Patients who complete a maximum test may be eligible for a heart transplant if peak $\dot{V}O_2$ is ≤14 mL/kg/min, or ≤12 mL/kg/min if on a beta blocker.[11]

Recipients waiting for heart transplantation are classified based on severity of disease. Patients in the worst medical condition (Status IA) are placed higher on the transplant recipient list. Table 40-2 outlines the criteria for each level of heart transplant recipient status.

Pretransplant management of the patient with heart failure is designed to preserve cardiac output until the transplant can be completed. Outpatient medical management includes medications and supplemental oxygen. Hospitalization may be needed for inotropic medication support such as dobutamine. The increased use of left or right ventricular assist devices (LVAD or RVADs) augments cardiac output and allows the patient a bridge to transplantation.

The main rehabilitation goal in the preoperative period is to prevent losses of physical function. Maintenance of range of motion, soft tissue extensibility, and muscle strength are suggested goals. Although patients with severe disease may be unable to participate in therapy, cardiac rehabilitation is an effective treatment for improving functional status of patients with significant heart failure and those with LVADs, whether or not transplantation is anticipated.[12,13] Recent literature demonstrates that medically supervised exercise training is both safe and effective at improving aerobic capacity and physical function in patients with LVAD devices awaiting heart transplantation.

Table 40-2 **Heart Transplant Recipient Status**

Status Level	Status Criteria
Status IA	Mechanical circulatory support for acute hemodynamic decompensation Mechanical circulatory support with objective medical evidence of significant device-related complications Continuous mechanical ventilation Continuous infusion of a single high-dose intravenous inotrope
Status IB	Patients require at least one of either of the following: a. Left or right ventricular assist device b. Continuous infusion of intravenous inotropes
Status II	Those patients not meeting Status IA or IB criteria

Source: http://optn.transplant.hrsa.gov/PoliciesandBylaws2/policies/pdfs/Policy_9.pdf

Lung Transplant and End-Stage Pulmonary Disease

Patients are referred for lung transplantation for end-stage pulmonary conditions. The primary diagnoses for adults requiring a lung transplant are severe chronic obstructive pulmonary disease (COPD) (44%), idiopathic pulmonary fibrosis (IPF) (17%), and cystic fibrosis (CF) (15%). Other conditions include pulmonary arterial hypertension (PAH). The guidelines for selection of patients for the lung transplant waiting list were updated by the ISHLT in 2006 and include specific criteria for the most common pulmonary conditions.[14,15] Within the disease-specific listing criteria for COPD, the guidelines include a BODE (body mass index, airflow obstruction, dyspnea, and exercise capacity) score of 7-10. The BODE is more useful than measures of airflow obstruction in predicting mortality from COPD; higher scores are associated with increased mortality.[16] Before 2005, patients who had accrued the most time on the waiting list were given priority for lung transplants. The change to a lung allocation score now gives priority for transplants to those patients who have a greater medical urgency for transplant. The lung allocation score is based on "(i) waitlist urgency measure (expected number of days lived without a transplant during an additional year on the waitlist), (ii) posttransplant survival measure (expected number of days lived during the first year posttransplant), and (iii) transplant benefit measure (posttransplant survival measure minus waitlist urgency measure)."[17] The urgency and survival measures are based on factors that predict risk for death in patients with lung transplant and include functional status as well as physiological measures. This change has increased the number of transplants for patients with IPF and slowed the number of transplants for COPD.[14]

Table 40-3 Preoperative Pulmonary Rehabilitation

Activity	Time	Specific Activities	Targeted Area Exercise and Intensity
Warm-up (group)	10 minutes	Active range of motion	Upper body Lower body Trunk
Individualized endurance program	10 to 30 minutes (may be done as intervals)	Cycle ergometer	25 to 30 watts
		Treadmill	0.8 to 1.5 mph, 0% to 5% grade
		Arm ergometer	0 to 25 watts (forward or backward)
Individualized strength program	15 to 20 minutes	1 set of 8-12 repetitions	Pulleys Theraband
		Upper extremities	Latissimus pull-downs Rhomboids Shoulder extension/ rotation Shoulder flexion Pectoral Triceps
		Lower extremities	Quadriceps Hip extensors Hip abductors
Cool-down (group)	10 minutes	Stretching (full-body) Breathing retraining Relaxation	

Idiopathic pulmonary fibrosis is characterized by scarring of lung parenchyma leading to decreased lung volumes and decreased diffusing capacity. Risk factors for mortality include the lung pathology, pulmonary function results, physical function from the 6-minute walk test, and respiratory failure.[14] Criteria for listing of patients with IPF include a decrease in FVC of 10% or more during 6 months and pulse oximetry less than 88% during a 6-minute walk test.[15] Patients with IPF waiting for lung transplant who walked less than 679 feet had higher mortality than those who walked longer distances.[18]

Recent advances in vasodilator therapy for patients with pulmonary artery hypertension and poor survival of patients with PAH after transplant have reduced the number of patients with PAH who receive lung transplants. The criteria for listing patients with PAH include an NYHA class III or IV status on the maximal vasodilator therapy and 6-minute walk test of less than 350 meters.[15]

In patients with cystic fibrosis, the predictors of mortality include declining FEV_1 and chronic infection. The current criteria for transplant include FEV_1 less than 30% of predicted, as well as other markers of declining pulmonary function.[19]

Pulmonary rehabilitation is an essential component of management of patients with chronic lung conditions even without transplant, and it is becoming an accepted requirement for patients awaiting lung transplantation. Clinical data from pulmonary rehabilitation programs suggest that patients with better physical function before transplant have improved posttransplantation outcomes.

The causes of exercise limitation in people with chronic lung conditions are both ventilatory and musculoskeletal. Muscle changes in pulmonary conditions include decreased muscle oxidative capacity and muscle weakness.[20] Reasonable goals for pretransplant rehabilitation include improvement in muscle strength in lower extremity musculature, functional upper extremity muscle strength and endurance, functional shoulder and chest wall range of motion, demonstration of coordinated diaphragmatic breathing with exercise and activities, and improved cardiovascular endurance. Because of the significant effect of immunosuppressive medications on muscle strength, a greater emphasis is placed on resistance training in a patient awaiting lung transplantation than in most typical pulmonary rehabilitation programs. An example of a preoperative pulmonary rehabilitation program is outlined in Table 40-3.

Patient Education

The pretransplant waiting period provides an ideal opportunity for patient education. Nursing generally provides much of the education regarding preoperative procedures, postoperative course, and medication. Rehabilitation teaching includes breathing training, airway clearance techniques, and activity progression.

Other Transplants

Patients awaiting other organ transplants may also be referred to physical therapy for treatment of musculoskeletal problems. Because of the level of metabolic abnormality in patients awaiting liver and kidney transplants, endurance training is difficult to perform. Other physical therapy interventions, however, may be used as appropriate (i.e., muscle strengthening, range of motion).

Surgical Implications

Surgical procedures have implications for the physical therapist in the areas of pain, abnormal hemodynamic responses, and movement patterns. The surgical approach for transplant is chosen to provide the surgeon the optimal working area and visual field. The choice of incision may affect patient comfort and function after surgery. Patients may experience pain in the area of the incision, and they may present with decreased muscle function and joint pain related to the muscles that were incised during surgery. The physical therapist should be familiar with the surgical incisions and their impact on rehabilitation. Other related complications from thoracic transplant include injury to the phrenic nerve, brachial plexus injury, and peroneal nerve injury secondary to prolonged positioning during surgery and recovery.

Heart transplants are usually performed through a median sternotomy incision and require cardiopulmonary bypass.[21] The native heart is excised, leaving a portion of the right atrium (atrial cuff), including the SA node. The left atrium of the donor heart is sutured to the recipient's atrial cuff and the major vessels reattached, starting with the pulmonary arterial vessels and followed by the aorta. Drainage tubes are placed in the pleural and mediastinal spaces and an epicardial pacing wire is placed before closure of the sternum. Total heart ischemic time is minimized, with less than 4 hours recommended. Finally, the two halves of the sternum are wired together, the new heart defibrillated, cardiopulmonary bypass discontinued, and the patient awakened.

Lung transplantation surgical incisions depend on whether a single- or double-lung transplant is to be performed. Single-lung transplants are performed through a standard posterolateral thoracotomy incision, made through the fifth rib. The latissimus dorsi and lower trapezius muscles are incised, as are the intercostal muscles at this level. If the rib at the surgical level fractures, it is resected so that the bone ends do not rub or puncture the lung. The serratus anterior muscle is preserved if at all possible, but the lateral portion of the rhomboid may be cut to allow more access for the surgeon. Postoperative pain and impaired upper quarter movement patterns may present significant problems for patients.

Double-lung transplants are performed as two single-lung transplants, in a technique referred to as bilateral sequential lung transplantation. The surgical incision extends from the midaxillary line under the submammary fold to the other midaxillary line and may or may not use a transverse sternotomy.[22] In this technique, called the clamshell incision, the pectoralis major is separated from the chest wall, and the serratus anterior may be incised.[23] Complications from this technique include sternal overlap if a transverse sternotomy is used.

Acute Phase Rehabilitation

The acute phase of rehabilitation begins in the intensive care unit and continues throughout the patient's hospital stay. Interventions are focused on facilitating normal cardiovascular and pulmonary function and increasing functional abilities in self-care and ambulation.

Heart Transplant Acute Management

Postoperative management of the patient following heart transplantation is similar to that of other cardiac surgeries. Patients experience hemodynamic instability, dysrhythmias, pulmonary hypertension, coagulopathies, and acute rejection. Factors that can lead to a complicated postoperative course include length of ischemic time and reperfusion injury. Prolonged ischemic time is associated with graft dysfunction.[24] Reperfusion injury is also associated with poor short-term outcomes.

Patients are weaned from mechanical ventilation within 24-36 hours, and chest tubes and pacing wires are removed after 2 days. During this time, there is a risk of acute cellular rejection. Acute cellular rejection is characterized by lymphocyte and myocyte infiltration into the cardiac muscle, resulting in dyspnea, fatigue, and heart failure. The symptoms of acute cellular rejection are often mild; therefore patients undergo cardiac biopsy at regular intervals to identify the presence of rejection. Biopsy specimens are obtained by inserting a catheter in the jugular or subclavian vein into the right atrium. Humoral rejection is observed in the first weeks or months after an organ transplant. Humoral rejection is considered an immune system response that results in inflammation and thickening of the endothelial lining of the cardiac vessels.

Current guidelines for management of patients with heart transplant include a recommendation for a multidisciplinary team that meets regularly.[25]

EXERCISE GUIDELINES

Goals of the acute phase of rehabilitation include the following: (1) regain normal postural cardiovascular responses (no postural hypotension) and (2) increase functional activities. The former is focused on the patient being able to tolerate changes in position, increase time in upright sitting, and transfer independently. Upper and lower extremity range of motion and strength need to be adequate to perform activities of daily living. An example of a cardiac rehabilitation program is presented in Table 40-4.

Specific issues for physical therapists include abnormal ECG and cardiovascular control. ECG readings may be normal because the donor heart has an intact conduction system, although the atrial cuff from the native heart may cause the ECG to have two P waves. Control of cardiovascular responses is altered because of cardiac denervation that occurs with surgery. When the donor heart is removed, the extrinsic nervous supply including vagus nerve and sympathetic trunk are severed. Consequently, there is no direct innervation to the heart to control heart rate response during change in position or exercise. Heart rate and stroke volume increase as a result of the effect of preload, as demonstrated by the Frank-Starling law, and through circulation of catecholamines. For the physical therapist, this means that heart rate and blood pressure respond more slowly to changes in position and exercise and require a longer time between position of activity changes. Other complications of heart transplant include sternum instability, infection, and pain.

In the rehabilitation process, median sternotomy precautions may need to be observed. Emerging evidence suggests that activity may be progressed more quickly than previously thought.[26] Principles of inpatient cardiac rehabilitation are followed in the postoperative period. Patient activity is progressed as long as a normal physiological response in achieved.

Lung Transplant Acute Management

Postoperative management of the patient following lung transplantation begins in the intensive care unit. After lung transplantation, patients are generally mechanically ventilated for 24 to 72 hours. Often, paralytic agents are used in this period so that ventilation can be optimized. Chest tubes are likely in place, and patients are medicated for pain. Infection

Table 40-4 University Hospital Cardiovascular Rehabilitation Supervised Exercise/Activity Plan for Surgical Patients

Step	METS	Exercise	Activity
1	1.5	Active/passive ROM, in bed for 5 reps Turn, cough, deep breathe, and use incentive spirometer q2-4 h	Partial self-care Feed self Use of bedside commode
2	1.5-2.0	Active ROM, sit on edge of bed for 5 reps Teach rating perceived exertion (RPE)	Partial/complete self-care Sitting bed bath Up in chair for meals
3	2.0	Walk 100 feet, slow pace Active ROM 10 reps	Complete self-care Incentive spirometer independently, TID
4	2.5	Walk 150 feet, average pace Teach pulse counting Warm-ups, standing for 10 reps	Use of bathroom with assistance May take warm shower after pacer wire removed
5	3.0-3.5	Walk 300 feet, average pace Walk down flight of stairs Instruct in home exercise	May stand at sink for ADLs Dressing independently
6	4.0	Walk up flight stairs Walk 500 feet, average pace Schedule submax ETT Enroll in phase II rehabilitation	All self-care independently

Guidelines for Exercise:
Patient HR to be 50 to 120 bpm
No significant arrhythmias
Exercise HR not more than 20 beats above rest
SBP <200, DBP <120 during exercise
No worsening ST changes
<10 to 15 DBP drop during exercise
RPE of 10 or less
No angina or other symptoms
Patient to complete entire step before advancing to next step

control is imperative; isolation rooms with negative-pressure ventilation are used, and respiratory isolation procedures are maintained.

Problems in the immediate lung transplantation period include ineffective airway clearance, poor gas exchange, and rejection. Hypotension and hypoxemia can lead to decreased blood flow at the site of anastomosis for the new lung, creating necrotic changes and impairment in airflow. Problems with airway clearance are related to the denervation of the transplanted lung, specifically the autonomic nervous system pathways. The lack of innervation leads to ineffective cough and ciliary clearance. Problems with gas exchange occur as a result of postoperative edema.

EXERCISE GUIDELINES

In the immediate postoperative period, the major goals are to prevent lung infection, optimize ventilation-perfusion ratio, increase time out of bed, and increase active range of motion on the surgical side. The primary goals are to mobilize the patient out of bed and increase daily activity. Patients are encouraged to be out of bed and walk in the hallway; in some cases, a stationary ergometer is used to increase endurance (ergometer can be brought to the room). Therapeutic interventions vary greatly. In general, an intervention may continue until an abnormal exercise response is reached. Abnormal responses include a decrease in heart rate or blood pressure with an increase in exercise, a decrease in oxygen saturation below recommended levels (88% to 90%), and/or symptoms of dizziness and diaphoresis.

Airway clearance is an essential component of acute care management. Many techniques are considered appropriate. Breathing training that targets diaphragm function is considered an essential component of acute management of the patient following lung transplantation. Suggested goals and interventions are shown in Table 40-5.

Posttransplant Outpatient Rehabilitation

Rejection

A common complication of organ transplantation is organ rejection. Acute rejection occurs within the first 6 months of transplantation, whereas chronic rejection remains a long-term problem. Rejection episodes are monitored closely, often with biopsy, and treated with a variety of immune suppressant medications.

Acute rejection is mediated by T cells. These T cells infiltrate the new organ allograft, and multiply, causing tissue destruction. Chronic rejection initially appears as hypertrophy of the intima in the transplanted organ and then progresses to fibrosis. In heart transplants, chronic rejection may also be seen as accelerated atherosclerosis. In lung transplants, chronic rejection appears in the airways as bronchiolitis obliterans. No effective treatment exists for chronic rejection.

Table 40-5 **Goals and Interventions for Acute Posttransplant Rehabilitation: Lung Transplant**

Problem	Goal	Interventions
Decreased secretion clearance	Independent secretion management Because the lungs are denervated, there is decreased sensation of secretions	Incentive spirometer Airway clearance techniques Assisted cough Positioning, single-lung: operative side up while side-lying to facilitate drainage; double-lung: avoid supine
Incisional pain	Pain management Postoperative pain related to surgical incision and decreased movement of muscles	Pain medication Active range of motion, shoulder girdle Positioning Mild heat Massage/soft tissue techniques
Abnormal postural hemodynamic responses	Normalize hemodynamic response (i.e., no postural hypotension, normal heart rate, respiratory rate, and blood pressure response to exercise)	Progressive mobilization from supine to sitting, sit in chair, walking in room Monitor HR, BP, RR, $Sa{O_2}$
Increased oxygen/ventilatory requirements	Adequate oxygenation without supplemental ($Sa{O_2}$ 94%-96% on room air) Normal vital capacity Diaphragmatic breathing	Instruction of diaphragmatic breathing Facilitation of diaphragmatic breathing Lateral costal expansion techniques (surgery side) Incentive spirometry
Decreased functional mobility	Independent activities of daily living (dressing, hygiene, shower, toilet) Need adequate shoulder range of motion to perform these activities	Active and active-assisted range of motion, shoulder Wand exercises Encourage and assist with activities of daily living (hygiene, shower, toilet)
Decreased exercise tolerance	Independent transfers Independent ambulation 500 feet Out of bed most of day	Daily schedule Assisted ambulation (room progressing to hallway) Bicycle in room, 2 minutes initially; progress to 10 minutes
Compromised nutrition	No supplemental feedings (IV)	Schedule rehabilitation around meals Medical management of nausea

Heart Transplant

After heart transplant, patients continue to experience decreased aerobic capacity and endurance, muscle atrophy, and decreased physical function. In addition, immune suppression increases the risk for infection and leads to loss of muscle and bone. Rejection remains a significant risk, and heart transplant patients are likely to acquire premature atherosclerosis. Despite these problems, aerobic capacity and physical function are amenable to rehabilitation.[27] Common long-term impairments are chest wall soreness, abnormal upper quarter movement patterns, and low back and knee pain from overuse. Once the patient leaves the hospital, rehabilitation looks much like phase II cardiac rehabilitation. The overall objective is to increase functional activity to within normal limits.

CARDIAC AND RESPIRATORY PHYSIOLOGY IN HEART TRANSPLANT

After transplantation, functional capacity is about 50% of the capacity of control subjects; abnormalities in heart rate, blood pressure, and ventilatory abnormalities also exist during this period. In posttransplant patients, peak heart rate is lower than in controls (156 versus 168 beats/minute),[28] although heart rate kinetics are not different.[29] In regard to long-term effects of heart transplantation on heart rate, some children who have received heart transplantation do acquire a normal heart rate response to exercise.[30] The ventilatory response to exercise is abnormal, as demonstrated by a decreased diffusing capacity.[31] However, there may be some peripheral limitations that contribute to decreased functional capacity; these include decreased capillary density in muscle.[32] A summary of how cardiac variables are affected by heart transplant is shown in Table 40-6.

SIGNS OF REJECTION

The primary signs and symptoms of rejection are flu-like symptoms, including low-grade fever and muscle aches. Dysrhythmias and bradycardia below 60 or relative bradycardia (decreased compared with patient's normal resting heart rate) are significant and should be reported to the physician immediately. Rejection episodes are monitored by biopsy. Exercise can continue if the rejection episode is mild or moderate as determined by biopsy.

EXERCISE AND THE HEART TRANSPLANT PATIENT

Exercise training is important for reversing the physiological abnormalities observed after heart transplant, returning patients to improved functional status, and preventing disability incurred from the immunosuppressant regimen. The outpatient phase of rehabilitation resembles phase II cardiac rehabilitation, which generally continues for 8 to 12 weeks, at which time the patient is encouraged to continue exercise on his or her own or at a fitness facility. ISHLT guidelines for care address health-related issues for patients after heart transplant. Hypertension after heart transplant should be treated to achieve the same goals as the general population, and

Table 40-6 Effect of Heart Transplant on Selected Cardiovascular Variables As Compared with Normal Age-Predicted Values

	Heart Rate	Stroke Volume	Blood Pressure	$\dot{V}o_2$
Rest	Lower than normal	Lower than normal with little change when shifting positions	+	NA
Exercise	Lower (approximately 15 beats less)	Decreased and late onset	+	May approximate normal with exercise training program

Box 40-2 Summary Guidelines for Posttransplant Cardiac Rehabilitation

- Use cardiac rehabilitation phase II protocols
- Heart rate is not best indicator of exercise intensity
- Increase warm-up and cool-down to 10 to 15 minutes
- RPE in conjunction with other physiological monitoring (e.g. RPP)
- No exercise when patient is in acute rejection episode (biopsy needed)
- Continue exercise in mild rejection

lifestyle modifications are the same as for others with cardiac risk factors.[25]Aerobic exercise and resistance training are recommended. Guidelines for exercise for the posttransplant cardiac patient are shown in Box 40-2.

After heart transplantation, there is no direct innervation to the heart to control heart rate response during exercise. Heart rate and stroke volume increase due to the effect of increased preload and through circulation of catecholamines. There is evidence that some sympathetic re-innervation can occur 1-2 years after transplant.[33] For the patient in phase II cardiac rehabilitation, this means that the warm-up and cool-down portions of exercise should be *slowly* increased to 10 to 15 minutes. Exercise intensity should not be determined by heart rate alone, because of the effects of denervation. In addition, rating of perceived exertion (RPE) scales remain an unreliable method for determining exercise intensity after heart transplant, because large inter-individual variations occur in the relationship of RPE and maximal oxygen consumption.[34] Although there is no strong clinical consensus about the optimal method for prescribing and monitoring exercise intensity for patients following heart transplant, ventilatory threshold, rate-pressure product (RPP), or a combination of RPE and physiological monitoring is recommended. Evidence suggests that patients with heart transplants can exercise at high intensity and achieve better functional outcomes than sedentary individuals without transplant.[35] Intensity set at 10% below anaerobic threshold produced significant increases in aerobic capacity.[36] Endurance and strength exercise can be performed in this rehabilitation stage, although upper extremity strengthening should not be started until after the sternum has healed. Treadmill, bike, arm ergometry, and indoor cross-country ski equipment are all appropriate choices.[37]

Cardiac rehabilitation can result in substantial increases in aerobic capacity with patients able to improve 20% to 50% over prerehabilitation levels. The mechanisms that contribute to increased aerobic capacity include increased maximal heart rate, improved ventilatory capacity, and improved peripheral muscle function.[38] Supervised exercise programs lead to greater increases in aerobic capacity than do home exercise programs (49% versus 18% improvement, respectively).[27] Resistance training has been used in patients following heart transplantation as an essential component of cardiac rehabilitation to improve physical function and prevent losses of muscle strength associated with corticosteroid use. Resistance training does appear to increase bone mineral density to nearly pretransplant levels.[39] Resistance training increases oxidative capacity of muscles[40] and also prevents adverse effects of corticosteroids and immune therapy on skeletal muscle.

Despite the evidence that cardiac rehabilitation is beneficial in increasing aerobic capacity and exercise capacity, scant literature exists to suggest that exercise training prevents transplant atherosclerosis. Early studies of patients after renal transplant, however, show promising results of exercise in preventing atherosclerosis.[41]

Lung Transplant

Patients who have received a lung transplant may be referred to physical therapy as early as 10 to 14 days after transplantation occurs. In the early stages of this postoperative outpatient phase, patients are medically labile and need once- or twice-a-week monitoring of their medical status. Rehabilitation should progress in this phase, but close communication with medical personnel is recommended because of the many medication changes. Blood levels of immunosuppressive drugs are monitored, along with metabolic function (fluid and electrolyte levels, kidney and liver function).

CARDIAC AND RESPIRATORY PHYSIOLOGY IN LUNG TRANSPLANT

After lung transplant, patients continue to experience decreased aerobic capacity and endurance, muscle atrophy, and decreased physical function. In addition, immune suppression increases the risk for infection and leads to loss of muscle and bone. Rejection remains a significant risk. Despite these problems, aerobic capacity and physical function are amenable to rehabilitation. Patients in the outpatient phase of rehabilitation begin at low levels of function and progress to having few functional limitations. Therapists need to adapt and progress the rehabilitation program appropriately. Because of the debilitating side effects of immunosuppressive medications, rehabilitation needs to be aggressive and preventive in nature. Rehabilitation can occur in a group setting and/or on

Box 40-3 Summary Guidelines for Posttransplant Lung Rehabilitation

- Keep $Sa{O_2}$ above 90%
- Add supplemental oxygen, if necessary, during treated acute rejection episodes
- Patient should wear mask when with people
- Increase resistance exercise program during prednisone bursts
- Evaluate for musculoskeletal dysfunction

an individual basis. General guidelines for posttransplant lung rehabilitation are shown in Box 40-3.

After transplantation, functional capacity remains between 40% and 60% of predicted oxygen uptake, whether the patient received a single- or double-lung transplant.[42] Although there are mild ventilatory abnormalities, the decreased $\dot{V}O_2$ is not well explained by the decrease in ventilation or by low oxygen saturation or anemia. Instead, several articles suggest that the main cause of decreased aerobic capacity is a peripheral muscle limitation. Problems in the periphery include decreased peripheral oxygen utilization, decreased mitochondrial capacity and decreased type I fibers, as well as decreased muscle power.[20,43]

SIGNS OF REJECTION

The primary symptoms of acute rejection are shortness of breath, exercise intolerance, and desaturation at rest or with exercise. Patients generally have a portable oximeter at home and may report episodes of desaturation. Rejection should be suspected and reported if a decrease in $Sa{O_2}$ of 4% to 5% for the same amount of activity is seen. Monitoring of ventilatory status should be the primary consideration of the therapist. Respiratory rate and oxygen saturation should be followed closely during exercise sessions.

EXERCISE AND THE LUNG TRANSPLANT PATIENT

Patients are generally excited about the improvement in shortness of breath and frequently surprised at the level of muscle weakness observed in the lower extremities. Once ventilation is no longer a limiting factor in function, other deficits emerge. In the initial stages of outpatient rehabilitation, patients may have multiple complaints about the side effects of medications and often generally do not feel well. Rehabilitation should continue through these periods of malaise. The overall objective of outpatient rehabilitation is to improve function to levels appropriate for the patient's age and interests. Usually, patients are closely followed by the medical staff for 2 to 3 months after transplant, and rehabilitation 2 to 3 times per week continues throughout this period. The most common impairments that limit function are decreased cardiopulmonary endurance, decreased muscle strength and endurance, range of motion limitations, and abnormal movement patterns of the shoulder or trunk. Impairments may be caused by the surgical procedure itself or as a result of years of abnormal muscle mechanics, posture, and decreased activity.

Aerobic exercise training for patients with lung transplantation provides substantial benefits in aerobic capacity. Frequency of exercise at least three times per week, intensity of 60% to 70% of heart rate maximum or RPE of 13 to 14, and duration of at least 30 minutes created significant increases in aerobic capacity.[42] Studies demonstrated an increase of aerobic capacity to 60% of prerehabilitation levels and decreased heart rate and ventilation for the same amount of submaximal exercise, indicating a training effect. After 6 to 12 weeks of training, $\dot{V}O_{2max}$ and $\dot{V}O_{2peak}$ increased as much as 14% over baseline testing and increased exercise time from 20 to 30 minutes.[42] The mechanisms by which aerobic capacity increases include decreased resting minute ventilation, suggesting increased efficiency of oxygen utilization. In addition, in two cohort studies, 6-MWD increased significantly.[20,44]

Peripheral muscle deconditioning contributes to decreased exercise ability and limited physical function. Lower extremity muscle strength can occur with resistance training. One study demonstrated a 35% increase in quadriceps force to almost 60% of that predicted after training, at 60% of 1-repetition maximum (1RM).[20] Lower extremity strengthening can begin early, but upper extremity resistive training should be delayed until wound and tissue healing is complete, generally about 6 weeks because of the delays in wound healing secondary to use of prednisone. Other important aspects of rehabilitation include posture reeducation, range of motion, and upper extremity movement patterns. Guidelines for outpatient physical therapy are provided in Table 40-7.

To improve physical function following lung transplantation, a pulmonary rehabilitation protocol may be used, or the therapist may creatively design a rehabilitation program. Except for delaying upper extremity strengthening for 6 weeks after surgery, no therapeutic interventions are contraindicated. For endurance training, stationary bicycles, treadmills, arm ergometers, indoor Nordic ski machines, rowers, and stair climbers may be used. Pulleys, weight equipment, free weights, resistive elastic bands, or gymnastic balls all may be appropriate for strengthening and facilitation of normal movement patterns. Because of the effects of prednisone, proximal muscle function must be addressed, and strengthening programs should be consistent with those designed to increase muscle force production, generally one set of 8 to 12 repetitions at 60% of 1RM. Once a patient has achieved a satisfactory level of function (determined by the therapist and patient), formal rehabilitation may be discontinued and the patient should participate in a community- or home-based rehabilitation program.

Community- or Home-Based Rehabilitation

Patients are generally followed at the transplant center until the medical staff is satisfied with patient progress. Return to home can occur at this point in time, whether or not rehabilitation goals have been met. For patients who have left their home community to wait for transplant, the transition to home frequently occurs at 3 months after transplant. The major goal of community-based rehabilitation is a return to normal function with minimal limitations. Therapists in rural settings and community hospitals may be involved with a transplant patient's plan of care in this phase. Therapists should be comfortable treating patients in many settings, skilled in addressing the common complications, and vigilant in watching for signs of rejection. In the initial stages of posttransplant rehabilitation, a supervised program is recommended. Hospital-based phase III cardiac rehabilitation

Table 40-7 Lung Transplant: Postoperative Outpatient Physical Therapy Management

Problem	Goal	Activity
Decreased aerobic capacity	Daily functional activities including leisure 30-minute aerobic exercise of moderate intensity (60%-70% $\dot{V}O_2$ max) at least 3 times/week Peak $\dot{V}O_2$ of 70%	Pulmonary rehabilitation Supervised aerobic exercise program with SaO_2 monitoring
Decreased lower extremity muscle strength Due to deconditioning and effects of prednisone	Functional muscle strength for sit to stand and stairs Leg press of 60% of body weight Manual muscle test, lower extremity muscle groups 5/5	Strength training program (1 set, 8-12 reps) Leg press Knee extension Hamstring curls
Abnormal upper extremity (shoulder girdle) mechanics for single-lung transplant due to thoracotomy incision	Able to perform all upper extremity activities in a normal fashion Range of motion to within functional limits muscle strength for function Muscle endurance for overhead activities	Strength training program (1 set 8-12 reps) Latissimus pull-down Shoulder retraction Fly Endurance training program (2-3 sets of 10 reps) Upper body ergometer
Abnormal coordination of breathing with activity or decreased diaphragm performance	Coordinate breathing with activity most of time Perform diaphragm breathing during exercise Demonstrate shortness of breath recovery techniques	Breathing training Breathing facilitation techniques

programs are appropriate, or patients may elect to exercise independently in a fitness facility. Some follow-up by the transplant center is important to encourage compliance in exercise programs. Once patients reach their desired level of fitness, a community-based program is appropriate for maintaining endurance, aerobic capacity, strength, and flexibility. Patients who participate in training can attain high levels of exercise performance, with an appropriate training regimen.[45]

Influence of Medications on Treatment

Rejection Issues

Although transplants prolong life, some health professionals believe that patients are merely exchanging one set of problems for another. For transplants to be successful, recipients must remain on powerful immunosuppressive drugs for the remainder of their lives. Some of these medications have crippling side effects. The effects of long-term prednisone are well known: osteoporosis, muscle weakness, and glucose intolerance. The long-term effects of cyclosporine and azathioprine affect the patient's ability to fight infection. Patients also need to manage medication side effects on a daily basis. It is these medications, however, that make for impressive survival rates.

Types of Medications

The drugs used to suppress the immune system are categorized as immunosuppressants. Each immunosuppressant targets a different component of the immune system, and multiple drugs are often required to prevent rejection of the transplanted organ. A side effect shared by all immunosuppressants is an increased risk for infection.

ANTILYMPHOCYTE ANTIBODIES

This class of medications includes the monoclonal or polyclonal antibodies to human lymphatic tissue. These antibodies have a powerful effect on decreasing T cell activity by causing cell death or movement of the T cells out of the vasculature. These drugs are most commonly used in treating acute rejection. Antithymocyte globulin (ATGAM [equine ATG] and Thymoglobulin [rabbit ATG]), muromonab-CD3 (Orthoclone OKT3), and daclizumab (Zenapax) are included in this category. Given intravenously, these drugs lead to flu-like symptoms and potentially unstable vital signs, mainly as a result of a significant increase in cytokine activity. Rehabilitation should not be provided during administration of these medications.

ANTIMETABOLITES

Medications in this class inhibit intracellular energy production and DNA synthesis pathways, preventing lymphocytes from proliferating. These drugs are most commonly used for long-term (maintenance) immune suppression. Azathioprine (Imuran) and mycophenolate mofetil (CellCept) are included in this category. Both of these drugs commonly cause gastrointestinal upset (nausea, vomiting, diarrhea, and abdominal pain). Intestinal absorption of these medications is easily affected by food intake or drug interactions (for example, antacids decrease absorption of CellCept). Aside from increasing a patient's risk for infection, these drugs may also cause bone marrow suppression (potentially resulting in anemia, thrombocytopenia, and leukopenia).

CORTICOSTEROIDS

Corticosteroids, such as prednisone and methylprednisolone, which are believed to block the production of interleukins and decrease the inflammatory response, have been a mainstay of organ transplant management for many years. Recently, however, corticosteroid-free immunosuppressive agent combinations have been tested; thus corticosteroids may have less of a role in maintenance immunosuppression in the future. Common adverse effects of corticosteroids include increased appetite, hypertension, diabetes, cataracts, delayed wound healing, muscle weakness, and osteoporosis. During the

Table 40-8 **Side Effects of Immunosuppressive Medications**

Medication Type	Trade Name	Action	Adverse effects
Antilymphocyte antibodies	ATGAM OKT3 Zenapax (daclizumab)	Mono- or polyclonal antibodies that cause T cell death or movement of T cells out of vasculature	Flu-like symptoms Unstable vital signs
Antimetabolites	Azathioprine (Imuran) Mycophenolate mofetil (CellCept)	Inhibits enzymes and prevents lymphocytes from proliferating	Blood: leukopenia, bone marrow suppression GI: pancreatitis Hepatic: toxicity
Corticosteroids	Prednisone	Block production of interleukins Stimulates protein breakdown	CNS: euphoria, insomnia Eyes: cataracts GI: hyperglycemia Skin: acne, delayed wound healing Muscle: weakness Bone: osteoporosis
Calcineurin inhibitors	Cyclosporine (Neoral) Tacrolimus (FK 506)	Decrease production of interleukins and T lymphocytes	Blood: leukopenia CNS: tremor, seizure Hepatic: toxicity Renal: toxicity

perioperative period, high doses of corticosteroids are initiated and then tapered to lower doses based on patient tolerance (with the goal of preventing acute rejection while minimizing side effects). Steroid therapy may be delayed until primary wound closure is certain (1 to 2 weeks), at which time the patient is begun on low-dose oral steroids. Acute rejection episodes are treated with high-dose oral or intravenous steroid pulses.

CALCINEURIN INHIBITORS

These drugs bind to proteins in the cells, decreasing the production of interleukin-2 or T lymphocytes. Cyclosporine (Neoral, Sandimmune) and tacrolimus (Prograf) are the most common of these drugs and are a main component of many immunosuppressant regimens. The main adverse effect is renal toxicity, which may be reversible if the dose is decreased. Cyclosporine is considered a nervous system irritant, leading to hand tremor and possible seizures. Therapists should be aware of these side effects. In addition, absorption of these drugs is affected by other medications and food intake. Serum concentrations of these drugs are increased with intake of grapefruit juice, as well as drugs such as erythromycin, diltiazem, and corticosteroids. Because of potential drug interactions, serum levels of these drugs are monitored closely. Table 40-8 summarizes the effects of common immunosuppressive medications.

Long-Term Complications of Transplant Management

Osteoporosis

Osteoporosis remains a prevalent and disabling problem for patients following organ transplantation surgery. Before transplant, the prevalence of osteoporosis is 37% in patients awaiting lung transplantation.[46] In the first year after transplant, a high incidence of vertebral and other atraumatic fractures occurs (between 8% and 65%), which can significantly limit physical function and complicate the posttransplantation rehabilitation course. Physical therapists have a role in identifying the physical limitations of osteoporosis and in prescribing appropriate exercise programs. Osteoporosis medications are considered essential components of care, and the addition of resistance exercise to a medication regimen does improve bone mineral density.[39]

Cardiac Allograft Vasculopathy

One of the most troubling long-term complications of heart transplantation is cardiac allograft vasculopathy, an accelerated form of coronary disease affecting cardiac arteries. Blockage of the arteries occurs, and the condition may be related to occurrences of acute rejection.[47] Physical therapists must continue to identify signs and symptoms of cardiac ischemia and refer patients for appropriate treatment. As preventive measures, patients may be on medications to lower cholesterol (statins) and to manage hypertension; these patients may be candidates for stenting or coronary artery bypass surgery as well. High-intensity exercise does appear to improve endothelial function and may decrease risk for cardiac events.[48]

Bronchiolitis Obliterans

Long-term chronic rejection of the transplanted lung results in a condition called bronchiolitis obliterans (BO). BO is the main problem seen in long-term survivors of lung transplantation. It results from lymphocyte infiltration into the basement membrane of the small airways, followed by migration through the intima into the respiratory mucosa. This process leads to epithelial damage and scarring, which may partially or fully occlude the small airways. As a complication of transplant, BO is usually irreversible. Because the primary pulmonary function affected is FEV_1, it is considered an obstructive lung condition. The diagnosis of BO is made through transbronchial biopsy.

Physical therapists working with long-term survivors of lung transplant may find that these patients demonstrate decreased lung function and symptoms of dyspnea with

Box 40-4 Long-Term Complications of Organ Transplant

- Accelerated atherosclerosis/hypertension/hypercholesterolemia
- Infections
- Cancers
- Osteoporosis
- Steroid myopathy with muscle weakness
- Glucose intolerance
- Nephrotoxicity
- Delayed wound healing

activity. The therapist, therefore, must continue to monitor ventilatory status and oxygen saturation in the lung transplant patient. Long-term complications of organ transplantation are summarized in Box 40-4.

Quality of Life

Although quality of life generally improves after heart and/or lung transplantation, many factors may influence that quality of life. Generally, patients report improved physical function, general health, and social functioning.[49] Despite these improvements, a decline in quality of life eventually occurs in long-term survivors. It is unclear whether this downturn is due to declines in physical condition or other social or psychological factors. Patients with lung transplantation generally have increased quality of life until the onset of bronchiolitis obliterans, which then causes a decline in quality of life.

Summary

Physical therapy has an important role in maintaining and improving functional levels of patients both before and after organ transplantation. Knowledge of cardiovascular and pulmonary physiology, along with the ability to analyze movement and function, allows rehabilitation professionals to maximize a patient's quality of life. The exciting field of organ transplant is growing quickly. New advances in long-term management of transplant recipients mean that rehabilitation professionals need to continue to develop and evaluate evolving approaches to care.

Review Questions

1. What are the psychological and social implications of organ transplant?
2. What is the role of pretransplant pulmonary rehabilitation?
3. How does the surgical incision affect the musculoskeletal function of a posttransplant patient?
4. What are the signs of organ rejection in the cardiac transplant patient? The lung transplant patient?
5. How is the rehabilitation of the heart transplant patient similar to and different from traditional cardiac rehabilitation?
6. How is the rehabilitation of the lung transplant patient different from other forms of pulmonary rehabilitation?
7. How do immunosuppressive drugs affect a patient's neuromuscular function? Muscle strength? Cardiopulmonary endurance?
8. What are the long-term complications of heart transplantation and of lung transplantation?

References

1. OPTN: Organ Procurement and Transplantation Network: Available at: http://optn.transplant.hrsa.gov/ [Accessed January 16, 2011].
2. Centers for Medicare & Medicaid Services: Centers for Medicare & Medicaid Services. Available at: http://www.cms.gov/ [Accessed January 16, 2011].
3. OPTN: Organ Procurement and Transplantation Network: Available at: http://optn.transplant.hrsa.gov/about/transplantation/matchingProcess.asp [Accessed January 24, 2011].
4. Nativi JN, Kfoury AG, Myrick C, et al: Effects of the 2006 U.S. thoracic organ allocation change: analysis of local impact on organ procurement and heart transplantation. *J Heart Lung Transplant* 29(3):235–239, 2010.
5. Kop WJ: Role of psychological factors in the clinical course of heart transplant patients. *J Heart Lung Transplant* 29(3):257–260, 2010.
6. OPTN: Organ Procurement and Transplantation Network: Available at: http://optn.transplant.hrsa.gov/policiesAndBylaws/nota.asp [Accessed January 24, 2011].
7. Burker EJ, Evon DM, Ascari JC, et al: Relationship between coping and depression in heart transplant candidates and their spouses. *Prog Transplant* 2006;16(3):215–221.
8. Stubblefield C, Murray RL: Waiting for lung transplantation: family experiences of relocation. *Pediatr Nurs* 28(5):501–504, 2002.
9. Goetzmann L, Klaghofer R, Wagner-Huber R, et al: Psychosocial vulnerability predicts psychosocial outcome after an organ transplant: results of a prospective study with lung, liver, and bone-marrow patients. *J Psychosom Res* 62(1):93–100, 2007.
10. Stehlik J, Edwards LB, Kucheryavaya AY, et al: The Registry of the International Society for Heart and Lung Transplantation: Twenty-seventh official adult heart transplant report—2010. *Journal of Heart and Lung Transplantation* 29(10):1089–1103, 2010.
11. Mehra MR, Kobashigawa J, Starling R, et al: Listing criteria for heart transplantation: International Society for Heart and Lung Transplantation guidelines for the care of cardiac transplant candidates—2006. *J Heart Lung Transplant* 25(9):1024–1042, 2006.
12. Laoutaris ID, Dritsas A, Adamopoulos S, et al: Benefits of physical training on exercise capacity, inspiratory muscle function, and quality of life in patients with ventricular assist devices long-term postimplantation. *Eur J Cardiovasc Prev Rehabil* 2010. Available at: http://www.ncbi.nlm.nih.gov/pubmed/20571404 [Accessed January 7, 2011].
13. Arena R, Humphrey R, Peberdy MA: Safety and efficacy of exercise training in a patient awaiting heart transplantation while on positive intravenous inotropic support. *J Cardiopulm Rehabil* 20(4):259–261, 2000.
14. Kreider M, Kotloff RM: Selection of candidates for lung transplantation. *Proc Am Thorac Soc* 6(1):20–27, 2009.
15. Orens JB, Garrity ER: General overview of lung transplantation and review of organ allocation. *Proc Am Thorac Soc* 6(1):13–19, 2009.
16. Celli BR, Cote CG, Marin JM, et al: The body-mass index, airflow obstruction, dyspnea, and exercise capacity index in chronic obstructive pulmonary disease. *N Engl J Med* 350(10):1005–1012, 2004.
17. OPTN policy_9.pdf. Available at: http://optn.transplant.hrsa.gov/PoliciesandBylaws2/policies/pdfs/policy_9.pdf [Accessed January 16, 2011].
18. Lederer DJ, Arcasoy SM, Wilt JS, et al: Six-minute-walk distance predicts waiting list survival in idiopathic pulmonary fibrosis. *Am J Respir Crit Care Med* 174(6):659–664, 2006.
19. Mayer-Hamblett N, Rosenfeld M, Emerson J, et al: Developing cystic fibrosis lung transplant referral criteria using predictors of 2-year mortality. *Am J Respir Crit Care Med* 166(12 Pt 1):1550–1555, 2002.
20. Maury G, Langer D, Verleden G, et al: Skeletal muscle force and functional exercise tolerance before and after lung transplantation: a cohort study. *Am J Transplant* 8(6):1275–1281, 2008.
21. Heart Transplantation: Cardiac Transplant Surgery. Available at: http://www.medscape.com/viewarticle/436544_6 [Accessed January 16, 2011].
22. Durrleman N: Clamshell and hemiclamshell incisions, *Multimedia Manual of Cardiothoracic Surgery, 2006*, 1867–1860. doi:10.1510/mmcts.2006.001867.

23. Spina A, Gatti G, Belgrano M, et al: Clamshell approach and partial cardiopulmonary bypass to repair a right aortic arch aneurysm. *J Cardiovasc Med (Hagerstown)* 10(11):859–860, 2009.
24. Stehlik J, Edwards LB, Kucheryavaya AY, et al: The Registry of the International Society for Heart and Lung Transplantation: Twenty-seventh official adult heart transplant report—2010. *Journal of Heart and Lung Transplantation* 29(10):1089–1103, 2010.
25. Costanzo MR, Costanzo MR, Dipchand A, et al: The International Society of Heart and Lung Transplantation Guidelines for the care of heart transplant recipients. *J Heart Lung Transplant* 29(8):914–956, 2010.
26. Brocki BC, Thorup CB, Andreasen JJ: Precautions related to midline sternotomy in cardiac surgery: a review of mechanical stress factors leading to sternal complications. *Eur J Cardiovasc Nurs* 9(2):77–84, 2010.
27. Karapolat H, Eyigör S, Zoghi M, et al: Comparison of hospital-supervised exercise versus home-based exercise in patients after orthotopic heart transplantation: effects on functional capacity, quality of life, and psychological symptoms. *Transplant Proc* 39(5):1586–1588, 2007.
28. Degre SG, Niset GL, De Smet JM, et al: Cardiorespiratory response to early exercise testing after orthotopic cardiac transplantation. *Am J Cardiol* 60(10):926–928, 1987.
29. Tomczak CR, Warburton DER, Riess KJ, et al: Pulmonary oxygen uptake and heart rate kinetics during the six-minute walk test in transplant recipients. *Transplantation* 2008;85(1):29–35.
30. Buendía Fuentes F, Martínez-Dolz L, Almenar Bonet L, et al: Normalization of the heart rate response to exercise 6 months after cardiac transplantation. *Transplant Proc* 42(8):3186–3188, 2010.
31. Habedank D, Ewert R, Hummel M, et al: Changes in exercise capacity, ventilation, and body weight following heart transplantation. *Eur J Heart Fail* 9(3):310–316, 2007.
32. Lanfranconi F, Borrelli E, Ferri A, et al: Noninvasive evaluation of skeletal muscle oxidative metabolism after heart transplant. *Med Sci Sports Exerc* 38(8):1374–1383, 2006.
33. Wong S, Carrault G, Kervio G, et al: Application of multiple correspondence analysis to assess the relation between time after transplantation and sympathetic activity in cardiac transplant recipient. *Conf Proc IEEE Eng Med Biol Soc* 4403–4406, 2008.
34. Shephard RJ, Kavanagh T, Mertens DJ, et al: The place of perceived exertion ratings in exercise prescription for cardiac transplant patients before and after training. *Br J Sports Med* 30(2):116–121, 1996.
35. Pokan R, Von Duvillard SP, Ludwig J, et al: Effect of high-volume and -intensity endurance training in heart transplant recipients. *Med Sci Sports Exerc* 36(12):2011–2016, 2004.
36. Tegtbur U, Busse MW, Jung K, et al: Time course of physical reconditioning during exercise rehabilitation late after heart transplantation. *J Heart Lung Transplant* 24(3):270–274, 2005.
37. Grady KL, Naftel DC, Young JB, et al: Patterns and predictors of physical functional disability at 5 to 10 years after heart transplantation. *J Heart Lung Transplant* 26(11):1182–1191, 2007.
38. Zoll J, N'Guessan B, Ribera F, et al: Preserved response of mitochondrial function to short-term endurance training in skeletal muscle of heart transplant recipients. *J Am Coll Cardiol* 42(1):126–132, 2003.
39. Braith RW, Magyari PM, Fulton MN, et al: Comparison of calcitonin versus calcitonin + resistance exercise as prophylaxis for osteoporosis in heart transplant recipients. *Transplantation* 81(8):1191–1195, 2006.
40. Braith RW, Magyari PM, Pierce GL, et al: Effect of resistance exercise on skeletal muscle myopathy in heart transplant recipients. *Am J Cardiol* 95(10):1192–1198, 2005.
41. Juskowa J, Lewandowska M, Bartłomiejczyk I, et al: Physical rehabilitation and risk of atherosclerosis after successful kidney transplantation. *Transplant Proc* 38(1):157–160, 2006.
42. Wickerson L, Mathur S, Brooks D: Exercise training after lung transplantation: a systematic review. *J Heart Lung Transplant* 29(5):497–503, 2010.
43. Reinsma GD, ten Hacken NHT, Grevink RG, et al: Limiting factors of exercise performance 1 year after lung transplantation. *J Heart Lung Transplant* 25(11):1310–1316, 2006.
44. Munro PE, Holland AE, Bailey M, et al: Pulmonary rehabilitation following lung transplantation. *Transplant Proc* 2009;41(1):292–295.
45. Patterson JA, Pitetti KH, Young KC, et al: Case Report on PWC of a Competitive Cyclist before and after Heart Transplant. *Medicine & Science in Sports & Exercise* 39(9):1447–1451, 2007.
46. Lakey WC, Spratt S, Vinson EN, et al: Osteoporosis in lung transplant candidates compared to matched healthy controls. *Clin Transplant* 2010. Available at: http://www.ncbi.nlm.nih.gov/pubmed/20482557 [Accessed January 15, 2011].
47. Raichlin E, Edwards BS, Kremers WK, et al: Acute cellular rejection and the subsequent development of allograft vasculopathy after cardiac transplantation. *J Heart Lung Transplant* 28(4):320–327, 2009.
48. Hermann TS, Dall CH, Christensen SB, et al: Effect of High Intensity Exercise on Peak Oxygen Uptake and Endothelial Function in Long-Term Heart Transplant Recipients. *Am J Transplant* 2011. Available at: http://www.ncbi.nlm.nih.gov/pubmed/21219582 [Accessed January 15, 2011].
49. Vasiliadis H, Collet J, Poirier C: Health-related quality-of-life determinants in lung transplantation. *J Heart Lung Transplant* 25(2):226–233, 2006.

VII

Chapter 41

The Patient in the Community

Donna Frownfelter and Jennifer M Ryan

KEY TERMS

Assisted living
Continuity of care
Home care
Managed care
Outpatient
Subacute hospitals
Skilled nursing and rehabilitation facilities
Transitional care units

CHAPTER OUTLINE

The role of the physical therapist in the community varies widely. Over the years, this role has changed in response to a range of factors, including epidemiological indicators of chronic conditions, advances in medical and surgical management, and policy changes. Lifestyle-related conditions and their associated comorbidity are health care priorities necessitating substantial community support, often for many years (Chapter 1). In addition, other chronic systemic conditions have well-documented cardiovascular and pulmonary consequences (Chapters 6 and 13). Policy changes during the 1980s resulted in the emergence of diagnostic-related groupings (DRGs), which led to patients being discharged from the hospital at more acute stages of illness. Further, the Balanced Budget Act of 1997[1] narrowed the criteria for those who qualified for prolonged inpatient postacute care, resulting in patients being transitioned home from extended care facilities sooner than they had been previously. The combination of these factors has changed the role of physical therapy in the community.

Physical therapy is provided in all inpatient care settings, including subacute hospitals, Medicare or another form of insured care skilled nursing settings, long-term acute care facilities, and rehabilitation facilities with transitional care units to facilitate functional progression so that patients are able to return home within days or weeks. Thus rehabilitation, by increasing the number of patients who return home, rather than remaining or being placed in facilities, is a way of reducing cost while maintaining care standards.[2] Changes in health care reimbursement from third-party payers affect patients' access to physical therapy services. Although such policy may be viewed as reducing physical therapy access, new paradigms of health care delivery and models of care for people with chronic conditions may emerge. Epidemiological indicators support patient-centered health care delivery systems and self-care and self-management approaches. The incorporation of self-management principles of practice can improve patients' quality of life and decrease hospitalization.[3-14] This chapter describes how physical therapists can facilitate the management of chronic conditions, particularly lifestyle-related conditions, when practicing in the community and home settings.

Because of dramatic increases in both patient longevity and prevalence of chronic illness, physical therapists see an ever-widening range of diagnoses in their patients in the community. Global aging is occurring at an unprecedented pace. Worldwide, the number of people age 65 and older is expected to increase from 500 million to 1 billion by 2030.[15] Physical therapist interventions unique to aging populations need to be considered in relation to the available resources, as well as the challenges that present in the community practice setting more often now that patients are living longer (Chapter 38). Chronic conditions that were previously associated with later stages in life are now presenting earlier in life as a result of changing lifestyle behaviors (Chapter 1). Also, the medical community has improved its ability to quickly and effectively manage complicated acute medical situations—premature births, heart failure, cancer. More patients are surviving diseases once considered fatal and consequently requiring more services to safely and effectively manage the morbidity issues that result. Medical interventions in intensive care units have improved greatly, thus decreasing mortality, but morbidity related to myopathy of critical illness, cognitive impairments, and mental health sequelae has been found to have a significant impact on patients' ability to resume their prior level of independence (Chapters 33-36).[16-21] These patients return home more often and more quickly than in the past, but they often do so accompanied by unresolved cardiovascular and pulmonary impairments. For patients who are too medically fragile to return home or to obtain sufficient medical care at skilled nursing facilities, specialty hospitals have become necessary. These hospitals make it possible for ventilator-dependent or ventilator-assisted patients to receive physical therapy longer and at less cost than an acute care hospital.[22]

Practicing physical therapy in the community is distinct from practicing in acute care. When people with chronic conditions are living in the community, their focus is on health promotion and optimal health, rather than recovery from an acute episode of a condition or surgical procedure or trauma with frequent changes in their functional status, as is seen in acute care. In the community setting, the patient's goals are less focused on safety and more on optimal health. Patients' participation is vital in order to understand their definition of optimal health. Consistent with values of autonomy and independence, shared decision making should always be used—including the patient and family/caregiver in decisions regarding the patient's care with guidance from the health care team.[14,23] This model is at times challenging for health care team members who may feel more comfortable continuing to use a method in which they prescribe a task and tell the patient what to do, with little collaboration. However, the expected level of practice of every physical therapist is evidence-based practice (EBP) in decision making and treatment. The three aspects of EBP are weighted comparably: external clinical evidence, patient circumstances, and individual clinical expertise.[24] In this approach to practice, the patient's goals and his or her ability to carry out an effective plan are important. A patient cannot carry out an effective plan unless he or she is taught how to identify problems and manage or avoid them in daily situations when health care professionals are not present. Patients need a targeted and tailored education to understand how to make the best decisions about their health and to appreciate their responsibility in their own health management.

Given these practice settings, cardiovascular and pulmonary concerns are often the highest priority. From the young to the old, primary and secondary cardiovascular and pulmonary issues are often the limiting factors in a patient's rehabilitation progress, thus, need to be addressed in the patient's standard physical therapy care. The focus in home and long-term care settings is to enable individuals to achieve optimal health in the environment in which they live. This chapter focuses on considerations specific to patients with cardiovascular and pulmonary dysfunction (as either primary pathology or secondary to other impairments) who require physical therapy at home or in a long-term care setting, such as a nursing home, skilled nursing facility, transitional or assisted living facility, adult day program, or outpatient setting.

Chronic Conditions and Self-Management

Many people at home or in long-term care have chronic conditions, often related to lifestyle behaviors. Regardless of whether these conditions are the diagnoses for which they are receiving physical therapy, the related activity limitations and participation restrictions can limit their abilities to participate and progress in their therapy. Chronic conditions can affect the person's physical capabilities, as well as his or her emotions, attitude, and motivation. Many patients with chronic conditions or functional decline lead full and rewarding lives, but doing so requires the active participation of the patient and the physical therapist to maintain the fullest level of function despite the changes. The choices patients make about their health care, exercises, and methods of self-management will largely determine their health-related quality of life (Chapter 1).

Though people with chronic conditions have multiple impairments requiring adaptation of their lifestyles and schedules, the majority still accomplish what they want and need to do each day. The goal is to augment their knowledge about their symptoms and enable them to work within a collaborative, self-advocacy, and self-help model with their health care team to achieve optimal health. Positive self-management involves a combination of positive emotional outlook, active involvement in decision making, and maintenance of a lifestyle that is as optimal as possible. The interprofessional team needs to engage the patient in his or her care decisions. The physical therapist needs to be caring and fully present with the patient. Although the physical therapist can provide the initial stimulus for the process, effective self-management comes only from within the patient. The physical therapist can continue to be a resource and provide interventions as needed, but the goal is for the patient to be his or her own case manager and decision maker, whenever possible, regarding health care and optimal function (Chapter 1).[14,23]

In the home or community setting, the person with a chronic condition needs to make several choices. How does he or she decide what will promote optimal function and health? What resources must be employed to meet these needs (e.g., a maintenance program), or does the person have the potential to improve to the extent that he or she can benefit from further professional services? Many people are discharged from the hospital without referral to home care or outpatient physical therapy to manage their chronic conditions. If they are referred to a pulmonary rehabilitation program, for example, what determines when they have completed the program? Financial support by private third-party payers and insurers is limited, influencing patients' decisions about which avenues to use to move further toward optimal health. Do they go to a health club or the local YMCA? Do they walk in a shopping mall or take yoga classes? Do they continue to pay privately for physical therapy, continue with a long-term pulmonary rehabilitation program, or simply exercise at home? The answers are as different as the people making the decision about what optimal health *is* in relationship to their personal circumstances. At times it may be a matter of trial and error; perhaps the patient's choice is not the same as that of a physician or other health care professional, but it is his or her decision and choice. A patient has the right to try, to succeed or fail, and make other decisions. He or she needs to know how to access the health care system if there are medical problems, and learning to do so must be an integral part of the patient education process.

Actively playing a role in decision making (i.e., self-management) empowers patients, making them more motivated, positive, active, and successful than passive patients who do only what the physical therapist and other health professionals advise.[23,25] A decrease in the number of visits allowed by third-party payers has forced a necessary change towards patient self-management and empowerment, which has led to improved efficiency and effectiveness in treatment. The promotion of positive self-management strategies for a more active, healthy lifestyle is one of the most important competencies of contemporary physical therapists.

The physical therapist facilitates this process by being caring, supportive, and respectful of patient goals and priorities. This has been referred to as a "healing presence," which may lead to a beneficial, therapeutic, positive experience for the patient.[26,27] The American Physical Therapy Association promoted this practice philosophy with the phrase "the science of healing, the art of caring."

Cardiovascular and Pulmonary Concerns in the Community

Patients with either chronic or acute conditions present with primary and/or secondary cardiovascular and pulmonary diagnoses at all levels of independence. Patients may have preexisting cardiovascular and pulmonary impairments such as asthma, hypertension, congestive heart failure, and comorbidities such as type 2 diabetes mellitus, obesity, and one or more types of cancer. Most patients will also have risk factors for one or more of these lifestyle-related conditions; thus risk factors need to be assessed and modified accordingly. Patients may have had problems such as hip fractures, joint replacements, CVAs, MIs, or some combination. The cardiovascular and pulmonary impairments related to the impairments and subsequent deconditioning associated with these conditions may be the limiting factor with respect to progression of physical therapy. These concerns need to be addressed so that the individual is able to reach his or her full rehabilitation potential.

One example is a patient with coronary artery disease, who is fully independent in his or her day-to-day activities but not at a maximal functional level because of limited education on how to further improve function. Another example is a patient who cannot resume his or her prior level of independent function after an acute bout of illness or hospitalization because of limits resulting from primary and/or secondary cardiovascular and pulmonary dysfunction. Both of these examples illustrate the resultant decrease in such patients' tolerance for, and ability to independently perform, activities of daily living. Because of these decreases, patients must acquire continued support to maintain their safety and improve their level of function. Those with the least ability to care for themselves after an acute bout of illness transfer into nursing homes or alternative long-term care, and those with higher levels of function move into assisted living facilities or return home with assistance and therapy. Such patients may present with decreased strength, endurance, and balance, leading to decreased independence, mobility, and activity level. Returning home with a decrease in independent functioning may be associated with negative emotions, which may further decrease appetite, activity level, motivation, and social/community interactions (Chapter 1).

Nursing homes, assisted living facilities, and senior housing offer residential services for those who can no longer care for themselves. Some facilities offer multiple levels of care within one system, ranging from independent living apartments to skilled-level care. For residents who live in independent apartments when they are well, the facility can offer temporary increased support from a skilled level of care with physical therapy and nursing support upon discharge from the hospital. The goal is for the patient to return to the least level of care with the highest level of independence. Physical therapy services can be utilized at all levels of care to improve independence and tolerance for daily activities to improve patient safety in the community. Patients living in residential facilities should be screened periodically to determine their readiness to benefit from further physical therapy intervention and enable them to live to their fullest capacity.

Functioning depends on the ability of the patient to maintain all of the components of oxygen transport to support activity. One example is a patient who fell in the parking lot of a hospital where she had been attending a pulmonary rehabilitation program. She was fitted with a long leg cast and discharged home. She reported being short of breath with sit-to-stand transfers, and soon she was hardly able to ambulate across the room with the standard walker she used before. When the physical therapist observed this patient using her bronchodilator metered-dose inhaler, she was using it improperly. After she was instructed on how to use the bronchodilator therapy effectively before activity, the patient's transfers and her walking ability improved markedly. She was able to coordinate her breathing with her activity, and her endurance further improved. Case reports and professional experiences such as this provide important information for the physical therapist to use in conjunction with the findings of research studies when planning and prescribing interventions for patients at home using evidence-based practice.[24]

Long-Term Care Facilities and Nursing Homes

Practicing in a long-term care facility as a physical therapist opens up an opportunity to work with an interprofessional health care team to carry out therapeutic goals during other tasks of the day. Aides, generalist and specialist nurses, respiratory therapists, occupational therapists, speech therapists, dietitians, and on-call physicians all interact with patients each day and are able to remind and encourage patients to follow through on their exercise and activity goals. In order for this to happen, it is necessary to communicate the importance of the patient's active participation throughout the day.

Therapeutic goals and treatment plans for patients should be designed with solicited input from the patient and family or significant other. Clear and achievable goals must be developed and revisited as the patient progresses or regresses in therapy. If the patient's goal is to transition to a more independent living facility (i.e., home or an assisted living facility), then the plan would be more aggressive than if the goal were to maximize function within the current living facility. In order to achieve the patient's goals, a holistic approach to care that is mindful of cognitive, psychological, and pathophysiological impairments should be used. As goals and interventions are determined, quality-of-life issues need to be considered in order to comprehensively address each patient's needs. To increase patients' ability to achieve their therapy goals, therapy sessions may need to be scheduled based on the time that is thought to be most efficient in relation to the patient's medication schedule and other events of the day, rather than the most convenient time that fits into the therapy schedule.

The patient's ability to participate in therapy may be driven by multiple system impairments. Nutritional concerns are a priority. It is important to monitor whether the patient is losing or gaining weight. Poor denture fit and the impact of medications on taste and appetite can affect the patient's ability to eat. The patient may be depressed, also limiting appetite. The patient may not want to drink because of difficulty getting to the bathroom independently. Determine whether the patient is taking a diuretic and whether he or she has urinary incontinence. Patients who have difficulty managing urination because of frequency or urgency may be less likely to drink sufficient fluids, increasing the risk for hypovolemia, hypotension, decreased cerebral perfusion, and falls.[28]

Patients with severe breathing problems, such as those with heart failure or COPD, can become extremely short of breath doing even such simple tasks as eating. Nurses and aides, as well as family and friends, can make observations about these occurrences. As much as 30% of $\dot{V}O_{2max}$ can be attributed to labored breathing, which places considerable metabolic demand on the patient simply to breathe, let alone the challenge of pausing breathing to eat. A nutrition consult can be initiated to assess the patient's caloric intake and supplement this intake if indicated.

Ineffective sleep can be a problem after surgery, trauma, or CVA. Multiple factors may be involved, but sometimes the problem is simply the fact that the required positions for sleep are driven by joint precautions or the need for joint and skin protection, rather than what is comfortable for the patient. Nurses and care staff can help by being receptive to positioning options that may increase the patient's chance for effective sleep but that still meet the criteria for joint and skin protection. If the patient has difficulty waking in the morning or has headaches or difficulty following directions, sleep apnea or other sleep disturbances need to be considered. A wide range of issues—incontinence, anxiety, depression, chronic pain, a busy environment outside the patient's door—may contribute to sleep deprivation and should be addressed.

Functional gains may be achieved sooner when physical therapy is incorporated into the patient's daily living with the help of the nurses and aides. This can improve physical capabilities by aiding the learning process, as well as increasing the number of repetitions performed for motor planning. For example, if the patient is taught to use ventilatory strategies with movement, such as inspiring when extending the trunk (Chapter 23), this should be communicated to other caregivers and encouraged during movements that extend the trunk, such as dressing. If the goal is for the patient to walk to meals, the physical therapist and caretakers can have the patient transition from walking as far as he or she can toward the dining room for one meal each day, then walking to two meals each day, and finally, to all meals. The next progression would be to set more functional goals, such as walking to daily activities, to social settings, to the car, and so on; thus walking is no longer associated only with therapy. In-services for nurses and care staff that help reinforce physical therapy interventions can be conducted individually and in formal classes. Instruction can be incorporated into the staff competencies upon hire and annually. One-on-one therapist/aide education sessions should not be replaced by the competencies; rather, they should occur as needed when unique patient needs arise. Educational opportunities such as this can help to make patient education more consistent.

When all facility programs collaborate to follow through with therapeutic goals, the patient's progress can be realized sooner. It may be helpful to make the activity department aware, for example, of patients who need extra time or help with oxygen in order to participate in activity programs. Events such as an open house for staff in the physical therapy department would allow staff members to visit and ask questions about physical therapy and to better understand what role they can serve. Offering educational materials about the physical therapy profession and patient information pamphlets may help the staff to better understand what physical therapists do for patients.

In many long-term care facilities, not all patients are on the present physical therapy caseload. Other staff members of the facility may have helpful input and suggestions for additional patients who may benefit from physical therapy. In addition to chart reviews and discussing patients with the staff, it is also helpful to screen for patients in the dining rooms, activity sessions, and halls.

Monitoring Cardiovascular and Pulmonary Status in the Long-Term Care Facility

Because of short hospital stays, patients in long-term care facilities may be less medically stable than patients in the past. With this increase in patient acuity, it is particularly important to monitor each patient's response to activity. Many long-term care and subacute facilities now provide pulse oximeters and portable electrocardiogram monitors because of increased patient acuity. In addition, physical therapists need to be competent in monitoring blood pressure and heart rates. Auscultation is highly recommended as a clinical competency (Chapter 15). When patients present with acute changes in their status, it is important to utilize any methods of telemedicine available to communicate their medical status to their primary care practitioner. Telemedicine can range from a formal program for AICD-pacer monitoring, for example, to using a secure Internet connection to send video or audio portions of a physical examination.[29,30]

During the initial evaluation, vital signs and oximetry are taken with the patient in supine or semi-Fowler's position for baseline, then in sitting and standing positions if orthostatic measurements are indicated. It is helpful to take the baseline resting blood pressure readings on both arms to ensure they are comparable. The arm with the higher reading should be used for recording and monitoring. If the two readings differ by more than 10 mm Hg on multiple recordings, cardiovascular pathology needs to be ruled out.

Vital signs and oximetry need to be evaluated before each physical therapy session and after intervention to assess the physiological response to exercise. Blood pressure and pulse should increase proportionally in relation to the activity (Chapter 18). An increase of 20% to 30% or 20 to 30 beats above resting heart rate would be within normal limits, with a recovery time of 5 to 10 minutes. These responses can be affected by medication; therefore it is vital to know what medications the patient is taking and to understand their impact on the vital sign response.

Many patients without primary cardiovascular and pulmonary diagnoses have abnormal responses to exercise, either as a result of a preexisting but undetected dysfunction or a more recent change. Each patient must be observed closely and measured objectively to be sure he or she is responding to exercise predictably. One example is a patient who was markedly deconditioned and obese prior to total knee arthroplasty. After the surgery, with short distance ambulation, she demonstrated a dramatic increase in HR without arrhythmias, an appropriate blood pressure response, and an increase in the work of breathing and accessory muscle use. If only the heart rate or the blood pressure had been used to determine therapeutic intervention limits, the exercise response may have been misinterpreted. Patients' response to exercise and intervention should be interpreted using their overall vital sign response. It is imperative to communicate the vital sign and exercise response to the primary care practitioner with as much information as possible to avoid inappropriate medication changes.

Physical Therapy in Home

Treating patients at home poses many challenges, one being the responsibility to help the patient return to the level of function before his or her illness. Gaining sufficient information from the prior level of care can expedite the care in the home. Some areas unique to home care are the need to continually assess and adapt treatment to the patient's living space, observing and anticipating safety concerns, and identifying creative ways to improve the patient's functional independence and quality of life.

Continuity of care is an essential component of quality health care, given the trend toward earlier and earlier hospital discharge. At minimum, acute care physical therapy addresses mobility, including safety, transfers, and household-distance ambulation as the patient recovers from an illness or procedure. Breathing exercises and positioning may be used in conjunction with functional mobility to facilitate movement and recovery. Patients are often unable to extrapolate their inpatient education to all of their home setting situations. Ideally, on discharge from acute care, patients should receive a home exercise program to help them with decision-making principles as well as exercises for them to perform. Decreased endurance due to recent insult/injury and bed rest during hospitalization and possible change in medication may compromise the potential of the patient to regain his or her premorbidity level of activity and function without appropriate follow-up care. A postacute exercise program designed for the specific needs of the patient and a complete review of the hospital stay should be communicated to the physical therapist in the community.

A patient's successful recovery from acute or long-term loss of independent function is often dependent on the availability of able caregivers. Patients who have a caregiver to help them can discharge home, rather than to a facility. Caregivers are often family, friends, or paid workers who provide this service. Caregivers should be educated to measure vital signs and monitor for changes in physical status, appetite, and behavior as part of their responsibility as the caregiver. Children with chronic illness whose parents can provide care, with or without nursing staff, often return home successfully. These children tend to integrate smoothly into the community, attend school, participate in recreation, function well, and report a high quality of life. Adult sons and daughters are often the caregivers of their parents. In such cases, these adult children may have children of their own, whose needs they are responsible for. This "sandwich generation" is often torn between caring for their aging parents and for their own children.[4] It is important for physical therapists to be sensitive to the needs of the patient and the limitations of the caregiver when determining the patient's safety at home. Many older adult patients remain independent at home, some of them amazing even the most seasoned clinicians with their inventiveness and the extent of their support systems. The physical therapist serves an integral role in teaching patients and families how to manage the impact of disease and elevate each patient's quality of life to the fullest extent.

Although a physical therapist makes numerous adaptations when treating patients at home, many physical therapy interventions performed in these settings are comparable to those prescribed for outpatients of similar ages and conditions. Activities to improve safety, strength, endurance, transfers, ambulation, and tolerance for activities of daily living (ADLs) are common, and often traditional methods such as supervised repetition of tasks (i.e., transfers and ADLs) are used as they would be elsewhere. Theraband products or nontraditional physical therapy equipment (e.g., water bottles as weights) may be indicated and prescribed based on the patient's needs and abilities. For patients whose activity tolerance waxes and wanes as a result of their chronic condition, water bottles or similar household objects can provide an inexpensive and readily adjustable tool to meet the patient's needs of any given day.

Education is especially important in home care. It can be directed to the patient, family, and caregivers and is especially important in ensuring the patient's safe and independent functioning when the physical therapist is not present. Safety and medical issues can arise unexpectedly. Patients and caregivers must be familiar with the signs and symptoms that indicate a change in their condition (e.g., weakness, discomfort/

pain, shortness of breath, changes in secretions, increased fatigue, inability to perform ADLs, depression, and loss of appetite). The physical therapist should gauge the patient's and/or caregiver's ability to interpret the medication schedule, understand the prescribed parameters for oxygen use, and recognize when to rest versus when to exercise. The therapist also needs to determine the patient's ability to self-monitor his or her sign and symptom response to activity (Chapters 17 and 18) both during therapy and during independent activities. Patients and their caregivers need to be able to monitor their cardiovascular and pulmonary status to prevent overexertion and accidents. Because of potential limits in learning, it is important to check the reliability and validity of each patient's self-assessments. Caregivers and family members can be taught how to monitor the patient's blood pressure, heart rate, and respiratory rate; they can also be taught to observe for changes in shortness of breath, amount and color of secretions, presence of dizziness or lightheadedness, color changes such as cyanosis or flushed skin, diaphoresis, changes in balance during ambulation, and changes in mental status—and to report such changes promptly to the physical therapist or physician. Patients and caregivers need to know how to manage signs and symptoms, as well as when to call 911 rather than simply calling the physician's office. If there are concerns about the patient's judgment and reasoning, which may cause gaps in the patient's learning, the physical therapist should adapt the education format accordingly.[14,31,32]

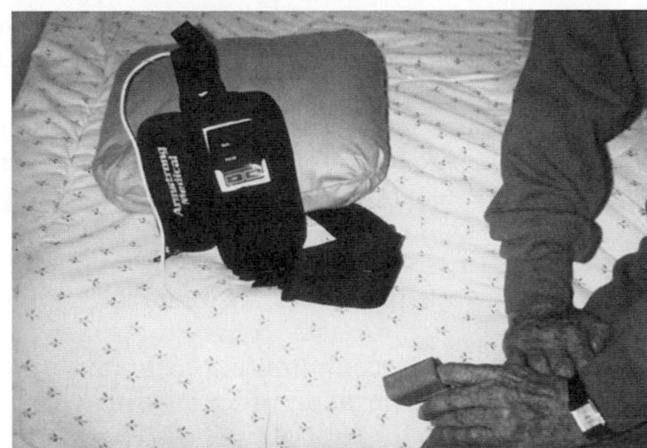

Fig. 41-1 Pulse oximeter.

Monitoring Cardiovascular and Pulmonary Status at Home

Because patients discharge to home in more acute states than they did in the past, physical therapists need to have a high level of clinical reasoning and measurement competencies commensurate with the needs of patients now being managed at home. Patients who are postoperative or who have had a recent decline in function may experience difficulty with breathing or endurance when performing ADLs. Without home-based physical therapy, the patient's full return to their premorbidity status can be jeopardized.

In the home-care setting, the physical therapist tends to be independent without the advantage of the health care team close by, even though support is available through nursing and home-care agencies. The physical therapist needs to be prepared to evaluate patients and their progress with minimal consultation and information from the management team. This specialized practice area requires foremost that physical therapists have the ability to practice independently. They often need to handle emergencies and crisis situations. As in other areas of health care, home-care practice requires physical therapists to have annually renewed health provider CPR certification. Knowledge about policies and procedures for handling emergencies, infection control, and safety is essential. Home-care physical therapists evaluate the need for referrals to other health professionals such as social workers, nursing staff, and occupational therapy. Unfortunately, problems such as abuse and neglect are not uncommon, particularly in the older adult population; thus health professionals in home care must be alert for such evidence. If the patient's condition declines or new conditions have arisen (for instance, the patient shares that he or she has been falling), the physical therapist may need to do preliminary medical screening and decide the appropriate intervention, including notification of the patient's referring provider. The patient's status needs to be monitored in relation to changes in diet, bowel and bladder habits, and mental status; such findings need to be included in frequent updates and reports to the referring practitioner. Home care is a challenging practice setting that requires astute clinical reasoning and observation skills.

By using equipment such as portable pulse oximeters (Figure 41-1) and blood pressure cuffs, along with physical examination (Chapters 6, 15, and 32), the physical therapist can do much to determine a patient's ability to safely perform exercise in the home setting, although there are limitations to the depth of such monitoring and examination. In rural and underserved areas, limited resources may restrict the use of 911 service to life-saving situations only. However, with advances in communication technology, patients and home therapists can gain access to care better than ever before. Advances in chronic disease management in relation to acute changes in status, maintenance care to avoid acute conditions, and research into chronic disease impact and management have come as greater bandwidth has improved the quality of visual and auditory communication.[29] According to the National Research Council Report in 2000,[33] the Internet is often used for health information websites but is only beginning to be explored for its potential value in clinical decision making, patient education, and clinical outcome improvement—all possible because of the sharing of resources by professionals, "immediate" access to specialists, and more timely adaptations in medication doses, among other advances.

Multiple articles have found limitations in health literacy can decrease a patient's ability to understand[14] prescription instructions, exercise programs, and appointment schedules. For example, in independent studies, Harmon and colleagues[13] and Sorensen and coworkers[32] noted that patients often do not adhere to their antihypertensive medication prescription regimen for a variety of reasons: a poor understanding of the importance of the medication, limited symptoms of hypertension, and a dislike of the side effects, complicated dosing rules, and financial constraints. This underscores the importance for physical therapists to clarify whether and how patients are taking their prescribed medication; only then can therapists determine whether their patients are sufficiently medicated to safely participate in an exercise program. Furthermore, ongoing communication between patients and their prescribing clinician needs to be fostered on a more frequent basis than is available through office visits.

The use of webcams has great potential as a communication tool for monitoring home-based exercise. This emerging resource provides patients with access to specialists that physical distance may preclude while also allowing more frequent patient interviews than would be possible with only face-to-face meetings. Webcam interviews are more revealing than phone conversations because they convey the patient's nonverbal, as well as verbal, communication. In this way, the webcam interview is similar to an office visit—perhaps even better because the patient's level of attention, or *inattention*, to self-care can often be more evident when the patient is in his or her own home.[30,34,35] Webcams can be used by physical therapists to access patients for review and upgrade of their home exercise program. In one study, pulmonary rehabilitation programs performed in an outpatient setting were compared with home programs with telemedicine access, and no statistical difference in outcomes was found.[36] Because of the convenience of the webcams, few patients in the study disliked them, but concern was raised about the potential for increased isolation. This concern would need to be addressed if webcams are to be used as a primary means of communication instead of face-to-face meetings. However, the use of a webcam *in addition* to vital sign response as a way of communicating a patient's response to exercise can help the home physical therapist to advocate for the patient's need for medical examination or medication adjustment more clearly than a phone call.

For patients with heart failure, the use of AICDs and biventricular pacemakers is more common because of advances in morbidity and mortality (Chapter 32). Emerging technology is available in some areas to allow the cardiologist not only to monitor a patient's heart rate and rhythm, but also to measure discrete changes in fluid retention that are evident before activity-limiting symptoms.[37,38] Changes in a patient's clinical examination, combined with interview questions regarding diet and bowel and bladder function, can help a clinician monitor changes in fluid retention and lab values. In cases in which a patient often presents with such symptoms, more sensitive monitoring should be used to better control the patient's disease if possible. No data point stands alone, so even when advanced telemedicine options are available, the AICD-communicated data should be analyzed in relation to the physical examination and the patient's interpretation of his or her symptoms.[39]

Regardless of whether or not telemedicine resources are available, physical therapists must continue to use their clinical reasoning skills and their patient's vital sign measurements and convey the information accordingly to achieve best-practice principles and to be the best advocates for their patients. An example that illustrates the importance of this concept involves a patient who was being monitored for his primary diagnosis post-CVA in a home-care setting. The patient demonstrated a new-onset profound fatigue and reported that his knees felt as though they would buckle. The patient had been progressing in his exercise program in each prior session without symptoms, but he had not been monitored. Once the patient expressed the feeling of weakness, however, the physical therapist recorded his vital signs at rest without symptoms and then again after the next walk with symptoms. The patient's blood pressure and heart rate dropped during the exercise. The physician was informed of all signs and symptoms as they correlated to the activity and the new presentation of weakness, which prompted the physician to order a blood test. The results showed that the patient did not have an appropriate blood level of digitalis. Medication was adjusted and the patient's signs, symptoms, and functional level improved. Had the physical therapist not checked the vital signs and instead continued to challenge the patient to work past his symptoms, serious consequences may have resulted. As another possibility, if the physical therapist had called the physician without objectively recorded signs to support the patient's symptoms, the physician may have had insufficient information to determine the best course of action and the patient may have continued to be untreated.

Special Monitoring Considerations for Patients on Oxygen

Oxygen therapy is usually prescribed for hypoxemia (low levels of oxygen in the arterial blood) or to relieve myocardial work such as in cases of severe myocardial infarction.

Typically, arterial blood gases are drawn at rest with no patient activity (unless specifically noted, as in an exercise test with a blood gas), so it is not a likely resource to use in the home setting. Generally, Medicare guidelines specify that a patient with an Spo_2 of 88% or less during activity or recovery be placed on home oxygen. This value is on the steep part of the oxyhemoglobin dissociation curve (Chapter 4). Because oxygen consumption increases proportionately with exercise, a patient may desaturate if oxygen transport is compromised to the extent that it is unable to compensate or respond appropriately to increased demand (Chapter 18). For example, if a patient is on oxygen at rest and the Spo_2 is 90%, he or she may desaturate because the red blood cells need to give up more oxygen to supply the exercising muscle. The patient will be short of breath, and oxygen saturation recorded with an oximeter will be abnormal. A drop below 90% is of concern.

The pulse oximeter reading is an indirect measure of arterial oxygen saturation. For otherwise healthy people, this value is at least 97% at rest, and it is clinically acceptable to maintain oxygen saturation at 90% or higher. This saturation corresponds with maintaining Pao_2 generally above 55 mm Hg; below 55 mm Hg, a dramatic drop in oxygen saturation is associated with a small drop in Pao_2 (Chapter 4).

Best practice in physical therapy requires a pulse oximeter for patients at home or in other facilities. If the facility or home-care agency does not have an oximeter, the medical equipment supplier can provide one.

Patients on oxygen at rest need to have their arterial saturation assessed. Oxygen is a drug, and thus needs to be ordered and prescribed appropriately. The prescription should be written with sufficient flexibility so that it can be adjusted to the patient's needs. A prescription is written to account for a range of liters of oxygen that is estimated to maintain a level of acceptable saturation. For example, the prescription may state to titrate the patient's oxygen to 4 L/min to maintain Spo_2 over 90%. This is true even for people who retain carbon dioxide and whose oxygen is carefully titrated to prevent a suppression of the hypoxic drive to breathe. Strategies are used to limit risk for CO_2 retention and increase ventilation, thereby improving signs and symptoms and reducing risk for desaturation (Chapters 29, 30, and 43).

Though patients may have oxygen established by another professional before the therapy evaluation, it is important to review a few parameters with the patient and caregiver during the course of physical therapy. First, ask patients to tell you their actual oxygen use versus what was prescribed. Next, ask whether they were instructed to adjust the level of oxygen with activity and whether they know how to adjust the dose. If they *do* adjust the oxygen level, what criteria do they use to determine that they need to adjust the dose?[31] Gaps in health literacy and awareness of risk factors can make it difficult for patients to manage their home oxygen safely.

Safety Considerations in the Home Setting

Any evaluation of a patient in a home setting involves an assessment of the patient's home layout and safety concerns. The risk for injury is increased if a patient needs to perform household tasks that trigger signs and symptoms such as overexertion. Several questions can help establish ways of adapting a patient's activity intensity and the physical environment, while also engaging the patient in decision making (Box 41-1).

Box 41-1 Suggested Questions for the Patient

- If the patient is on oxygen, does he or she have a gas stove? Do close relatives, friends, or caretakers smoke? Signs need to be posted to warn about the danger of smoking and flames around oxygen. Patients who smoke need to have this reinforced.
- Does the layout of the home need to be altered to decrease the energy expenditure? Helping patients improve the efficiency of their home layout can improve their safety and independence.
- Patients with chronic primary and secondary cardiovascular and pulmonary conditions who live alone need to make provisions if they have medical emergencies. Does the patient have an alert necklace device or a cell phone that he or she can carry in a pocket? What procedure will be followed? Does the patient know how and when to contact 911 for help? Are there neighbors or family that can regularly check on the patient?
- Does the patient have a multi-level home? Is there a bathroom on all levels? If there is not a bathroom on each floor, can the patient ascend/descend the stairs safely and in a timely manner or does a commode need to be available on some levels?
- Does the patient have the proper adaptive equipment and assistive devices? The use of a rolling walker may improve a patient's walking endurance, allowing them to walk farther without activity-stopping symptoms. Grab bars in bathrooms and toilet seat risers may be needed to reduce energy cost.
- Has the patient modified the intensity and duration of instrumental ADLs, such as laundry and dishes, or is a caretaker available if the patient does not have sufficient endurance to perform such activities?
- Is the patient's bed and bedroom furniture designed to allow safe and efficient transfers into and out of bed?

Home-care agencies often provide the support of a social worker to help patients identify resources available to them. A physician's referral may be needed, and the service is generally covered under Medicare. Although these guiding questions are not exhaustive, they provide a basis for part of the assessment and evaluation.

Exercise and Activity at Home

For patients managed at home, the baseline tolerance for activity and exercise is often low, particularly in those with primary and secondary impairments of the cardiovascular and pulmonary systems. Establishing an exercise program with these patients can be challenging, especially when the patient is inactive or has attempted exercise before with unsuccessful or unpleasant results. Exercise is then less likely to be effective as a therapeutic intervention, and another approach may be necessary to address the patient's need for increased activity for functional and health reasons.

The physical therapist needs to consult with the patient so that exercise is incorporated into daily activities and interests that the patient enjoys, such as playing with grandchildren, gardening, walking, or visiting family and friends (which may involve walking to and from the car, as well as several transfers).

The frequency and intensity of these activities may be minimal initially and increase commensurate with improvement in conditioning. The patient's program is progressed accordingly in conjunction with feedback from the patient. Self-monitoring (perceived exertion and heart rate) and input from the patient should be encouraged. Some patients purchase their own oximeters and use them to monitor their saturation at rest and during activity.

The physical therapist ensures that patients can perform the exercises and ADLs safely and independently (with the appropriate device or caregiver support) while properly and accurately monitoring their own condition and modifying the intensity or distance appropriately with fewer and fewer prompts from the physical therapist. Once patients do this reliably, they or she can pursue activities of their choice, which hastens progression of therapy goals. Also, patients who actively participate in their own rehabilitation will more likely be effective in generalizing the skills learned to their daily life.

Home Oxygen

Home oxygen devices include oxygen concentrators, tanks, and liquid oxygen systems (Figure 41-2, *A*, and Chapter 43). Multiple extensions of oxygen tubing may be needed to enable patients to navigate throughout their homes—for instance, going to the bathroom, maneuvering in the kitchen, and walking to the living room (Figure 41-2, *B*). Although the presence of oxygen in the home is a safety concern that the home-care physical therapist needs to address, long tubing allows for proper oxygen delivery. Compensated flow meters measure the amount of oxygen that reaches the patient, and problems such as kinks are shown by a reduced flow reading. Some portable oxygen systems, particularly demand oxygen systems, may not deliver the amount expected (Figure 41-2, *C*). Thus a pulse oximeter is needed to ensure that the patient's

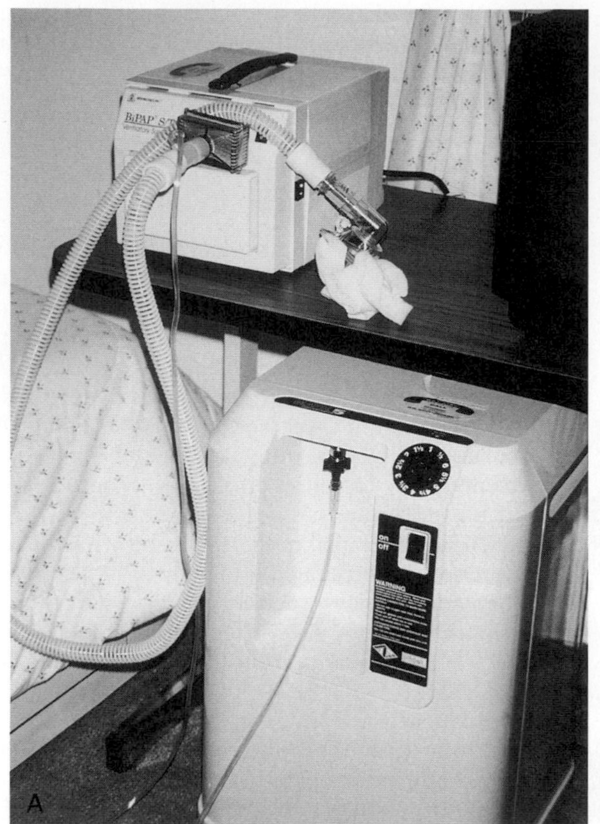

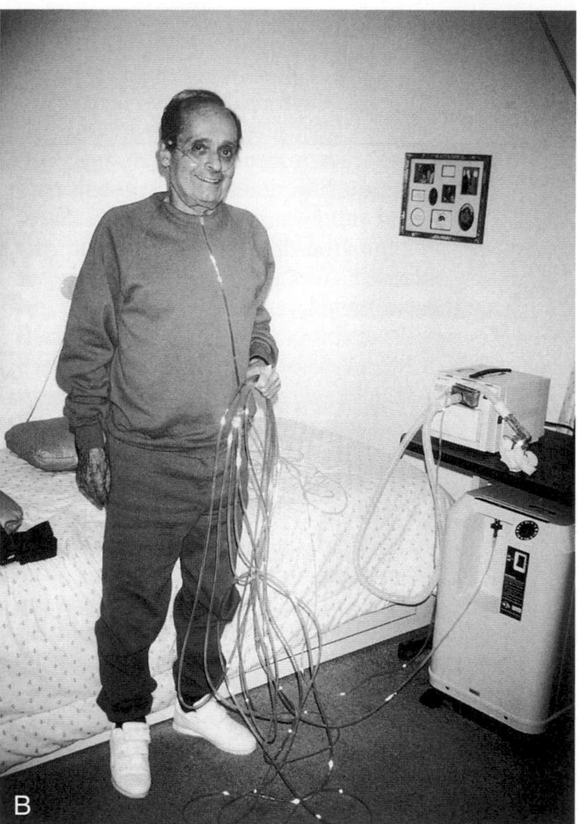

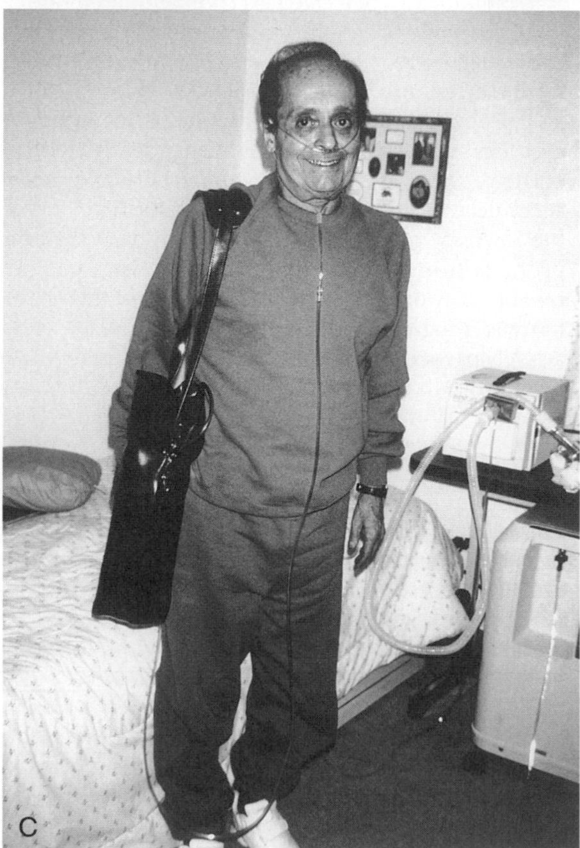

Fig. 41-2 A, Oxygen concentrator. **B,** Oxygen tubing can be a safety hazard. **C,** Portable demand oxygen system.

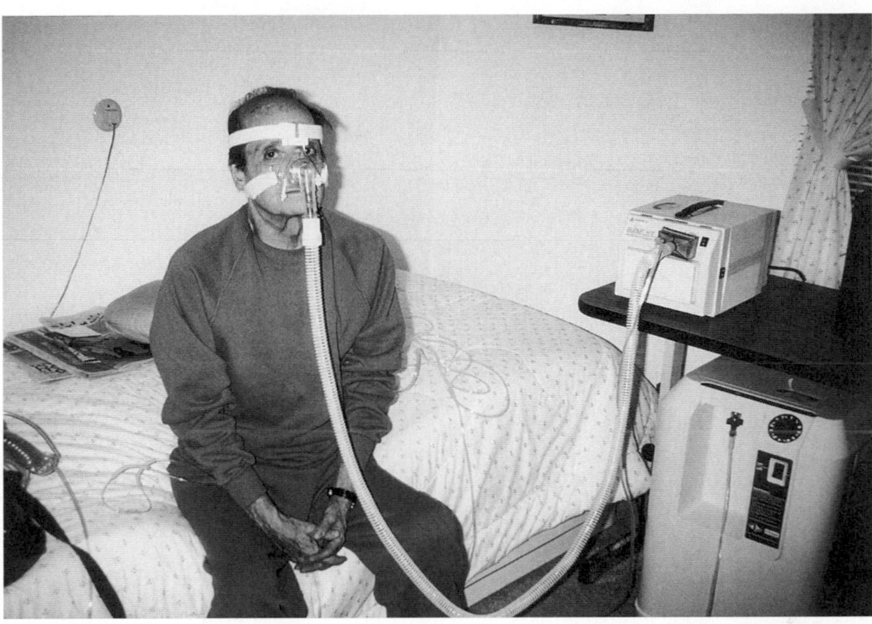

Fig. 41-3 Nasal CPAP machine.

arterial saturation is acceptable. Patients are taught to coil the tubing or use a similar strategy to minimize the risk for tripping. To minimize the need for long lengths of tubing, some patients use more than one tank or concentrator.

Patients with sleep apnea may use nocturnal nasal continuous positive airway pressure (CPAP) (Figure 41-3) or biphasic continuous positive airway pressure (Bi-PAP), which provides varying levels of ventilator assistance at night. A Bi-PAP machine allows the patient to rest and assists ventilation by providing pressure support on inspiration and exhalation. The patient is encouraged to use the machine at night in particular. Although the patient may have difficulty adjusting to the nasal CPAP, he or she will adapt to the assistance and appreciate its benefits.

Documentation

Functional outcomes consistent with the ICF have become as important as outcomes associated with limitation of function and structure (Chapters 7 and 17). Both short- and long-term goals are linked to functional outcomes that enable patients to be safe and as mobile, functional, and independent as possible in the care setting in which they live. The Guide to Physical Therapist Practice (published by the American Physical Therapy Association) defines practice patterns within the cardiovascular and pulmonary areas to use as a reference to establish goals and treatment plans.[40] Goals for patients with cardiovascular and pulmonary conditions, primary or secondary, are typically more detailed than, for example, being able to walk a specific number of feet with a particular device. Goals should also include quantifiable measures of quality—for example, rating of perceived exertion, dyspnea scores, and demonstration of symptom management during functional tasks.

Documentation needs to show progress toward the functional outcomes that the physical therapist has developed with the patient. The cardiovascular and pulmonary systems need to be optimized for the patient to reach maximal outcomes. When functional outcomes are met, the patient is reassessed to determine whether he or she can accomplish more or whether active therapies in the home or long-term care setting need to be replaced with a maintenance program. Patients with chronic conditions should be reexamined periodically to determine whether changes in their disease warrant further therapy. Patients may also progress to a higher level of function that could be managed at an outpatient level of care.

Documentation is the basis for reimbursement. Third-party payers read therapist documentation to determine the examination findings, evaluation, and plan of intervention for the patient. These notes are their primary means of determining a patient's overall status, including functional outcomes and quality of life. For patients who require long-term physical therapy, thorough and accurate documentation is vital to communication with third-party payers to increase the likelihood that patients will be able to receive the services they need. Teamwork that includes the patient in the decision making and goal planning has become a focus of optimal management in recent years.[23] Written and verbal communication is vital to the exchange of information and the targeted and timely progression of care to meet patients' ongoing and often-changing needs. One rule of thumb must always be remembered: "If it wasn't written, it wasn't done."

Support for People in the Home or Community

An important part of achieving optimal health upon returning home or settling into a new living facility is having the necessary social and emotional supports. Hospital stays or new functional limitations can often cause patients to think of themselves only as patients, solely defined by their medications, symptoms, and diagnoses. Family and friends can help prevent this. Close social ties help to keep patients connected to memories and situations that define them as individuals.

Support can also be found with people who have similar diagnoses or limitations. Support groups and networks are

Box 41-2 Patient-Friendly COPD Websites*

- National Emphysema COPD Association (NECACommunity.org)
- Self-care, sharing of information for people with COPD (COPD-ALERT.org)
- American College of Chest Physicians (chestnet.org)
- American Lung Association (lungsusa.org/diseases)
- Canadian Lung Association (lung.ca/copd)
- Harvard University Medical School, COPD and pulmonary disease (intellihealth.com)
- Medical information site geared to patients (medicinenet.com/lungs/focus)
- National Heart, Lung and Blood Institute (nhlbi.nih.gov/health/public/lung)
- Information on alpha-1-antitrypsin deficit (alphaone.org)

*This is a partial listing of some websites for people with chronic diseases and their families or caregivers. Numerous other helpful informational sites are available. This is meant as a starting point. Many links to other resources will be found by accessing these websites.

often formed in the community and, increasingly, on the Internet. Such groups can be important resources for patients, regardless of the support they receive from family and friends. Peers in these groups may be the only people who fully understand what the patient is going through; support from these peers, as well as the opportunity for the patient to support others in return, can help inspire physical and emotional gains.

Peer groups, in person or over the Internet, can be valuable resources to help patients with chronic conditions make choices concerning their health and life situations.[41-46] Many websites and blogs offer free information or may request a nominal fee for membership for patients, health professionals, and supporters to receive newsletters and information in the mail. They host grassroots efforts such as conferences and informational sessions on self-care management and patient empowerment. These support groups publish newsletters that discusses research and provide tips from people living with chronic conditions to help share evidence-based information. These organizations inform people that they are not alone and steer them towards resources that can help with decision making as they strive for optimal health.

Many patient-friendly websites are available for people with COPD and other common chronic conditions, all of which are easily accessed through various search engines or by exploring the links sections of related websites. **Box 41-2** lists examples of websites that may be helpful to people with chronic conditions and their families or caregivers.

Therapeutic Goals for Home-Care Patients with Cardiovascular and Pulmonary Dysfunction

To be independent at home, patients with cardiovascular and pulmonary dysfunction should strive toward achieving all of the following:

- Understand the dysfunction or condition and how it results in the changes in signs and symptoms that affect daily functioning.
- Acquire the necessary adaptive equipment and assistive devices for use in the home and community.
- Acknowledge functional limitations (e.g., do not push limits without monitoring responses) to ensure safety.
- Adhere to medication regimens and the direction of physicians and other health professionals. Discuss what is working well—and what is not—and collaborate to find better solutions and interventions.[14,32]
- Arrange for caregivers to safely and consistently provide assistance as needed.
- Learn preventative care strategies (e.g., prevent pulmonary infections and do not increase salt/water intake if on cardiac precautions or taking steroids).
- Learn ventilatory strategies to increase comfort and function (Chapter 23).
- Learn to self-monitor for signs of impending difficulty (e.g., increased shortness of breath, swelling in ankles, productive cough, changes in mucus, decreased urine output, or rapid weight gain of 2-3 pounds per day).
- Pace activities and use energy conservation strategies and rest periods to accomplish more with less physiological demand.
- Optimize nutrition and hydration and notify health professionals about increases or decreases in weight.
- Seek referral to a dietitian as needed to understand the impact of food choice on health and function if knowledge deficits are affecting health promotion.
- Develop a social support network to provide emotional support when needed.
- Increase general exercise both in terms of a specific exercise program and in completing the necessary tasks of the day to continue functional gains.

Summary

The physical therapist can promote optimal health for patients with chronic and short-term illnesses who live in various community settings. A patient's path to optimal health involves patient education on effective methods of self-monitoring during activity, adherence to medication regimen, and use of multiple available resources to achieve a higher functional level. Education methods using shared decision making[23] can improve patient risk factor reduction, nutrition, and overall functional level more effectively and efficiently than methods in which the patient is not actively part of the solution. People living with chronic conditions can live more safely and independently at home if given sufficient education in a format in which they can understand the goals and expectations before them. As health professionals, physical therapists recommend modifications of patients' home environments and offer tools to use to best achieve their functional independence and fit their lifestyle based on the best available research. Patients' participation in such recommendations is vital to improve the degree and longevity of their progress toward optimal health. If patients are to be successful in living independently in the home setting, they need to be independent in their judgments and activities. Physical therapists must respect patients' choices and decisions, while sharing their own experience, therapeutic judgment, and expertise. The home setting can be a particularly rewarding practice experience, although at times it can be challenging. One thing is certain—if you ask a patient where he or she wants to be, the answer is almost always the same: "There's no place like home!"

Review Questions

1. What are some common problems patients in the community may experience?
2. What role do preexisting cardiovascular and pulmonary conditions play in a new diagnosis or trauma (e.g., CVA or hip fracture)?
3. What are some common and unique situations or concerns particular to patient care delivery in (a) a nursing home, (b) an assisted living center, and (c) home care?
4. What role can a physical therapist play in optimizing the patient's self-management in each of the settings listed in the previous question?
5. Describe how cardiovascular and pulmonary function can be monitored in long-term care and in home care.
6. What instructions and considerations should be provided for a patient on oxygen?
7. How can caregivers and family members be incorporated into the management of patients with chronic conditions in the home and in a long-term care setting?

References

1. United States Department of Health and Human Services, www.HHS.gov.
2. Carson, 1999
3. Epping-Jordan JE, Pruitt SD, Bengoa R, et al: Improving the quality of health care for chronic conditions. *Quality Safe Heath Care* 13:299–305, 2004.
4. Guinn MJ: A daughter's journey promoting geriatric self-care: promoting positive health care interactions. *Geriatric Nursing* 2595:267–271, 2004.
5. Hainsworth T: A new model of care for people who have long-term conditions. *Nursing Times* 101:L28–L29, 2005.
6. Holman H, Lorig K: Patient self-management: a key to effectiveness and efficiency in care of chronic disease. *Public Health Report* 119:239–243, 2004.
7. Hughes S: Promoting self-management and patient independence. *Nursing Standard* 19:L47–L52, 2004.
8. Jerant AF, Levich B, Balsbaugh T, et al: Walk a mile in my shoes: a chronic illness care workshop for first year students. *Family Medicine* 37:L21–L26, 2005.
9. Marks R, Allegrante JP, Lorig K: A review and synthesis of research evidence for self-efficacy-enhancing interventions for reducing chronic disability: implications for health education practice (part I). *Health Promotion Practice* 6:37–43, 2005.
10. Monninkhof E, van der Aa M, van der Valk P, et al: A qualitative evaluation of a comprehensive self-management programme for COPD patients: effectiveness from the patients' perspective. *Patient Education Counseling* 55:177–184, 2004.
11. O'Donnell DE, Aaron S, Bourbeau J, et al: State of the art compendium: Canadian Thoracic Society recommendations for the management of chronic obstructive pulmonary disease. Canadian Respiratory *Journal* 11(Suppl B):7B–59B, 2004.
12. Tanner EK: Chronic illness demands for self-management in older adults. *Geriatric Nursing* 25:313–317, 2004.
13. Harmon G, Lefante J, Krousel-Wood M: Overcoming barriers: the role of providers in improving patient adherence to antihypertensive medications. *Curr Opin Cardiol* 21:310–315, 2006.
14. Gold DT, McClung B: Approaches to patient education: emphasizing the long-term value of compliance and persistence. *Am J of Med* 119(4A):32S–37S, 2006.
15. National Institute on Aging, 2007
16. Needham, 2008
17. Needham, 2010
18. Herridge, et al, 2003
19. Hopkins, et al, 2005
20. Desai, 2011
21. Iwashyna, 2010
22. Senoff, 2000
23. Légaré F, Stacey D, Brière N, et al: A conceptual framework for interprofessional shared decision making in home care: protocol for a feasibility study. *BMC Health Services Research* 11:23–30, 2011.
24. Guyatt G. 1992
25. Weston, 2001
26. Authier P: Being present—the choice that re-instills caring. *Nursing Administration* 28:276–279, 2004.
27. McDonough-Means SI, Kreitzer MJ, Bell IR: Fostering a healing presence and investigating its mediators. *Journal of Alternative and Complementary Medicine* 10(Suppl 1):S25–S41, 2004.
28. Pedelty L, Gorelick PB: Management of hypertension and cerebrovascular disease in the elderly. *The Amer J of Med* 121(8A):S23–S31, 2008.
29. Ackerman M, Locatis C: Advanced networks and computing in health care. *J Am Med Inform Assoc* 18:523–528, 2011.
30. Pols J: The wonderful world of webcams: About Active Gazes and Invisible Technologies. *Sci, Tech and Human Values* 36(4):451–473, 2011.
31. Neri M, Melani AS, Miorelli AM, et al: Long-term oxygen therapy in chronic respiratory failure: a multicenter Italian study on oxygen therapy adherence. *Resp Med* 100:795–806, 2006.
32. Sorensen L, Stokes JA, Purdie DM, et al: Medication management at home: medication risk factor prevalence and inter-relationships. *J Clin Pharm and Therapeutics* 31:485–491, 2006.
33. National Research Council Report in 2000
34. Morgan DG, Crossley M, Kirk A, et al: Evaluation of telehealth for preclinic assessment and follow-up in an interprofessional rural and remote memory clinic. *Journal of Applied Gerontology* 30(3):304–331, 2011.
35. Turner, 2004
36. Maltais F, Bourbeau J, Shapiro S, et al: Effects of home-based pulmonary rehabilitation in patients with chronic obstructive pulmonary disease. *Ann Intern Med* 149:869–878, 2008.
37. Brachmann J, Böhm M, Rybak K, et al: Fluid status monitoring with a wireless network to reduce cardiovascular-related hospitalizations and mortality in heart failure: rationale and design of the Optilink HF Study (Optimization of heart failure management using OptiVol fluid status monitoring and CareLink). *Eur Heart Journal* 13:796–804, 2011.
38. Santini M, Ricci RP, Lunati M, et al: Remote monitoring of patients with biventricular defibrillators through the CareLink system improves clinical management of arrhythmias and heart failure episodes. *Journal of Interventional Cardiac Electrophysiology* 24(1):53–61, 2009 Jan.
39. Andersen T, Bjørn P, Kensing F, et al: Designing for collaborative interpretation in telemonitoring: re-introducing patients as diagnostic agents. *Int J Med Informatics* 80:112–126, 2011.
40. Guide to PT Practice, 2003
41. Anhoj J, Jensen AH: Using the Internet for life style changes in diet and physical activity: a feasibility study. *Journal of Medical Internet Resources* 6:33, 2004.
42. Gunnarsdottir, 2004
43. Jamison, 2004
44. Lieberich, 2004
45. Nguyen HQ, Carrieri-Kohlman V, Rankin SH, et al: Is Internet-based support for dyspnea self-management in patients with chronic obstructive pulmonary disease possible? Results of a pilot study. *Heat & Lung* 34:51–62, 2005.
46. Wentland DJ, et al: The effectiveness of Web-based vs. non-Web based intervention on a meta-analysis of behavioral change outcomes. *Journal of Medical Internet Resources* 6:40, 2003.

Part VIII

Related Aspects of Cardiovascular and Pulmonary Physical Therapy

PART VIII OUTLINE

Body Mechanics: Positioning and Moving Patients

BJ Lehecka, Donna Frownfelter, and Mary Massery

KEY TERMS

Body mechanics
Dependent patients
Lifting and moving
"Positioning for success"
Ventilation

CHAPTER OUTLINE

Body mechanics can be defined as the efficient use of one's body as a machine and locomotive entity. When working with critically ill or chronically dependent patients, physical therapists frequently change patients' body positioning before and during treatments to facilitate ventilatory potential and improve patient outcomes. Therapists and nurses attempting to position or move dependent patients need to understand and use proper body mechanics.[1-5] This knowledge is necessary to maximize treatment outcomes and to reduce biomechanical stress and trauma for the patient and for those working directly with the patient. Low back pain is the most common cause of work-related disability among employees younger than 46 years, and nurses and physical therapists account for over half of the annual prevalence of low back pain among health care personnel.[6,7] Positioning and moving dependent patients is an art that is quite different from working with a patient who can move independently and assume any given position with ease. In this chapter, the principles of body positioning and moving dependent patients are discussed.

Positioning for Optimal Ventilation

Because of the three-dimensional nature of breathing, one of the therapist's most important goals is to facilitate chest excursion in all three planes of ventilation: anterior-posterior, superior-inferior, and lateral.[8] This can be accomplished by improving the length-tension relationships of the muscles used in inspiration.[9,10] Massery[8] reasons that proper positioning to enhance inspiratory muscles will accomplish the following:

1. Improve the length-tension relationship of the accessory ventilatory muscles involved in that posture.
2. Incorporate a passive stretch of the chest wall.
3. Use the natural coordination of the trunk-chest wall movement with inspiration and exhalation patterns to maximize movement.

The following are some common improvements that can be incorporated into normal positioning.

Supine Position

All activity is performed within the field of gravity. Patients in a supine position may find breathing difficult because they must overcome gravity to move the chest wall with each breath. Using towel rolls or pillows to facilitate a better position may improve the patient's ventilation, both its ease and capacity. Positioning alternatives, however, need to be applied with each patient's comfort and tolerance in mind.

Upper chest expansion can be increased by removing pillows from under the patient's head to increase thoracic extension. This will increase the length-tension relationship of the neck accessory muscles (scalene and sternocleidomastoid muscles). Increased movement will be noted in the upper chest in the superior and anterior planes.[8] Further anterior expansion may be achieved with a towel roll placed longitudinally at the vertebral spine to open the anterior chest of a patient who tends toward excessive flexion of the trunk (Figure 42-1, *A*).

If the patient needs support under the head to achieve a neutral chin tuck to protect swallowing ability, a thin pillow or horizontal towel roll under the occiput can be used (Figure 42-1, *B*).

External rotation of the shoulders with the scapulae in a neutral or retracted position will stretch the pectoralis and intercostal muscles. This may improve lateral and anterior chest wall movements.[10,11] If a patient has full range of motion (ROM) and is comfortable with the arms placed overhead or in full flexion/abduction/external rotation for maximal stretch, this is the optimal position for potential maximal excursion of the anterior chest wall (Figure 42-1, *C*). If there are major shoulder limitations, moderate shoulder abduction with forearm supination may be the best position available to facilitate chest excursion. Whenever significant limitations are found, the therapist should try to modify the position to accommodate the patient's needs and achieve optimal ventilation.

Side-Lying Position

Side-lying is an optimal position that may improve breathing patterns. At the same time, medical professionals should continue to heed the need for prescriptive rather than routine patient positioning. In side-lying, gravity is eliminated for anterior expansion and the diaphragm moves freely, particularly the upper hemi-diaphragm, which is not having to shift the abdominal contents as much as the lower hemi-diaphragm. Such a position may be optimal for preterm infants who, when placed in a side-lying or prone position, have been shown to have fewer stress behaviors, resulting in longer periods of sleep with less fussiness and crying.[12] However, side-lying positions can also result in decreased forced vital capacity and forced expiratory volume lung measurements and may not be optimal for patients with risks for cardiopulmonary compromise.[13] A specific example of the need for prescriptive rather than routine positioning of a patient in side-lying involves a patient with pneumonia or atelectasis. If a patient has right lower lobe pneumonia or atelectasis, side-lying on the unaffected left side will improve oxygenation. Conversely, side-lying with the affected side down will cause a decrease in oxygenation (differential shunt) because a patient with decreased ventilation receives more perfusion to the down lung with more shunting.

In side-lying, the patient's hips and knees should be flexed and supported for comfort. The upper extremities can be moved up and away from the body to allow for free movement of the upper chest wall. A pillow can be used to support the upper arm anteriorly, or the patient can be placed in a three-quarter supine position with a pillow behind the back to support the uppermost arm. If the patient has full ROM and is comfortable, a butterfly position of the arms can be used. This tends to expand the rib cage, lengthen the pectoral muscles, and facilitate inspiration.

Prone Position

Prone positioning can improve oxygenation with minimal untoward effects in several patient populations, including those who are critically ill and medically unstable, such as preterm infants, patients with acute respiratory distress syndrome (ARDS), and patients with hypoxemic acute respiratory failure.[12,14-23] Oxygenation is improved with prone positioning when compared with supine positioning via more homogenous lung inflation and alveolar ventilation,[24] but some cases with concomitant difficulties have been reported. One instance of severe hypotension was noted in a child with scoliosis, pectus excavatum, and neurofibromatosis who presented for a spinal fusion. It is recommended that sternal pressure be avoided in patients with chest wall deformities.[25] Early enteral nutrition is poorly tolerated in critically ill patients receiving invasive mechanical ventilation in the prone position. Medication can be given to enhance gastric emptying and prevent vomiting. Feeding the patient in the prone position becomes challenging if the patient is mechanically ventilated as well.[26]

When a patient is mechanically ventilated and has numerous tubes and monitors, turning him or her to the prone position takes planning and is staff intensive. Although turning a patient prone may be difficult, reviews of related studies report that prone positioning may reduce the absolute mortality of severely hypoxemic ARDS patients by approximately 10% in addition to improving their oxygenation by 27%-39%. However, the reviews also suggest that long-term prone positioning can expose patients with less severe ARDS to unnecessary increased risks for pressure ulcers, endotracheal tube obstruction, and chest tube dislodgement.[24,27] Thus body positioning requires careful prescription of not only the specific positions, but also the time the patient spends in those positions, which is largely response dependent.

Upright Postures

Upright postures create challenges to breathing by adding the components of balance and an unsupported spinal column. Many patients, however, spend prolonged periods of time in their wheelchairs or in other situations in which they are sitting or standing. Patients with poor trunk support may sit in a slumped position, which decreases tidal volume and minute ventilation. Approximating erect upright sitting postures may improve pulmonary function and better breathing support for functional activities.

Pelvic alignment is a key component to optimal posture. A relatively anterior tilted pelvis in healthy, flexible adults may reduce the kyphotic curve in the thoracic spine, adduct the scapulae toward a neutral position, produce a more neutral or externally rotated upper-extremity position, and pull the head back into a neutral chin tuck.[28,29] The anterior tilt of the pelvis may improve upper-extremity ROM and ventilation. Attending to this one consideration may be all that is needed to improve the breathing capacity of some patients, allowing them to continue to advance in their exercise programs or rehabilitation. Further benefit may be achieved with a lumbar roll.

Another simple means of attaining an anterior pelvic tilt in sitting is to have the patient lean forward over his or her legs, then slide a towel roll horizontally just behind the ischial

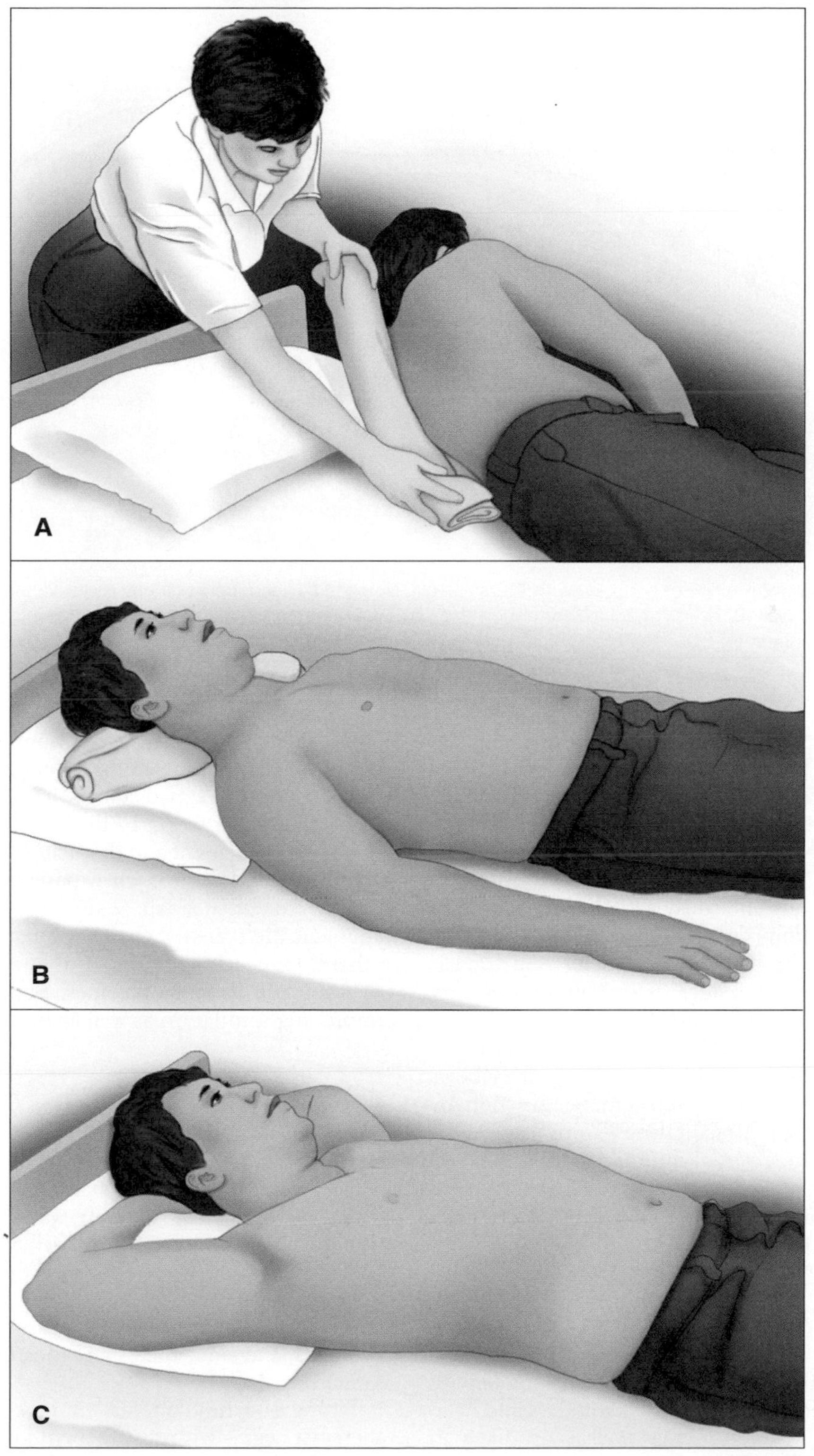

Fig. 42-1 A, Placement of a vertical towel roll. **B,** Increased openness of the anterior chest wall with the vertical thoracic towel roll and the occipital towel roll combined. **C,** Butterfly position with a thoracic towel roll to open the anterior chest.

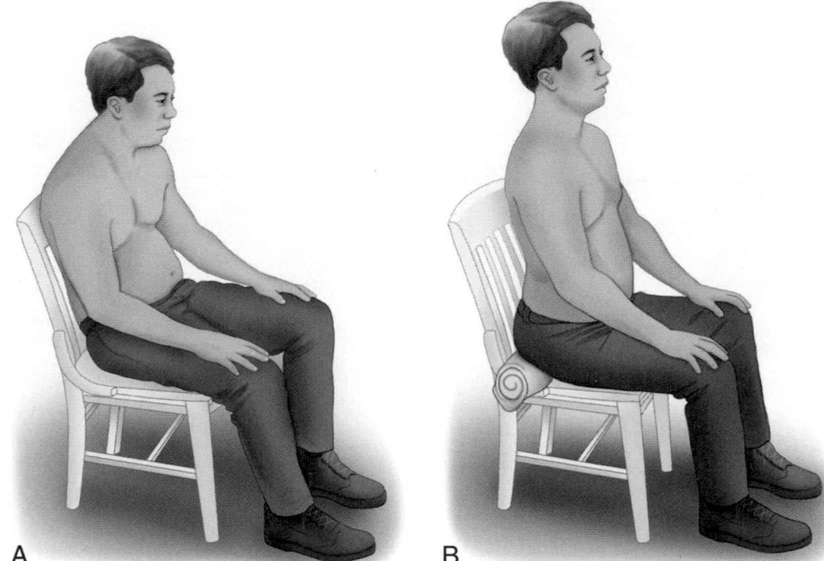

Fig. 42-2 A, Unsupported upright position of a patient with T1 paraplegia. Note the posterior pelvic tilt and excessive thoracic kyphosis with resulting collapse of the anterior chest wall. **B,** Ischial towel roll to support the pelvis in anterior tilt in a patient with T1 paraplegia. Note the changes in the thoracic spine and open anterior chest wall, as well as improved head and neck alignment.

tuberosities, which can prevent the pelvis from tilting posteriorly (Figure 42-2).[30] This can be well tolerated by patients with intact sensation and a pelvis that is at least minimally mobile. For patients with neurological impairment who have impaired sensation or less pelvic mobility, a wedge can be substituted; however, some sliding may occur.

In addition to a relatively anteriorly tilted pelvis, a posture of anterior trunk inclination (forward-lean) with arm bracing has been shown to increase ventilatory capacity.[31] Such positioning has resulted in higher values of maximal respiratory pressures and respiratory muscle endurance in patients with chronic obstructive pulmonary disease.[32] This forward-lean position with arm bracing posture (as in sitting with elbows on knees or a table) improves diaphragmatic function by reducing abdominal tension,[33] facilitating expiratory muscle action (such as that of the external oblique abdominis), and enabling arm and shoulder girdle muscles (such as the pectorals and serratus anterior) to act more effectively as accessory muscles of inspiration.[34]

Neutral Alignment of the Head and Shoulders

A vertical or horizontal towel roll may also be used with wheelchair positioning to better align the shoulders and head into neutral position. The anterior chest wall is also likely to be less compressed in this position.

A neutral head and neck position is important for patients with impaired speech volume or endurance and for patients with swallowing or aspiration impairments. A neutral chin tuck may optimize the length-tension relationship of the vocal folds, minimize vocal strain, and improve protective airway reflexes.[8] Vertical head alignment may also help to reduce airway resistance and maintain normal breathing rates, thereby helping to ensure optimal contribution from the diaphragm without compensation from chest wall inspiratory muscles.[35]

It is vital to evaluate the positioning of the patient's shoulders. Internal rotation of the shoulders and scapular protraction may restrict expansion of the upper chest. On the other hand, external rotation of the shoulders may increase upper chest wall movement and thoracic extension.[11] Clinically, lung volumes may improve when patient positioning is carefully considered. Often small, seemingly insignificant changes may augment the patient's clinical outcomes in conjunction with other therapeutic activities. If unattended, these small factors may impede patient outcomes. Body positioning is vital to improving ventilation as well as functional skills.

Lifting and Moving Dependent Patients

There have been changes in the concepts and principles of lifting. As discussed, the body was historically thought of in terms of a machine. Improper mechanics of lifting was thought to place disproportionate load on the discs. The key components of lifting were to "keep it close," "bend the knees," and "lift with the legs." Over 20 years ago, a shift in thought occurred, and since then spinal posture has been the focus of safe lifting.[36]

Lifting is a fundamental human activity. In practice, the therapist begins with slightly bent knees and the patient rears backward as the therapist extends his or her knees and starts to lift the patient's gluteal area first. Injuries seem to occur with the back in flexion. The rationale for a therapist having strong core muscles is to promote safe lifting. Abdominal strength is necessary to support the pelvis during lifting. Commercially available lumbar and abdominal elastic supports are widely used. These provide additional abdominal wall support, as well as serving as a reminder to the therapist to lift safely. Care needs to be taken to ensure these supports are worn properly and replaced when worn out. Another lifting principle is maintaining the lordotic lumbar curve when lifting. This technique is used by weight lifters.

Lifting techniques may need to be modified because of factors such as limited space (e.g., small hospital rooms), clothing issues, or health conditions of the health care team members (e.g., degenerative knee joints).

A primary consideration when applying appropriate body mechanics during lifting is proper posture and balance (body stability), specifically with respect to the relationship between gravity, posture, and body stability (Figure 42-3). Gravitational force is exerted in a vertical direction down toward the earth's center. In addition, that point in a patient or object at which all of its mass is centered is called the center of gravity (the point at which the patient's maximum weight is concentrated). When standing, the body's center of gravity is located at approximately 55% of the body's total height from the ground: in the pelvic cavity, slightly anterior to the upper part of the sacrum. The lower a person's center of gravity, the greater his or her body stability. Consequently, when the body lifts a patient or an object, muscular effort needs to increase sufficiently to maintain stability and lift against the force of gravity because the lifter's center of gravity is displaced toward the object. Therefore the therapist can conserve energy and maintain stability by bearing the weight of the patient (or object) as close to his or her own center of gravity as possible. This allows the lifter maximum concentration of energy toward movement of the patient and minimal stress or injury. To facilitate a lift, the bed should be adjusted so that the lifter can reach the patient comfortably. Usually, adjusting the bed to the lifter's hip level is adequate. This places the patient close to the lifter's center of gravity.

Most lifting should be done with the legs (knees) as opposed to lifting with the arms and back to minimize biomechanical strain (Figure 42-4). Whenever there is a question about a single therapist's ability to lift a patient alone, assistance should be obtained either from another health care professional or by an assistive device such as a mechanical lift.[37]

Another consideration in lifting is the base of support of the lifter. The base of support is defined as the area between the feet, which provides the body's stability. The wider the base of support, the greater the body's stability. To expand on this point, it is necessary to define the line of gravity and its relationship to body stability. The line of gravity is an imaginary line passing through the center of gravity of an object and perpendicular to the surface on which the object (body) rests (see Figure 42-3). The closer the line of gravity passes to the center of the base of support, the greater the body's (object's) stability. Muscular effort is directly related to the distance that the line of gravity is shifted from the base of support.[38]

The guidelines for patient lifting are summarized below.

- The lower your center of gravity, the wider your base of support, and the nearer the line of gravity falls to

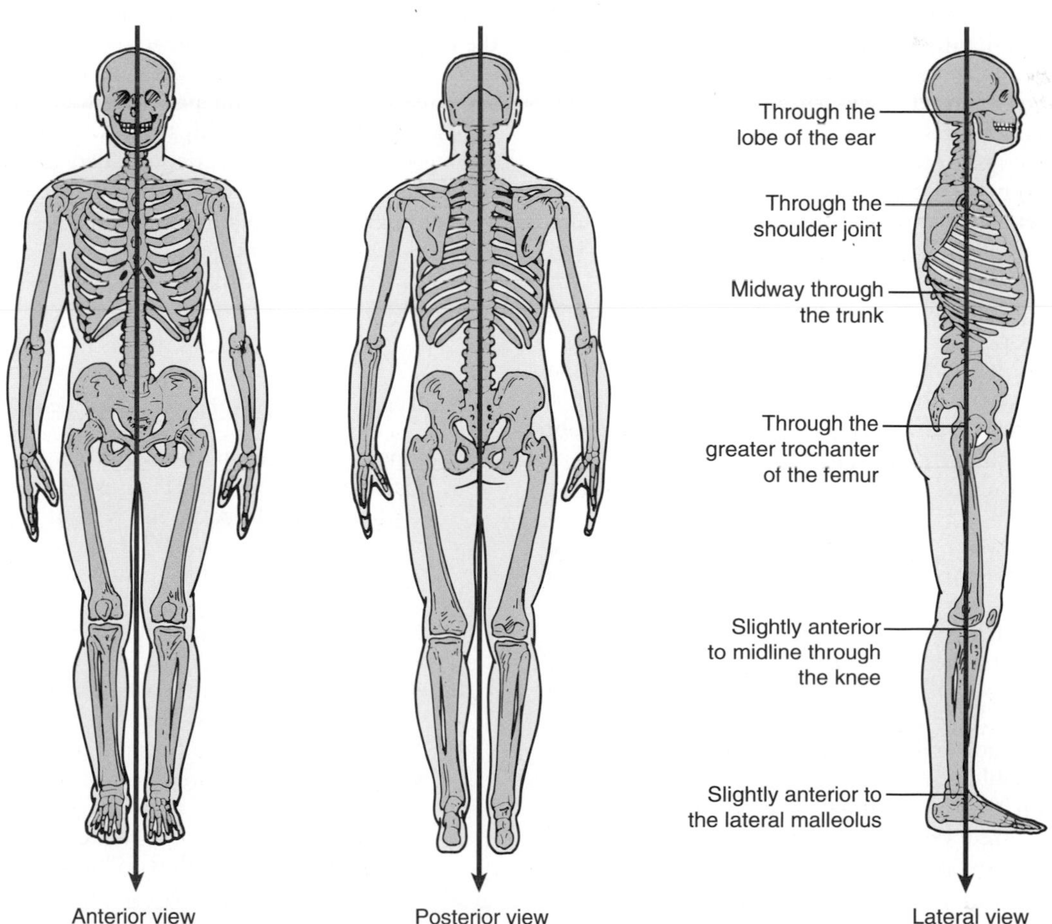

Fig. 42-3 The line of gravity passes through the center of gravity and the base of support to maintain body stability. *(From Cameron MH, Monroe LG: Physical rehabilitation: Evidence-based examination, evaluation, and intervention, St Louis, 2008, Saunders.)*

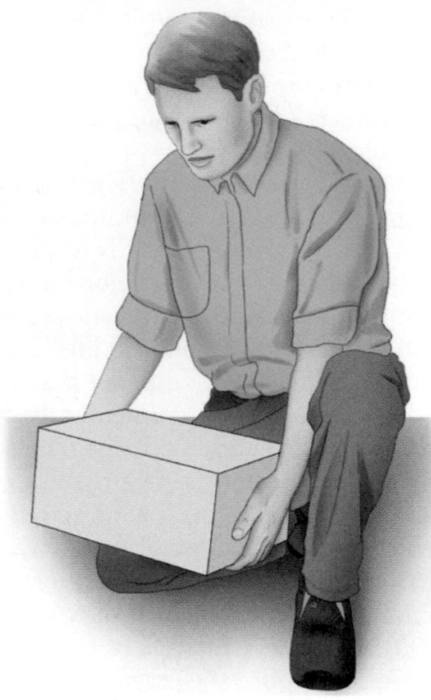

Fig. 42-4 Reach work level by bending the knees and hips rather than the back. Lift with the legs! This can also be done with a full double-knee squat similar to techniques by weightlifters.

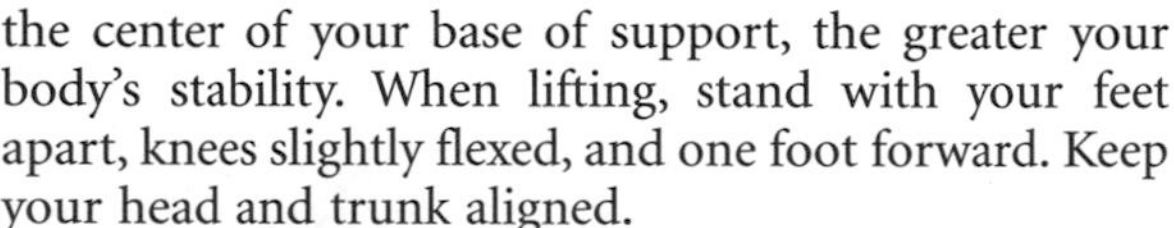

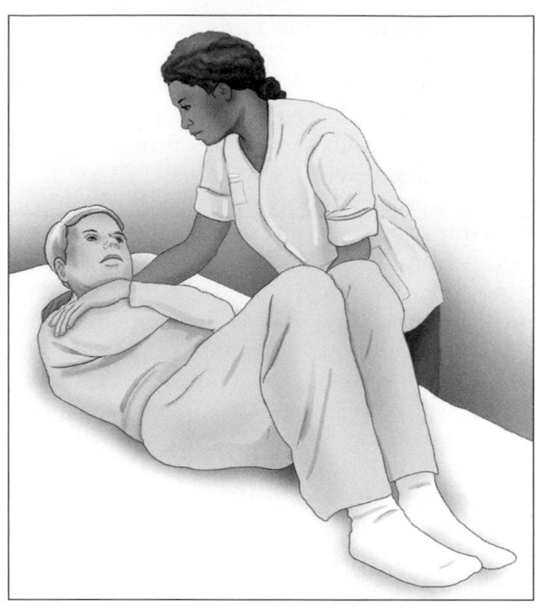

Fig. 42-5 The patient should be prepared for a position change: knees bent, arms crossed over chest, and head lifted up to reduce friction between the patient's body and the bed.

the center of your base of support, the greater your body's stability. When lifting, stand with your feet apart, knees slightly flexed, and one foot forward. Keep your head and trunk aligned.

- When a body is used as a machine, the external weight on which it works displaces the body's center of gravity in the direction of the weight being lifted. To conserve energy and maintain stability, carry the weight as close to your center of gravity as possible. Lower your hips to the level of the surface supporting the weight you plan to lift by flexing your hips and knees. Adjust the bed as high or low as you need for comfortable and efficient work.
- The effort required to perform an activity depends on the weight of the object to be lifted. Know your limits. Do not attempt to lift alone if you have any doubt about your ability to do so.
- Other general tips for lifting are as follows (see Figure 42-4):
  - Lift with your legs. Keep legs in a position that permits them to supply most of the force for shifting your trunk.
  - Do not attempt to lift with your arms and back.
  - When lifting, avoid rotation of the spine. Shift your feet into a position that supports the patient's weight shift when moving or lifting the patient.
  - Stabilize your body against a stationary object whenever possible.
  - For efficiency, coordinate the move by using a synchronized verbal expression that is understood by therapists and patient—for instance, "one, two, three, lift."

One additional consideration must be noted—moving against the resistance of friction. Friction is defined as a force that opposes the movement of one object over the surface of another. Friction is reduced as the amount of surface-area contact between two objects is reduced.

When moving a patient side to side or up and down in bed, the therapist or nurse attempts to reduce the contact between the patient's body surface and the bed. The use of a turning sheet placed just above the patient's shoulders and extending to just below the patient's hips will help reduce such friction. Strategies for shifting a patient in bed include crossing the patient's arms over his or her chest or abdomen, having the patient flex the knees and hips, and asking the patient to flex the neck and raise the head as he or she is lifted (if the patient is unable to do this, the therapist or nurse can assist) (Figure 42-5).

Moving Dependent Patients

I. Moving the patient up or down.[39-40]
  A. Using a turning sheet (Figures 42-6).
    1. Sheet should cover the patient from shoulders to hips.
    2. Gather sheet material as close to the patient's body as possible.
    3. Hold at shoulders and hips with a flexion pattern (see Figure 42-6, *B*).
    4. Cross patient's arms over his or her chest; have the patient flex knees and hips.
    5. Ask the patient to raise his or her head if possible.
    6. Synchronize action by counting "one, two, three, lift."
    7. Shift weight from one leg to the other rather than lifting up and pulling on back.
  B. Without a turning sheet (up or down), more than one lifter may be needed.
    1. Follow basic procedure: cross patient's arms, ask patient to lift head, flex knees and hips.

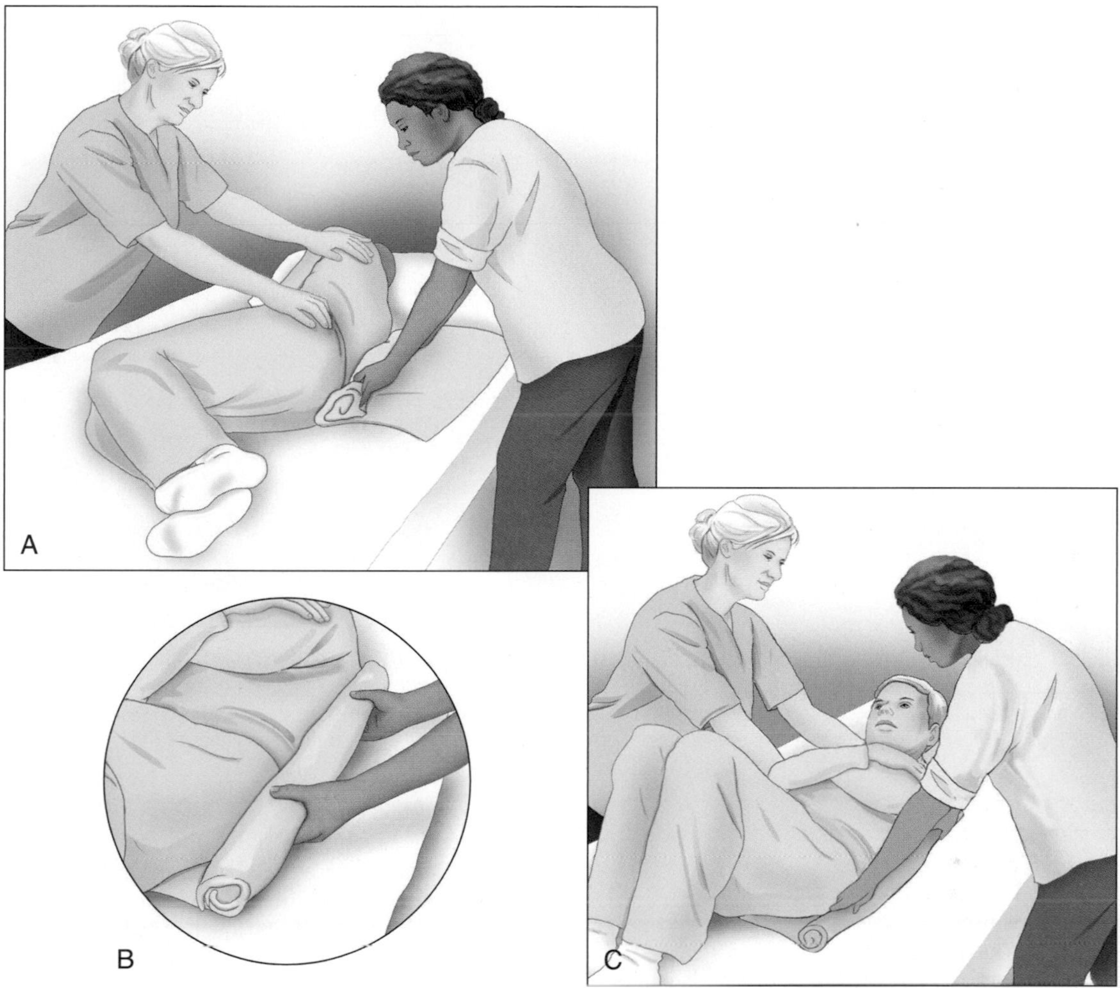

Fig. 42-6 A, To insert the draw sheet, the patient is turned onto his or her side and the half-rolled draw sheet is tucked under the patient (from just above the shoulders to just below the hips). The patient rolls over the draw sheet and it is pulled out behind him or her. **B,** The draw sheet should be rolled close to the patient's body. A flexion hand grip at the patient's shoulders and hip is most efficient. **C,** Moving the patient toward the head of the bed. The patient is prepared. The therapist is positioned to move toward the head of the bed in order to shift his or her body weight to move the patient.

2. The therapist places his or her hands and forearms under the patient's shoulders and hips.
3. If patient is extremely heavy or tall, another person can bend knees and assist.

II. Moving the patient to the side of the bed.
A. With turning sheet.
1. Cross patient's arms and other body parts toward the side to which the patient is to be moved.
2. Therapist places his or her hands at the patient's hips and shoulder on material close to the patient's body.
3. One therapist pushes, and the other pulls.

B. Without turning sheet.
1. Both therapists stand on the desired side.
2. One therapist's forearms go under the patient's shoulder; the other's go under the patient's hips.
3. Synchronize action by counting "one, two, three, pull."

III. Turning the patient onto his or her side.
A. With turning sheet (to right side) (Figure 42-7).
1. Move the patient supine to the opposite side of the turn (e.g., if turning onto right side, move the patient to the left side of the bed).
2. Bring the patient's right arm to the side at a 90-degree angle up and away from the body.
3. Place the patient's left arm across the chest.
4. Place the patient's left leg over the right leg.
5. Pull the sheet at the patient's back to turn.

B. Without turning sheet (to right side).
1. Move patient to opposite side (therapist's hands and forearms under patient's shoulders and hips).
2. Use steps 2, 3, and 4 above.
3. Roll patient to right side by pushing or pulling patient's left shoulder and left hip.

IV. Turning the patient prone (e.g., roll to right side) (Figure 42-8).
A. With or without turning sheet.
1. Move the patient to the opposite side of the bed from the side toward which he or she is turning.
2. Cross the patient's left arm and left leg over the body.

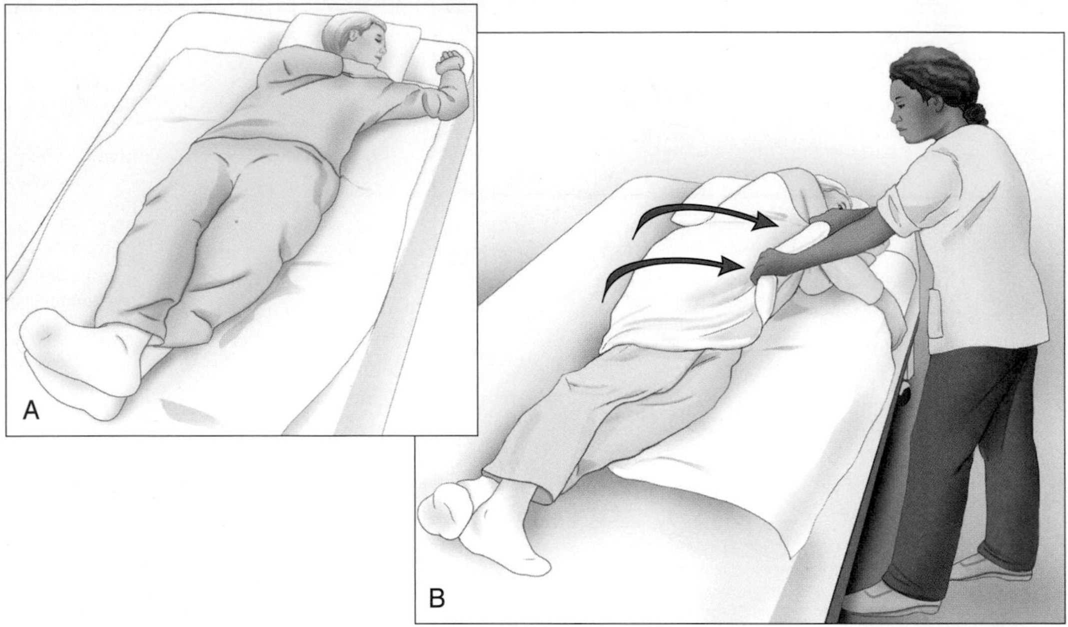

Fig. 42-7 A, Preparation for the patient to turn onto his or her left side: move the patient to the right side of the bed, position his or her left arm up to the side at a 90-degree angle, cross the right leg and arm over his or her body, and turn the patient's head to the left. **B,** A one-person turn to the right side using a draw sheet. The patient's body position is the same as for the turn to the side. The therapist is positioned with one foot forward, the other back. The therapist pulls the sheet with his or her hands positioned at the hips and shoulders of the patient.

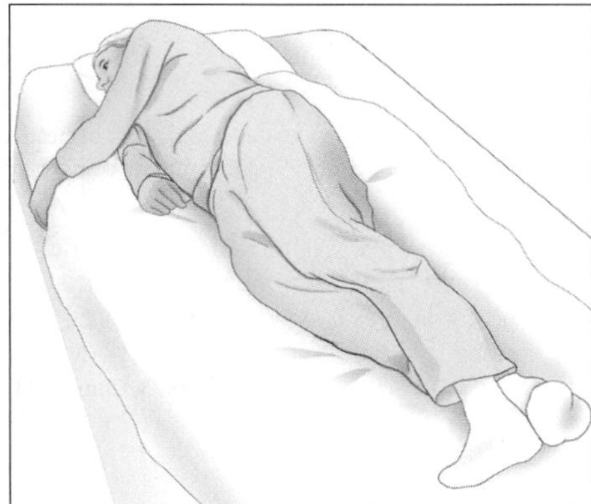

Fig. 42-8 Positioning the patient prone (example: rolling to the right side). The patient's right arm is tucked in at his or her side with the left arm and leg crossed over.

3. Tuck in patient's right hand and arm at the body side as close as possible.
4. Push or pull on the patient's hips and shoulders to turn.
5. Free both arms; do not allow the patient to lie on the arm or hand.
6. A pillow may be placed under the patient's hips and lower legs to bend the knee and relieve strain of the patient's back at the lumbar spine.

Summary

Positioning and moving patients are integral functions of physical therapy. To be effective for the patient and safe for both the patient and practitioner, these functions need to be considered as clinical skills and performed systematically. Therapists and nurses need to analyze their physical activities in relation to the principles of efficient movement and the proper application of body mechanics before moving a patient. A "tube index," counting and identifying each technical attachment (e.g., IV, Foley catheter, arterial blood gas stent, or chest tubes), should be taken before moving a patient. Extra care needs to be taken to prevent dislodging important medical equipment—it could be a life-threatening situation if ventilator tubing in a patient were inadvertently extubated. The practical application of body mechanics has the potential not only to conserve energy and minimize strain to muscles and joints but also to enable the patient to be moved with the least discomfort or pain. Such strategies will help protect members of the health care team directly involved with positioning and moving the patient, as well as maximize patient safety.

Review Questions

1. What factors would determine the number of staff members needed to position a patient who is mechanically ventilated into a prone position?
2. How can changing a patient's position affect ventilation?
3. How can the therapist use towel rolls and easily accessible equipment to improve a patient's position and potential for improved ventilation?
4. What ventilation/perfusion changes occur when a patient is turned from the "affected" side down to the "unaffected" side down?
5. Can positioning be considered a clinical competency when it accomplishes a treatment goal? Discuss.
6. How could positioning to reach a therapeutic goal be documented?

References

1. McConnell EA: Using proper body mechanics. *Nursing* 32:17, 2002.
2. Hefti KS, Farnham RJ, Docken L, et al: Back injury prevention: a lift team success story. *AAOHN J* 51:246–251, 2003.
3. Karahan A, Bayraktar N: Determination of the usage of body mechanics in clinical settings and the occurrence of low back pain in nurses. *International Journal of Nursing Studies* 41:67–74, 2004.
4. Neil C: Body management in nursing. *Nursing Times* 55:163, 1959.
5. Fuerst E, Wolff L: *Fundamentals of nursing*, ed 4, Philadelphia, 1969, J.B. Lippincott.
6. Edlich RF, Winters KL, Hudson MA, et al: Prevention of disabling back injuries in nurses by the use of mechanical patient lift systems. *J Long Term Eff Med Implants* 14(6):521–533, 2004.
7. Carter C, Stratton C, Mallory D: Yoga to treat nonspecific low back pain. *AAOHN J* 59(8):355–361, 2011.
8. Massery M, et al. Chest wall excursion and tidal volume change during passive positioning in cervical spinal cord injury [abstract]. *Cardiopulmonary Physical Therapy* 8:27, 1997.
9. Crosbie WJ, Myles, S: An investigation into the effect of postural modification on some aspects of normal pulmonary function. *Physiotherapy* 7:311–314, 1985.
10. Kendall FP, McCreary EK, Provance PG: *Muscles testing and function*, Baltimore, 1993, Williams & Wilkins.
11. Ishii M, Matsuo Y, et al: Optimizing forced vital capacity with shoulder positioning in a mechanically-ventilated patient with amyotrophic lateral sclerosis. *Cardiopulmonary Physical Therapy Journal* 15:12–16, 2004.
12. Grenier IR, Bigsby R, Vergara ER, et al: Comparison of motor self regulatory and stress behaviors of preterm infants across body positions. *American Journal of Occupational Therapy* 57:289–297, 2003.
13. Manning F, Dean E, Ross J, et al: Effects of side lying on lung function in older individuals. *Phys Ther* 79(5):456–466, 1999.
14. Oczenski W, Hormann C, Keller C, et al: Recruitment maneuvers during prone positioning in patients with acute respiratory distress syndrome. *Critical Care Medicine* 33:54–61, 2005.
15. Vollman KM: Prone positioning in the patient who has acute respiratory distress syndrome: the art and science. *Critical Care Nursing Clinics of North America* 16:319–336, 2004.
16. Piedalue F, Albert RK: Prone positioning in acute respiratory distress syndrome. *Respiratory Care Clinics of North America* 9:495–509, 2003.
17. Harcombe CJ: Nursing patients with ARDS in the prone position. *Nursing Standard* 18:33–39, 2004.
18. Guerin C, Gaillard S, Lemasson S, et al: Effects of systematic prone positioning in hypoxemic acute respiratory failure: a randomized controlled trial. *Journal of the American Medical Association* 292:2379–2387, 2004.
19. Gainnier M, Michelet P, Thirion X, et al: Prone position and positive end-expiratory pressure in acute respiratory distress syndrome. *Critical Care Medicine* 31:2719–2726, 2003.
20. Patroniti N, Bellani G, Pesenti A: Nonconventional support of respiration. *Curr Opin Crit Care* 2011 Aug 5. 2011. [Epub ahead of print]
21. Papazian et al: Comparison of prone positioning and high-frequency oscillatory ventilation in patients with acute respiratory distress syndrome. *Crit Care Med* 33(10):2162–2171, 2005.
22. Jolliet P, Bulpa P, Chevrolet JC: Effects of the prone position on gas exchange and hemodynamics in severe acute respiratory distress syndrome. *Crit Care Med* 26(12):1977–1985, 1998.
23. Wright AD, Flynn M: Using the prone position for ventilated patients with respiratory failure: a review. *Nurs Crit Care* 16(1):19–27, 2011.
24. Gattinoni L, Carlesso E, Taccone P, et al: Prone positioning improves survival in severe ARDS: a pathophysiologic review and individual patient meta-analysis. *Minerva Anestesiol* 76(6):448–454, 2010.
25. Alexianu D, et al: Severe hypotension in the prone position in a child with neurofibromatosis, scoliosis and pectus excavatum presentation for posterior spinal fusion. *Anesth Analg* 98:3334–3335, 2004.
26. Reignier J, Thenoz-Jost N, Fiancette M, et al: Early enteral nutrition in mechanically ventilated patients in the prone position. *Critical Care Medicine* 32:94–99, 2004.
27. Sud S, et al: Prone ventilation reduces mortality in patients with acute respiratory failure and severe hypoxemia: systematic review and meta-analysis. *Intensive Care Med* 36(4):585–599, 2010.
28. Woodhall-McNeal AP: Changes in posture and balance with age. *Aging* 4:219–225, 1992.
29. Borello-France DP, Burdett RG, Gee ZL: Modification of sitting posture of patients with hemiplegia using seat boards and backboards. *Physical Therapy* 68:68–71, 1988.
30. Johnson G: Functional orthopedics I. San Ansellmo, Calif: Institute of Physical Art. Chicago: Course presentation June 8–11, 1989, 1989.
31. Banzett RB, Topulos GP, Leith DE, et al: Bracing arms increases the capacity for sustained hyperpnea. *Am Rev Respir Dis* 138(1):106–109, 1988.
32. Cavalheri V, Camillo CA, Brunetto AF, et al: Effects of arm bracing posture on respiratory muscle strength and pulmonary function in patients with chronic obstructive pulmonary disease. *Rev Port Pneumol* 16(6):887–891, 2010.
33. Barach AL: Chronic obstructive lung disease: postural relief of dyspnea. *Arch Phys Med Rehabil* 55(11):494–504, 1974.
34. Kera T, Maruyama H: The effect of posture on respiratory activity of the abdominal muscles. *J Physiol Anthropol Appl Human Sci* 24(4):259–265, 2005.
35. Segizbaeva MO, Pogodin MA, Lavrova IN, et al: [Effect of head-down tilt on respiratory responses and human inspiratory muscles activity]. *Fiziol Cheloveka* 37(2):52–59, 2011. [Article in Russian]
36. Is there a right way to lift? *Physical Therapy Forum* 4:23, 1985.
37. Rantz M, Courtial D: *Lifting, moving and transferring patients: a manual*, St Louis, 1977, Mosby.
38. Rauch B: *Kinesiology and applied anatomy*, Philadelphia, 1971, Lea & Febiger.
39. Roper N: *Principles of nursing*, ed 2, New York, 1973, Churchill Livingstone.
40. Lewis L: *Fundamental skills in patient care*, Philadelphia, 1976, J.B. Lippincott.

VIII

Chapter 43

Respiratory Care Practice Review

Donna Frownfelter

KEY TERMS

Interprofessional approach to pulmonary patients
Aerosol
Oxygen therapy
Low-flow systems
High-flow systems
Portable oxygen systems
Continuous positive airway pressure (CPAP)
Positive airway pressure
Biphasic positive pressure ventilation (BIPAP)
Respiratory modalities
Humidity and aerosol therapy
Incentive spirometry
Mechanical ventilation
Noninvasive mechanical ventilation
Alarm management and precautions

CHAPTER OUTLINE

Proper care of the pulmonary patient involves an interprofessional team approach for optimal patient outcomes. In order to maximize patient care, each team member should have a working knowledge of the scope of practice of every other professional on the team. As respiratory therapists, physical therapists, occupational therapists, speech therapists, physicians, and nurses apply their expertise in providing care for pulmonary patients, it becomes evident that coordinated teamwork is essential for patients to reach their full potential. The purpose of this chapter is to provide an overview of respiratory care principles and modalities frequently encountered in various settings for the other health care professionals who collaborate with physical therapists. Also discussed is the physical therapist's interaction with various modalities and pieces of equipment. A knowledge and comfort level with respiratory care modalities and equipment will relieve anxiety and promote effective and safe interventions. Physical therapists focus on patient interventions routinely; however, they need to know exactly why each patient is receiving respiratory treatment, why particular monitoring systems are chosen, and why patients respond to various interventions that are utilized.

Oxygen Therapy

The atmosphere contains 20.95% oxygen, the most essential element needed to sustain human life. Oxygen exerts a partial pressure of 159.6 mm Hg at sea level (dry air) and approximately 97 mm Hg (Torr) in arterial blood. The normal range, as measured by arterial blood gas (ABG) analysis, is 80 to 100 mm Hg (Torr). Under normal circumstances, oxygen molecules travel from the atmosphere to the mitochondria at the cellular level, where it is used to produce ATP in a process called aerobic metabolism (oxygen transport mechanisms). The oxygen transport pathway involves the airways and lungs, heart and peripheral vasculature, and the muscle tissue in which the mitochondria reside. Any process that inhibits the transport of oxygen from the atmosphere to the cellular level can cause hypoxemia, decreased patient function, and, ultimately, death.

When oxygen is prescribed, it should be considered a drug. A particular dosage must be ordered by a set prescription. In general, physical therapists do not instruct patients to increase or decrease medication they are taking without a physician's order. Some practices have standing orders that allow the health care team to change oxygen settings by following a standardized protocol. For example, a prescription may be for 1 L/min of oxygen by nasal cannula at rest titrated up to 6 L/min to keep oxygen saturation above 90%. Although higher-flow oxygen cannulas can deliver increased liter flow, it is more standard in practice to increase titration according to a prescribed protocol.

Patients with cardiovascular and pulmonary impairments frequently need oxygen supplementation.[1] Respiratory care practitioners and the nursing staff are generally responsible for administration of this drug under a physician's order. Therapists have a variety of methods from which to choose to deliver oxygen in the most effective way (individual methods are discussed later in this chapter). Long-term oxygen therapy for patients with chronic obstructive pulmonary disease (COPD) who are hypoxemic has been reported to improve quality of life and life expectancy.[2-5] However, even though the benefits of long-term oxygen therapy have been established, U.S. congressional mandates for competitive bidding and caps in rental agreement programs have led to cutbacks. As a consequence, the dose of oxygen and its mode of delivery may need to be modified at rest and during activity.[6] This is an issue of significant concern. As practitioners working with patients requiring oxygen, physical therapists need to advocate for their patients to ensure that they receive appropriate oxygen therapy.

The purpose of oxygen therapy is to treat and prevent hypoxemia, excessive work of breathing, and excessive myocardial work.[7] Although individual oxygen appliances offer suggested guidelines regarding oxygen administration, the only way to ensure effective delivery from a given device is by blood gas monitoring of PaO_2 (partial pressure of oxygen in the arterial blood) or monitoring hemoglobin saturation by oximetry. Medicare and third-party payers have specific indications for oxygen therapy. These indications may differ and physical therapists need to identify these in the practice setting and provide the documentation required for patients to receive the oxygen they need. Initially, a patient may need oxygen only with higher levels of activity or exercise; that needs to be documented by an exercise test that shows desaturation by oximetry. As a patient's disease progresses, continuous oxygen may be indicated. Careful monitoring of patients will determine when the need for continuous oxygen occurs. Oxygen therapy is usually administered by one of two methods: low-flow or high-flow systems.

Low-Flow Systems

A low-flow oxygen system is one that is not intended to meet the total oxygen requirements of the patient (does not deliver atmospheric oxygen concentration to the patient). For example, using a normal minute ventilation (minute ventilation = tidal volume [TV] × respiratory rate [RR]) of 8 L/min (500 mL × 16 breaths per minute) with a patient receiving 1 L/min of oxygen, the patient is breathing 8 L/min but the device only provides 1 L/min. Thus 7 L/min are contributed from room air. Each time there is a change in the patient's breathing pattern, tidal volume, and respiratory rate, the fraction of inspired oxygen (FiO_2) may also change. Ideally, for efficient use of a nasal cannula, the patient should have a normal tidal volume, respiratory rate, and breathing pattern. This is often not the case, but the cannula is used because it is well tolerated by the patient. This method of oxygen delivery is not used when a specific concentration of oxygen is needed.[8]

Nasal Cannulas

The nasal cannulas (also called nasal prongs) are one of the most common low-flow devices encountered because of low expense and high patient compliance (Figure 43-1). This device supplies an FiO_2 of approximately 24% to 40% oxygen with flow rates from 1 L/min to 6 L/min. Flow rates greater than 6 L/min can cause nasal mucosal irritation and drying. The approximate liter flow and resultant FiO_2 values are shown in Table 43-1.

Nasal cannulas deliver 100% oxygen; however, this percentage significantly lessens as the oxygen mixes with inspired air from the room. The amount of oxygen delivered depends on the flow rate and the ventilatory pattern of the patient. A larger minute volume (TV × RR) would dilute the oxygen at any given flow rate and cause a greater decrease in the percentage delivered to the lungs. In other words, the faster and deeper a patient breathes, the more diluted the oxygen becomes. On the other hand, if a patient has a low minute volume, the oxygen percentage delivered increases.[7] If precise control of FiO_2 is needed, the nasal cannula should not be used.[9] In these cases a high-flow system (i.e., a Venturi mask) may be used.

Skin integrity, especially behind the ears, needs to be evaluated because the pressure of the cannula can cause skin breakdown. Patients at times will pull on the cannula or take the oxygen off. It is important to check for skin breakdown behind the ears, especially if patients are not able to communicate.

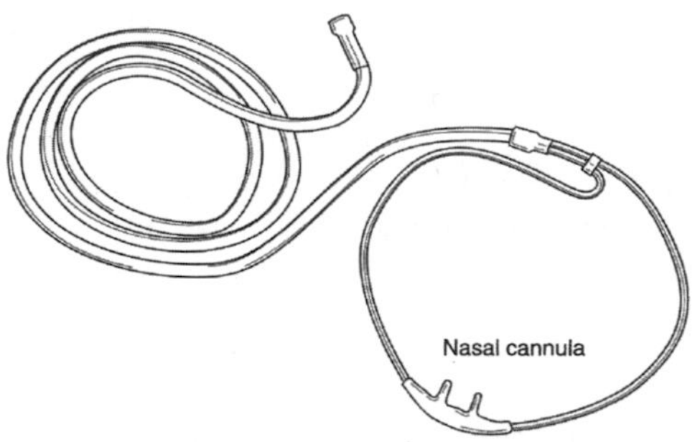

Fig. 43-1 Oxygen cannula.

Table 43-1 Approximate Liter Flow and Resultant FiO_2 Values

Flow (L/min)	FiO_2 (%)
1	24
2	28
3	32
4	36
5	40
6	44

Adapted from the American College of Sports Medicine: *Guidelines for exercise testing and prescription,* ed 6, Philadelphia: Lippincott, Williams & Wilkins, 2000.

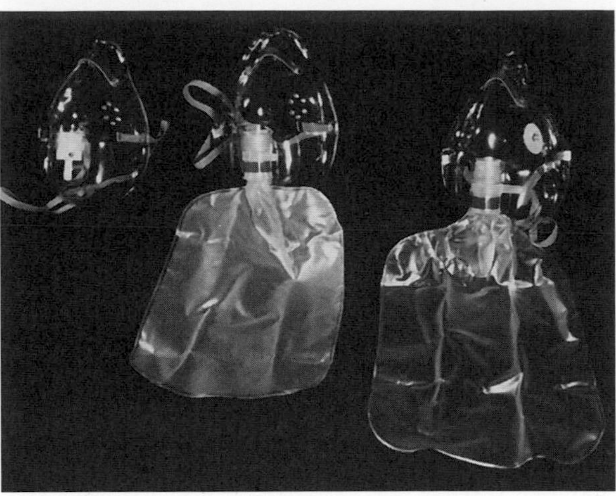

Fig. 43-2 From left to right: Mask without bag, partial rebreathing bag, nonbreathing bag. Note the valves on the mask and at the junction between the mask and bag.

Mouth-breathing by patients using a nasal cannula typically causes concern from some of the health care team. This concern, however, may be unnecessary. If the nasal passages are unobstructed, then oxygen is able to collect in the oral and nasal cavity (anatomical reservoir). On inspiration, the oxygen collected in this area is drawn into the airways and lungs. If a patient with a nasal cannula is mouth-breathing, the practitioner should ensure the nasal passages are unobstructed. If there is concern that the patient is not receiving adequate oxygen, a blood gas or oxygen saturation measurement should be obtained. If this is not feasible, or if the patient is unable to breathe through the nose, it may be appropriate to switch the patient to a mask.

The patient should be encouraged to breathe through the nose to receive maximum benefit from the nasal cannula; however, mouth breathing does not mean the patient will not receive appropriate oxygen.[10] Clinically, it is found that some patients who mouth-breathe do so because of nasal polyps, sinus congestion, deviated septum, or other physical issues. If the work of breathing is increased when the patient tries to breathe through the nose, it may be counterproductive.

Simple Mask

The simple mask is another commonly used low-flow oxygen-delivery device. It can deliver from 40% to 60% oxygen, depending on the flow rate and the patient's ventilatory pattern. This device requires a flow rate of 5 to 6 L/min to prevent rebreathing carbon dioxide and excessive respiratory work.[11] As with the nasal cannula, this type of oxygen delivery method should not be used if precise control of oxygen concentration (FiO_2) is required because the simply mask is still considered a low-flow oxygen system.

Partial Rebreathing Mask

The partial rebreathing mask is basically a mask with a reservoir bag attached. The oxygen source supplies the bag with 100% oxygen, which then mixes with exhaled anatomical dead-space air that has not taken place in gas exchange. This exhaled air is rich in oxygen. The exhaled air that has taken place in gas exchange and contains CO_2 is vented through the open port on each side of the mask. This mask can deliver oxygen concentrations from 70% to more than 80%. It requires flows between 7 and 10 L/min to keep the bag from fully collapsing during inspiration.[7]

Nonrebreathing Mask

Another low-flow delivery device, the nonrebreathing mask, also contains a bag reservoir, but it can deliver up to 100% oxygen. This mask has valves on the reservoir bag and side vents. This feature prevents ambient air mixing on inspiration and exhaled air mixing on expiration. For this mask to operate effectively, a good seal between the patient's face and the mask must be achieved. The bag should partially deflate during inspiration (Figure 43-2).

Transtracheal Oxygen Catheter

Another form of low-flow oxygen delivery is the transtracheal oxygen catheter. This has been used for pediatric and adult patients.[12,13] It is a cannula that is surgically placed into the trachea via a small incision between the second and third tracheal rings. Generally these devices are used by patients at home who need continuous oxygen therapy. Transtracheal oxygen catheters are more efficient than nasal cannulas, and they have a high patient acceptance rate with low complications.[14] Because the oxygen is administered directly into the trachea, 50% less oxygen is needed.[7] For people who use portable oxygen systems and for those who require high oxygen flow rates, transtracheal oxygen catheters may be beneficial.[15] The catheter can be covered by the patient's clothing and is therefore cosmetically appealing. Complications such as plugging of the catheter and subcutaneous emphysema have been reported.[16,17] These complications may be avoided with proper care of the catheter, good hydration, and maintenance as directed by the patient's health care team. The transtracheal procedure is not routine in many practice settings; thus if a patient is interested in this form of oxygen therapy, it is wise to find a team that has done the procedure frequently enough to become highly skilled at it.

High-Flow Systems

A high-flow oxygen delivery system delivers a specific oxygen concentration (FiO_2) despite the patient's ventilatory pattern. This system delivers atmospheric oxygen pressure to the patient, which means that the entire volume that is breathed is delivered through the device. A patient requires oxygen delivered at specific FiO_2 of 50% to keep the arterial oxygen and oxygen saturation at a safe level, then a high-flow system is the method of choice. If a patient has CO_2 retention and a hypoxic drive to breathe, a high-flow system with an exact FiO_2 can be used. This is often the case when a patient with COPD who is a CO_2 retainer has pneumonia and goes into respiratory failure. The physician wants to provide adequate oxygen to the patient and avoid having to mechanically ventilate. The ideal choice would be a high-flow device at a lower FiO_2 to prevent CO_2 retention while not reducing the hypoxic drive to breathe. Unfortunately, patient tolerance of the high-flow oxygen-delivery mask, which covers both the nose and mouth, is often less than optimal. Patients who are acutely ill and very dyspneic or those who have decreased cognitive awareness may tolerate the mask, but as these patients begin to improve, they may have a claustrophobic reaction to the mask and the high flow of gas.

Venturi Mask

The Venturi mask is a common method of delivering high-flow oxygen concentrations from 24% to 50%. This mask operates via the Venturi principle, which provides for a mixing of 100% oxygen and entrained ambient air. The oxygen flows though a narrow orifice at a high velocity, causing a subatmospheric pressure. This drop in pressure is what causes the ambient air to be entrained through a port. The size of the port determines the amount of air that is entrained, thus the percentage of oxygen delivered. The Venturi mask has a rotating air entrainment port that allows the health care provider to "dial in" the desired FiO_2 (Figure 43-3). Flow rates of 40 to 80+ L/min provide minute ventilation at rates that are higher than those the patient could breathe without assistance; consequently, the mask provides the entire inspired atmosphere to the patient. This means that regardless of the patient's respiratory rate, tidal volume, or breathing pattern, the oxygen delivery (FiO_2) will be consistent.

Mechanical aerosol systems also operate via air entrainment, but the mask is connected to the aerosol unit by large-bore tubing to allow a specific FiO_2 to be delivered with high humidity (Figure 43-4). Although drainage bags are usually attached to the tubing to collect condensation, the tubing must be monitored for possible pooling of water, which causes flow obstruction to the patient. If partial obstruction occurs, a mild back pressure results in the tubing, causing less air entrainment. This means that a higher concentration of oxygen results and potentially a higher dosage of oxygen than desired may be delivered to the patient.

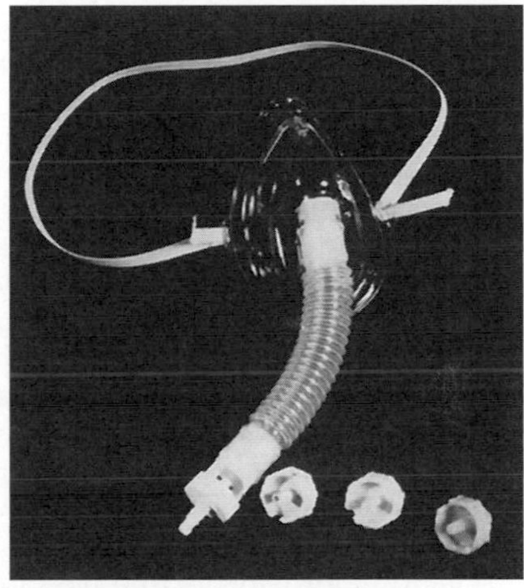

Fig. 43-3 Venturi mask.

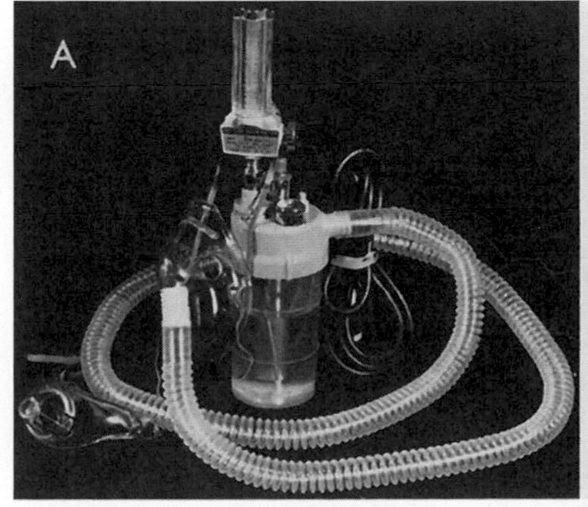

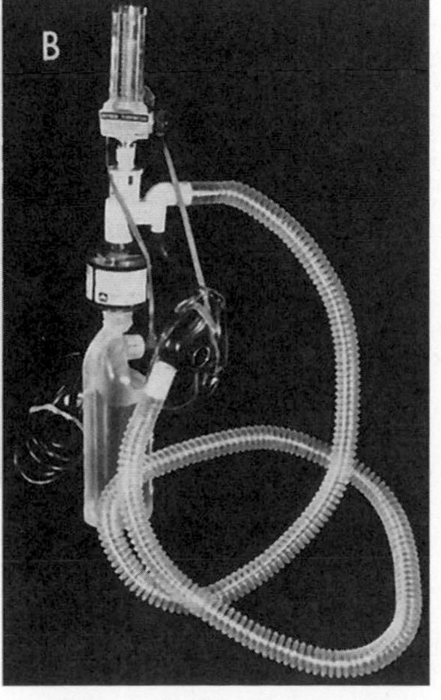

Fig. 43-4 A, Heated aerosol. **B,** Nebulizers.

Portable Oxygen

As health care continues to move out of the hospital setting and into the home, more health care practitioners will provide care to patients who require oxygen in their homes. When this is the case, it is essential that a sign be posted about the use of oxygen in the home. Patient teaching before hospital discharge should include a discussion of safety concerns—for example, not cooking with a gas stove, not smoking, and allowing anyone to smoke in the home (or anywhere around the patient). In addition, it must be made clear to the patient that oxygen is considered a prescription medication and thus the amount of oxygen delivered should not be changed unless ordered by the doctor.

Oxygen is most commonly provided in the home for those patients with long-term oxygen needs, usually patients with COPD who are hypoxemic. Generally 1 to 2 L/min is prescribed via nasal cannula, but the flow rate will depend on the patient's need.

Home oxygen-delivery systems include high-pressure oxygen cylinders, low-pressure liquid oxygen,[18] and oxygen concentrators.[8] Additional options include continuous flow versus demand or pulsed oxygen delivery.[19-21] There are also a number of oxygen-conserving devices from which to choose.[22] When a continuous system is changed to either a demand or pulsed system, or when a new oxygen-conserving device is started, the patient must be monitored carefully. Clinical experience has shown that some patients may not tolerate the same liter flow with a pulsed system, and oximetry and perceived exertion must be evaluated when there is any change in oxygen delivery. The oxygen delivery may not be as effective as a continuous flow device when changing to a pulsed oxygen system. Unfortunately, there is no mandate for clinical testing of the devices before they come to market, so documented effectiveness of one versus another in clinical use is not available.[23]

Heliox, a combination of 21% oxygen and 79% helium, has been used in acute care for patients who have upper airway obstruction and increased work of breathing (spontaneously breathing patients, as well as those on a ventilator). However, use of heliox has not been widespread because of its cost, which has been estimated to be 13 times that of oxygen. Heliox for portable oxygen and home use has been documented as effective for patients with asthma and COPD. It has been shown to decrease airway resistance and decrease the work of breathing and has also been effective with patients who have increased mucus secretions. Studies have demonstrated an increase in patients' ability to exercise using heliox; however, it has not been shown to significantly decrease dyspnea.[24-26]

High-pressure oxygen tanks are not used as frequently as are low-pressure tanks, but they are used in some settings. High-pressure tanks come in various sizes. The larger ones, such as the H and K sizes, are used as a base unit or reservoir. Long oxygen tubing connected to these tanks allows for patient mobility. Smaller tanks (such as E cylinders) are used for portability and can provide up to 3 hours of use depending on the liter flow of oxygen. Some systems allow for the smaller tank to be refilled by transferring gas from the larger reservoir tank. The primary concern with the high-pressure tanks is guarding them against tipping over. They must be well tied and secured because if a tank tips over or falls, the neck that holds the regulator could break. If this happens, the high pressure inside can propel the tank at a very high velocity, causing damage to surrounding structures and posing a danger to anyone around. The tanks are usually tied to a bed, put in a standard box, or secured on a portable wheeled cart. Thus the high-pressure tanks are difficult to move and maneuver, especially up and down stairs, making their use less than optimal for most patients, especially those who wish to be more active. In terms of cost, the high-pressure tanks are less expensive overall, but deliveries and replacements need to occur regularly.

Liquid oxygen, a low-pressure oxygen delivery method, tends to be more convenient than the high-pressure oxygen tanks, especially for active patients on oxygen. The canisters are lightweight and allow patients to be away from the home reservoir for up to 8 hours. The downside is that liquid oxygen costs more and, with heavy use, the reservoirs may need to be filled up to twice a week. If high flows are needed, these units are not recommended.

Oxygen concentrators are commonly used in the home health setting, especially because Medicare offers coverage for these devices (Figure 43-5). They are electrically powered and create oxygen by drawing ambient air across a semipermeable membrane, separating oxygen from nitrogen. They generally operate at 2 L/min and provide FiO_2 90% oxygen output. Long oxygen tubing, up to 50 feet, allows patients extra mobility. Patients using concentrators should have a back-up device, such as a portable tank, in case of a power outage. In addition, the electrical power company should be notified of any patient who is using oxygen by concentrator so that the patient's location is designated as a high priority for backup and restoration of power if an outage occurs.

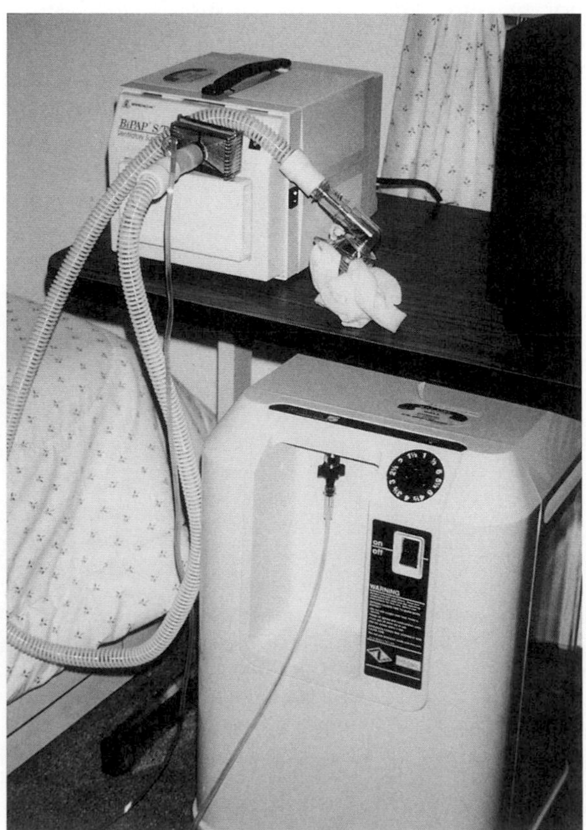

Fig. 43-5 Oxygen concentrator.

The local fire department should also be informed of any patient who is on oxygen therapy, especially if the patient is limited physically. Oxygen devices will not "explode," but oxygen does support combustion. As noted, high-pressure tanks, if knocked over, have a tremendous force due to the pressurized oxygen and there have been reports of these tanks going through walls. Firefighters, or any emergency personnel, should be informed that oxygen is in use so that in the case of a fire or other emergency, they are aware of this potential danger.

Continuous (Constant) Positive Pressure Breathing

Continuous positive airway pressure (CPAP) is oxygen delivered with pressure above atmospheric pressure (i.e., positive airway pressure). Whereas normally during the respiratory cycle there is a negative pressure during inspiration, the pressure curve in CPAP is always above atmospheric pressure (positive pressure) on the airways.

CPAP may be used to improve oxygenation[27,28] in patients for whom the usual means of oxygen delivery is not effective or for those with obstructive sleep apnea.[29] Sleep apnea and COPD often occur together; recently, recognition of when "overlap syndrome" occurs there is higher mortality than either disease process alone.[30] CPAP has also been used to help the transition of weaning patients from mechanical ventilation,[31] including infants who have had cardiac surgery. CPAP can help stabilize these infants and normalize their spontaneous breathing pattern.[32] It has also been useful in the management of respiratory distress in premature babies and decreases the need for invasive mechanical ventilation.[33] Early intervention using CPAP in older patients with cardiogenic pulmonary edema has also been effective.[34] Quality-of-life predictors have been shown to be positive a year after initiation of CPAP; improvement was noted at 3 months after initiation of CPAP and continued at 1 year.[35,36]

Patients who are mouth breathers may have difficulty adjusting to CPAP, thus rendering it less effective in these cases. Those with moderate to severe sleep-disordered breathing have been found to be less adherent to CPAP therapy than are who are nose breathers. This is related to a leak that compromises the CPAP.[37]

Use of Oxygen to Improve Exercise

Oxygen has been shown to increase exercise performance in patients with COPD who have moderate to severe airflow obstruction and mild hypoxemia at rest.[38-40] It has also been shown to benefit patients with COPD who are nonhypoxemic at rest.[41,42] Breathlessness is the most common symptom that limits exercise tolerance. Oxygen supplementation will often provide an increased driving pressure of oxygen, which allows the patient to decrease the work of breathing.[43] Peripheral muscle weakness has been found in many patients with COPD. Improving exercise tolerance will result in improved muscle strength and endurance. Another consideration, if hyperoxia is not enough, is the use of noninvasive positive pressure (NPPV). This is still somewhat controversial and requires more study, but in this author's clinical opinion, NPPV can be very beneficial.[44] As previously discussed in this chapter, heliox has been shown to improve exercise tolerance in patients with asthma and COPD who have upper airway obstruction, inflammation, and increased mucus secretions.

Noninvasive ventilation will be discussed later in the chapter, but it is interesting to note that in some pulmonary rehabilitation programs it is being used in addition to supplemental oxygen with very positive results. The combination of oxygen and noninvasive ventilation was shown to be better than supplemental oxygen alone.[45] The rationale for this improvement when using both oxygen and noninvasive ventilation is that in patients with severe COPD, the ventilatory muscles can be "unloaded" and this may promote higher levels of exercise.[46]

Additional Respiratory Modalities

Incentive Spirometry

Incentive spirometry (IS), also called sustained maximum inspiration (SMI), is a visual and/or audio feedback device that encourages slow, deep inspiration (Figure 43-6). Generally this treatment is performed frequently, up to every hour, and its purpose is to treat and prevent atelectasis and pneumonia, especially in postoperative patients who are considered a high risk for postoperative complications.[47-51] In many acute care settings, IS is done routinely. Several articles challenge the routine use of IS and have found that the addition of IS added no benefit to breathing exercise postoperatively.[52-55] In a study of patients scheduled for lung resection, when a combination of inspiratory muscle training and IS was performed before and after lung resection, there were significant lung function improvements in FEV_1 that were higher postoperatively than preoperatively.[52]

There may be potential benefits to using IS with patients with neuromuscular and musculoskeletal impairments as

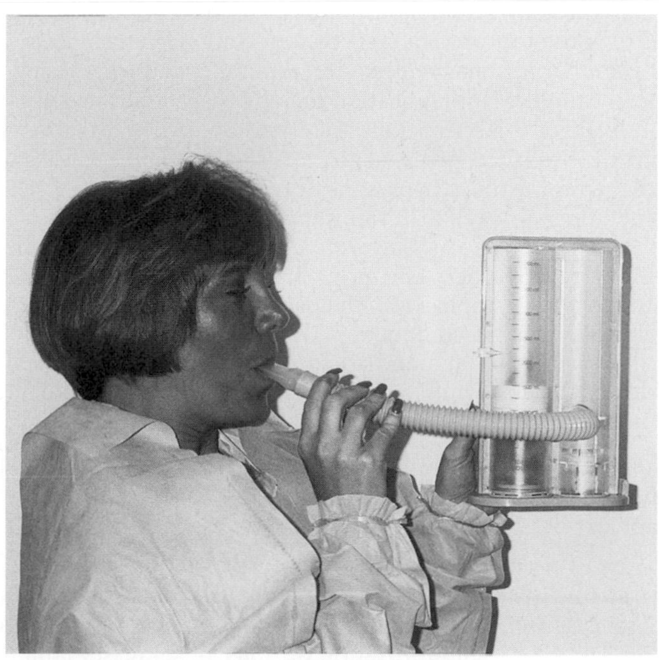

Fig. 43-6 Incentive spirometry device in use.

well. They often demonstrate a decreased vital capacity and decreased chest wall mobility. IS devices encourage deep breathing and a sustained inspiration. During the sustained inspiration, collateral ventilation can occur as well-ventilated areas of the lung equilibrate with areas that are poorly ventilated. This is an area for future research, perhaps combining inspiratory muscle training and IS.

Many commercial incentive spirometers are available. Some are focused on volume, others on flow rates. Regardless of the type, the importance of patients using them should be stressed. Patients with COPD may have these devices prescribed when they are undergoing surgical procedures. Care must be taken not to have patients continue to use them when the acute episode is over. Patients with COPD have air trapping, which can be made worse by using an incentive spirometer and will not take deeper breaths needed to prevent respiratory problems post op when they have pain.

Airway Clearance Devices

Several airway clearance devices are currently available. These are discussed fully in Chapter 21.

Humidity and Aerosol Therapy

Humidity Therapy

Under normal circumstances, when inhalation takes place, air becomes 100% saturated with water vapor before entering the lower airway tracts below the carina. This humidification process is important to mucus production, ciliary activity, and a healthy respiratory tract. When this normal humidification process is interfered with, such as in patients with endotracheal or tracheostomy tubes, other methods of adding moisture to the respiratory system must be employed.

Humidification is the addition of water vapor in its molecular form to a gas. When a dry gas is administered to a patient (e.g., via a nasal cannula), some type of humidification appliance is used to prevent unnecessary complications. Flows of 2 L/min or less may not require humidification when using a nasal cannula. Humidification therapy is also indicated in the presence of thick tenacious secretions and when an artificial airway is in place. Artificial airways, such as endotracheal and tracheostomy tubes, bypass the normal humidification system (the upper airway); therefore supplementation is essential.[56]

There are basically two types of humidifiers. Bubble-through humidifiers are those that are generally used with simple oxygen appliances. The passover type of humidifier is usually found in conjunction with a mechanical ventilator. Both bubble-through and passover humidifiers are available for ventilators,[57] and they are usually heated to warm the humidified air to body temperature before it enters the airway.[7]

Aerosol Therapy

An aerosol is created when a suspension of liquid or solid particles exists in a gas. Two common forms of aerosol medication delivery in the clinical setting are the small-volume nebulizer (SVN) and the metered-dose inhaler (MDI). A bland aerosol is administration of water or saline solution to the patient's lungs.[58]

In general the goals of aerosol therapy are to hydrate dried retained secretions, to improve cough efficiency, to restore and maintain function of the mucociliary escalator, to deliver medications, and to humidify gases delivered through artificial airways. The MDI is strictly used for medication delivery (see Chapter 45).

Other forms of aerosol delivery are the spinning disk (such as in a room humidifier or mist) and the ultrasonic nebulizer. Both of these are electrically powered as opposed to the SVN, which is pneumatically powered (Figure 43-7).[59]

A key element in aerosol delivery is particle size. The size of the aerosol particle will determine its ability to penetrate the airway before depositing or raining out. The therapeutic range is considered 1 micron, with the smaller range of particles having the greatest penetrating ability. The larger particles deposit sooner. If they are greater than 5 microns, then the chances of entry into the airway are less. The particles may deposit in the nose and proximal airway. The greatest amount of alveolar deposition (95% to 100%) occurs in the 1 to 2 micron range. On the other hand, aerosol particles smaller than 1 micron are so stable that they may not deposit at all.[7]

Although particle size is important in determining appropriate deposition, a patient's ventilatory pattern is probably more important in that it is the more variable and controllable of the two. Gravity also plays a factor, and it too can be used to benefit particle deposition. Patients should be sitting up as much as possible while taking slow, deep breaths with a short 3- to 4-second inspiratory hold. Mouth breathing is encouraged if aerosol therapy is delivered by mask. Nasal breathing may filter out particles of optimal size. Not all patients will be able to achieve this position and ventilatory pattern, and the therapist must modify accordingly.

Comparisons between the ability of SVNs and MDIs to deliver medications have found that the MDI is either equal in efficacy or outperforms nebulizers. Significant cost savings are also realized by those institutions that recognize MDI usage as an effective means of aerosol medication delivery over SVN.[60]

To further enhance the efficacy of the MDI treatment, the recommendation is that a spacer or holding chamber may be attached to hold the aerosol particles before inhalation. This

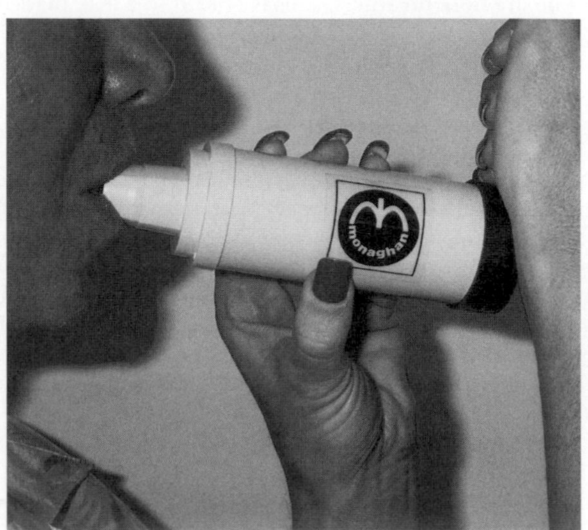

Fig. 43-7 Commonly used spacer device.

device allows greater drug particle deposition to the airways and reduces oropharyngeal deposition.[61] Ventilator patients who are receiving drug aerosol therapy also receive greater benefit from an in-line MDI with a holding chamber compared with a jet nebulizer.[62]

Aerosol-Therapy Precautions

It should be mentioned that there are hazards associated with aerosol therapy. Bronchospasm may occur as the smooth muscles of the bronchial passages react to foreign particles entering the lung. Shortness of breath and respiratory distress may also occur as a result of dried retained secretions swelling and occluding portions of the lung. Cross contamination is a concern in that aerosol devices may harbor organisms that can be transmitted to patients. Frequent equipment changes and proper sterilization and cleaning techniques are key in preventing this occurrence.

Intermittent Positive Pressure Breathing

Intermittent positive pressure breathing (IPPB) continues to be used in some settings, but there is little evidence to support its efficacy as a treatment modality.[58]

This particular technology was developed during World War II to assist pilots breathing in unpressurized cabins at high altitudes. IPPB subsequently became a very popular respiratory therapy device in the 1960s and 1970s (Figure 43-8). Its use began to decline in the 1980s. In 1983 the National Heart, Lung, and Blood Institute reported that IPPB has limited therapeutic benefit. This clinical trial is only one of several studies that show IPPB is an outmoded medical technology. Research dating back to the 1950s questions the efficacy of this device.[63]

The purpose of the IPPB machine is to increase alveolar ventilation, improve the ventilation-perfusion ratio, mobilize and facilitate expectoration of thick secretions, decrease the work of breathing, and deliver aerosolized medications. It is a pressure-cycled ventilator that, when triggered by a patient's inhalation, delivers ambient air or oxygen to the patient until a preset pressure is reached. It is basically a lung expansion device that helps deliver an increased tidal volume. IPPB is used for a variety of pulmonary conditions, and treatment sessions usually last 10 to 15 minutes.

The modality of IPPB comes into question in the clinical setting because it has not been shown to provide benefits over that of other simpler respiratory treatment methods. It also introduces potential complications and hazards that the other treatments do not. Typically, IPPB has been used to treat asthma, COPD, and postoperative atelectasis; however, other therapies, such as IS, airway clearance techniques and devices, and aerosol therapy, tend to prevail as the treatment of choice over IPPB, which is virtually no longer used. This discussion is included because IPPB is the precursor to mechanical ventilation.

Although the use of IPPB is questionable in regard to its clinical efficacy, it may be a beneficial form of treatment in acute asthma or COPD that is refractory to standard therapy, atelectasis that has not responded to simpler therapy, and the prevention of respiratory failure in patients with kyphoscoliosis and neuromuscular disorders.[64]

Mechanical Ventilation

Many disease states that lead to cardiac and/or respiratory failure will require mechanical ventilation to support the patient's effort to ventilate and oxygenate (Figure 43-9). Patients receiving mechanical ventilator support can be found in many settings, from the acute care hospital to skilled nursing facilities and home care. Children needing continuous mechanical ventilation who live in the home and community need to be integrated into the school system and community recreational facilities. Patients with acute exacerbations of disorders such as emphysema, COPD, and chronic bronchitis may require mechanical ventilation and are generally seen in hospital intensive care units and weaned before they are discharged home. Patients with disorders requiring long-term ventilation, such as spinal cord injury, brain injury, and certain neuromusculoskeletal diseases, may be found receiving mechanical ventilation in rehabilitation hospitals, the home, or a long-term care facility. According to the American Association for Respiratory Care (AARC), the scope of practice for the respiratory therapist has expanded to include anywhere that patients with respiratory disease present. Therapists currently practice in hospitals, long-term care, pulmonary rehabilitation, patients' homes, and pulmonary physicians' offices.

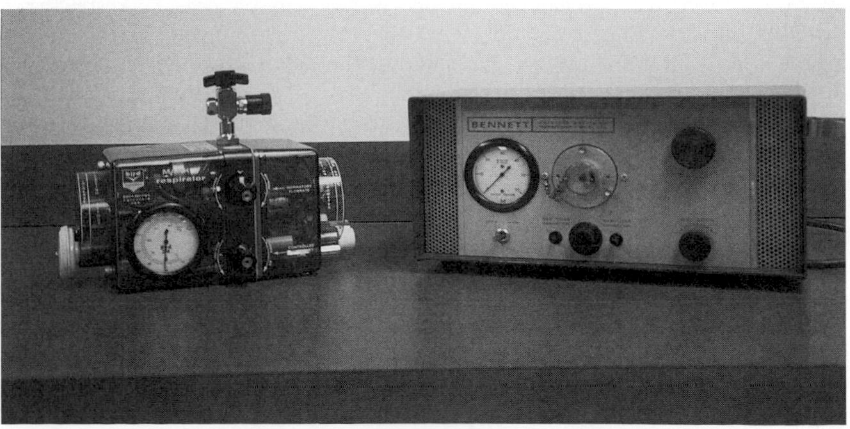

Fig. 43-8 Left to right: Bird Mark machine, Bennett AP-5 IPPB machine.

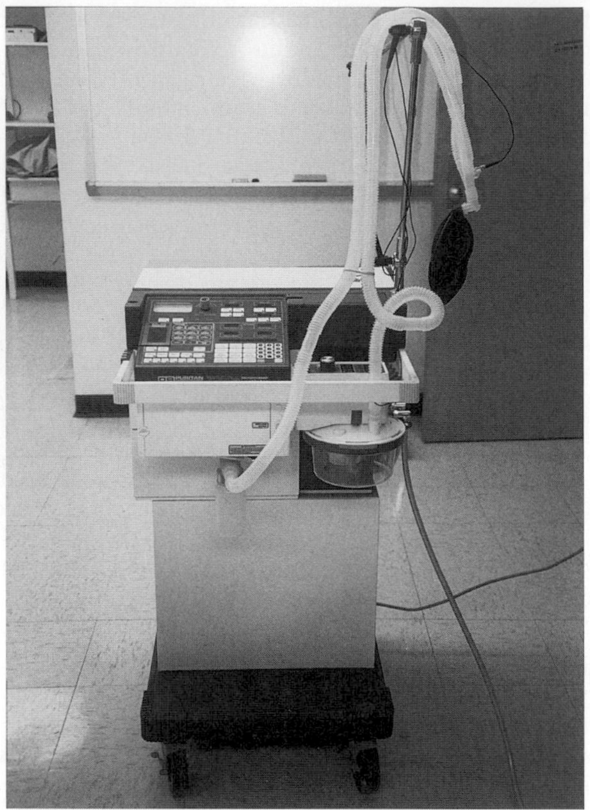

Fig. 43-9 Puritan Bennett 7200a microprocessor driven ventilator.

Mechanical ventilator assistance in the past was provided primarily by machines that deliver preset volume and/or positive pressure breaths to the patient. Positive pressure ventilation is the opposite of normal physiological ventilation in that normal ventilation occurs when negative pressure, created by contraction of the diaphragm, causes air to enter the lungs. Whereas normal inspiration occurs by pulling air into the lungs, ventilators push air into the lungs (positive pressure) or apply pressure to the airways and thus increase ventilation. This is important because the thoracic cavity becomes an area of higher pressure, which may create adverse cardiovascular and hemodynamic events. Monitoring of heart rate and blood pressure is vital when patients are placed on a mechanical ventilator to make sure there are not cardiovascular compromises with increase in pressure and/or volume in the lungs.

Over the past 20 years there has been an increase in the use of noninvasive mechanical ventilation (NIMV) in patients with respiratory failure to avoid the risks involved with intubation. It is becoming the standard "first line therapy in several situations" in acute care.[65]

Several other patient populations have also been supported and their health and sleep improved through the use of NIMV, among them patients with end-stage Duchenne muscular dystrophy, cystic fibrosis, and other neuromuscular dysfunction. In patients with Duchenne MD the pulmonary function data are monitored and the patient may be started on NIMV only at night, progressing to continuous ventilation as needed.[66] This has also been shown to prolong life and eliminate the need for tracheostomy in these patients needing ventilation.[67] In patients with cystic fibrosis, as the disease process progresses, a heavier workload is placed on the respiratory muscles. The patient will often develop a rapid, shallow breathing pattern that results in decreased alveolar ventilation. NIMV may reduce respiratory muscle work of breathing and improve gas exchange. It can decrease oxygen desaturation during exercise and airway clearance and help in patient recovery following an exacerbation. More data are needed to evaluate long-term benefits and criteria for the use of NIMV in people with cystic fibrosis.[68]

Invasive Versus Noninvasive Mechanical Ventilation

Invasive mechanical ventilation involves the insertion of an artificial airway into the trachea that attaches to ventilator tubing. Noninvasive mechanical ventilation (NIV) is delivered by a nasal or facial mask that attaches to a positive airway pressure BiPAP machine. Patient preferences are observed in an attempt to have them feel comfortable and increase adherence to using NIV. In one study of 60 patients with acute respiratory failure being treated with NIV, no preference between the standard oronasal mask and a total face mask was found.[69] Noninvasive mechanical ventilation is growing in use, especially for acute exacerbations of COPD. It has been used primarily for patients with acute hypercapnic ventilatory failure, but its use is now expanding to larger populations. Benefits of NIV include a reduction in the need for intubation, a decrease in complication rate, and a reduced length of hospitalization. One factor in the success of NIV is the early delivery of ventilation in patients with respiratory failure.[70]

In a study involving medical-surgical intensive care units in North American, South America, Spain, and Portugal, 1638 patients were studied who were receiving mechanical ventilation. The median age of study patients was 61 years. Indications for mechanical ventilation were acute respiratory failure (66%), acute exacerbation of COPD (14%), coma (10%), and neuromuscular disorders (10%). Mechanical ventilation was administered via endotracheal tube in 75%, tracheostomy tube in 24%, and facial mask in 1% of patients. A total of 47% of patients were ventilated on an assist-control mode and 46% were ventilated with synchronized intermittent mandatory ventilation (SIMV), pressure support, or a combination of both modes.[71] In North America it seems that, clinically, the trend toward NIV is growing significantly.[72-74]

Patients with chest wall restriction such as severe kyphoscoliosis also benefit from NIV. Ventilation and oxygenation go hand in hand. If the chest wall is not moving, ventilation is decreased. Just giving oxygen to patients with severe thoracic restriction will not bring them to optimal respiratory function. The NIV provides improved ventilation that will improve patient function and endurance.[75]

BiPAP is a noninvasive form of ventilation that uses a tightly fitted oronasal mask that delivers positive pressure at two different levels, one for inspiration and another for exhalation, both of which are above atmospheric pressure. It may also be referred to as pressure release ventilation. Indications for BiPAP include signs of respiratory failure or chronic respiratory failure in patients with severe COPD, increased work of breathing, patients with neuromusculoskeletal impairments that limit ventilation and thus oxygenation, and sleep disordered breathing. Use of BIPAP has improved outcomes in terms of less daytime fatigue and improved activity levels. In addition, it may be used as a bridge for patients such as those at the end stage of cystic fibrosis who need lung transplants.[76,77]

It is important to assess skin integrity because the pressure from the strap on the face and around the head can cause skin breakdown. This is an important consideration to discuss with the patient.

Modes of Mechanical Ventilation for Positive Pressure Ventilation (Invasive Mechanical Ventilation)

The physician and respiratory therapist have a wide variety of choices from which to select the most appropriate method of ventilation for a given patient. Terms defining properties of mechanical ventilation can be confusing. Choosing the appropriate mode of ventilation is at times considered more of an art than a science. There are basic fundamental starting points for mechanical ventilation; then the variable modes are adjusted to optimize each individual patient's needs. Before describing the modes of ventilation, the following terms are defined.

Trigger. Variable that causes a breath to be delivered by the ventilator. A patient may inhale, causing the ventilator circuit pressure to drop to a preset number (i.e., less than 1 or 2 cm H_2O). This is called a pressure trigger. Some ventilators are volume and flow triggered.

Flow rate. The speed at which the ventilator breath is delivered. This parameter is usually measured in liters per minute.

Frequency. Refers to the number of breaths delivered over time (e.g., 10 breaths per minute).

Spontaneous breath. Breathing through the ventilator circuit without assistance.

The following are descriptions of common current ventilator modes.[78]

Controlled mechanical ventilation (CMV) or total support of ventilation. The control mode is now a lesser-used method of ventilation and generally requires the patient to be sedated and paralyzed. The ventilator delivers all breaths at a preset frequency, volume or pressure, and flow rate. The patient cannot take spontaneous breaths or trigger the machine. This mode may be used when total control of ventilation is needed (e.g., during surgery, in patients with high-level quadriplegia).

Assist control (AC) or partial support of ventilation. The patient receives a preset pressure or volume, frequency or number of breaths, and flow rate. In between machine-cycled breaths, the patient can trigger the machine to deliver another breath at the preset parameters. All breaths are machine delivered. No spontaneous breathing can occur.

Assisted mechanical ventilation. This mode is similar to AC; however, there is no set frequency. The patient triggers the machine at will to deliver a set pressure or volume at a set flow rate.

Intermittent mandatory ventilation (IMV). As the ventilator delivers a set mandatory frequency and volume or pressure, the patient is allowed to take spontaneous breaths between cycles. The problem with this mode is that the breath is delivered without regard to the patient's breathing cycle. This has usually been replaced by an improved method, synchronous intermittent mandatory ventilation (SIMV).

SIMV. This mode synchronizes the machine-delivered breaths (IMV) with the patient's spontaneous breaths. In IMV the machine may cycle a breath before the patient can completely exhale a spontaneous breath. If no inspiratory effort is present, the machine delivers the mandatory breaths. Usually, the preset number of breaths is low, allowing more effort with support on the part of the patient.

CPAP. The patient allows the patient to spontaneously breathe and has a preset level of pressure that is constantly maintained during the whole respiratory cycle. This method of positive pressure support can also be achieved through use of commercially available pneumatically powered units that hook directly into the oxygen wall outlet. A tight-fitting mask is secured around the patient's mouth and nose, and a preset pressure and oxygen percentage is delivered.

BiPAP. A noninvasive form of mechanical ventilation usually delivered through a tight-fitting oronasal mask. There are different pressures for inspiration and exhalation, which are always above atmospheric levels. Inspiratory pressure is higher than expiratory pressure.

Airway pressure release ventilation (APRV). This may also be called pressure release ventilation. The patient is allowed to spontaneously breathe with a set amount of CPAP. If additional ventilation is required, the CPAP will be dropped periodically, releasing the pressure, causing the patient to exhale. When the exhalation is complete, CPAP is restored. Proponents of this mode claim that by allowing the patient control, patient comfort and compliance are high.

Pressure support ventilation (PSV). When using pressure support, the patient is allowed to breathe spontaneously, triggering a preset amount of inspiratory support until the flow rate reaches a minimal level of preset pressure in the airway. The patient controls the frequency, tidal volume, and inspiratory time. This mode is often used in conjunction with SIMV. This mode is also popular because of high patient compliance. The pressure is set for safe levels, and the volume is variable. When the patient breathes in, the volume continues until the preset pressure is reached. That is the end of inspiration.

Mandatory minute ventilation (MMV). The patient is allowed to breathe spontaneously; however, a minimal level of minute ventilation will be achieved through ventilator-assisted breaths. This is usually accomplished by using PSV.

Volume-assured pressure support (VAPS). This is one of the newest modes of ventilation. It allows the patient to breathe spontaneously in the PSV mode and monitors each breath's tidal volume. If the breath is not going to reach the set volume, the ventilator will hold the flow rate constant and increase the pressure until the desired volume is reached.

Alarm Management and Precautions

When patients are using mechanical ventilators, it is inevitable that alarms will sound. Alarms are important indicators of a change in patient condition or a machine malfunction. All alarms should be recognized and valued as excellent sources of information. If alarms are silenced or ignored without interpretation, patient fatalities may result. Alarms should not be turned off. When therapy is being delivered, the alarms are a valuable tool. Therapists, however, need to realize they are treating the patient, not the machine. If an alarm sounds during a therapy treatment, stop the intervention and wait a few seconds to see whether the alarm stops. Before continuing therapy, identify which alarm went off and evaluate why. If it is not clear why the alarm sounded, contact the respiratory care practitioner or the patient's nurse immediately.

The most common alarms are those that monitor high and low pressure, FiO_2, apnea, disconnection, and volume. The high-pressure alarm is the one that sounds most commonly when the patient is receiving physical therapy. This alarm indicates that more than the preset pressure is needed to deliver the volume of ventilation. Generally, if the high-pressure alarm continues to sound, the patient should be checked for secretions. Suctioning can remedy this problem. The ventilator tubing should also be checked for possible occlusion from compression or excessive water buildup (Figure 43-10). High-pressure alarms may also sound in the case of bronchospasm or breath holding. Do not use strong resistance exercise with patients on mechanical ventilation because they may hold their breath and perform a Valsalva maneuver, which will cause increased circuit pressure to deliver the tidal volume to the patient. Low pressure alarm may signify a leak in the ventilator circuitry or a disconnection from the machine. Before turning a patient or performing upper extremity exercise, make sure there is clearance and ease of movement in the ventilator circuit tubing to prevent it from coming off during the interventions. In one case (in an unnamed medical center's intensive care unit) a patient's low-pressure alarm sounded and the patient was bagged while the cause was evaluated. The source was a disconnection that occurred when a new employee from the housekeeping department unplugged the ventilator to use the plug for a cleaning machine. When the low-pressure alarm sounds, first consider that the patient is not being ventilated.

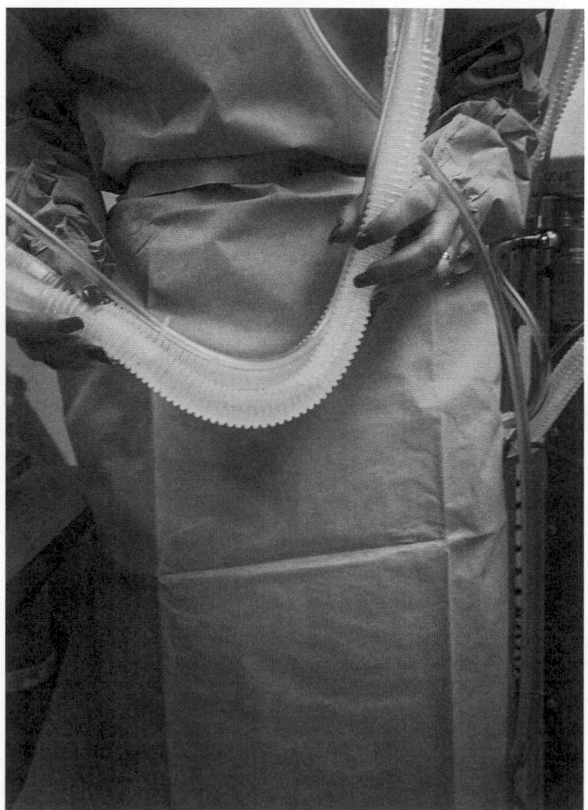

Fig. 43-10 Condensation build-up in ventilator tubing—a potential hazard.

If you are unfamiliar with a particular ventilator and an alarm sounds that you are unable to identify and/or remedy, first ensure the patient is not in any extra distress. Assess the overall appearance of the patient and, most important, the rise and fall of the patient's chest as the ventilator cycles. If the patient does not appear to be receiving breaths, immediate action should be taken to remove the ventilator from the patient and begin manual ventilation with a self-inflating bag. The respiratory care practitioner should be called to rectify the situation. When the problem is resolved, the patient should be returned to the mechanical ventilator.

Another significant precaution to take when working with a patient on a ventilator is to watch for condensation in the tubing that could accidentally be poured directly into the patient's lungs, especially during turning. When moving a patient who is using a ventilator, plan ahead by securing all lines, wires, and tubing. Follow the appropriate procedure for emptying any water from the ventilator tubing before moving the patient. If the patient aspirates water from ventilator tubing, it can be fatal.

Weaning from Mechanical Ventilation

Weaning is generally initiated when the reason for placing the patient on mechanical ventilation is reversed. Several factors need to be evaluated. Is there adequate ventilation and oxygenation? During weaning, the work required by the patient to breathe may increase and oxygen may need to be titrated appropriately. Hemodynamic stability must be monitored. Using CPAP during weaning may provide the bridge necessary to wean with less stress and decreased ventilatory demand. In general in patients who are receiving mechanical ventilation, the ventilator is discontinued and then the artificial airway is evaluated and removed. In some patients with neuromuscular and musculoskeletal issues, however, ventilator weaning by lung expansion with NIV and decannulation will be a better solution.[79]

Some patients with neuromusculoskeletal concerns may use other mechanical means of ventilation, such as a pneumobelt.[80] The pneumobelt is a noninvasive device placed over the abdomen. It has a bladder that inflates and mechanically puts pressure on the abdomen, thereby causing exhalation. When the bladder deflates, the diaphragm descends and inspiration occurs. Another negative pressure device used to help patients with neurological deficits is the chest cuirass, which resembles a turtle shell placed over the chest wall. Negative pressure is applied to the chest wall, which elevates the thorax to provide inspiration and then releases to allow for exhalation. The benefits of these mechanical aids are that the patient does not need an artificial airway and he or she is provided with a more physiological means of ventilation. They are well received by many people with neurological impairments.

Role of the Physical Therapist

The physical therapist can have a significant role in keeping the patient who is mechanically ventilated from having decreased aerobic capacity by helping the patient perform aggressive mobilization (see Chapters 18, 19, and 20), exercise, airway clearance techniques, and breathing strategies and interventions (see Chapters 21, 22, and 23). The physical therapist can also play a role in finding optimal positions to support the patient who is being weaned. Therapists who have been working on breathing strategies can be a source of comfort and encouragement for the patient during the weaning periods. Active mobilization early in the course of mechanical ventilation will result in more successful outcomes.

Evidence now supports the use of early physical and occupational therapy by giving patients sedation breaks and rousing patients to exercise. This has been shown to result in better functional outcomes at discharge, fewer ventilator days, and fewer days of delirium compared with standard ventilator treatment without waking patients for therapy.[81,82]

Summary

Physical therapists need to understand the basic equipment and principles of respiratory care in order to optimize the functional outcomes of their patients. The interprofessional team approach is vital in acutely ill patients. Working in collaboration with respiratory care practitioners and nurses will maximize interventions and improve patient outcomes.

Review Questions

1. Why does a high-flow system provide the most accurate oxygen delivery?
2. What circumstances will drive the physician to order a low-flow system when a high-flow system would be optimal?
3. Why do low-flow oxygen masks require a certain minimum-liter flow (i.e., 5 to 10 L/min for a simple mask)?
4. How does noninvasive mechanical ventilation improve exercise performance?
5. Which ventilator monitor would alert the therapist that the patient has become disconnected from the machine?
6. If the high-pressure alarm sounds during a patient treatment with resistance to the lower extremity, how can the intervention be changed?
7. What parameters should a physical therapist use when exercising a patient who is mechanically ventilated?
8. What is the role of the physical therapist in the interprofessional health care team that cares for patients who are receiving NIMV?

References

1. AARC Clinical Practice Guidelines: Oxygen therapy for adults in the acute care facility. *Respiratory Care* 46:717–720, 2002.
2. Web JG, Haas CF: Long term oxygen therapy for COPD: improving longevity and quality of life in hypoxemic patients. *Postgrad Medicine* 103:143–144, 147–148, 153–155, 1998.
3. Petty TL: Controversial indications for long term respiratory care: long term oxygen therapy. *Monaldi Archives of Chest Disease* 54:58–60, 1999.
4. Dunne PJ: The demographics and economics of long term oxygen therapy. *Respiratory Care* 45:223–228, 2000.
5. DesRosiers A, Russo R: Long term oxygen therapy. *Respiratory Care Clinic of North America* 6:625–644, 2000.
6. Christopher KL, Porte P: Long-term Oxygen Therapy. *Chest* Rdb;139(2):430–434, 2011.
7. Kacmarek RM, Mack CW, Dimas S: *The essentials of respiratory care*, ed 3, St Louis, 1990, Mosby.
8. Burton GG, Hodgkin JE, Ward JJ: *Respiratory care a guide to clinical practice*, ed 3, Philadelphia, 1991, JB Lippincott.
9. Bazuaye EA, Stone TN, Corris PA, et al: Variability of inspired oxygen concentration with nasal cannulas. *Thorax* 47:609–611, 1992.
10. Dunlevy CL, Tyl SE: The effect of oral versus nasal breathing on oxygen concentrations received from nasal cannulas. *Respiratory Care* 37:357–360, 1992.
11. Jensen AG, Johnson A, Sandstedt S: Rebreathing during oxygen treatment with face mask: the effect of oxygen flow rates on ventilation. *Acta Anaesthesiologica Scandinavica* 35:289–292, 1991.
12. Christopher KL: Transtracheal oxygen catheters. *Clinical Chest Medicine* 24:489–510, 2003.
13. Preciado DA, Thatcher G, Panitch HB, et al: Transtracheal oxygen catheters in a pediatric population. *Ann Otol Rhinol Laryngol* 111:310–314, 2002.
14. Christopher KL, Spofford BT, Petrun MD, et al: A program for transtracheal oxygen delivery: assessment of safety and efficacy. *Annals of Internal Medicine* 107:802–808, 1987.
15. Jackson M, King MA, Wells FC, et al: Clinical experience and physiologic results with an implantable intratracheal oxygen catheter. *Chest* 102:1413–1418, 1992.
16. Veen JC, Stolk J, Dijkman JH: Complications in the use of the subcutaneous tunnelled intratracheal oxygen catheter. *Netherlands Journal of Medicine* 48:8–10, 1996.
17. Rothe TB, Frey JG, Ciobanu TD, et al: Dangerous complication of transtracheal oxygen therapy with the SCOOP system. *Pneumologie* 50:700–702, 1996.
18. Kampelmacher MJ, Cornelisse PB, Alsbach GP, et al: Accuracy of oxygen delivery by liquid oxygen canisters. *European Respiratory Journal* 12:204–207, 1998.
19. Tiep BL, Barnett J, Schiffman G, et al: Maintaining oxygenation via demand oxygen delivery during rest and exercise. *Respiratory Care* 47:887–892, 2002.
20. Garrod R, Bestall JC, Paul E, et al: Evaluation of pulsed dose oxygen delivery during exercise in patients with severe chronic pulmonary disease. *Thorax* 54:242–244, 1999.
21. Johann U, Fichter J, Sybrecht GW: Efficacy of demand oxygen delivery systems in patients with chronic obstructive lung disease. *Pneumologie* 55:306–310, 2001.
22. McCoy R: Oxygen-conserving techniques and devices. *Respiratory Care* 45:95–103, 2000.
23. Palwai A, Skowronski M, Coreno A, et al. Critical comparisons of the clinical performance of oxygen conserving devices. *Am J Respir Crit Care Med* 181(10):1061–1071, 2010 May 15.
24. Valli G, Paoletti P, Savi D, et al. Clinical use of Heliox in asthma and COPD. *Monaldi Arch Chest Dis* 3(67):159–164, 2007 Sept.
25. Palange P: Lighter than air: Heliox breathing improves exercise tolerance in COPD. *Eur Respir Rev* 19(115):1–3, 2010, Mar 1.
26. Hunt T, Williams MT, Frith P, et al: Heliox, dypsnoea and exercise in COPD. *Eur Respir Rev* 19(115):30–38, 2010 Mar 1.
27. Squadrone V, Coha M, Cerutti E, et al: Continuous positive airway pressure for treatment of postoperative hypoxemia: a randomized controlled trial. *Journal of the American Medical Association* 293:589–595, 2005.
28. American Association for Respiratory Care (AARC): www.aarc.org, 2004.
29. Skinner MA, Kingshott RN, Jones DR, et al: Elevated posture for the management of obstructive sleep apnea. *Sleep Breath* 8:193–200, 2004.
30. Owens RL, Malhotra A: Sleep disordered breathing and COPD: the overlap syndrome. *Respir Care* 55(10):1333–1336, 2010 Oct.
31. Halliday HL: What interventions facilitate weaning from the ventilator? A review of the evidence from systematic reviews. *Paediatric Respiratory Review* 5(Suppl A):S347-S352, 2004.
32. Imanaka H, Takeuchi M, Tachibana K, et al: Changes in respiratory pattern during continuous positive airway pressure in infants after cardiac surgery. *Journal of Anesthesiology* 18:241–249, 2004.
33. Upadhyay A, Deorari AK: Continuous positive airway pressure: a gentler approach to ventilation. *Indian Pediatrics* 41:459–469, 2002.

34. L'Her E, Duquesne F, Girou E, et al: Noninvasive continuous positive airway pressure elderly cardiogenic pulmonary edema patients. *Intensive Care Medicine* 30:882–888, 2004.
35. Lloberes P, et al: Predictive factors of quality of life improvements and continuous positive airway pressure use in patients with sleep apnea-hypopnea syndrome:study at 1 year. *Chest* 126:1241–1247, 2004.
36. Buttner A, Ruhle KH: Quality of life before and during CPAP. *Pneumologie* 58:651–659, 2004.
37. Bachour A, Maasilta P: Mouth breathing compromises adherence to nasal continuous positive airway pressure therapy. *Chest* 126:1248–1254, 2004.
38. Fujimoto K, Matsuzawa Y, Yamaguchi S, et al: Benefits of oxygen on exercise performance and pulmonary hemodynamics in patients with COPD with mild hypoxemia. *Chest* 122:457–463, 2002.
39. Snider G: Enhancement of exercise performance in COPD patients by hyperoxia. *Chest* 122:1830–1837, 2002.
40. Brusasco V, Pellegrino R: Oxygen in the rehabilitation of patients with chronic obstructive pulmonary disease: an old tool revisited. *American Journal of Respiratory Critical Care Medicine* 168:1021–1022, 2003.
41. Emtner M, Porszasz J, Burns M, et al: Benefits of supplemental oxygen in exercise training in nonhypoxemic chronic obstructive pulmonary disease patients. *American Journal of Respiratory Critical Care Medicine* 168:1034–1042, 2003.
42. Jolly EC, Di Boscio V, Aguirre L, et al: Effects of supplemental oxygen during activity in patients with advanced COPD without severe resting hypoxemia. *Chest* 120:437–443, 2001.
43. AARC Clinical Practice Guidelines: Exercise testing for evaluation of hypoxemia and/or desaturation. *Respiratory Care* 46:514–522, 2001.
44. Ambrosino N, Strambi S: New strategies to improve exercise tolerance in chronic obstructive pulmonary disease. *European Respiratory Journal* 24:313–322, 2004.
45. Borghi-Silva A, Mendes RG, Toldeo AC, et al: Adjuncts to physical training of patients with severe COPD: oxygen or noninvasive ventilation? *Respir Care* 55(7):885–894, 2010 Jul.
46. DeBacker LA, Ides K, Daems D, et al: Pulmonary rehabilitation and non-invasive ventilation in COPD. *Acta Clin Belg* 65(5):330–335, 2010 Set–Oct.
47. AARC Clinical Practice Guidelines: Incentive spirometry. *Respiratory Care* 36:1402–1403, 1991.
48. Lezon K: Teaching incentive spirometry. *Nursing* 29:60–61, 1999.
49. Pullen RL: Teaching bedside incentive spirometry. *Nursing* 33:24, 2003.
50. Hall JC, et al: Prevention of respiratory complications after abdominal surgery: a randomized clinical trial. *British Medical Journal* 312:148–152, 1996.
51. King MS: Preoperative evaluation. *American Family Physician* 62:308–311, 2000.
52. Weiner P, Man A, Weiner M, et al: The effect of incentive spirometry and inspiratory muscle training on pulmonary function after lung resection. *Journal of Thoracic Cardiovascular Surgery* 113:552–557, 1997.
53. Crowe JM, Bradley CA: The effectiveness of incentive spirometry with physical therapy for high-risk patients after coronary artery bypass surgery. *Physical Therapy* 77:260–268, 1997.
54. Gosselink R, et al: Incentive spirometry does not enhance recovery after thoracic surgery. *Critical Care Medicine* 28:679–683, 2000.
55. Overend TJ, Anderson CM, Lucy SD, et al: The effect of incentive spirometry on postoperative pulmonary complications: a systematic review. *Chest* 120:971–978, 2001.
56. Frownfelter DL: *Chest physical therapy and pulmonary rehabilitation an interdisciplinary approach*, ed 2, St Louis, 1987, Mosby.
57. AARC Clinical Practice Guidelines: Humidification during mechanical ventilation. *Respiratory Care* 37:887–890, 1992.
58. American Association for Respiratory Care (AARC): www.aarc.org, 2003.
59. Branson RD, Seger SM: Bronchial hygiene techniques. In Kacmarek RM, Stoller JK, editors: *Current respiratory care*, Philadelphia, 1988, B.C. Decker.
60. Orens KD, Kester L, Fergus LC, et al: Cost impact of metered dose inhalers versus small volume nebulizers in hospitalized patients: the Cleveland Clinic experience. *Respiratory Care* 36:1099–1104, 1991.
61. Ashworth HL, Wilson CG, Sims EE, et al: Delivery of propellant soluble drug from a metered dose inhaler. *Thorax* 46:245–247, 1991.
62. Fuller HD, Dolovich MB, Posmituck G, et al: Pressurized aerosol versus jet aerosol delivery to mechanically ventilated patients: comparison of dose to the lungs. *American Review of Respiratory Disease* 141:440–444, 1990.
63. Duffy SQ, Farley DE: The protracted demise of medical technology: the case of intermittent positive pressure breathing. *Medical Care* 30:718–734, 1992.
64. Handelsman H: Intermittent positive pressure breathing (IPPB) therapy. *Health Technology Assessment Reports* 1:1–9, 1991.
65. Aboussouan LS, Ricaurte B: Noninvasive positive pressure ventilation: Increasing use in acute care. *Cleve Clin J Med* 77(5):307–316, 2010 May.
66. Hamada S, Ishikawa Y, Aoyagi T, et al. Indicators for ventilator use in Duchenne Muscular Dystrophy. *Respir Med* 2010, Dec 29 Epub ahead of print.
67. Bach JR, Martinez D: Duchenne Muscular Dystrophy End Stage Respiratory Muscle Failure: Prolongation of Survival by Noninvasive Interventions. *Respir Care* 2011 Feb 11 (EPub ahead of print).
68. Fauroux B: Noninvasive ventilation in cystic fibrosis. *Expert Rev Respir Med* 4(1):39–46, 2010 Feb.
69. Ozsancak A, Sidhorn S, Liesching RN, et al: Evaluation of the total face mask for noninvasive ventilation to treat acute respiratory failure. *Chest* 139(5):1034–1041, 2011 May, Feb 17 (EPub ahead of print).
70. Brochard L: Mechanical ventilation: invasive versus noninvasive. *European Respiratory Journal* 47(Suppl):31S–37S, 2003.
71. Esteban A, Anzueto A, Alia I, et al: How is mechanical ventilation employed in the intensive care unit? An international utilization review. *American Journal of Respiratory Critical Care Medicine* 161:1450–1458, 2000.
72. Antonelli M, Pennisi MA, Conti G: New advances in the use of noninvasive ventilation for acute hypoxaemic respiratory failure. *European Respiratory Journal* 22(Suppl 42):65s–71s, 2003.
73. Wysocki M, Antonelli M: Noninvasive mechanical ventilation in acute hypoxaemic respiratory failure. *European Respiratory Journal* 18:209–220, 2001.
74. Reference deleted in proofs.
75. Schonhofer B, Wallstein S, Wiese C, et al: Noninvasive mechanical ventilation improves endurance performance in patients with chronic respiratory failure due to thoracic restriction. *Chest* 119:1371–1378, 2001.
76. Padman R, et al: Noninvasive mechanical ventilation for cystic fibrosis patients at end stage disease. *Pediatric Pulm A* 232:297, 1992.
77. Hill AT, et al: Nasal intermittent positive pressure ventilation in cystic fibrosis, more than a bridge to transplantation? *Pediatric Pulmonology* 285:259, 1995.
78. Branson RD, Chatburn RL: Technical description and classification of modes of ventilator operation. *Respiratory Care* 37:1026–1044, 1992.
79. Bach JR, Goncalves M: Ventilator weaning by lung expansion and decannulation. *American Journal of Physical and Medical Rehabilitation* 83:560–568, 2004.
80. Reference deleted in proofs.
81. Jakob SM, Takala J: Physical and occupational therapy during sedation stops. *The Lancet* 373(9678):1824–1826, May 5-June 2009.
82. Schweickert W, Pholhman M, Pholman A, et al: Early physical and occupational therapy in mechanically ventilated, critically ill patients: a randomised control trial. *The Lancet* 373(9678):1874–1882, 30 May–June 2009.

Chapter 44

VIII

Care of the Patient with an Artificial Airway

Donna Frownfelter and Lisa Sigg Mendelson

KEY TERMS

Airway clearance
Artificial airway
Open and closed suctioning systems
Suctioning technique
Tracheostomy
Tracheostomy tube/cuff

CHAPTER OUTLINE

An artificial airway is a tube inserted in the trachea either through the mouth or nose or by a surgical incision. Artificial airways have been known to medical science for 3000 years. George Washington ultimately died of upper airway obstruction because his physicians could not agree on the use of tracheostomy. It was not until 1909, when Chevalier Jackson published his classic paper on tracheotomy,[1] that this procedure gained some acceptance. The procedure did not become a highly specialized technique in patient care until the invention of modern tracheostomy tubes and the development of intermittent positive-pressure ventilators. In today's clinical practice, artificial airways have the following four basic purposes: to bypass upper airway obstruction, to assist or control respirations over prolonged periods, to facilitate the care of chronic respiratory tract infections, and to prevent aspiration of oral and gastric secretions. Multiple disease processes and traumatic problems can require an artificial airway, but each situation, simple or complex, can fit into one or several of these categories (Box 44-1).

Indications of Need

The respiratory care team can play a vital role in recognizing patient need for a tracheostomy by noting physiological changes that indicate respiratory distress.[2] Cardinal signs of dangerous airway obstruction are stridor and chest wall retractions. Early clinical signs may include restlessness, agitation, tachycardia, confusion, motor dysfunction, and decreased oxygen saturation on pulse oximetry. These signs may be accompanied by headache, flapping tremor, audible wheezing, congestion, and diaphoresis. Cyanosis from impaired oxygenation of the blood is a late, ominous sign.

In children, restlessness is due to the lack of oxygen unless another factor (e.g., thirst) is clearly evident. Extreme fatigue and an inability to sleep indicate impending danger. Apprehension, restlessness, and mental confusion at any age may be taken as early signs of hypoxemia.

Complications of Tracheostomy

Depending on the patient's impairment, selection of the appropriate airway is made by considering the following factors: What is the best means of accomplishing the goal? Is it an emergency or a controlled, determined situation? Will the airway be needed for long-term care? In general, oral endotracheal tubes are inserted in emergencies. They are the quickest and easiest tubes to insert, even for relatively

Box 44-1 Disease Processes That Could Require an Artificial Airway Because of Respiratory Insufficiency

- Primary lung disease (e.g., emphysema, chronic bronchitis, pulmonary fibrosis, cystic fibrosis, severe pneumonia, burned lung, and toxic inhalation)
- Systemic disease with secondary lung involvement (e.g., cardiac failure, renal failure [fluid overload], and multiorgan system failure)
- Neuromuscular disease (e.g., polio, Guillain-Barré syndrome, myasthenia gravis, use of muscle relaxants, and tetanus)
- Central nervous system depression (e.g., drugs, postanesthesia, metabolic coma, cerebrovascular accident, meningitis, and central nervous system tumors)
- Trauma (e.g., head/neck/chest surgery or injuries)
- Diseases complicated by extremes of age (e.g., premature infant or older adult)
- Mechanical obstruction (e.g., upper airway infection, laryngeal paralysis, tumor, edema, bleeding, foreign body, and thyroid malignancy)
- Recurrent aspiration (e.g., glottic incompetence, occlusive diseases of the esophagus, and swallowing disorders of various causes)

From Selecky PA: Tracheostomy—a review of present-day indications, complications, and care, *Heart Lung* 3:272-283, 1974.

untrained personnel. A nasotracheal tube will generally replace the oral endotracheal tube for a long-term intubation. The nasal tube is more efficient in that it is better secured, allows the patient to eat, is easier to suction, and is generally more comfortable for the patient.

There are certain complications with nasotracheal tubes. Among these are sinus blockage and pain, vocal cord damage, and pressure necrosis to the cartilaginous structure of the nose. To reduce these complications, the airway should be evaluated daily. The tube should be removed as quickly as possible when the indication for intubation is reversed. If there appears to be a need for a more long-term airway, however, a tracheostomy should be considered. The procedure should not be taken lightly because many additional complications may occur.

Complications of tracheostomy can be surgical, postoperative, or physiological. Complications that occur at the time of the operation are more frequently direct results of the surgical procedure itself. Delayed complications may result directly or indirectly from surgery, postoperative care, or the abrupt physiological changes resulting from tracheostomy. Objectives of caring for the patient after a tracheostomy are to maintain patency of the tube, cleanliness of the wound site, and good aeration of the lungs, as well as to observe any changes in the patient's vital signs and oxygenation by pulse oximetry.

In patients with artificial airways, the normal physiological mechanism for adding moisture to the air via the nasal mucosa is bypassed. Therefore supplemental humidification is extremely important to protect the mucosa from drying and crusting, which results in obstruction.

The dressing under the tracheostomy tube and tracheostomy ties should be changed when they become soiled because dried blood and other secretions near the incision can encourage bacterial growth. The incision should be checked frequently for bleeding. The skin may be cleaned with half-strength hydrogen peroxide and sterile saline when a new dressing is applied. The dressing should be folded into place, never cut. This eliminates the possibility of lint or frayed threads being aspirated. Commercially prepared dressings best meet these criteria.

When changing the tapes that hold the tube in place, it is best to have one nurse hold the tube in place while another replaces the old tapes. An angle is cut at the end of the tape to facilitate its placement through the flange of one side of the tube. The tape is then threaded through the back of the tracheostomy tube and through the other flanged opening and tied securely with a square knot placed on one side of the patient's neck. One finger should be placed under the twill tape while tying it; this will prevent the tape from being tied too tight.

Pneumothorax can occur immediately after tracheostomy because of laceration of the mediastinal pleura at the time of or within 24 hours of surgery (this arises often in children and patients with chronic obstructive lung disease). Other problems include air embolism, aspiration, and subcutaneous and mediastinal emphysema. Recurrent laryngeal nerve damage or posterior tracheal penetration may occur but is uncommon.

Postoperative Physiological Complications

Attentive nursing care is the single most essential factor in postoperative tracheostomy management. Vigilant monitoring and observation by the entire respiratory care team is of vital importance.

Patients with an artificial airway are understandably apprehensive and have special communication needs. They should be reminded that their inability to speak is only temporary. These patients must be reassured that they will be monitored frequently and can trust and depend fully on the health care team to attend to their needs. If alert, patients must be equipped with a signal light or bell, paper and pencil, magic slate, or picture board for communication.

Airway obstruction is the foremost complication that exists postoperatively for the patient who has undergone tracheostomy. Tracheal secretions are the major source of obstruction, particularly if they are excessive or viscous. When using a cuffed tube, acute obstruction might occur from overinflating the cuff, which allows it to balloon over the end of the tube. Other causes of obstruction are dislodgement of the tube into a false tract anterior to the tube tracheal opening, and kinking of softened plastic cannula.

Tracheobronchitis, inflammation of the trachea and bronchus, is a complication resulting primarily from irritation due to incorrect suctioning technique and the presence of a foreign body in the trachea.

Crusting is a common and complex problem that may result from inadequate humidification of inspired air or patient dehydration. In many instances, ulceration of the tracheal mucosa results from irritation by the airway or incorrect suctioning. This ulcerated area becomes infected with various organisms and is virtually covered by crust. Further suctioning removes the crust, causing discharge of serum and bleeding. The discharge produces a wet eschar that is covered with mucus. Because of the drying effect of air passing over this mass, a hard crust can form. The development of this crust in the trachea might eventually produce a mass large enough to completely plug the tracheal cannula and almost completely obstruct the trachea. Cases have been cited in which an entire cast of the tracheobronchial tree has been removed.

Other physiological complications may be related to the following: hypoxemia developing before or during the procedure and resulting in an uncontrollable patient, cardiac arrest, and increased myocardial sensitivity to adrenalin; alkalosis developing from rapid carbon dioxide washout after establishment of the airway, resulting in myocardial fibrillation and apnea; and cardiac failure, resulting in profuse bronchorrhea caused by pulmonary edema and shock.

A less commonly known physiological complication is related to lack of good oral care. This means the patient with an artificial airway should have his or her teeth brushed at least twice a day (if this is not possible, the green disposable oral swabs can be used) to decrease potential pathogens as *Staphylococcus aureus* or gram-negative rods.

Chronic complications cited by Dailey and colleagues (1992)[3] include the following: infection at the surgical site, aspiration, aerophagia, persistent stoma, and tracheal stenosis.

Postoperative Mechanical Complications

Dislocation of the tube may result from unsatisfactory nursing care, poor attention to the airway during positioning, or ventilator tubing pulling on the airway. If the tracheostomy tube tapes are not kept tight and tied with a square knot or if they become loose as a result of subcutaneous emphysema or edema, the tube may be coughed out of the trachea and become lodged in the tissues of the neck and obstruct the airway. In pediatric patients, stay sutures are frequently used to prevent dislodgement of the tracheostomy tube. These sutures are valuable during recannulization of the tube if it comes dislodged before a tract has been well established. Stay sutures will prevent entry into a false tract. Advantages of this technique include the following: rapid replacement of blocked or displaced tubes, improved exposure of the trachea at surgical intervention, firm anchoring of the trachea at the moment of incision, decreased trauma associated with extubation, and uniform tracheostomy technique for all ages.

Dislodgement of the outer cannula or required removal before a tract has been well established (usually 5 to 10 days) again requires diligence and quick action by the nurse. No attempt at reinsertion should be made without adequate light, satisfactory tissue retraction, tracheal hook, and a Trousseau's dilator. A Trousseau's dilator and tracheal hook should be readily available. A spare tracheostomy tube of the correct size should be kept at the patient's bedside at all times. Should the tube be coughed out, the nurse uses the Trousseau's dilator to hold the wound apart while summoning the physician. Tragedies have occurred from inserting the tube into the soft tissues of the neck or mediastinum because of a dislodged cannula and the frantic efforts to replace it. Once the tracheostomy tract has been firmly established, the tube can be replaced by the nurse on written order of the physician.

Tracheostomy Tubes

Metal Tubes

Tracheostomy tubes are of two basic types: metal and polyvinyl chloride (hard and soft). Metal tubes are no longer commonly used, but some patients with long-standing metal tracheostomies may prefer not to switch to a polyvinyl chloride tube. Metal tubes can be made of either stainless steel or sterling silver and are composed of the following three parts: an outer cannula that fits into the tracheal incision, an inner cannula that fits into the outer cannula, and an obturator that facilitates insertion of the tube. These three parts constitute a metal tracheostomy set and are not interchangeable with the parts of any other set. Before the outer cannula is inserted into the tracheal incision, the obturator is placed inside. The lower end of the obturator protrudes from the end of the outer cannula and facilitates its insertion into the trachea. This is the only purpose of the obturator. The protruding end of the obturator obstructs the lumen of the outer cannula. When the obturator is removed, it is immediately replaced with the inner cannula. If one part is lost or damaged, the entire set is useless. Therefore each part, including the obturator, must be accounted for carefully. Care should be exercised in handling sterling silver tubes because silver is easily dented.

The inner cannula should always be inspected to be sure it is clean and clear of secretions before it is reinserted. Mucus that has dried inside the inner cannula cannot be cleaned by merely rinsing it with water. The cannula should be soaked in hydrogen peroxide, scrubbed with a tracheostomy brush, and rinsed with saline to be sure all secretions have been removed. If a silver inner cannula becomes discolored, it may be cleaned with silver polish.

To prevent dislodgement, lock the inner cannula into position after reinsertion. The locking mechanism is different with each tube, and the therapist should become familiar with the types used. If the inner cannula is not locked, it may come out if the patient has a forceful exhalation or position change. It is vital that the inner cannula be reinserted quickly if the patient is on mechanical ventilation, especially if the patient is on full support.

Polyvinyl Chloride (Plastic) Disposable Tubes

The development of plastic tracheostomy tubes brought about three major improvements that account for their widespread use: application of silicone to the inner surface of the plastic tube minimizes crusting and adherence of secretions; it is easier to attach a safe, dependable, permanent inflatable cuff to the plastic tube that cannot slip off and occlude the tracheal opening; and lower costs allow the tube to be disposable. Plastic tubes, unlike metal sets, generally have interchangeable parts. The tubes come with and without cuffs.

The cuffed tracheostomy tube is primarily used in conjunction with a positive-pressure ventilator to form a closed system (Figure 44-1). It is also used to reduce the possibility of aspiration because of absent reflexes, protective laryngeal reflexes, or pharyngeal reflexes. The inflatable cuff is located around the lower portion of the tube and, when inflated, seals the trachea from most airflow except through the tube itself (see Figure 44-1). The cuff, usually made of pliable plastic, is inflated by injecting air into the fine-bore tubing. A small pilot balloon is

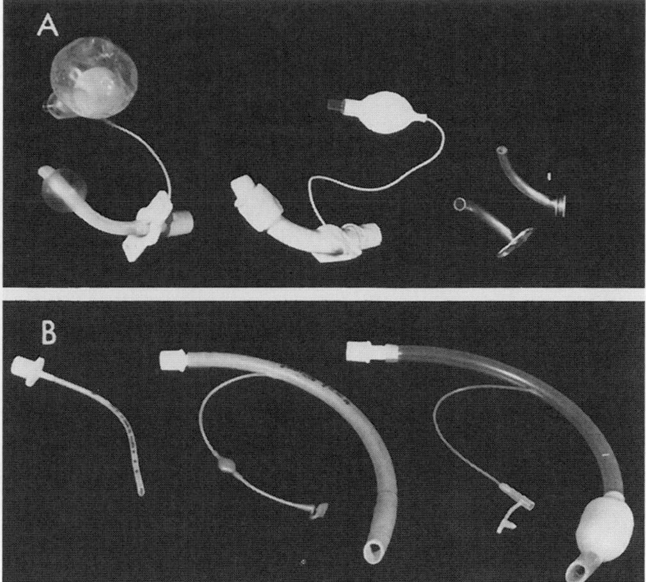

Fig. 44-1 A, Cuffed adult tracheostomy tubes, uncuffed pediatric tracheostomy tube *(far left).* **B,** Cuffed adult endotracheal tubes, uncuffed pediatric endotracheal tube *(far left).*

located proximally in the tubing and indicates that the cuff is inflated. The inflation end of the cuff and the balloon must be checked before insertion of the tube into the trachea to be certain that there are no leaks. The Luer valve inflation port to the pilot balloon is self-sealing. Some Luer valves have a relief valve when pressure exceeds 25 mm Hg.

Cuff Inflation

There are two commonly used methods of cuff inflation: minimal air leak, in which a small amount of air escapes on inspiration; and minimal occlusive volume, in which just enough air is placed in the cuff to stop air from escaping on inspiration. According to Crabtree Goodnough (1988)[4], the minimal leak cuff technique may produce less injury than the minimal occlusive volume inflation technique. Regardless of which technique is used, the pressure of the cuff should be checked every 4 to 8 hours and the pressures documented. With continued research and monitoring of tracheal cuff pressures, potential tracheal injury can be prevented.

Once the cuff is inflated, the only route for air exchange is through the patient's tracheostomy tube; therefore careful observation of the patient is essential. If the patient is on mechanical ventilation, observation is essential. Alarms are always to be in the "on" position when a patient is being mechanically ventilated. Some means of resuscitation, such as a manual resuscitation bag with mask, must be available at the bedside to ventilate the patient in case the tracheostomy tube comes out or is dislodged.

Considerable emphasis has been given to the incidence of tracheal ischemia and resulting stenosis from the use of a cuffed tube. Tracheal ischemia results from the pressure of the cuffed tube against the tracheal wall, which heals with scar formation and thereby leads to subsequent stenosis. This complication can be reduced or eliminated by minimal air leak or minimal occlusive volume. For the minimal occlusive volume, the cuff must be inflated to eliminate any air leak on inspiration. Cuff pressures should be monitored and documented every 4 to 8 hours to prevent tracheal injury. The recommended cuff pressure is 15 to 25 mm Hg. The cuff is inflated until there is no air leak between the wall of the trachea and the cuff, and then a small amount of air is released to allow only a slight air leak between the walls of the trachea and the cuff. This reduces the pressure of the cuff, still allows the ventilator to function properly, and reduces the likelihood of tracheal ischemia. Any difficulty in properly inflating the cuffed tracheostomy tube should be reported to the physician immediately.

If the tracheotomized patient is conscious, he or she may attempt to speak. If the cuff is properly inflated, the patient will be aphonic because no air can pass over the vocal cords. If the patient needs to speak, the cuff can be deflated, and the patient may be given a sterile dressing to hold over the tube. This will allow him or her to speak and also clear secretions by rapid exhalation (simulated cough).

To prevent the formation of crusts, inspired air must be continuously and adequately humidified by means of nebulizing equipment. The equipment used for this purpose can be a possible source of infection. Ideally, the nebulizer and tubing should be changed every 8 hours—at the very least, once every 24 hours.

The Communitrache I is a tracheostomy tube that permits the removal of secretions above the inflation cuff without nasotracheal suctioning. The other benefit to this tracheostomy tube is the patient's ability to communicate, especially while on a ventilator. When the patient is weaned from the ventilator, a fenestrated tube may be used. The term *fenestrated* comes from the French word *fenestre,* meaning "window." There is a window (fenestration) in the outer cannula. When the tube is used for speaking, the cuff is deflated, the inner cannula is removed, and an external plug is inserted to cap the tracheostomy tube to allow the patient to speak. The cuff must be deflated when the cap is in place. If the cuff is inflated, the patient is unable to breathe air into the lungs and will exhibit immediate distress. If a patient with a fenestrated tube needs to be suctioned, the inner cannula must be replaced so that the suction catheter does not enter the fenestration and cause injury to the tracheal wall mucosa.

Other Airway Devices

The Olympic tracheostomy button is used as an interim airway after tracheostomy tube removal (Figure 44-2). This method is another example of weaning a patient from the tracheostomy tube but still maintaining the stoma should a tracheostomy be again needed. Patients that may benefit most from this device are those with chronic obstructive pulmonary disease (COPD). This is one method used to facilitate secretion removal after hospitalization when it becomes necessary because of the disease process. The Olympic tracheostomy button allows the tracheostomy patient the opportunity to reestablish an unobstructed airway and at the same time allows the patient to speak.

Many other speaking tracheostomy tubes are available.[5] Airway clearance needs to be optimized before a speaking valve is used. If a patient has increased secretions, he or she may find it difficult to tolerate the procedure. A benefit of the

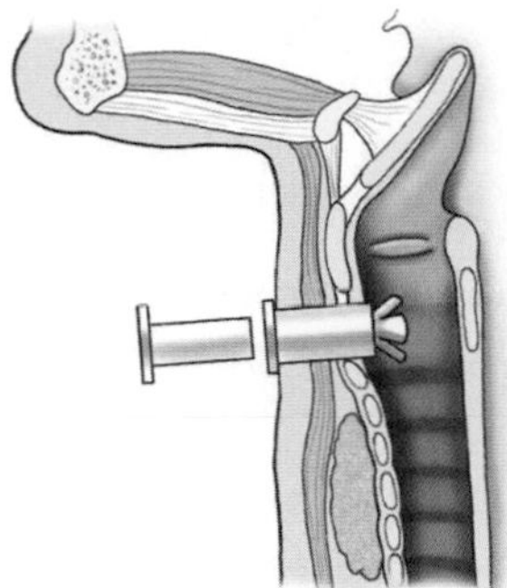

Fig. 44-2 Dimensions and actual positioning of an Olympic tracheostomy button. *(From Pierson DJ, Kacmarek RM.* Foundations of respiratory care, *Churchill Livingstone, 1992, Edinburgh.)*

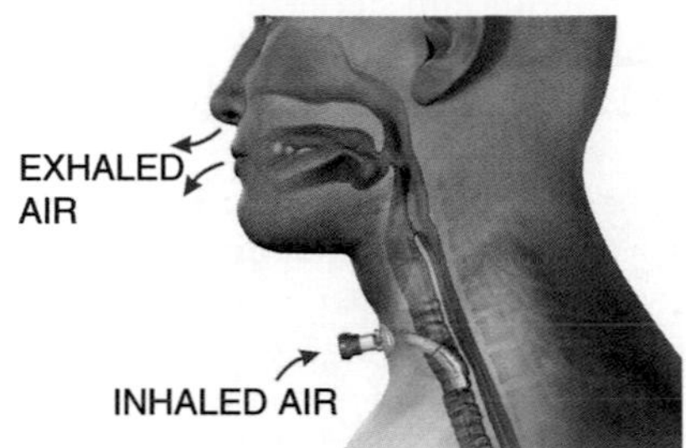

Fig. 44-3 The Passy-Muir Valve. This valve attaches to a standard 15-mm tracheostomy adapter. It allows inspiration via the valve, but exhalation must occur via the upper airway. *(Courtesy Passy-Muir.)*

valve, however, is that the patient may be able to simulate coughing and promote mobilization of upper airway secretions.

One common speaking valve is the Passy-Muir Swallowing and Speaking valve (Figure 44-3). The Passy-Muir is a one-way valve that allows inspiration only and redirects exhalation through the upper airway. It is important to note that the cuff must be deflated when using the valve, or a cuffless tracheostomy tube may be used. Breath stacking exercises (taking a few breaths in without exhaling) can be used to get more air into the lungs before exhalation. Using the valve, the upper airway muscles gradually recover, allowing for transition to a fenestrated tube or a smaller size tracheostomy tube and thereby preparing the patient for eventual decannulation.[6] Another benefit may be an improved ability to swallow. Also, some patients claim that they can taste their food again, which may promote improved nutrition and hydration.[7,8]

The management of major airway obstruction by tracheal tumor, external compression, or tracheal disease below the thoracic inlet still presents difficult problems. The Montgomery T tube is a bifurcated silicone rubber stent designed to preserve patency of the airways in a patient with injury to the trachea or main stem bronchi (Figure 44-4). When the T tube is in place, the patient breathes normally through the nose and mouth and can speak. The T tube is helpful in long-term therapy to alleviate obstruction or during reconstructive surgery. This device does not cause any adverse tissue reaction on a long-term basis, according to Montgomery.[9,10]

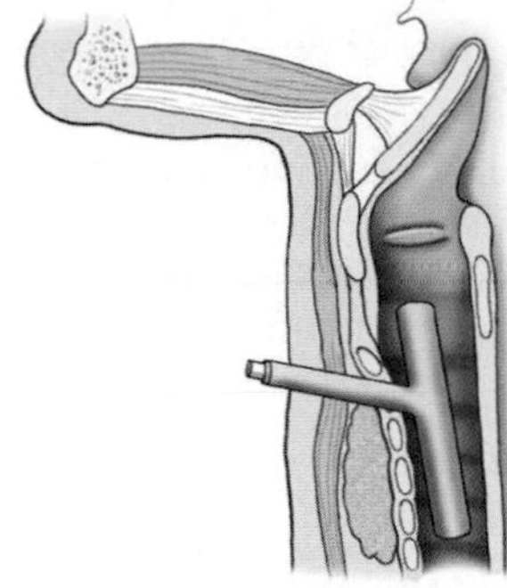

Fig. 44-4 The Montgomery T tube. *(From Montgomery WW: Manual care of the Montgomery silicone tracheal T tube,* Ann Otol, Rhinol & Laryngol *89 [Suppl 73]:3, 1980.)*

Table 44-1 The Three Phases of Suctioning

Before suctioning	Patient assessment and preparation, as well as hyperoxygenation, are essential. Proper catheter size will be discussed later in the chapter.
During suctioning	Awareness of the appropriate depth of insertion is essential, and time limits for the procedure must be observed. A decision must be made as to how many passes of the catheter will be needed. Monitoring of the patient by ECG and pulse oximetry will demonstrate the patient's tolerance of the procedure.
After suctioning	The patient needs to be reassured and positioned comfortably. Reconnection to the ventilator or previous level of equipment must be completed in cases of open-system suctioning.

Airway Care

Normally, the mucociliary escalator and the cough reflex provide airway clearance. When these mechanisms fail, suctioning of the airways, manual cough assistance, or the cough machine is indicated. Suctioning does have potential hazards, but it should be a safe procedure with proper guidance and care.[11] Health care professionals also need to protect themselves during open system suctioning. This procedure can cause dissemination of particle droplets in the immediate area. Ng and colleagues (1999)[12] studied 50 consecutive suctioning procedures with intubated patients using an open system (i.e., the mechanical ventilator tubing is removed from the tracheostomy or endotracheal tube to suction the patient). Visible droplets were scattered from 25 to 168 cm from the artificial airway. When they were cultured, the same bacteria aspirated grew on the agar plates. This highlights how important it is for the person performing the suction procedure to use protective eyewear and to take necessary precautions.[12]

Suctioning

When preparing to suction, three phases should be considered (Table 44-1)[13,14]:

1. Preparation before suctioning
2. The actual suctioning procedure
3. Postsuctioning

Open Versus Closed Suctioning Systems

Patients on mechanical ventilators may be suctioned by disconnecting the ventilator tubing and suctioning (open system), or suctioning may be done directly in-line with the ventilator tubing (closed system). Studies have shown that a closed system maintains better physiological stability, less oxygen desaturation, and fewer dsyrhythmias.[15-18]

Suction Procedure

Proper explanation of the suctioning technique to the patient helps allay apprehension and enhance cooperation. Medicate the postoperative patient before suctioning to decrease the pain of coughing. Always maintain a calm and reassuring manner.

Maintain aseptic technique throughout the entire procedure. Use sterile gloves and a sterile, disposable catheter for each suctioning.

Position the patient properly unless contraindicated. Nasotracheal and/or pharyngeal suctioning should be done with the patient in Fowler position, 60 to 70 degrees (Figure 44-5, *A*), or semi-Fowler position, approximately 45 degrees, with the neck hyperextended (Figure 44-5, *B*). The supine position is best for the patient with tracheostomy or endotracheal tubes (Figure 44-5, *C*).

Pharyngeal suctioning may be necessary before deflating the cuffed tracheostomy tube. The nurse should not suction the pharynx and then the trachea with the same catheter; however, the trachea may be suctioned first and then the pharynx with the same catheter.

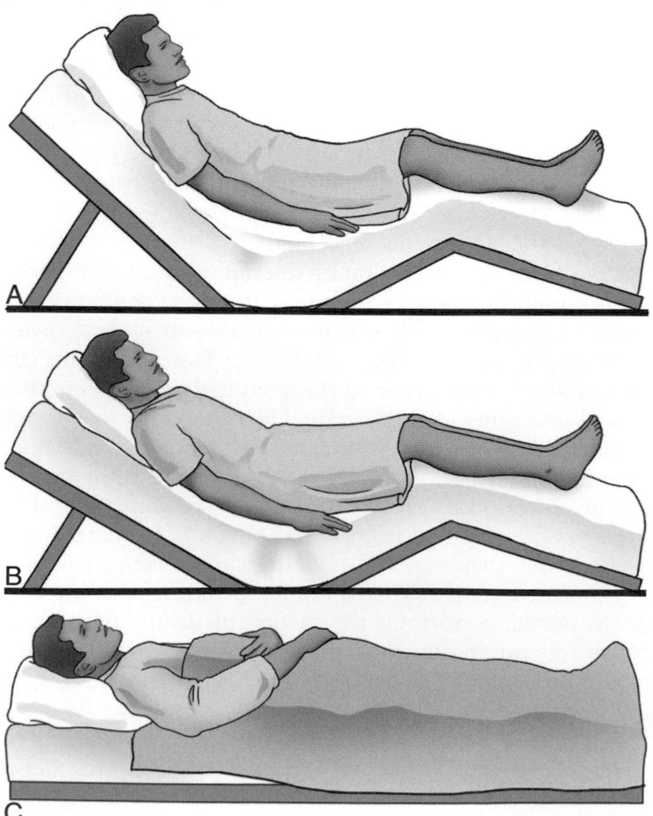

Fig. 44-5 Positioning for suction. **A,** Fowler's position. **B,** Semi-Fowler's position. **C,** Supine position.

Duration of suctioning is very important. Each suctioning procedure should last no longer than 5 to 10 seconds to avoid hypoxia.

Prolonged suctioning may result in precipitating a dysrhythmia or cardiac arrest. A good way to judge the elapsed time is to hold one's own breath and be guided by the development of discomfort. This is most important for the patient who depends on ventilatory assistance.

Use the lowest possible vacuum settings (below 120 mm Hg) that will still support suctioning the tracheostomy tube. The higher the setting is raised, the greater the risk for trauma to the tracheal mucosa. Caution should be exercised to avoid kinking the suction tubing or catheter. When negative pressure is excessive and released suddenly, inadvertent removal of portions of tracheal mucosa may occur.

Insertion of the suction catheter should be done gently, using aseptic technique and sterile gloves. Goggles are used as part of universal precautions if there is any danger of coughed-out secretions. The catheter should first be moistened in sterile saline or with a water-soluble gel. Suction is not applied while the catheter is passed down into the trachea. Proper insertion of the catheter will stimulate coughing when it contacts the carina (Figure 44-6, *A*). It is then immediately withdrawn one cm before suction is applied (Figure 44-6, *B*). Do not force the catheter up and down while suctioning. Suction is applied only while the catheter is being withdrawn. Rotating the catheter during withdrawal results in suctioning a larger area and increases the surface contact of the trachea and tracheostomy tube (Figure 44-7).

Left main-stem bronchus aspiration is more difficult because of the anatomical arrangement of the bronchus. It was formerly thought that left bronchial aspiration was facilitated by turning the patient's head to the right. Studies by Kirimli and colleagues (1970)[19] and Panacek and colleagues (1989)[20] indicate that left bronchial aspiration is best accomplished by using a Coudé tip catheter. After its insertion into the trachea, the curved tip should be positioned to point toward the left main-stem bronchus. Even so, insertion is difficult, and auscultation by stethoscope is necessary to thoroughly access the suctioning.

Right main-stem bronchus aspiration is the usual method because of the more direct alignment of this bronchus with the trachea. This can almost always be carried out with a straight tracheal catheter. The deeper suction would rarely be indicated; generally when the catheter hits the carina, it is withdrawn before suctioning.

Excessive suctioning can be harmful. Use judgment to determine just how often a patient requires suctioning. It should not be routine; rather, it should be based on the need of the patient.[21,22] Assessment by auscultation and patient clinical observations should be used to determine the need for suctioning. Suction only when it is needed.[23] Allow the patient to rest and breathe between each insertion of the suction catheter and, if necessary, ventilate the patient for a few minutes before further suctioning. Remember that each suctioning attempt removes air as well as secretions. Hyperoxygenation with 100% oxygen has been suggested to provide better results and fewer complications. Hyperventilation was previously encouraged, but studies have shown that it is not necessary; hyperoxygenation is the important factor.[24,25]

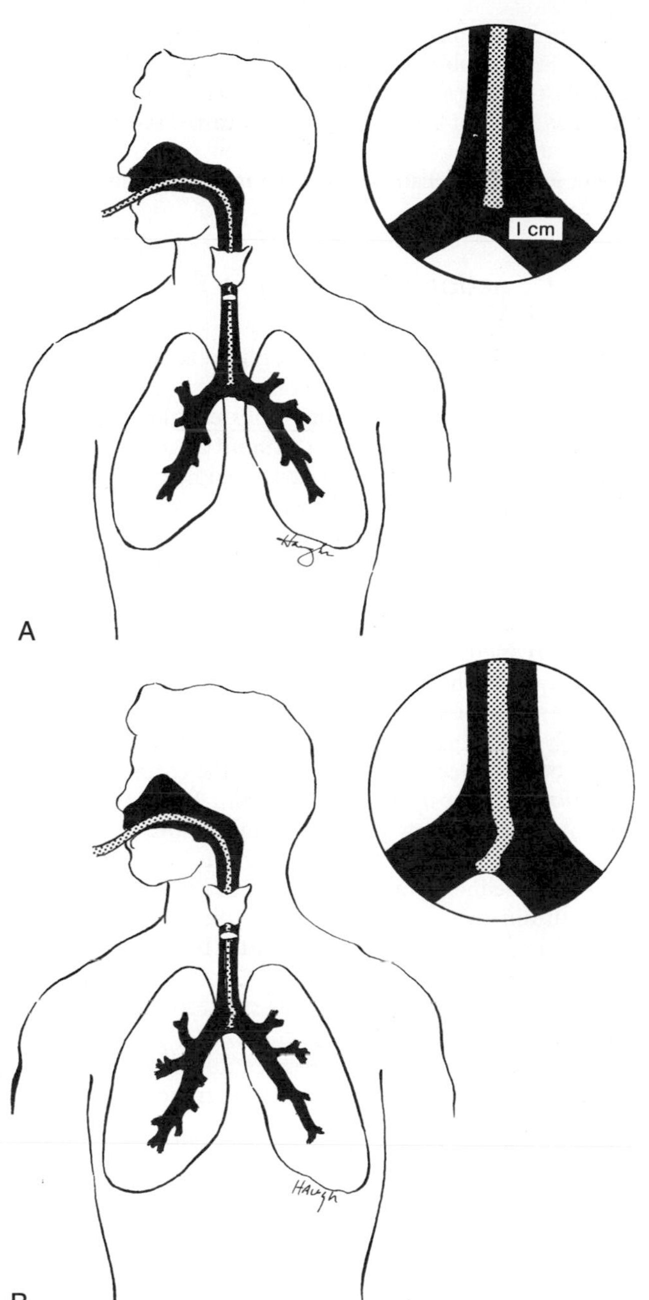

Fig. 44-6 Suctioning procedures. **A,** The catheter will stimulate coughing when it contacts the carina (in a patient with cough reflex). **B,** The catheter is withdrawn 1 cm after it reaches the carina, before applying suction.

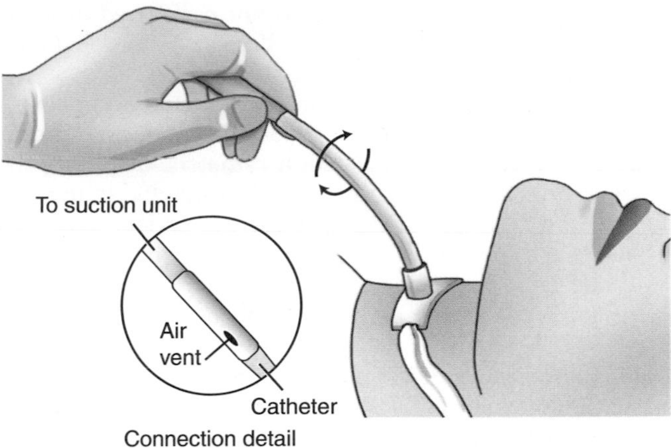

Fig. 44-7 The catheter is rotated during withdrawal in order to suction a larger surface area.

Complications

Complications from tracheal suctioning include hypoxemia, cardiac dysrhythmia, bronchospasm, and infection.

HYPOXIA

Suctioning can lead to hypoxemia because oxygen is removed from the airways, and this could lead to tissue hypoxia. To minimize this problem, patients should be given preoxygenation with 100% oxygen for three to five breaths. This can be done on the ventilator without disconnection.

CARDIAC DYSRHYTHMIA

Cardiac dysrhythmias, such as premature ventricular contractures, bradycardia, and tachycardia, can be diminished by hyperoxygenating the patient with 100% oxygen. If any dysrhythmias occur on the monitor, the suctioning procedure should be discontinued momentarily to allow the patient to stabilize and increase his or her oxygen level.

BRONCHOSPASM

Bronchospasm may be effectively prevented by administration of a bronchodilator, such as albuterol, before suctioning.

INFECTION

Infection can be decreased by maintaining sterile techniques with sterile gloves and sterile catheters when suctioning.

Suctioning Artificial Airways

Nasopharyngeal Airways

When frequent, aggressive nasopharyngeal suctioning is indicated in a patient who is comatose, a nasopharyngeal airway (NPA) will lessen the trauma of frequent passage of the catheter. The NPA is a soft latex material that provides easy access to the trachea for nasopharyngeal suctioning. The nasal and pharyngeal mucosa are protected, and the procedure thus becomes more comfortable to the patient. In addition, a fiberoptic bronchoscope may be passed through the airway if the procedure is indicated.

Endotracheal or Tracheostomy Suctioning

Sterile technique is followed for endotracheal and tracheostomy suctioning. Usually no lubrication is necessary, although it may be used if there is difficulty passing the catheter.

Sterile Suctioning

The technique for correct sterile suctioning of artificial airways is perhaps the most important and vital segment of care for the patient because it removes secretions that would otherwise obstruct the airway. If suctioning is not performed properly, it can cause physiological or psychological trauma to the patient.

The equipment necessary for proper sterile suctioning includes the proper mechanical apparatus, connecting tubing, sterile gloves, sterile saline, suction catheters, dressings, and goggles as indicated with universal precautions. It must be remembered that during suctioning, the patient's only air passage is being partially occluded. Thus the suction catheter should never be larger than one-half the diameter of the tube opening; if it is larger, it may completely occlude the patient's air passage.

One method for determining the size of the catheter used for suctioning is to double the size of the tracheostomy tube in place and add 2. For example, if the patient has a #6 tube, the calculation would be as follows: 6 + 6 = 12, 12 + 2 = 14. Therefore a 14-F catheter would be the largest catheter that could be used to suction the #6 tracheostomy. See Table 44-2 for a correlation of tracheostomy sizes to catheter sizes.

The catheter used for pharyngeal suctioning should never be used for subsequent suctioning of the artificial airway, but using an artificial airway suction catheter for pharyngeal suction is acceptable. Aseptic technique is absolutely necessary to minimize the risk for infection, and ideally, only disposable catheters should be used.

Suctioning may be necessary every few minutes when the patient initially returns from surgery because there is an increase in secretions, which is usually the result of irritation of the endotracheal tube plus a reflex mechanism initiated by the surgical trauma. Usually, by paying attention to the patient's color, respiratory rate, lung sounds, and oxygen saturation on pulse oximetry, the nurse or therapist can determine the amount of secretions present. Excessive mucus in the trachea or large bronchi is usually indicated by coarse, rattling sounds. Fine bubbling sounds usually suggest fluid located more peripherally (i.e., in the alveolar spaces). If accumulated secretions are not cleared, they can cause respiratory and cardiac rates to increase; effective oxygen and carbon dioxide transfer is impaired, causing cyanosis to appear and low-grade fever to develop.

Table 44-2 The Pediatric Tracheostomy Card

Tracheostomy Size	Recommended Catheter Size
Pediatric tubes	
00 PT	6.5 F
0 PT	6.5 F
1 PT	8 F
2 PT	8 F
3 PT	10 F
4 PT	10 F
Neonatal tubes	
00 NT	6.5 F
0 NT	6.5 F
1 NT	6.5 F
Single cannula tracheostomy (SCT) tubes	
5 SCT	10 F
6 SCT	12 F
7 SCT	14 F
8 SCT	14 F

From Warnoch C, Porpora K: A pediatric trache card: transforming research into practice, Pediatric Nursing *20:186-188, 1994.*

General Suctioning Procedure for an Artificial Airway

The procedure for suctioning an artificial airway begins after the clinician has taken all of the same appropriate procedure preparatory measures, including sterile technique procedures, as are required when suctioning without an artificial airway.

- Hyperoxygenate with 100% oxygen for three to five breaths with manual resuscitation bag.
- Place the patient's neck in extension.
- Lubricate the catheter with sterile saline or water-soluble gel.
- Place the catheter (without suction) upward and backward in short increments. Continue until an obstruction (the carina) is reached.
- When the carina is stimulated, the patient will generally cough unless his or her reflexes are obtunded.
- Pull the catheter back slightly from the carina; then apply suction with no more than 120 mm Hg pressure as the catheter is withdrawn in a rotating motion.
- Aspiration time should be within 10 to 15 seconds total. A good guideline is for the therapist to hold his or her own breath during suctioning (because the patient is also not breathing). This gives the therapist a better sensitivity for what the patient is experiencing.
- Allow the patient to rest for several seconds and preoxygenate the patient again.
- Check the patient's breath sounds and repeat the procedure, if necessary, to remove more secretions.
- Suction pharynx.
- Observe the patient and monitor for any dysrhythmias.
- Use pulse oximetry to monitor desaturation.

Instillation of Saline

Saline instillation is not recommended. Studies have shown that it is ineffective and can cause reflex and uncomfortable airway responses (i.e. cough, bronchospasm). Also, the saline instillation potentiates infection. It is not a recommended practice.[26,27]

Extubation/Decannulation

Extubation or decannulation is the removal of the artificial airway. In general, this is done when the reason for establishing the artificial airway no longer exists. In certain cases the artificial airway may be removed to facilitate airway clearance and aspiration. This can be prevented with thorough attention and care of the tracheostomy tube.[28,29] The patient is aided in gradually relearning normal breathing through his or her upper respiratory tract before the tube is removed. This can be a time of considerable fear and anxiety for patients because they have learned they can breathe safely through their tracheostomy, and they may become apprehensive when asked to breathe in a normal manner. The relearning process can be accomplished under the physician's direction by reducing the lumen of the tube for a day or two or by partially obstructing the tube's outer opening for increasing lengths of time. Eventually the patient is able to tolerate the complete occlusion of the tracheostomy opening. This is sometimes difficult and similar to breathing through a straw.

When occluding the tracheostomy opening with a cuffed tube, the cuff must be deflated first. Failure to do this will result in total obstruction of the patient's airway as the tube opening is occluded.

Fenestrated tubes are excellent for weaning the patient from the tracheostomy tube. They are probably more effective than using cuff tubes; furthermore, they do not actually increase the airway resistance, as do cuffed tubes. Fenestrated tubes also allow the patient to talk and attempt to cough to mobilize secretions. Other methods used in decannulation include the Olympic tracheostomy button and the Passy-Muir valve. The Olympic tracheostomy button allows the airway to remain patent for suctioning and reinsertion of a tracheostomy tube should it become necessary. The Passy-Muir valve allows for normal recovery of the upper airway muscle, making it possible to reduce the size of the tracheostomy tube, leading to eventual plugging and decannulation. Careful observation and documentation of the patient's ability to ventilate must be done when any of these devices are used in the decannulation process.

Close supervision should continue after extubation. After a tracheostomy tube is removed, the skin edges are usually taped together with butterfly strips for a few days until the wound heals. During healing, air will escape through the wound and reduce the effectiveness of the patient's cough. The patient should be instructed that the noise from the partially closed trachea is normal, and small secretions should be removed from this area. The patient should be taught and instructed to hold a sterile dressing firmly over the incision when coughing until the opening heals.

Summary

Artificial airways are commonly used, so the health care team needs to be proficient at using them and comfortable working with patients who have them. Precautions need to be observed and techniques consistently applied to prevent respiratory tract infections and unplanned decannulation. Training and orientation need to be thorough so that suctioning procedures are safe for the patient and the health care team. Knowing the indications for the artificial airway will help identify when the airway is no longer needed. For patients who require lifelong use of tracheostomy tubes, the patient, family, and care-taker need to be instructed in the airway clearance and cleaning procedures.

Review Questions

1. What physiological changes occur with surgical placement of a tracheostomy tube?
2. Discuss possible psychosocial concerns of patients with an artificial airway.
3. When would a speaking valve be indicated? What is the cuff position?
4. How does the patient-care team prepare the patient with a tracheostomy for self-care?
5. Compare emergency care, acute care, and long-term care for a patient with upper airway obstruction and tracheostomy placement.

References

1. Jackson C: Tracheostomy. *Laryngoscope* 18:285–290, 1909.
2. St. John RE, Malen JF: Contemporary issues in adult tracheostomy management. *Critical Care Nursing Clinics North America* 16:413–430, 2004.
3. Dailey RH, Simon B, Young GP, et al: Airway maneuvers. In *The airway emergency management*. St Louis, 1992, Mosby.
4. Crabtree Goodnough SK: Reducing tracheal injury and aspiration. *Dimension of Critical Care Nursing* 7:324–331, 1988.
5. Fitsimones L: Tracheostomy and ventilator speaking valves. *Vital Signs* April:6–8, 2003.
6. Pierson DJ, Kacmarek RM: *Foundations of respiratory care*. New York, 1992, Churchill Livingstone.
7. Elpern EH: Effect of the Passy-Muir valve on pulmonary aspiration in adults with tracheostomies. *Chest* 116(4-S2):365S, 1999.
8. Lichtman SW, Birnbaum IL, Sanfilippo MR, et al: Effect of a tracheostomy speaking valve on secretions, arterial oxygenation and olfaction: a quantitative evaluation. *Journal of Speech and Hearing Research* 38:549–555, 1995.
9. Wahidi MM, Ernst A: The Montgomery T-tube tracheal stent. *Clinical Chest Medicine* 24:437–443, 2003.
10. Montgomery WW: Manual of care of the Montgomery silicone tracheal T-tube. Annals of Otology, *Rhinology and Laryngology* 89(Suppl 73):3, 1989.
11. Dean B: Evidence-based suction management in accident and emergency vital component of airway care. *Accident and Emergency Nursing* 5:92–98, 1997.
12. Ng KS, Kumarasinghe G, Inglis TJ: Dissemination of respiratory secretions during tracheal tube suctioning in an intensive care unit. *Annals of the Academy of Medicine Singapore* 28:178–1821999.
13. Day T, Farnell S, Wilson-Barnett J: Suctioning: a review of current research recommendations. *Intensive Critical Care Nursing* 18:79–89, 2002.
14. AARC Clinical Practice Guideline: Nasotracheal suctioning—revision and update. Irving, Tex: American Association for Respiratory Care, 2004
15. Kalyn A, Blatz S, Feuerstake S, et al: Closed suctioning of intubated neonates maintains better physiologic stability: a randomized trial. *Journal of Perinatology* 23:218–222, 2003.
16. Lee CK, Ng KS, Tan SG, et al: Effect of different endotracheal suctioning systems on the cardiorespiratory parameters of ventilated patients. *Annals of the Academy of Medicine Singapore* 30:239–244, 2001.
17. Johnson KL, Kearney PA, Johnson SB, et al: Closed versus open endotracheal suctioning: costs and physiologic consequences. *Critical Care Medicine* 22:658–666, 1994.
18. Grossi SA: Closed endotracheal suction system for the prevention of hypoxemia. *Rev Esc Enferm USP* 29:25–33, 1995.
19. Kirimli B, King JE, Pfaeffle HH: Evaluation of tracheobronchial suction technique. *Journal of Thoracic and Cardiovascular Surgery* 59:340–344, 1970.
20. Panacek EA, Albertson TE, Rutherford WF, et al: Selective left endobronchial suctioning in the intubated patient. *Chest* 95:885–887, 1989.
21. Wood CJ: Endotracheal suctioning: a literature review. *Intensive Critical Care Nursing* 14:124–136, 1998.
22. Gilbert M: Assessing the need for endotracheal suction. *Paediatric Nursing* 11:14–17, 1999.
23. Carroll P: Safe suctioning PRN. *RN* May:32–37, 1994.
24. Grapp MJ: Endotracheal suctioning: ventilator vs. manual delivery of hyperoxygenation breaths. *American Journal of Critical Care* 5:192–197, 1996.
25. Pritchard M, Flenady W, Woodgate P: Preoxygenation for tracheal suctioning in intubated, ventilated newborn infants. *Cochrane Database System Review* 3:CD000464, 2001.
26. McKelvie S: Endotracheal suctioning. *Nursing in Critical Care* 3:244–248, 1998.
27. Akgul S, Akyolcu N: Effects of normal saline on endotracheal suctioning. *Journal of Clinical Nursing* 11:826–830, 2002.
28. Ross 2003
29. Bach JR: Indications for tracheostomy and decannulation of tracheotomized ventilator users. *Monaldi Archives of Chest Disease* 50:223–227, 1995.

VIII

Chapter 45

Respiratory and Cardiovascular Drug Actions

Stacy J. Laack and Arthur V. Prancan

KEY TERMS

Angiotensin-converting enzyme inhibitors
Adrenergic drugs
Alpha-adrenergic blockers
Anticholinergics
Anticholinesterase drugs
Antileukotrienes
Angiotensin II receptor blockers
Beta-adrenergic blockers
Calcium-channel blockers
Cardiovascular reflex
Cholinergic drugs
Corticosteroids
Diuretics
Mediator inhibitors
Metered dose inhalers
Methylxanthines
Mucolytics/expectorants
Multi-dose powdered inhaler
Obstructive airway disease

CHAPTER OUTLINE

The respiratory and cardiovascular systems have many built-in mechanisms for controlling their functions during health and disease. In healthy individuals, both systems act quickly and positively to maintain proper functioning under the most complicated conditions. Even during trauma or disease, these systems often overcome distress and regain normal function. Disease sometimes alters the physiology of respiration or circulation to the extent that the homeostatic mechanisms are no longer effective. In such a case, a drug with the appropriate action becomes necessary to restore normal physiological function.

Before a drug can be used effectively, the system it is to modify must be understood. How the mechanism of the drug action relates to the biological system must be clear before an effect can be predicted.

This chapter describes much of the basic respiratory and cardiovascular physiology that underlies the action of the drugs presented, with the goal of elucidating the relationship between basic physiology and the drug mechanism of action (Table 45-1). Some of the trade names of the medications mentioned in the text will be changing, but the generic names will remain the same. Not all pharmacological interventions for the respiratory and cardiovascular systems are covered. Certainly, no attempt has been made to describe the pharmacology of other systems or disease states. For further study, any of the texts listed in the reference section at the end of the chapter are highly recommended.

Table 45-1 **Respiratory and Cardiovascular Drugs**

Sympathetic neurotransmission	Adrenergic (sympathomimetic) drugs	Norepinephrine Epinephrine Isoproterenol Phenylephrine and metaraminol Ephedrine Amphetamine Beta$_2$-receptor stimulants
	Alpha-adrenergic blocking drugs	Phentolamine Phenoxybenzamine Prazosin, doxazosin, and terazosin
	Beta-adrenergic blocking drugs	Propranolol Metoprolol and atenolol
	Sympatholytic drugs	Reserpine Guanethidine Methyldopa and clonidine
Parasympathetic neurotransmission	Cholinergic drugs	Acetylcholine Bethanecol Carbachol Pilocarpine
	Anticholinesterase drugs	Physostigmine Neostigmine Edrophonium Donepezil, rivastigmine, and galantamine
	Cholinergic blocking drugs	Atropine Ipratropium and tiotropium Homatropine and cyclopentolate Dicyclomine Trihexyphenidyl HCL and benztropine mesylate Trimethaphan and mecamylamine
Special considerations	Adrenergic (sympathomimetic) drugs	Epinephrine Ephedrine Albuterol, metaproterenol, terbutaline, pirbuterol, formoterol, and salmeterol
	Anticholinergics	Ipratropium and tiotropium
	Methylxanthines	Theophylline and aminophylline
	Corticosteroids	Budesonide, flunisolide, fluticasone, and triamcinolone
	Mediator inhibitors	Cromolyn sodium and nedocromil sodium
	Antileukotrienes	Zileuton, zafirlukast, and montelukast
	Mucolytics and expectorants	Acetylcysteine Guaifenesin

Autonomic Pharmacology

This section introduces the basic aspects of drug action related to both components of the autonomic nervous system: sympathetic and parasympathetic. For both systems, synthesis, storage, and release of the chemical neurotransmitter are described to emphasize the places in the metabolic scheme where drugs can intervene. The sites of action for the adrenergic (sympathetic) and cholinergic (parasympathetic) transmitters and blockers are also described.

The autonomic nervous system controls all of the bodily functions over which the individual has no voluntary control (and which the individual might not control well given the opportunity). These functions include regulation of respiratory airway diameter, respiratory secretions, blood vessel diameter, heart rate, intestinal motility, and pupil size, among many others. It is easy to see that it might take more than the talents of a well-trained expert to keep an active person functioning day and night.

The sympathetic nervous system is the half of the autonomic system that takes a dominant role in the cardiovascular and respiratory systems when bodily activity is necessary. This includes actions such as increasing ventilation capacity, elevating blood pressure, and shunting blood flow to the skeletal muscles. Classically, the sympathetic component of the autonomic nervous system has been called the fight-or-flight system. The other half of the autonomic system is called the parasympathetic nervous system. This system is most important in maintaining the "less exciting" functions of the body, such as digestion, salivation, and urination. In some organs the two systems work in a complementary way to provide very fast and very fine control. For example, the size of the pupil responds quickly to a change in light intensity. The parasympathetic system actively functions to decrease the size of the opening while the sympathetic system relaxes, thereby causing a quick decrease in pupil size. If the light is turned down, the opposite occurs just as quickly. This is a good example of the antagonistic action of the two components of the autonomic nervous system.

Some organs, however, have only one innervation. Much of the arterial blood vessel network is controlled only by sympathetic nerves, whereas gastric secretion and gastric motility are primarily regulated by the parasympathetic system.

Sympathetic Neurotransmission

Sympathetic nerves transport impulses from the vasomotor center in the medulla of the brain through the spinal cord and out to the smooth muscle, heart muscle, and secretory cells. These tissues have receptor sites that will accept the norepinephrine released from the nerve ending. Norepinephrine, also called noradrenalin, is synthesized in the nerve ending only in the sympathetic neurons. It is stored in the terminal until an electric impulse reaches the terminal; then it is released into the synapse.

The norepinephrine molecule attaches to a receptor molecule on a cell surface in the immediate vicinity of its release. This drug-receptor combination causes a biological change, such as stimulation of the pacemaker cells in the heart to fire more frequently (increased heart rate). The effect is terminated when the norepinephrine is reabsorbed into the nerve terminal. About 90% of the released norepinephrine is taken back into the neuron, where it is either restored into granules for future release or destroyed by the enzyme monoamine oxidase (MAO).

There are two types of sympathetic receptors: alpha and beta. The alpha-receptor is found in the arterioles, and the beta-receptor is found in the arterioles, heart, and bronchioles. Stimulation of the alpha-receptor in the arteriole causes vasoconstriction, which results in increased blood pressure. Stimulation of the beta-receptor in the arteriole causes vasodilation and lowered blood pressure. Some drugs stimulate both receptors, and in those cases the effect will be determined by the degree of alpha or beta activity of the drug. One example is norepinephrine. It has 90% alpha activity and 10% beta activity, and it always causes vasoconstriction. Epinephrine is 50% alpha and 50% beta and may cause a rise or drop in blood pressure.

Stimulation of the beta-receptor in the heart results in increased heart rate (HR) (beats per minute) and increased stroke volume (SV) (number of milliliters of blood the left ventricle pumps out into the aorta every time it contracts). Incidentally, the combination of HR and SV changes is another way to express cardiac output (CO) (milliliters of blood pumped per minute):

$$\text{beats/min (HR)} \times \text{mL/beat (SV)} = \text{mL/min (CO)}$$

This expression, cardiac output, is a common one, and it constitutes half of the blood pressure regulation equation: $CO \times TPR = BP$, where CO is cardiac output, TPR is total peripheral resistance, and BP is blood pressure. TPR is determined by vasoconstriction or vasodilation in the arterioles. For example, vasoconstriction increases resistance; therefore TPR and BP go up.

Stimulation of smooth muscle beta-receptors will relax these tissues wherever they are found. Respiratory airway smooth muscle will decrease tension when the beta-receptor is activated by beta-acting drugs like epinephrine or isoproterenol. The functional result will be an increase in air flow because of a larger airway diameter, otherwise referred to as bronchodilation. Likewise, blood vessels respond to beta-acting drugs by dilating as well, allowing a greater rate of flow. In this case, TPR has decreased and blood pressure will drop.

Adrenergic (Sympathomimetic) Drugs

Norepinephrine

As mentioned previously, norepinephrine (Levarterenol, Levophed) is a mixed-activity drug (90% alpha, 10% beta). It stimulates beta-receptors in the heart, which results in an increase of heart rate and stroke volume (increased cardiac output). In the arterioles, norepinephrine causes vasoconstriction via the alpha-receptor, resulting in increased total peripheral resistance. The total effect is an increase in blood pressure. Norepinephrine has little effect on the bronchioles. This drug is given only intravenously, and it is reserved for use in hypotensive emergencies to raise blood pressure, therefore preserving blood supply to the brain and heart. The natural sympathetic compounds are known as catecholamines.

Epinephrine

Epinephrine (Adrenalin) is also a mixed-activity drug (50% alpha, 50% beta). It is naturally produced in the adrenal medulla and can be released during sympathetic nervous system activation. When this occurs, it acts as a circulating hormone, stimulating both alpha- and beta-receptors. This drug will increase heart rate and stroke volume and may slightly increase or decrease total peripheral resistance at the arterioles. In any case, cardiac output always goes up; blood pressure may go up or down slightly.

In the bronchioles, epinephrine exerts a dramatic dilating effect that is mediated by the beta-receptor. Epinephrine can be administered by inhalant aerosol to reverse a bronchoconstrictive episode. It is also administered intramuscularly and subcutaneously to treat asthma and anaphylactic reactions to an allergic response, cardiac arrest, heart block, and as a mild vasoconstrictor to keep local anesthetics at the injection site.

Isoproterenol

Isoproterenol (Isuprel) is a synthetic compound that has 100% beta activity. This means that it can increase heart rate and stroke volume to produce a great rise in cardiac output, and it stimulates the beta-receptor on the arterioles to cause a profound vasodilation. The final result can be a high cardiac output with low blood pressure. This drug improves blood circulation in shock patients by increasing local blood flow (vasodilation) and elevating cardiac output. Isoproterenol has been useful for treating acute asthmatic conditions because of its bronchodilating action; however, it is seldom used currently, because new safer, $beta_2$ selective drugs have been developed.

Phenylephrine and Metaraminol

Both phenylephrine (Isophrin, Neo-Synephrine) and metaraminol are powerful and prolonged stimulators of alpha-receptors. The action is directly on the receptor site itself. The response to the administration of either of these drugs is a rise in blood pressure because of vasoconstriction accompanied by a reflex bradycardia, which causes a decrease in cardiac output. Reflex alterations of cardiovascular function are explained later in this chapter. The primary usefulness of these drugs is in various hypotensive states. Phenylephrine is used as a nasal decongestant, mydriatic, and for the relief of paroxysmal atrial tachycardia. Phenylephrine affords relief from tachycardia because it increases blood pressure and evokes the cardiovascular reflex that is marked by high vagal tone and bradycardia.

Ephedrine

Ephedrine has both alpha and beta activity as direct effects, and it also causes release of epinephrine and norepinephrine. Its pharmacological actions are similar to epinephrine, with the main exception that the duration of action of ephedrine is longer. Ephedrine increases cardiac output and vascular resistance, resulting in increased blood pressure. Ephedrine also causes bronchial muscle relaxation, which is less potent than that of epinephrine but has a longer duration. Although this drug has been useful in controlling milder cases of bronchoconstriction, it is also seldom used since the development of new $beta_2$ selective drugs.

Amphetamine

Amphetamine (Dextroamphetamine, Dexedrine) drug has pharmacological properties related to the catecholamines because it causes release of norepinephrine from the nerve terminal. Amphetamine has both alpha- and beta-receptor activity, although indirectly, through its release of norepinephrine. The usual cardiovascular response is an increase in blood pressure often accompanied by a reflex bradycardia. Amphetamine also has potent central nervous system (CNS) activity. It is a stimulant of the medullary respiratory center, and it can antagonize drug-related central nervous system depression. Respiratory depression often accompanies overdoses of CNS depressant drugs and this effect may be overcome by amphetamine. This drug is usually used for its CNS effects and not for peripheral cardiovascular or respiratory effects.

$Beta_2$-Receptor Stimulants

As mentioned above, there are several drugs that act primarily at the $beta_2$ smooth muscle receptor site, causing selective actions in the bronchioles and arterioles but not in the heart (Box 45-1). These drugs will produce a bronchodilation without increasing cardiac output. This particular lack of cardiovascular effect makes them safer than drugs like isoproterenol or ephedrine in treatment of bronchial asthma. This class of drugs is currently part of the mainstay of treatment for asthma and chronic obstructive pulmonary disease (COPD).

Alpha-Adrenergic Blocking Drugs

The alpha-adrenergic blocking class of drugs should not be used as monotherapy because of their propensity to cause fluid retention. When combined with diuretics, there is no evidence to contraindicate their use. Diuretics are drugs that act on the kidney to increase the formation of urine, therefore decreasing blood volume and fluid accumulation.

Box 45-1 $Beta_2$-Receptor Stimulants

- Albuterol (Proventil, Ventolin)
- Metaproterenol (Alupent, Metaprel)
- Terbutaline (Brethine, Bricanyl)
- Isoetharine (Bronkosol, Bronkometer)
- Pirbuterol (Maxair)
- Bitolterol (Tornalate)
- Formoterol (Foradil)*
- Salmeterol (Serevent)*

*Formoterol and salmeterol are used primarily in combination with inhaled steroids for long-term use.

Phentolamine

Phentolamine (Regitine) is a competitive alpha-receptor blocker. Its action is reversible. This drug prevents the hypertensive effect of norepinephrine and reverses the blood pressure elevating effect of epinephrine (epinephrine reversal). Epinephrine reversal looks like an isoproterenol effect with high cardiac output and low blood pressure. Phentolamine may be used clinically as a vasodilator. It is useful in the emergency treatment of hypertensive patients who have pheochromocytoma, which is a tumor that grows most commonly on the adrenal glands. The tumor produces epinephrine and norepinephrine and may be responsible for one aspect of a clinical hypertension.

Phenoxybenzamine

Phenoxybenzamine (Dibenzyline) is also an alpha-adrenergic blocking agent. It has effects similar to phentolamine in the cardiovascular system, but it is less reversible. This is the drug of choice for preoperative management of pheochromocytoma. This drug is gaining some usefulness in the treatment of shock syndromes characterized by high vascular tone.

Prazosin, Doxazosin, and Terazosin

Prazosin (Minipress), doxazosin (Cardura), and terazosin (Hytrin) are $alpha_1$ selective for arterioles and venules and are the most useful drugs in this class to deal with hypertension. They also have a dilatory effect on urethral smooth muscle and are therefore useful agents in males with enlarged prostates. Although they act by vasodilation, these drugs exert minimal reflex tachycardia because they do not potentiate the vasomotor center and the increased venous capacitance reduces venous return and cardiac output.

Beta-Adrenergic Blocking Drugs

The beta-blocker class of drugs is highly effective for the treatment of hypertension. They are commonly prescribed in conjunction with diuretics. The following drugs are just a few examples of the many beta-blockers available.

Propranolol

Propranolol is a beta-adrenergic blocker. This drug occupies the beta-receptor sites of the heart, the blood vessels, and the bronchioles. It prevents the beta-adrenergic effect usually seen with drugs such as epinephrine, norepinephrine, and isoproterenol. In the arterioles, when epinephrine is given after propranolol, the usual mixed alpha and beta effect is eliminated, leaving only an alpha-adrenergic action. This causes profound vasoconstriction, allowing greater increase in blood pressure than is normally seen with epinephrine alone. In the heart the beta-receptors are blocked, and because there are no alpha-adrenergic receptors in this organ, all effects of catecholamine drugs on the heart are effectively eliminated, allowing the vagal influence on the heart to predominate. Propranolol decreases the heart's requirement for oxygen because it blocks the cardiac stimulant action of norepinephrine. In the respiratory system the administration of propranolol results in bronchoconstriction. This effect is increased dramatically in patients who are susceptible to asthma. The main use for propranolol is in conditions related to hypertension and tachycardia, where a decrease in cardiac output is beneficial.

Metoprolol and Atenolol

Metoprolol (Lopressor) and atenolol (Tenormin) are beta-adrenergic antagonists that have been designed to be cardioselective. This offers an advantage in safety when a beta-blocker must be used in patients with asthma because this disease would be aggravated if respiratory beta-receptors were blocked. The natural beta-adrenergic agonist, epinephrine, is a bronchodilator, and an important class of bronchodilating drugs acts at bronchiolar beta-adrenergic receptors.[1]

Sympatholytic Drugs

The sympatholytic drugs are highly effective as antihypertensive agents; however, their clinical utility is limited by their side-effects profile.

Reserpine

Reserpine is an alkaloid of *Rauwolfia serpentina,* also known as the Indian snake root plant. Many commercial preparations of this compound are available, but it is widely sold as the simple plant extract. This compound depletes norepinephrine from the nerve endings in the various tissues of the body that produce and store norepinephrine, including the brain. The depletion takes several days to accomplish, and it may take several weeks to restore catecholamine levels to normal after therapy is discontinued. During this time, there is a decrease in catecholamine response to sympathetic stimulation. Blood pressure in humans does not drop dramatically with therapeutic doses of reserpine, but when reserpine is used in combination with diuretics or other antihypertensive agents, a significant antihypertensive effect is obtained. Reserpine is used in this way to treat essential hypertension. One serious side effect related to reserpine use is the behavioral modification that can result in severe depression and suicide.

Guanethidine

Guanethidine (Ismelin) is an adrenergic neuron-blocking agent that works by replacing norepinephrine in the nerve terminal. Norepinephrine is usually taken up by the nerve terminal after its discharge and is reused to maintain granule concentrations. Guanethidine takes the place of norepinephrine in the granules and prevents the reuptake of norepinephrine, thereby causing its metabolism outside of the neuron and its eventual depletion. The result on the cardiovascular system of this action is postural hypotension. The patient is unable to control blood pressure by sympathetic activity. This drug is no longer commonly used in the treatment of hypertension.

Methyldopa and Clonidine

Methyldopa (Aldomet) and clonidine (Catapres) decrease the activity of the sympathetic nervous system at its control center in the brain. The consequence is a total decrease in sympathetic activity in the heart and blood vessels, which leads to a reduction in blood pressure. These agents are primarily used as second- and third-line treatments because of adverse side effects such as sedation, dry mouth, postural hypotension, impotence, and rebound hypertension. However, methyldopa remains the drug of choice for nonemergent hypertension in pregnancy. Clonidine comes in a patch form (transdermal administration), which is a longer-acting preparation that decreases the deleterious side effect of rebound hypertension.

Parasympathetic Neurotransmission

The center for parasympathetic control is the vagal nucleus in the medulla. The vagus nerves pass through the spinal cord and out to the heart, the smooth muscle, and exocrine glands (salivary glands and pancreas). In all of these tissues, acetylcholine (ACh) is released from the nerve terminals and combines with receptor sites to cause an effect such as bradycardia (slowing of the heart) or an increase in gastric motility. ACh is found in many parts of the central and peripheral nervous system. ACh is the only transmitter used in the parasympathetic system. It is used to transmit impulses from the nerve that comes out of the spinal cord to the nerve that finally reaches the cells in the organ being affected. This connection is called a ganglion and exists in both sympathetic and parasympathetic systems. ACh is also the neurotransmitter that makes the connection between the voluntary (somatic) nerves and the skeletal muscle.

There are two types of receptors in the central and peripheral nervous systems. ACh affects both, but some drugs affect only one and not the other. These two types of receptors are called nicotinic and muscarinic, named after the drugs that selectively stimulate them. Nicotine stimulates only those receptors in the ganglia and at the neuromuscular junction. The muscarinic receptor site is found everywhere that a parasympathetic nerve terminal synapses at a tissue. The biological effects usually attributed to the parasympathetic nervous system, such as bradycardia, salivation, and bronchoconstriction, are produced when the muscarinic receptors are stimulated. It is also possible to stimulate muscarinic receptors indirectly with a nicotinic drug by activating the parasympathetic ganglia. In a similar way, it is possible to stimulate the entire sympathetic nervous system. The neurotransmitter at the sympathetic ganglia is ACh, and it affects nicotinic receptor sites there. One of the toxic effects of ACh (and similar-acting drugs) is hypertension with tachycardia, which is the result of stimulation of the sympathetic postganglionic fibers.

To better understand the action of ACh and related drugs, let us consider the synthesis, release, and inactivation of this transmitter. ACh is synthesized inside the nerve terminal from acetyl-CoA and choline. The ACh is then stored in granules and released out into the synapse when an action potential reaches the terminal. The ACh molecule attaches to a receptor site, muscarinic or nicotinic, or to the enzyme that breaks it apart. Combination with the receptor site results in biological action, and coupling with the enzyme ends in destruction. The enzyme, acetylcholinesterase, is found at all cholinergic synaptic sites. A nonspecific variety of the enzyme is also prevalent in many other tissues. It too will break down ACh. The final action of either enzyme is the production of acetic acid and choline. The acetic acid is washed away for further metabolism, and the choline is reabsorbed into the nerve terminal for resynthesis to ACh.

Cholinergic Drugs

Acetylcholine

ACh is the endogenous cholinergic transmitter that accounts for nicotinic and muscarinic actions within the autonomic nervous system (Table 45-2). It is rapidly hydrolyzed by acetylcholinesterase and the nonspecific cholinesterase and therefore has a short duration of action if administered parenterally. Therefore, in general, this drug is not very efficacious.

Bethanecol

Bethanecol (Urecholine) is a synthetic choline ester that is not destroyed as easily as ACh by cholinesterase enzymes. It is useful in treating patients with urinary retention and paralytic ileus, and it is administered orally or subcutaneously. The side effects and toxicities for this drug are the same as those for ACh. Because the drug is not given intravenously, however, cardiac and respiratory effects are minimized.

Table 45-2 Effects of Acetylcholine

Nicotinic effects	Stimulation of parasympathetic ganglia, causing occurrence of all muscarinic effects Stimulation of sympathetic ganglia, causing increase in vascular resistance and cardiac output to produce hypertension Stimulation of the neuromuscular junction (NMJ) at the skeletal muscle (muscle contraction and movement)
Muscarinic effects	Bradycardia Salivation Pinpoint pupils Bronchial constriction Gastric and intestinal hypermotility Increased gastric acid and mucous secretion Facilitated urination
Toxic effects*	Diarrhea Urinary incontinence Bradycardia Bronchoconstriction Excessive salivation CNS excitement Respiratory collapse

*With all of these toxic effects, atropine, a competitive muscarinic blocker, is the antidote of choice.

Carbachol

Carbachol (Carcholin) is a mixed nicotinic and muscarinic drug because it releases ACh from the nerve ending, producing the expected cholinergic effects at all receptor sites. The drug has been used for treatment of glaucoma (applied topically), paralytic ileus, and urinary retention (orally and subcutaneously).

Pilocarpine

Pilocarpine (Pilocar) is a cholinomimetic that is useful in ophthalmology as an antiglaucoma agent. Cholinergic compounds decrease intraocular pressure by relieving the obstruction to the canal of Schlemm, a drainage circuit for the eye. Miosis (pinpoint pupils) is one feature of cholinergic therapy and may be beneficial to glaucoma treatment because the muscular base of the relaxed iris may contribute to the drainage block. Another use of pilocarpine (Salagen) is to promote salivary flow in patients with a ganglionic blockade.

Anticholinesterase Drugs

Before proceeding to specific anticholinesterase drugs, it is important to understand the basic mechanism of action for these compounds. Acetylcholinesterase is the enzyme responsible for destroying ACh at the various nerve junctions where it is released. The class of drugs that interfere with this function is called the anticholinesterases. These drugs attach to the enzyme and thereby block the enzymatic hydrolysis of ACh, causing ACh to accumulate outside of the nerve ending. This results in a greater response than normal to any cholinergic nerve stimulation. Some of these anticholinesterases are relatively short-acting compounds and are therapeutically important, whereas others are extremely long-lasting and potent compounds that are important only as poisons. The long-acting compounds have been used as insecticides and as nerve gases in chemical warfare. The therapeutically useful anticholinesterases are beneficial in problems related to the eye, intestine, and the skeletal neuromuscular junction (NMJ). In these applications, these drugs increase the amount of ACh available for activity, an effect that is especially important in cases in which the synthesis or release of ACh is lower than normal, as in myasthenia gravis.

There is great medical interest in the toxicology of the anticholinesterases, especially the extremely potent irreversible anticholinesterases. Toxicity due to these compounds is not uncommon and is often severe. When a toxic irreversible anticholinesterase, such as diisopropylfluorophosphate (DFP) or sarin, is ingested, inhaled, or absorbed across the skin, a great variety of toxic cholinergic effects are seen. The first effects seen after exposure to an anticholinesterase are often ocular and respiratory effects. In the eyes, marked miosis is produced quickly. In the respiratory system, bronchoconstriction and bronchial secretions combine to produce tightness in the chest and wheezing. Gastrointestinal symptoms include nausea, vomiting, cramps, and diarrhea. Other muscarinic effects are severe salivation, involuntary defecation and urination, sweating, lacrimation, bradycardia, and hypotension.

Further effects of anticholinesterases are related to nicotinic functions of ACh. These include skeletal muscle twitching, weakness, and paralysis. CNS effects include depression of the respiratory and cardiovascular control centers, leading to respiratory collapse. At the time of death, respiratory paralysis is evident, caused by a combination of bronchoconstriction, bronchosecretions, respiratory muscle paralysis from overstimulation, and CNS/control center depression. The treatment of this toxicity is closely related to preserving respiratory function. Administration of atropine, a muscarinic blocker, will effectively decrease bronchoconstriction and secretion. Another drug, pralidoxime (Protopam), is used to reactivate the acetylcholinesterase. It is most effective shortly after exposure to the toxic agent because it breaks down the anticholinesterase so it can be removed from the enzyme site. Additional measures are related to physiological support of the patient. Maintenance of an airway, artificial respiration, and oxygen administration are important therapeutic applications for these patients.[2]

Physostigmine

Physostigmine (Eserine) is useful in glaucoma and in selected therapeutic measures where a cholinergic effect is beneficial. It can also be used as an antidote for various anticholinergic agents. It functions as an indirect cholinomimetic by blocking the acetylcholinesterase.

Neostigmine

Neostigmine (Prostigmine) is useful in patients with nonobstructive paralytic ileus to increase tone and motility of the small and large intestines. It is also useful for stimulating skeletal neuromuscular junction (NMJ). Neostigmine is used for treating myasthenia gravis because it indirectly increases ACh at the NMJ and it acts directly at the nicotinic receptor site itself. Myasthenia gravis is marked by subnormal response to ACh, resulting in skeletal muscle weakness. Neostigmine temporarily restores muscle strength.

Edrophonium

Edrophonium (Tensilon) is a very short-acting anticholinesterase. It is primarily useful as a diagnostic agent in myasthenia gravis to reveal, for a few minutes, whether the dose of neostigmine is appropriate. A longer-acting drug would risk a serious cholinergic toxicity if the neostigmine dose was already at the therapeutic limit.

Donepezil, Rivastigmine, and Galantamine

Donepezil (Aricept), rivastigmine (Exelon), and galantamine (Reminyl) increase ACh levels, which are found to be decreased in patients with Alzheimer disease. These drugs are not only efficacious in improving cognition but are found to improve activities of daily living and other neuropsychiatric symptoms. However, none of these have been proven to slow the disease progression. Donepezil (Aricept) is currently most often prescribed due to the advantage of once-a-day dosing.

Cholinergic Blocking Drugs

Cholinergic antagonists block the various receptor sites where ACh is a transmitter. There are specific blocking drugs for each type of ACh receptor. Atropine blocks all cholinergic action right at the muscarinic receptor site on smooth muscle, exocrine glands, and myocardium. The cholinergic antagonist curare works only at the neuromuscular junction to block the nicotinic effect of ACh, resulting in paralysis of skeletal muscle. Still another type of nicotinic blocker is the ganglionic blocker hexamethonium, which blocks both sympathetic and parasympathetic ganglia by occupying the ACh receptor there. These drugs are useful wherever sympathetic or parasympathetic tone needs to be decreased. It is possible to selectively inhibit cholinergic effects in the body to produce a desired effect or to eliminate an undesirable effect. Because of this selectiveness, cholinergic antagonists have widespread use in many areas of medicine.

Atropine

Atropine is an extract from the plant *Atropa belladonna,* also known as the deadly nightshade. Another plant extract, scopolamine, has action similar to atropine. Atropine works by establishing a competitive blockage at the muscarinic receptor site, which is the effector at all tissues innervated by the parasympathetic nervous system. This blockade is selective for the tissue effect of the parasympathetic system and does not counteract the nicotinic ganglionic effects or the nicotinic effects at the NMJ.

Because heart rate is controlled by both sympathetic and parasympathetic tone, atropine will eliminate the parasympathetic effect on the heart, allowing the sympathetic system to increase heart rate and stroke volume to cause an increase in cardiac output. In fact, tachycardia may occur after atropine administration. In cases where bradycardia exists because of high vagal tone, atropine can be used to reverse this depression.

In the respiratory tract, atropine is a bronchodilator. It is also possible to delay respiratory depression associated with anesthetic, tranquilizing, and anticholinesterase drugs by using atropine, either as a pretreatment agent or as an antidote during overdose.

Atropine is used widely as pre-anesthetic medication to prevent bronchiolar secretions and laryngeal spasm, as well as bradycardia. A more general medical use for atropine exists as an emergency tool. It is the antidote of choice for all cholinergic toxicities.[3]

One of the most important clinical uses for atropine is in the gastrointestinal (GI) tract as an antiulcer and antispasmodic agent. This drug acts to decrease motility in the GI tract so that other antiulcer agents can remain in contact with the GI mucosa longer, and it is possible that it also decreases acid secretion. Other problems related to hypermotility of the GI tract are treated with atropine, mainly to decrease gastric muscle activity during treatment of conditions such as cramping and diarrhea.

In ophthalmology, atropine is useful for producing mydriasis, which is pupillary dilation. It is contraindicated in glaucoma patients because it may precipitate an acute attack.

Atropine itself is also capable of producing toxic effects, including mydriasis, tachycardia, dry mouth, constipation, and urinary retention. Effects related to the CNS are also apparent and include initial sedation followed by delirium and hallucinations, leading to a coma. In severe toxicities the patient convulses and experiences severe respiratory depression, which may be the final course. Anticholinesterase drugs, such as physostigmine and neostigmine, are effective antidotes for atropine because they increase the amount of ACh that will compete with atropine for the receptor site.

Ipratropium and Tiotropium

Ipratropium (Atrovent) is a synthetic analog of atropine and is more frequently used than atropine in the treatment of asthma. It has also proved useful in the treatment of COPD. It is administered in aerosolized form. This route provides the advantage of maximal concentration at the bronchial target tissue with limited systemic effects. Tiotropium (Spiriva) is a long-acting anticholinergic, exhibiting bronchodilation in the lungs with indications for COPD. Like ipratropium, it exerts site-specific effects. Tiotropium is a dry powder that is inhaled.

Homatropine and Cyclopentolate

Homatropine (Novatrin) and cyclopentolate (Cyclogyl) are anticholinergic drugs related in action to atropine. They are useful in ophthalmology to produce mydriasis.

Dicyclomine

Dicyclomine (Bentyl) is considered very useful in the gastrointestinal tract to decrease secretions and motility. It is sometimes called a chemical vagotomy.

Trihexyphenidyl HCL and Benztropine Mesylate

Trihexyphenidyl HCL (Artane) and benztropine mesylate (Cogentin) are primarily antiparkinson drugs that enter the CNS to reverse the imbalance between the cholinergic and dopaminergic systems in this disease. They have some of the same side effects as atropine.

Trimethaphan and Mecamylamine

Trimethaphan (Arphonad) and mecamylamine (Inversine) are currently the only ganglionic blockers available in the United States. They block the ACh receptor site in the ganglia in both the sympathetic and parasympathetic nervous systems. Because of their blocking action at the sympathetic ganglion, these drugs will produce a postural hypotension. They will also decrease cholinergic effects at the parasympathetic effector sites because they block the ganglia for the entire parasympathetic nervous system as well. This means that a patient may experience blurred vision, dry mouth, and tachycardia, as well as other atropine-like peripheral effects. They have been surpassed by many other drugs to control hypertension. Their only remaining use is occasionally for the initial control of blood pressure in patients with an aortic dissection who have preexisting contraindications to other drugs. Another clinical use is to induce controlled hypotension during surgery to minimize blood loss.

Cardiovascular Reflex

The cardiovascular reflex involves many of the components of the autonomic nervous system to maintain a normal blood pressure. This mechanism is important for maintaining blood pressure within certain limits during all phases of physical activity. Even the simple act of standing from a seated position requires prompt compensation by this reflex system. If in some way this reflex is interrupted, a condition known as orthostatic hypotension will exist. A common manifestation of this condition is fainting upon standing because of inadequate blood flow to the brain. This section is devoted to the functional aspects of the reflex after a change in blood pressure.

Carotid Baroreceptors

Neuronal elements, known as baroreceptors, exist in the sinus of the carotid arteries supplying the brain. These are stretch receptors that fire electrical impulses at a rate directly related to blood pressure. As the pressure in the artery increases, the vessel wall (and baroreceptor) stretches, causing an increase in the receptor firing rate. Conversely, a decrease in blood pressure results in a decrease in stretch receptor firing rate. This firing rate signal is sent directly to the brain, where the vasomotor center and vagal nucleus respond to it.

Functional Reflex

As an example to demonstrate this reflex, let us assume we have just experienced a loss of blood pressure. The carotid baroreceptors shorten and slow their firing. This message is then delivered to the brain, and the vasomotor center responds by increasing sympathetic nerve activity. This control always responds to information regarding blood pressure in the carotid artery by directly opposing the baroreceptors. If the pressure had risen, the baroreceptors would have increased their firing rate and the vasomotor center would have responded by slowing the sympathetic nerve firing rate. Because blood pressure in this example is low, the vasomotor center increases sympathetic nerve firing, resulting in increased release of norepinephrine from the nerves that reach the heart and arterioles. Norepinephrine increases the heart rate and stroke volume, thereby producing an increase in cardiac output. In the arterioles, norepinephrine stimulates the alpha-receptors, producing vasoconstriction, which results in increased resistance and ultimately raised blood pressure. A third component of the sympathetic nervous system can be involved during sympathetic activation: epinephrine released from the adrenal medulla also increases cardiac output. Meanwhile the vagal nucleus responds to the decreased baroreceptor firing by decreasing its own activity. The vagus nerve to the heart releases less ACh, allowing the sympathetic effect to predominate. The total effect becomes an increase in blood pressure, which is the response required to return the systemic pressure to normal. If the original pressure alteration had been an increase to above normal blood pressure, the opposite reflexive actions would have occurred to return pressure to a normal range. The predominant effect would have been an increase in vagal nerve tone to release high amounts of ACh at the heart, causing a dramatic slowing of heart rate accompanied by a decrease in stroke volume. This combination produces a decrease in cardiac output. The sympathetic system would have responded to the increased baroreceptor firing by decreasing firing in all sympathetic nerves, thereby decreasing norepinephrine and epinephrine release. All of these factors combine to decrease blood pressure to normal.[2]

Other Drug Classes Used in the Treatment of Hypertension

As mentioned in the previous sections, many drugs have the potential to affect blood pressure, cardiac output, heart rate, etc. Many studies have been done to establish appropriate guidelines for patients with hypertension, which is an important risk factor for heart disease and stroke. The Antihypertensive and Lipid Lowering Treatment to Prevent Heart Attack Trial (ALLHAT) found that it takes at least two medications of different classes to treat most cases of mild hypertension, and three to four medications for those with severe hypertension.[4] The latest Joint National Committee JNC report (2003)[5] recommends starting patients on a two-drug regimen in which one of the drugs is a diuretic. There are many types of diuretics, all classified according to which part of the kidney is affected and what type of action is performed. Some examples are hydrochlorothiazide (HCTZ) (HydroDIURIL), furosemide (Lasix), and spironolactone (Aldactone). In addition to the diuretics and beta-blockers discussed previously, there are angiotensin-converting enzyme (ACE) inhibitors, angiotensin II receptor blockers (ARBs), calcium-channel blockers, and many drugs that combine two of these classes. These drugs are commonly used for the treatment of hypertension but are also used in heart failure and other heart diseases. Recently, more focus has been put on hypertension in the context of overall cardiovascular risk and the importance of the long view. Evidence from the Anglo-Scandinavian Cardiac Outcomes Trial (ASCOT)[6] shows that in addition to blood pressure lowering medications, cholesterol-lowering medications (such as the statins) should be considered as part of primary therapy in certain patients.

ACE inhibitors and ARBs affect a cascade of events that ultimately leads to an increase in blood pressure. This is known as the renin-angiotensin system. The endogenous components of this system effect vascular tone and thereby affect blood pressure. Renin is an enzyme produced by the kidneys and released in response to changes in blood pressure. When renin is circulated throughout the blood stream, it comes in contact with angiotensinogen, which is synthesized by the liver and circulates throughout the body. The angiotensinogen is then converted to angiotensin I. With the aid of ACE, angiotensin I is converted to angiotensin II, which has vasoconstricting effects. Bradykinins are inflammatory mediators that are also broken down by ACE. ACE inhibitors block the enzyme and do not allow angiotensin I to be converted or bradykinins to be broken down.[7] Excessive bradykinins can cause many systemic effects, one of them being chronic cough. Some patients need to be taken off their ACE inhibitor for that reason. Two examples of the many ACE inhibitors commonly used are enalapril (Vasotec) and lisinopril (Prinivil). There has been a significant debate over the recommendation for first-line drugs in the treatment of hypertension. Some feel beta-blockers should be used, and others feel ACE inhibitors are a better first line medication, but most agree that both should be used in combination with diuretics. Many ongoing studies continue to address those options. The JNC guidelines primarily are responsible for publishing these recommendations, and healthcare providers should frequently check for updates by going to the National Institute of Health (NIH) website (http://www.nih.gov/) and searching for "JNC Guidelines."

Another class of drugs known as the ARBs has helped eliminate chronic cough as well as many other side effects. ARBs work by blocking the receptor to which angiotensin II binds. Therefore angiotensin II is not able to exert its vasoconstrictive effects on the body, and the result is a decrease in blood pressure. Some examples of ARBs are losartan (Cozaar), candesartan (Atacand), and valsartan (Diovan).

Calcium-channel blockers are another class of drugs used to treat HTN, but these are unrelated to the renin-angiotensin system. There are calcium channels on the cardiac myocytes that, when activated, increase heart rate and contractility as well as vasoconstriction. Therefore when these channels are blocked, the opposite occurs: heart rate, contractility, and vasodilation decrease. In addition to the treatment of hypertension, calcium-channel blockers can be used in heart failure and other heart diseases. Some examples of calcium-channel blockers are diltiazem (Cardizem), nifedipine (Procardia-XL), and verapamil (Calan).

The ACE inhibitors, ARBs, and calcium-channel blockers have many side effects and contraindications that are not discussed here but can be reviewed in any of the texts listed in this chapter's references. Although these drug have different mechanisms of action, they all work toward reducing blood pressure and decreasing the risk for heart damage.

Drugs Used in Obstructive Airway Disease

Patients suffering from asthma or COPD (emphysema or chronic bronchitis) may have an obstructed airway for several reasons. Acute asthmatic obstruction and some chronic airway obstructions are due to bronchial smooth muscle contraction, which results in a smaller diameter airway. Inflamed passageways, which are swollen because of edema, may also constitute an airway obstruction. A further complication seen in many respiratory diseases is the thickening and collection of secretions that cannot be eliminated from the respiratory tree and subsequently block the airway. In this section, the various drugs that can reverse smooth muscle contraction, inflammatory edema, and collection of secretions are presented.

A variety of therapeutic mechanisms are useful against this collection of obstructive conditions. The single most effective mechanism for relief of smooth muscle spasm is the aerosolized beta$_2$ activity that is available in some of the adrenergic agents. Other useful mechanisms aim at potentiating the beta activity of adrenergic agents, decongesting the inflamed airway, and in a broader approach, generally stabilizing cells that can release mediators of the disease, thereby lowering the severity of the disease. The following drugs will be discussed in regard to their actions in obstructive airway disease.

Adrenergic (Sympathomimetic) Drugs

Epinephrine

The muscle-relaxant bronchodilator effect attributed to the beta-adrenergic sympathomimetic compounds is most commonly required for asthmatic or allergic emergencies. During a severe exacerbation of asthma, when a patient is unable to coordinate aerosolized treatments, epinephrine can be given via subcutaneous routes. It is commonly used in systemic anaphylactic reactions as well. As mentioned earlier, epinephrine has 50% beta-adrenergic activity and exerts a great bronchodilating effect. Epinephrine may cause an anxiety reaction in a patient, along with headache, palpitations, and respiratory difficulty. It can also cause serious cardiac reactions (dysrhythmias), which have resulted in death.[3]

Ephedrine

Ephedrine is a sympathomimetic that acts by liberating norepinephrine and epinephrine from storage sites, in addition to possibly directly affecting adrenergic receptors. Its usefulness and side effects are similar to those of epinephrine. Because of the development of more efficacious and $beta_2$-selective agonists, it is used infrequently in the treatment of asthma.

Albuterol, Metaproterenol, Terbutaline, Pirbuterol, Formoterol, and Salmeterol

Albuterol (Proventil, Ventolin), metaproterenol (Alupent, Metaprel), terbutaline (Brethine, Bricanyl), pirbuterol (Maxair), and salmeterol (Serevent) are isoproterenol analogs that are specific $beta_2$-receptor agonists. They therefore exert most of their action on respiratory or vascular smooth muscle but have little effect on the heart. They are useful compounds for selectively relaxing bronchial smooth muscles in asthma and COPD. The major advantage of these drugs is that their action on the heart is minimal or absent, and their potential for inducing cardiac toxicities is correspondingly reduced. Although these beta agonists can be given orally, they are most often given by inhalation, which minimizes their systemic absorption and potential for side effects. Formoterol (Foradil) and salmeterol (Serevent) are long-acting $beta_2$ agonists and are recommended to be used in combination with an inhaled steroid for the treatment of asthma (i.e., budesonide/formoterol [Symbicort] and fluticasone/salmeterol [Advair]).

Anticholinergics

Ipratropium and Tiotropium

Ipratropium (Atrovent), mentioned earlier in this chapter, is a synthetic analog of atropine used for its bronchodilatory effects. It is commonly used in conjunction with a $beta_2$ agonist to provide effective control in chronic stable asthma and in acute exacerbations of asthma. It has also proved useful in the treatment of symptomatic COPD. Response to the medication varies widely from patient to patient; this is attributed to the difference in parasympathetic tone in individuals. Because it is delivered in aerosolized form, ipratropium provides maximal concentration at the bronchial target tissue with limited systemic effects. As mentioned before, tiotropium (Spiriva) is a new anticholinergic on the market also used in patients with COPD. This drug can be taken in once-a-day doses and is indicated only for maintenance treatment. It is dispensed in a powder form from a multi-dose powder inhaler.

Methylxanthines

Methylxanthines have effects similar to the catecholamines in the respiratory and cardiovascular systems. This similarity in effect may be due to the elevation of cyclic adenosine monophosphate (AMP.) Both the catecholamines and methylxanthines are known to produce elevated cyclic AMP levels in the tissues they stimulate. The catecholamines activate adenylate cyclase, the enzyme that converts adenosine triphosphate (ATP) to cyclic AMP. The newly formed cyclic AMP exerts its effects on the local tissue (e.g., bronchial muscle relaxation) and is inactivated by the enzyme phosphodiesterase. The methylxanthines inhibit phosphodiesterase, conserving cyclic AMP and thereby promoting its effects. Additional actions of methylxanthines may be direct smooth muscle relaxation, which could increase airway diameter, and antagonism of adenosine, which is bronchoconstricting.

Theophylline and Aminophylline

Theophylline and aminophylline are structurally very similar to caffeine. Treatment with either of these drugs is recommended only for patients with moderate or severe persistent asthma who are receiving other controller medications, such as inhaled steroids or antileukotrienes, but whose asthma is still not adequately controlled. These drugs are given orally or intravenously and can be used in the inpatient or outpatient setting. In either situation, drug levels in the blood must be monitored because of the toxic effects and the difference in metabolism among patients. Theophylline and aminophylline are not frequently used since advancements have been made in other asthma therapies.

Corticosteroids

The antiinflammatory steroids (prednisone, methylprednisolone, and beclomethasone) are related to the naturally occurring glucocorticoid cortisol. Many compounds have been synthetically derived to produce a variety of antiinflammatory potencies. The usefulness of corticosteroids in treating respiratory diseases depends on the ability of these drugs to depress the symptoms of inflamed tissue. The mechanism of action for the drugs, however, has not clearly been defined. Some specific effects of corticosteroids that relate to the antiinflammatory action are decreased capillary dilation and permeability, as well as stabilization of lysosomal membranes in white blood cells. In addition, these compounds decrease the synthesis of compounds that can promote broncho-obstructive disease—prostaglandins and leukotrienes. The long-term use of the corticosteroids is recommended only after other measures fail. The reason for this caution is that they produce serious side effects and permanent changes if used for 2 weeks or longer. After one week of corticosteroid therapy, behavioral changes and acute peptic ulcers may be observed. When longer therapy is instituted and adrenal suppression occurs, however, the patient requires supplemental corticosteroid therapy until normal adrenal cortex function is restored. This state of insufficiency may last for as long as several months after suppression. Most patients who receive corticosteroids for long-term therapy develop a condition called Cushing's syndrome. It is characterized by wasting of muscles because of protein breakdown and by redistribution of fat from the extremities to the face and trunk. Eventually these patients develop osteoporosis and diabetes. Other serious complications are peptic ulcers, psychosis, glaucoma, intercranial hypertension, and growth retardation. The time to onset of these side effects can be prolonged and their severity minimized by applying dosing strategies that provide antiinflammatory benefit in the lung at low systemic doses. Corticosteroids can be given at low doses in alternate-day administration or by inhalation in a form that is not systemically absorbed.

Budesonide, Flunisolide, Fluticasone, and Triamcinolone

In the treatment of persistent asthma, inhaled steroids are shown to be effective and safer treatments. They do not modify the progression of the disease; however, they improve the day-to-day symptoms. Some examples of these are budesonide (Pulmicort), flunisolide (Aerobid), fluticasone (Flovent), and triamcinolone (Azmacort). Oral steroids such as methylprednisolone or prednisone are reserved for acute exacerbations of asthma. In a life-threatening situation, intravenous methylprednisolone can be given and then switched to oral administration and tapered off over 2 to 3 weeks. If the patient is not on an inhaled steroid at the time, one is initiated. In rare cases when a patient has continued difficulty controlling asthma, the steroids can be taken every other day. This type of treatment is not routinely recommended because of the deleterious side effects of chronic steroid use. In the treatment of severe COPD with multiple exacerbations, evidence shows that inhaled steroids in combination with beta$_2$ agonists reduce the frequency and severity of the exacerbations. As mentioned in the previous section, an example of a steroid/beta$_2$ agonist is fluticasone/salmeterol (Advair). As in the treatment of asthma, oral steroids (methlyprednisolone, prednisone) are reserved for acute exacerbations of COPD, and usually patients are sent home on a short, tapered course.[8]

Mediator Inhibitors

Cromolyn Sodium and Nedocromil Sodium

Cromolyn sodium and nedocromil sodium can prevent asthma attacks that are normally triggered by specific stimulants, such as exercise or allergen exposure. The mechanism of action is presumed to be regulation of mast cell mediator release and eosinophil recruitment, therefore inhibiting responses to allergen challenge and exercise-induced bronchospasm. These drugs are administered by inhalation and are frequently used in the pediatric population and/or when a specific stimulant is identified. The antileukotrienes are becoming more popular for nonsteroid long-term treatment of asthma, slowly replacing this class of drugs.[8]

Antileukotrienes

Zileuton, Zafirlukast, and Montelukast

Leukotrienes are eicosanoids that are prevalent in many body tissues. In the lungs they are potent bronchoconstrictors that can be up to 1000 times more potent than histamine. They also are responsible for increasing mucus production and they enhance eosinophil and basophil influx into the airways. The development of the class of drugs referred to as antileukotrienes works in two ways. They are classified as either leukotriene-synthesis inhibitors (zileuton) or leukotriene-receptor antagonists (zafirlukast and montelukast). These drugs have been shown to improve lung function and reduce asthma symptoms, thereby lessening the need for rescue B_2-agonist therapy. They are used as alternatives to low-dose inhaled steroids in patients with mild persistent asthma. Continued studies are investigating more uses for this class of drugs. For example, montelukast (Singulair) is commonly used for patients with allergies who do not have asthma. These drugs are dispensed in oral form.

Mucolytics and Expectorants

Acetylcysteine

Acetylcysteine (Mucomyst) is a mucolytic that acts by breaking the chemical bonds that hold together the large protein structure that contributes to the viscosity of mucus. Mucolytics are inhaled to liquify mucus so that it can be moved out of the bronchial tract to prevent airway obstruction. Side effects associated with these drugs are bronchospasm, nausea, and vomiting. Acetylcysteine also inactivates the penicillin antibiotics and is contraindicated in their presence. Mucolytics are used in conjunction with other medications in COPD or asthma, but they are most commonly used in patients with upper respiratory illnesses. They are usually administered by inhalation.

Guaifenesin

Guaifenesin (Mucinex) is an expectorant that acts by increasing production of respiratory secretions, therefore encouraging their ejection and making coughs more productive. It can be used in chronic disease but is most commonly used in acute respiratory illnesses. It is dispensed in oral form. The primary side effect is gastrointestinal upset.

Drug Inhalation Devices

Most drugs administered by inhalation in respiratory disease are delivered by pressurized metered-dose inhalers (MDI) (Figure 45-1) or nebulizers. MDIs rely on pressurized chlorofluorocarbon or hydrofluoroalkane propellants to deliver very small drug particles (less than 5-micron diameter) into the airway. Each activation of the metered valve allows an

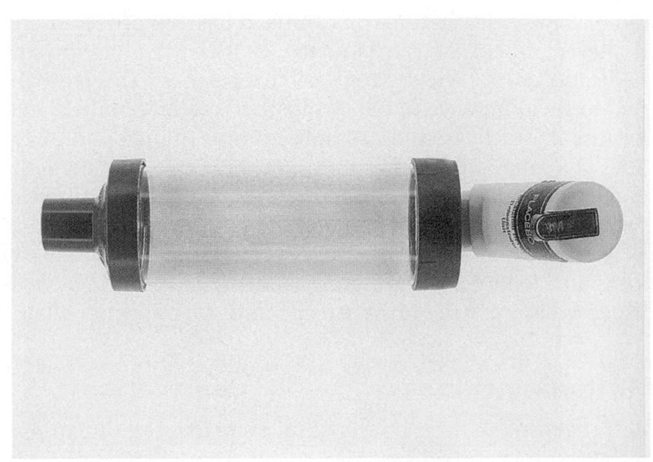

Fig. 45-1 Metered-dose inhaler (MDI) with spacer.

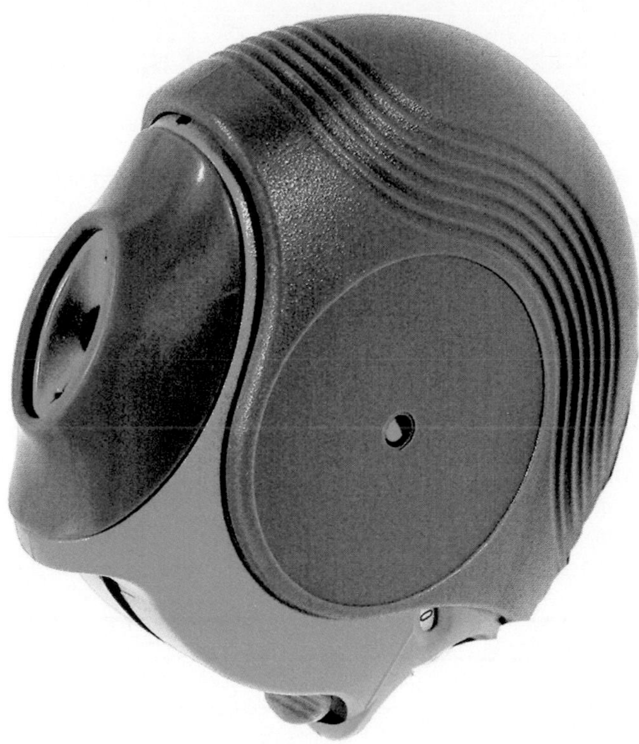

Fig. 45-2 Multi-dose powder inhaler.

accurately determined volume (dose) of propellant and drug mixture to be released at a high velocity. As of 2010, most CFC based MDIs have been removed from the market in attempts to protect the environment.[9] A nebulizer is a machine that delivers the drug after it has been aerosolized with room air. One important advantage of a nebulizer is that the patient does not need hand/breathing coordination, which is further discussed below. The nebulizer, however, is not portable like an MDI and is more expensive than an MDI.

The delivery of drugs to the site of action in the airway by any type of inhalation is inefficient, and therefore, correct technique in MDI use is an important concern. The MDI will allow delivery of 20% of the metered drug to the airway if the patient correctly coordinates the proper rate of inhalation with activation of the device and then adequately holds his or her breath before exhalation. Unfortunately, it is estimated that 50% or fewer patients manage the drug delivery correctly. In response, patient education on correct MDI technique is an important part of therapy, and additional devices, called spacers, have been developed to allow success with variations in technique. The spacers come in various configurations, but they all provide a chamber between the patient and the MDI, which can be charged with the drug-propellant mixture that is then inhaled without concern for critical timing. Patients with poor MDI technique should benefit from the addition of a spacer (see Figure 45-1).

An alternative to the MDI, for patients who have difficulty with the inhalation technique, is the single-dose or multi-dose powder inhaler (Figure 45-2). This device offers a drug compounded into a fine powder that is delivered from a container on simple inhalation by the patient. Coordination of drug delivery is simple and not a problem because only inspiration by the patient drives powder delivery to the airway. The method offers the same or lower efficacy of drug delivery (6% to 20%) when compared with MDI. Also, a relatively high airflow is needed to suspend the powder properly. Therefore young children and the older adults may not benefit from this type of device. Overall, studies have shown that if the patient uses the correct technique, each of the delivery devices provides similar outcomes.[10]

Summary

This chapter describes the basic respiratory and cardiovascular physiology that underlies pharmacological considerations of drug prescription for people with heart and lung conditions. The actions of common drugs are presented. The relationship between physiology and the mechanisms of action of these drugs is highlighted. Medications for hypertension and chronic airway disease are given special consideration. Finally, drug inhalation devices are reviewed because it is important that physical therapists understand these devices and their proper use for effective outcome.

Review Questions

1. Why is it important to have an understanding of the system that a drug is to modify?
2. Describe the function of beta-blockers, diuretics, ACE inhibitors, and ARBs in the treatment of high blood pressure.
3. What is the cardiovascular reflex, and why is it important to physical therapists?
4. What is the pharmacologic rationale for treatment of patients with obstructive airway disease?
5. Why is a patient's compliance with medications a concern of the physical therapist?

References

1. Goldman L, Ausiello D, editors: *Cecil textbook of medicine*, ed 22, Pennsylvania, 2004, Saunders.
2. Hardman J, Gilman AG, Limbird L, Rall TW, editors: *The pharmacological basis of therapeutics*, New York, 2001, McGraw-Hill.
3. Tintinalli JE, editor: *Emergency medicine: a comprehensive study guide*, New York, 2004, McGraw-Hill.
4. Davis BR, Furberg CD, Jackson TW, Jr, et al: ALLHAT: setting the record straight. *Annals of Internal Medicine* 141:39–46, 2004.
5. National Heart, Lung, and Blood Institute: *The seventh report of the Joint National Committee on Prevention, Detection, Evaluation, and Treatment of High Blood Pressure (NIH Publication No. 03-5233)*, Washington, DC, 2003, U.S. Government Printing Office.
6. Sever P, Dahlof B, Poulter N, et al: ASCOT Steering Committee Members. Potential synergy between lipid-lowering and blood-pressure-lowering in the Anglo-Scandinavian Cardiac Outcomes Trial. *Eur Heart J* 27 (24):2982–2988, 2006 Dec.
7. Katzung BG, editor: *Basic and clinical pharmacology*, ed 9, New York, 2004, McGraw-Hill.
8. Fanta CH: Asthma. *New England Journal of Medicine* 360(10):1002–1014, March 2009.
9. McPhee SJ, Papadakis MA, editors: *Lange 2010 current medical diagnosis & treatment*, ed 49, New York, 2010, McGraw-Hill.
10. Dolovich MB, Ahrens RC, Hess DR, et al: American College of Chest Physicians, & American College of Asthma, Allergy, and Immunology. Device selection and outcomes of aerosol therapy: evidence-based guidelines: American college of chest physicians/American college of asthma, allergy, and immunology. *Chest* 127:335–371, 2005.

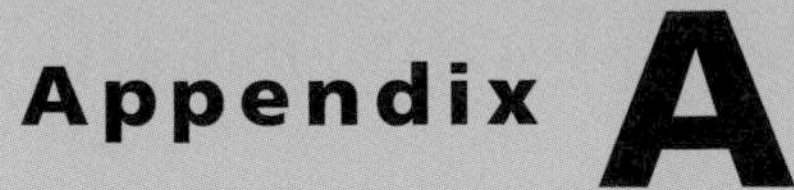

Elements of International Standards for a Cardiac Rehabilitation Program

	Cardiac Rehabilitation Program
Aims	Increase functional capacity Return to safe vocational and recreational activities Restore patients to active and productive lifestyle Improve health-related quality of life Increase ischemic threshold and decrease signs and symptoms such as angina Decrease fear of angina, disease progression, and premature mortality Offset deleterious psychological and physiological effects of bedrest/acute incidence Support mental health and minimize anxiety and depression Risk factor reduction through patient and family education and lifestyle-related health behavior change Prevent progression of atherosclerosis and cardiovascular disease Promote reversal of atherosclerosis and cardiovascular disease Reduce risk of re-infarction and sudden death Develop and help patient implement a safe and effective home exercise/activity program Communication: Provide feedback to referring physician regarding efficacy of medical management
Setting	Inpatient and outpatient Outpatient physical therapy clinic Fitness and wellness facilities School or community gymnasium
Target Population	Medical patients—for example, after myocardial infarction, cardiomyopathy, heart failure Surgical patients—for example, after coronary artery bypass surgery, valve replacement, left ventricular assist device, heart transplant, heart/lung transplant Patients with cardiac dysrhythmias and pacemakers Patients with peripheral vascular disease Primary/secondary prevention for people with risk profiles for vascular disease (cardiovascular and cerebrovascular conditions)
Recruitment of Potential Participants	Physician, cardiac care manager, and physical therapist referrals Community health and wellness fairs Advertising, social media, and marketing programs
Components of Cardiac Rehabilitation/Secondary Prevention Programs (available on-site or through referral to satellite facility)	Patient assessment Physical activity counseling Exercise training Weight management Nutritional counseling Lipid management Hypertension management Smoking cessation Type 2 diabetes mellitus management Psychosocial management

	Cardiac Rehabilitation Program
Initial Intake and Assessment	Patient medical history and chart review Assessment of patient's goals and readiness for lifestyle modification Symptom assessment Cardiac risk assessment and risk stratification Physical examination and system review Diagnostic tests—for example, ECG, scans (pulmonary function and oximetry may be included) Vascular assessment (cardiac, cerebrovascular, and peripheral) Musculoskeletal assessment Nutrition assessment Psychosocial assessment Exercise testing assessment
Program Time Frame for Phase 2 Outpatient Cardiac Rehabilitation	Low-risk patients: 6-18 sessions or 30 days post-event or post-procedure Moderate-risk patients: 12-18 sessions or 60 days post-event or post-procedure High-risk patients: 18-30 sessions or 90 days post-event or post-procedure Frequency of outpatient visits: May vary greatly based on patient access to cardiac rehabilitation program, patient resources, and individual program structure

Personnel	Medical director
	Program director
	Patient care coordinator
	Cardiac rehabilitation specialists
	  Physical therapist or nurse professional with specialization in cardiovascular and pulmonary care
	Health care consultants
	  Dietitian or nutritionist
	  Diabetes counselor
	  Psychologist
	  Social worker or counselor
	  Health educator
	  Occupational therapist
	  Pharmacist
	  Other exercise specialists

Exercise Assessment	Pretest procedures
	  Informed consent
	  Patient orientation and instructions
	  Resting ECG
	  Resting vital signs
	Exercise test modalities and protocols
	  Standard and modified Bruce treadmill protocol
	  Standard and modified Balke-Ware treadmill protocol
	  USAFSAM treadmill protocol
	  Incremental cycle ergometer protocol
	  Treadmill or cycle ergometer ramping protocols
	  Individualized, mode-specific protocols
	  Standardized submaximal exercise testing protocols
	  Clinical submaximal exercise tolerance test
	  Vocational job simulation tests
	Exercise testing measures
	  Heart rate and blood pressure
	  Monitoring of signs or symptoms of cardiovascular compromise
	  Oximetry
	  ECG monitoring
	  Rating of perceived exertion, dyspnea, angina, fatigue, claudication pain
	  Ventilation gas analysis to measure oxygen uptake, anaerobic threshold, and minute ventilation
	Exercise testing with imaging modalities
	  Radionuclear imaging stress test
	  Exercise echocardiography
	Staff qualifications and medical supervision requirements

Training Interventions	Aerobic or endurance conditioning exercise Resistance exercise training Flexibility exercise Relaxation exercise Job simulation training

Continued

	Cardiac Rehabilitation Program
Education	Individualized to each patient's needs based on diagnosis, health status, comorbidities, lifestyle, and vocational/recreational/home environment Delivery methods and considerations Cultural appropriateness Literacy appropriateness Small group classes One-on-one consultation sessions Printed material for self-study Online education sessions One-on-one consultation during exercise training sessions Educational content Normal cardiovascular anatomy and physiology Pathophysiology of vascular conditions (cardiac, cerebrovascular, and peripheral) Interpretation of medical tests and procedures General principles of self-management of chronic heart conditions Cardiovascular medications Reduced periods of sedentary activity Exercise and physical activity Nutrition and weight management Risk factors for vascular conditions (cardiac, cerebrovascular, and peripheral) Stress reduction and relaxation techniques
Self-Management	Home-based cardiac rehabilitation programs Home program with outpatient initial evaluation and follow-up Internet-based home exercise and monitoring Internet-based interactive education Social support network
Outcomes	Patient-centered outcomes Increase in peak oxygen consumption or physical work capacity Reduction in symptoms such as angina or exertional dyspnea Risk factor modification, including smoking cessation, improved blood pressure, blood glucose control, lipid profile, body weight, and body composition Improved functional performance Return to work and recreational activities Increased home- and community-based physical activity Improved health-related quality of life Medication compliance and needs Program performance measures Patient satisfaction Patient adherence Decreased health care utilization Mortality and morbidity statistics
Facility Considerations	Adequate floor space for activities Emergency access and regularly tested emergency call system Adequate temperature and humidity control Clean water source for hydration Patient privacy and confidentiality of patient records Toilet, locker, and shower facilities
Equipment Considerations	High-quality, commercial-grade exercise equipment Aerobic training equipment Treadmill, upright and recumbent cycle ergometer, elliptical trainer Combined arm/leg ergometer, arm cycle ergometer Walking track Resistance training equipment Weight machines, weight pulleys Resistance bands, cuff/hand weights Free weights—dumbbells and barbells Testing and monitoring equipment Calibrated treadmill, cycle ergometer, and other exercise machines if available Electrocardiographic monitoring system Sphygmomanometer Cardiology-grade stethoscope Rating scales for perceived exertion, dyspnea, angina, fatigue, claudication pain Calibrated weight scale Regular scheduled maintenance and calibration

	Cardiac Rehabilitation Program
Emergency Management	Emergency resuscitation equipment and crash cart Appropriate cardiac life support training and certification by all staff members Appropriate medical supervision Emergency policies and procedures Regular emergency procedure in-services and drills
Quality Control	Regular review of detailed policy and procedure manuals Evaluation of staff performance Evaluation of client satisfaction Evaluation of program outcomes Review of medical records and documentation Facility and program review by mandatory regulatory agencies

Bibliography

American Association of Cardiovascular and Pulmonary Rehabilitation: *Guidelines for cardiac rehabilitation and secondary prevention programs*, ed 4, Champaign, Ill., 2004, Human Kinetics.

American Association of Cardiovascular and Pulmonary Rehabilitation: *Cardiac rehabilitation resource manual*, Champaign, Ill., 2006, Human Kinetics.

Balady GJ, Ades PA, Comoss P, et al: Core components of cardiac rehabilitation/secondary prevention: a statement for healthcare professionals from the American Heart Association and the American Association of Cardiovascular and Pulmonary Rehabilitation. *Circulation* 102:1069–1073, 2008.

British Association for Cardiac Rehabilitation: Standards and core components for cardiac rehabilitation, 2007.

Goble AJ, Worcester MUC: *Best practice guidelines for cardiac rehabilitation and secondary prevention*, Victoria, Australia, 1999, Department of Human Services Victoria.

Scottish Intercollegiate Guidelines Network (SIGN): *Cardiac rehabilitation: A national clinical guideline*, SIGN Publication No. 57, Edinburgh, Scotland, 2002, Scottish Intercollegiate Guidelines Network.

Wenger NK, Froelicher ES, Smith LK, et al: Cardiac rehabilitation, Clinical Practice Guideline Number 17, Rockville, Md., U.S. Department of Health and Human Services, Public Health Service, Agency for Health Care Policy and Research and the National Heart, Lung, and Blood Institute. AHCPR Publication No. 96-0672. October 1995.

Appendix B

Elements of International Standards for a Pulmonary Rehabilitation Program

	Pulmonary Rehabilitation Program
Aims	Reduce symptoms (particularly breathlessness) to manageable levels Optimize functional capacity Increase participation in vocational and recreational activities Improve health-related quality of life Reduce health care costs through stabilizing or reversing disease symptoms Support mental health and minimize anxiety and depression Reduce risk factors through patient and family education and behavior change Develop and help patient implement a safe and effective home exercise/activity program Communication: Provide feedback to referring physician regarding efficacy of medical management
Setting	Inpatient and outpatient Outpatient physical therapy clinic Fitness and wellness facilities School or community gymnasium May be combined with cardiac rehabilitation program
Target Population	Patients with chronic lung conditions, including cystic fibrosis, asthma, bronchiectasis, bronchiolitis obliterans, and restrictive lung conditions such as interstitial pulmonary fibrosis Patients with associated activity and participation limitations due to respiratory symptoms Patients with chronic lung conditions after acute exacerbations Surgical patients after thoracic surgery, lung reduction surgery, or lung transplant
Recruitment of Potential Participants	Physician, pulmonary care manager, and physical therapist referrals Advertising, social media, and marketing programs Community health and wellness fairs
Components of Pulmonary Rehabilitation Programs (available on-site or through referral to satellite facility)	Patient assessment Physical activity counseling Smoking cessation Exercise training Psychosocial management Weight management Nutritional counseling Lipid management Hypertension management Diabetes management
Initial Intake and Assessment	Patient medical history and chart review Assessment of patient's goals and readiness for lifestyle modification Symptom assessment Physical examination and system review Diagnostic tests—for example, pulmonary function testing, oximetry, ECG, cardiac testing Vascular assessment (cardiac, cerebrovascular, and peripheral) Musculoskeletal assessment Nutrition assessment Psychosocial assessment Exercise testing assessment

	Pulmonary Rehabilitation Program
Program Time Frame for Outpatient Pulmonary Rehabilitation	6-12 weeks of participation in pulmonary rehabilitation results in significant benefits in program outcomes Longer pulmonary rehabilitation programs produce greater sustained benefits than do shorter programs Frequency of outpatient visits may vary based on patient access to pulmonary rehabilitation program, patient resources, and individual program structure
Personnel	Medical director Program director Patient care coordinator Pulmonary rehabilitation specialists Physical therapist, respiratory therapist, or nurse professional with specialization in pulmonary care Health care consultants Dietitian or nutritionist Psychologist Social worker or counselor Health educator Occupational therapist Pharmacist Other exercise specialists
Exercise Assessment	Objectives Measure exercise capacity to determine baseline for exercise prescription, outcome assessment, and goal setting Detect exercise-induced hypoxemia Screen for exercise-induced bronchoconstriction Screen for signs or symptoms suggestive of cardiac disease Pretest procedures Informed consent Patient orientation and instructions Pulmonary function testing Resting oximetry Resting dyspnea score Resting vital signs Resting ECG Administration of inhaled bronchodilator medicine if prescribed Exercise test modalities and protocols 6-minute walking test Incremental shuttle test Endurance shuttle walk Incremental maximal treadmill protocols, such as the standard or modified Bruce treadmill protocol, Balke-Ware, or USAFSAM treadmill protocol Incremental cycle ergometer protocol Treadmill or cycle ergometer ramping protocols Individualized, mode-specific protocols Standardized submaximal exercise testing protocols Clinical submaximal exercise tolerance test Vocational job simulation tests Exercise testing measures Oximetry Heart rate and blood pressure Monitoring of signs or symptoms of cardiovascular compromise ECG monitoring Rating of dyspnea, perceived exertion, angina, fatigue, etc. Ventilator gas analysis to measure oxygen uptake, anaerobic threshold, and minute ventilation Staff qualifications and medical supervision requirements
Training Interventions	Aerobic or endurance conditioning exercise Resistance exercise training Flexibility exercise Respiratory muscle training Relaxation exercise Job simulation training

Continued

	Pulmonary Rehabilitation Program
Education	Individualized to each patient's needs based on diagnosis, health status, comorbidities, lifestyle, and vocational/recreational/home environment, etc. Delivery methods and considerations Cultural appropriateness Literacy appropriateness Small group classes One-on-one consultation sessions Printed material for self-study Online education sessions One-on-one consultation during exercise training sessions Educational content Normal pulmonary anatomy and physiology Pathophysiology of chronic lung conditions Interpretation of medical tests and procedures Pulmonary medications and respiratory devices General principles of self-management of chronic lung conditions Breathing control strategies Secretion clearance techniques Reduced periods of sedentary activity Exercise and physical activity Nutrition and weight management Risk factors for respiratory conditions and smoking cessation Stress reduction and relaxation techniques
Self-Management	Home-based pulmonary rehabilitation programs Home program with outpatient initial evaluation and follow-up Internet-based home exercise and monitoring Internet-based interactive education Social support network
Outcomes	Patient-centered outcomes Increase in physical work capacity or peak oxygen consumption Symptom reduction Risk factor modification including smoking cessation, improved blood pressure, blood glucose control, lipid profile, body weight, and body composition Improved functional performance Increased home- and community-based physical activity Improved health-related quality of life Medication compliance and needs Program performance measures Patient satisfaction Patient adherence Decreased health care utilization Mortality and morbidity statistics
Facility Considerations	Adequate floor space for activities Low-traffic hallway for walk tests Emergency access and regularly tested emergency call system Adequate temperature and humidity control Clean water source for hydration Patient privacy and confidentiality of patient records Toilet, locker, and shower facilities
Equipment Considerations	High-quality, commercial-grade exercise equipment Aerobic training equipment Treadmill, upright, and recumbent cycle ergometer, elliptical trainer Combined arm/leg ergometer, arm cycle ergometer Walking track Resistance training equipment Weight machines, weight pulleys Resistance bands, cuff/hand weights Free weights—dumbbells and barbells Testing and monitoring equipment Calibrated treadmill, cycle ergometer, and other exercise machines if available Electrocardiographic monitoring system Sphygmomanometer Cardiology-grade stethoscope Rating scales for perceived exertion, dyspnea, angina, fatigue, pain Calibrated weight scale Oxygen with delivery apparatus Regular scheduled maintenance and calibration

	Pulmonary Rehabilitation Program
Emergency Management	Emergency resuscitation equipment and crash cart Appropriate cardiac life support training and certification by all staff members Appropriate medical supervision Emergency policies and procedures Regular emergency procedure in-services and drills
Quality Control	Regular review of detailed policy and procedure manuals Evaluation of staff performance Evaluation of client satisfaction Evaluation of program outcomes Review of medical records and documentation Facility and program review by mandatory regulatory agencies

Bibliography

Abramson MJ et al: COPDX: an update of guidelines for the management of chronic obstructive pulmonary disease with a review of recent evidence. *Med J Australia* 184:342–334, 2006.

American Association of Cardiovascular and Pulmonary Rehabilitation: *Guidelines for pulmonary rehabilitation programs*, ed 4, Champaign, Ill., 2011, Human Kinetics. 2011.

Marciniuk DD et al: Optimizing pulmonary rehabilitation in chronic obstructive pulmonary disease—practical issues: A Canadian Thoracic Society Clinical Practice Guideline. *Can Resp J* 17:159–168, 2010.

Nici L et al: American Thoracic Society/European Respiratory Society Statement on Pulmonary Rehabilitation. *Amer J Respir Crit Care Med* 173:1390–1413, 2006.

Ries AL et al: Pulmonary rehabilitation. Joint ACCP/AAVCPR evidence-based clinical guidelines. *Chest* 131:4S–42S, 2007.

Troosters T et al: Pulmonary rehabilitation in chronic obstructive pulmonary diseases. *Amer J Respir Crit Care Med* 172:19–38, 2005.

Appendix C

Exercise Testing and Prescription Considerations for People with Primary Cardiovascular, Pulmonary, and Endocrine Conditions

Basal activity and exercise status consistent with maximal health condition: *To the greatest extent possible*, to be physically active throughout each day and engage in structured exercise, depending on an individual's basal physical activity demands (for example, a heavy laborer may be sufficiently fit and not in need of a structured exercise program; on the other hand, for a sedentary office clerk, a structured exercise program may be a high priority).

Requirements for deriving maximal health benefits from being physically active throughout each day:

- Decreased periods of sedentary activity (particularly screen-based activities such as television viewing and computer use)
- Increased periods of regular physical activity of low to moderate intensity (ideally integrated into ADL, stairs, foot/cycle transportation, and occupation, as well as recreation and leisure)

Requirements for deriving maximal health benefits from a structured exercise program for an apparently healthy person; parameters may be approximately in individuals with mild signs and symptoms of chronic conditions:

- Stretching:
  - 5-10 min after warm-up/cool-down before and after each exercise (e.g., aerobic and strengthening)
- Aerobic:
  - F(requency): 3-5 days/week
  - I(ntensity): Moderate to high
  - T(ype): Aerobic walking, cycling, jogging, hiking, rowing, dancing
  - T(ime): 20-40 min
- Strengthening:
  - F(requency): 2-3 days/week
  - I(ntensity): Low to moderate weights; 40%-70% capacity; one repetition maximum
  - T(ype): Weights, bands, pulleys, weight-training equipment
  - T(ime): 3 sets of 8-15 repetitions maximum

Note: Regarding the guidelines below, exercise parameters are modified based on individual differences in age, body weight, baseline conditioning level, pathologies and their severities, comorbidities and their severities, and other factors extracted from the assessment, physical examination, and laboratory investigations.

CARDIOVASCULAR CONDITIONS: HYPERTENSION (MEDICALLY CONTROLLED)	
Baseline Considerations	Age and wellness (based on a standardized outcome measure) Health status and potential education outcomes (smoking, nutrition, general profiles of daily physical activity and prolonged sedentary activity, structured exercise, sleep status, and stress) Mental health BP profile and responsivity to body position change, exercise, and rest and recovery Condition severity and adequacy of control Comorbidities and their severities (including bone health and musculoskeletal symptoms/deformity) Multisystem review, including heart, CNS, kidneys, vision, hearing Secondary complications, such as involvement of the brain, heart, kidneys Medical management and response Medications that augment or attenuate exercise responses Psychosocial considerations: Social network and support system Health literacy Self-efficacy Readiness to change lifestyle-related health behavior
Assessment and Outcome Evaluation	Blood work profile, including Hgb, HgbA1c, lipids, homocysteine, and blood glucose Electrolytes and fluid balance ECG Adherence to medication Change in blood pressure profile Reduction or cessation of medication BMI WHR Adherence to a healthy diet (e.g., DASH diet, Mediterranean diet) Status of activity and participation Sleep quality and quantity Stress Patient's health knowledge and literacy with special reference to high BP, medication types, and medication use Resting HR, BP, RPP, RR, RPE, and exercise test responses, including recovery
Exercise Prescription Parameters: Special Considerations	Goal: To achieve optimal basal physical activity and exercise status (to be physically active and participate in a structured exercise program) and to reduce BP Adequate BP control Avoidance of excessive increases (secondary to extreme weight or effort such as in isometric contractions and breath holding) Close monitoring of HR, BP, and RPP Depending on the medications being taken and the patient's responses, objective parameters may be blunted and subjective parameters (such as exertion) may be more valid indicators of exercise intensity Optimal weight control Aerobic: F: 2-5 times/day I: Light to moderate T: Rhythmic whole body exercise; primarily legs with less arm work, particularly heavy resistance or isometric work T: 15-30 min, at minimum Progress as needed commensurate with reduction in resting and exercise BPs; typically, the more severe the hypertension, the shorter and more frequent sessions may be effective; less severe hypertension may respond to a daily bout of moderate continuous aerobic exercise Progress in accordance with musculoskeletal adaptation as well as cardiovascular and respiratory adaptations As resting and exercise BPs drop in response to increased volume of physical activity, intensity can progressively increase and frequency decrease Emphasize self-monitoring of HR and BP during home program, and indications for modifying activity Other activities—brisk leisure activities such as gardening, dancing; stress-reducing activities such as yoga, meditation, and tai chi (possibly gardening for some people)
Potential Pre-exercise or Concurrent Interventions Initiated and/or Supported by the Physical Therapist	Smoking cessation Optimize nutrition Fluid balance Specialized diets (e.g., DASH diet) Salt restriction Weight control Body composition Sleep hygiene Relaxation Stress reduction Biofeedback Education regarding regular use of medication Partner with physician to reduce or eliminate medication as nondrug interventions take effect Partner with other health professionals as needed (e.g., nutritionist)

Continued

CARDIOVASCULAR CONDITIONS: ANGINA (MEDICALLY CONTROLLED)	
Baseline Considerations	Age and wellness (based on a standardized outcome measure) Health status and potential education outcomes (smoking, nutrition, general profiles of daily physical activity and prolonged sedentary activity, sleep status, and stress) Mental health Condition severity, medical management, and response Comorbidities and their severities (including bone health and musculoskeletal symptoms/deformity) Multisystem review to assess atherosclerosis throughout body systems Medications that augment or attenuate exercise responses Psychosocial considerations: Social network and support system Health literacy Self-efficacy Readiness to change lifestyle-related health behavior
Assessment and Outcome Evaluation	Risk factor review to target risk factor modification Blood work profile, including Hgb, HgbA1c, lipids, homocysteine, and blood glucose Adherence to medication Change in angina profile Reduction or cessation of medication BMI WHR Adherence to a healthy diet (e.g., DASH diet, Mediterranean diet) ECG Status of activity and participation Sleep quality and quantity Stress Patient's health knowledge and literacy with special reference to angina and related symptoms, medication types, and medication use Resting HR, BP, RPP, RR, RPE, and exercise test responses, including recovery
Exercise Prescription Parameters: Special Considerations	Goal: To achieve optimal basal physical activity and exercise status (to be physically active and participate in a structured exercise program) and to reduce the signs and symptoms of angina and prevent future episodes Avoidance of excessive increases (secondary to extreme weight or effort such as in isometric contractions and breath holding) Aerobic: F: 5 days/week I: Moderate intensity; depending on disease lability or severity 40%-80% HRR (Karvonen formula if severe) or 60%-80% peak exercise capacity within anginal threshold Progress in accordance with musculoskeletal adaptation as well as cardiovascular and respiratory adaptations Emphasize self-monitoring of signs and symptoms and indications for modifying activity Other activities—brisk symptom-free performance of leisure activities; may include yoga, meditation, and tai chi
Potential Pre-Exercise or Concurrent Interventions Initiated and/or Supported by the Physical Therapist	Smoking cessation Optimize nutrition Lipid control Salt restriction Weight control Sleep hygiene Relaxation Stress reduction Use of anti-angina medication Education regarding avoiding anginal threshold Liaison with physician to reduce or eliminate medication as nondrug interventions take effect Liaison with other health professionals as needed (e.g., nutritionist)

CARDIOVASCULAR CONDITIONS: MYOCARDIAL INFARCTION	
Baseline Considerations	Age and wellness (based on a standardized outcome measure) Health status and potential education outcomes (smoking, nutrition, general profiles of daily physical activity and prolonged sedentary activity, sleep status, and stress) Mental health Condition severity, medical management, and response Comorbidities and their severities (including bone health and musculoskeletal symptoms/deformity) Cardiovascular, cerebrovascular, and metabolic risk factors Pulmonary function Medications that augment or attenuate exercise responses Psychosocial considerations: Social network and support system Health literacy Self-efficacy Readiness to change lifestyle-related health behavior

Assessment and Outcome Evaluation	Risk factor review to target risk factor modification Hgb, HgbA1c, lipids, homocysteine, and blood glucose Fluid and electrolyte balance Presence of peripheral edema Baseline fatigue and breathlessness Adherence to medication Change in angina profile Reduction or cessation of medication BMI WHR Adherence to a healthy diet (e.g., DASH diet, Mediterranean diet) ECG Status of activity and participation Fatigue Sleep quality and quantity Stress Frequency and causes of visits to physician and hospital Patient's health knowledge and literacy with special reference to MI and related symptoms, medication types, and medication use Resting HR, BP, RPP, RR, RPE, and exercise test responses, including recovery; SpO_2 should remain within normal limits
Exercise Prescription Parameters: Special Considerations	Goal: To achieve optimal basal physical activity and exercise status (to be physically active and participate in a structured exercise program) and to help reverse MI signs and symptoms and prevent future episodes Avoidance of excessive increases (secondary to extreme weight or effort such as in isometric contractions and breath holding) Aerobic: F: 5 days/week I: Moderate intensity (70%-85% peak exercise capacity); if severe heart damage, begin at 40% T: Whole body rhythmic continuous exercise T: 20 to 40 min Strengthening: F: 2-3 days/week I: 3 sets, 30% to 60% capacity, 8-15 estimated repetitions maximum T: Weights, dumbbells, pulleys, bands T: Contractions performed deliberately with rest and recovery time between sets Emphasize self-monitoring of signs and symptoms and indications for modifying activity Progress in accordance with musculoskeletal adaptation as well as cardiovascular and respiratory adaptations Other activities—brisk leisure activities (may include yoga, meditation, and tai chi)
Potential Pre-Exercise or Concurrent Interventions Initiated and/or Supported by the Physical Therapist	Smoking cessation Optimize nutrition Lipid control Salt restriction Weight control Sleep hygiene Relaxation Stress reduction Liaison with physician to reduce or eliminate medication as nondrug interventions take effect Liaison with other health professionals as needed (e.g., nutritionist)
CARDIOVASCULAR CONDITIONS: STENTS/BYPASS SURGERY	
Baseline Considerations	Age and wellness (based on a standardized outcome measure) Health status and potential education outcomes (smoking, nutrition, general profiles of daily physical activity and prolonged sedentary activity, sleep status, and stress) Mental health Condition severity, medical management, and response Comorbidities and their severities (including bone health and musculoskeletal symptoms/deformity) Medications that augment or attenuate exercise responses Psychosocial considerations: Social network and support system Health literacy Self-efficacy Readiness to change lifestyle-related health behavior

Continued

Assessment and Outcome Evaluation	Risk factor review to target risk factor modification Blood work profile, including Hgb, HgbA1c, lipids, homocysteine, and blood glucose Fluid and electrolyte balance Baseline fatigue and breathlessness Peripheral edema Adherence to medication Change in blood pressure profile Reduction or cessation of medication Musculoskeletal status, including chest wall symmetry and trunk strength (absence of surgical residua) BMI WHR Adherence to a healthy diet (e.g., DASH diet, Mediterranean diet) ECG Status of activity and participation Sleep quality and quantity Stress Frequency and causes of visits to physician and hospital Patient's health knowledge and literacy with special reference to cardiac signs and symptoms, related medication types, and medication use Resting HR, BP, RPP, RR, RPE, and exercise test responses, including recovery; SpO_2 should remain within normal limits
Exercise Prescription Parameters: Special Considerations	Goal: To achieve optimal basal physical activity and exercise status (to be physically active and participate in a structured exercise program) and to reverse and prevent cardiac signs and symptoms Aerobic: F: 5 days/week I: Moderate intensity (70%-85% peak exercise capacity) if little comorbidity; reduce intensity if severe cardiac muscle damage T: Whole body rhythmic exercise T: 20 to 40 min Strengthening (>6 weeks after surgery): F: 2-3 days/week I: 3 sets, 30% to 60% capacity, 8-15 estimated repetitions maximum T: Weights, dumbbells, pulleys, bands T: Contractions performed deliberately with rest and recovery time between sets Emphasize self-monitoring of signs and symptoms and indications for modifying activity Progress in accordance with musculoskeletal adaptation as well as cardiovascular and respiratory adaptations Other activities—brisk leisure activities (may include yoga, meditation, and tai chi)
Potential Pre-Exercise or Concurrent Interventions Initiated and/or Supported by the Physical Therapist	Smoking cessation Optimize nutrition Lipid control Salt restriction Weight control Sleep hygiene Relaxation Stress reduction Minimize indications for "re-do" surgeries Liaison with physician to reduce or eliminate medication as nondrug interventions take effect Liaison with other health professionals as needed (e.g., nutritionist)
CARDIOVASCULAR CONDITIONS: VALVE REPLACEMENT	
Baseline Considerations	Age and wellness (based on a standardized outcome measure) Health status and potential education outcomes (smoking, nutrition, general profiles of daily physical activity and prolonged sedentary activity, sleep status, and stress) Mental health Condition severity, medical management, and response Comorbidities and their severities (including bone health and musculoskeletal symptoms/deformity) Medications that augment or attenuate exercise responses Psychosocial considerations: Social network and support system Health literacy Self-efficacy Readiness to change lifestyle-related health behavior

Assessment and Outcome Evaluation	Risk factor review to target risk factor modification Blood work profile, including Hgb, HgbA1c, lipids, homocysteine, and blood glucose Fluid and electrolyte balance Adherence to medication Change in blood pressure profile Reduction or cessation of medication Musculoskeletal status, including chest wall symmetry and trunk strength (absence of surgical residua) BMI WHR Adherence to a healthy diet (e.g., DASH diet, Mediterranean diet) ECG Status of activity and participation Sleep quality and quantity Stress Patient's health knowledge and literacy, related medication types, and medication use if indicated Resting HR, BP, RPP, RR, RPE, and exercise test responses, including recovery; Spo_2 should remain within normal limits
Exercise Prescription Parameters: Special Considerations	Goal: To achieve optimal basal physical activity and exercise status (to be physically active and participate in a structured exercise program) and to maximize fitness and health Aerobic: F: 5 days/week I: Moderate intensity (70%-85% peak exercise capacity) T: Whole body rhythmic continuous exercise T: 20 to 40 min Strengthening (>6 weeks after surgery): F: 2-3 days/week I: 3 sets, 30% to 60% capacity, 8-15 estimated repetitions maximum T: Weights, dumbbells, pulleys, bands T: Contractions performed deliberately with rest and recovery time between sets Emphasize self-monitoring of signs and symptoms and indications for modifying activity Progress in accordance with musculoskeletal adaptation as well as cardiovascular and respiratory adaptations Other activities—brisk leisure activities, including yoga, meditation, and tai chi
Potential Pre-Exercise or Concurrent Interventions Initiated and/or Supported by the Physical Therapist	Smoking cessation Optimize nutrition Lipid control Salt restriction Weight control Sleep hygiene Relaxation Stress reduction Liaison with other health professionals as needed (e.g., nutritionist)
CARDIOVASCULAR CONDITIONS: HEART FAILURE	
Baseline Considerations	Age and wellness (based on a standardized outcome measure) Health status and potential education outcomes (smoking, nutrition, general profiles of daily physical activity and prolonged sedentary activity, sleep status, and stress) Quality of life Mental health, anxiety, and depression Condition severity, medical management, and response Comorbidities and their severities (including COPD, type 2 diabetes mellitus, and renal disease, as well as how these are being managed; bone health and musculoskeletal symptoms/deformity) Cardiovascular, cerebrovascular, and metabolic risk factors Pulmonary function Ventilatory support (e.g., supplemental O_2 and nighttime CPAP) Medications that augment or attenuate exercise responses Psychosocial considerations: Social network and support system Health literacy Self-efficacy Readiness to change lifestyle-related health behavior

Continued

Assessment and Outcome Evaluation	Risk factor review to target risk factor modification Blood work profile, including Hgb, HgbA1c, lipids, homocysteine, and blood glucose Adherence to medication Fluid and electrolyte balance Peripheral edema BMI WHR Baseline breathlessness and fatigue Adherence to a healthy diet (e.g., DASH diet, Mediterranean diet) ECG Status of activity and participation Sleep quality and quantity Stress Patient's health knowledge and literacy with special reference to heart failure (worsening/improving signs and symptoms), medication types, and medication use Resting HR, BP, RPP, RR, RPE, SpO_2, and exercise test responses, including recovery
Exercise Prescription Parameters: Special Considerations	Frequent periods of paced activity interspersed between sitting and rest periods guided by symptoms (i.e., within breathing tolerance to avoid exacerbating cardiopulmonary congestion) Stretching: Low-level warm-up/cool-down commensurate with goal activity or exercise Aerobic: F: Several times daily I: 40% to 80% HRR or less (Karvonen formula), guided by responses and avoidance of cardiopulmonary congestion T: Gently paced physical activity and aerobic walking T: From a couple to several minutes of exercise interspersed with rests guided by recovery (increasing length of exercise duration with reduced duration of rests between) Strengthening (Note: The responsivity of muscle exposed to chronic hypoxia secondary to chronic heart failure and associated myopathy has not been well documented; assess and monitor the individual's response): F: Daily (if moderately severe); 2-3 times/week (if less severe or well tolerated) I: Low-level resistance (arms and legs) coordinated with breathing control; commensurate with tolerance and avoidance of strain and cardiopulmonary congestion T: Weights, dumbbells T: 3 sets of 5-10 estimated repetition maximum contractions performed deliberately with rest and recovery time between sets Other activities—restorative rest and activity-to-rest pacing
Potential Pre-Exercise or Concurrent Interventions Initiated and/or Supported by the Physical Therapist	Smoking cessation Optimize nutrition Lipid control Salt restriction Weight control Relaxation Sleep hygiene Stress reduction Liaison with other health professionals as needed (e.g., nutritionist)
CARDIOVASCULAR CONDITIONS: PERIPHERAL VASCULAR DISEASE	
Baseline Considerations	Age and wellness (based on a standardized outcome measure) Health status and potential education outcomes (smoking, nutrition, general profiles of daily physical activity and prolonged sedentary activity, sleep status, and stress) Mental health Condition severity Comorbidities and their severities (including heart disease, cerebrovascular disease, and type 2 diabetes mellitus, as well as how these are being managed; bone health and musculoskeletal symptoms/deformity) Medications that augment or attenuate exercise responses Psychosocial considerations: Social network and support system Health literacy Self-efficacy Readiness to change lifestyle-related health behavior

Assessment and Outcome Evaluation	Risk factor review to target risk factor modification Multisystem review, particularly with respect to systemic atherosclerosis Blood work profile, including Hgb, HgbA1c, lipids, homocysteine, and blood glucose Adherence to medication BMI WHR Adherence to a healthy diet (e.g., DASH diet, Mediterranean diet) ECG Status of activity and participation Sleep quality and quantity Stress Patient's health knowledge and literacy with special reference to atherosclerosis and its multisystemic effects, medication types, and medication use Resting HR, BP, RPP, RR, RPE, and exercise test responses, including recovery; Spo_2 should remain within normal limits Claudication pain: VAS (0-10); ideally returning to 0 within several minutes of exercise cessation
Exercise Prescription Parameters: Special Considerations	Goal: To achieve optimal basal physical activity and exercise status (to be physically active and participate in a structured exercise program) and to reduce claudication discomfort and potential for arterial narrowing elsewhere, including the coronary vessels Aerobic: F: Depending on severity from several times to once daily I: Set below claudication threshold OR at threshold (if no cardiac involvement or symptoms); patient adjusts walking pace to make claudication discomfort manageable (objectify on the VAS scale) while ensuring gait is not changed T: Aerobic walking (preferable) or cycling; rhythmic continuous alternating extremity exercise T: Up to 40 min, beginning with several minutes that are tolerable with rest periods between (guided by claudication recovery time); with vascular collateralization adaptation to exercise, periods and intensity of exercise will increase and rest periods or reduced intensity bouts will decrease) Other activities—activity-rest pacing may be an effective strategy to push into claudication zone
Potential Pre-Exercise or Concurrent Interventions Initiated and/or Supported by the Physical Therapist	Smoking cessation Optimize nutrition Lipid control Salt restriction Weight control Sleep hygiene Relaxation Stress reduction Wound surveillance and care Intermittent claudication management Liaison with physician to reduce or eliminate medication as nondrug interventions take effect Liaison with other health professionals as needed (e.g., nutritionist)
PULMONARY CONDITIONS: ASTHMA	
Baseline Considerations	Age and wellness (based on a standardized outcome measure) Health status and potential education outcomes (smoking, nutrition, general profiles of daily physical activity and prolonged sedentary activity, sleep status, and stress) Mental health Condition severity, medical management, and response Comorbidities and their severities (including bone health and musculoskeletal symptoms/deformity) Medications that augment or attenuate exercise responses Psychosocial considerations: Social network and support system Health literacy Self-efficacy Readiness to change lifestyle-related health behavior
Assessment and Outcome Evaluation	Lifestyle risk factor review as a basis for lifestyle modification Pulmonary function profile (volumes, capacities, and flow rates) within 3 months Vascular screen as indicated based on lifestyle and family history—blood work profile, including Hgb, HgbA1c, lipids, homocysteine, and blood glucose Adherence to medication Change in asthmatic attacks (frequency, severity, recovery, and recovery time) Reduction or cessation of medication BMI WHR Adherence to a healthy diet (e.g., DASH diet, Mediterranean diet) ECG Status of activity and participation Sleep quality and quantity Stress Patient's health knowledge and literacy with special reference to asthma triggers and attenuators (self-management strategies and their effectiveness), breathing distress, and medication types and use Resting HR, BP, RPP, RR, Spo_2, and breathlessness and exercise test responses, including recovery

Continued

Exercise Prescription Parameters: Special Considerations	Goal: To achieve optimal basal physical activity and exercise status (to be physically active and participate in a structured exercise program) and to reduce asthmatic attack frequency and severity and increase recovery Activity/exercise-rest pacing Stretching: Chest wall mobility stretching exercises in three planes of movement Upper extremity and shoulder girdle movements in three planes of movement Stretching coordinated with breathing control strategies as indicated Aerobic: F: Daily I: Below disabling breathlessness threshold (objectify on VAS scale) and/or Spo_2 <90%; coordinate with breathing control and premedicate as needed, allowing sufficient time for meds to reach peak effectiveness; avoidance of disabling wheezing; coordinate with breathing control strategies depending on condition severity T: Rhythmic progressively continuous exercise (e.g., walking, jogging, cycling, rowing) T: Shorter, more frequent periods for more severe asthma; for less severe asthma, use longer, less frequent periods of exercise that may approximate 20 to 40 min; cut back intensity or rest if breathlessness unmanageable and/or Spo_2 <90%; reinitiate exercise after recovery and stabilization of breathlessness and Spo_2 recovery for several minutes Other activities—daily walking; stress the oxygen transport pathway at a consistent level
Potential Pre-Exercise or Concurrent Interventions Initiated and/or Supported by the Physical Therapist	Smoking cessation Optimize nutrition Salt restriction Weight control Sleep hygiene Relaxation Stress reduction Allergy surveillance and education Asthmatic attack management Liaison with physician to reduce or eliminate medication as nondrug interventions take effect Liaison with other health professionals as needed (e.g. nutritionist)
PULMONARY CONDITIONS:	**CHRONIC BRONCHITIS**
Baseline Considerations	Age and wellness (based on a standardized outcome measure) Health status and potential education outcomes (smoking, nutrition, general profiles of daily physical activity and prolonged sedentary activity, sleep status, and stress) Mental health Condition severity, medical management, and response Comorbidities and their severities (including bone health and musculoskeletal symptoms/deformity) Medications that augment or attenuate exercise responses Psychosocial considerations: Social network and support system Health literacy Self-efficacy Readiness to change lifestyle-related health behavior
Assessment and Outcome Evaluation	Lifestyle risk factor review as a basis for lifestyle modification Pulmonary function profile (volumes, capacities, and flow rates) within 3 months Vascular screen as indicated based on lifestyle and family history—blood work profile, including Hgb, HgbA1c, lipids, homocysteine, and blood glucose Immune status Adherence to medication Change in exacerbations (frequency, severity, recovery, and recovery time) Reduction or cessation of medication BMI WHR Adherence to a healthy diet (e.g., DASH diet, Mediterranean diet) ECG Status of activity and participation Sleep quality and quantity Stress Patient's health knowledge and literacy with special reference to infection and bronchitis triggers and attenuators (self-management strategies), breathing distress, medication types, and medication use Resting HR, BP, RPP, RR, Spo_2 (as indicated), breathlessness and exercise test responses, including recovery

Exercise Prescription Parameters: Special Considerations	Goal: To achieve optimal basal physical activity and exercise status (to be physically active and participate in a structured exercise program) and to reduce infections and exacerbations and speed recovery in the event of an exacerbation Activity/exercise-rest pacing Stretching: Chest wall movements as well as extremity muscles and joints in three planes of movement; coordinate with breathing control strategies as indicated Aerobic: F: Daily for less severe disease; more frequent bouts of exercise for more severe symptoms and disease I: Guided by breathlessness tolerance (objective on VAS 0-10); intermittent exercise and rest as needed (e.g., 2-3 min tolerable exercise to 1 min of rest) and coordinated with breathing control strategies as indicated T: Continuous rhythmic walking, cycling, rowing movements T: If frequent bouts, then shorter periods; less frequents bouts, longer periods of exercise; as patient adapts to exercise stimulus, frequent short exercise bouts progress to less frequent longer exercise bouts
Potential Pre-Exercise or Concurrent Interventions Initiated and/or Supported by the Physical Therapist	Smoking cessation Optimize nutrition Salt restriction Weight control Sleep hygiene Relaxation Stress reduction Infection control Breathing control Liaison with physician to reduce or eliminate medication as nondrug interventions take effect Liaison with other health professionals as needed (e.g., nutritionist)
PULMONARY CONDITIONS: EMPHYSEMA	
Baseline Considerations	Age and wellness (based on a standardized outcome measure) Health status and potential education outcomes (smoking, nutrition, general profiles of daily physical activity and prolonged sedentary activity, sleep status, and stress) Mental health Condition severity, medical management, and response Comorbidities and their severities (including bone health and musculoskeletal symptoms/deformity) Medications that augment or attenuate exercise responses Psychosocial considerations: Social network and support system Health literacy Self-efficacy Readiness to change lifestyle-related health behavior
Assessment and Outcome Evaluation	Lifestyle risk factor review as a basis for lifestyle modification Pulmonary function profile (volumes, capacities, and flow rates; potentially, V/Q scan, closing volume, and diffusing capacity) within 3 months Respiratory muscle strength and endurance General muscle strength and endurance Use of home oxygen (mode, delivery, and concentration) Vascular screen—blood work profile, including Hgb, HgbA1c, lipids, homocysteine and blood glucose, and red and white blood cell counts, platelets ECG Involvement of right and left sides of the heart Peripheral swelling Immune status Respiratory muscle strength and endurance General muscle strength and endurance Adherence to medication Change in exacerbations (frequency, severity, recovery, and recovery time) Reduction or cessation of medication BMI WHR Adherence to a healthy diet (e.g., DASH diet, Mediterranean diet) Status of activity and participation Sleep quality and quantity (use of nocturnal noninvasive ventilation, such as CPAP) Stress Patient's health knowledge and literacy with special reference to infection and exacerbation triggers and attenuators (self-management strategies), breathing distress, and medication types and use Resting HR, BP, RPP, RR, Spo_2, breathlessness and exercise test responses, including recovery

Continued

Exercise Prescription Parameters: Special Considerations	Goal: To achieve optimal basal physical activity and exercise status (to be physically active and participate in a structured exercise program) and to reduce episodes of breathlessness, improve recoverability, and reduce exacerbations and visits to physician and hospital Activity/exercise-rest pacing Monitor upper extremity exercises to ensure muscle work does not compete with the work of breathing and compound breathlessness Stretching: Upper extremity, shoulder, and chest wall movements (trunk forward flexion, side flexion, extension, and rotation to either side), as well as extremity muscles and joints in three planes of movement Coordinate with breathing control strategies as indicated based on condition severity Aerobic: F: Daily for less severe disease; for more severe symptoms and disease, use more frequent short bouts of exercise throughout the day I: Guided by breathlessness tolerance (objective on VAS 0-10); intermittent exercise and rest as needed (e.g., 2-3 min tolerable exercise to 1 min of rest to stabilize Spo_2 and breathing demands) and coordinated with breathing control strategies and medication as indicated T: Rhythmic whole body exercise; may need to be supported if symptoms are severe (ergometer handle bar); may need to support shoulder girdle; single leg exercise (e.g., ergometer cycling) may reduce respiratory demand and produce more work T: If frequent bouts, then shorter periods; less frequents bouts, then longer periods of exercise; rest periods between bouts of exercise based on physiologic recovery of Spo_2, RR, HR, BP and RPP, and breathlessness Strengthening (Note: The responsivity of muscle exposed to chronic hypoxia secondary to chronic respiratory dysfunction and associated myopathy has not been well documented; assess and monitor the individual's response): F: Daily if severe symptoms (light intensity) to 2-4 days/week if mild to moderate symptom severity I: Light if severe symptoms; if mild to moderate symptoms, 20%-60% capacity, estimated 1 repetition maximum T: Weights, dumbbells, bands T: 3 sets of 5-12 estimated repetitions maximum Breathing control and oxygen or medications as needed to promote exercise endurance and maintain Spo_2 within acceptable limits Avoidance of excessive increases (secondary to extreme weight or effort such as in isometric contractions and breath holding) Close monitoring of HR, BP, RPP, Spo_2 Optimal nutrition and weight control Emphasize self-monitoring of signs and symptoms and indications for modifying activity
Potential Pre-Exercise or Concurrent Interventions Initiated and/or Supported by the Physical Therapist	Smoking cessation Optimize nutrition Salt restriction Weight control Sleep hygiene Relaxation Stress reduction Infection control Breathing control Liaison with physician to reduce or eliminate medication as nondrug interventions take effect Liaison with other health professionals as needed (e.g., nutritionist)
PULMONARY CONDITIONS: INTERSTITIAL PULMONARY FIBROSIS	
Baseline Considerations	Age and wellness (based on a standardized outcome measure) Health status and potential education outcomes (smoking, nutrition, general profiles of daily physical activity and prolonged sedentary activity, sleep status, and stress) Mental health Condition severity, medical management, and response Comorbidities and their severities (including bone health and musculoskeletal symptoms/deformity) Medications that augment or attenuate exercise responses Psychosocial considerations: Social network and support system Health literacy Self-efficacy Readiness to change lifestyle-related health behavior

Assessment and Outcome Evaluation	Lifestyle risk factor review as a basis for lifestyle modification Pulmonary function profile (volumes, capacities, and flow rates; potentially, V/Q scan, closing volume, and diffusing capacity) within 3 months Vascular screen as indicated based on lifestyle and family history—blood work profile, including Hgb, HgbA1c, lipids, homocysteine, and blood glucose Adherence to medication Change in infection rate Reduction or cessation of medication In severe cases, use of home oxygen (mode, delivery, and concentration) Respiratory muscle strength and endurance General muscle strength and endurance BMI WHR Adherence to a healthy diet (e.g., DASH diet, Mediterranean diet) ECG Status of activity and participation Sleep quality and quantity Stress Patient's health knowledge and literacy with special reference to triggers and attenuators of respiratory distress (self-management strategies and their effectiveness), medication types, and medication use Resting HR, BP, RPP, RR, Spo_2 (as indicated), breathlessness and exercise test responses, including recovery Exercise desaturation profile
Exercise Prescription Parameters: Special Considerations	Goal: To achieve optimal basal physical activity and exercise status (to be physically active and participate in a structured exercise program) and to reduce episodes of breathlessness and associated desaturation, infection rate, and visits to physician and hospital Stretching: Chest wall mobility and upper extremity and should girdle mobility (three planes of movement) Aerobic: F: Daily (light intensity) if severe symptoms; 3-5 days/week if mild or moderate symptoms I: Guided by breathlessness tolerance (visual analog scale 0-10) and in some patients Spo_2 >90% T: Whole body continuous rhythmic aerobic exercise; rest periods as needed for physiologic recovery of breathlessness and Spo_2 to comfortable and acceptable limits T: If severe symptoms, several minutes interspersed with rest periods for recovery; if mild to moderate symptoms, longer periods of continuous exercise Strengthening: F: Daily if severe symptoms (light intensity); 2-4 days/week if mild to moderate symptom severity I: Light if severe symptoms; if mild to moderate symptoms, 20%-60% capacity, estimated 1 repetition maximum T: Weights, dumbbells, bands T: 3 sets of 5-12 estimated repetitions maximum
Potential Pre-Exercise or Concurrent Interventions Initiated and/or Supported by the Physical Therapist	Smoking cessation Optimize nutrition Salt restriction Weight control Sleep hygiene Relaxation Stress reduction Liaison with other health professionals as needed (e.g., nutritionist)
PULMONARY CONDITIONS: LUNG CANCER	
Baseline Considerations	Age and wellness (based on a standardized outcome measure) Health status and potential education outcomes (smoking, nutrition, general profiles of daily physical activity and prolonged sedentary activity, sleep status, and stress) Mental health, anxiety and depression Condition severity (stage), including metastases (sites and severity), medical management (chemotherapy and radiation) and response Comorbidities and their severities (including bone health and musculoskeletal symptoms/deformity) Medications that augment or attenuate exercise responses Psychosocial considerations: Social network and support system Health literacy Self-efficacy Readiness to change lifestyle-related health behavior

Continued

Assessment and Outcome Evaluation	Lifestyle risk factor review as a basis for lifestyle modification Pulmonary status and consistency over the recent past Vascular screen as indicated based on lifestyle and family history—blood work profile, including Hgb, HgbA1c, platelets, red and white blood cell counts, lipids, homocysteine, and blood glucose Immune status Discomfort/pain profile Fatigue profile ECG Adherence to medication Reduction or cessation of medication BMI WHR Adherence to a healthy diet (e.g., DASH diet, Mediterranean diet) Status of activity and participation Sleep quality and quantity Stress Patient's health knowledge and literacy with special reference to cancer, treatment, responses (self-management strategies for countering treatment side effects and their effectiveness), medication types, and medication use Resting HR, BP, RPP, RR, Spo_2 (as indicated), breathlessness, fatigue and discomfort/pain, and exercise test responses, including recovery
Exercise Prescription Parameters: Special Considerations	Goal: To achieve optimal basal physical activity and exercise status (to be physically active and participate in a structured exercise program) and to improve tolerance for activities of daily living, activity and participation, and overall quality of life Guided by enjoyment as well as physical parameters Guided by Hgb, platelet, and white blood cell counts when undergoing treatment Minimize discomfort/pain and undue fatigue and breathlessness Stretching: Whole body stretching program Aerobic (Note: If patient undergoing radiation therapy or chemotherapy, coordinate exercise program with patient's status on any given day): F: Multiple times daily if severe symptoms, within limits of tolerance (light intensity) I: Guided by breathlessness tolerance (visual analog scale 0 to 10); intermittent exercise and rest as needed (e.g., 2 to 3 min tolerable exercise followed by 1 min of rest) T: Gentle aerobic walking, ergometer cycling, or rowing with breathing control T: From several minutes with rests as indicated to 20-30 min of continuous exercise as tolerated Strengthening: F: Daily if severe symptoms (light intensity); 2-4 days/week if mild to moderate symptom severity I: Light if severe symptoms; if mild to moderate symptoms, 20%-60% capacity, estimated 1 repetition maximum T: Weights, dumbbells, bands T: 3 sets of 5-12 estimated repetitions maximum
Potential Pre-Exercise or Concurrent Interventions Initiated and/or Supported by the Physical Therapist	Smoking cessation Optimize nutrition Salt restriction Weight control Sleep hygiene Relaxation Stress reduction Support group Palliative care Liaison with other health professionals as needed (e.g., nutritionist)
ENDOCRINE AND METABOLIC CONDITIONS: TYPE 1 DIABETES MELLITUS (CONTROLLED)	
Baseline Considerations	Age and wellness (based on a standardized outcome measure) Health status and potential education outcomes (smoking, nutrition, general profiles of daily physical activity and prolonged sedentary activity, sleep status, and stress) Mental health Condition severity, medical management, and response Comorbidities and their severities Medications that augment or attenuate exercise responses Psychosocial considerations: Social network and support system Health literacy Self-efficacy Readiness to change lifestyle-related health behavior

Assessment and Outcome Evaluation	Lifestyle risk factor review as a basis for lifestyle modification Multisystem assessment to establish the multisystemic signs and symptoms of the diabetes Vascular screen as indicated based on lifestyle and family history—blood work profile, including Hgb, HgbA1c, lipids, homocysteine, and blood glucose Adequacy of medical control over the years (degree of lability with exercise and stress) Cardiovascular function Peripheral vascular function CNS and autonomic nervous system function Muscle function Vision and hearing Wounds, healing, and healing rate Adherence to healthy diet (e.g., DASH diet, Mediterranean diet) Status of activity and participation Sleep quality and quantity Stress Patient's health knowledge and literacy with special reference to diabetes, treatment, responses (self-management strategies for countering treatment side effects and their effectiveness), medication types, and medication use Resting HR, BP, RPP, RR, Spo_2 (as indicated), RPE, and exercise test responses, including recovery
Exercise Prescription Parameters: Special Considerations	Goal: To achieve optimal basal physical activity and exercise status (to be physically active and participate in a structured exercise program) and to maximize oxygen transport, collateralization to improve blood flow, and tissue perfusion Sugar source available throughout exercise; patient should develop exceptional self-monitoring skills Abrasions of extremities are to be avoided Patient knowledge of how to inspect extremities for abrasions; proper use of socks and footwear; recognition that modifications of exercise are indicated if any abrasions occur and to promote healing Adjust carbohydrate load to metabolic demands May need to check blood glucose levels during an exercise bout (at least initially) May have abnormal ANS responsivity; need to be closely assessed and monitored in regard to exercise responses, at least initially Subjective responses (breathlessness) may be blunted; closely assess and monitor, at least initially Angina awareness may be blunted; if patient has history of angina, closely assess and monitor Aerobic: F: 3-7 days/week I: 50%-80% HRR (Karvonen formula) T: Aerobic walking and/or cycling (steady work rate) T: 20-40 min Strengthening: As tolerated; low-intensity multiple repetitions can improve and regulate glucose metabolic activity of peripheral muscle Other activities—stress the oxygen transport pathway at a consistent level to minimize extreme fluctuations in blood glucose; always have a sugar source at hand
Potential Pre-Exercise or Concurrent Interventions Initiated and/or Supported by the Physical Therapist	Smoking cessation Optimize nutrition Salt restriction Weight control Sleep hygiene Relaxation Stress reduction Wound surveillance and care Liaison with physician to reduce or eliminate medication as nondrug interventions take effect Liaison with other health professionals as needed (e.g., nutritionist)
ENDOCRINE AND METABOLIC CONDITIONS: TYPE 2 DIABETES MELLITUS (CONTROLLED)	
Baseline Considerations	Age and wellness (based on a standardized outcome measure) Health status and potential education outcomes (smoking, nutrition, general profiles of daily physical activity and prolonged sedentary activity, sleep status, and stress) Mental health Condition severity, medical management, and response Comorbidities and their severities (including heart, peripheral vascular, renal, vision and hearing; bone health and musculoskeletal symptoms/deformity) Medications that augment or attenuate exercise responses Psychosocial considerations: Social network and support system Health literacy Self-efficacy Readiness to change lifestyle-related health behavior

Continued

Assessment and Outcome Evaluation	Lifestyle risk factor review as a basis for lifestyle modification (atherosclerosis is accelerated with type 2 diabetes mellitus) Multisystem assessment to establish the multisystemic signs and symptoms of the diabetes Vascular screen as indicated based on lifestyle and family history—blood work profile, including Hgb, HgbA1c, lipids, homocysteine, and blood glucose Cardiovascular function Peripheral vascular function CNS and autonomic nervous system function Muscle function Vision and hearing Hemoglobin HgbA1c Wounds and healing Adherence to healthy diet (e.g., DASH diet, Mediterranean diet) Status of activity and participation Sleep quality and quantity Stress Patient's health knowledge and literacy with special reference to diabetes, treatment and responses (self-management strategies for countering treatment side effects and their effectiveness), medication types, and medication use Resting HR, BP, RPP, RR, Spo_2 (as indicated), RPE and exercise test responses, including recovery
Exercise Prescription Parameters: Special Considerations	Goal: To achieve optimal basal physical activity and exercise status (to be physically active and participate in a structured exercise program) to maximize oxygen transport, collateralization to improve blood flow, and tissue perfusion Sugar source available throughout exercise; patient should develop exceptional self-monitoring skills Avoidance of abrasions to extremities Patient knowledge of how to inspect extremities for abrasions; proper use of socks and footwear; recognition that modifications of exercise are indicated if any abrasions occur and to promote healing Adjust carbohydrate load to metabolic demands May need to check blood glucose levels during an exercise bout (at least initially) May have abnormal ANS responsivity; need to be closely assessed and monitored in regard to exercise responses, at least initially Subjective responses (breathlessness) may be blunted; closely assess and monitor, at least initially Angina awareness may be blunted; if patient has history of angina, closely assess and monitor Aerobic: F: Daily I: 50%-80% HRR (Karvonen formula) T: Aerobic walking and/or cycling (steady work rate) T: 20-60 min Strengthening: As tolerated; low-intensity multiple repetitions can improve and regulate glucose metabolic activity of peripheral muscle Other activities—stress the oxygen transport pathway at a consistent level to minimize extreme fluctuations in blood glucose; always have a sugar source at hand
Potential Pre-Exercise or Concurrent Interventions Initiated and/or Supported by the Physical Therapist	Smoking cessation Optimize nutrition Salt restriction Weight control Sleep hygiene Relaxation Stress reduction Wound surveillance and care Liaison with physician to reduce or eliminate medication as nondrug interventions take effect Liaison with other health professionals as needed (e.g., nutritionist)

BMI, Body mass index; *WHR,* waist-to-hip ratio; *HR,* heart rate; *BP,* blood pressure, *HRR,* heart rate reserve; *RR,* respiratory rate; *Spo_2,* arterial saturation assessed with the pulse oximeter; *DASH diet,* Dietary Approaches to Stop Hypertension diet; *VAS,* visual analog scale.

Bibliography

American Cancer Society: ACS Guidelines on Nutrition and Physical Activity for Cancer Prevention. www.cancer.org/Healthy/EatHealthyGetActive/ACSGuidelinesonNutritionPhysicalActivityforCancerPrevention/index; Retrieved March 2011.

American College of Sports Medicine: *ACSM's Guidelines for Exercise Testing and Prescription*, ed 8, Philadelphia, 2010, Lippincott Williams & Wilkins.

American Diabetes Association: Food and Fitness, www.diabetes.org/food-and-fitness/fitness/; Retrieved March 2011.

American Heart Association: AHA Guidelines, www.heart.org/HEARTORG/GettingHealthy/PhysicalActivity/American-Heart-Association-Guidelines_UCM_307976_Article.jsp; Retrieved March 2011.

Dean E, editor: Physical therapy in the 21st century: A new evidence-informed practice paradigm and implications. *Physiotherapy Theory and Practice* (Special Issue) 25:327–462, 2009.

Donnely JE, Blair S, Jakicic JM, et al: Appropriated physical intervention strategies for weight loss and prevention of weight regain for adults. *Med Sci Sports Exerc* 41:459–471, 2009.

Olin JW, Allie DE, Belkin M, et al: 2010 performance measures for adults with peripheral artery disease: A Report of the American College of Cardiology

Foundation/American Heart Association Task Force on Performance Measures, the American College of Radiology, the Society for Cardiac Angiography and Interventions, the Society for Interventional Radiology, the Society for Vascular Medicine, the Society for Vascular Nursing, and the Society for Vascular Surgery. *J Vasc Nurs* 29:23–60, 2010.

Pescatello LS, Franklin BA, Fagard R, et al: American College of Sports Medicine position stand. Exercise and hypertension. *Med Sci Sports Exerc* 36:533–553, 2004.

U.S. Department of Health and Human Services: Physical Activity Guidelines for Americans, www.health.gov/PAGuidelines/pdf/paguide.pdf; Retrieved March 2011.

Warburton DER, Katzmarzyk PT, Rhodes RE, et al: Evidence-informed physical activity guidelines for Canadians. *Applied Physiology, Nutrition, and Metabolism* 32(S2E):S16–S68, 2007.

Appendix D

Exercise Testing and Prescription Considerations for People with Nonprimary Heart, Lung, and Endocrine Conditions

Basal activity and exercise status consistent with maximal health condition: *To the greatest extent possible*, to be physically active throughout each day and engage in structured exercise, depending on an individual's basal physical activity demands (for example, a heavy laborer may be sufficiently fit and not in need of a structured exercise program; on the other hand, for a sedentary office clerk, a structured exercise program may be a high priority).

Requirements for deriving maximal health benefits from being physically active throughout each day:

- Decreased periods of sedentary activity (particularly screen-based activities such as television viewing and computer use)
- Increased periods of regular physical activity of low to moderate intensity (ideally integrated into ADL, stairs, foot/cycle transportation, and occupation, as well as recreation and leisure)

Requirements for deriving maximal health benefits from a structured exercise program for an apparently healthy person; parameters may be approximately in individuals with mild signs and symptoms of chronic conditions:

- Stretching:
  - 5-10 min after warm-up/cool-down before and after each exercise (e.g., aerobic and strengthening)
- Aerobic:
  - F(requency): 3-5 days/week
  - I(ntensity): Moderate to high
  - T(ype): Aerobic walking, cycling, jogging, hiking, rowing, dancing
  - T(ime): 20-40 min
- Strengthening:
  - F(requency): 2-3 days/week
  - I(ntensity): Low to moderate weights; 40%-70% capacity; one repetition maximum
  - T(ype): Weights, bands, pulleys, weight-training equipment
  - T(ime): 3 sets of 8-15 repetitions maximum

Note: Regarding the guidelines below, exercise parameters are modified based on individual differences in age, body weight, baseline conditioning level, pathologies and their severities, comorbidities and their severities, and other factors extracted from the assessment, physical examination, and laboratory investigations.

NEUROMUSCULAR CONDITIONS: STROKE	
Baseline Considerations	Age and wellness (based on a standardized outcome measure) Health status and potential education outcomes (smoking, nutrition, general profiles of daily physical activity and prolonged sedentary activity, structured exercise, sleep status, and stress) Mental health (well-being, life satisfaction, anxiety, depression) BP profile and responsivity to body position change, exercise, and rest and recovery Condition severity and adequacy of control Comorbidities and their severities (including bone health and musculoskeletal symptoms/deformity) Secondary complications (e.g., involvement of the brain, heart, kidneys) Medical management and response Medications that augment or attenuate exercise responses Psychosocial considerations: Social network and support system Health literacy Self-efficacy Readiness to change lifestyle-related health behavior
Assessment and Outcome Evaluation	Lifestyle risk factor review to target risk factor modification Multisystem status: cardiovascular, pulmonary (spirometry in moderate to severe cases), musculoskeletal (muscle symmetry, flaccidity, spasticity, gait, chest wall symmetry, and functional integrity), neurological (including balance; swallowing and choking status), and endocrine (type 2 diabetes mellitus risk factors/manifestations, in particular) Blood work profile, including Hgb, HgbA1c, lipids, homocysteine, and blood glucose Adherence to medication Change in blood pressure profile and general hemodynamic status ↓ Or cessation of medication BMI WHR Adherence to a healthy diet (e.g., DASH diet, Mediterranean diet) Status of activity and participation Sleep quality and quantity Stress Patient's health knowledge and literacy with special reference to risk factors for vascular conditions, triggers for worsening and lessening symptoms, medication types, and medication use Resting HR, BP, RPP, RR, RPE, Spo_2 (as indicated), and exercise test responses, including recovery
Exercise Prescription Parameters: Special Considerations	Goal: To achieve optimal basal physical activity and exercise status (to be physically active and participate in a structured exercise program) for fitness, health promotion, prevention and amelioration of lifestyle-related conditions Adequate control of BP and/or blood coagulability Avoidance of excessive increases (secondary to extreme weight or effort such as in isometric contractions and breath holding) Minimize activities that unduly aggravate spasticity Close monitoring of HR, BP, RPP, RR, ECG, and Spo_2 (as indicated); breathlessness and discomfort/pain in some patients (VAS 0-10) Guide progression of exercise program also based on recovery of objective and subjective exercise parameters Optimal weight control Optimal selection and use of walking aids and devices Stretching: Muscles and joints daily, and pre-exercise as indicated Aerobic: F: 2-5 times daily if moderately severe disability/deformity; daily if mild to moderately severe disability/ deformity I: if light to moderate, 40%-80% HRR (Karvonen formula if severe involvement); 60%-75% age-predicted maximum HR if mild to moderate severe disability/deformity T: continuous rhythmic whole body exercise; primarily legs with less arm work, particularly heavy resistance or isometric (walking, ergometer cycling); use of body harness on a treadmill with supervision may be effective in some patients to help restore some bilateral symmetric muscle activation and balance T: 15-30 min at least Strengthening: F: 2-3 days/week I: low to moderate weight, 40%-70% capacity, estimated one repetition maximum (avoid undue strain, breath holding, and intensity that increases spasticity) T: weights, dumbbells, pulleys, bands T: 3 sets of 8-15 repetitions Other activities: Bilateral activities commensurate with capacity Progress as needed commensurate with reduction in resting HR, BP, and RPP; typically, with more severe disability/deformity, shorter and more frequent sessions may be effective; less severe signs and symptoms may respond to a daily bout of moderate continuous aerobic exercise Progress in accordance with musculoskeletal adaptation as well as cardiovascular and respiratory adaptations Resting and exercise HR and BP may drop in response to increased volume of physical activity, intensity

Continued

Potential Pre-Exercise or Concurrent Interventions Initiated and/or Supported by the Physical Therapist	Smoking cessation Optimize nutrition Specialized diets (e.g., DASH diet, Mediterranean-type diet) Salt restriction Weight control Sleep hygiene Relaxation Stress reduction Education regarding regular use of medication Liaison with other health professionals as needed (e.g., nutritionist)
NEUROMUSCULAR CONDITIONS: PARKINSON SYNDROME	
Baseline Considerations	Age and wellness (based on a standardized outcome measure) Health status and potential education outcomes (smoking, nutrition, general profiles of daily physical activity and prolonged sedentary activity, structured exercise, sleep status, and stress) Mental health and cognitive well-being (life satisfaction, anxiety, depression) Condition severity and adequacy of control Comorbidities and their severities (including bone health and musculoskeletal symptoms/deformity) Secondary complications (e.g., involvement of the brain, heart, kidneys) Medical management and response Medications that augment or attenuate exercise responses Psychosocial considerations: Social network and support system Health literacy Self-efficacy Readiness to change lifestyle-related health behavior
Assessment and Outcome Evaluation	Lifestyle risk factor review to target risk factor modification Multisystem status: CNS (sensorimotor status), cardiovascular, pulmonary, musculoskeletal (muscle symmetry, rigidity, spasticity, gait and coordination, chest wall symmetry and functional integrity), neurological (including balance; swallowing and choking status), and endocrine (type 2 diabetes mellitus risk factors/manifestations, in particular) Blood work profile, including Hgb, HgbA1c, lipids, homocysteine, and blood glucose Adherence to medication ↓ Or cessation of medication (exercise can improve L-dopa effectiveness) BMI WHR Adherence to a healthy diet (e.g., DASH diet, Mediterranean diet) Status of activity and participation Sleep quality and quantity Stress Patient's health knowledge and literacy with special reference to risk factors for lifestyle-related conditions, triggers for worsening and lessening symptoms, medication types, and medication use Resting HR, BP, RPP, RR, RPE, Spo_2 (as indicated), and exercise test responses, including recovery
Exercise Prescription Parameters: Special Considerations	↓ Periods of sedentary activity (particularly screen-based activities such as TV viewing and computer use) ↑ Periods of regular physical activity Premedication to reduce rigidity may be beneficial Stretching: Whole body ROM, particularly spine and shoulder and pelvic girdles (daily) Aerobic: F: daily (shorter, more frequent sessions throughout the day with increased severity and disability) I: low to moderate, within subjective limits of coordination and comfort T: whole body (e.g., walking, aquatic, ergometer) T: 10-30 min; with intermittent rests and recovery as needed Strengthening: Guided by biomechanical considerations such as not exacerbating rigidity Other activities: Of interest to the patient (yoga, tai chi, dancing)
Potential Pre-Exercise or Concurrent Interventions Initiated and/or Supported by the Physical Therapist	Smoking cessation Optimize nutrition Specialized diets (e.g., DASH diet) Salt restriction Weight control Sleep hygiene Relaxation Stress reduction Education regarding regular use of medication Liaison with physician to reduce or eliminate medication as nondrug interventions take effect Liaison with other health professionals as needed (e.g., nutritionist)

NEUROMUSCULAR CONDITIONS: MULTIPLE SCLEROSIS	
Baseline Considerations	Age and wellness (based on a standardized outcome measure) Health status and potential education outcomes (smoking, nutrition, general profiles of daily physical activity and prolonged sedentary activity, structured exercise, sleep status, and stress) Cognitive status and mental health (well-being, life satisfaction, anxiety, depression) BP profile and responsivity to body position change, exercise, and rest and recovery Condition severity and adequacy of control Comorbidities and their severities (including bone health and musculoskeletal symptoms/deformity) Secondary complications—involvement of the brain, heart, kidneys (continence status) Medical management and response Medications that augment or attenuate exercise responses Psychosocial considerations: Social network and support system Health literacy Self-efficacy Readiness to change lifestyle-related health behavior
Assessment and Outcome Evaluation	Lifestyle risk factor review to target risk factor modification Multisystem status: CNS (sensorimotor status), cardiovascular, pulmonary, musculoskeletal (muscle symmetry, spasticity, gait and coordination, chest wall symmetry and functional integrity), neurological (including balance; swallowing and choking status) and ANS status (response to position change), and endocrine (type 2 diabetes mellitus risk factors/manifestations, in particular), renal (continence) Monitor disease progression (peaks and troughs) Blood work profile, including Hgb, HgbA1c, lipids, homocysteine, and blood glucose Adherence to medication Change in blood pressure profile and general hemodynamic status ↓ Or cessation of medication BMI WHR Adherence to a healthy diet (e.g., DASH diet, Mediterranean diet) Status of activity and participation Sleep quality and quantity Stress Patient's health knowledge and literacy with special reference to risk factors for lifestyle-related conditions, triggers for worsening and lessening symptoms, medication types, and medication use Resting HR, BP, RPP, RR, RPE, Spo_2 (as indicated), and exercise test responses, including recovery
Exercise Prescription Parameters: Special Considerations	↓ Periods of sedentary activity (particularly screen-based activities such as TV viewing and computer use) ↑ Periods of regular physical activity Consider morning exercise program to maximize higher energy time of day Stretching: Whole body gentle stretching regime Aerobic: F: daily (shorter, more frequent sessions throughout the day with increased severity and disability) I: low to moderate, within subjective limits of coordination and comfort (VAS 0-10) T: whole body (e.g., walking, aquatic, ergometer) T: 10-30 min; with intermittent rests and recovery as needed Strengthening: Guided by biomechanical considerations such as not exacerbating incoordination Other activities: Of interest to the patient (yoga, tai chi, dancing)
Potential Pre-Exercise or Concurrent Interventions Initiated and/or Supported by the Physical Therapist	Smoking cessation Optimize nutrition Specialized diets (e.g., DASH diet) Salt restriction Weight control Sleep hygiene Relaxation Stress reduction Education regarding regular use of medication Liaison with physician to reduce or eliminate medication as nondrug interventions take effect Liaison with other health professionals as needed (e.g., nutritionist)

Continued

NEUROMUSCULAR CONDITIONS: CEREBRAL PALSY	
Baseline Considerations	Age and wellness (based on a standardized outcome measure) Health status and potential education outcomes (smoking, nutrition, general profiles of daily physical activity and prolonged sedentary activity, structured exercise, sleep status, and stress) Mobility status (wheelchair dependency) Cognitive and mental health (well-being, life satisfaction, anxiety, depression) BP profile and responsivity to body position change, exercise, and rest and recovery Condition severity and adequacy of control Comorbidities and their severities (including bone health and musculoskeletal symptoms/deformity) Secondary complications, (e.g., involvement of the brain, heart, kidneys) Medical management and response Medications that augment or attenuate exercise responses Psychosocial considerations: Social network and support system Health literacy Self-efficacy Readiness to change lifestyle-related health behavior
Assessment and Outcome Evaluation	Lifestyle risk factor review to target risk factor modification Multisystem status: cardiovascular, pulmonary, musculoskeletal (muscle symmetry, flaccidity, spasticity, gait, chest wall symmetry and functional integrity), neurological (including balance; swallowing and choking status), and endocrine (type 2 diabetes mellitus risk factors/manifestations, in particular) Blood work profile, including Hgb, HgbA1c, lipids, homocysteine, and blood glucose Adherence to medication Change in blood pressure profile and general hemodynamic status ↓ Or cessation of medication BMI WHR Adherence to a healthy diet (e.g., DASH diet, Mediterranean diet) Status of activity and participation Sleep quality and quantity Stress Consistent with cognitive capacity, patient's health knowledge and literacy with special reference to risk factors for lifestyle-related conditions, medication types, and medication use (or, knowledge of the primary caregiver) Resting HR, BP, RPP, RR, RPE, Spo_2 (as indicated), and exercise test responses, including recovery
Exercise Prescription Parameters: Special Considerations	↓ Periods of sedentary activity (particularly screen-based activities such as TV viewing and computer use) ↑ Periods of regular physical activity Focus on exercise effects of functional activities Coordinate activity intensity with minimizing spasticity and discoordination as much as possible Stretching: Gentle active, active assisted, or assisted movements (all planes), particularly muscles with excessive tone Aerobic: Commensurate with capacity F: daily (shorter, more frequent sessions throughout the day with increased severity and disability) I: low to moderate, within subjective limits of coordination and comfort T: whole body (e.g., walking, aquatic, ergometer) T: 10-30 min; with intermittent rests and recovery as needed Strengthening: Guided by biomechanical considerations such as not exacerbating spasticity Other activities Of interest to the patient (yoga, tai chi, dancing)
Potential Pre-Exercise or Concurrent Interventions Initiated and/or Supported by the Physical Therapist	Smoking cessation Optimize nutrition Specialized diets (e.g., DASH diet) Salt restriction Weight control Sleep hygiene Relaxation Stress reduction Education regarding regular use of medication Liaison with physician to reduce or eliminate medication as nondrug interventions take effect Liaison with other health professionals as needed (e.g., nutritionist)

NEUROMUSCULAR CONDITIONS: SPINAL CORD INJURY (HIGH)	
Baseline Considerations	Age and wellness (based on a standardized outcome measure) Health status and potential education outcomes (smoking, nutrition, general profiles of daily physical activity and prolonged sedentary activity, structured exercise, sleep status, and stress) Mental health (well-being, life satisfaction, anxiety, depression) BP profile and responsivity to body position change, exercise, and rest and recovery Condition severity and adequacy of control Comorbidities and their severities (including bone health and musculoskeletal symptoms/deformity) Secondary complications—involvement of the brain, heart, kidneys (continence status) Medical management and response Medications that augment or attenuate exercise responses Psychosocial considerations: Social network and support system Health literacy Self-efficacy Readiness to change lifestyle-related health behavior
Assessment and Outcome Evaluation	Lifestyle risk factor review to target risk factor modification Multisystem status: cardiovascular, pulmonary (baseline spirometry and respiratory muscle strength and endurance measures), musculoskeletal (muscle symmetry, flaccidity, spasticity, gait, spinal alignment, chest wall symmetry and functional integrity), neurological (including balance; swallowing and choking status), and endocrine (type 2 diabetes mellitus risk factors/manifestations, in particular) Blood work profile, including Hgb, HgbA1c, lipids, homocysteine, and blood glucose Adherence to medication Change in blood pressure profile and general hemodynamic status ↓ Or cessation of medication BMI WHR Adherence to a healthy diet (e.g., DASH diet, Mediterranean diet) Status of activity and participation Sleep quality and quantity Stress Patient's health knowledge and literacy with special reference to living and aging with a spinal cord injury, risk factors for lifestyle-related conditions, triggers for worsening and lessening symptoms, medication types, and medication use Resting HR, BP, RPP, RR, RPE, Spo_2 (as indicated), and exercise test responses, including recovery
Exercise Prescription Parameters: Special Considerations	↓ Periods of sedentary activity (particularly screen-based activities such as TV viewing and computer use) ↑ Periods of regular physical activity Minimize overuse; incorporate activity-rest regimen Focus on exercise effects of functional activities Assess ANS involvement to determine the validity of exercise responses to exercise; establish a meaningful baseline of responsivity of the patient Stretching: Whole body, particularly of paretic or paralyzed muscles and involved joints Avoid overstretching and traumatizing affected muscles, fragile connective tissue, and joints Aerobic: F: alternate days I: 60%-80% HRR (Karvonen formula) provided adequate ANS responsiveness to maintain HR and BP T: upper extremity (avoiding stress) cycling T: 5-10 min with a few minutes recovery between, progressing to 30-40 min without rest (provided no musculoskeletal strain) Strengthening: As tolerated for upper extremities Use breathing control Minimize overuse muscle and chronic stress on other soft tissues; allow at least a day of rest between exercise days
Potential Pre-Exercise or Concurrent Interventions Initiated and/or Supported by the Physical Therapist	Smoking cessation Optimize nutrition Specialized diets (e.g., DASH diet) Salt restriction Weight control Sleep hygiene Relaxation Stress reduction Education regarding regular use of medication Liaison with physician to reduce or eliminate medication as nondrug interventions take effect Liaison with other health professionals as needed (e.g., nutritionist)

Continued

NEUROMUSCULAR CONDITIONS: SPINAL CORD INJURY (LOW)	
Baseline Considerations	Age and wellness (based on a standardized outcome measure) Health status and potential education outcomes (smoking, nutrition, general profiles of daily physical activity and prolonged sedentary activity, structured exercise, sleep status, and stress) Mental health (well-being, life satisfaction, anxiety, depression) BP profile and responsivity to body position change, exercise, and rest and recovery Condition severity and adequacy of control Comorbidities and their severities (including bone health and musculoskeletal symptoms/deformity) Secondary complications—involvement of the brain, heart, kidneys (continence status) Medical management and response Medications that augment or attenuate exercise responses Psychosocial considerations: Social network and support system Health literacy Self-efficacy Readiness to change lifestyle-related health behavior
Assessment and Outcome Evaluation	Lifestyle risk factor review to target risk factor modification Multisystem status: cardiovascular, pulmonary, musculoskeletal (muscle symmetry, flaccidity, spasticity, gait, chest wall symmetry and functional integrity), neurological (including balance; swallowing and choking status), and endocrine (type 2 diabetes mellitus risk factors/manifestations, in particular) Blood work profile, including Hgb, HgbA1c, lipids, homocysteine, and blood glucose Adherence to medication Change in blood pressure profile and general hemodynamic status ↓ Or cessation of medication BMI WHR Adherence to a healthy diet (e.g., DASH diet, Mediterranean diet) Status of activity and participation Sleep quality and quantity Stress Patient's health knowledge and literacy with special reference to living and aging with a spinal cord injury, risk factors for lifestyle-related conditions, triggers for worsening and lessening symptoms, medication types, and medication use Resting HR, BP, RPP, RR, RPE, Spo_2 (as indicated), and exercise test responses, including recovery
Exercise Prescription Parameters: Special Considerations	↓ Periods of sedentary activity (particularly screen-based activities such as TV viewing and computer use) ↑ Periods of regular physical activity Minimize overuse; incorporate activity-rest regimen Focus on exercise effects of functional activities Assess ANS involvement to determine the validity of exercise responses to exercise; establish a meaningful baseline of responsivity of the patient Stretching: Whole body, particularly of paretic or paralyzed muscles and involved joints Avoid overstretching and traumatizing affected muscles, fragile connective tissue, and joints Aerobic: F: alternate days I: 60%-80% HRR (Karvonen formula) provided adequate ANS responsiveness to maintain HR and BP T: upper extremity (avoiding stress) cycling T: 5-10 min with a few minutes recovery between progressing to 30-40 min without rest (provided no musculoskeletal strain) Strengthening: As tolerated for upper extremities Use breathing control Minimize overuse muscle and chronic stress on other soft tissues; allow at least a day of rest between exercise days
Potential Pre-Exercise or Concurrent Interventions Initiated and/or Supported by the Physical Therapist	Smoking cessation Optimize nutrition Specialized diets (e.g., DASH diet) Salt restriction Weight control Sleep hygiene Relaxation Stress reduction Education regarding regular use of medication Liaison with physician to reduce or eliminate medication as nondrug interventions take effect Liaison with other health professionals as needed (e.g., nutritionist)

NEUROMUSCULAR CONDITIONS: POST POLIOMYELITIS SYNDROME	
Baseline Considerations	Age and wellness (based on a standardized outcome measure) Health status and potential education outcomes (smoking, nutrition, general profiles of daily physical activity and prolonged sedentary activity, structured exercise, sleep status, and stress) Mental health (well-being, life satisfaction, anxiety, depression) BP profile and responsivity to body position change, exercise, and rest and recovery Condition severity and adequacy of control Comorbidities and their severities (including bone health and musculoskeletal symptoms/deformity) Secondary complications—involvement of the brain, heart, kidneys (continence status) Medical management and response Medications that augment or attenuate exercise responses
Assessment and Outcome Evaluation	Lifestyle risk factor review to target risk factor modification Multisystem status: cardiovascular, pulmonary, musculoskeletal (muscle symmetry, flaccidity, spasticity, gait, chest wall symmetry and functional integrity, muscle and joint pain), neurological (including balance; swallowing and choking status), and endocrine (type 2 diabetes mellitus risk factors/ manifestations, in particular) Blood work profile, including Hgb, HgbA1c, lipids, homocysteine, and blood glucose Ventilator support (garments, bed, CPAP, O_2) Adherence to medication Change in blood pressure profile and general hemodynamic status ↓ Or cessation of medication BMI WHR Adherence to a healthy diet (e.g., DASH diet, Mediterranean diet) Status of activity and participation Sleep quality and quantity Stress Patient's health knowledge and literacy with special reference to living and aging with the effects of poliomyelitis, risk factors for lifestyle-related conditions, triggers for worsening and lessening symptoms, medication types, and medication use Resting HR, BP, RPP, RR, RPE, SpO_2 (as indicated), and exercise test responses, including recovery
Exercise Prescription Parameters: Special Considerations	↓ Periods of sedentary activity (particularly screen-based activities such as TV viewing and computer use) ↑ Periods of regular physical activity Plan exercise program for mornings to maximize energy levels (avoid contributing to some patients hitting the "polio wall" in the afternoon) Stretching: Whole body, particularly of paretic or paralyzed muscles and involved joints Avoid overstretching and traumatizing affected muscles, fragile connective tissue, and joints Aerobic: F: daily with recovery I: intensity within limits of discomfort/pain and fatigue that recovers within a few hours of discontinuation of exercise; guided by capacity to recover satisfactorily without undue fatigue, discomfort/pain in a few hours of exercise cessation; activity-rest regimen as indicated with recovery being a defining factor T: walking or ergometer T: intermittent exercise (e.g., 5-10 min with 1-2 min rest between bouts, up to 30-60 min continuous with fewer rests) Strengthening: Differentiate weak muscle from chronically fatigued muscle (from chronic overuse); weak muscle needs conditioning and fatigued muscle needs judicious rest F: daily to 2-3 days/week; target unaffected deconditioned, and polio-affected muscles that can recover (absence of prolonged muscle fatigue) I: low (gauged by capacity for recovery and by discomfort/pain and fatigue) T: weights, dumbbells, bands, pulleys T: 3 sets of 8-12 repetitions (starting at 4-6) Alternate days provided muscle and subjective recovery has occurred
Potential Pre-Exercise or Concurrent Interventions Initiated and/or Supported by the Physical Therapist	Smoking cessation Optimize nutrition Specialized diets (e.g., DASH diet) Salt restriction Weight control Sleep hygiene Relaxation Stress reduction Education regarding regular use of medication Liaison with physician to reduce or eliminate medication as nondrug interventions take effect Liaison with other health professionals as needed (e.g., nutritionist)

Continued

NEUROMUSCULAR CONDITIONS: MUSCULAR DYSTROPHY	
Baseline Considerations	Age and wellness (based on a standardized outcome measure) Health status and potential education outcomes (smoking, nutrition, general profiles of daily physical activity and prolonged sedentary activity, structured exercise, sleep status, and stress) Mental health (well-being, life satisfaction, anxiety, depression) BP profile and responsivity to body position change, exercise, and rest and recovery Condition severity and adequacy of control Comorbidities and their severities (including ventilatory status; bone health and musculoskeletal symptoms/deformity) Secondary complications—involvement of the brain, heart, kidneys (continence status) Medical management and response Medications that augment or attenuate exercise responses Spinal alignment and symmetry Pulmonary function, including respiratory muscle status Ventilatory support (e.g., supplemental O_2 and nighttime CPAP) Medications that augment or attenuate exercise responses
Assessment and Outcome Evaluation	Lifestyle risk factor review to target risk factor modification Multisystem status: cardiovascular, pulmonary (baseline spirometry and respiratory muscle strength and endurance), musculoskeletal (muscle symmetry, strength, flaccidity, gait if ambulatory, chest wall symmetry and functional integrity), neurological (including balance; swallowing and choking status), and endocrine (type 2 diabetes mellitus risk factors/manifestations, in particular) Blood work profile, including Hgb, HgbA1c, lipids, homocysteine, and blood glucose Necessity for ventilatory (daytime and/or CPAP) and O_2 support Adherence to medication Change in blood pressure profile and general hemodynamic status ↓ Or cessation of medication BMI WHR Adherence to a healthy diet (e.g., DASH diet, Mediterranean diet) Status of activity and participation Sleep quality and quantity Stress Patient's health knowledge and literacy with special reference to progression of muscular dystrophy, risk factors for lifestyle-related conditions, triggers for worsening and lessening symptoms, medication types, and medication use Resting HR, BP, RPP, RR, RPE, SpO_2 (as indicated), and exercise test responses, including recovery
Exercise Prescription Parameters: Special Considerations	↑ Periods of regular movement Avoidance of prolonged periods of unaltered movement or body position (including chest wall) Aids and devices Wheelchair (manual or electric) Stretching: 10 minutes after warm-up/cool-down Aerobic: F: 3 to 5 times a week I: moderate intensity (40%-80% of HRR; Karvonen formula) T: aerobic walking if ambulatory; gentle low intensity exercise in sitting and supine/prone if no undue respiratory distress T: 20-40 min Strengthening: F: 2 or 3 times a week I: low to moderate weight, 40%-70% capacity, estimated one repetition maximum T: weights T: 3 sets of 8 to 15 repetitions
Potential Pre-Exercise or Concurrent Interventions Initiated and/or Supported by the Physical Therapist	Smoking cessation Optimize nutrition Specialized diets (e.g., DASH diet or Mediterranean-type diet) Salt restriction Weight control Sleep hygiene Relaxation Stress reduction Liaison with other health professionals as needed (e.g., nutritionist)

MUSCULOSKELETAL CONDITIONS: OSTEOPOROSIS	
Baseline Considerations	Age and wellness (based on a standardized outcome measure) Health status and potential education outcomes (smoking, nutrition, general profiles of daily physical activity and prolonged sedentary activity, structured exercise, sleep status, and stress) Mental health (well-being, life satisfaction, anxiety, depression) BP profile and responsivity to body position change, exercise, and rest and recovery Condition severity and adequacy of control Comorbidities and their severities (including bone health and musculoskeletal symptoms/deformity) Secondary complications—involvement of the brain, heart, kidneys (continence status) Medical management and response Medications that augment or attenuate exercise responses Fracture history Balance and stumbling/falling history
Assessment and Outcome Evaluation	Lifestyle risk factor review to target risk factor modification Multisystem status: CNS (neuropathies), cardiovascular, pulmonary, musculoskeletal, including baseline bone mineral density (examine factors that contribute to patient's osteoporosis diet, lack of exercise, ethnicity, gender; gait, chest wall symmetry and functional integrity, posture and postural curvatures consistent with vertebral compression fractures, balance and coordination), endocrine (type 2 diabetes mellitus risk factors/manifestations, in particular), renal status Movement efficiency Movement economy Blood work profile, including Hgb, HgbA1c, lipids, homocysteine, and blood glucose Adherence to medication Change in blood pressure profile and general hemodynamic status ↓ Or cessation of medication BMI WHR Adherence to a healthy diet (e.g., DASH diet, Mediterranean diet) Status of activity and participation Sleep quality and quantity Stress Patient's health knowledge and literacy with special reference to living with osteoporosis, principles of calcium balance, risk factors for lifestyle-related conditions, triggers for worsening and lessening symptoms, medication types, and medication use Resting HR, BP, RPP, RR, RPE, Spo_2 (as indicated), and exercise test responses, including recovery Medications (past or current use of long-term steroids) Supplement use (Ca and vitamin D)
Exercise Prescription Parameters: Special Considerations	↓ Periods of sedentary activity (particularly screen-based activities such as TV viewing and computer use) ↑ Periods of regular physical activity Note: Ensure safety from loss of balance and falling Hip protectors during exercise if risk factors are high Stretching: 10 min after warm-up/cool-down Aerobic: F: daily I: moderate intensity (70%-85% of peak exercise capacity) T: weight bearing with a lower extremity rotation movement to knees, hips, and ankles; aerobic walking, cycling, jogging, hiking, dancing T: 20-40 min Strengthening: F: 2-3 times/week I: low to moderate weight, 40%-70%, one repetition maximum T: weights T: 3 sets of 8 to 15 repetitions Core strength; include spinal extension exercises Other activities: activities that create rotational stress on lower extremity joints augment osteoblast activity (e.g., dancing)
Potential Pre-Exercise or Concurrent Interventions Initiated and/or Supported by the Physical Therapist	Smoking cessation Optimize nutrition Specialized diets (e.g., DASH diet) Salt restriction Restrict caffeine and alcohol Weight control Sleep hygiene Relaxation Stress reduction Education regarding regular use of medication Liaison with physician to reduce or eliminate medication as nondrug interventions take effect Liaison with other health professionals as needed (e.g., nutritionist)

Continued

COLLAGEN/CONNECTIVE TISSUE CONDITIONS: SYSTEMIC LUPUS ERYTHEMATOSUS	
Baseline Considerations	Age and wellness (based on a standardized outcome measure) Health status and potential education outcomes (smoking, nutrition, general profiles of daily physical activity and prolonged sedentary activity, structured exercise, sleep status, and stress) Mental health (well-being, life satisfaction, anxiety, depression) BP profile and responsivity to body position change, exercise, and rest and recovery Condition severity and adequacy of control Comorbidities and their severities (including bone health and musculoskeletal symptoms/deformity) Secondary complications—involvement of the brain, heart, kidneys (continence status) Medical management and response Medications that augment or attenuate exercise responses
Assessment and Outcome Evaluation	Lifestyle risk factor review to target risk factor modification Multisystem status: CNS (neuropathies), cardiovascular, pulmonary (baseline spirometry), musculoskeletal (arthralgia, muscle symmetry, flaccidity, spasticity, gait, chest wall symmetry and functional integrity), neurological (including balance; swallowing and choking status), and endocrine (type 2 diabetes mellitus risk factors/manifestations, in particular) Blood work profile, including Hgb, HgbA1c, lipids, homocysteine, and blood glucose Cardiac dysfunction and ECG (associated dysrhythmias) Adherence to medication ↓ Or cessation of medication BMI WHR Adherence to a healthy diet (e.g., DASH diet, Mediterranean diet) Status of activity and participation Sleep quality and quantity Stress Patient's health knowledge and literacy with special reference to living and aging with lupus, risk factors for lifestyle-related conditions, triggers for worsening and lessening symptoms, medication types, and medication use Resting HR, BP, RPP, RR, RPE; SpO_2 (as indicated), and subjective pain and fatigue status; and exercise test responses, including recovery Muscle function (complaints of weakness and delayed recovery) Fatigue Discomfort/pain
Exercise Prescription Parameters: Special Considerations	↓ Periods of sedentary activity (particularly screen-based activities such as TV viewing and computer use) ↑ Periods of regular physical activity Stretching: Gentle whole body and joint stretching daily; yoga, tai chi Aerobic: F: alternate days I: moderate activity commensurate with desaturation, RR, and fatigue and discomfort/pain levels T: aerobic (e.g., walking, aquatic, ergometer) T: 10-40 min with rest intervals as needed; goal to reduce number and length of rests Strengthening: F: 2-3 times/week I: Low-to-moderate weight T: weights, dumbbells, pulleys, bands T: 3 sets of 8-15 repetitions Other activities: yoga
Potential Pre-Exercise or Concurrent Interventions Initiated and/or Supported by the Physical Therapist	Smoking cessation Optimize nutrition Specialized diets (e.g., DASH diet) Salt restriction Weight control Sleep hygiene Relaxation Stress reduction Education regarding regular use of medication Liaison with physician to reduce or eliminate medication as nondrug interventions take effect Liaison with other health professionals as needed (e.g., nutritionist)

COLLAGEN/CONNECTIVE TISSUE CONDITIONS: SCLERODERMA	
Baseline Considerations	Age and wellness (based on a standardized outcome measure) Health status and potential education outcomes (smoking, nutrition, general profiles of daily physical activity and prolonged sedentary activity, structured exercise, sleep status, and stress) Mental health (well-being, life satisfaction, anxiety, depression) BP profile and responsivity to body position change, exercise, and rest and recovery Condition severity and adequacy of control Comorbidities and their severities (including bone health and musculoskeletal symptoms/deformity) Secondary complications—involvement of the brain, heart, kidneys (continence status) Medical management and response Medications that augment or attenuate exercise responses

Assessment and Outcome Evaluation	Lifestyle risk factor review to target risk factor modification Multisystem status: cardiovascular, pulmonary (baseline spirometry and desaturation profile; and respiratory muscle strength and endurance as indicated), musculoskeletal (muscle symmetry, flaccidity, spasticity, gait, chest wall symmetry and functional integrity), neurological (including balance; swallowing and choking status), and endocrine (type 2 diabetes mellitus risk factors/ manifestations, in particular) Blood work profile, including Hgb, HgbA1c, lipids, homocysteine, and blood glucose Cardiac dysfunction and ECG (associated dysrhythmias) Adherence to medication ↓ Or cessation of medication BMI WHR Adherence to a healthy diet (e.g., DASH diet, Mediterranean diet) Status of activity and participation Sleep quality and quantity Stress Patient's health knowledge and literacy with special reference to living and aging with scleroderma, risk factors for lifestyle-related conditions, triggers for worsening and lessening symptoms, medication types, and medication use Resting HR, BP, RPP, RR, RPE, Spo_2 (as indicated), and exercise test responses, including recovery Muscle function (complaints of weakness and delayed recovery) Fatigue Discomfort/pain
Exercise Prescription Parameters: Special Considerations	↓ Periods of sedentary activity (particularly screen-based activities such as TV viewing and computer use) ↑ Periods of regular physical activity Stretching: Gentle whole body and joint stretching daily; yoga, tai chi Aerobic: F: alternate days I: moderate activity commensurate with desaturation, RR, and fatigue levels T: aerobic (e.g., walking, aquatic, ergometer) T: 10-40 min with rest intervals as needed; goal to reduce number and length of rests Strengthening: F: 2-3 times/week I: low-to-moderate weight T: weights, dumbbells, pulleys, bands T: 3 sets of 8-15 repetitions maximum
Potential Pre-Exercise or Concurrent Interventions Initiated and/or Supported by the Physical Therapist	Smoking cessation Optimize nutrition Specialized diets (e.g., DASH diet) Salt restriction Weight control Sleep hygiene Relaxation Stress reduction Education regarding regular use of medication Liaison with physician to reduce or eliminate medication as nondrug interventions take effect Liaison with other health professionals as needed (e.g., nutritionist)
COLLAGEN/CONNECTIVE TISSUE CONDITIONS: ANKYLOSING SPONDYLITIS	
Baseline Considerations	Age and wellness (based on a standardized outcome measure) Health status and potential education outcomes (smoking, nutrition, general profiles of daily physical activity and prolonged sedentary activity, structured exercise, sleep status, and stress) Mental health (well-being, life satisfaction, anxiety, depression Condition severity and adequacy of control BP profile and responsivity to body position change, exercise, and rest and recovery Comorbidities and their severities (including bone health and musculoskeletal symptoms/deformity) Secondary complications—involvement of the brain, heart, kidneys (continence status) Medical management and response Medications that augment or attenuate exercise responses

Continued

Assessment and Outcome Evaluation	Lifestyle risk factor review to target risk factor modification Multisystem status: CNS (neuropathies), cardiovascular, pulmonary (baseline spirometry and respiratory muscle strength and endurance), musculoskeletal (muscle symmetry, flaccidity, spasticity, gait, chest wall symmetry and functional integrity), neurological (including balance; swallowing and choking status), and endocrine (type 2 diabetes mellitus risk factors/manifestations, in particular) Blood work profile, including Hgb, HgbA1c, lipids, homocysteine, and blood glucose Fatigue profile Discomfort/pain profile Adherence to medication Change in blood pressure profile and general hemodynamic status ↓ Or cessation of medication BMI WHR Adherence to a healthy diet (e.g., DASH diet, Mediterranean diet) Status of activity and participation Sleep quality and quantity Stress Patient's health knowledge and literacy with special reference to living and aging with ankylosing spondylitis, risk factors for lifestyle-related conditions, triggers for worsening and lessening symptoms, medication types, and medication use Resting HR, BP, RPP, RR, RPE, SpO_2 (as indicated), and exercise test responses, including recovery
Exercise Prescription Parameters: Special Considerations	↓ Periods of sedentary activity (particularly screen-based activities such as TV viewing and computer use) ↑ Periods of regular physical activity Coordinated with exacerbations as indicated Stretching: Gentle whole body and joint ROM daily; be guided by discomfort/pain; gentle mobility exercise Aerobic: F: 3-5 days/week I: moderate activity commensurate with desaturation, RR, and fatigue and discomfort/pain levels T: aerobic (e.g., walking, aquatic in heated pool, ergometer) T: 10-40 min with rest intervals as needed; goal to reduce number and length of rests Strengthening: F: 2-3 times/week I: Low-to-moderate weight T: weights, dumbbells, pulleys T: 3 sets of 8-15 repetitions maximum Other activities: yoga, tai chi
Potential Pre-Exercise or Concurrent Interventions Initiated and/or Supported by the Physical Therapist	Smoking cessation Optimize nutrition Specialized diets (e.g., DASH diet) Salt restriction Weight control Sleep hygiene Relaxation Stress reduction Education regarding regular use of medication Liaison with physician to reduce or eliminate medication as nondrug interventions take effect Liaison with other health professionals as needed (e.g., nutritionist)
COLLAGEN/CONNECTIVE TISSUE CONDITIONS: RHEUMATOID ARTHRITIS	
Baseline Considerations	Age and wellness (based on a standardized outcome measure) Health status and potential education outcomes (smoking, nutrition, general profiles of daily physical activity and prolonged sedentary activity, structured exercise, sleep status, and stress) Mental health (well-being, life satisfaction, anxiety, depression) Condition severity and adequacy of control Comorbidities and their severities (including bone health and musculoskeletal symptoms/deformity) Secondary complications—involvement of the brain, heart, kidneys (continence status) Medical management and response Medications that augment or attenuate exercise responses

Assessment and Outcome Evaluation	Lifestyle risk factor review to target risk factor modification Multisystem status: CNS (neuropathies), cardiovascular, pulmonary (restrictive profile and effusion risk), musculoskeletal (muscle symmetry, flaccidity, spasticity, gait, chest wall symmetry and functional integrity), neurological (including balance; swallowing and choking status), and endocrine (type 2 diabetes mellitus risk factors/manifestations, in particular) Blood work profile, including Hgb, HgbA1c, lipids, homocysteine, and blood glucose Discomfort/pain profile Fatigue profile Adherence to medication Change in blood pressure profile and general hemodynamic status ↓ Or cessation of medication BMI WHR Adherence to a healthy diet (e.g., DASH diet, Mediterranean diet) Status of activity and participation Sleep quality and quantity Stress Patient's health knowledge and literacy with special reference to living and aging with rheumatoid arthritis, risk factors for lifestyle-related conditions, triggers for worsening and lessening symptoms, medication types, and medication use Resting HR, BP, RPP, RR, RPE, SpO_2 (as indicated), and exercise test responses, including recovery Muscle function (complaints of weakness and delayed recovery)
Exercise Prescription Parameters: Special Considerations	↓ Periods of sedentary activity (particularly screen-based activities such as TV viewing and computer use) ↑ Periods of regular physical activity If severe signs and symptoms, focus on functional activity primarily Activity-rest balance Pacing and energy conservation Stretching: Gentle whole body and joint stretching daily; yoga, tai chi Aerobic: F: alternate days I: moderate activity commensurate with desaturation, RR, and subjective parameters of discomfort/pain and fatigue levels—VAS (0-10) low for discomfort/pain as tolerated (<3), and VAS; SOB 3-5 T: aerobic (e.g., walking, ergometer, and aquatic exercise in warm/hot water) T: 10-40 min with rest intervals as needed; goal to reduce number and length of rests Strengthening: F: 2-3 times/week I: low-to-moderate weight T: weights, dumbbells, pulleys T: 3 sets of 8-15 repetitions maximum
Potential Pre-Exercise or Concurrent Interventions Initiated and/or Supported by the Physical Therapist	Smoking cessation Optimize nutrition Specialized diets (e.g., DASH diet) Salt restriction Weight control Sleep hygiene Relaxation Stress reduction Education regarding regular use of medication Liaison with physician to reduce or eliminate medication as nondrug interventions take effect Liaison with other health professionals as needed (e.g., nutritionist)
CHRONIC RENAL INSUFFICIENCY	
Baseline Considerations	Age and wellness (based on a standardized outcome measure) Health status and potential education outcomes (smoking, nutrition, general profiles of daily physical activity and prolonged sedentary activity, structured exercise, sleep status, and stress) Mental health (well-being, life satisfaction, anxiety, depression) Condition severity and adequacy of control Comorbidities and their severities (including bone health and musculoskeletal symptoms/deformity) Secondary complications—involvement of the brain, heart, kidneys (continence status) Medical management and response Medications that augment or attenuate exercise responses Dialysis candidate

Continued

Assessment and Outcome Evaluation	Lifestyle risk factor review to target risk factor modification (particularly heart disease, high BP, and diabetes) Multisystem status: cardiovascular, pulmonary, musculoskeletal (muscle symmetry, flaccidity, spasticity, gait, chest wall symmetry and functional integrity), neurological (including balance; swallowing and choking status), endocrine (type 2 diabetes mellitus risk factors/manifestations, in particular), and renal status Fluid and electrolyte balance Blood work profile, including Hgb, HgbA1c, lipids, homocysteine, and blood glucose Dyspnea profile Fatigue profile Adherence to medication ↓ Or cessation of medication BMI WHR Adherence to a healthy diet (e.g., DASH diet, Mediterranean diet) Status of activity and participation Sleep quality and quantity Stress Patient's health knowledge and literacy with special reference to living and aging with chronic renal insufficiency, its associated risk factors and risk factors for lifestyle-related conditions in general, triggers for worsening and lessening symptoms, medication types, and medication use Resting HR, BP, RPP, RR, RPE, Spo_2 (as indicated), and exercise test responses, including recovery
Exercise Prescription Parameters: Special Considerations	↓ Periods of sedentary activity (particularly screen-based activities such as TV viewing and computer use) ↑ Periods of regular physical activity Progress based on serial and frequent monitoring; patient needs to be proficient at self-monitoring Stretching: Gentle whole body and joint stretching daily; yoga, tai chi Aerobic: F: walking daily (non-dialysis days if applicable); ergometer (dialysis days if applicable); commensurate with capacity I: low to moderate based on subjective tolerance and well-being on any given day T: cycle ergometry preferable for monitoring and physical support if on dialysis T: intermittent exercise protocol (e.g., 5 min of exercise, followed by 1 min of rest; progress to 60 min continuous) Strengthening: Gentle whole body and joint stretching daily; yoga, tai chi
Potential Pre-Exercise or Concurrent Interventions Initiated and/or Supported by the Physical Therapist	Smoking cessation Optimize nutrition Specialized diets (e.g., DASH diet) Salt restriction Weight control Sleep hygiene Relaxation Stress reduction Renal status Mental status Fatigue Muscle comfort
ENDOCRINE AND METABOLIC CONDITIONS: OVERWEIGHT AND OBESITY	
(Note: Overweight and obesity are frequently coupled with preclinical or frank type 2 diabetes mellitus, so the special considerations for each condition apply.)	
Baseline Considerations	Age and wellness (based on a standardized outcome measure); quality of life Health status and potential education outcomes (smoking, nutrition, general profiles of daily physical activity and prolonged sedentary activity, sleep status, and stress) Mental health (anxiety and depression) Body image Condition severity, medical management and response Comorbidities and their severities Cardio/cerebrovascular and metabolic risk factors Medications that augment or attenuate exercise responses Psychosocial considerations: Social network and support system Health literacy Self-efficacy Readiness to change lifestyle-related health behavior

Assessment and Outcome Evaluation	Lifestyle risk factor review (particularly metabolic syndrome and obstructive sleep apnea) as a basis for lifestyle modification Vascular screen as indicated based on lifestyle and family history: Blood work profile, including Hgb, HgbA1c, lipids, homocysteine, and blood glucose Adequacy of medical control over the years (degree of lability with exercise and stress) Body composition measures (e.g., skin fold measurements, BMI, and WHR) Cardiovascular function Peripheral vascular function CNS and autonomic nervous system function Muscle function and musculoskeletal status/deformity Adherence to healthy diet (e.g., DASH diet, Mediterranean diet) Status of activity and participation Sleep quality and quantity (use of modalities such as CPAP) Stress and self-management strategies Patient's health knowledge and literacy with special reference to weight control and associated conditions, risk factors for lifestyle-related conditions in general (addressing weight will mitigate risk factors for a wide range of lifestyle-related conditions including musculoskeletal conditions), triggers for worsening and lessening symptoms, medication types, and medication use Resting HR, BP, RPP, RR, (Spo_2 as indicated particularly in morbid obesity), RPE and exercise test responses, including recovery
Exercise Prescription Parameters: Special Considerations	Goal: To achieve optimal basal physical activity and exercise status (to be physically active and participate in a structured exercise program) and to maximize oxygen transport, collateralization to improve blood flow and tissue perfusion Restructuring prolonged periods of sedentary activity Caution: Exercise in accordance with cardiac, respiratory, or musculoskeletal limitations (limit undue work of breathing or work of the heart, as well as musculoskeletal strain) and appropriately monitor depending on extent and severity of secondary comorbidity Walking aid may be required that relieves potential musculoskeletal strain Ensure physical activity and exercise program are being maintained by healthy nutrition and salt restriction Stretching: Whole body stretching to prepare the individual to what may be unfamiliar activity Aerobic: F: 2-3 time/day; as frequently as possible for morbidity obese I: low to moderate to minimize musculoskeletal strain, yet elicit an aerobic response that burns maximal number of calories in a given period To lose weight: 250-300 min/week To prevent weight regain: 150 min/week T: Whole body continuous rhythmic aerobic exercise; "aquacize" (water height adjusted to level of patient's tolerance—pressure of water on chest wall can restrict ventilation, level maintained at leg or abdomen level) T: 10-min bouts with rests to recover; to 60 min continuous exercise without rests Strengthening (Note: Objective is multiple repetitions at low intensity to burn calories): F: 1-2 times/day I: low intensity, 20%-60%, repetitions maximum T: weights, dumbbells, pulleys T: 3 sets of 10-20 repetitions performed deliberately Other activities: sports, gym activities of interest and intrinsically motivating to the individual; consider leisure time activities that are metabolically demanding (gardening, cleaning, walking)
Potential Pre-Exercise or Concurrent Interventions Initiated and/or Supported by the Physical Therapist	Smoking cessation Optimize nutrition Specialized diets (e.g., DASH diet and Mediterranean-type diets) Salt restriction Weight control Sleep hygiene Relaxation Stress reduction Counseling

BMI, Body mass index; *WHR,* waist-to-hip ratio; *HR,* heart rate; *BP,* blood pressure, *HRR,* heart rate reserve; *RR,* respiratory rate; *Spo2,* arterial saturation assessed with the pulse oximeter; *DASH diet,* Dietary Approaches to Stop Hypertension diet; *VAS,* visual analog scale.

Bibliography

Dean E, editor: Physical therapy in the 21st century: A new evidence-informed practice paradigm and implications. *Physiotherapy Theory and Practice* (Special Issue) 25:327–462, 2009.

Evans N, Forsyth E: End-stage renal disease in people with type 2 diabetes: Systemic manifestations and exercise implications. *Physical Therapy* 84:454–463, 2004.

Johansen KL: Exercise and dialysis. *Hemodialysis International* 12:290–300, 2008.

Appendix E

Common Complementary Therapies

MANUAL THERAPIES

Myofascial Release

Myofascial release is a manual therapy that utilizes energy from the therapist along with mechanical pressure of the hands to "release" fascia that is constricted. As taught by John F. Barnes, PT,[101] this therapy includes release, unwinding, and rebounding as a triad of approaches that releases "stuck" fascia to further enhance the flow of chi, which is thought to travel over the fascia much like electrons of energy travel over copper wire.

Craniosacral Therapy

Developed by John Upledger, DO, FAAO, craniosacral therapy is a manual therapy that uses light touch to balance energy flow, in part by balancing the flow of the cerebral spinal fluid as it circulates around the meninges of the cranium and down the spinal column. Those who have attempted to criticize this technique by asserting that the cranial plates are fused in adulthood and thus cannot move are now conceding that electron microscope pictures of the cranial sutures reveal blood vessels and fascia that may indicate that the plates are not fused.

Rosen Method Body Work

Founded by Marion Rosen, PT, Rosen method body work is a form of hands-on therapy, the goal of which is to enhance relaxation and emotional awareness by helping the patient identify holding patterns and assisting in the release of the physical and emotional tension, thereby allowing more of the "true self" to emerge and facilitating healing.

Rolfing, Soma, Neuromuscular Therapy, Hellerwork

Rolfing was first developed by Ida Rolf, PhD, and is sometimes referred to as structural integration. This approach uses a deep connective tissue massage to loosen fascial restrictions and line up the structure of bones, muscles, and organs so that the body/mind has a more vertical relation to gravity. After 10 prescribed sessions, it is reasoned that the body is more in alignment and can heal itself. Soma, Hellerwork, and neuromuscular therapy are slight variations on this same theory.

Massage

Massage is the manipulation of tissue through the skin with the intention of bringing about a change in the present condition of the mind/body. Massage from a mechanistic perspective may be intended to move fluid from the extremities to the core or simply to mechanically break up fibrocystic nodules in muscle. Massage from an energy-based intention is carried out with similar physical maneuvers, but the intention of the practitioner is to influence the body energy, or chi, to flow so that the mind/body can then heal itself; thus manual techniques are less vigorous and more gentle.

Osteopathic Medicine

In contrast to allopathic medicine, osteopathic medicine stresses the importance of holistic health, nutrition, and joint mobilization to maintain proper balance and homeostasis. At one time, curricula in osteopathic medical schools were quite different from that in allopathic schools and thus deemed inferior. Over time, osteopathic schools have become more rigorous and similar to allopathic medical schools and have increased in stature and reputation in Western medicine.

Chiropractic Medicine

Chiropractic medical education is oriented toward the belief that illness and disease result from vertebral misalignment and that regular manipulation can maintain flow of energy to organs and the body/mind, thus maintaining health.

MIND/BODY INTERVENTIONS

Psychotherapies, Hypnosis

The approach to healing taken by psychotherapies and hypnosis suggests that bringing to awareness incorrect or harmful ways of thinking about something and using this insight to change the way one thinks can remove blocks in energy flow and open up, for example, improved neurotransmitter flow. PET scans have shown that cognitive therapy and serotonin reuptake inhibitors work in similar ways to change synaptic transmission, resulting in the patient feeling better.

Meditation

With meditation the emphasis is on purposely shifting awareness away from logical, left-brain thought (some call the ceaseless left-brain chatter "monkey mind") to the rhythmical flow of the breath, or the peace of a pleasant sound, thus closing off the stream of worry about the past and fear about the future. Meditation lowers stress by lowering cortisol levels, thus balancing blood pressure and other physiological responses to stress.

Mindfulness meditation is sometimes called Vipassana meditation and has been developed very successfully as a stress reducer by Jon Kabat-Zinn. It comes from the Buddhist tradition.

Transcendental meditation (TM) stems from the Hindu tradition and emphasizes focused concentration on a mantra that is given to a person after a period of initiation. Maharishi University in Fairfield, Iowa was founded by Maharishi Mahesh Yogi, the person most known for bringing TM to the United States. All campus personnel at Maharishi University meditate regularly.

Imagery

Imagery purposefully replaces stressful thought with images that enhance relaxation, thus affecting the ANS. One can use imagery alone or participate in a group led by a person suggesting an imagery exercise.

Prayer for Self

Prayer for the self involves quieting the mind and purposefully intending communication with the transcendent, or God, for the well-being of the self.

Support Groups

Support groups allow the individual to meet with others and share experiences to lessen the feeling of powerlessness. Religious groups can be included in this category.

Dance, Music Therapy, and Art Therapy

Dance, music, and art therapy work by altering the existing flow of energy by movement, pulling up creative feelings, and unleashing "stuck" energy by focusing concentration outward.

Neurolinguistic Psychology

Originally named neurolinguistic programming, neurolinguistic psychology is a psychotherapeutic approach that brings to awareness ways in which the use of certain words, body postures, and eye movements reveal "stuck" energy, thus allowing a person to choose a way in which to think and move that will enhance energy flow and bring a more relaxed state.

Biofeedback

Biofeedback involves the use of external monitoring devices that record autonomic and cortical nervous system and muscle action, so that a person can, through thought, change the reading on the monitor and thus alter the body/mind function. External monitors include EMG and oscilloscopes that quantify thermal energy.

Yoga

Yoga is an eight-fold path, comprising eight separate activities that emphasize physical, mental, and spiritual elements that enhance union of body and mind. Yoga means union. The most widely known yogic practice is hatha yoga, which features a variety of physical postures and exercises called asanas. Meditative asanas stress alignment of the spine with the head and focus on proper breathing. Therapeutic asanas, such as the cobra and shoulder stand, feature elongation of fascia and soft tissue. Both are done with discipline, awareness, and relaxed openness and thus help to stimulate prana—or life energy or chi.

Pilates

Named for its founder, Joseph Pilates, this is an exercise system that aims to facilitate successful movement with less effort, less fatigue, and greater movement awareness retention. Often using equipment such as the Clinical Reformer and the Cadillac, the practitioner can manipulate gravity, the base of support, the length of levers, and the center of gravity with a series of springs and slings to assist or resist smooth movement.

Tai Chi

Tai chi is a mind/body exercise that features slow, controlled, nonimpact movement that gently moves the center of the mind/body mass over the base of support without loss of balance. It is an ancient physical art form that was developed by families in China as a way of defending the household from attack and passed on from generation to generation. The specific form of tai chi used would carry the family name, such as Chin, Yang, Wu, Chuan, etc. These are further condensed, at times, into short forms. Tai chi develops both mind and body as the movement and breath facilitate the proper balance between the yin and yang energies, reducing yang and increasing yin and thus contributing to the healthy flow of chi.

MOVEMENT AWARENESS

Feldenkrais Method

The Feldenkrais method was developed by Moshe Feldenkrais, a physicist and judo expert athlete. When told an injury he sustained would require fusing his knee, Feldenkrais developed a way of thinking that emphasized being able to purposely choose how he might move to protect his knee and avoid fusion. He adapted. He then identified habitual movements and helped others to recognize endless options for adapting to a particular blockage or restriction in a movement, avoiding pain or perception of strain and thus avoiding reflex muscle splinting. Two strategies, awareness through movement (ATM) and functional integration (FI), are used in class "lessons." ATM is mainly verbal and visual; FI adds positioning, contact, and pressure.

Alexander Technique

The Alexander technique was developed by Frederick Matthias Alexander, who used himself in a single-case research design. Alexander discovered how habitual positions in the body affect movement and organ function. Through consciously inhibiting automatic ways of holding positions, we can choose to act in healthier ways. By integrating proper awareness and attention, movement can bring the mind and body into harmony and meet goals of efficient function. Alexander teachers assist students to learn by using touch to bring the student's awareness to areas of tension, inhibiting habitual use and facilitating a redistribution of postural tone, thus providing a different kinesthetic experience. In this way it is somewhat similar to the Feldenkrais method, without words.

Trager Approach

Developed by Milton Trager, MD, the Trager Approach uses a process of rhythmic "rocking, fluffing, jiggling, lengthening, and shimmering" motions to trigger tissue relaxation reflexively.

ENERGY WORK

Traditional Chinese Medicine

Traditional Chinese medicine is an entire health care system made up of various specific practices or approaches. Rather than treating disease, this approach looks for underlying systems of imbalance and patterns of disharmony in each individual and treats the whole patient by influencing the flow of chi along meridians. It features pulse and tongue diagnosis, acupuncture, qi gong, herbal medicine, and tui na, a form of massage that combines acupressure, massage, and deep tissue manipulation.

Acupuncture, Acupressure

Acupuncture and acupressure are modalities of traditional Chinese medicine in which various points along meridians or pathways are stimulated by way of very fine needles (acupuncture) or by way of touch or tapping (acupressure). This mechanical stimulation of the various points is hypothesized to facilitate the flow of electrons along the fascia, thus opening up blocked energy and facilitating the flow of chi.

Reflexology

Reflexology posits that organs and body parts are represented as zones on the feet; the practice works by way of stimulating the corresponding zone with a constant deep pressure for 1 or 2 minutes. Energy, circulation, and nerve impulses are stimulated, raising the vitality of the body and restoring homeostasis and flow of chi.

Qi Gong

An aspect of traditional Chinese medicine, qi gong (pronounced chee-kung) ranges from simple positions to rather complicated movements that emphasize, at the same time, rhythmic breathing and deep relaxation in order to facilitate the flow of chi. In external qi gong a master projects or emits his or her own chi to serve to heal another. Internal qi gong is breathing without movement to enhance self-healing and self-maintenance (meditation is sometimes referred to as internal or quiescent qi gong). Dynamic qi gong includes movement; as such, tai chi is often classified as dynamic qi gong.

Therapeutic Touch

Developed by Delores Krieger and Dora Kunz, therapeutic touch is sometimes referred to as an energetic therapy and sometimes as a manual therapy. The therapist's hands are used, but they do not come in contact with the skin. Instead the therapist "smoothes" the energy field surrounding the mind/body, thus gaining access to the flow of energy by way of the ethereal body or energetic field surrounding the mind/body.

BIOELECTROMAGNETICS/ENERGY WORK

Laser

Cold laser, or soft laser, uses a beam of low-intensity laser to initiate a series of enzymatic reactions and bioelectrical events that stimulate the natural healing process at the cellular level. It is often used to stimulate acupuncture points.

TENS Units

Although transcutaneous electrical neuromuscular stimulation (TENS) is most commonly used to block noxious pain stimulus in physical therapy, TENS units have been shown to stimulate the production of the neurotransmitters and thus increase flow.

Pulsed Electromagnetic Field Therapy

Pulsed electromagnetic field therapy uses small, battery-powered pulse generators to produce a magnetic field that induces currents to flow in nearby tissues, "jump starting" bone repair.

Magnets

The use of magnets involves magnetized substances against the skin or close to the skin (as in a cloth packet) to bring about a physiochemical or physiological effect. Monopolar magnets have only one pole (north or south) in contact with the skin, whereas bipolar magnets have both north and south poles in contact. Strength of the magnets is measured in gauss units. The literature on magnets has been confusing, in part because of inconsistent meanings of the terms *north pole* and *south pole* and inadequate true measures of magnet strength by manufacturers.

Reiki

Reiki (pronounced ray-kee) is a healing system from Japan (*rei,* meaning "universal" or "omnipresent," and *ki,* meaning "life force" or "energy"). A Reiki practitioner channels the universal life force through the hands to promote energy balancing, healing, and a state of well-being. The universal life force energy can be transmitted through direct touch or by "intending" its transmission from a distance. The belief is that the life force has intelligence and will flow to where it is needed.

Distant Healing Prayer

In distant healing prayer, focused attention is given to the person being prayed for with the intention of causing a positive outcome to result. In intercessory prayer, healing is requested for the self or for others. Directed prayer specifies a particular outcome that is desired. Nondirected prayer intends only that God's will be done in the life of the subject. At the heart of this method is the concept of nonlocal mind, or the belief that a person's consciousness is not limited to distance or time and that individuals can influence the world at a distance through their focused thoughts.

HERBAL APPROACHES

Homeopathic Medicine

Homeopathic medicine is an approach to health and healing developed by Samuel Hahnemann, MD. This practice suggests that reactions to diluted tinctures of natural substances (herbs that cause symptoms similar to those of the disease) can be used to treat disease.

Naturopathy

Naturopathy is a holistic system of healing that requires practitioners to complete a 4-year medical degree. Naturopathic doctors study herbal medicine, homeopathy, osteopathy, nutrition, and some forms of physical therapy as part of their curriculum, which is geared to prepare holistic diagnosticians and therapists.

Bibliography

This appendix is summarized from the following texts.

Burton Goldberg Group, editors: *Alternative medicine—the definitive guide*, Fife, Wash., 1995, Future Medicine Publishing, Inc.

Davis CM, editor: *Complementary therapies in rehabilitation/holistic approaches for prevention and wellness*, Thorofare, N.J., 1997, SLACK, Inc.

Davis CM, editor: *Complementary therapies in rehabilitation/holistic approaches for prevention and wellness*, ed 2, Thorofare, N.J., 2004, SLACK, Inc.

Glossary

Acid-base balance: A condition that exists when the net rate at which the body produces acids or bases equals the net rate at which acids or bases are excreted. The result of acid-base balance is a stable concentration of hydrogen ions in body fluids. The amount of acid or base in the arterial blood is measured by pH.

Acidosis: A process causing acidemia, which is a blood pH of less than 7.38.

Acoustic airway clearance: Form of airway clearance using acoustic vibrations to clear secretions from the lungs.

Active cycle of breathing technique: Technique for clearing bronchial secretions in patients with asthma, consisting of repeated cycles of three ventilatory phases: breathing control, thoracic expansion exercises, and the forced expiration technique.

Acute exacerbation of chronic airflow limitation: An increase in the severity of the signs and symptoms of chronic airflow limitation, usually triggered by infection, inflammation, or increased sputum production.

Acute lung injury: Injury to the lung characterized by a clinical spectrum of parenchymal lung dysfunction resulting from multiple etiologies and leading to alveolar capillary membrane leaking (high protein content). Mild-to-moderate injury results in noncardiogenic edema, and severe injury results in adult respiratory distress syndrome. The hallmarks of worsening lung injury include refractory hypoxemia, right-to-left shunt, and reduced lung compliance.

Adrenergic drugs: Class of drugs acting on the sympathetic nervous system.

Adult respiratory distress syndrome (ARDS): A respiratory syndrome characterized by respiratory insufficiency and hypoxemia. Triggers include aspiration of a foreign body, cardiopulmonary bypass surgery, gram-negative sepsis, multiple blood transfusions, oxygen toxicity, trauma, pneumonia, and other respiratory infection.

Aerosol: Nebulized particles suspended in a gas or air.

Airway clearance: The removal of mucus and foreign material from the airways.

Airway-clearance deficits: Deficits in the ability to remove mucus and foreign material from the airways.

Alveolar proteinosis: A disorder marked by the accumulation of plasma proteins, lipoproteins, and other blood components in the alveoli of the lungs. The cause is unknown and clinical symptoms vary, although only the lungs are affected. Some patients are asymptomatic, whereas others show dyspnea and an unproductive cough.

Alveolar ventilation: The volume of inspired air that reaches the alveolar level and participates in gas exchange, measured by PCO_2.

Alveolitis: An allergic pulmonary reaction to the inhalation of antigenic substances characterized by acute episodes of dyspnea, cough, sweating, fever, weakness, and pain in the joints and muscles lasting from 12 to 18 hours. Recurrent episodes may lead to chronic obstructive lung disease with weight loss, increasing exertional dyspnea, and interstitial fibrosis.

Anesthesia: The absence of normal sensation, especially sensitivity to pain, as induced by an anesthetic substance or by hypnosis or as occurs with traumatic or pathophysiological damage to nerve tissue.

Angina (often angina pectoris): A paroxysmal thoracic pain caused most often by myocardial anoxia as a result of atherosclerosis of the coronary arteries. The pain usually radiates down the inner aspect of the left arm and is frequently accompanied by a feeling of suffocation and impending death. Attacks of angina pectoris are often related to exertion, emotional stress, and exposure to intense cold.

Ankylosing spondylitis: A chronic inflammatory disease of unknown origin, first affecting the spine and adjacent structures and commonly progressing to eventual fusion (ankylosis) of the involved joints. In addition to the spine, the joints of the hip, shoulder, neck, ribs, and jaw are often involved. Physical therapy aids in keeping the spine as erect as possible to prevent flexion contractures. In advanced cases, surgery may be performed to straighten a badly deformed spine.

Arrhythmia: An abnormal heart rhythm represented by an irregularity of the timing or appearance of the ECG tracing. This term is often used synonymously with dysrhythmia.

Arterial blood gas: A test to evaluate the acid-base balance and partial pressures of oxygen and carbon dioxide in the arterial blood.

Arteriovenous-oxygen difference (a-vO_2 difference): The difference between the oxygen content in arterial blood versus venous blood.

Artifact: Extraneous deflection of the ECG waveform caused by movement or electrical interference. Artifact may be mistaken for a dysrhythmia.

Artificial airway: A plastic or rubber device that can be inserted into the upper or lower respiratory tract to facilitate ventilation or the removal of secretions.

Assessment: An evaluation or appraisal of a condition.

Assisted cough: Physical assistance with coughing, provided either by the patient or an assistant.

Asthma: A respiratory disorder characterized by recurring episodes of paroxysmal dyspnea, wheezing on expiration/inspiration because of constriction of the bronchi, coughing, and viscous mucoid bronchial secretions. Treatment may include elimination of the causative agent, hyposensitization, aerosol or oral bronchodilators, beta-adrenergic drugs, methylxanthines, and short-term use of corticosteroids.

Atelectasis: An abnormal condition characterized by the collapse of lung tissue, preventing the respiratory exchange of carbon dioxide and oxygen. Symptoms may include diminished breath sounds, a mediastinal shift toward the side of the collapse, fever, and increasing dyspnea.

Atherosclerosis: A common arterial disorder characterized by yellowish plaques of cholesterol, lipids, and cellular debris in the inner layers of the walls of large and medium-sized arteries. The vessel walls become thick, fibrotic, and calcified, and the lumen narrows, resulting in reduced blood flow to organs normally supplied by the artery. Antilipidemic agents do not reverse atherosclerosis, but a diet low in cholesterol, calories, and saturated fats, adequate exercise, and the avoidance of smoking and stress may help prevent the disorder.

Athletic heart syndrome: Cardiovascular adaptation to intense exercise in athletes.

Autogenic drainage: An "antidyspnea" technique based on quiet expirations in a relaxed state and without use of postural drainage positions.

Blood: The liquid pumped by the heart through all the arteries, veins, and capillaries. Blood is composed of a clear yellow fluid (called plasma), the formed elements, and a series of cell types with different functions. The major function of the blood is to transport oxygen and nutrients to the cells and remove carbon dioxide and other waste products from the cells for detoxification and elimination.

Body mechanics: Using one's body effectively to prevent injury.

Bradycardia: An abnormally slow heart rate.

Bradypnea: A decreased respiratory rate under 10 breaths per minute.

Bronchiectasis: An abnormal condition of the bronchial tree characterized by irreversible dilatation and destruction of the bronchial walls. Symptoms of bronchiectasis include a constant cough productive of copious purulent sputum, hemoptysis, chronic sinusitis, clubbing of fingers, and persistent moist, coarse rales. Treatment includes mobilization, frequent postural drainage, antibiotics, and, rarely, surgical resection of the affected part of the lungs.

Bronchiolitis: An acute viral infection of the lower respiratory tract that occurs primarily in infants under 18 months of age, characterized by expiratory wheezing, respiratory distress, inflammation, and obstruction at the level of the bronchioles.

Bronchitis: An acute or chronic inflammation of the mucous membranes of the tracheobronchial tree. Acute bronchitis is characterized by a productive cough, fever, hypertrophy of mucus-secreting structures, and back pain. Most common in adults, it is often a complication of cystic fibrosis in children. Treatment includes the cessation of cigarette smoking, avoidance of airway irritants, the use of expectorants, and postural drainage. Currently, prophylactic antibiotics, steroids, and desensitization therapy are not recommended.

Bronchopulmonary dysplasia: An iatrogenic condition observed in neonates that resembles chronic airflow limitation and is associated with positive pressure mechanical ventilation and oxygen therapy.

Burns: An injury to tissues of the body caused by heat, electricity, chemicals, radiation, or gases in which the extent of the injury is determined by both the amount of exposure of the cell to the agent and the nature of the agent. Treatment of burns includes pain relief, careful asepsis, prevention of infection, maintenance of the balance of body fluids and electrolytes, and good nutrition. Severe burns of any origin may cause shock, which is treated before the wound.

Cardiac output (Q): The amount of blood ejected from the heart into the aorta each minute.

Cardiac rehabilitation: A supervised program of progressive exercise, psychological support, and education or training to enable a patient who has had a myocardial infarction to resume the activities of daily living on an independent basis. Special training may be needed to adapt the patient to a new occupation and lifestyle.

Cardiac silhouette: Outline of the heart visible on a chest radiograph.

Cardiopulmonary failure: Progressive insufficiency of cardiopulmonary function resulting in significant impairment of cardiac output and/or ventilation that cannot be adequately compensated without ventilatory support.

Cardiopulmonary function: Integrated function of the heart and lungs.

Cardiopulmonary unit: The heart and lungs, which function interdependently as a unit.

Catabolic: Relating to catabolism, which is the breaking down in the body of complex chemical compounds into simpler compounds, often accompanied by the liberation of energy.

Cellular respiration: The processes involved with cellular metabolism, including energy transfer, oxygen utilization, and carbon dioxide production.

Cerebral palsy: A motor function disorder caused by a permanent, nonprogressive brain defect or lesion present at birth or shortly thereafter. Early identification of the disorder facilitates the handling of infants with cerebral palsy and the initiation of an exercise and training program. Treatment is individualized and may include the use of braces, surgical correction of deformities, speech therapy, and various indicated drugs, such as muscle relaxants and anticonvulsants.

Childhood asthma: Reversible airway hyperreactivity and edema affecting children that is often triggered by dust or animals. It is hallmarked by narrowing of the airways, wheezing, shortness of breath, accessory muscle use, and impaired oxygenation.

Cholinergic drugs: Class of drugs acting on the parasympathetic nervous system.

Chronic airflow limitation: A more precise term for chronic obstructive pulmonary disease (e.g., chronic bronchitis and emphysema).

Chronic bronchitis: Lung condition characterized by the presence of a chronic productive cough for at least 3 months in each of 2 successive years.

Chronic renal insufficiency: Impaired function of the kidneys manifested by impaired blood urea nitrogen, creatinine clearance, and reduced urinary output. Renal insufficiency may precipitate renal failure.

Clinical decision making: The process of making decisions based on a thorough history, assessment, integration of the results of laboratory tests and investigations, and the patient's needs and wants.

Complementary therapy: Holistic, mind/body, or energy-based therapy techniques used by physical therapists to complement (usually not replace) traditional therapy techniques. Also known as alternative therapies, alternative medicine, or integrative therapies.

Complications with coughing: Complications associated with an impaired cough (e.g., impaired mucociliary transport, mucus accumulation, pulmonary aspiration, and increased risk for infection).

Computed tomography: Diagnostic tool using ionizing radiation to generate pictures as "slices" through the patient in the axial plane. CT allows for rapid scanning in much more detail than a radiograph.

Congestive heart failure (CHF): An abnormal condition that reflects impaired cardiac pumping, caused by myocardial infarction, ischemic heart disease, or cardiomyopathy. Failure of the ventricle to eject blood efficiently results in volume overload, chamber dilatation, and elevated intracardiac pressure. Retrograde transmission of increased hydrostatic pressure from the left heart causes pulmonary congestion; elevated right heart pressure causes systemic venous congestion and peripheral edema.

Connective tissue dysfunction: Impaired function of connective tissue observed in connective tissue and vascular collagen conditions.

Continuity of care: The provision of continuous care from one setting to another (e.g., inpatient to outpatient facilities).

Continuous positive airway pressure: Oxygen delivery system in which pressure is maintained on the airways above atmospheric pressure.

Control of breathing: The central and peripheral regulation and control mechanisms of breathing.

Control of the heart: The central and peripheral regulation and control mechanisms of the heart.

Controlled breathing: Teaching a patient ventilatory strategies to exert cognitive control over ineffective breathing patterns.

Coronary artery disease: Any one of the abnormal conditions that may affect the arteries of the heart and produce various pathological effects, especially the reduced flow of oxygen and nutrients to the myocardium. Any of the coronary artery diseases, such as coronary atherosclerosis, coronary arteritis, or fibromuscular hyperplasia of the coronary arteries, may produce the common characteristic symptom of angina pectoris. Studies over the last 30 years confirm that coronary atherosclerosis occurs most frequently in populations with regular diets high in calories, total fat, saturated fat, cholesterol, and refined carbohydrates. Other risk factors include cigarette smoking, hypertension, serum cholesterol levels, coffee intake, alcohol intake, deficiencies of vitamins C and E, water hardness, hypoxia, carbon monoxide, social overcrowding, heredity, climate, and viruses.

CoughAssist machine: A commercially produced noninvasive machine used for airway clearance. Earlier versions of this product were known as the Cofflator and the Mechanical In-Exsufflator (MI-E).

Cough pump: The integrated thoracic and abdominal mechanisms involved in cough resulting in forced expiration and evacuation and clearance of the airways.

Cough stages: The stages of cough include maximal inspiration, closure of the glottis, increased intraabdominal pressure, opening of the glottis, and forced expiration.

Cough: A sudden, audible expulsion of air from the lungs. Coughing is preceded by inspiration—the glottis is partially closed, and the accessory muscles of expiration contract to expel the air forcibly from the respiratory passages. Coughing is an essential protective response that serves to clear the lungs, bronchi, or trachea of irritants and secretions or to prevent aspiration of foreign material into the lungs. It is a common symptom of diseases of the chest and larynx. Because the function of coughing is to clear the respiratory tract of secretions, it is important that the cough bring out accumulated debris. When it does not, because of weakness or inhibition of the force of the cough caused by pain, instruction and assistance in effective coughing and deep-breathing exercises are required.

Crackles: Discontinuous, low-pitched lung sounds. Crackles occur predominantly during inspiration. Also known as rales.

Cystic fibrosis: An inherited disorder of the exocrine glands that causes exocrine gland production of abnormally thick secretions of mucus, elevation of sweat electrolytes, increased organic and enzymatic constituents of saliva, and overactivity of the autonomic nervous system. The glands most affected are those in the pancreas, the respiratory system, and the sweat glands. Because there is no known cure, treatment is directed at the prevention of respiratory infections, which are the most frequent cause of death. Mucolytic agents and bronchodilators are used to help liquefy the thick, tenacious mucus. Physical therapy measures, such as exercise, postural drainage, and breathing exercises, can also dislodge secretions. Life expectancy in cystic fibrosis has improved markedly over the past several decades, and with early diagnosis and treatment, most patients can be expected to reach adulthood.

Dead space: The amount of lung in contact with ventilating gases but not in contact with pulmonary blood flow. Alveolar dead space refers to alveoli that are ventilated by the pulmonary circulation but not perfused. Anatomical dead space is an area in the trachea, bronchi, and air passages containing air that does not reach the alveoli during respiration. Physiological dead space is an area in the respiratory system that includes the anatomical dead space together with the space in the alveoli occupied by air that does not contribute to the oxygen-carbon dioxide exchange.

Denervation of heart: The transplanted heart initially loses its innervation (i.e., it is denervated and relies on exogenous catecholamines for cardiac acceleration and deceleration).

Dependent patients: Patients who are unable to help themselves.

Depolarization: Changes in ionic concentrations across muscle cell membranes leading to contraction of the cell.

Diabetes: A clinical condition characterized by the excessive excretion of urine. The excess may be caused by a deficiency of antidiuretic hormone (ADH), as in diabetes insipidus, or it may be the polyuria resulting from the hyperglycemia occurring in diabetes mellitus.

Diagnosis: Specific analysis of the patient's health problem(s).

Diaphragmatic breathing pattern: Involves teaching patients with COPD how to relax the accessory muscles and perform controlled diaphragmatic breathing.

Diffusion: The process in which solid, particulate matter in a fluid moves from an area of higher concentration to an area of lower concentration, resulting in an even distribution of the particles in the fluid. No energy is required.

Diuretics: Drugs that act on the kidney to increase the formation of urine, therefore decreasing blood volume and fluid accumulation.

Documentation: Written material associated with the history, the compilation of laboratory reports and investigations, and the results of clinical assessment.

Dyspnea: The sensation of difficulty in breathing.

Echocardiography: Evaluation of cardiac structure and function by using the properties of sound. Quantitative and qualitative measurements can be derived. The most common types include two-dimensional, Doppler, and transesophageal.

Ectopic focus: A beat or rhythm that does not originate in the SA node. Also known as pacemaker.

Ejection fraction: The amount of ventricular volume ejected with each heart beat. Expressed as a percentage, ejection fraction is determined by the following equation: [(end-diastolic volume − end-systolic volume) × 100]/end-diastolic volume.

Electrocardiogram (ECG): The tracing produced by the sequential depolarization and repolarization of myocardial cells as detected by surface electrodes placed on the skin.

Electrocardiographic monitoring: Electrocardiographic monitoring involving electrode placement on the chest wall and on the limbs for a 12-lead ECG. Such monitoring provides a tracing of the electrical activity of the heart.

Electromechanical coupling: The coupling of electrical and mechanical events of the heart to effect cardiac output.

Electromyographic (EMG) power spectrum: Electromyography is the process of recording the electrical activity of muscle on a cathode-ray oscilloscope. The electromyographic (EMG) power spectrum is the full range of electrical activity of the muscle.

Emphysema: Lung condition characterized by an abnormal, permanent enlargement of the air spaces distal to the terminal bronchioles accompanied by destruction of their walls.

Endocardial cushion defect: Any cardiac defect resulting from the failure of the endocardial cushions in the embryonic heart to fuse and form the atrial septum.

Endocrine function: The function of the endocrine glands responsible for normal physiological function.

Evidence-informed practice: Practice indicated or informed by epidemiological indicators and prioritized on that basis, e.g., premature death and prolonged morbidity from lifestyle-related conditions.

Evidence-based practice: Evidence for specific interventions based on scientific evaluation and appraisal.

Exercise blood gases: Blood gases taken before, during, and after exercise to determine the effect of exercise on oxygen transport.

Exercise prescription: Intervention plan based on the patient's presentation, history, premorbid status and conditioning level, lab and investigative reports related to physiological reserve capacity, the exercise test, and the goals of the exercise prescription.

Exercise stress: Physical stress imposed by movement (i.e., mobilization and exercise).

Exercise testing: A series of select tests and procedures aimed at evaluating a patient's physical health. Exercise testing is the first step in exercise prescription.

Exercise: (1) The performance of any physical activity for the purpose of conditioning the body, improving health, or maintaining fitness, or as a means of therapy for correcting a deformity or restoring the organs and bodily functions to a state of health. (2) Any action, skill, or maneuver that exerts the muscles and is performed repeatedly in order to develop or strengthen the body or any of its parts. (3) To use a muscle or part of the body in a repetitive manner to maintain or develop its strength. The physical therapist constantly assesses the patient's needs and provides the proper type and amount of exercise, taking into account the patient's physical or mental limitations. Exercise has a beneficial effect on each of the body systems, although in excess it can lead to the breakdown of tissue and cause injury.

Expiratory reserve volume (ERV): The maximum volume of gas that can be expired from the resting expiratory level.

Extracorporeal life support: Life support with artificial heart and lung, commonly called extracorporeal membrane oxygenation (ECMO). ECMO is a temporary means of providing partial or total life support; it stabilizes the patient by regulating gas exchange and perfusion.

Extrinsic factors: Factors related to the patient's care that contribute to cardiopulmonary dysfunction and impaired gas exchange.

Fluid and electrolyte status: The status of blood volume and distribution, and the status of electrolyte balance in the body; fluid balance often has a direct effect on electrolytes.

Forced expiratory volume in 1 second (FEV_1): Amount of air expired in 1 second during a forced exhalation after a maximal inhalation.

Forced vital capacity (FVC): Total amount of air exhaled during a forced exhalation after a maximal inhalation.

Function optimization: Optimal functioning of the patient as a whole person based on optimal physiological functioning at an organ system level.

Functional residual capacity: Volume of gas in the lungs at the end of a normal expiration. Functional residual capacity is equal to the residual volume plus the expiratory reserve volume.

Gas exchange: The movement of oxygen and carbon dioxide between the pulmonary capillary blood and the alveolar tissue and between the systemic capillary blood and peripheral tissue cells.

Gastrointestinal dysfunction: Abnormal function of the gastrointestinal system.

Gravitational stress: Stress imposed on the human body by gravity and its physiological effects.

Gravity: The heaviness or weight of an object resulting from the universal effect of the attraction between any body of matter and any planetary body. The force of the attraction depends on the relative masses of the bodies and on the distance between them.

Head injury: Any traumatic damage to the head resulting from blunt or penetrating trauma of the skull. Blood vessels, nerves, and meninges can be torn; bleeding, edema, and ischemia may result.

Health According to the World Health Organization, health is a complete state of physical, social, and emotional wellbeing; rather than being the objective of living health is conceptualized as a resource for everyday life.

Health behavior: An action taken by a person to maintain, attain, or regain good health and to prevent illness. Health behavior reflects a person's health beliefs. Some common health behaviors are exercising regularly, eating a balanced diet, and obtaining necessary inoculations.

Health Literacy: A person's ability to comprehend health information and use that information to make informed decisions about one's health and medical care.

Heart: The muscular, cone-shaped organ, about the size of a clenched fist, that pumps blood throughout the body and beats normally about 70 times per minute by coordinated nerve impulses and muscular contractions. Enclosed in pericardium, the heart rests on the diaphragm between the lower borders of the lungs, occupying the middle of the mediastinum. The sinoatrial node of the heart sets the rate. Other factors affecting the heartbeat are emotion, exercise, hormones, temperature, pain, and stress.

Heart-lung interdependence: The heart and lung are structurally and functionally interdependent and form a cardiopulmonary unit.

Hemiplegia: Paralysis of one side of the body.

Hemodynamic status: Status of the heart and its capacity to effect blood movement to perfuse the tissues of the body.

Henderson Hasselbach equation: Equation demonstrating how H^+ concentration results from the dissociation of carbonic acid and the interrelationship of the blood acids, bases, and buffers.

Hibernating myocardium: Contractile dysfunction of the myocardium resulting from prolonged ischemia, appearing as a regional wall motion abnormality.

High-frequency chest wall oscillation: A large-volume, variable-frequency air-pulse delivery system that can be used by patients with obstructive lung disease to promote mucus clearance.

HIPAA guidelines: Federal guidelines in the United States that protect the confidentiality of health information (also known as personal protected health information, or PHI). Acronym stands for Health Insurance Portability and Accountability Act.

Holistic approach: An interventional philosophy that considers both the body and the mind as contributors to health and/or intervention.

Home care: A health service provided in the patient's place of residence for the purposes of promoting, maintaining, or restoring health or minimizing the effects of illness and disability.

Humidity: Pertaining to the level of moisture in the atmosphere, the amount varying with the temperature. The percentage is usually represented in terms of relative humidity, with 100% being the point of air saturation or level at which the air can absorb no additional water.

Hyaline membrane disease: Disease of the newborn, characterized by airless alveoli, inelastic lungs, more than 60 respirations a minute, nasal flaring, intercostal and subcostal retractions, grunting on expiration, and peripheral edema. This is also called respiratory distress syndrome (RDS) of the newborn.

Hypercapnia: The presence of an abnormally large amount of carbon dioxide in the circulating blood.

Hyperpnea: Rapid, shallow breathing.

Hyperresonant: Lung sound with a very low pitch and prolonged duration.

Hypertension: A common, often asymptomatic disorder characterized by elevated blood pressure persistently exceeding 140/90 mm Hg. Patients with high blood pressure are advised to follow a low-sodium, low-saturated-fat diet, reduce calories to control obesity, exercise, avoid stress, and take adequate rest.

Hypoxemia: A low level of oxygen in the blood, often characterized by a PaO_2 of less than 80 mm Hg.

Immune function: Function of the immunological system and its components to effect optimal immunological protection.

Immunological dysfunction: Abnormal function of the immunological system.

Immunosuppression: Of or pertaining to a substance or procedure that lessens or prevents an immune response.

Incentive spirometry: A visual and/or audio feedback device that encourages slow, deep inspiration. Also known as sustained maximum inspiration (SMI).

Inspiratory capacity (IC): Maximum volume of gas that can be inhaled from the resting expiratory level. Equal to the sum of the tidal volume and the inspiratory reserve volume, it is measured with a spirometer.

Inspiratory muscle training: Resistance ventilatory training designed to increase the strength and endurance of the inspiratory muscles.

Inspiratory reserve volume: Maximum volume of gas that can be inspired from the end-tidal inspiratory level.

Inspiratory resistance breathing: A method of respiratory muscle training that includes normal ventilation with added external threshold loading on inspiration and consists of 15 to 30 minutes of training five days per week. External loading is increased from 30% of maximal inspiratory pressure to 60% of maximal inspiratory pressure as the patient's tolerance increases.

Intermittent positive pressure breathing (IPPB): A form of assistive or controlled respiration produced by a ventilatory apparatus in which compressed gas is delivered under positive pressure into the patient's airways until a preset pressure is reached. Passive exhalation is allowed through a valve, and the cycle begins again as the flow of gas is triggered by inhalation. This is also called intermittent positive pressure ventilation (IPPV).

Interstitial pulmonary fibrosis: A classification of restrictive lung disease including conditions that result in a final common pathway of bouts of chronic lung infection and irreversible fibrosis.

Intervention prescription: Intervention plan consisting of optimal interventions and intervention parameters identified for each problem.

Intraaortic balloon counterpulsation: Procedure for assisting left ventricular function and coronary perfusion that involves inserting a balloon into the femoral artery. The inflation and deflation of the balloon is synchronized with the ECG such that the balloon inflates during diastole and deflates during systole.

Intracardiac pressures: Pressures within the chambers of the heart. Optimal movement of blood through the heart depends on pressure gradients throughout the heart. Normal pressures within each heart chamber are within a restricted range.

Intracranial pressure monitoring: Invasive monitoring instituted to measure changes in cranial pressure usually resulting from increased volume of the brain because of injury, bleeding, fluid accumulation, or an intracranial mass.

Intrinsic factors: Factors that are related to a patient's personal characteristics and that affect the patient's care.

Isocapnic hyperpnea: A method of respiratory muscle training that includes high ventilation with low external loading consisting of sustained periods of hyperpnea lasting 15 to 30 minutes daily for several weeks with the addition of carbon dioxide to maintain a normal level.

Jacobsen's progressive relaxation exercise: A technique involving contraction followed by relaxation to progressively relax muscle groups.

Kidneys: A pair of bean-shaped urinary organs in the dorsal part of the abdomen, one on each side of the vertebral column. The kidneys produce and eliminate urine through a complex filtration network and reabsorption system comprising more than 2 million nephrons. All the blood in the body passes through the kidneys about 20 times every hour but only about one-fifth of the plasma is filtered by the nephrons during that period. The kidneys remove water as urine and return water that has been filtered to the blood plasma, thus helping to maintain the water balance of the body. Hormones, especially the antidiuretic hormone (ADH) produced by the pituitary gland, control the function of the kidneys in regulating the water content of the body.

Kyphoscoliosis: An abnormal condition characterized by an anteroposterior curvature and a lateral curvature of the spine. It occurs in children and adults and can be associated with cor pulmonale.

Late sequelae of poliomyelitis: Late effects of poliomyelitis that may occur in poliomyelitis survivors 30 to 35 years after onset. These effects include disproportionate fatigue, weakness, pain, reduced endurance, choking and swallowing problems, altered temperature sensitivity, and psychological problems.

Learning theory: A group of concepts and principles that attempts to explain the learning process. One concept, Guthrie's contiguous conditioning premise, postulates that each response becomes permanently linked with stimuli present at the time so that contiguity rather than reinforcement is a part of the learning process.

Lifestyle-related behaviors: Behavioral choices a person makes related to lifestyle, e.g., smoking, nutrition, and physical activity.

Lifestyle-related conditions: Conditions significantly related to lifestyle behaviors, e.g., smoking-related conditions, high blood pressure, stroke, type 2 diabetes mellitus, obesity, and cancers.

Liver: Largest gland of the body and one of its most complex organs. More than 500 of its functions have been identified. It is divided into four lobes, contains as many as 100,000 lobules, and is served by two distinct blood supplies. Some of the major functions performed by the liver are the production of bile by hepatic cells, the secretion of glucose, proteins, vitamins, fats, and most of the other compounds used by the body, the processing of hemoglobin for vital use of its iron content, and the conversion of poisonous ammonia to area.

Lung cancer: Pulmonary malignancy attributable to cigarette smoking in 50% of cases. Lung cancer develops most often in scarred or chronically diseased lungs and is usually far advanced when detected because metastases may precede the detection of the primary lesion in the lung. Symptoms of lung cancer include persistent cough, dyspnea, purulent or blood-streaked sputum, chest pain, and repeated attacks of bronchitis or pneumonia. Surgery is the most effective treatment, but only one half of cases are operable at the time of diagnosis and of these 50% are not resectable. Thoracotomy is contraindicated if metastases are found in contralateral or scalene lymph nodes. Irradiation is used to treat localized lesions and unresectable intrathoracic tumors and as palliative therapy for metastatic lesions. Radiotherapy may also be administered after surgery to destroy remaining tumor cells and may be combined with chemotherapy.

Lung capacities: Lung volumes that consist of two or more of the four primary nonoverlapping volumes. Functional residual capacity is the sum of residual volume and expiratory reserve volume. Inspiratory capacity is the sum of the tidal volume and inspiratory reserve volume. Vital capacity is the sum of the expiratory reserve volume, the tidal volume, and the inspiratory reserve volume. Total lung capacity, at the end of maximal inspiration, is the sum of the functional residual capacity and the inspiratory capacity.

Lung compliance: Volume change per unit of pressure change in the lungs.

Lung volume: Volume of the lungs that may be compartmentalized into component volumes and capacities.

Lungs: Pair of light, spongy organs in the thorax, constituting the main component of the respiratory system. The two highly elastic lungs are the main mechanisms in the body for inspiring air, from which oxygen is extracted for the arterial blood system, and for exhaling carbon dioxide, which is dispersed from the venous system.

Magnetic resonance imaging: Diagnostic tool using magnetic energy to create detailed views of anatomy. MRI images provide better views of soft tissues than CT scans, but MRI scans are more expensive and time-consuming (a chest CT can be done in less than a minute; an MRI takes about an hour).

Malnutrition: Any disorder of nutrition. It may result from an unbalanced, insufficient, or excessive diet or from the impaired absorption, assimilation, or use of foods.

Managed care: Health care system in which there is administrative control over primary health care services in a medical group practice. Redundant facilities and services are eliminated and costs are reduced. Health education and preventive medicine are emphasized. Patients may pay a flat fee for basic family care but may be charged additional fees for secondary care services of specialists.

Measurement: The determination, expressed numerically, of the extent or quantity of a substance, energy, or time.

Mechanical ventilation: Use of artificial mechanical means to support ventilation.

Metabolic demand: The energy and oxygen demands of the body required to support metabolism. Metabolic demand fluctuates depending on the activity level of the individual, the presence of illness and increased temperature, and the requirements of healing and repair.

Method: A technique or procedure for producing a desired effect, such as a surgical procedure, a laboratory test, or a diagnostic technique.

Mind/body therapy: Movement, and verbal and nonverbal communication, with the mind/body open up new pathways for thought and thereby unblock what might be blocked energy flow, or chi. The treatment of stress involves mind/body therapeutic techniques.

Minute ventilation (VE): Amount of air inspired in 1 minute. It is the product of tidal volume and respiratory rate.

Mobilization: Therapeutic and prescriptive application of low-intensity exercise in the management of cardiopulmonary dysfunction, usually in acutely ill patients. The primary goal of mobilization is to exploit the acute effects of exercise to optimize oxygen transport.

Morbid obesity: Excess of body fat that threatens normal bodily functions, such as respiration.

Mucous blanket: Normal layer of mucus lining the bronchopulmonary tree. This blanket provides a medium through which foreign material and bacteria can be wafted centrally by the cilia for eventual removal by coughing or swallowing.

Multiple sclerosis (MS): A progressive disease characterized by disseminated demyelination of nerve fibers of the brain and spinal cord. It begins slowly, usually in young adulthood, and continues throughout life with periods of exacerbation and remission.

Multisystem assessment: Assessment of multiple organ systems based on clinical examination and investigative laboratory reports.

Such assessment helps identify all factors that contribute to deficits in oxygen transport.

Muscle endurance: Ability to sustain repetitive contraction against a given load.

Muscle strength: Maximum force that a muscle can develop with maximal stimulation.

Muscular dystrophy (MD): A group of genetically transmitted diseases characterized by progressive atrophy of symmetrical groups of skeletal muscles without evidence of involvement or degeneration of neural tissue.

Myocardial infarction: Necrosis of a portion of cardiac muscle caused by obstruction in a coronary artery from either atherosclerosis or an embolus. Also called a heart attack.

Needs assessment: Assessment of the patient's specific physical, functional, and psychological needs.

Nocturnal ventilation: Selective use of mechanical ventilation during the night. Patients with cardiopulmonary dysfunction are at greater risk during the night when they are recumbent and the respiratory drive is depressed.

Obesity: Abnormal increase in the proportion of fat cells, mainly in the viscera and subcutaneous tissues of the body. Obesity may be exogenous or endogenous. Hyperplastic obesity is caused by an increase in the number of fat cells in the increased adipose tissue mass. Hypertrophic obesity results from an increase in the size of the fat cells in the increased adipose tissue mass.

Objective: (1) A goal. (2) Of or pertaining to a phenomenon or clinical finding that is observed; not subjective. An objective finding is often described in health care as a sign, as distinguished from a symptom, which is a subjective finding.

Obstructive lung disease: Classification of lung disease referring to airflow limitation secondary to obstruction and increased airway resistance (e.g., chronic bronchitis and emphysema).

Osteoporosis: A disorder characterized by abnormal rarefaction of bone, occurring most frequently in postmenopausal women, in sedentary or immobilized individuals, and in patients on long-term steroid therapy. The disorder may cause pain, especially in the lower back, pathological fractures, loss of stature, and various deformities.

Outpatient: A patient, not hospitalized, who is being treated in an office, clinic, or other ambulatory care facility.

Oxygen (O_2): Tasteless, odorless, colorless gas essential for human respiration.

Oxygen consumption ($\dot{V}O_2$): The difference between the amount of inspired oxygen and the amount of oxygen exhaled. The difference between inspired and expired oxygen is a primary measure of aerobic fitness.

Oxygen delivery ($\dot{D}O_2$): Delivery of oxygen to the tissues of the body; an essential component of oxygen transport.

Oxygen desaturation: Desaturation of oxygen from the hemoglobin molecule in the blood in response to a reduction of tissue oxygen levels.

Oxygen saturation: Measurement of the amount of oxygen attached to a hemoglobin molecule.

Oxygen transport pathway: Pathway for oxygen delivery to the tissues from the ambient air: through the airways and lungs, across the alveolar capillary membrane, into the pulmonary circulation through the chambers of the heart via the peripheral and regional circulation to the tissues and the mitochondria where oxygen is used in cellular respiration.

Oxygen transport: Process by which oxygen is absorbed in the lungs by the hemoglobin in circulating deoxygenated red cells and carried to the peripheral tissues. The process is made possible because hemoglobin has the ability to combine with oxygen present at a high concentration, such as in the lungs, and to release this oxygen when the concentration is low, such as in the peripheral tissues.

Oxyhemoglobin dissociation: Dissociation of oxygen from the hemoglobin molecule in peripheral tissues when the concentration of oxygen is low.

Paradoxical breathing: Paradoxical movements of the chest wall during normal breathing; sometimes clinically referred to as belly breathing, see-saw breathing, or reverse breathing.

Parenchyma: The tissue of an organ, as distinguished from supporting or connective tissue.

Parkinson's disease: A slowly progressive, degenerative, neurological disorder characterized by resting tremor, pill rolling of the fingers, a masklike expression, shuffling gait, forward flexion of the trunk, loss of postural reflexes, and muscle rigidity and weakness. It is usually an idiopathic disease of people over 60 years of age, although it may occur in younger people, especially after acute encephalitis or carbon monoxide or metallic poisoning, particularly by reserpine or phenothiazine drugs.

Partial pressure of gases: Pressure exerted by an individual gas, a percent of the total pressure of gases.

Patent ductus arteriosus (PDA): An abnormal opening between the pulmonary artery and the aorta caused by failure of the fetal ductus arteriosus to close after birth. The defect, which is seen primarily in premature infants, allows blood from the aorta to flow into the pulmonary artery and recirculate through the lungs, where it is reoxygenated and returned to the left atrium and left ventricle, causing an increased workload on the left side of the heart and increased pulmonary vascular congestion and resistance.

Pediatric cardiac rehabilitation: Specialized cardiac rehabilitation for children instituted in the chronic stage of heart disease or after cardiovascular surgery when the patient is through the acute phase.

Pediatric pulmonary rehabilitation: Specialized pulmonary rehabilitation for children instituted in the subacute or chronic stages of lung disease or after thoracic surgery when the patient is through the acute phase.

Perfusion: Passage of a fluid through a specific organ or an area of the body.

Perioperative complications: Complications before, during, and after surgery.

Peripheral circulation: The systemic circulation, which excludes the circulation to the heart and lungs (the central circulation).

Peripheral vascular disease: Any abnormal condition that affects the blood vessels outside the heart and the lymphatic vessels.

Pneumonia: An acute inflammation of the lungs, usually caused by inhaled pneumococci of the species *Streptococcus pneumoniae*. The alveoli and bronchioles of the lungs become plugged with a fibrous exudate. Pneumonia may be caused by other bacteria, as well as by viruses, rickettsiae, and fungi.

Positron emission scans: Tomographic scans using positron emitting radionuclides. The tracers used are often taken up in the metabolic pathways of the tissues being studied (e.g., oxygen metabolism or glucose metabolism).

Post polio syndrome: A collection of symptoms present in survivors of poliomyelitis. New delayed symptoms include disproportionate fatigue, increased weakness, deformity, pain, reduced endurance, breathing and swallowing problems, and respiratory insufficiency.

Postural drainage: A passive technique in which the patient is placed in positions that allow gravity to assist with the drainage of secretions from the bronchopulmonary tree. Also known as bronchial drainage.

Prescription: An order for medication, therapy, or a therapeutic device given by a properly authorized person to a person properly authorized to dispense or perform the order. A prescription is usually in written form and includes the name and address of the patient, the date, the [4]+ symbol (superscription), the medication prescribed (inscription), directions to the pharmacist or other dispenser (subscription), directions to the patient that must appear on the label, the prescriber's signature, and in some instances, an identifying number.

Prevention: Any action directed toward preventing illness and promoting health to avoid the need for secondary or tertiary health care.

Primary cardiopulmonary dysfunction: Cardiopulmonary dysfunction resulting from a primary condition of the heart, lungs, or both.

Pulmonary circulation: Blood flow through a network of vessels between the heart and the lungs for the oxygenation of blood and removal of carbon dioxide.

Pulmonary development: Anatomical and physiological development of the cardiopulmonary system during normal growth and development.

Pulmonary rehabilitation: Rehabilitation of cardiopulmonary dysfunction including the acute, subacute, and chronic phases of the disease or after thoracic surgery. The long-term management includes a comprehensive program of exercise, ventilatory support, additional airway clearance interventions as needed, nutrition, stress reduction, smoking cessation, pacing and energy conservation, vocational rehabilitation, sexual rehabilitation, and education.

Quality care: Provision of holistic care in which the needs and wants of the patient are considered.

Radiolucent: Pertaining to the darkest areas on a radiograph film.

Radiopaque: Pertaining to dense areas of material (i.e., metal) on a radiographic film; these areas will appear opaque.

Recumbency: The state of lying down or leaning against something.

Reflex cough: A cough stimulated reflexively.

Reliability: The extent to which a test measurement or a device produces the same results with different investigators, observers, or administration of the test over time. If repeated use of the same measurement tool on the same sample produces the same consistent results, the measurement is considered reliable.

Residual volume: Volume of air remaining in the lung after a maximal expiration.

Resources: Services, personnel, and treatment options that can be drawn on to maximize treatment delivery and effectiveness.

Respiratory failure: Inability of the cardiac and pulmonary systems to maintain an adequate exchange of oxygen and carbon dioxide in the lungs. Respiratory failure may be oxygenation or hypercapnic. Treatment of respiratory failure includes maximizing ventilation, clearing the airways by suction, bronchodilators, or tracheostomy, antibiotics for infections usually present, anticoagulants for pulmonary thromboemboli, and electrolyte replacement in fluid imbalance. Oxygen may be administered in some cases; in others it may further decrease the respiratory reflex by removing the stimulus of a decreased elevated level of oxygen.

Respiratory mechanics: The physical properties of the lung, including resistance and compliance characteristics.

Respiratory muscle fatigue: Loss in the capacity of a muscle under load to develop force or velocity that is reversible by rest.

Respiratory muscle weakness: Chronic loss in the capacity of a rested muscle to generate force.

Respiratory muscles: Muscles that produce volume changes of the thorax during breathing. The inspiratory muscles include the hemidiaphragms, external intercostals, scaleni, sternomastoids, trapezius, pectoralis major, pectoralis minor, subclavius, latissimus dorsi, serratus anterior, and muscles that extend the back. The expiratory muscles are the external intercostals, abdominals, and the muscles that flex the back.

Restrictive lung disease: Category of lung disease involving restriction of the lung parenchyma and characterized by stiffness (reduced compliance) and reduced lung volume.

Rheumatoid arthritis: A chronic, destructive, sometimes deforming collagen disease that has an autoimmune component. Rheumatoid arthritis is characterized by symmetric inflammation of the synovium and increased synovial exudate, leading to thickening of the synovium and swelling of the joint.

Rhonchi: Lung sound with a low but continuous pitch. Snoring is a term used to describe its quality.

Risk factors: Factors that cause a person or a group of people to be particularly vulnerable to an unwanted, unpleasant, or unhealthful event. Examples include immunosuppression, which increases the incidence and severity of infection, and cigarette smoking, which increases the risk for developing a respiratory or cardiovascular disease.

Routine body positioning: Routine use of body positioning in the management of patients to minimize the negative effects of static positioning and maximize comfort. The purposes of routine body positioning are distinct from the specific goals of prescriptive body positioning, which are related to optimizing particular components of cardiopulmonary function and gas exchange.

Sandifer's syndrome: A condition marked by posturing in infants of thoracic extension and right head rotation in supine position. This posturing may be mistaken initially for a neuromuscular lesion; the infant may use this posturing to move away from the noxious stimulus of reflux experienced whenever he or she moves into a flexed thoracic posture of head turning and lateral thoracic bending to the left.

Scleroderma: A relatively rare autoimmune disease affecting the blood vessels and connective tissue. The disease is characterized by fibrous degeneration of the connective tissue of the skin, lungs, and internal organs, especially the esophagus, digestive tract, and kidneys. Scleroderma is most common in middle-aged women.

Secretion management: Management of airway secretions.

Sedation: An induced state of quiet, calmness, or sleep, as by means of a sedative or hypnotic medication.

Sepsis and multiorgan system failure: Overwhelming systemic infection and pathogens leading to failure within multiple organ systems.

Shock: An abnormal condition of inadequate blood flow to the body's peripheral tissues, with life-threatening cellular dysfunction, hypotension, and oliguria. The condition is usually associated with inadequate cardiac output, changes in peripheral blood flow resistance and distribution, and tissue damage. Causal factors include hemorrhage, vomiting, diarrhea, inadequate fluid intake, or excessive renal loss, resulting in hypovolemia.

Skilled nursing and rehabilitation facilities: An institution or part of an institution that meets criteria for accreditation established by the sections of the Social Security Act that determine the basis for Medicaid and Medicare reimbursement for skilled nursing care, including rehabilitation and various medical and nursing procedures.

Spinal cord injury: Disruptions of the spinal cord, often associated with extensive musculoskeletal involvement. Common spinal cord injuries are vertebral fractures and dislocations, such as those commonly experienced by individuals involved in car accidents, airplane crashes, or other violent impacts. Such trauma may cause varying degrees of paraplegia and quadriplegia.

Stable angina: Anginal pain that is well-controlled, medically stable, and has a predictable activity/exercise threshold.

Status asthmaticus: An acute, severe, and prolonged asthma attack. Hypoxia, cyanosis, and unconsciousness may follow. Treatment includes bronchodilators given intravenously or by aerosol inhalation, corticosteroids, controlled positive pressure ventilation, sedation, frequent therapy, and emotional support. A bronchodilator may be given by aerosol inhalation from a ventilator.

Stroke volume (SV): The amount of blood ejected from the ventricles during systole.

Stunned myocardium: Contractile dysfunction of the myocardium as a result of an acute episode of ischemia that persists even after perfusion has returned to normal.

Subacute hospitals: Hospitals that specialize in the management of nonacute conditions.

Subjective: (1) Pertaining to the essential nature of an object as perceived in the mind rather than to a thing in itself. (2) Existing only in the mind. (3) That which arises within or is perceived by the individual, as contrasted with something that is modified by external circumstances or something that may be evaluated by objective standards.

Suctioning: Use of mechanical airway suctioning that uses a catheter and negative pressure to remove oropharyngeal or airway secretions when the patient is unable to spontaneously or voluntarily take deep breaths and cough effectively.

Supraventricular: Pertaining to a feature or event occurring superior to the ventricles of the heart.

Surgery: The branch of medicine concerned with diseases and trauma requiring operative procedures.

Syncytium: The arrangement of cells, as in the myocardium, such that stimulation of one cell causes stimulation of adjacent cells, thus causing an action potential to spread from the initial focus.

Systemic disease: Dysfunction or condition affecting one or more systems.

Systemic inflammatory response syndrome (SIRS): Loss of local control or an overly active response that results in an exaggerated systemic response.

Systemic lupus erythematosus (SLE): A chronic inflammatory disease affecting many systems of the body. The pathophysiology of the disease includes severe vasculitis, renal involvement, and lesions of the skin and nervous system. The primary cause of the disease has not been determined; viral infection or dysfunction of the immune system has been suggested. Adverse reaction to certain drugs also may cause a lupus-like syndrome. SLE occurs four times more often in women than in men.

Tachycardia: Abnormally rapid heart rate.

Tachypnea: Increased respiratory rate over 20 breaths per minute.

Tactile fremitus: Vibrations of spoken words palpable when the therapist's hands are placed on the patient's chest wall.

Thallium-201 scan: A radionuclide scan that evaluates myocardial perfusion. The tracer is taken up in the myocardium based on perfusion of the area. This agent can be used for rest studies, exercise stress studies, and pharmacological stress studies.

Thoracic cavity: The cavity enclosed by the ribs, the thoracic portion of the vertebral column, the sternum, the diaphragm, and associated muscles.

Thoracic surgery: The branch of medicine that deals with disease and injuries of the thoracic area by manipulative and operative methods.

Throat clearing: Spontaneous elicitation of a cough-like maneuver to clear secretions or an obstruction from the oropharynx that may be threatening the upper airway.

Tidal volume (TV): Amount of air inhaled and exhaled during normal ventilation. Inspiratory reserve volume, expiratory reserve volume, and tidal volume make up vital capacity.

Total lung capacity (TLC): Volume of gas in the lungs at the end of a maximum inspiration. It equals the vital capacity plus the residual capacity.

Tracheobronchial tree (TBT): Anatomic complex that includes the trachea, the bronchi, and the bronchial tubes. It conveys air to and from the lungs.

Tracheostomy tube/cuff: A tube/cuff that is positioned directly through the trachea in the neck to provide a functioning airway that bypasses the nares and oropharynx.

Tracheostomy: An opening through the neck into the trachea through which an indwelling tube may be inserted.

Transitional care units: Settings that specialize in providing care between the acute, subacute, and long-term stages of a patient's illness.

Transitional circulation: A transition from one type of blood vessel to another on moving peripherally through the circulation.

Treatment selection and prioritization: The process of selecting treatments and then prioritizing the order in which these treatments are administered. This process is based on the relative contribution of the pathogenesis that each treatment addresses with respect to oxygen transport deficiencies.

Trunk-ventilation interaction: Interrelationship of the shape and movement of the trunk or chest wall on alveolar ventilation. Trunk and ventilation interaction depends on body positioning and movement.

Tuberculosis: A chromic granulomatous infection caused by an acid-fast bacillus, mycobacterium tuberculosis, generally transmitted by the inhalation or ingestion of infected droplets and usually affecting the lungs, although infection of multiple organ systems occurs.

Type I fiber: Type of skeletal muscle fiber that is also called slow-twitch and is suitable for sustained tonic activity (e.g., the maintenance of posture or breathing, which require resistance to fatigue).

Type IIA fiber: Type of skeletal muscle fiber that is used for short-term, fast, powerful activity in which endurance to fatigue is not required; also called fast-twitch fiber.

Validity: Extent to which a device measures what it is intended to measure.

Valvular heart disease: An acquired or congenital disorder of a cardiac valve, characterized by stenosis and obstructed blood flow or by valvular degeneration and regurgitation of blood.

Ventilation and perfusion matching: Matching of ventilation and perfusion in the lungs. Optimal ventilation and perfusion matching occurs in the midzones of the upright lung, where the ratio is 0.8 to 1.0.

Ventilation: Process by which gases are moved into and out of the lungs.

Ventilation-perfusion scan: Two scans that are used to assess patients for the presence of pulmonary emboli. Criteria (BIELLO or PIOPED) are used to determine whether matched defects present with high, intermediate, or low probability of pulmonary embolus.

Ventilatory strategies: Teaching patients to control breathing with the use of ventilatory patterns (e.g., combining inspiration with trunk extension and exhalation with trunk flexion).

Vital capacity (VC): A measurement of the amount of air that can be expelled at the normal rate of exhalation after a maximum inspiration, representing the greatest possible breathing capacity. The vital capacity equals the inspiratory reserve volume plus the tidal volume plus the expiratory reserve volume.

Work of breathing: Total amount of effort required to expand and contract the lungs; the physiological "cost" of breathing. Generally, quiet breathing consumes 2% to 3% of the oxygen consumption and requires 10% of the vital capacity. If a greater amount is used, one would say the work of breathing is increased.

Index

Note: Page numbers followed by "b" indicate boxes; "f" figures, "t" tables.

M

O